GOMELLA AND HAIST'S
Clinician's Pocket Reference

12th EDITION

EDITED BY

LEONARD G. GOMELLA, MD, FACS

The Bernard W. Godwin Professor of
Prostate Cancer
Chairman, Department of Urology
Sidney Kimmel Medical College
Senior Director Clinical Affairs,
Sidney Kimmel Cancer Center
Vice President for Urology, Jefferson Health
Thomas Jefferson University
Philadelphia, Pennsylvania

STEVEN A. HAIST, MD, MS, FACP, FCPP

Professor of Medicine
Department of Internal Medicine
University of Kentucky College of Medicine
Lexington, Kentucky, and
Associate Dean and Professor of Medicine
University of Kentucky College of Medicine—
Northern Kentucky Campus
Highland Heights, Kentucky

**Based on a program developed in 1979
at the University of Kentucky College of Medicine
Lexington, Kentucky
by th~~e Class of 1980~~**

T0175982

Mc
Graw
Hill

New York   Chicago   San Francisco   Lisbon   London   Madrid   Mexico City
Milan   New Delhi   San Juan   Seoul   Singapore   Sydney   Toronto

Gomella and Haist's Clinician's Pocket Reference, 12th Edition

1 2 3 4 5 6 7 8 9   DSS   26 25 24 23 22

ISBN 978-0-07-160282-2
MHID 0-07-160282-8

Notice

Medicine is an ever-changing science. As new research and clinical experience broaden our knowledge, changes in treatment and drug therapy evolve. The authors and the publisher of this work have checked with sources believed to be reliable in their efforts to provide information that is complete and generally in accord with the standards accepted at the time of publication. However, in view of the possibility of human error or changes in medical sciences, neither the editors nor the publisher nor any other party who has been involved in the preparation or publication of this work warrants that the information contained herein is in every respect accurate or complete, and they disclaim all responsibility for any errors or omissions or for the results obtained from use of the information contained in this work. Readers are encouraged to confirm the information contained herein with other sources. For example and in particular, readers are advised to check the product information sheet included in the package insert of each drug they plan to administer to be certain that the information contained in this work is accurate and that changes have not been made in the recommended dose or in the contraindications for administration. This recommendation is of particular importance in connection with new or infrequently used drugs.

This book was set in AGaramond Pro by MPS Limited.
The editor was Jason Malley.
The production supervisor was Catherine Saggese.
Project management was provided by Poonam Bisht, MPS Limited.
This book is printed on acid-free paper.

Library of Congress Control Number: 2021950136

To: Tricia, Leonard, Patrick, Sam, Andrew, Michael, Kristi, Adam, and Maisie

To: Meg, Sarah (Kit), and Will

To: Our students, residents, and fellows who over the years challenged us and inspired us to be better clinicians and teachers

"We don't drive the trucks; we only load them."

Nick Pavona, MD
UKMC Class of 1980

Contents

Editorial Board

Sarah Boden, MD, PharmD
University of Kentucky College of Medicine Class of 2020, Lexington, Kentucky and Resident, Department of Anesthesiology, Brigham and Women's Hospital, Boston, Massachusetts

Lydia Glick, MD
Urology Research Scholar, Department of Urology, Thomas Jefferson University, Philadelphia, Pennsylvania, Sidney Kimmel Medical College Class of 2021, Thomas Jefferson University, Philadelphia, Pennsylvania, Resident, Department of Medicine, Baylor College of Medicine, Houston, Texas

Michael G. Gomella, DDS
University of Maryland School of Dentistry Class of 2021, University of Maryland, Baltimore, Maryland, Resident, Department of Dentistry, Evanston Hospital, North Shore University Health System, Evanston, Illinois

Timothy Han, MD
Urology Research Scholar, Department of Urology, Thomas Jefferson University, Philadelphia, Pennsylvania, Chicago Medical School Class of 2021, Rosalind Franklin University of Medicine and Science, Chicago, Illinois, Resident, Department of Urology, Loyola University, Chicago, Illinois

Mitchell Jacobs, MD
University of Kentucky College of Medicine Class of 2021, Lexington, Kentucky and Researcher, Department of Ophthalmology, University of Kentucky College of Medicine, Lexington, Kentucky

Joon Yau Leong, MD
Sidney Kimmel Medical College Class of 2020, Thomas Jefferson University, Philadelphia, Pennsylvania, Resident, Department of Urology, Thomas Jefferson University Hospital, Philadelphia, Pennsylvania

John "Jay" Ogunkeye, MD
Rush Medical College Class of 2021, Rush University, Chicago, Illinois, Resident, Department of Urology, Stanford, University, Stanford, California

Seth Teplitsky, MD
Sidney Kimmel Medical College Class of 2020, Thomas Jefferson University, Philadelphia, Pennsylvania, Resident, Department of Urology, University of Kentucky Medical Center, Lexington, Kentucky

Contributors

Babak Abai, MD, FACS
Associate Professor, Department of Surgery, Sidney Kimmel Medical College, Thomas Jefferson University, Philadelphia, Pennsylvania

Vaneet Arora, MD, MPH, D (ABMM)
Associate Professor of Pathology and Laboratory Medicine, Associate Director, Clinical Microbiology, Department of Pathology and Laboratory Medicine, University of Kentucky College of Medicine , Lexington, Kentucky and Director, Kentucky State Public Health Laboratory, Frankfort, Kentucky

A.E. Baker, PA-C, MS
Physician Assistant Program Director, West Chester University, West Chester, Pennsylvania

Alison L. Bailey MD, FACC, FAACVPR
Affiliated Associate Professor of Medicine, University of Tennessee Health Science Center; Chief, Cardiology, Centennial Heart at Parkridge and Physician Director, Cardiovascular Disease, HCA Healthcare, Chattanooga, Tennessee

Oksana H. Baltarowich, MD, FAIUM, FSRU
Professor of Radiology, Director, Medical Student Education, Department of Radiology, Sidney Kimmel Medical College, Thomas Jefferson University, Philadelphia, Pennsylvania

Rachel Belfer, MD
Sidney Kimmel Medical College Class of 2019, Thomas Jefferson University, Philadelphia, Pennsylvania and Resident, Department of Psychiatry, Montefiore Medical Center, Bronx, New York

Timothy P. Brigham, MDiv, PhD
Chief of Staff and Chief Education and Organizational Development Officer, Accreditation Council for Graduate Medical (ACGME), Chicago, Illinois

Brian P. Calio, MD
Resident, Department of Urology, Thomas Jefferson University Hospital, Philadelphia, Pennsylvania

Anne E. Lizardi-Calvaresi, DNP, CRNP, RNFA
Director of Clinical Operations, Urology Nurse Practitioner, Department of Urology, Sidney Kimmel Cancer Center, Thomas Jefferson University, Philadelphia, Pennsylvania

Mark B. Chaskes, MD, MBA
Resident, Department of Otolaryngology-Head and Neck Surgery, Thomas Jefferson University Hospital, Philadelphia, Pennsylvania

Mitchell Conn, MD, MBA
Professor of Medicine, Division of Gastroenterology and Hepatology, Sidney Kimmel Medical College and Director of Operational Efficiency and Productivity, Jefferson Digestive Diseases Institute, Thomas Jefferson University, Philadelphia, Pennsylvania

Caitlyn Costanzo, MD
Assistant Professor, Sidney Kimmel Medical College, Division of Colon and Rectal Surgery, Department of Surgery, Thomas Jefferson University Hospital, Philadelphia, Pennsylvania

William Denk, MD
Resident, Department of Anesthesiology, Thomas Jefferson University Hospital, Philadelphia, Pennsylvania

Amy Gewirtz, MD
Professor of Pathology and Laboratory Medicine, Department of Pathology and Laboratory Medicine, University of Kentucky College of Medicine, Lexington, Kentucky

Vanessa Gleason, PharmD, BCCCP
Advanced Practice Pharmacy Specialist-Surgical Intensive Care Unit, Department of Pharmacy, Thomas Jefferson University Hospital, Philadelphia, Pennsylvania

Lydia Glick, MD
Urology Research Scholar, Department of Urology, Thomas Jefferson University, Philadelphia, Pennsylvania, Sidney Kimmel Medical College Class of 2021, Thomas Jefferson University, Philadelphia, Pennsylvania and Resident, Department of Medicine, Baylor College of Medicine, Houston, Texas

Andrew A. Gomella, MD
Resident, Department of Radiology, Thomas Jefferson University Hospital, Philadelphia, Pennsylvania

Leonard G. Gomella, MD, FACS
The Bernard W. Godwin Professor of Prostate Cancer, Chairman, Department of Urology, Sidney Kimmel Medical College, Senior Director Clinical Affairs, Sidney Kimmel Cancer Center, Vice President for Urology, Jefferson Health, Thomas Jefferson University, Philadelphia, Pennsylvania

Michael G. Gomella, DDS
University of Maryland School of Dentistry Class of 2021, University of Maryland, Baltimore, Baltimore, Maryland, Resident, Department of Dentistry, Evanston Hospital, North Shore University Health System, Evanston, Illinois

Patrick T. Gomella, MD, MPH, EMT-P
Assistant Professor, Department of Urology, Sidney Kimmel Medical College, Sidney Kimmel Cancer Center, Thomas Jefferson University, Philadelphia, Pennsylvania

Tricia Lacy Gomella, MD
Assistant Professor of Pediatrics Part-Time, Department of Pediatrics, Johns Hopkins University School of Medicine, Baltimore, Maryland

Patrick J. Greaney, Jr. MD, FACS
Assistant Professor, Sidney Kimmel Medical College, Division of Plastic Surgery, Department of Surgery, Thomas Jefferson University Hospital, Philadelphia, Pennsylvania

Ritu Grewal, MD
Associate Professor, Department of Medicine, Sidney Kimmel Medical College, Thomas Jefferson University, Philadelphia, Pennsylvania

Rakesh Gulati, MD, MRCP
Clinical Professor of Medicine, Division of Nephrology, Department of Medicine, Sidney Kimmel Medical College, Thomas Jefferson University, Philadelphia, Pennsylvania

Steven A. Haist, MD, MS, FACP, FCPP
Professor of Medicine, Department of Internal Medicine, University of Kentucky College of Medicine, Lexington, Kentucky and Associate Dean and Professor of Medicine, University of Kentucky College of Medicine-Northern Kentucky Campus, Highland Heights, Kentucky

Timothy Han, MD
Urology Research Scholar, Department of Urology, Thomas Jefferson University, Philadelphia, Pennsylvania, Chicago Medical School Class of 2021, Rosalind Franklin University of Medicine and Science, Chicago, Illinois, Resident, Department of Urology, Loyola University

Andrew R. Hoellein, MD, MS, FACP
Professor of Medicine, Division of General Internal Medicine, Department of Internal Medicine, University of Kentucky College of Medicine, Lexington, Kentucky

Elizabeth G. Holt, MD
Associate Professor of Medicine and Director of Endoscopy, Division of Digestive Diseases & Nutrition, Department of Internal Medicine, University of Kentucky College of Medicine, Lexington, Kentucky

Colin Huntley, MD
Assistant Professor, Sidney Kimmel Medical College, Department of Otolaryngology-Head and Neck Surgery, Thomas Jefferson University Hospital, Philadelphia, Pennsylvania

Gerald A. Isenberg, MD, FACS
Professor and Vice Chair for Education, Professor of Surgery, Sidney Kimmel Medical College,
Thomas Jefferson University, Philadelphia, Pennsylvania

Rose Jung, PharmD, MPH, BCPS
Adjunct Associate Professor, Department of Academic Medical Education, University of
Kentucky, College of Medicine-Northern Kentucky Campus, Highland Heights, Kentucky

Goni Katz-Greenberg, MD
Transplant Nephrology Fellow, Department of Medicine, Thomas Jefferson University Hospital,
Philadelphia, Pennsylvania

Costas D. Lallas, MD, FACS
Professor and Vice Chair of Education, Department of Urology, Sidney Kimmel Medical College,
Sidney Kimmel Cancer Center, Thomas Jefferson University, Philadelphia, Pennsylvania

Kathryn Landers, MD
Resident, Department of Otolaryngology-Head and Neck Surgery, Thomas Jefferson University
Hospital, Philadelphia, Pennsylvania

Joon Yau Leong, MD
Sidney Kimmel Medical College Class of 2020, Resident, Department of Urology, Thomas
Jefferson University Hospital, Philadelphia, Pennsylvania

Yair Lev, MD
Assistant Professor, Sidney Kimmel Medical College, Department of Medicine, Jefferson Heart
Institute, Thomas Jefferson University Hospital, Philadelphia, Pennsylvania

Joseph F. Majdan, MD, FACP, FCPP
Associate Professor, Department of Medicine, Director of Clinical Proficiency Remediation,
Sidney Kimmel Medical College, Thomas Jefferson University, Philadelphia, Pennsylvania

Fred William Markham, MD
Professor, Department of Family and Community Medicine, Sidney Kimmel Medical College,
Thomas Jefferson University, Philadelphia, Pennsylvania

Aaron Martin, MD
Gastroenterology Fellow, Department of Medicine, Division of Gastroenterology and
Hepatology, Thomas Jefferson University Hospital, Philadelphia, Pennsylvania

Morgan H. McCoy, MD, PhD
Assistant Professor of Pathology and Laboratory Medicine, Department of Pathology and
Laboratory Medicine, University of Kentucky College of Medicine, Lexington, Kentucky

John A. Morris, Jr. MD, FACS
Professor of Surgery and Biomedical Informatics, Associate Chief of Staff, Vanderbilt Medical
Center, and Chief Medical Officer, Vanderbilt Health Affiliated Network, Vanderbilt University
Medical Center, Nashville, Tennessee

Alana Murphy, MD, FACS
Associate Professor, Department of Urology, Sidney Kimmel Medical College, Thomas Jefferson
University, Philadelphia, Pennsylvania

Jessica Freyer Most, MD
Assistant Professor, Department of Medicine, Jane & Leonard Korman Respiratory Institute,
Thomas Jefferson University Hospital, Philadelphia, Pennsylvania

Miguel Paniagua, MD, FACP, FAAHPM
Adjunct Professor of Medicine, Palliative Care Program, Perelman School of Medicine, University of Pennsylvania, Philadelphia, Pennsylvania

Alexis R. Peedin, MD
Assistant Professor, Sidney Kimmel Medical College, Department of Pathology, Anatomy & Cell Biology, Thomas Jefferson University Hospital, Philadelphia, Pennsylvania

Charles A. Pohl, MD, FAAP
Chancellor, Center City Campus and Vice Provost of Student Affairs, Thomas Jefferson University and Vice Dean of Student Affairs and Professor of Pediatrics, Sidney Kimmel Medical College, Thomas Jefferson University, Philadelphia, Pennsylvania

Michael J. Pucci, MD, FACS
Associate Professor of Surgery, Department of Surgery, Sidney Kimmel Medical College, Thomas Jefferson University, Philadelphia, Pennsylvania

J. Patton Robinette, MD
Resident, Department of Orthopedic Surgery, Duke University Health System, Durham, North Carolina

David W. Rudy, MD
Professor of Medicine, Division of General Internal Medicine, Department of Internal Medicine, University of Kentucky College of Medicine, Lexington, Kentucky

Eric S. Schwenk, MD, FASA
Associate Professor of Anesthesiology and Orthopedic Surgery, Sidney Kimmel Medical College, Thomas Jefferson University, Philadelphia, Pennsylvania

Francis G. Serio, DMD, MS, MBA, Doctor of Public Service (Hon.)
Associate Dental Director, Greene County Health Care, Inc. Pamlico Dental Services, Bayboro, North Carolina

John M. Spandorfer, MD, FACP
Professor of Medicine, Roger B. Daniels, Associate Dean for Professionalism in Medicine, Sidney Kimmel Medical College, Thomas Jefferson University, Philadelphia, Pennsylvania

Michael R. Sperling, MD
Baldwin Keyes Professor of Neurology, Vice Chair for Research, Director, Jefferson Comprehensive Epilepsy Center, Sidney Kimmel Medical College, Thomas Jefferson University, Philadelphia, Pennsylvania

Benjamin J. Stahr, MD
Pathologist/Dermatopathologist, Sonic Health Care, Greensboro Pathology Division and Pathologist, Moses Cone Healthcare System, Greensboro, North Carolina and Assistant Clinical Professor of Dermatology, University of North Carolina, Chapel Hill, North Carolina

Luis Cesar Suarez Rodriguez, MD
Assistant Professor, Department of Surgery, Mount Sinai Morningside and Mount Sinai West, Icahn School of Medicine, New York, New York

Seth Teplitsky, MD
Sidney Kimmel Medical College Class of 2020, Thomas Jefferson University, Philadelphia, Pennsylvania and Resident, Department of Urology, University of Kentucky Medical Center, Lexington, Kentucky

William Tester, MD, FACP
Clinical Professor of Medical Oncology, Sidney Kimmel Cancer Center, Thomas Jefferson University, Philadelphia, Pennsylvania

Jessica L. Tomaszewski, MD, FAAP
Clinical Associate Professor, Department of Pediatrics, Thomas Jefferson University,
Philadelphia, Pennsylvania and Pediatric Hospitalist, Nemours Children's Health System,
Wilmington, Delaware

Tanya J. Uritsky, PharmD, CPE
Opioid Stewardship Coordinator, Co-Chair Penn Medicine Opioid Task Force, Department of
Pharmacy, Hospital of the University of Pennsylvania, Philadelphia, Pennsylvania

Eugene R. Viscusi, MD
Professor of Anesthesiology, Sidney Kimmel Medical College, Chief of Pain Medicine, Director,
Acute Pain Management, Thomas Jefferson University Hospital, Philadelphia, Pennsylvania

Preface

Long time contributors and fans of the "Clinician's Pocket Reference" will note the cover no longer identifies this as the "Famous Scut Monkey Book." In 40 years of publication of this manual no one has ever expressed concern or have been offended by the "Scut Monkey" character portrayal. In our new world of heightened sensitivities, the term "Scut Monkey Book" is not a prominent feature in this edition. However, the historical references to the "Scut Monkey," which has always been considered an energetic, fun, and positive symbol of medical training, have been maintained in the introductory portions of the book as well as in the back-cover image. The editors and publisher appreciate everyone's understanding and hope we have made it clear the "Scut Monkey" is only portrayed in a very positive light.

Since 1979, students, residents, practicing physicians, nurses, nurse practitioners, PA's and other allied health professionals have turned to the "Scut Monkey Book" for learning the essential information on basic patient care. The *Clinician's Pocket Reference* is based on the University of Kentucky manual entitled *So You Want to Be a Scut Monkey: Medical Student's and House Officer's Clinical Handbook*. The "Scut Monkey" program at the University of Kentucky College of Medicine was first held in the summer of 1979 and was developed by the Class of 1980 to help ease the sometimes frustrating transition from the preclinical to the clinical years of medical school. Based on detailed surveys from the University of Kentucky and 44 other medical schools, the essential information and skills that students should be familiar with at the start of their clinical years was developed.

The "Scut Monkey" program was developed around this core and consisted of a simple reference manual and a series of workshops conducted at the start of the third year. Held originally as a pilot program for the University of Kentucky College of Medicine Class of 1981, the program has become an annual event. Each new fourth-year class traditionally takes the responsibility of orienting the new third-year students in basic skills. The program is successful because it was developed and taught *by students for other students*. The 40th "Scut Monkey Day" was held on June 21, 2019 in Lexington. Students have been the main source of feedback for the book, critical to its longevity. Information on the rising third-year "Scut Monkey" orientation program is available from Charles H. "Chipper" Griffith, III, MD, MSPH, Vice Dean for Education at the University of Kentucky College of Medicine in Lexington (cgrif00@uky.edu). Over the years, similar programs, sometime referred to as "boot camps," for new students and interns have appeared.

Over the last 11 editions, the book has been continually updated to reflect the dynamic changes in medical education and patient care. An attempt is made to cover the most frequently asked basic management questions that are normally found in many different sources such as procedure and lab manuals, and the extensive resources on the internet. This book is not meant as a substitute for specialty-specific reference manuals; the core information presented is the essential foundation for the new medical student or healthcare provider beginning to learn hands-on patient care. While some key pediatric content is presented, the focus of the book is on general concepts in adult medicine.

Our goal is to represent common medical practices around the country and internationally. Over the years, contributors from many different medical centers have enhanced the content of the book. The *Clinician's Pocket Reference* has been translated into foreign languages, including Japanese, Chinese, Korean, Indonesian, Portuguese, and Spanish. The "Scut Monkey Book" was honored to have been asked by Warner Brothers, the producers of the TV show "ER," to be one of the prop books used on their series. The book has also been a topic of conversation concerning medical education on National Public Radio (NPR). Medical students on the TV show "Scrubs" were lovingly referred to as "scut monkeys" by Dr. Cox in the "My Bed Banter and Beyond" episode.

With the explosion in online resources, downloadable apps, and many new pocket manuals, we thought the Scut Monkey would be laid to rest after the 11th edition was published in 2007. Over the years, feedback to the publisher and the desire for the book to be updated for a new generation of students has increased. The core content of the book is so enduring that the sales of the book continued to be strong even with a 2007 publication date. It was our pleasure to not only update the manual but also add new content to reflect the changes in contemporary healthcare education. Sections on multidisciplinary healthcare teams, palliative care, and outpatient medical management are just a few of the new chapters. Due to the rapid FDA drug approval process and the extensive resources available for online drug updates, we removed the general drug prescribing section of the book to allow for expansion of core clinical elements.

The 12th edition was updated during the 2020–2021 Covid-19 corona virus pandemic. Sections on lab testing, personal protection equipment (PPE), and cardiopulmonary resuscitation were updated to the latest information available at that time of publication. The 12th edition also received a major upgrade in terms of illustrations. The tremendous McGraw Hill Medical "AccessMedicine" online reference was a most valuable resource and we are appreciative of the opportunity to use many fine images from that resource.*

---

*https://accessmedicine.mhmedical.com/

A word of eternal gratitude to the past Deans and administration of the University of Kentucky College of Medicine: Drs. Kay Clawson, Terry Leigh, and Roy Jarecky, and the then very young faculty member Dr. Richard Braen, who took a chance and supported a group of third-year medical students who wanted to try to do something a little bit different way back in 1978. Thanks also to the hundreds of past contributors, early edition co-editor Dr. Michael Olding, and readers who have helped to establish the "Scut Monkey Book" as one of the enduring references for students and residents. Every medical student at the University of Kentucky College of Medicine since 1979 has received a courtesy copy of this book as a small token of Drs. Gomella and Haist's appreciation for UK's dedication to producing outstanding and caring physicians who serve patients in the Commonwealth and beyond.

We would like to express special thanks to our respective wives Tricia and Meg and our children for their patience and long-term support of the "Scut Monkey" project. Our appreciation to McGraw-Hill, for keeping this book as one of their high priority publications. Many faculty, house staff and students from the University of Kentucky College of Medicine and the Sidney Kimmel Medical College of Thomas Jefferson University contributed critical 12th edition updates. Other faculty, residents, and students from a dozen other medical centers were valued contributors to this edition. Many of these colleagues have been involved with the "Scut Monkey" for many years over many editions.

As always, we look forward to your comments and suggestions as the creation of the essential content of the book would be impossible if we did not receive feedback from our readers. We hope this book will not only help you learn some of the basics of the art and science of medicine but also allow you to care for your patients in the best way possible.

Leonard G. Gomella, MD, FACS
Philadelphia, Pennsylvania
leonard.gomella@jefferson.edu

Steven A. Haist, MD, MS, FACP, FCPP
Highland Heights, Kentucky
steven.haist@uky.edu

Visit our website www.thescutmonkey.com for additional *Clinician's Pocket Reference* content.

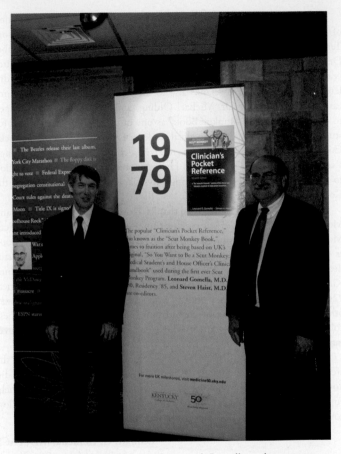

Drs. Steve Haist and Leonard Gomella at the
University of Kentucky College of Medicine 50th
anniversary celebration in 2010 at a display in honor of the
"Clinicians Pocket Reference," part of history at UKMC.

Professional Health and Wellness: "Be a Grace Note"

Becoming a physician is to embark on a journey of transformation that produces an almost alchemical change in identity; from a person who **wishes to be** a physician, into a person who **is** a physician. It is a journey where one walks the path of mastery moving from novice to expert, becoming a new person along the way. It's a journey of "Awe" that is trodden on a pathway as arduous and wondrous as any quest described in old myths and ancient legends.

"Awe" is an interesting word. It contains both the feeling of a surprising sense of reverence and wonder, and a powerful, overwhelming feeling of dread. In fact there are two words that have the same definition yet have very different meanings: "awesome" and "awful." The entomology of both mean "full of awe," yet one is about feeling sheer overwhelming joy and the other about feelings related to dread, despair, and disaster.

Medical students, fellows, and practicing physicians live in a world filled with awe in all its various forms and with all its continuum of meaning: it is like balancing on a tight rope: awesome on one side, awful on the other. Becoming a physician is no ordinary adventure. It is easy to get lost on this journey. The steepness of the climb and the responsibility one has for the lives and health of patients feel overwhelming and exhausting at times. Endless hours of studying; long hours in the hospital or other clinical settings; running toward what others run away from; disease, emotional distress, difficult sights and smells, death, dying. All this and the need for continual peak performance are but a few things that make this path so very difficult.

Walking this path can lead to a life that is wonderful, rewarding, and deeply meaningful. Few individuals are as privileged as physicians to connect with people at the nexus of the most meaningful junctures of their lives, shepherding them through births, sickness, healing, tears of joy and sorrow, and toward health and cure. Physicians touch hearts and lives in ways that few can imagine. Yet, if we don't attend to our own lives and hear the cries of our own souls, the consequences can be dramatic and tragic.

In fact, Lotte Dyrbye, MD, MHPE, FACP, and colleagues (Dyrbye et al. 2014) found that at orientation, medical students are psychologically healthier than their age comparison peers while shortly thereafter levels of their stress rate and burnout go up.

Srijan Sen, MD, PhD, and colleagues (Sen et al., 2010) have found that interns at orientation across specialties have rates of depression of 3.9% and those rates rose to over 25% at three months and stayed constant for the rest of the year. The burnout rate of practicing physicians exceeds that of the general population (Shanafelt et al., 2019). And most tragic of all, it is estimated that up to 400 physicians at all stages of the profession take their own lives by suicide annually.

The nation has taken notice of the potential toll the journey can exact and has taken steps to address the issue. The Institute for Healthcare Improvement's concept of the Triple Aim has been expanded by some to include a fourth element: Attaining Joy at Work. The National Academy of Medicine has established an Action Collaborative on Clinician Well-Being to provide tools and inspiration to prevent caregiver suicide, burnout, depression, and stress and to increase well-being and joy in practice.

Thomas J. Nasca, MD, MACP, CEO, and President of the ACGME, has noted:

1. Physicians who care for themselves provide better care for others.
2. They are less likely to make errors or leave the profession.
3. Habits of practice to promote well-being and resilience need to be cultivated across the continuum.
4. A healthy learning environment will lead to improved health care for both providers and patients.

The importance of attending to the "**you**" along this path of mastery cannot be overstated. You _must_ pay attention to you … as much as you do to your patients if you want to become the physician your patients truly want and truly need. In order to do that while you are working so hard and learning so much, there are at least three areas you need to focus on with intent and vigilance:

1. Taking care of "you."
2. Connecting with others.
3. Connecting to meaning.

Taking care of "you" is both a confession and a task. It starts with admitting you are human, and you have the same human psychological, physiological, and emotional needs that any human has. Recognizing this truth, you need to make sure that to the best of your ability, you attend to these needs. Taking the time to take your own "pulse" relative to self-care is vitally important. Exercising, eating nutritiously, sleeping when you can, learning and practicing letting-go techniques like meditation, yoga, mindfulness, that elicit what Harvard physician Herbert Benson, MD, called the relaxation response. You also need to practice challenging thoughts that distort reality and might otherwise prevent you from reaching your goals by leading to self-defeating behavior like maladaptive perfectionism and imposter syndrome. It is important to celebrate your strengths and work toward increasing them. It is equally important to acknowledge your flaws and work toward reducing them. Appreciate who you are and the uniqueness you bring to the profession. Grow, develop, and cultivate mastery. Reduce the urge to punish yourself for being human. You know the golden rule: "Do unto others as you would have them do unto you." Turn it around—"Do unto yourself as you would do to others." Most important, never, ever hesitate to reach out when you need help, support, and care. It is not a sign of weakness to reach out. Rather it is a sign of strength and maturity. No one has ever walked the path of mastery without falling and needing help and assistance to rise again.

This brings us to the second point, the importance of connection. Research has shown that human connection and positive social relationships are crucial to joy and well-being and that one of the most insidious features of burnout is loneliness. Connection has been found to be one of the most important factors in work happiness and satisfaction. It is important that you create and nurture positive connections with colleagues, role models, faculty, healthcare team members, friends, loved ones, helpers, and so on; seek those with whom you can interact with at the deepest levels, sharing your joys, frustrations, dreams, and fears in order to create the network of support that you'll need to walk this path and navigate it well. It's also important that you be that colleague, role model, and friend to others in your life in order to begin to shatter the code of silence, and help create the connected environment that fosters the health of individuals, teams, programs, and institutions, in order to better care for the patients you serve.

The third element is crucially important. Victor Frankel reminds us in his seminal work *Man's Search for Meaning* that the primary positive motivation in life is found through meaning. A psychiatrist and contemporary of Sigmund Freud, Frankel survived a horrific experience in Auschwitz, a concentration camp, during World War II. From intense reflection on his bitter experience, he concluded that meaning, described as giving ourselves over to something greater than our self, is essential to surviving and thriving in one's circumstances. When the journey gets long and starts to weigh on your soul, it is important to remind yourself (in self-reflection or with others) why you began this journey in the first place. Perhaps it was the healing connection with patients, the calling to do something special for the world, the desire to join with others in what are citadels of awe. To be where people take their first breaths ... and their last ... Where people cry tears of joy for a baby born, a cure found, a wound healed. Where people cry tears of sorrow for life altered, a cure not yet discovered, a loved one's fate. This is what it means to be in a place of awe. In every instance you are there in your white coat (metaphorically or otherwise), no matter your specialty, caring for someone every step of the way. A touch of concern, a kind word, a compassionate presence; you are a symbol of hope and love. In the broadest sense of the term, your presence with your patients is to stand on holy ground.

All of us are writing a narrative with our lives, authoring a novel, a play, a short story with "me" as the protagonist. Only rarely does the pen get shared. The sharing of the pen to help co-author the books of your patients' lives comes during the most thunderously meaningful time of Awe in their lives. That co-author will be you. You will help write the next sentence; the next paragraph; the next chapter. That gift you give and that you receive is what it means to work as a physician. I can't think of any job more deeply meaningful than that.

It is now time to embark on this journey. This book will help you in both concrete and profound ways. It contains an essential roadmap for success. Remember as you walk this wonderfully transformative road to **take care of yourself**, **connect with others** and stay focused on the North Star; in essence, the **meaning** of medicine in your life.

I leave you with this. LaSalle Leffall, MD, was one of the most important physicians of our time. A master surgeon, a master educator, and among other achievements, the first African-American President of the American College of Surgeons and the American Cancer Society. He was a Full Professor and Chairman of the Department of Surgery at Howard University's College of Medicine. He died on May 25, 2019 at the age of 89. I had the great pleasure to meet, share a meal, and talk with him at a white coat ceremony in the early part of the century, and he shared a story with us that I have never forgotten and that I will paraphrase here. Not only was Dr. Leffall a surgeon's surgeon and a beloved master physician to his patients and colleagues, he was also a great lover of jazz. One day he was listening to a recording of John Coltrane with his good friend, the jazz great, Cannonball Adderly. At the end of the piece Cannonball Adderly asked Dr. Leffall a question. "Did you hear that?" Dr. Leffall exclaimed, "Oh yes. What a wonderful record". Cannonball Adderley replied somewhat quizzically, "No I mean - did you hear **that**; the grace note?" "What's a grace note?" responded Dr. Leffall. Cannonball Adderly replied something like this (I may not recall the exact words). "A grace note is one extra note that the musician puts in the measure that does not affect the rhythm of the measure. It's a beautiful gift, a little something extra, just to delight the soul of the listener." Dr. Leffall told us that day that this is a metaphor for what it means to be a physician; to be a grace note to your patients by doing your best, and then adding that little extra something to let your patients know you genuinely care **about** them, not just **for** them. I ask you to extend the metaphor as you take this arduous next, yet extremely rewarding and wonderful journey. Be a grace note … to your colleagues, to all members of the healthcare team, to your faculty, to your patients, and to yourself. If everyone who has read this far in this books forward commits to being a grace note, the "awful" times become not only bearable but also can galvanize a community, and the "awesome" times become transcendent.

Be a Grace note. Happy reading. Have a wonderful joyous journey.

Timothy P. Brigham, M.Div, PhD.

References

1. Dyrbye L, West C, Satele D, et al. Burnout Among U.S. Medical Students, Residents and Early Career Physicians Relative to the General U.S. Population. Acad. Med 2014;89(3):443–51

2. Sen S, Krazler H, Krystal J, et al. A Prospective Cohort Study Investigating Factors Associated with Depression During Medical Internship. Arch Gen Psychiatry 2010;67(6):557–65

3. Shanafelt T, West C, Sinstig C, et al. Changes in Burnout and Satisfaction with Work-Life Integration in Physicians and the General Working Population Between 2011 and 2017. Mayo Clin Proc 2019;94(9):1681–94

An Introduction to Clinical Medicine*

The transition from the preclinical years to the clinical years of medical school is an important time. Understanding the new responsibilities and the general ground rules can ease this transition. Here we provide a brief introduction to clinical medical training for the new student on the wards or in the clinic.

THE HIERARCHY

Most services have some or all of the following team members.

The Intern

In some programs, the intern is also known as the first-year resident. This person has the day-to-day responsibilities of patient care. This duty, combined with a total lack of seniority, usually serves to keep the intern in the hospital more than the other members of the team and may limit his or her teaching of medical students. Any question you have concerning details in the evaluation of the patient, for example, whether Mrs. Pavona gets a complete blood count this morning or this evening, is usually referred first to the intern.

The Resident

The resident is a member of the house staff who has completed at least 1 year of postgraduate medical education. The most senior resident is typically in charge of the overall conduct of the service and is the person you might ask a question such as "What might cause Mrs. Pavona's white blood cell count to be 142,000?" You might also ask your resident for an appropriate reference on the subject or perhaps to arrange a brief conference on the topic for everyone on the service. A surgical service typically has a chief resident, a physician in the last year of residency who usually runs the day-to-day activities of the

---

*Editor's Note: This "So You Want to be a Scut Monkey" section was originally written by Nick Pavona, MD UKMC Class of 1980 and was based on a concept by Epstein A, Frye T (eds.): "So You Want to Be a Toad," College of Medicine, Ohio State University, Columbus, Ohio. While much has changed in professional education over the last 40 years, some concepts are enduring. We include this original work, with a few important updates over the years, to help capture the original spirit of the University of Kentucky College of Medicine Scut Monkey project.

service. On medical services the chief resident is usually an appointee of the chair of medicine who is serving an additional year and functions as junior faculty; they primarily have administrative and teaching responsibilities and may function as an attending either on the wards or in clinic.

The Attending Physician

The attending physician is also called simply "The Attending," and on nonsurgical services, "the attending." (*Note:* Before we get any more letters—yes, this is a joke!) This physician has completed postgraduate education and has become a member of the teaching faculty. He or she is usually already board-certified in a specialty but may be newly trained and preparing to take their boards, thus they are "board eligible." The attending is morally and legally responsible for the care of all patients whose charts are marked with the attending's name. All major therapeutic decisions made about the care of these patients are ultimately the responsibility of the attending. In addition, this person is responsible for teaching and evaluating the house staff and medical students. You might ask this member of the team, "Why are we treating Mrs. Pavona with busulfan?"

The Fellow

The fellow is a physician who has completed his or her residency and elected to do extra study in a subspecialty field, such as nephrology, high-risk obstetrics, or surgical oncology. This person may or may not be an active member of the team and may not be obligated to teach medical students but usually is happy to answer any questions you may ask. You might ask this person to help you read Mrs. Pavona's bone marrow smear.

Physician Extenders

Nurse practitioners and physician assistants are being incorporated into the healthcare system, including important roles in academic medical centers. Their responsibilities vary by service, hospital, and state regulation. These professionals are critical members of the team and excellent resources for both students and patients. You might ask them about Mrs. Pavona's discharge plans.

TEAMWORK

The medical student, in addition to being a member of the medical team, must interact with members of the professional team of nurses, dietitians, pharmacists, social workers, physician assistants, nurse practitioners, and all others who provide direct care for the patient. Good working relations with this group of professionals can make your work go more smoothly; bad relations with them can make your rotation miserable.

Nurses are generally good-tempered but are overworked in most systems. Like most human beings, they respond favorably to polite treatment. Leaving a mess in a patient's room after a procedure, standing by idly while a 98-lb licensed practical nurse struggles to move a 350-lb patient onto the chair scale, and obviously listening to three ringing telephones while room call lights flash are acts guaranteed not to please. Do not let anyone talk you into being an acting nurse's aide or ward secretary, but try to be polite and help when you can.

You will occasionally meet a staff member who is having a bad day, and you will be able to do little about it. Returning hostility is unwarranted at these times, and it is best to avoid confrontations except when necessary for the appropriate care of the patient.

When faced with ordering a diet for your first sick patient, you might be confronted with the limitation in your education in nutrition. Fortunately, dietitians are available, and you should never hesitate to call one.

In matters concerning drug interactions, side effects, individualization of dosages, alterations of drug dosing in different disease states, and equivalence of different brands of the same drug, it never hurts to call the pharmacist. Most medical centers have PharmD residents who follow inpatients on a given floor or service and who will gladly answer any questions and they are an excellent resource for additional references and all matters of medications.

YOUR HEALTH AND A WORD ON "AGGRESSIVENESS"

In your months of curing disease both day and night, it becomes easy to ignore your own right to keep yourself healthy. With the implementation of the Accreditation Council for Graduate Medical Education (ACGME) guidelines on resident duty hours on July 1, 2003 (www.acgme.org), the numerous bad examples of medical and surgical interns working on 3 hours of sleep a night and eating most of their meals from vending machines have been reduced dramatically. Despite the hit, the hospitals have taken on sales of candy bars, do not let anyone talk you into believing that you are not entitled to decent meals and sleep. Even though the ACGME rules do not apply to students, many medical school have adopted their own duty hour policies, often similar to those of the ACGME. If you offer yourself as a sacrifice, it will be a rare rotation on which you will not become one. On the other hand, try to extend yourself when the need arises. The house staff will appreciate it, and because the house staff usually has significant input into your grade, your efforts may be reflected in an outstanding grade on the rotation.

You may have the misfortune someday of reading an evaluation that says you were not "aggressive enough." This notion is enigmatic to everyone. Does it mean that the student refused to attempt to start an intravenous line after eight previous failures? Does it mean that the student was not consistently the first to shout out the answer over the mumbling of fellow students on rounds? Whatever constitutes "aggressiveness" must be a dubious virtue at best.

A more appropriate virtue might be **assertiveness in obtaining your education**. Ask **good** questions, read about your patient's illness, review the basics of a procedure before going to the OR or being present for a bedside procedure, participate actively in your patient's care, take an interest in other patients on the service, and have the house staff show you procedures and review your chartwork. This approach avoids the need for victimizing your patients and comrades, as the definition of *aggression* suggests.

ROUNDS

Rounds are meetings of all members of the service for discussing the care of the patient. Rounds occur daily and are of three kinds.

Morning Rounds

Also known as "work rounds," morning rounds take place anywhere from 6:00 to 9:00 A.M. on most services and are attended by residents, interns, and students and in some hospitals and services, the attending physician. Morning rounds are the time for discussing what happened to the patient during the night, the progress of the patient's evaluation or therapy or both, the laboratory and radiologic tests to be ordered for the patient, and, last but not least, talking with and evaluating the patient. Know about your patient's most recent laboratory reports and progress; this is a chance for you to look good.

Ideally, differences of opinion and glaring omissions in patient care are politely discussed and resolved at morning rounds. Writing new orders, filling out consultation forms, and making telephone calls related to the patient's care are best done right after morning rounds. Discharge planning is an essential part of all morning rounds.

Attending Rounds

Attending rounds vary greatly depending on the service and on the nature of the attending physician. The same people who gathered for morning rounds are at attending rounds, as is the attending. At this meeting, patients are often seen again (especially on the surgical services); significant new laboratory, radiographic images, and physical findings are described (often by the student caring for the patient); and new patients are formally presented to the attending (often by the medical student).

The most important priority for the student on attending rounds is to **know the patient**. Be prepared to concisely tell the attending what has happened to the patient. Also, be ready to give a brief presentation of the patient's illness, especially if it is unusual. The attending will probably not be interested in minor details that do not affect therapeutic decisions. In addition, the attending will probably not wish to hear a litany of normal laboratory values, only the pertinent ones, such as "Mrs. Pavona's platelets are still 350,000/mL in spite of her bone marrow disease." You do not have to tell everything you know on rounds, but you must be prepared to do so. You might be asked! (The essential components of the patient presentation can be found in Chapter 8, "Patient Presentations and Safe Handovers".)

Disputes among house staff and students are usually bad form on attending rounds. For this reason, the unwritten rule is that any differences of opinion not previously discussed should not be raised initially in the presence of the attending.

Check-out or Evening Rounds

Formal evening rounds on which the patients are seen by the entire team a second time are typically done only on surgical and pediatric services. Other services, such as medicine, often have check-out with the resident on call that evening (sometimes called "card rounds" and these meetings must be face-to-face and follow an institutional protocol to help assure patient safety through efficient handovers. This is also reviewed in Chapter 8 "Patient Presentations and Safe Handovers"). Expect to convene for check-out rounds between 3:00 and 7:00 P.M. on most days.

All new data are presented by the person who collected the test results (often the student). Orders are again written, laboratory tests desired for early the next day are requested, and those on call, compile a "scut list" of work to be done that night and a list of patients who need close attention. To comply with the ACGME directive regarding an 80-hour work week, many services have adopted "night-float" coverage systems. The interns and residents caring for your patients overnight will meet with the team at evening sign-out rounds. These cross-coverage strategies call for clear, concise communication essential during handovers.

BEDSIDE ROUNDS

Bedside rounds are basically the same as other rounds except that tact is at a premium. The first consideration at the bedside must be for the patient. If no one else on the team says "Good morning" and asks how the patient is feeling, do it yourself; this is not a presumptuous act on your part. Keep this encounter brief and then explain to the patient that you will be talking about him or her for a while. Most patients treated this way feel flattered by the attention and listen with interest.

Certain points of a hallway presentation are omitted in the patient's room. The patient's race and gender are usually apparent to all and do not warrant inclusion in your first sentence.

The patient must *never* be called by the name of the disease, e.g., Mrs. Pavona is not "a 45-year-old CML (chronic myelogenous leukemia)" but "a 45-year-old *with* CML." The patient's general appearance need not be reiterated. Descriptions of evidence of disease must not be prefaced by words such as *outstanding* or *beautiful*. Mrs. Pavona's massive spleen is not beautiful to her, and it should not be to the physician or student either.

At the bedside, keep both feet on the floor and keep hands out of your pockets (unless briefly looking for something). These actions convey impatience and disinterest to the patient and other members of the team. It is poor form to carry beverages or food into the patient's room. There has been a renewed focus on effective provider-patient communication and often a member of the team may sit in a chair when speaking directly with the patient to be at the same eye level.

Although you will probably never be asked to examine a patient during bedside rounds, it is still worthwhile to know how to do so considerately. Bedside examinations are often done by the attending at the time of the initial presentation or by one member of a surgical service on postoperative rounds. First, warn the patient that you are about to examine the wound or affected part. Ask the patient to uncover whatever needs to be exposed rather than boldly removing the patient's clothes yourself. If the patient is unable to do so alone, you may do it, but remember to explain what you are doing and ask if it is OK with the patient if you (fill in the blank… "Listen to your abdomen, examine your incision, etc."). Remove only as much clothing or expose no more of the patient as is necessary, and always use the bedsheet to provide as much privacy as possible. Remember to promptly cover the patient again. In a shared room, remember to pull the curtain.

Bedside rounds in the intensive care unit call for as much consideration as they do in any other room. That still, naked person on the bed may not be as "out of it" as the resident (or anyone else) believes and may be hearing every word you say. Again, exercise discretion in discussing the patient's illness, plan, prognosis, and personal character as it relates to the disease.

Remember that patient information with which you are entrusted as a healthcare provider is confidential. There is a time and place to discuss sensitive information, and public areas such as elevators or cafeterias are not the appropriate location for these discussions.

READING

Time for reading is at a premium on many services, and it is therefore important to use that time effectively. Unless you can remember everything you learned in the first 20 months of medical school, you will probably want to review the basic facts about the disease that brought your patient into the hospital. These facts are most often found in the same core texts or references that got you through the pre-clinical years (and not Pathoma or other test prep book). Unless specifically directed to do so, avoid the temptation to log on to PUBMED to find all the latest articles on a disease you have not read about for the last 7 months; you do not have the time.

The appropriate time to use PUBMED is when a therapeutic dilemma arises and only the most recent literature will adequately inform the team. You may wish to obtain some direction from the attending, the fellow, or the resident before plunging online on your only Friday night off this month.

Ask the residents and your fellow students which pocket manuals, websites, or downloads they found most useful for a given rotation. Many schools provide specific handouts or textbooks for use on the various services.

THE WRITTEN HISTORY AND PHYSICAL

Much has been written on how to obtain a useful medical history and perform a thorough physical examination, and there is little to add here. Three things worth emphasizing are your own physical findings, your impression, and your own differential diagnosis.

Trust and record your own physical findings, even if other examiners have written things different from those you found. You just may be right, and if not, you have learned something from it. Avoid the temptation to copy another examiner's findings as your own when you are unable to do the examination yourself. Still, it would be an unusually cruel resident who would make you give Mrs. Pavona her fourth rectal examination of the day, and in this circumstance you may write "rectal per resident." *Do not do this routinely just to avoid performing a complete physical examination. Check with the resident first.*

Although not always emphasized in physical diagnosis, your clinical impression is probably the most important part of your write-up. Reasoned interpretation of the medical history and physical examination findings is what separates physicians from the computers touted by the tabloids as their successors. Judgment is learned only by boldly stating your case, even if you are wrong more often than not.

The differential diagnosis is your impression and should include only entities that you consider when evaluating your patient. Avoid including every possible cause of your patient's ailments. List only those that you are seriously considering, and include in your plan what you intend to do to rule in or rule out each one. Save the exhaustive list for the time your attending asks for all the causes of a symptom, syndrome, or abnormal laboratory value.

THE PRESENTATION

The object of the presentation is to *briefly* and *concisely* (usually in a few minutes) describe your patient's reason for being in the hospital to all members of the team who do not know the patient and the patient's story. Unlike the write-up, which contains all the data you obtained, the presentation may include only the pertinent positive and negative evidence of a disease and its course in the patient. It is hard to get a feel for what is pertinent until you have seen and done a few presentations yourself and listen carefully to the presentations of other students and the interns.

Practice is important. Try never to read from your write-up, because doing so, often produces dull and lengthy presentations. Most attendings will allow you to carry note cards, but this method can also lead to trouble unless the content is carefully edited. Presentations are given in the same order as a write-up: identification, chief concern*, history of the present illness, past medical history, family history, psychosocial history, review of systems, physical examination, laboratory and x-ray data, clinical impression, and plan. These and truly relevant items from other parts of the interview often can be and should be added to the history of the present illness. Finally, the length and content of the presentation vary greatly according to the wishes of the attending and the resident, but you will learn quickly what they do and do not want. Always ask at the start of a new service the expectations regarding the length of your presentations. Oral presentations are reviewed in Chapter 8.

RESPONSIBILITY

Your responsibilities as a student should be clearly defined on the first day of a rotation by either the attending or the resident. Ideally, this enumeration of your duties should also include a list of what you might expect concerning teaching, assessment of clinical skills and presentations, and all the other things you are paying many thousands of dollars a year to learn.

On some services, you may feel like a glorified unit secretary (clinical rotations are called "clerkships" for good reason!), and you will not be far from wrong. This is *not* why many of you are going into debt for +$200,000. The scut work should be divided among the house staff and students.

You will frequently be expected to call for a certain piece of laboratory data or to go review an x-ray with the radiologist. You may then mutter under your breath, "Why waste my time? The report will be in the chart later that day or the next morning!" You will feel less annoyed in this situation if you consider that every piece of data ordered is vital to the care of your patient and, if abnormal, this information may need to be acted upon immediately!

Outpatient clinic experiences are incorporated into many rotations. The same basic rules and skill set necessary for in-patient care can be easily transferred to the outpatient setting. The student's responsibility, again, can be summarized in three words: **know your patient**. The entire service relies to a great extent on a well-informed presentation by the student. The better informed you are, the more time is left for education, and the better your evaluation will be. A major part of becoming a physician is learning responsibility.

ORDERS

Orders are the physician's instructions to nurses and other members of the professional staff concerning the care of the patient. These instructions may include the frequency of assessment of vital signs, administration of medications, respiratory care, laboratory and radiologic studies, and nearly anything else that you can imagine.

There are many formats for writing concise admission, transfer, and postoperative orders. Some services may have a precisely fixed set of routine

---

*The term "Chief Complaint" is being replace by the term "Chief Concern".

orders, but others leave you and the intern to your own devices. It is important in each case to avoid omitting instructions critical to the care of the patient. Although you will be confronted with a variety of lists and mnemonics, ultimately it is helpful to devise your own system and commit it to memory. Why memorize? Because when you are an intern and it is 3:30 A.M., you may overlook something if you try to think it out. One system for writing admission or transfer orders uses the mnemonic "A.A.D.C. VAAN DISSL," which is discussed in Chapter 7 "Chartwork."

The word *stat* is the abbreviation for the Latin word *statim*, which means "immediately." When added to any order, it puts the requested study in front of all the routine work waiting to be done. Ideally, a stat order is reserved for the truly urgent situation, but in practice it is often inappropriately used. Most of the blame for this situation rests with physicians who either fail to plan ahead or order stat lab results when routine studies would do.

Student orders usually require a co-signature from a physician, although at some institutions students are allowed to order routine laboratory studies. Do not ask a nurse or pharmacist to act on an unsigned student order; it is illegal for them to do so.

The service intern is responsible for most orders. The amount of interest shown by the resident and the attending varies greatly, but ideally you will review with the intern the orders for routinely admitted patients. Have the intern show you how to write/enter orders for a few patients. In the days of the paper chart, students could write orders themselves and review them with the intern. Unfortunately, this important part of learning basic patient care is a thing of the past as most medical centers have made the transition from paper charts to electronic medical records and now many medical centers exclude students from some aspects of the electronic medical record. From a safety standpoint, the opportunity to work with standard order sets is a good thing for patient care. There is also good news here since CMS (Centers for Medicare & Medicaid Services) now recognize students charting in the electronic medical record and this documentation can be used for billing. The note must be endorsed by a licensed provider. Even if your hospital uses computerized orders, take the opportunity to watch the intern or resident entering the orders when you admit patients.

THE DAY

The events of the day and the effective use of time are two of the most distressing enigmas encountered in making the transition from preclinical to clinical education. For example, there are no typical days on surgical services because the operating room schedule prohibits making rounds at a regularly scheduled time every day. The following suggestions will help on any service.

1. Schedule special studies early in the day. The free time after work rounds is usually ideal for this task. Also, call consultants early in the morning. Often they can see your patient on the same day or at least early the next day.

2. Take care of all your business in the radiology department in one trip unless a given problem requires viewing a film promptly. You must avoid making as many separate trips as you have patients.

3. Make a point of knowing when certain services become unavailable, for example, for electrocardiograms, contrast-study scheduling, and phlebotomy. Be sure to get these procedures done while it is still possible to do so rather than waiting until the next day.

4. Make a daily work or "scut"† list, and write down laboratory results as soon as you obtain them. Few people can keep all the daily data in their heads without making errors.

5. Arrange your travels around the hospital efficiently. If you have patients to see on four different floors, try to take care of all their needs, such as drawing blood, removing sutures, writing progress notes, and calling for consultations, in one trip. Geographic localization of patients in some hospital systems have made this much easier.

6. Strive to work thoroughly but quickly. If you do not try to get work done early, you never will (this is not to say that you will succeed even if you do try). There is no sin in leaving at 5:00 P.M. or earlier if your obligations are *completed* and the supervising resident has dismissed you.

The focus of most clinical education for medical students and other health professional has traditionally been in the in-patient hospital setting. Increasingly, understanding care of the patient in the outpatient setting has become as important. Chapter 3 "Introduction to Outpatient Clinical Medicine" provides a nice overview of the important aspects of outpatient care.

A PARTING SHOT

The clinical years are when all the years of premed study in college and the first 2 years of medical school suddenly come together. We recognize that there are many variations today on when medical students transition to actual hands on patient care but that transition will invariably happen. Trying to tell you everything there is about being a clinical clerk is similar to trying to teach someone to swim on dry land. The insider terms for describing new clinical clerks ("scut monkey," "scut dog," "torpedoes" and "toads") have varied from medical center to medical center and always with a lighthearted spirit. These expressions describing the new clinical clerk acknowledge that the transition, a rite of passage, into the next phase of physician training has occurred.

We hope that this "So You Want to Be a Scut Monkey" introduction to clinical medicine and the information contained in this book will give you a good start as you enter the "hands-on" phase of becoming a successful and respected physician or other professional member of the healthcare team.

---

†Although the origin of how the word *scut* (real definition: the tail of a hare) entered the medical jargon is obscure, we like to think it represents an acronym for "**s**ome **c**ommon **u**nfinished **t**ask" or "**s**ome **c**linically **u**seful **t**raining."

The Professional Journey:
A Dean's View of Medical Education

1

INTRODUCTION

The landscape of healthcare has undergone tremendous changes over the past several decades, especially with the explosion of medical information and discovery, innovative solutions, and technologic advances, which, in turn, have improved the health outcomes and safety of our patients and their communities. The physician remains the steward of the healthcare team who must encompass the necessary knowledge base and skills to not only deliver high quality medical care, but also respond to the disruptors facing the evolving healthcare environment. Medical schools have been modifying their curriculum to keep pace with the ever-changing clinical environment. In fact, 84% of the 124 medical schools surveyed in 2017–18 were either planning for or were implementing change, or had completed implementation of a new curriculum in the last three years.[1]

DISRUPTORS IN HEALTHCARE

1. **Patient individuality.** Beliefs and superstitions, access to care, economic status, family interactions and pressures, environmental stressors, and the political climate.
2. **Shared governance of care.** Shift toward shared decisions between the patient, their family, if the patient so chooses, and the medical team.

Original chapter by Charles A. Pohl, MD

1

3. **Patient trust.** Patients are satisfied with their physician but not with the health system.
4. **Patient safety.** Reports note that medical error accounts for a significant number of deaths daily.
5. **Fragmented care and limited resources.**
6. **Competing information on care.** Multiple unregulated sources of information on the Internet.
7. **Exponential expansion of medical knowledge and scientific discovery.** Clinicians are challenged to assimilate and apply the ever-expanding amount of medical information. By 2020–21, the amount of medical-related knowledge will double in less than 100 days.
8. **Rapid explosion of technology and innovation in the delivery of care.** Digital health is now augmenting care by assisting in decision-making, patient engagement, altering health behaviors, scientific discovery, and reengineering of the healthcare system.
9. **Physician wellness.** Provider wellness is now linked to quality of care, patient safety, and overall satisfaction by both clinicians and their patients.
10. **Steady state of change in medicine.**

OVERVIEW OF MEDICAL EDUCATION IN THE UNITED STATES

The intent of medical education is to provide future physicians with the core knowledge and skills to be competent specialists in a chosen field and the ability to adapt to the ever-evolving healthcare environment. The goal of every medical student is to become a competent physician who practices safe and effective medicine. To reach this goal, aspiring clinicians must be licensed to practice medicine by one of the 71 state medical and osteopathic boards in the United States and its territories. The requirements for medical licensure vary from medical board to medical board.

One licensure requirement for every graduate of a Liaison Committee on Medical Education (LCME)–accredited allopathic medical school in the United States and Canada and any graduate of an international medical school wishing to practice in the United States is to successfully complete the United States Medical Licensing Examination (USMLE). The USMLE is co-owned by the National Board of Medical Examiners (NBME) and the Federation of State Medical Boards (FSMB). The sole purpose of USMLE is for medical licensure; despite this, over the years, there have been a number of secondary uses of the examinations, such as for residency selection, promotion to the third year of medical school, and as a graduation requirement from medical school. USMLE currently consists of three examinations: Step 1, Step 2 Clinical Knowledge (CK), and Step 3.

The Step 2 Clinical Skills (CS) examination was suspended in May of 2020 because of the COVID-19 pandemic. On January 26, 2021, the NBME and the FSMB announced that the Step 2 CS examination would be discontinued and there are no plans to modify or replace the examination. International medical graduates must have obtained "the equivalent of the MD degree from a medical school outside the US and Canada that is listed in the World Directory of Medical Schools … and [they must] obtain ECFMG Certification"[2] before they can sit for Step 1, Step 2 CK, and Step 3. To be eligible to take Step 3, you must pass Step 1 and Step 2 CK, and you must have graduated from an allopathic or osteopathic medical school that is LCME or American Osteopathic Association (AOA)–accredited, respectively, or be an international medical graduate meeting the requirements above. It is recommended that you complete or be near completion of one postgraduate year of training before taking Step 3.

The USMLE Step 1 test is a comprehensive, standardized examination to assess whether examinees "understand and can apply important concepts of the sciences basic to the practice of medicine, with special emphasis on principles and mechanisms underlying health, disease, and modes of therapy."[2] Step 2 CK assesses an examinee's "ability to apply medical knowledge, skills, and understanding of clinical science essential for the provision of patient care under supervision and includes emphasis on health promotion and disease prevention."[3] The purpose of Step 3 is to assess "whether … [the examinee] can apply medical knowledge and understanding of biomedical and clinical science essential for the unsupervised practice of medicine, with emphasis on patient management in ambulatory settings."[4] Step 3 is administered over two days and day 2 includes computer-based simulations.

The Comprehensive Osteopathic Medical Licensing Exam (COMLEX-USA) is the licensing exam administered by the National Board of Osteopathic Medical Examiners for graduates of osteopathic medical schools. Although the USMLE is the required exam for licensure of all allopathic physicians, it may also be taken in place of the COMLEX-USA for osteopathic physicians. COMLEX-USA is designed to assess the osteopathic medical knowledge and clinical skills considered essential for osteopathic generalist physicians to practice medicine without supervision. The exam is a three-level sequence that tests knowledge and skills in two dimensions. Dimension 1 addresses the patient presentation, while Dimension 2 addresses physician tasks. COMLEX-USA scores are reported numerically for Level 1, Level 2-CE, and Level 3, while Level 2-PE is scored as pass/fail.[5]

1

Core principles of medical education in the United States and Canada include:

1. **Overall mission.**
   a. Assure that medical school graduates possess the knowledge, skills, and attitudes to become competent physicians
   b. Provide broad-based exposure (e.g., basic and clinical medical sciences; generalized care, critical care, and subspecialty care)
   c. Promote and cultivate professional behavior
   d. Instill skills in lifelong learning, patient advocacy, cost-effective care, teaching, and leadership
2. **Desired outcomes (key qualities for the doctors of tomorrow).**
   a. **Discipline-specific knowledge and skills**
   b. **Social intelligence** (communication skills, cultural sensitivity and community stewardship, perseverance, teamwork, resilience, emotional intelligence, grit, empathy, and compassion)
   c. **Augmented intelligence** (comfort with complexity, tolerance of ambiguity, creativity, design thinking, data analytics, and leadership)
3. **Entrustable Professional Activities (EPAs) and Core Competencies**. The Association of American Medical Colleges (AAMC) developed the EPAs in 2014 "to provide expectations for both learners and teachers that include 13 activities that all medical students should be able to perform upon entering residency, regardless of their future career specialty."[6] The EPAs are designed to be competency based, and two examples include EPA 1, "Gather a History and Perform a Physical Examination," and EPA 13, "Identify System Failures and Contribute to a Culture of Safety and Improvement."[5] Each of the EPAs has key functions with related competencies and expected behaviors. Additionally, most medical schools have adopted a competency-based framework similar to the Accreditation Council for Graduate Medical Education (ACGME) core competencies that were initially developed in 1999.[7] The core competencies include patient care, medical knowledge, practice-based learning and improvement, interpersonal and communication skills, professionalism, and systems-based practice.[7] The key functions and related competencies within the EPA framework are based on the ACGME core competencies with the addition of two new competencies: "Interprofessional Collaboration" and "Personal and Professional Development." An example of how the EPAs and competencies are tied together is EPA 13—two key functions relate to systems-based practice; two relate to practice-based learning and improvement; and each one relates to knowledge of practice, interpersonal and communication skills, professionalism, and personal and professional development.[6] The use of these frameworks helps ensure all graduates, regardless of the medical school, have met the minimal competency needed to enter residency and to be successful residents. Within this framework are the following:

a. A continuum of core competencies. Initially general exposure and introduction of skills, with increasing specialty exposure and complexity of problems as well as patient care responsibility and clinical oversight

b. More emphasis on individual variation by implementing individual learning plans (ILPs) to remediate lagging skills

4. **Responsibility of the medical team members in patient care in the academic setting.** (Note that there are usually other health professional students on the care team. See Chapter 4, Interdisciplinary Healthcare Teams.)

   a. **Medical student** – directly supervised
   b. **Intern (first-year resident)** – supervised; manages patient care and provides education
   c. **Senior resident** – supervises patient care and educates the team
   d. **Faculty member** – team manager who is ultimately responsible for patient care and education of all learners

CHOOSING A RESIDENCY PROGRAM

Factors in choosing a specialty and residency program include:

1. **Competitiveness.**
   a. **Specialty competitiveness.** It is important to understand the variation among specialties. Resources include the National Resident Matching Program (NRMP) Results and Data: Main Residency Match, at available nrmp.org (overview of the residency match process, highlighting the popularity and success of specialties). Information for ophthalmology can be found at https://www.aao.org/medical-students/residency-match-basics. Urology information can be found at the American Urological Association website (auanet.org) and the Society of Academic Urologists site (sauweb.org). These are both early match specialties.
   b. **One's competitiveness for a specialty.** Factors include the medical school's academic performance in the basic science courses and clinical clerkships, the USMLE Step 1 (see below) and Step 2 CK scores, class rank in medical school, participation in research, letters of recommendation, and Alpha Omega Alpha (AOA) membership. No earlier than January 1, 2022 USMLE Step 1 will become pass/fail.[8] This change will have significant ripple effects. The timing of when a student takes Step 1, how residencies select fourth-year medical students for postgraduate training, and the information medical schools provide residencies about their students will likely change in ways impossible to predict.

   A cohort of four medical schools required their students to take Step 1 after their third year of medical school. The result of this change was a modest 2.7-point increase in scores across the schools. However, the most important finding was a marked decrease in the failure rate, a decrease by a factor of 7 (2.87–0.39%).[9] After Step 1 becomes pass/fail, residency programs may use Step 2 CK scores in place of Step 1 scores for determining who to invite for interviews and/or where to place applicants on their program's NRMP rank list. Also, some residency programs or specialties may decide to use another examination for these same purposes. Hopefully, residency programs will explore ways to more holistically evaluate applicants than through the use of a single test score. Furthermore, medical schools will need to find ways to make the medical school performance evaluation for each of their students more meaningful. While the change to pass/fail for Step 1 is a welcome change by most everyone, there are many questions left unanswered.

Resources to gauge one's strengths and weaknesses within a specialty include NRMP's Charting Outcomes in the Match (nrmp.org), NRMP Program Directors Survey (nrmp.org), and AAMC Careers in Medicine (aamc.org).

    c. **Program competitiveness.** Medical school specialty-specific advisors and student affairs staff can provide helpful advice.

2. **Personal preferences.** Consider factors that affect one's quality of life, educational goals, and future career options.

    a. **Location of the program.**

    b. **Learning style and type of program.** Learning in university programs occurs by evaluating and caring for a large volume of patients, while community programs allow for more time to augment the patient experience with book learning. The American Medical Association's website Fellowship and Residency Electronic Interactive Database–FREIDA Online (ama-assn.org/ama/pub/education-careers/graduate-medical-education/freida-online.page) is a good resource for specific information on individual programs.

3. **Compatibility with the healthcare team.**

4. **Restrictions.** For example, couples matching and geographical restrictions.

APPLYING TO A U.S. RESIDENCY PROGRAM (SPECIALTY TRAINING)*

The applicant pool for U.S. residency training continues to grow, exceeding the number of available positions. Therefore, one needs to be strategic in the application process. Program directors scrutinize each applicant's academic portfolio, extracurricular accomplishments, and unique characteristics and

---

*Note that the 2020 pandemic altered many of these routine residency application activities. For many in the 2020–21 residency application cycle, virtual open houses and video interviews were commonplace.

interests to identify candidates who they feel will be successful physicians in their specialty as well as the best fit for their particular program. Typically, 95% of U.S. senior medical students successfully obtain a position, while only 60% of graduates who attend international schools are successful. In aggregate, program directors report that the most important factors in select-ing a candidate for an interview include clinical grades, letters of recommen-dation, the personal statement, and the USMLE Step 1 score (refer to the NRMP Program Directors Survey at nrmp.org). Obviously, the importance of Step 1 results will diminish greatly when the outcome changes from a three-digit score to a binary pass/fail.[9] The Step 2 CK score may replace the Step 1 score as a means to measure medical knowledge across applicants from different schools, or there may be a more holistic way of assessing applicants.

THE COMPONENTS OF THE RESIDENCY SELECTION PROCESS

1. **Curriculum vitae (CV).** A snapshot of one's academic and extracurricular accomplishments while highlighting unique interests and characteristics. The content should emphasize leadership ability and scholarly activity as well as specialty-specific skills. Surgical fields, for example, prefer activi-ties that demonstrate manual dexterity (e.g., carpentry, video gaming), while primary care fields prefer humanistic activities (e.g., community outreach programs with the underserved or tutoring). The information must be grammatically correct, accurate, and self-explanatory.
2. **Academic transcripts.** Provided in a secure fashion by the school.
3. **USMLE scores.** Most residency programs require a USMLE transcript of all applicants. Once an applicant provides an authorized release, the transcript is provided to residency programs through the Electronic Residency Application Service (ERAS). The transcript includes results for each examination taken, including all attempts. The result of a Step 1 attempt will be reported as pass/fail beginning no earlier than January 2022.[8] Step 2 CK scores are reported as a three-digit score. The NRMP Charting Outcomes (nrmp.org) provide mean USMLE Step scores for students matching in a specific specialty.
4. **Personal statement.** Opportunity to express a variety of thoughts, feel-ings, or facts about one's self, career aspirations, and/or passions. It is the least structured piece of the application and should engage the reader, tell a story about you, and not exceed one page. As with the CV, a personal statement is another opportunity for the applicant to highlight scholarly and community outreach activities, leadership experience, and ability to get along with others and work on a team and to demonstrate competen-cies in skills sought by the particular specialty. Careful attention should be directed at proper grammar, correct spelling, and complete sentences,

1

as residency programs will interpret careless mistakes as the type of care that you will give to their patients.

5. **Institutional letter.** In the United States, every allopathic medical school submits an institutional letter (i.e., the Medical School Performance Evaluation [MSPE]) with a student's application. This is an LCME requirement (LCME standard 11.4). It is an evaluation rather than a letter of recommendation that candidly describes a student's unique background, scholarly work, and ability to function in the clinical setting. Residency programs value this evaluation because it provides an independent overview and summary of the strengths and weaknesses of the student.

6. **Letters of recommendation (LORs).** LORs are a residency program's way to gain further insight into an applicant's professional behavior, clinical competence including clinical decision-making, team interaction, and ability to perform a specialty-specific task and to work independently. These letters augment the clerkship evaluations. They should be written by faculty members who have directly observed the trainee in patient care and have positive feelings toward his or her ability to be a successful resident. Programs typically require either three or four LORs, and it is optimal to obtain at least two letters within the desired specialty unless the program indicates differently. In some instances, an LOR from a department chair, a core clerkship faculty such as internal medicine, or a faculty member from a different discipline may be required. It is important for the applicant to meet with the letter writer, if possible, and supply a copy of an updated CV and personal statement. Additionally, the applicant should "waive the right to review the LOR" to assure the program that the LOR is unbiased.

7. **The residency interview.** Interviews are required by all U.S. residency programs to allow the applicant and the programs to become better acquainted and assess their compatibility.** While this process can be very intimidating for the interviewee, it is important to be oneself and explore areas of the program that one finds interesting and/or are not self-explanatory on the program's website. The program, on the other hand, will talk about its unique qualities, answer and clarify questions by the interviewee, confirm the legitimacy of an applicant's CV, and evaluate a candidate's communication and language skills. The program will expect the applicant to be familiar with his or her own CV; be punctual, interested, and engaged; answer questions honestly; and dress professionally. It is important to be polite with everyone, make eye contact, and be honest and confident. The interview day typically lasts 3–4 hours, where you will meet with the program director, various faculty, and, most importantly, the residents. Please keep in mind that the interview begins the moment the applicant makes contact with the program to schedule the interview. Candidates have adversely affected their chances of getting an interview or of matching with a program by how they treat the departmental staff on the phone or in person. Always be on your best behavior!

**Due to the COVID-19 pandemic many programs have gone to virtual online interviews. It is expected that the in-person process will resume in the future; although some hybrid virtual and in-person interviews have been proposed.

THE MATCH

The match is a legally binding process that pairs the applicant with a residency program. The candidates and the programs submit a rank list in February that prioritizes a ranking of programs and examinees, respectively. The computer program makes the pairing in a confidential way (refer to nrmp.org, sfmatch.org, and auanet.org). The residency applicant should always rank programs in order of their preference, regardless of the likelihood of matching in a particular program, because the match algorithm always favors the applicant's rank order list (ROL) over a residency program's ROL. It is important to include on your rank list any program that you are willing to go to because you don't want to regret leaving off a program if you end up not matching. On the other hand, do not include any program that you would not want to attend and you would rather NOT match than attend the particular program. Additionally, the NRMP allows couples to link their rank lists to help medical students who have a significant other in the same class to continue their training in the same location.

The match process includes 1-year positions for those who are also applying to programs that require a separate preliminary year, in addition to residency positions in almost every specialty. Ophthalmology and urology do not participate in the NRMP and have separate and earlier matches. Also, those students who are on a military scholarship (U.S. Air Force, Army, and Navy) must participate in the military and the NRMP match programs. The military match is also an early match, and if you do not match within a military residency, you will be allowed to participate in the NRMP if your branch of the military is not in need of physicians in the specialty you are seeking.

So what happens if you do not match through the NRMP? There are several options for those fourth-year medical students who do not match. The first question to ask yourself: Are there available unmatched positions in the specialty I desire for my career path? If the answer is no, you need to decide whether you are still committed to the career path you were seeking. If you are, you could consider bolstering your resume during the next year to make yourself a more competitive residency candidate, such as participating in research in the specialty. If there is another specialty that you are interested in pursuing that has unfilled positions, you can participate in the second match, Supplemental Offer and Acceptance Program (SOAP) through NRMP. Unmatched candidates are able to view the list of unfilled programs traditionally on Monday morning of match week. On Monday afternoon, participants can apply for the unmatched positions, and interviews are conducted between Monday afternoon and Wednesday morning (telephone/Zoom/in person). Three rounds are conducted, and open positions are updated after each round. If an applicant has multiple offers in one round, they can accept only one position, and once they have accepted the position, all others are automatically rejected.

USEFUL RESOURCES

- Careers in Medicine (aamc.org/students/medstudents/cim)
- The Education Commission for Foreign Medical Graduates (ecfgme.org)
- FREIDA Online (ama-assn.org/ama/pub/education-careers/graduate-medical-education/freida-online.page)
- Military Match (https://www.medicineandthemilitary.com/officer-and-medical-training/residency-and-match-day)
- The National Board of Medical Examiners (nbme.org)
- The National Resident Matching Program (nrmp.org)
- Pohl, CA. Ask the Advisor Column in Choices, The Careers in Medicine Newsletter of the Association of American Medical Colleges, January 2010
- The San Francisco Matching Program (sfmatch.org) for ophthalmology
- Spandorfer J, Pohl CA, Rattner S, and Nasca T (eds). *Professionalism in Medicine: The Case-based Guide for Medical Students*. Cambridge University Press, London, 2010
- The Supplemental Offer and Acceptance Program (SOAP) (http://www.nrmp.org/wp-content/uploads/2015/09/SOAP-FAQ-Schools.pdf)

References

1. https://www.aamc.org/data-reports/curriculum-reports/interactive-data/curriculum-change-us-medical-schools, accessed March 22, 2021.
2. https://www.usmle.org/step-1/, accessed March 22, 2021.
3. https://www.usmle.org/step-2-ck/, accessed March 22, 2021.
4. https://www.usmle.org/step-3/, accessed March 22, 2021.
5. https://www.nbome.org/exams-assessments/comlex-usa/bulletin/. Accessed March 19, 2021.
6. https://www.aamc.org/what-we-do/mission-areas/medical-education/cbme/core-epas, accessed March 20, 2021.
7. Holmboe ES, et al. *The Milestones Guidebook*. Chicago, IL: Accreditation Council for Graduate Medical Education; 2016, available at http://www.acgme.org/Portals/0/MilestonesGuidebook.pdf?ver¼2016-05-31-113245-103, accessed March 19, 2021.
8. https://www.usmle.org/incus/. Accessed March 19, 2021.
9. Jurich D, et al. Moving the United States Medical Licensing Examination Step 1 After Core Clerkships: An Outcome Analysis. *Acad Med* 2019;94(3):371–377.

Professionalism in Healthcare

2

- ➤ Patient Welfare
- ➤ Patient Autonomy
- ➤ Social Justice
- ➤ Professional Competence
- ➤ Honesty with Patients
- ➤ Patient Confidentiality
- ➤ Appropriate Relations with Patients
- ➤ Just Distribution of Finite Resources

Over the last three decades, there has been an emphasis on the understanding and teaching of professionalism in both practice and education. Accrediting bodies such as the Liaison Committee on Medical Education (LCME) and Accreditation Council for Graduate Medical Education (ACGME) have expectations that trainees in medical school and residency programs will have training in medical professionalism.

Medical specialty organizations have issued statements and position papers with the expectation that practicing physicians and educators will uphold and teach the tenets of professionalism. The Physician Charter is the most cited example, having been endorsed by over 100 medical organizations. In the charter (see Table 2-1), there are three fundamental principles and ten professional responsibilities that comprise the elements of medical professionalism.

The American College of Physicians periodically publishes an updated Ethics Manual—the seventh edition was published in 2019. The updates include new or expanded topics to address changes in technology and the practice of medicine such as telemedicine ethics, electronic health records, and precision medicine and genetics.

The following eight sections illustrate excerpts from the Physician Charter along with related challenges that physicians may have while trying to adhere to the charter's principles.

PATIENT WELFARE

The principle of patient welfare is based on a dedication to serving the interest of the patient. Altruism contributes to the trust that is central to the physician–patient

Original chapter by John Spandorfer, MD

2

Table 2-1. The Physician Charter

THREE FUNDAMENTAL PRINCIPLES
Primacy of patient welfare
Patient autonomy
Social justice
TEN PROFESSIONAL RESPONSIBILITIES (COMMITMENTS)
Commitment to professional competence
Commitment to honesty with patients
Commitment to patient confidentiality
Commitment to maintaining appropriate relations with patients
Commitment to improving quality of care
Commitment to improving access to care
Commitment to a just distribution of finite resources
Commitment to scientific knowledge
Commitment to maintaining trust by managing conflicts of interest
Commitment to professional responsibilities

Source: Medical Professionalism Project 2002. (Annals of Internal Medicine, 5 February 2002;136:243–6).

relationship. Market forces, societal pressures, and administrative exigencies must not compromise this principle.

While recognizing the need to serve the interests of their patients, physicians also need to be aware of their own well-being and balance how to prioritize patient care while avoiding burnout. Physicians should become adept at collaborating with other members of the healthcare team to maximize efficient and effective care. This collaboration with other healthcare workers helps to ease the burden on any individual physician while ensuring the needs of the patient are met.

PATIENT AUTONOMY

Physicians must have respect for patient autonomy. Physicians must be honest with their patients and empower them to make informed decisions about their treatment.

Physicians may struggle with how much detail to disclose about an abnormal shadow on a radiograph and whether to mention every possible adverse event of a recommended surgical procedure or medication. When deciding what to disclose, physicians should be aware of the reasonable person standard. This standard directs physicians to provide the amount of information that a reasonable person would want in order to make a decision regarding their health.

SOCIAL JUSTICE

The medical profession must promote justice in the healthcare system, including the fair distribution of healthcare resources. Physicians should work actively to eliminate discrimination in healthcare, whether based on race, gender, socioeconomic status, ethnicity, religion, or any other social category.

Physicians may work for a practice that does not accept certain lower-reimbursing insurances such as Medicaid or in academic medical centers where patients with such insurances may be referred to the "resident clinic" for ambulatory care. While physicians in these settings may be aware of and struggle with the perceived dichotomy of care, they should advocate for health policies—at their institution and nationally—that ensure that all patients are able to receive appropriate care regardless of socioeconomic class.

PROFESSIONAL COMPETENCE

Physicians must be committed to lifelong learning and be responsible for maintaining the medical knowledge and clinical and team skills necessary for the provision of quality care. More broadly, the profession as a whole must strive to see that all of its members are competent and must ensure that appropriate mechanisms are available to accomplish this goal.

Physicians should be empowered to give respectful and nonpunitive feedback to colleagues who are not delivering appropriate care.

HONESTY WITH PATIENTS

Physicians must ensure that patients are completely and honestly informed before the patient has consented to treatment and after treatment has occurred. Physicians should also acknowledge that in healthcare, medical errors that injure patients do sometimes occur. Whenever patients are injured as a consequence of medical care, patients should be informed promptly because failure to do so seriously compromises patient and societal trust.

Physicians should not only disclose patient care errors but also ensure patients have learned of errors related to the care of other patients. Concern about liability should never interfere with error disclosure to patients.

PATIENT CONFIDENTIALITY

Earning the trust and confidence of patients requires that appropriate confidentiality safeguards be applied to disclosure of patient information. Fulfilling the commitment to confidentiality is more pressing now than ever before, given the widespread use of electronic information systems for compiling patient data and an increasing availability of genetic information. Physicians recognize, however, that their commitment to patient confidentiality must occasionally yield to overriding considerations in the public interest (for example, when patients endanger others).

When talking about patients outside the clinical setting, care must be taken to avoid including any identifying information (protected health information). Moreover, there needs to be justification for sharing such information. Appropriate justification for discussing nonidentifying patient information includes discussions that have educational value or that can be beneficial to the physician or student in order to better understand or process emotional responses to care.

APPROPRIATE RELATIONS WITH PATIENTS

Given the inherent vulnerability and dependency of patients, certain relationships between physicians and patients must be avoided. In particular, physicians should never exploit patients for any sexual advantage, personal financial gain, or other private purpose.

Physicians and students may be asked personal questions by patients or may want to disclose personal information about themselves to patients. Care should be taken to disclose only information that may benefit the therapeutic relationship. An example would be the doctor who is a former smoker sharing the success of tobacco cessation with a patient considering a decision to quit smoking. Gifts from patients should never interfere with how care is delivered. When being offered a gift, the physician should assess the value of the gift and whether accepting the gift will change the patient-physician relationship. One must avoid favored treatment based on a gift.

JUST DISTRIBUTION OF FINITE RESOURCES

While meeting the needs of individual patients, physicians are required to provide healthcare that is based on the wise and cost-effective management of limited clinical resources. The physician's professional responsibility for appropriate allocation of resources requires scrupulous avoidance of superfluous tests and procedures.

Many examples of such cost-effective care are described in the "Choosing Wisely" campaign. Physicians who are aware of the American Board of Internal Medicine's "Choosing Wisely" campaign guidelines often struggle to avoid less cost-effective care or lower-value care, as they may succumb to patient pressures (e.g., ordering an MRI for acute back pain without alarm symptoms) or long-held practices (e.g., daily labs for many inpatients). "Choosing Wisely" is an initiative of the American Board of Internal Medicine Foundation that promotes patient-physician conversations about unnecessary medical tests and procedures (https://www.choosingwisely.org/). Many specialty organizations have endorsed these recommendations.

Further Reading

ABIM Foundation; ACP-ASIM Foundation; European Federation of Internal Medicine. Medical Professionalism in the New Millennium: A Physician Charter. *Ann Intern Med* 2002;136:243–246.

Sulmasy LS, et al. American College of Physicians Ethics Manual. *Ann Intern Med* 2019;170(Supplement):S1–32.

Introduction to Outpatient Clinical Medicine

3

A trend in healthcare today is moving patient care to the outpatient setting. In order for students to successfully navigate this change, they must understand the differences in dynamics between outpatient and inpatient settings. Compared to the inpatient setting where the patients are available for evaluation over an extended period, the outpatient clinical environment is much more fast paced; students need to be able to evaluate, diagnose, and design a treatment plan under a time constraint. The volume of patients seen over a given period is also much greater than that of inpatient services. The general principles of outpatient care discussed here are similar for all medical, pediatric, and surgical disciplines.

UNDERSTANDING YOUR ROLE

The first step for a student to become a successful member of the outpatient team is to understand their role. If you put the welfare of your patients first and use that as your guide, you are more likely to have a positive experience. In your role as a student, you will quickly become very close to many of your patients. You are likely to have more time to give to your patients than the residents or attendings, who might be caring for their patients in 15- to 20-minute intervals. You will often hear important details of the patient's health that the attending or resident is unaware of. Students are often seen as less threatening to patients and thus more comfortable opening up to you. The history you gather might provide an opportunity to really improve your patient's health. You should not underestimate the important role you can play for your patients.

Original chapter by Fred Markham, MD and Rachel S. Belfer, MD

It is important that you constantly think of ways to improve your clinical skills and basic medical knowledge. Rotations are a time to think about your growth as a student, a clinical learner, a team member, and a healthcare provider. Set aside time every week to reflect on your progress. Think critically about what you enjoyed in a given week as well as about ways in which you can improve as a learner and as a team member. The more you invest in your development, the more interested you will be in your patient encounters. This enthusiasm will likely be apparent to your supervisor. While self-reflection is key to a successful experience, it is also important to internalize feedback from other members of the team. You should regularly ask for feedback from residents and attendings with whom you work. In a busy office session, it is important to arrange a few minutes at least each week to receive feedback. If you feel like you are struggling with some aspect of your performance, you should arrange a time to discuss your concerns with your supervising clinician.

TEAMWORK

According to Dr. Fred Markham, "As I orient students to their outpatient experience, I tell them that they will be successful when I think that it will be a better day for me and my patients when I see that they are working with me. This means they are working hard to be as useful as possible to the team." The successful students know the major health issues of each patient they are responsible for. They review consultations, know the recent lab work, and recognize vital signs and physical exam changes. It is also important to get to know the team with whom you will be working. Introduce yourself to the nurses on your team, the social workers in the office, and the front desk personnel. Know the practical details such as where the social work office is and what the best way is to contact the social worker. Volunteer, with the permission of your supervising provider, to contact other resources that will help your patient. These are the people who are working to make the day run smoothly, and they deserve your respect. They are a great resource and will help you care for your patients. A successful student also understands the value of creating collaborative relationships with other medical students. Your fellow students will have much to teach you, and you will help them. The wonderful thing is that the harder you work for the team, the better doctor you become. An overview of the modern interdisciplinary healthcare team is provided in Chapter 4.

THE ELECTRONIC HEALTH RECORD

Almost all outpatient offices have moved to electronic health records (EHRs), and successful medical practices are increasingly dependent on skillful use of the EHR. You should start practicing how to navigate the EHR before you begin the outpatient experience, as this will enable you to be ready to use the EHR on the first day of the rotation. Although the integration of the EHR in healthcare organizations should ideally incorporate inpatient and outpatient medical records, this may not always be the case. Furthermore, even fully integrated EHR systems may present different interfaces based on the site of service. Learn the system, such as how to view a trend summary, such as the patient's blood pressure, weight, or K^+. Knowing the latest data on your patient will lead to better care. If you do not know the lab results, never "assume they are normal" or make up the results, as this is very dangerous and will damage your credibility with your team. You must learn how to document your history and physical findings and how you will write orders as a resident. Remember that the way you and your team document encounters will likely affect billing and payment. Additionally, future payments from insurance companies for meeting quality goals will depend upon careful documentation in the EHR.

READING

At the beginning of your clinical rotation, the wide variety of problems seen in an outpatient primary care office can seem daunting. In reality, the vast majority of patients present with a small number of common diseases. Make a practice of setting aside time each evening to read about the common diseases that you encounter. This is key to improving and building upon your knowledge base. Many online resources and basic textbooks can help you master the basic pathophysiology and treatment options for the common diseases you encounter. More uncommon diseases might require a deeper dive into the literature, but during your early stages of clinical experiences, it is better to master the basics before spending too much time on esoteric issues. You may want to break down some of these more common diseases in a manageable way. For example, read about the treatment of diabetic neuropathy one night and how to manage diabetic foot ulcers the next night. Think about how these different readings fit together. There are often 10–15 minutes of downtime while you wait for the attending. Use this time to read up on pathophysiology and treatment guidelines to further increase your knowledge base. Always remember that when you are in the setting of patient care, only use your electronic device such as a cellphone to access clinically relevant information. Do not text or communicate personal information when caring for patients unless it is an emergency. It is useful and very courteous to announce to your attending when you are using your device to help the patient.

PROFESSIONALISM IN THE OUTPATIENT SETTING

The term professionalism encompasses many aspects of the physician's role and is conveyed through your behavior. First, a physician wants to convey a tone of respectful caring and professional competence. This starts with

3

the way you dress. Your white coat should be clean and your identification badge should be easily seen. Make sure to follow your medical school's dress code. Be careful to clean your hands before and after each patient encounter using the sink in the room or the disinfectant available outside the examining room. In order to set the stage for a therapeutic interaction, introduce yourself as a medical student, ask how the patient would like to be addressed, and explain your role in the patient's care. Always acknowledge the presence of others in the room and understand their relationship to the patient. Be sure to make the atmosphere in the room as comfortable and pleasant as possible for the patient in regard to their physical and emotional comfort. As you enter the patient's room, try to sense the mood of the patient. If the patient seems to be in emotional or physical distress, you should delay focusing on the EHR and instead focus on the patient's distress. Documentation in the EHR takes a secondary role to your connection with the patient.

Your interactions with both patients and colleagues are essential for a positive therapeutic relationship. Making up data, deliberately recording inaccurate data in the EHR, and stating you did an exam when you did not perform it are ethically and professionally wrong. Each of these can harm your patient and will damage your reputation. Do not lie when asked a question to which you do not know the answer. You are not expected to know the correct answer to all difficult questions the first time you are asked. But you are expected to learn and know the answer the next time the question is raised. This is essential to being a good medical student and future physician. From this point on, you represent your medical school and your profession. This is true in all your interactions, even when outside a clinical setting. Do not discuss patients outside of the office in public locations such as hallways, elevators, or cafeterias. Protecting confidential patient information is a key part of professionalism. An overview of professionalism in healthcare is discussed in detail in Chapter 2.

A TYPICAL OUTPATIENT CLINIC DAY

Outpatient clinical rotations are often unique and based on various aspects of your school. Students will usually be assigned to work with a resident or an attending either for a whole day or a half day. That primary care doctor might have 10–14 patients scheduled with office visits lasting 15–20 minutes. A new patient visit will usually take a bit more time than an established patient. There is much to be accomplished in this short time. Careful preparation on your part enhances your learning. With regard to the EHR, it is worthwhile to try to do a quick review of the records of patients being seen that day before you start with the attending or resident with whom you are working. Obtain an overview of their history, review important diagnoses and what happened during the last visit, and check what routine preventive measures need to be performed going forward. A very important, and often overlooked, aspect of the outpatient visit is reviewing the current medication list with patients. Often medications get changed after hospital stays or by other providers, and not knowing these changes can lead to dangerous outcomes. Ask the attending or resident you are working with how they want you to present the patients you encounter. For example, do they want to introduce you to the patient, or is it okay if you get started seeing a patient on your own if they are busy? How detailed and how much time should your presentations take? Should the presentation be done in a private area outside the patient's exam room or in the patient's room? How should you notify them when you are done seeing the patient? Are there parts of the EHR that you can complete while waiting for the attending? How can you be most helpful for them?

WELLNESS

Throughout the rotation you should set aside time to reflect on your experiences. These reflections may range from formal discussions with the rest of your cohort to diary entries or informal conversations with peers. You should reflect on how you felt during different patient encounters and interactions with your attending or resident. Review knowledge gaps that became evident to you during the day and your general feeling about your rotation experiences. Incorporating time for reflection will provide you with the opportunity to critically think about your performance and will allow you to find ways to incorporate your own wellness into daily practice. At times you may feel that your clinical education does not fully incorporate wellness values that you are trying to promote for your patients. Your busy lifestyle may prevent you from getting the proper exercise, rest, and diet that you are recommending for your patients. Try to set realistic goals for yourself while realizing that you may need to adjust your expectations. Setting unrealistic goals for yourself by demanding perfection in all aspects of your life can be exhausting, can hinder your curiosity, and can interfere with teamwork.

Summary Thoughts

- Remain self-aware and do not underestimate the importance of common sense in the clinical setting.
- Some stress as you enter clinical medicine can work to your advantage, as it can help focus your learning and enhance your performance.
- You should be well versed about your patients and their problems. You will likely be surprised by how much better care patients receive because you listen to and care for them.

- Be professional and honest in all of your interactions, both with patients and the members of your team. Maintain empathy and use it to comfort your patients.
- Be as gentle and forgiving of yourself as you are of your patients.
- In clinical medicine an amazing journey awaits you. Take time to reflect on all that you see and learn. Enjoy the journey!

Selected References

Drolet BC, et al. A Comprehensive Medical Student Wellness Program—Design and Implementation at Vanderbilt School of Medicine. *Acad Med.* 2010;85(1):103–110.

Kligler B, et al. Becoming a Doctor: A Qualitative Evaluation of Challenges and Opportunities in Medical Student Wellness During the Third Year. *Acad Med.* 2013;88(4):535–540.

Yanes AF. The Culture of Perfection: A Barrier to Medical Student Wellness and Development. *Acad Med* 2017;92(7):900–901.

Interdisciplinary Healthcare Teams

4

- ➤ Introduction to Interdisciplinary Care
- ➤ Advanced Practice Providers (APP)
- ➤ Entry-Level Nursing Providers
- ➤ Mental Health and Psychosocial Support Professionals
- ➤ Rehabilitation Professionals
- ➤ Pharmacy Professionals
- ➤ Additional Allied Health Professionals

INTRODUCTION TO INTERDISCIPLINARY CARE

The complexity involved with providing healthcare continues to increase. In order to reduce the intricacy of healthcare delivery, an improved model of patient care has evolved that involves an interdisciplinary team working collaboratively to set goals, make decisions, share resources, and distribute responsibilities. The expansion of scope of practice and the increased options for sub-specializations within the various healthcare fields lend themselves to increased need and opportunity for collaboration. Increased engagement with the patient and their family, enhanced patient experiences and outcomes, increased efficiency, and better utilization of resources are benefits of this approach. The sharing of expertise and workload among care team members increases professional satisfaction, encourages innovation, and enriches the learning environment by enabling practitioners to learn new skills and approaches with the ultimate goal to improve patient care.

During training and beyond you will likely interact with a variety of healthcare professionals who will address a variety of the physical, emotional, psychological, and social needs of the patient. In order to optimize the team-based approach, it is crucial that all members have a thorough understanding of the credentials, education, role, and scope of practice of each healthcare professional.

Original chapter by Anne E. Calvaresi, DNP, CRNP, RNFA, and Amy Baker, PA-C

4

In most clinical settings the term healthcare "providers" or "practitioners" includes individuals who are trained as Doctors of Medicine or Osteopathy (MD or DO), Doctors of Dental Medicine (DMD) or Doctors of Dental Surgery (DDS), Doctors of Podiatric Medicine (DPM), and Doctors of Optometry (OD). In addition, chiropractors, nurse practitioners, midwives, physician assistants, clinical psychologists, and clinical social workers who are given authority by the state in which they practice may be classified as providers. Any other healthcare professionals from whom an employee's group plan accepts claims for insurance payments may also qualify as healthcare providers. Additional interdisciplinary healthcare professionals include a broad group: athletic trainers, audiologists, clinical nurse specialists, community health workers, dietitians, dental hygienists, nutritionists, emergency medical technicians, paramedics, healthcare administrators, medical assistants, medical coders, medical laboratory scientists, medical prosthetic technicians, medical transcriptionists, nurses, nurse anesthetists, physical therapists, occupational therapists, paramedics, traditional registered pharmacists, pharmacy technicians, phlebotomists, physical therapists, radiographers, medical radiation dosimetrists, medical physicists, radiation therapists, recreational therapists, respiratory therapists, speech-language pathologists, surgical assistants, surgical technologists, and others.

Traditional naturopaths and licensed naturopathic doctors (ND/NMD) work to heal through natural substances (food, herbs, water) and are uncommon in academic medical centers. The education of these two providers is very different with their scope of practice and status varying from state to state. In some states there are no regulations regarding naturopathic practice. A state-licensed Doctor of Naturopathic Medicine is a primary care provider who is trained to diagnose and prescribe, while a traditional naturopath is not able to do either.

A larger number of healthcare professionals who also support patient care may not be discussed here. These other healthcare professionals with specialized training may engage with the interdisciplinary team and offer essential support roles to the patient and the healthcare team.

You may encounter many of these healthcare workers in the inpatient and outpatient setting, and their degree designations are summarized in Table 4-1. A review of some of the more common healthcare professionals you may encounter as you strive to deliver quality interdisciplinary care is noted next.

ADVANCED PRACTICE PROVIDERS (APP)

This group of providers has advanced education and training in order to provide care to patients with physician supervision; collaboratively with physicians; or independently depending on education, experience, and scope of practice as defined by state law. Many of these providers are advanced practice nurses who have education and training beyond basic nursing.

Table 4-1. Professional Degrees and Professional Designations Commonly Encountered in Healthcare

AA	Associate of Arts
AAS	Associate of Applied Science
AD	Associate's Degree
ADN	Associate's Degree in Nursing
AEC	Associate in Emergency Care
ANP	Adult Nurse Practitioner
APNP	Psychiatric Nurse Practitioner
APRN	Advanced Practice Registered Nurse
APSW	Association of Psychiatric Social Workers
AS	Associate of Science
BA	Bachelor of Arts
BCOP	Board Certified Oncology Pharmacist
BH	Bachelor of Health
BN	Bachelor of Nursing
BPharm	Bachelor of Pharmacy
BPsych	Bachelor of Psychology
BS	Bachelor of Science
BSc	Bachelor of Science
BSN	Bachelor of Science in Nursing
BSPT	Bachelor of Science in Physical Therapy
BSW	Bachelor of Social Work
CAGS	Certificate of Advanced Graduate Study
CASAC	Certified Alcoholism & Substance Abuse Counselor
CCM	Certificate in Case Management
CGC	Certified Genetic Counselor
CNM	Certified Nurse-Midwife
COSC	Certified Orthopaedic Surgery Coder
CPC	Certified Professional Coder
CPC-I	Certified Professional Coding Instructor
CPFT	Certified Pulmonary Function Technologist
CPhT	Certified Pharmacy Technician
CPMA	Certified Professional Medical Auditor
CPPM	Certified Physician Practice Manager
CRNA	Certified Registered Nurse Anesthetist
CRT	Certified Respiratory Therapist

(Continued)

Table 4-1. Professional Degrees and Professional Designations Commonly Encountered in Healthcare (*Continued*)

CVT	Cardiovascular Technician
DD	Doctor of Divinity
DDS	Doctor of Dental Surgery
Dipl Psych	Diploma in Psychology
DMD	Doctor of Medicine in Dentistry
DMin	Doctor of Ministry
DNP	Doctor of Nursing Practice
DNS (DNSc)	Doctor of Nursing Science
DO	Doctor of Osteopathic Medicine
DPA	Doctor of Public Administration
DPH	Doctor of Public Health
DPM	Doctor of Podiatric Medicine
DPT	Doctor of Physical Therapy
DSW	Doctor of Social Work
DTh	Doctor of Theology
DVM	Doctor of Veterinary Medicine
EdD/DEd	Doctor of Education
FAAD	Fellow of the American Academy of Dermatology
FAAEM	Fellow of the American Academy of Emergency Medicine
FAAFP	Fellow of the American Academy of Family Physicians
FACC	Fellow of the American College of Cardiologists
FACCP	Fellow of the American College of Chest Physicians
FACE	Fellow of the American College of Endocrinology
FACEP	Fellow of the American College of Emergency Physicians
FACFAS	Fellow of the American College of Foot and Ankle Surgeons
FACG	Fellow of the American College of Gastroenterology
FACHE	Fellow American College of Healthcare Executives
FACOG	Fellow of the American College of Obstetrics and Gynecologists
FACOS	Fellow of the American College of Osteopathic Surgeons/Fellow of the American College of Orthopedic Surgeons
FACP	Fellow of the American College of Physicians
FACS	Fellow of the American College of Surgeons
FAIUM	Fellow American Institute of Ultrasound in Medicine
FASPS	Fellow of the American Society of Podiatric Surgeons
FFPHM	Fellow Faculty of Public Health Medicine
FFR	Fellow Faculty of Radiologists

Table 4-1. Professional Degrees and Professional Designations Commonly Encountered in Healthcare (*Continued*)

FHM	Fellow in Hospital Medicine
FICS	Fellow of the International College of Surgeons
FNP	Family Nurse Practitioner
FPMRS	Female Pelvic Medicine and Reconstructive Surgery
FRCPSC	Fellow of the Royal College of Physicians and Surgeons of Canada
FRCS	Fellow of the Royal College of Surgeons
FSCAI	Fellow of the Society for Cardiovascular Angiography and Interventions
FSTS	Fellow of the Society of Thoracic Surgeons
GNP	Geriatric Nurse Practitioner
JD	Doctor of Jurisprudence (Lawyer)
LCSW	Licensed Clinical Social Worker
LICSW	Licensed Independent Clinical Social Worker
LMFT	Licensed Marriage and Family Therapist
LMHC	Licensed Mental Health Counselor
LPC	Licensed Professional Counselor
LPN	Licensed Practical Nurse
LVN	Licensed Vocational Nurse
MA	Master of Arts/Medical Assistant
MBA	Master of Business Administration
MBBS/MB ChB	Bachelor of Medicine, Bachelor of Surgery (Latin: Medicinae Baccalaureus, Baccalaureus Chirurgiae); often used for medical degrees in the United Kingdom and India
MC	Master of Counseling
MD	Medical Doctor
MEd	Master of Education
MHS	Master of Health Science
MMHC	Master of Management in Health Care
MMin	Master of Ministry
MMS	Master of Management Studies
MPAS	Master of Physician Assistant Studies
MPH	Master in Public Health
MPsych	Master of Psychology
MPT	Master of Physical Therapy
MRCOG	Member Royal College of Obstetricians and Gynecologists
MRCS	Member of the Royal College of Surgeons

(*Continued*)

Table 4-1. Professional Degrees and Professional Designations Commonly Encountered in Healthcare (*Continued*)

MS	Master of Science/Master of Surgery
MSEd	Master of Science in Education
MSN	Master of Science in Nursing
MSPT	Master of Science in Physical Therapy
MSSW	Master of Science in Social Work
MSW	Master of Social Work
MTh	Master of Theology
ND/NMD	Naturopathic Doctors (ND/NMD)
NP	Nurse Practitioner
OD	Doctor of Optometry
OSW-C	Oncology Social Worker Board Certified
OT	Occupational Therapist
PA	Physician Assistant/Pathology Assistant
PA-C	Physician Assistant certified by the National Commission of Certification of PAs
PharmD	Doctor of Pharmacy
PhD/DPhil	Doctor of Philosophy (Doctorate/Advanced degree)
Psych	Psychologist
PsyD	Doctor of Psychology
PT	Physical Therapist
RCIS	Registered Cardiovascular Invasive Specialist
RD	Registered Dietitian
RDCS	Registered Diagnostic Cardiac Sonographer
RDMS	Registered Diagnostic Medical Sonographer
RDN	Registered Dietitian Nutritionist
RN	Registered Nurse
RNFA	Registered Nurse First Assistant (Operating room)
RPFT	Registered Pulmonary Function Technologist
RPh	Registered Pharmacist
RPSGT	Registered Polysomnographic Technologist
RRT	Registered Respiratory Therapist
ScD	Doctor of Science
SLP	Speech-Language Pathologist
SScD	Doctor of Social Science
ThD	Doctor of Theology

Physician assistants[*] **(PAs)** have completed an undergraduate bachelor's degree and an additional 24–36-month certificate, master's, or doctoral-level physician assistant program in the medical model of education. They work in hospitals, operating rooms, and outpatient offices to examine, diagnose, and treat patients in nearly every medical subspecialty. State laws determine the scope of practice and requirements for supervision, which may include supervisory or collaborative agreements with a physician. PAs have prescriptive privileges in all 50 states. PA-C indicates certification by the National Commission of Certification of PAs.

Certified nurse-midwives (CNMs) or Certified midwives (CMs) hold a 4-year bachelor's degree, typically in nursing, followed by advanced training in midwifery. Minimum education requirements for this specialty include a bachelor's degree, completion of a certificate, master's, or doctoral training program in midwifery, and passing a national certification exam. CNMs and CMs provide prenatal, postnatal, labor and delivery, gynecologic, and primary care for women in hospitals, birth centers, and at home. Other types of midwives, such as certified professional midwives (CPMs), have less formal training and a much narrower scope of practice.

Certified registered nurse anesthetists (CRNAs) are licensed registered nurses with advanced training, including master's or doctoral degrees, having completed an anesthesia-based program of 24–26 months. Additionally, they must pass a national certification exam. They work with other care providers, including obstetricians, surgeons, dentists, and anesthesiologists, to deliver anesthesia to patients.

Clinical nurse specialists (CNSs) are licensed registered nurses with advanced training, including master's or doctoral degrees, with a specialized focus in various areas of nursing. They may work in direct patient care, administration, education, research, or training, or as case managers.

Nurse practitioners (NP, CRNP, APN, APRN) and Doctors of Nursing Practice (DNP) are registered nurse professionals with additional clinical training, most often with a master's or doctoral degree. Nurse practitioners may have specific training in specialties including family health, adult/gerontology, pediatrics, OB/GYN, or others but can be found practicing in any specialty. They are trained to evaluate, diagnose, and treat patients in a variety of settings. State laws determine the scope of practice and requirements for supervision, which may include direct supervision by a licensed physician or physician collaboration agreements, although in some states, no physician supervision is required. Prescription authority also varies by state.

Registered nurse first assistant (RNFA) is a perioperative registered nurse who functions as a first assistant during surgical operations. The role will vary based on the institution and the surgeon. Many academic teaching hospitals do not regularly use RNFAs due to the presence of surgical residents and fellows.

---

[*]The designation of Physician's Associate is being considered by some organizations.

4

ENTRY-LEVEL NURSING PROVIDERS

Registered nurses (RNs) are nurses with an associate's (2-year) or bachelor's (4-year) degree in nursing. They may work in a variety of settings such as the intensive care unit, emergency department, labor and delivery, home healthcare, in the operating room, or as a staff nurse in the hospital or in the ambulatory setting.

Licensed practical nurses (LPNs) perform a variety of tasks typically under the supervision of an RN. They are qualified to administer medications, check vital signs, and give injections. LPNs are licensed and must complete a state-approved educational program, which takes around 1–2 years to complete.

Medical assistants (MAs) have a scope of practice that varies by state, with most states having no specific regulations or any specific training mandates. Many facilities require state certification. These healthcare providers usually have on-the-job training or enroll in a certificate program that provides basic medical skills instruction. They carry out a wide variety of duties under the supervision of a physician and work most commonly in the outpatient setting. Their duties include administrative (computer applications, appointment scheduling, insurance forms, etc.) and clinical duties such as medical history taking, vital signs, basic point-of-care testing, phlebotomy, administering medications, and assisting with physical exams and procedures.

Nursing assistants/associates (CNAs) and Patient care technicians (PCTs) have a scope of practice and training requirements that vary by state. These healthcare providers usually have on-the-job training or enroll in a certificate program that provides basic instruction in skills related to completion of supporting activities of daily living. They function in hospitals, long-term care facilities, and rehabilitation centers to supplement nursing care by providing basic care to patients such as bathing, dressing, feeding, and obtaining vital signs.

MENTAL HEALTH AND PSYCHOSOCIAL SUPPORT PROFESSIONALS

Clinical psychologists evaluate and treat patients with acute and chronic psychological trauma and illness. They must complete 4–5 years of training following their undergraduate studies and have completed an internship, followed by licensure. They work with patients to manage psychological disorders that include but are not limited to mood and anxiety disorders, addiction, and adjustment disorders.

Licensed professional counselors (LPCs) are mental health service providers with a master's degree who are trained to work with individuals, families, and groups in treating mental, behavioral, and emotional problems and disorders. LPCs make up a large percentage of the workforce employed in community mental health.

Pastoral care services are available in hospital and long-term care settings. Chaplains or spiritual care professionals assist patients with their spiritual needs. Chaplains are usually required to have a degree in counseling and theology and are typically ordained and endorsed by their religious organization. Many chaplains work in an interfaith environment using a nondenominational approach to counsel, minister, and provide spiritual guidance to patients and families. The pastoral care team may also include lay providers who have specific training in the area of pastoral support. The pastoral care team can also serve as a source of emotional support to the medical team.

Social workers support patients of all ages in many different settings, including hospitals, schools, detention centers, rehabilitation centers, and nursing homes. They counsel patients and advocate for patient services, including financial, behavioral, health, and social services. Licensed clinical social workers typically have completed at least a master's degree with significant fieldwork as required by each state and have passed a licensure exam to become a licensed clinical social worker (LCSW). They may further specialize in areas such as oncology and be board certified, with some achieving doctoral status.

REHABILITATION PROFESSIONALS

Occupational therapists (OTs) work with other members of the patient care team to optimize patients' abilities to carry out daily activities and to reach maximum activity levels and independence. They work with patients across the lifespan to learn, relearn, or master activities of daily living. They work in hospitals, long-term care facilities, rehabilitation centers, schools, and homes. They complete a bachelor's degree followed by either a master's degree or doctoral degree (OTD) and have passed a national certification exam.

Physical therapists (PTs) work with patients to optimize function, independence, activity, and movement for patients with injuries or limitations. They work in hospitals, rehabilitation centers, long-term care facilities, outpatient clinics, and homes with patients of all ages. In the past, a physical therapist's education involved a master's degree program, and today a 3-year Doctor of Physical Therapy (DPT) degree is required before sitting for the national certification exam.

Recreation therapists (RTs) work with patients to promote functional outcomes, increased activity levels, and independence. They incorporate a vast array of interventions and therapies to obtain these outcomes, including movement, dance, and music. They work with patients of all ages in a variety of settings, including hospitals, rehabilitation centers, and schools, and must have completed at least a bachelor's degree and internship and have passed a national certification exam.

Speech-language pathologists (SLPs) have completed a bachelor's degree and now require a master's degree in order to be licensed and certified. These providers work in hospitals, long-term care facilities, rehabilitation centers, schools, and homes to prevent, assess, diagnose, and treat speech, language, social communication, cognitive-communication, and swallowing disorders in children and adults.

PHARMACY PROFESSIONALS

Pharmacists (PharmD) graduating today in the United States are required to complete a 4-year PharmD/Doctor of Pharmacy program after 2–4 years of undergraduate coursework. The traditional "Registered Pharmacist" or RPh training has been replaced by the PharmD. Pharmacists ensure optimal medication treatment by providing guidance to practitioners about appropriate pharmacotherapeutic selections, ensuring appropriate medication doses, limiting drug interactions, and answering patient and provider questions regarding medications. They can work in both inpatient and outpatient settings. There are additionally an increasing number of pharmacists with state-regulated prescriptive authority and the ability to administer immunizations. Many PharmDs will do an additional 1–2 years of residency training in such specialized areas as oncology, ambulatory care, critical care, infectious disease, pediatrics, and drug information.

Pharmacy technicians work in a variety of inpatient and outpatient pharmacy settings to support the role of the pharmacist. Training and licensure are not standardized from state to state, and training programs vary in length. Most training programs require a high school diploma or GED as a prerequisite.

ADDITIONAL ALLIED HEALTH PROFESSIONALS

Case managers and more specifically hospital case managers evaluate a patient's needs and available resources as part of the discharge planning process. Case managers are often nurses who work to find the safest, most efficient, and most economical way of meeting the patient's needs with input from the family as part of discharge planning. Case managers also work in a variety of outpatient settings.

Genetic counselors evaluate and counsel an individual or family on the risk of inherited medical conditions. They may evaluate patients in the prenatal, newborn/pediatric, adult, or oncology settings. Training requires completion of a master's degree and passing a board examination to become a certified genetic counselor (CGC). Some states require genetic counselors to have a license to practice (LCGC).

Registered dietitians (RD) complete a bachelor's degree in nutrition with standards meeting the American Dietetic Association requirements. They must also have completed practical education experience and passed a national exam. RDs help patients obtain maximum health benefits through dietary plans designed for specific disease states, including renal disease, diabetes, hypercholesterolemia, heart disease, food allergies/intolerances, and obesity.

Respiratory therapists (RTs) and Registered respiratory therapists (RRTs) evaluate and treat patients with respiratory disease and lung injury. They also manage patients requiring mechanical ventilation. They have completed either an associate's or bachelor's degree in respiratory therapy and have passed a national examination.

References

American Association of Nurse Anesthetists – www.aana.com.
American Academy of Nurse Practitioners – www.aanp.org.
American Academy of Physician Assistants – www.aapa.org.
American Association for Respiratory Care – www.aarc.org.
American College of Nurse-Midwives – www.acnm.org.
American Dietetic Association – www.eatright.org.
American Occupational Therapy Association – www.aota.org.
American Pharmacist's Association – www.pharmacist.com.
American Podiatric Medical Association – www.apma.org.
American Psychological Association – www.apa.org.
American Speech-Language-Hearing Association (ASHA) https://www.asha.org.
American Therapeutic Recreation Association – http://www.atra-tr.org/about.htm.
Careers in Psychology – https://careersinpsychology.org.
Cornell Law – https://www.law.cornell.edu/cfr/text/29/825.125.
Grant RW, et al. *Interdisciplinary Collaborative Teams in Primary Care: A Model Curriculum and Resource Guide*. San Francisco, CA: Pew Health Professions Commission; 1995.
National Association of Clinical Nurse Specialists – www.nacns.org.
https://www.verywellhealth.com.
https://study.com/articles/Hospital_Chaplain_Job_Description_and_Education_Requirements.html.

The Language of Healthcare

5

- ➤ Outpatient Coding/Billing
- ➤ Inpatient Coding/Billing
- ➤ Medicare, Medicaid, and Managed Care
- ➤ Classification Systems Used in Healthcare
  - ➢ International Classification of Diseases (ICD)
- ➢ Current Procedural Terminology (CPT)
- ➢ Diagnosis Related Group (DRG)
- ➢ Diagnostic and Statistical Manual of Mental Disorders (DSM)

Transitioning from the classroom to entering the world of patient care involves applying concepts of anatomy, physiology, pharmacology, clinical exam skills, and other important principles learned in the early years of medical school. Developing sound clinical skills is of paramount importance, but in our complex healthcare system, understanding the administrative structure that directs and oversees the system and how this affects patient care is equally important. Understanding these basic concepts will help provide healthcare professional students with an increased understanding of how to provide patients with optimum care. While these concepts that we have called the "language of healthcare" may not be a focus of medical students' and other healthcare providers' education, it is critical to have a general understanding of these concepts, as they provide a framework on how healthcare services are provided in the United States.

OUTPATIENT CODING/BILLING

- The evaluation and management (E&M or "E and M") patient visit is the foundation of most physician practices. Based on the characteristics of the office visit or hospital encounter (length, complexity, consultation, etc.), the practitioner chooses the correct Current Procedural Terminology (CPT) code (see page 41) for an E&M visit.
- CPT codes 99201 through 99205 are used for new patients (NPV) and 99211 through 99215 for returning or established patients (EPV).

Original chapter by Costas Lallas, MD, FACS

5

Consultation codes are 99241–99245. In general, the higher the number in each coding group, the more complex the evaluation. These higher codes are associated with higher billing and in turn higher payment to the provider. Additionally, consultations are billed at a higher rate. Practitioners must justify the level of billing in the patient encounter in order to be compensated completely (see full discussion on CPT below).

- A consultation is a type of E&M service provided at the request of another physician or appropriate source to either recommend care for a specific condition or problem or to determine whether to accept responsibility for ongoing management of the patient's entire care *or* for the care of a specific condition or problem. In order to qualify as a consultation, the practitioner must document the three Rs: request, rendering of the service, and report back. Notably, Medicare and some commercial carriers do not currently recognize consultation codes.

- As the level of provider billing increases, so does the relative value unit (RVU). The RVU is a measure of value used in the U.S. Medicare reimbursement formula for physician services. It is routinely used to measure physician productivity and is often linked to overall compensation by the provider's employer. This information is useful when comparing physicians of the same specialty. Within specialties there are percentiles associated with RVUs over a set time period, such as 90th percentile for RVUs in a year by a cardiologist.

- Once the practitioner submits a bill, it is prepared by the billing staff as a claim.

- Each claim contains the patient information (their demographic information and medical history) and the procedures performed (in CPT or HCPCS codes) if appropriate (see page 41). Claims also have provider information listed via a National Provider Index (NPI) number: a unique 10-digit identification number issued to U.S. healthcare providers by the Centers for Medicare and Medicaid.

- Each CPT code is paired with a diagnosis code, known as an ICD code, that demonstrates the medical necessity. The International Coding of Diseases (ICD) was originally designed as a healthcare classification system, providing a uniform system of diagnostic codes for classifying diseases (see page 40). ICD incudes classifications of a wide variety of signs, symptoms, abnormal findings, Ifconcerns, social circumstances, and external causes of injury or disease. The current generation of ICD codes is the ICD-10.

- In the case of high-volume third-party payers, like Medicare or Medicaid, billers can submit the claim directly to the government payer. If, however, a biller is not submitting a claim directly to these large payers, they will most likely go through a clearinghouse.

- A clearinghouse is a third-party organization or company that receives and reformats claims from billers and then transmits them to payers such as private insurance companies.

- Once a claim reaches a payer, it undergoes a process called adjudication. In this process, a payer evaluates a medical claim and decides whether the claim is valid, is compliant with submission guidelines, and, if so, how much of the claim the payer will reimburse the provider.

- A claim may be accepted, denied, or rejected. An *accepted* claim is one that the payer agrees to cover. In the case of *rejected* claims, the biller may correct the claim and resubmit it, whereas a *denied* claim is one where the payer refuses to process payment for the medical services rendered.
- The payer will next send a report to the provider/biller, detailing what and how much of the claim they are willing to pay and why. This often differs from the fees listed in the initial claim. The payer usually has a contract with the provider that stipulates the fees and reimbursement rates for a number of procedures, as well as a day of in-hospital care.
- If the patient has secondary insurance, the biller takes the difference between what was billed minus reimbursed from the primary insurance for the approved claim and sends it to the patient's secondary insurance.
- If there are any discrepancies, the biller/provider will enter into an appeal process with the payer.
- Once the payer has agreed to pay the provider for a portion of the services on the claim, the remaining amount is passed on to the patient.
- A biller may include an explanation of benefits (EOB) with the final statement. This can be useful in explaining to patients why certain procedures were covered while others were not.
- If the patient is delinquent in their payment or if they do not pay the full amount, it is the responsibility of the biller to ensure that the provider is properly reimbursed for their services. This may involve contacting the patient directly, sending follow-up bills, or, in worst-case scenarios, enlisting a collection agency.

INPATIENT CODING/BILLING

- An inpatient is an individual who has been officially admitted to the hospital under a physician's order. This usually requires a 2-day stay or longer than 24 hours. The patient will remain classified as an inpatient until 1 day before discharge.
- Examples of inpatient facilities include acute and long-term care hospitals, skilled nursing facilities, hospices, and home health services.
- Original Medicare inpatient claims are paid under Part A, whereas outpatient claims are paid under Medicare Part B (see below).
- Inpatient medical coding is reported using ICD-10-CM (Clinical Modification) and ICD-10-PCS (Procedure Coding System) codes, which result in payments based on Medicare Severity-Diagnosis Related Groups (MS-DRGs) (see page 42). Reimbursement is based primarily on the DRG.
- In an inpatient facility, medical coders must determine the principal diagnosis for the admission, as well as present on admission (POA) indicators on all diagnoses.
- Diagnoses listed as "probable," "suspected," "likely," and other such terms may be coded when documented as existing at the time of discharge and no definitive diagnosis has been established. This is in contrast to outpatient coding, where these diagnoses are not permitted.

5

MEDICARE, MEDICAID, AND MANAGED CARE

- Medicare is a U.S. federal health insurance program for people 65 and older, people under 65 with certain disabilities, and people of all ages with end-stage renal disease. Medicare is partly funded by payroll taxes from most employers, employees, and all people who are self-employed. The Medicare program offers basic coverage to help pay for things like doctor visits, hospital stays, and surgeries.
- Medicare is overseen by the government organization known as the Center for Medicare & Medicaid Services (CMS). This program is federally funded primarily through wage taxes.
- Medicare is broken out into four parts: A, B, C, and D. Parts A and B are known as original Medicare. This is the most basic coverage you can get. Parts C and D are available through private or "supplemental" health plans.
  - o Part A (hospital coverage): Covers items such as inpatient hospital stays, home healthcare, and skilled nursing facility care.
  - o Part B (medical coverage): Covers items such as doctor visits, outpatient services, and diagnostic screenings.
  - o Part C (Medicare Advantage): Medicare Advantage plans are a type of Medicare health plan offered by a private company that contracts with Medicare to provide all Part A and Part B benefits, with most offering some prescription drug coverage. These plans must provide the same coverage as original Medicare and can also offer extra benefits. The most common types of Medicare Advantage plans are health maintenance organization (HMO) plans, preferred provider organization (PPO) plans, and private fee-for-service (PFFS) plans.
  - o Part D (prescription drug coverage): Only offered through private health Medicare Advantage plans. The Medicare Part D "donut hole" or "coverage gap" markedly decreased in 2020 with changes in the amount the patient paid while in the gap. The patient enters the donut hole when total drug costs reach $4,130 in the year. By design, while in the coverage gap, the patient is responsible for 25% of the drug costs. Previously most or all of the cost was the responsibility of the patient. In all Part D plans, after the patient has paid $6,550 in out-of-pocket costs for covered drugs, the patient leaves the donut hole and enters "catastrophic coverage." The patient then pays the greater amount of either 5% or $3.70 for generic medications and $9.20 for brand-name drugs. There is no maximum amount or cap on how much one will pay. Once the year ends, the cycle resets and the costs are adjusted for the new year.
  - o There is a "Medicare loophole" that concerns people who need skilled nursing care after being hospitalized for a health issue. Such care is covered by Medicare, but only if the person has been formally admitted to the hospital as an inpatient for at least 3 days. Outpatients are not covered by Medicare for subsequent nursing needs, and people

admitted to hospitals as outpatients will not be covered by Medicare if they need to be transferred to a skilled nursing facility.

- Medicaid is the United States' public health insurance program for people with low income. The Medicaid program covers one in five low-income Americans, and the vast majority of Medicaid enrollees lack access to other affordable health insurance.
  o Medicaid is financed jointly by the federal government and states. The federal government matches state Medicaid spending.
  o In addition to low-income individuals, Medicaid covers children who are impoverished or with special healthcare needs, nonelderly adults with disabilities, and the elderly.
  o Medicaid participates in managed care plans that provide for the delivery of Medicaid health benefits and additional services through contracted arrangements between state Medicaid agencies and managed care organizations (MCOs) that accept a set per member per month (capitation) payment for these services.
  o The WIC (Women, Infants, Children) program is related in that it safeguards the health of low-income pregnant, postpartum, and breast-feeding women, infants, and children up to age 5 who are at nutritional risk by providing nutritious foods to supplement diets, information on healthy eating (including breastfeeding promotion and support), and referrals to healthcare. Unlike Medicaid, which is managed by CMS, WIC is managed by the U.S. Department of Agriculture.
- Managed healthcare plans are an alternative to traditional healthcare plans and provide a health insurance policy to individual members of a group or employer (called a sponsor). These plans allow sponsors to negotiate reduced rates for their policyholders with hospitals, medical service providers, and physicians by including them in the network.
  o Health Maintenance Organization (HMO): Specific providers must be used by the employee for the reduced fees to be provided to their medical insurance plan. In an HMO plan, you have the least flexibility but will likely have the easiest claims experiences, since the network takes care of putting in the claims for you.
  o Preferred Provider Organization (PPO): Members can choose the physician they want to see instead of being solely restricted to the HMO providers. A member can choose between a member or nonmember provider.
  o Point of service (POS): Members can choose their own physician, who has previously agreed to provide services at a discounted fee. The member would have to use the chosen physician as a gateway first before moving on to a specialist.
  o Exclusive provider network (EPO): The member of the plan can choose from the providers within the network and does not have to work with a primary care physician. However, any service taken outside of the network may not be covered.

CLASSIFICATION SYSTEMS USED IN HEALTHCARE

International Classification of Diseases (ICD)

The World Health Organization (WHO) previously created the International Classification of Diseases (ICD), and it is recognized as the international "standard diagnostic tool for epidemiology, health management and clinical purposes." ICD-10 came into use gradually in the United States in different settings and was fully implemented in 2015, with ICD-11 scheduled to come into use in 2022. ICD-10-CM (clinical modification) incorporates a further level of detail needed for more specific disease classification and allows assigning diagnostic and procedure codes associated with inpatient, outpatient, and physician offices. It has been widely adopted by government and private insurance carriers.

The system consists of more than 68,000 codes, compared to approximately 13,000 ICD-9-CM codes in the prior version. ICD-10-CM codes have the potential to reveal more about quality of care to better understand complications, design care and algorithms, and improve the tracking of outcomes. ICD-10-CM codes may consist of up to seven characters, with the seventh-digit extensions representing visit encounter or sequelae for injuries and external causes. ICD-10-CM consists of new features and greater specificity. Sample ICD-10-CM codes are outlined in Table 5-1 to illustrate this increased detail over the ICD-9-CM. Figure 5-1 provides a framework for the six or seven characters usually seen with an ICD-10 code. However, an ICD-10 can have as few as three characters, all representing the category.

Table 5-1. Sample ICD-10 CM System Notations

Sample ICD-10 CM System Notations*

Combination Codes for Conditions and Common Symptoms

- I25.110, Arteriosclerotic heart disease of native coronary artery with unstable angina pectoris
- K50.013, Crohn's disease of small intestine with fistula
- K71.51, Toxic liver disease with chronic active hepatitis with ascites

Combination Codes for Poisonings and the External Cause

- T39.011, Poisoning by aspirin, accidental (unintentional)
- T39.012, Poisoning by aspirin, intentional self-harm
- T39.013, Poisoning by aspirin, assault
- T39.014, Poisoning by aspirin, undetermined

Laterality

- C50.212, Malignant neoplasm of upper-inner quadrant of left female breast
- H02.835, Dermatochalasis of left lower eyelid
- I80.01, Phlebitis and thrombophlebitis of superficial vessels of right lower extremity
- L89.213, Pressure ulcer of right hip, stage III

---

*https://library.ahima.org/doc?oid=106177#.XfAjd-hKibg. Accessed February 2, 2020.

ICD-10-CM Code Format

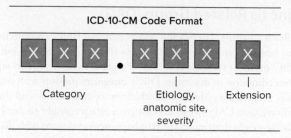

Category   Etiology,   Extension
             anatomic site,
             severity

Figure 5-1. ICD-10-CM code format.

5

Current Procedural Terminology (CPT)

CPT is a medical code set published and copyrighted by the American Medical Association (AMA), used to report medical, surgical, and diagnostic procedures and services to a variety of entities, such as insurance companies and accreditation organizations. There are several sections of the CPT code, with Section 1 most commonly used by physicians to submit billing for services. It is broken down as follows:

- Evaluation and Management: 99201 – 99499
- Anesthesia: 00100 – 01999; 99100 – 99140
- Surgery: 10021 – 69990
- Radiology: 70010 – 79999
- Pathology and Laboratory: 80047 – 89398
- Medicine: 90281 – 99199; 99500 – 99607

As an example using an E&M code, a physician who sees an inpatient consultation for 40 minutes and performs basic history and physical evaluations, codes CPT Code 99252. An office or other outpatient visit for the E&M of a new patient with a history, detailed examination, and medical decision-making of low complexity uses CPT Code 99203.

HCPCS (Healthcare Common Procedure Coding System) is a set of healthcare procedure codes based on CPT. It was designed to provide a standardized coding system in order to describe specific items and services that are provided when healthcare is delivered. It is a necessary form of coding for Medicare, Medicaid, and other health insurance programs in order to ensure that insurance claims are processed efficiently. CPT is largely private, with the American Medical Association the copyright owner, and the AMA does not wish to give away the codes freely. However, according to the Health Insurance Portability and Accountability Act of 1996, everyone must have access to HCPCS codes.

Diagnosis Related Group (DRG)

The DRG is a patient classification system that standardizes prospective payment to hospitals and encourages the use of cost containment initiatives. The DRG payment typically covers all charges associated with an inpatient stay from admission to discharge. DRGs categorize patients with respect to diagnosis, surgical procedures, comorbidities, complications, and discharge status. Every year, CMS (Medicare) assigns a relative weight to every DRG. The relative weight determines the reimbursement associated with that DRG and reflects the patient's severity of illness and cost of care during hospitalization. A higher relative weight is associated with a longer length of stay, greater severity of illness, and higher reimbursement. For example, DRG 189 (respiratory failure) has a relative weight of 1.2353 and DRG 312 (syncope) has a relative weight of 0.8015.[1]

Diagnostic and Statistical Manual of Mental Disorders (DSM)

The DSM is a taxonomic and diagnostic tool published by the American Psychiatric Association (APA). DSM-5 (the most recent version published in 2018) contains the most up-to-date criteria for diagnosing mental disorders, along with extensive descriptive text, providing a common language for clinicians to communicate about their patients and perform research studies.

Reference

1. https://acphospitalist.org/archives/2019/05/coding-corner-the-abcs-of-drgs.htm, accessed 3/20/2020.

The History and Physical Examination | 6

HISTORY AND PHYSICAL EXAMINATION, ADULT

First, some general comments about the initial history and physical (H&P) in particular, and medical records in general. The H&P write-up provides others on your team, and in the future, other healthcare providers caring for your patient, a record of the current hospitalization. Your H&P usually becomes part of the medical record and after review and sign-off by a senior physician, it becomes part of this living and breathing document. After your H&P is added to the chart, along with other H&Ps from the attending, resident, and intern, progress notes are added each day, as well as notes from consultants and other healthcare providers such as nurses, dieticians, and physical therapists. Whether an electronic medical record or an "old" paper-based record that is often scanned into the electronic health record (EHR), the patient chart is a legal document and needs to

---

Chapter update by Steven Haist, MD, MS, Leonard Gomella, MD, Jessica Tomaszewski, MD, Michael Gomella, DDS, and Francis Serio, DMD

be treated as such. Your H&P, along with any other documentation added to the chart, should be legible, and the content should be clear and concise. Some outpatient practices may have their own format to document basic patient information.

Some important comments: The medical record is never a place to verbally "spar" with other physicians or services because of differences of opinion in the care of a patient. And just as important, the language used in our patient notes may introduce biases that may affect the care provided by future healthcare workers, and ultimately can adversely affect the health of the patient. Avoid the use of quotations around potentially sensitive subjects, such as alcohol use and behavior that could be interpreted in a negative light, such as "verbally abusive to the on-call doctor."[1]

The details, style, and length of a written history and physical exam will likely vary with the patient's particular problem(s) and are typically based on the service to which the patient is admitted. Here we describe the general approach to the history and physical exam in an adult admitted to a general medical service. A sample general adult write-up can be found on page 120. This chapter also highlights some specialty-specific key elements (obstetrics, ophthalmology, others) that may be helpful based on the admitting service or the patient's clinical presentation. Information on the history and physical for pediatric patients is found on page 105 with a sample pediatric admission history and physical write-up on page 126.

Practical pointers for the H&P:
- Before interacting with and examining the patient, practice hand hygiene. Also, gloves should be worn when it is anticipated that the examiner will encounter blood or other potentially infectious materials. Consider the need for additional personal protective equipment (PPE) based on the clinical setting and the patient's history and follow your institutional guidelines for PPE use.
- Introduce yourself and your role in the medical care team.
- Ask the patient for their preferred name or title and use such.
- If others are participating in the session (interpreter, caregiver, parent with a child), include the patient in the process as much as possible, e.g., look at and address the patient, not the interpreter.
- Use the interview skills you were taught during your first or second year of medical school.
- Keep questions clear and concise. Avoid presumptive or leading questions.
- In general, avoid medical jargon and abbreviations.
- Try not to interrupt the patient when they answer questions. It is appropriate to have the patient clarify their statements if needed.
- As much as possible, maintain eye contact with the patient. Be mindful of your facial expressions, body language, and tone of voice.
- A seated position at the same eye level (if possible) facilitates the interaction and can communicate interest and concern.
- Be an attentive listener.
- Explain maneuvers during the physical exam. Be mindful and sensitive when exposing body parts for the exam. Use a sheet for proper draping if necessary.

- After the H&P is completed, explain the next steps. Ask, "May I answer any questions for you?"

History (Adult)

Identification: Name, age, gender (see Table 6-13, page 120), preferred pronouns, referring physician, informant (e.g., patient, relative, old chart), and reliability of the informant.

Chief Concern: State the current problem in the patient's words.

History of the Present Illness (HPI): Defines the present illness by quality; quantity; setting; anatomic location and radiation; time course, including when the illness began; whether the concern is progressing, regressing, or steady; whether the concern is of constant or intermittent frequency; and aggravating, alleviating, and associated factors. The information should be in chronologic order, including diagnostic tests done before admission. Record related history, including previous treatment for the problem, risk factors, and pertinent negative results. Include family history and psychosocial history pertinent to the chief concern. Other significant ongoing problems should be included in the HPI in a separate section or paragraph. For instance, if a patient with poorly controlled diabetes mellitus (DM) comes to the emergency department because of chest pain, the HPI should first include information regarding the chest pain followed by a detailed history of the DM. If the DM is diet controlled or otherwise well controlled, the history of the DM may be placed in the past medical history.

Past Medical History (PMH): Current medications, including over-the-counter (OTC) medications, vitamins, and herbal agents; allergies (drug and other, as well as specific allergy manifestations); operations; hospitalizations; blood transfusions, including when and how many units and the type of blood product; trauma; and stable current and past medical problems unrelated to the HPI. Adult patients: Ask about DM; hypertension (HTN); coronary artery disease (CAD), myocardial infarction (MI); peripheral vascular disease (PVD); cerebrovascular accident (CVA); transient ischemic accident (TIA); ulcer disease; asthma; peptic ulcer disease (PUD); emphysema; gout; thyroid, liver, and kidney disease; bleeding disorders; cancer; tuberculosis (TB); hepatitis; and sexually transmitted infections (STIs). Also ask about routine health maintenance. The questions for this category depend on the age and gender of the patient but can include the last Pap smear; screening for human papillomavirus (HPV), human immunodeficiency virus (HIV), hepatitis C, *Chlamydia trachomatis*, and *Neisseria gonorrhoeae*; breast exam; date and result of last mammogram; diphtheria/tetanus/acellular pertussis (DTaP), pneumococcal (PCV-13 and/or PPSV23), influenza, COVID-19, hepatitis B, hepatitis A, HPV, meningococcal and meningococcal B, and varicella zoster vaccinations; stool samples for occult blood; sigmoidoscopy or colonoscopy; cholesterol, high-density lipoprotein (HDL) cholesterol, triglycerides, calculated low-density lipoprotein (LDL) cholesterol; inquiry about functioning smoke alarms on each floor at home, guns in the house and storage, and use of seat belts.

Family History: Age, status (alive, dead) of blood relatives and medical problems of blood relatives (ask about cancer, especially breast, ovarian, colon, thyroid, and prostate; TB; asthma; CAD; MI; HTN; CVA; PVD; thyroid disease; kidney disease; PUD; DM; bleeding disorders; sickle cell disease, thalassemia, or any other anemias; glaucoma; macular degeneration; and psychiatric disorders, including depression, bipolar disorder, schizophrenia, and alcohol or substance abuse). Diagram a family tree if it will be helpful (see Figure 6-3, pages 61-62.).

Psychosocial (Social) History: Stressors (financial, significant relationships, work and/or school, health) and support (family, friends, significant other, clergy); lifestyle risk factors (alcohol, drugs, tobacco, and caffeine use; diet; exercise; exposure to environmental agents; and sexual history [many clinicians will inquire about sexual history as part of the review of systems]); patient profile (may include marital status and children, sexual orientation; present and past employment; financial support and insurance; education; religion; hobbies; beliefs; living conditions); for veterans include military service history, service-related medical conditions, including traumatic brain injury, post-traumatic stress disorder, permanent physical disabilities, and care provided by the Veterans Administration.

Review of Systems (ROS):

General: Weight loss, weight gain, fatigue, insomnia, hypersomnia, weakness, appetite, fever, chills, night sweats

Skin: Rashes, pruritus, bruising, dryness, skin cancer or other lesions, nail changes; changes in hair (see also Dermatologic Descriptions, page 71)

Head: Trauma, headache, tenderness, dizziness, syncope

Eyes: Vision, changes in visual field, glasses, photophobia, blurring, diplopia, spots or floaters, halos, inflammation, discharge, dry eyes, excessive tearing, history of cataracts or glaucoma, last eye exam, use of glasses, contacts, or corrective surgery (see also Ophthalmology Key Elements, page 90)

Ears: Hearing changes, use of hearing aids, tinnitus, pain, discharge, vertigo, history of ear infections (see also Otolaryngology Key Elements, page 101)

Nose: Sinusitis or rhinitis, epistaxis, hay fever, sinus drainage, obstruction, history of trauma/fracture, polyps, changes in or loss of sense of smell

Throat: Bleeding gums; dental history (last checkup, etc.); ulcerations or other lesions on tongue, gums, buccal mucosa; changes in or loss of sense of taste (especially in patients with suspected COVID-19); hoarseness; surgery (tonsillectomy) (see also Otolaryngology Key Elements, page 101)

Neck: Thyroid disease, goiter, masses, adenopathy, history of cervical spine disease

Respiratory: Chest pain; dyspnea; cough; amount and color of sputum; hemoptysis; history of pneumonia, influenza, and pneumococcal vaccinations; TB exposure; positive purified protein derivative (PPD) or interferon gamma release assay; Bacillus Calmette–Guérin (BCG) vaccination for persons born outside the United States; last chest x-ray (CXR); pulmonary function tests (PFTs) or other pulmonary tests

Cardiovascular (CV): Chest pain, orthopnea, trepopnea, platypnea, dyspnea on exertion (DOE), paroxysmal nocturnal dyspnea (PND), history of murmur, claudication, peripheral edema, palpitations, last electrocardiogram (ECG), history of stress test, cardiac procedures (e.g., cath, stent)

Gastrointestinal (GI): Abdominal pain, dysphagia, heartburn, nausea, vomiting, diarrhea, constipation, hematemesis, indigestion, melena, hematochezia, hemorrhoids, change in stool shape and color, jaundice, fatty food intolerance, PUD, history of liver disease, pancreatic disease, gallbladder disease, previous GI procedures

Genitourinary (GU): Frequency, urgency, hesitancy, dysuria, hematuria, polyuria, polydipsia, nocturia, incontinence, change in urinary stream, lower abdominal or flank pain

Male GU: Urethral discharge; sterility; erectile dysfunction; testicular pain or scrotal mass; circumcision status; penile lesions; sexual history, including frequency of intercourse, number of partners, sexual orientation and satisfaction, history of STIs; sexual problems or concerns

Endocrine: Polyuria, polydipsia, polyphagia, glycosuria, excessive thirst, change in weight, temperature intolerance, edema, excessive sweating, hormone therapy, changes in hair or skin texture, change in hair distribution, pigment changes

Musculoskeletal: Arthralgia, arthritis, myalgias, joint swelling, redness, tenderness, limitations in range of motion (ROM), back pain, musculoskeletal trauma, gout

Peripheral Vascular: Varicose veins, intermittent claudication, history of thrombophlebitis (deep or superficial)

Hematology: Anemia, history of transfusion, bleeding tendency, easy bruising, petechia, lymphadenopathy

Neuropsychiatric: Syncope; seizures; weakness or paralysis; change in sensation, paresthesias; vertigo, ataxia, or coordination problems; tremor; history of psychiatric disorder, depression, mania, schizophrenia; alterations in memory, mood, or sleep pattern, anhedonia, loss of energy, sense of hopelessness, decreased ability to concentrate, change in weight or appetite, family history of depression or suicide; hallucinations; delusions; if symptoms of depression inquire further about thoughts or plans to harm themselves or others and history of suicide attempt; emotional disturbances; drug and alcohol use or misuse/abuse (if appropriate, consider the Mental Status Exam, see page 113)

Obstetrical/Gynecological (OB/GYN): Gravida/para/abortions; age at menarche; last menstrual period (frequency, duration, flow); dysmenorrhea; spotting; menopause; contraception; sexual history, including history of STIs, frequency of intercourse, number of partners, sexual orientation and satisfaction, and dyspareunia. (see also page 87 for Gynecology and page 88 for Obstetric Key Elements)

Physical Examination (Adult)

General: Mood, gender. State if patient is in distress or is assuming an unusual position, such as sitting up leaning forward (position often seen in patients with acute exacerbation of chronic obstructive pulmonary disease [COPD] or pericarditis). Note if patient appears markedly older or younger than stated age.

Vital Signs: Temperature (note if oral, rectal, axillary, or ear; for conversion of temperatures from Fahrenheit to Celsius and vice versa, see Appendix, Temperature Conversion, Table A-12, page 1087; also see Temperature Considerations on page 54. Pulse/heart rate (HR) (note if regular, regularly irregular, irregularly iregular); respirations (note if there is an abnormal pattern); blood pressure (BP) (note body position for BP and HR) (also see Blood Pressure Measurement Techniques and Guidelines, page 54 and Tables 6-1 and 6-2, page 57); and for body mass index (BMI) (weight in kilograms / height in meters squared) see Appendix, Body Mass Index (BMI), page 1044 and Table A-2, page 1047. If concerned about volume depletion (e.g., GI bleeding, pancreatitis, diarrhea, vomiting, other causes) or autonomic insufficiency, or if the patient reports dizziness or syncope, include BP and heart rate supine and also after the patient has been standing for 2–3 minutes. If standing is not tolerated, then have the patient sit in a chair or on the examining table.

Skin: Color, rashes, eruptions, scars, tattoos, moles, hair pattern; nails, color, pitting, clubbing (see Dermatologic Descriptions, page 71 and locations of common skin lesions in Figure 6-5, page 71).

Lymph Nodes: Specify location (head and neck, supraclavicular, epitrochlear, axillary, inguinal), size, tenderness, mobility, consistency.

Head, Eyes, Ears, Nose, and Throat (HEENT):

Head: Size and shape, tenderness, trauma, bruits.

Hair: Texture, signs of infection or vitamin deficiency.

Eyes: Lids; position of eyes in orbits; conjunctiva; sclera; pupil size, shape, reactivity to light directly and indirectly; extraocular muscle movements; visual acuity (e.g., 20/20); visual fields; fundoscopic exam (disc color, size, margins, cupping, spontaneous venous pulsations, hemorrhages, exudates, nicking [see also Ophthalmology Key Elements page 90]).

Ears: **Pinna:** tenderness, lesions, piercings, discharge. **Otoscopic findings:** external canal, tympanic membrane (intact, dull or shiny, bulging, motility, fluid or blood, injected). See Figure 6-17, page 103, for the anatomy of the external ear, and Figure 6-18, page 104, for the tympanic membrane. Hearing screen: finger rub, whisper test, Weber and Rinne tests (see page 102).

Nose: Symmetry; inspection for obstruction, lesions, exudate, inflammation; palpation over frontal, maxillary, and ethmoid sinuses.

Throat: Lips, teeth (see also Figure 6-4, page 70), gums, tongue, pharynx (lesions, erythema, exudate, tonsillar size, presence of crypts).

Neck: ROM, tenderness by palpation or with movement, jugular venous distension (JVD), lymph nodes, thyroid examination, palpation of anterior neck, check for carotid bruits and hepatojugular reflux (HJR). Record JVD in relation to the number of centimeters vertically above or below the sternal angle, such as "1 cm above the sternal angle," rather than "no JVD."

Chest: Configuration and symmetry of movement with respiration; intercostal retractions; palpation for tenderness, fremitus, and chest wall expansion; percussion (include diaphragmatic movement with tidal breathing and full inspiration); breath sounds, note any adventitious sounds (rales/crackles, rhonchi, wheezes, rubs). If indicated: vocal fremitus, whispered pectoriloquy, egophony (found with consolidation).

Heart: Rate and regularity, inspection, and palpation of precordium for point of maximal impulse, apical impulse, and thrills; auscultation at the apex, lower left sternal border (LLSB), and right and left second intercostal spaces with the diaphragm and apex and LLSB with the bell. Also at the apex with the bell with patient in the left lateral decubitus position and at the left third and fourth intercostal spaces with diaphragm with the patient sitting up, leaning forward, and fully exhaled. For a more complete description of S_1 and S_2 and where best to hear various heart sounds including murmurs, see Figure 6-2, page 58, and Table 6-3, pages 59–60.

Breast: Inspection for nipple discharge, inversion, excoriations and fissures, and skin dimpling or flattening of the contour; palpation for masses, tenderness; gynecomastia in men and boys. Men do get breast cancer (~1% of all new breast cancer diagnoses and breast cancer deaths). (See Figure 6-1, page 50–51, for description of a complete breast exam.)

Abdomen: Shape (scaphoid, flat, distended, obese); examination for scars; auscultation for bowel sounds and bruits; percussion for tympani and masses; liver size (span measured in right midclavicular line; estimated by percussion or using the scratch test [place the stethoscope over the liver in the mid-clavicular line between the eighth and ninth or ninth and tenth ribs; listen as you lightly stroke a finger nail against the skin in the horizonal or transverse plane moving from mid-abdomen superiorly, the sound will drastically change in intensity when you are over the inferior border of the liver and continue superiorly with stroking the nail against the skin until the sound decreases in intensity marking the superior border of the liver]); costovertebral angle (CVA) tenderness; palpation for tenderness (if present, check for rebound tenderness);

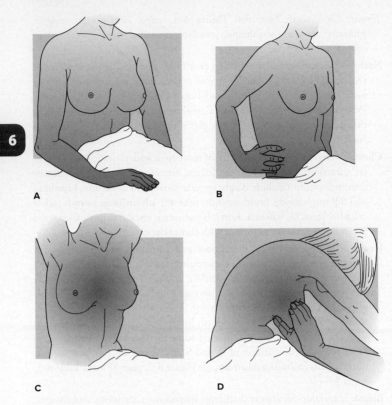

Figure 6-1. Breast examination by the physician or other qualified provider. A: Patient is sitting, arms at sides. Perform visual inspection in good light, looking for lumps or for dimpling or wrinkling of skin. B: Patient is sitting, hands pressing on hips so that pectoralis muscles are tensed. Repeat visual inspection. C: Patient is sitting, arms above head. Repeat visual inspection of breasts and perform visual inspection of axillae. D: Patient is sitting and leaning forward, hands on examiner's shoulders, the stirrups, or her own knees. Perform bimanual palpation, paying particular attention to the base of the glandular portion of the breast. E: Patient is sitting, arms extended 60–90 degrees. Palpate axillae. F: Patient is supine, arms relaxed at sides. Perform bimanual palpation of each portion of the breast (usually each quadrant, but smaller sections for unusually large breasts). Repeat examinations C, E, and F with patient supine and arms above head. G: Patient is supine, arms relaxed at sides. Palpate under the areola and nipple with the thumb and forefinger to detect a mass or test for expression of fluid from the nipple. H: Patient is either sitting or supine. Palpate supraclavicular areas. (Reproduced with permission from DeCherney AH, Nathan L, Laufer N, Roman AS, eds. *Current Diagnosis & Treatment: Obstetrics & Gynecology*, 12e, New York, NY: McGraw-Hill; 2019.) (*continued next page*)

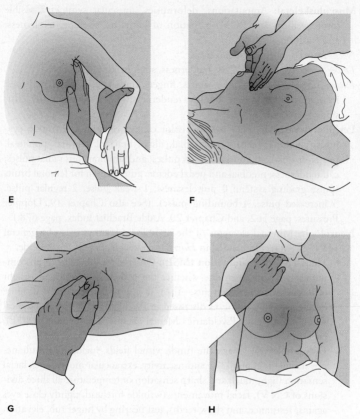

6

Figure 6-1. (Continued)

assess for ascites, hepatomegaly, splenomegaly; guarding, inguinal adenopathy.

Male Genitalia: Note if circumcised or uncircumcised. Inspection for penile lesions (condyloma, vesicles, skin abnormalities), scrotal swelling, testicles (size, tenderness, masses, varicocele), and hernia; transillumination of testicular masses (must confirm with ultrasound).

Pelvic Exam (Women and Girls): See Chapter 19, page 629.

Rectal: Inspection and palpation for hemorrhoids, fissures, skin tags, sphincter tone, masses; presence or absence of stool; test stool for occult blood; in men grade prostate size from small (1+) to massively enlarged (4+); note any nodules, tenderness.

6

Musculoskeletal: Amputations, deformities, muscular symmetry, visible joint swelling, and ROM; palpation of joints for swelling, tenderness, and warmth.

Neck: Inspection, ROM, tenderness

Lower back: Inspection, ROM, tenderness, straight leg raising

Extremities: Shoulders, elbows, wrists, fingers, hips, knees, ankles, and toes: inspection, ROM, joint stability, tenderness, muscle tone/atrophy, effusions, crepitation

Peripheral Vascular: Hair pattern; color change of skin; varicosities; cyanosis; clubbing; palpation of radial, ulnar, brachial, femoral, popliteal, posterior tibial, and dorsalis pedis pulses; and simultaneous radial pulses; calf tenderness; pretibial and pedal edema; auscultation for femoral bruits (pulse grading system: 0 pulselessness, 1 weak pulse, 2 regular pulse, 3 increased pulse, 4 bounding pulse). (See also Chapter 19, Doppler Pressures, page 562, and Chapter 20, Ankle Brachial Index, page 678.)

Neurologic: Minimal elements of the neurologic exam as part of a general H&P and as recommended in *Harrison's Manual of Medicine*[1] include:

- **Mental Status Examination (MSE):** Observe for difficulties with communication and determine whether the patient has recall and insight into recent and past events. Then if appropriate, perform a more detailed screening MSE as discussed in Psychiatric History and Physical Examination and Psychiatric Mental Status Examination (MSE), page 113.

- **Cranial Nerves:** Check the fundi, visual fields, including simultaneous stimulation, pupil size and reactivity, extraocular movements, facial sensation (light touch and sharp sensation or temperature all three divisions of CN V), facial movements (wrinkle forehead, tightly close eyes against resistance, and show teeth), test hearing by finger rub, elevation of palate and uvula by saying "Ah," shoulder shrug and turning head against resistance, and observe tongue and tongue movement.

- **Motor:** Strength of upper and lower extremities: test arm flexion and extension, wrist flexion and extension, and hand grip and finger abduction, hip flexion, leg flexion and extension, foot flexion and extension, and flexion of the toes.

- **Sensory:** Ask whether the patient can feel light touch and sharp sensation or temperature of a cool object distal, mid, and proximal upper and lower extremities bilaterally. Check double simultaneous stimulation using light touch on the hands.

- **Coordination and Gait:** Test rapid alternating movements of the hands and feet and the finger-to-nose maneuver. Observe the patient while he or she is walking along a straight line, walking on toes, on heels, and heel to toe. Observe patient with heels and toes together with eyes open and then closed. Observe for pronator drift with eyes closed.

- **Reflexes:** Biceps, triceps, patellar, and Achilles reflexes.

Additional details can be found in Neurology Key Elements, pages 75–87, including dermatomes and cutaneous nerve innervations; see Figure 6-6A and B, pages 80 and 81.

Database: Laboratory tests, imaging, and other available diagnostic testing results.

Problem List: See the example problem list on page 124. Include entry date of problem, date of problem onset, problem number. In the initial problem list, the order of the problem number is in the order of severity. After the initial list is generated, add problems chronologically. List problem by status: active or inactive.

Assessment: Discussion with a differential diagnosis of each current problem followed by the plan for each problem. The assessment is more than just a listing of problems. Provide rationale for your primary diagnosis and your differential based on the history, physical and diagnostic testing.

Plan: Additional laboratory and diagnostic tests, medical treatment, consults, etc.

If not an electronic health record, then legibly sign the H&P and note your title. Record the date and time with each entry.

TEMPERATURE CONSIDERATIONS

Body temperature can be measured by oral, rectal, axillary, or tympanic (ear) methods, and the temperature readings can vary with the device used (follow the instructions to obtain an accurate reading). General concepts concerning body temperature:

- Mean normal adult oral temperature is 96.5–99.5°F (36.0–37.5°C), with lowest levels at ~4 A.M. and highest at ~6 P.M. Based on historical studies, the normal adult oral temperature is 98.6°F (37°C). A recent study that crowdsourced 5,038 oral temperatures from 329 subjects found the mean oral temperature to be 97.7°F or 36.5°C.[2]
- Rectal temperatures are 0.5–1°F (0.3–0.6°C) higher than oral on average but are variable. In the study by Barnett et al., the range is from almost 3°F (1.8°C) higher than the oral temperature to 0.7°F (0.4°C) lower than oral temperature. Tympanic (ear) temperature is 0.5–1°F (0.3–0.6°C) higher than an oral. In the study by Barnett et. al, tympanic temperature varies greatly, 1.5°F (0.9°C) lower than rectal temperature to 2.0°F (1.2°C) higher than rectal temperature.[3]
- Axillary temperature is usually 0.5–1°F (0.3–0.6°C) lower than oral.
- Forehead/temporal scanner reading is usually 0.5–1°F (0.3–0.6°C) lower than an oral temperature.
- Normally body temperature decreases with age; elderly patients normally can drop to 97.6°F (36.4°C).
- A temperature over 100.4°F (38°C) orally is generally described as a fever in adults.

6

- Hypothermia is considered 95°F (35°C) or lower.
- Hyperpyrexia is considered 106°F (41.1°C) or higher (usually from a non-infectious cause such as malignant hyperthermia, serotonin syndrome, environmental hyperthermia).
- Rectal temperature is the most accurate method for checking a young child's temperature.
- Plastic strip thermometers have limited utility, as they measure skin temperature, not body temperature.
- Fever has many causes, including bacterial, viral, fungal, and protozoan infections; medications (many antibiotics, anticonvulsants, chemotherapeutic drugs, GI medications, and many other medications and syndromes associated with medications such as severe hemolysis with glucose-6-phosphate deficiency [G6PD], serotonin syndrome, neuroleptic malignant syndrome, malignant hyperthermia, and drug reaction with eosinophilia and systemic symptoms [DRESS]); malignancy (lymphoma, acute myeloid leukemia [AML], renal cell, hepatic, lung, and pancreatic carcinomas, others), rheumatologic diseases (systemic lupus erythematosus [SLE], temporal arteritis, rheumatoid arthritis, polymyositis/dermatomyositis, polyarteritis nodosa, others), thrombotic thrombocytopenic purpura (TTP), hypothalamic disorders, thyroid storm, adrenal insufficiency, deep vein thrombosis/pulmonary embolism (DVT/PE), acute myocardial infarction, inflammatory bowel disease, environmental hyperthermia, transfusion reactions, hematomas, and factitious.
- For every 1°F increase in temperature above 99° expect an increase in pulse by about 10 beats per minute (BPM). In certain infections you see a temperature–pulse dissociation (pulse does not increase or increase to the degree expected). Temperature–pulse dissociation classically occurs in *Mycoplasma pneumoniae*, *Salmonella typhi*, *Plasmodium falciparum*, and *Campylobacter fetus*.
- The pattern of a fever may point toward the etiology. Sustained fever (little variation throughout the day) can be from *Streptococcus pneumoniae*, hypothalamic injury, others; remittent fever (an increase of at least 1°F each day from a baseline that is above normal and does not return to normal) can be caused by malignancy, endocarditis, others; relapsing or recurrent fever (fever with at least 1 day of normal temperatures between fevers) is caused by nonfalciparum *Plasmodium,* Hodgkin lymphoma, others); and intermittent or quotidian fever (a wide variation each day with the high temperature usually in the afternoon) is from *Plasmodium falciparum*, *Mycobacterium tuberculous*, endocarditis, and others.[4]

BLOOD PRESSURE MEASUREMENT TECHNIQUES AND GUIDELINES

There is a clear association between HTN and coronary artery and cerebrovascular diseases. **Hypertension is defined as systolic blood pressure (BP) >120 mm Hg or diastolic BP >80 mm Hg in adults.**

- In 2018 the American Heart Association (AHA) and the American College of Cardiology (ACC) published new blood pressure guidelines. (See Table 6-1 for citation.)
- In 2020 the United States Preventive Services Task Force (USPSTF) recommended hypertension screening for adults aged 18 years or older with office-based blood pressure measurement (OBPM). Before starting treatment, blood pressure measurements should be obtained outside of the clinical setting for diagnostic confirmation. The recommendations for blood pressure testing in the office:

6

1. Encourage the patient to avoid caffeine, exercise, and smoking for 30 minutes before the measurement.
2. Direct the patient to use the bathroom before the reading and not to talk during the reading.
3. Measure BP after 5 minutes of rest with the patient seated, feet resting on the floor, and arm at heart level. BP should be measured in both arms. Significant differences (>10 mm each arm) are associated with subclavian stenosis, aortic coarctation, and overall signify an increased likelihood of peripheral vascular disease and cardiovascular risk.
4. The lower end of the BP cuff should be 2–3 cm above the antecubital fossa. The entire blood pressure cuff should be over skin. Do not roll the shirt sleeve up, as this can restrict blood flow.
5. Two BP methods: Auscultatory method and oscillometric method
   - **Auscultatory method** with a traditional BP cuff and using the stethoscope bell (the last sounds heard are the Korotkoff sounds, which are low pitched) placed over the brachial artery. Manually inflate the cuff to 30 mm Hg greater than systolic BP previously estimated by disappearance of pulse with palpation of the radial or brachial artery. Slowly release the pressure (2 mm Hg decrease/second); systolic BP is when you hear the first of two consecutive beats. With continual lowering of the cuff pressure, the diastolic BP is when the sound goes from being muffled to no longer audible with the bell of the stethoscope.
   - **Oscillometric method** uses electronic sensors and is becoming commonplace where the device automatically inflates and deflates and displays the BP.
6. Take the average of two readings separated by 2 minutes. Elevated readings on three separate days are required for a diagnosis of HTN.
7. Blood pressure cuff width influences the pressure readings. The narrow cuffs require more pressure, and the widest cuff less pressure, to occlude the brachial artery for determination of systolic pressure. The result is that too narrow a cuff may produce a large overestimation of systolic pressure and too wide a cuff may underestimate the systolic pressure. The 2017 ACC/AHA/AAPA/ABC/ACPM/AGS/APhA/ASH/ASPC/NMA/PCNA Guideline for the Prevention, Detection, Evaluation and Management of High Blood Pressure in Adults in the

Journal of the American College of Cardiology recommendations cuff size based on arm circumference:

- 22–26 cm, small adult cuff, 12 × 22 cm
- 27–34 cm, adult cuff, 16 × 30 cm
- 35–44 cm, large adult cuff, 16 × 36 cm
- 45–52 cm, adult thigh cuff, 16 × 42 cm

8. **Ambulatory blood pressure monitors** are worn by the patient for at least 24–48 hours. The device acquires a blood pressure every 15–30 minutes during the day and every 60 minutes at night, and the reading intervals can be customized. Some sources suggest this is the reference standard to confirm the diagnosis of HTN and can be used to titrate antihypertensive medications. The latest guidelines also stress the importance of home BP measurements by patients.

9. BP classification and measurement guidelines for adults are shown in Table 6-1 and measurement techniques by physical location Table 6-2, page 57.

10. Avoid taking BP in an arm with an IV, dialysis shunt, pervious lymph node dissection, or injury.

11. In **children** 1–10 years old, reference for systolic BP can be calculated as follows: Lower limits (fifth percentile): 70 mm Hg, + (child's age in years × 2); typical (fiftieth percentile): 90 mm Hg, + (child's age in years × 2).

Heart Murmurs and Extra Heart Sounds

Figure 6-2 and Table 6-3, on pages 58 and 59, graphically represent and describe heart sounds and common heart murmurs with detailed physical examination findings.

FAMILY HISTORY AND PEDIGREE

A family medical history provides insight into the conditions that may be common in a family. Constructing a formal pedigree can be used as a diagnostic tool and help guide decisions about genetic testing for the patient and other family members. This can also identify a variety of potential health problems (e.g., heart disease, diabetes, cancer, early-onset Alzheimer disease) that an individual may be at increased risk for developing. Early identification of increased risk may allow steps to be taken such as lifestyle changes, medical interventions, and increased disease surveillance. Genetic counselors can be most helpful in assessing a variety of inherited genetic diseases. Commonly used in the setting of childhood genetic diseases, many other important conditions can be inherited. One common example is breast cancer, where up to 10% are hereditary and may be caused by inherited mutations in genes such as *BRCA1* or *BRCA2*. The U.S. Preventive Services Task Force

Table 6-1. Guidelines for Blood Pressure Management in Adults

CLASSIFICATION OF BLOOD PRESSURE IN ADULTS (BP)			
Category	SBP (mmHg)		DBP (mmHg)
Normal	<120	and	<80
Elevated	120–129	and	<80
Hypertension, stage 1	130–139	or	80–89
Hypertension, stage 2	≥140	or	≥90
*Hypertensive urgency/ emergency	>180	or	>120

SBP = systolic blood pressure; DBP = diastolic blood pressure
*Emergency = target organ damage: stroke, MI, unstable angina, ARF, acute CHF, papilledema, eclampsia, dissecting aortic aneurysm, hypertensive encephalopathy.
Based on update of JNC7 published online in 2017 in *Hypertension*. (Whelton PK, et al. Hypertension. 2018;71: e13–e115).

6

Table 6-2. Blood Pressure Measurement Techniques Based on Location

Method	Notes
In-office	Two readings, 1–2 min apart, sitting in chair, relaxed, both feet on the floor, with proper cuff size and no clothing between skin and cuff, arm supported at heart level. Confirm elevated reading contralateral arm.
Ambulatory BP monitoring (ABPM)	Indicated for evaluation of "white coat hypertension." Better than office BP as measured by long-term CVD outcomes. Absence of 10–20% decrease in BP during sleep may indicate increased cardiovascular disease risk.
Home/self BP Monitoring (often more practical than ABPM)	Provides information on response to therapy. May help improve adherence to therapy and is useful for evaluating "white coat hypertension."

(USPSTF) recommends awareness of family history patterns associated with an increased risk for *BRCA* mutations as an example of the increasing role of genetic testing and personalized medicine. This record of genetic and medical information is often more useful in visual form than in list form (see Figure 6-3A, page 61, for standard pedigree nomenclature and an example of a *BRCA1* inheritance pattern in Figure 6-3B, page 62). Key concepts in preparing a medical pedigree include the following:

- The proband is usually the first person in the family who has come to medical attention.

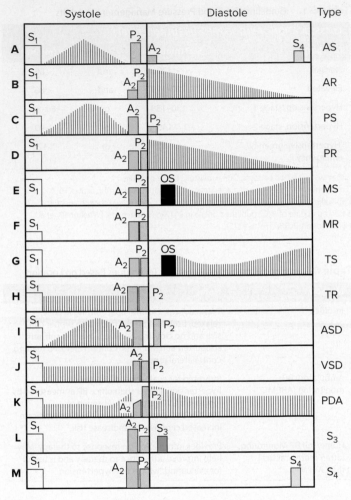

Figure 6-2. Graphic representation of common heart murmurs and heart sounds. Table 6-3, page 59, indicates abbreviations and further descriptions. Height of box indicates intensity of heart sound; hatched lines indicate pattern of murmur. S_1: Occurs at beginning of systole and is closure of the mitral (M_1) and tricuspid (T_1) valves. Normally, T_1 is heard only at the LLSB. S_1 is loudest at the apex. S_2: Occurs at end of systole and is closure of the aortic (A_2) and pulmonic valves (P_2). P_2 is best heard at the L second ICS. S_2 is loudest at R second ICS. The L second ICS is where to listen for splitting of A_2 and P_2. At end inspiration with tidal breathing there is more pronounced splitting of the A_2 and P_2 sounds (they are farther apart than at end expiration). With normal physiology M_1 occurs before T_1; A_2 occurs before P_2.

Table 6-3. Heart Murmurs and Extra Heart Sounds[a]

Type[b]	Description
A. Aortic stenosis (AS)	Heard best at second ICS. Systolic (medium-pitched) crescendo–decrescendo murmur with radiation to the carotid arteries. A_2 decreased, ejection click and S_4 heard at apex with the bell. Paradoxical splitting of S_2. Narrow pulse pressure, delayed carotid upstroke, and left ventricular hypertrophy (LVH) with lift at apex.
B. Aortic regurgitation (AR)	Heard best at LLSB at third and fourth ICS with patient sitting up, leaning forward, and fully exhaled. Diastolic (high-pitched) decrescendo murmur. Often with LVH. Widened pulse pressure, bisferiens pulse, de Musset sign, Traube sign, Quincke sign, and Corrigan pulse may be seen with chronic aortic regurgitation. S_3 and pulsus alternans often present with acute aortic regurgitation.
C. Pulmonic stenosis (PS)	Heard best at left second ICS. Systolic crescendo–decrescendo murmur. Louder with inspiration. Click often present. P_2 delayed and soft if severe. Right ventricular hypertrophy (RVH) with parasternal lift.
D. Pulmonic regurgitation (PR)	Heard best at left second ICS. Diastolic decrescendo murmur. Louder with inspiration. RVH usually present.
E. Mitral stenosis (MS)	Localized at the apex. Diastolic (low-pitched rumbling sound) murmur heard with the bell in the left lateral decubitus position at the PMI. With increased or decreased S_1. Opening snap (OS) heard best at apex with diaphragm. Increased P_2, right-sided S_4, left-sided S_3 often present. RVH with parasternal lift may be present.
F. Mitral regurgitation (MR)	Heard best at apex. Holosystolic (high-pitched) murmur with radiation to axilla. Soft S_1, may be masked by murmur. S_3 and LVH often present. Midsystolic click suggests mitral valve prolapse.
G. Tricuspid stenosis (TS)	Heard at the LLSB and 4th ICS. Presystolic-diastolic low pitched sound heard best with the bell. OS heard at the LLSB/4th ICS, murmur/OS increase with increased blood flow across the value (inspiration, leg raising)
H. Tricuspid regurgitation (TR)	Heard best at LLSB. Holosystolic (high-pitched) murmur. Increases with inspiration. Right-sided S_3 often present. Large V wave in jugular venous pulsations.
I. Atrial septal defect (ASD)	Heard best at LLSB. Systolic (medium-pitched) murmur. Fixed splitting of S_2 and RVH, often with left- and right-sided S_4.
J. Ventricular septal defect (VSD)	Heard best at LLSB. Harsh holosystolic (high-pitched) murmur. S_1 and S_2 may be soft.

6

(continued)

Table 6-3. Heart Murmurs and Extra Heart Sounds[a] (*Continued*)

Type[b]	Description
K. Patent ductus arteriosus (PDA)	Heard best at left first and second ICS. Continuous, machinery (medium-pitched) murmur. Increased P_2 and ejection click may be present.
L. Third heart sound (S_3)	Early diastolic sound caused by rapid ventricular filling. Heard with bell. Left-sided S_3 heard at apex, right-sided S_3 heard at LLSB. Left-sided S_3 can be normal in young people, also seen in pregnancy, thyrotoxicosis, mitral regurgitation, and congestive heart failure. Right-sided S_3 occurs with right ventricular failure.
M. Fourth heart sound (S_4)	Late diastolic sound caused by a noncompliant ventricle. Heard with bell. Left-sided S_4 heard at apex, right-sided S_4 heard at LLSB. Left-sided S_4 seen with hypertension, aortic stenosis, and myocardial infarction. Right-sided S_4 seen with pulmonic stenosis and pulmonary hypertension.

[a] Refer to Figure 6-2 for graphic representations of murmurs and other heart sounds (page 58).
[b] Capital letters preceding type of murmur refer to graphs in Figure 6-2.

- First-degree relatives (parents, siblings), second-degree relatives (aunts, uncles, grandparents), and third-degree relatives (first cousins, great grandparents) all are from the same side of the family as the patient.
- Obtain a three-generational history at minimum and data from both sides of the family if possible.

PHYSICAL SIGNS, SYMPTOMS, AND EPONYMS

Allen Test: (See Chapter 19, page 526.)

Angle of Louis: "Sternal angle" where the manubrium joins the sternum. Site where costal cartilages of rib two articulate with the sternum.

Apley Test; Apley Grind Test: Determination of meniscal tear in the knee by grinding the joint manually.

Argyll Robertson Pupil: Bilaterally small, irregular, unequal pupils that react to accommodation but not to light. Seen with tertiary syphilis.

Asterixis: Extension of wrists causes flapping motion; hepatic encephalopathy, Wilson disease, other metabolic diseases.

Athetosis: Slow, distal, writhing, involuntary movements with a propensity to affect the arms and hands (this represents a form of dystonia with increased mobility); seen in Huntington disease.

Auspitz Sign: Pinpoint bleeding after removal of a psoriasis scale.

Austin Flint Murmur: Late diastolic mitral murmur; associated with aortic regurgitation with a normal mitral valve.

Babinski Sign: Extension of the large toe with stimulation of the plantar surface of the foot instead of the normal flexion; should be performed with

Standard Pedigree Nomenclature

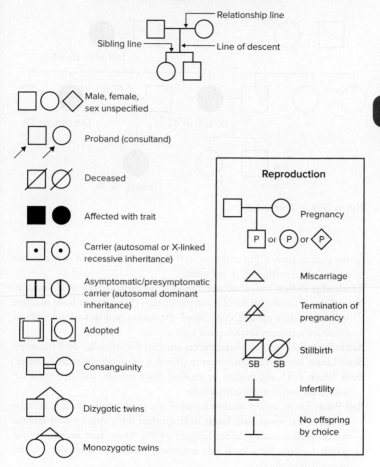

Figure 6-3. A: Basic elements used to construct a family history and pedigree. (From Cancer Genetics Risk Assessment and Counseling [PDQ]; https://www.ncbi.nlm.nih.gov/books/NBK65817/figure/CDR0000062865__1237/. Accessed May 25, 2020.) B: Illustrative example of a pedigree showing some of the classic features of a family with a *BRCA1* pathogenic variant across three generations, including affected family members with breast cancer or ovarian cancer and a young age at onset. *BRCA1* families may exhibit some or all of these features. As an autosomal dominant syndrome, a *BRCA1* pathogenic variant can be transmitted through maternal or paternal lineages, as depicted in the figure. (From the Genetics of Breast and Gynecologic Cancers [PDQ]; https://www.ncbi.nlm.nih.gov/books/NBK65767/figure/CDR0000062855__2585/. Accessed May 25, 2020.)

6

Classic *BRCA1* Pedigree

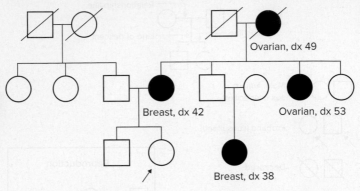

Figure 6-3.   (Continued)

the patient supine, hip and knee at 0 degrees; indicative of upper motor neuron disease (normal in neonates).

Bainbridge Reflex: Increased heart rate due to increased right atrial pressure.

Barre Sign: (Pronator drift) The patient extends their arms in front of them with the palms up and eyes closed. Pronation and downward drift of either arm suggests corticospinal tract disease.

Battle Sign: Ecchymosis behind the ear associated with basilar skull fractures.

Beau Lines: Transverse depressions in nails due to previous systemic disease.

Beck Triad: JVD, diminished or muffled heart sounds, and decreased BP associated with cardiac tamponade.

Bell Palsy: Lower motor neuron lesion of the facial nerve affecting muscles of upper and lower face. Easily distinguished from upper motor lesions, which predominately affect muscles of the lower face because upper motor neurons from each side innervate muscles on both sides of the upper part of the face.

Bell Phenomenon: Also called the palpebral-oculogyric reflex movement of the eyeballs in an upward direction when the eyelids are forcefully closed. A normal finding may not be appreciated until there is paralysis of the facial nerve (i.e., Guillain-Barre syndrome post viral neuropathy).

Bergman Triad: Altered mental status, petechiae, and dyspnea associated with fat embolus syndrome.

Biot Breathing: Abruptly alternating apnea and equally deep breaths (seen with brain injury).

Bisferiens Pulse: Double-peaked pulse seen in severe chronic aortic regurgitation.

Bitot Spots: Small scleral white patches suggesting vitamin A deficiency.

Blumberg Sign: Pain felt in the abdomen when steady constant pressure is quickly released (seen with peritonitis).

Blumer Shelf: Palpable hardness on rectal examination due to metastatic cancer of the rectouterine pouch (pouch of Douglas) or rectovesical pouch.

Bouchard Nodes: Hard, nontender, painless nodules in the dorsolateral aspects of the proximal interphalangeal joints associated with osteoarthritis, caused by hypertrophy of the bone.

Branham Sign: Abrupt slowing of the heart rate with compression of the feeding artery (seen with large atrioventricular [A-V] fistulas).

Brudzinski Sign: Flexion of the neck causing flexion of the hips (seen in meningitis).

Castell Point/Sign: Point is most inferior interspace in the left anterior axillary line. Percussion in this location (splenic percussion sign) is usually tympanic with a deep breath. Dullness to percussion suggests splenomegaly.

Chadwick Sign: Bluish color of cervix and vagina, seen with pregnancy.

Chandelier Sign: Extreme pain elicited with movement of the cervix during bimanual pelvic examination (indicates pelvic inflammatory disease [PID]).

Charcot Triad: Right upper quadrant pain, fever and chills, and jaundice associated with cholangitis.

Cheyne–Stokes Respiration: Repeating cycle of a gradual increase in depth of breathing followed by a gradual decrease to apnea (seen with central nervous system [CNS] disorders, uremia, some normal sleep patterns).

Chorea: Rapid, semi-purposeful, graceful, dancelike, nonpatterned, involuntary movements involving distal or proximal muscle groups. When the movements are of large amplitude and predominantly proximal in distribution, the term "ballism" is used. Huntington disease and acute rheumatic fever ("Sydenham chorea").

Chvostek Sign: Facial spasm elicited by tapping over the facial nerve, indicating hypocalcemia (tetany). May be normal finding in some patients.

Corrigan Pulse: Large-volume carotid pulsation from severe aortic regurgitation (actually seen rather than felt).

Cullen Sign: Ecchymosis around the umbilicus associated with severe intraperitoneal bleeding (seen with ruptured ectopic pregnancy and hemorrhagic pancreatitis).

Cushing Triad: Hypertension, bradycardia, and irregular respiration associated with increased intracranial pressure.

Darier Sign: Erythema and edema elicited by stroking of the skin, indicating mastocytosis; similar to dermatographism ("skin writing").

Doll Eyes: Conjugated movement of eyes of comatose patients in one direction as head is briskly turned in the other direction. Tests oculocephalic reflex indicating intact brainstem.

Drawer Sign: Forward (or backward) movement of the tibia with pressure, indicating laxity or a tear in the anterior (or posterior) cruciate ligament.

Dupuytren Contracture: Proliferation of fibrosis tissue of the palmar fascia resulting in contracture of the fourth and/or fifth digits; often bilateral. May be hereditary or seen in patients with chronic alcoholic liver disease or seizures.

Duroziez Sign: To-and-fro murmur when stethoscope is pressed over the femoral artery, indicating aortic regurgitation.

Dystonia: Involuntary, patterned, sustained, or repeated muscle contractions often associated with twisting movements and abnormal posture; writer's cramp, blepharospasm, torticollis.

Electrical Alternans: Beat-to-beat variation in the electrical axis (seen in large pericardial effusions), suggesting impending hemodynamic compromise.

Erb Palsy/Erb–Duchene Palsy: Brachial plexus injury at childbirth or adult trauma. Arm hangs limply from the shoulder with flexion of the wrist and fingers due to weakness of muscles innervated by cervical roots C5 and C6; most infants recover.

Essential Tremor: High-frequency tremor with sustained posture (e.g., outstretched arms, worsened with movement or when anxious). Commonly familial and improves with alcohol use.

Ewart Sign: Dullness to percussion, increased fremitus, and bronchial breathing beneath the angle of the left scapula, indicating pericardial effusion.

Fong Lesion/Syndrome: Autosomal dominant anomalies of the nails and patella associated with renal abnormalities.

Frank Sign: Fissure of the ear lobe; may be associated with coronary artery disease, diabetes mellitus, and hypertension.

Galant Reflex: See page 86.

Gibbus: Angular convexity of the spine due to vertebral collapse (associated with osteoporosis or metastasis).

Gregg Triad: Cataracts, heart defects, and deafness with congenital rubella.

Grey Turner Sign: Ecchymosis in the flank associated with retroperitoneal hemorrhage.

Grocco Sign: Triangular area of paravertebral dullness, opposite side of a pleural effusion.

Heberden Nodes: Hard, nontender, painless nodules on the dorsolateral aspects of the distal interphalangeal joints associated with osteoarthritis. Results from hypertrophy of the bone.

Hegar Sign: Softening of the distal uterus. Reliable early sign of pregnancy.

Hill Sign: Femoral artery pressure 20 mm Hg greater than brachial pressure (seen in severe aortic regurgitation).

Hoffman Sign/Reflex: A positive Hoffman sign is indicative of an upper motor neuron lesion affecting the upper extremity in question. For the reflex, hold the patient's middle finger between the examiner's thumb and index finger. Ask the patient to relax their fingers completely and, using your thumbnail, press down on the patient's fingernail and move downward until your nail "clicks" over the end of the patient's nail. Normally, nothing occurs. A positive Hoffman response is when the other fingers flex transiently after the "click." Repeat this maneuver multiple times on both hands.

Hollenhorst Plaque: Cholesterol plaque on retina seen on funduscopic examination (associated with amaurosis fugax).

Homan Sign: Calf pain with forcible dorsiflexion of the foot (associated with DVT); has poor sensitivity and specificity.

6

Horner Syndrome: Unilateral miosis, ptosis, and anhidrosis (absence of sweating). From destruction of ipsilateral superior cervical ganglion often caused by lung carcinoma, especially squamous cell carcinoma.

Intention Tremor: Slow zig-zag motion when pointing or extending towards a target.

Janeway Lesion: Erythematous or hemorrhagic lesion seen on the palm or sole with subacute bacterial endocarditis.

Jendrassik Maneuver: Used during assessment of reflexes (patella and Achilles tendon). The examiner asks the patient to bend their arms in front of their upper body, interlock their fingers, and then the patient is asked to pull the hands apart as strongly as possible (isometric contraction). Leads to a significantly stronger reflex response.

Joffroy Reflex: Inability to wrinkle the forehead when bending head and looking up (seen in hyperthyroidism).

Kayser–Fleischer Ring: Brown pigment lesion due to copper deposition (seen in Wilson disease).

Kehr Sign: Left shoulder and left upper quadrant pain associated with splenic rupture.

Kernig Sign: Inability to completely extend the leg when the thigh is flexed at a right angle, caused by inflammation of the meninges (seen with meningitis).

Klumpke Palsy: Traction or tear of C8–T1 nerve roots often during birth or motor vehicle accident (MVA) injury in adults. Finger and wrist flexion ("claw hand").

Koplik Spots: White papules on buccal mucosa opposite molars (seen in measles).

Korotkoff Sounds: Low-pitched sounds resulting from vibration of the artery, detected when measuring BP with the bell of a stethoscope. The last Korotkoff sound is a more accurate estimate of the true diastolic BP than is diastolic BP measured with the diaphragm of the stethoscope.

Kussmaul Respiration: Deep, rapid respiratory pattern (seen in coma or diabetic ketoacidosis [DKA]).

Kussmaul Sign: Paradoxical increase in jugular venous pressure (JVP) on inspiration (seen in constrictive pericarditis, mediastinal tumor, right ventricular infarction, acute cor pulmonale, and congestive heart failure).

6

Kyphosis: Excessive rounding of the thoracic spinal convexity, associated with aging, especially in women.

Lachman Test: With the patient supine and the knee flexed at about 20 to 30 degrees, stabilize the patient's thigh by putting your knee under their thigh; with one hand, press the thigh onto your thigh and with the other hand grasp the proximal tibia and pull it anteriorly; excessive anterior movement compared to the other knee suggests an anterior cruciate ligament (ACL) tear; Lachman test is more sensitive than the anterior drawer test for detecting an ACL tear.

Lasègue Sign/Straight-Leg-Raising Sign: Pain in the distribution of the nerve root with the patient's leg extended in the supine position and gently passively raising the leg; suggests lumbar disk disease.

Levine Sign: Clenched fist over the chest while describing chest pain (associated with angina and acute myocardial infarction [AMI]).

Lhermitte Sign: Neck flexion results in a "shock sensation" (seen in multiple sclerosis and cervical spine problems).

List: Lateral tilt of the spine; usually associated with herniated disk and muscle spasm.

Lordosis: Accentuated normal concavity of the lumbar spine, normal in pregnancy.

Louvel Sign: Coughing or sneezing causes pain in the leg with DVT.

Marcus Gunn Pupil: Dilation of pupils with swinging flashlight test. Results from unilateral optic nerve disease. Normal pupillary response is elicited when light is directed from the normal eye and a subnormal response when light is quickly directed from the normal eye into the abnormal eye. When light is directed into the abnormal eye, both pupils dilate rather than maintain the previous degree of miosis.

McBurney Point/Sign: Point located one-third of the distance from the anterosuperior iliac spine to the umbilicus on the right. (Tenderness at the site is associated with acute appendicitis.)

McMurray Test: Palpable or audible click on the joint line produced by external rotation of the foot, suggesting medial meniscal injury.

Möbius Sign: Inability to maintain convergence, seen in thyrotoxicosis.

Moro Reflex (Startle Reflex): Abduction of hips and arms with extension of arms when infant's head and upper body are suddenly dropped several inches while being held. Normal reflex in early infancy.

Murphy Sign: Severe pain and inspiratory arrest with palpation of the right upper quadrant during deep inspiration (associated with cholecystitis).

Musset or de Musset Sign: Rhythmic nodding or movement of the head with each heartbeat, caused by blood flow back into the heart secondary to aortic regurgitation.

Myerson Sign: See page 85.

Myoclonus: Sudden, brief (<100 ms), jerklike, arrhythmic muscle twitches. Hiccups, metabolic abnormalities such as liver and renal failure.

Nikolsky Sign: Elicited in blistering diseases to determine whether the epidermis is adherent to the underlying dermis. A finger or rounded object such as a pencil eraser is used to rub or rotate the skin with a mild shearing effect. Seen in severe cases of erythema multiforme, epidermolysis bullosa, pemphigoid, and variegate porphyria.

Obturator Sign: Hypogastric pain elicited by flexion and internal rotation of the thigh in cases of inflammation of the obturator internus (present with pelvic abscess and appendicitis).

Ortolani Test/Sign: Sign: hip click that suggests congenital hip dislocation. Test: with the infant supine, point the legs toward you and flex the legs to 90 degrees at the hips and knees.

Osler Node: Tender, red, raised lesions on the hands or feet; seen with infective endocarditis.

Pancoast Syndrome: Carcinoma involving apex of lung, resulting in arm and/or shoulder pain from involvement of brachial plexus and Horner syndrome from involvement of the superior cervical ganglia.

Pastia Lines: Linear striations of confluent petechiae in axillary folds and antecubital fossa, seen in scarlet fever.

Phalen Test: Prolonged maximum flexion of wrists while opposing dorsum of each hand against each other. A positive test result is pain and tingling in the distribution of the median nerve; seen in carpal tunnel syndrome.

Psoas Sign (Iliopsoas Test): Flexion against resistance or extension of the right hip, producing pain; seen with inflammation of the psoas muscle (present with appendicitis).

Pulsus Alternans: Fluctuation of pulse pressure with every other beat (seen in aortic stenosis and congestive heart failure [CHF]).

Queckenstedt Test: Compression of the internal jugular vein during lumbar puncture to determine patency of the subarachnoid space; normal result is immediate increase in cerebrospinal fluid (CSF) pressure.

Quincke Sign: Alternating blushing and blanching of the fingernail bed after light compression (seen in chronic aortic regurgitation).

Radovici Sign: Chin contractions caused by scratching of the palm; a frontal release sign.

Raynaud Phenomenon/Disease: Pain and tingling in fingers after exposure to cold with characteristic color changes of white to blue and then often red. May be seen with scleroderma and SLE or be idiopathic (Raynaud disease).

Resting Tremor: Uncontrolled movement of distal appendages (most noticeable in hands), tremor alleviated by intentional movement. Occurs at rest; "pill rolling tremor" with Parkinson disease.

Rinne and Weber Tests: A test for hearing loss. See page 102.

Romberg Test: The patient stands with heels and toes together with arms outstretched and palms facing up or down or with arms at sides. The examiner lightly taps the patient, first with the patient's eyes open and

6

then with the patient's eyes closed. A positive result is the patient's loss of balance. Loss of balance with the eyes open indicates cerebellar dysfunction. Normal balance with eyes open and loss of balance with eyes closed indicate loss of position sense. Used to test position sense and cerebellar function.

Roth Spots: Oval retinal hemorrhages with a pale central area occurring in patients with bacterial endocarditis.

Rovsing Sign: Pain in the right lower quadrant (RLQ) with deep palpation of the left lower quadrant (LLQ) (seen in acute appendicitis).

Schmorl Node: Degeneration of the intervertebral disk resulting in herniation into the adjacent vertebral body.

Scoliosis: Lateral curvature of the spine.

Sentinel Loop: A single dilated loop of small or large bowel, usually secondary to localized inflammation such as pancreatitis.

Sister Mary Joseph Sign/Node: Metastatic cancer to umbilical lymph node.

Stellwag Sign: Infrequent ocular blinking.

Tietze Syndrome: Inflammation and swelling of the cartilage where ribs connect to sternum (costochondritis). Characterized by chest pain and pain on palpation.

Tic: Brief, repeated, stereotyped muscle contractions that can often be suppressed for a short time. These can be simple and involve a single muscle group or complex and affect a range of motor activities.

Tinel Sign: Radiation of an electric shock sensation in the distal distribution of the median nerve elicited by percussion of the flexor surface of the wrist when fully extended (seen in carpal tunnel syndrome).

Traube Sign: Booming or pistol shot sounds heard over the femoral arteries in chronic aortic regurgitation.

Tremor: Rhythmic oscillation of a body part due to intermittent muscle contractions.

Trendelenburg Test: Patient shifts weight from one leg to the other while being observed from behind; a pelvic tilt to opposite side suggests hip disease and weakness of the gluteus medius muscle. A normal pelvis does not tilt.

Trousseau Sign: Carpal spasm produced by inflation of a BP cuff above the systolic pressure (~ 20 mm Hg) for 2–3 minutes, indicates hypocalcemia or migratory thrombophlebitis associated with cancer.

Turner Sign: See Grey Turner sign.

Unterberger Test: The patient is asked to walk on the same spot with their eyes closed for 50 paces. A positive test is when the patient rotates more than 45 degrees around his or her central axis. This suggests vestibular impairment or a cerebellar lesion.

Virchow Node (Signal or Sentinel Node): A palpable, left supraclavicular lymph node; often first sign of a GI neoplasm, such as pancreatic or gastric carcinoma.

von Graefe Sign: Lid lag associated with thyrotoxicosis.

Weber and Rinne Tests: A test for hearing loss. See page 102.

Whipple Triad: Hypoglycemia, CNS, and vasomotor symptoms (i.e., diaphoresis, syncope); relief of symptoms with glucose (associated with insulinoma).

HISTORY AND PHYSICAL EXAMINATION: SPECIALTY CONSIDERATIONS

Dental Examination

The dental examination is an often-overlooked part of the general H&P. The patient may have an intraoral problem contributing to the overall medical condition (i.e., inability to eat because of a toothache, abscess, or ill-fitting denture in a patient with poorly controlled diabetes) for which a dental consult may be necessary. Loose dentures can compromise manual maintenance of an open airway. In addition, in an emergency in which intubation is necessary, complications can occur if the clinician is unfamiliar with the oral structures.

The patient may be able to give some dental history, including recent toothaches, abscesses, loose teeth or dentures, and any dental procedures (e.g., root canal). Be sure to ask whether the patient is wearing a removable partial denture (partial plate), which should be removed before intubation. Because lost dentures are a chief dental concern of hospitalized patients, take care not to misplace the removed prosthesis.

Perform a brief dental examination with a gloved hand, two tongue blades, and a flashlight. Look for obvious inflammation, erythema, edema, or ulceration of the gingiva (gums) and oral mucosa. Gently tap on any natural teeth to test for sensitivity. Place each tooth between two tongue blades and push gently to check for looseness. This step is especially important for the maxillary anterior teeth, which serve as the fulcrum for the laryngoscope blade. Note abnormal dental findings and request the appropriate consults. Many diseases, including acquired immunodeficiency disease (AIDS), STIs, pemphigus, pemphigoid, allergies, uncontrolled diabetes, leukemia, and others, may first manifest themselves in the mouth.

Hospitalized patients often have difficulty cleaning their teeth or dentures. Add this care to the daily orders if indicated. Patients who will be receiving head and neck radiation must be examined and treated for any tooth extractions or dental infections before initiation of radiation therapy. Extractions after radiation to the maxilla and particularly the mandible can lead to osteoradionecrosis, a condition that can be difficult to control.

Eruption of Teeth

The eruption of teeth may be of great concern to new parents. Parents often think something is developmentally wrong with a child if teeth have not appeared by a certain age. The timing of tooth eruption varies tremendously. Factors contributing to this variation include family history, ethnic background, vitality during fetal development, position of teeth in the arch, size

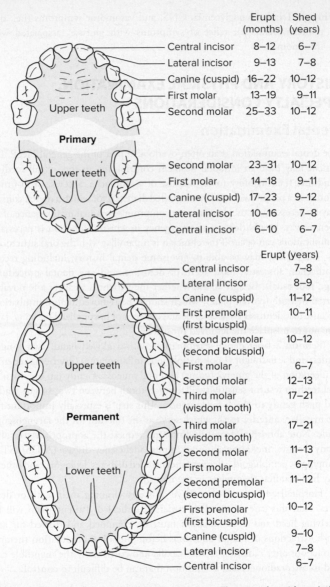

	Erupt (months)	Shed (years)
Central incisor	8–12	6–7
Lateral incisor	9–13	7–8
Canine (cuspid)	16–22	10–12
First molar	13–19	9–11
Second molar	25–33	10–12

Upper teeth

Primary

Lower teeth

Second molar	23–31	10–12
First molar	14–18	9–11
Canine (cuspid)	17–23	9–12
Lateral incisor	10–16	7–8
Central incisor	6–10	6–7

	Erupt (years)
Central incisor	7–8
Lateral incisor	8–9
Canine (cuspid)	11–12
First premolar (first bicuspid)	10–11
Second premolar (second bicuspid)	10–12
First molar	6–7
Second molar	12–13
Third molar (wisdom tooth)	17–21

Upper teeth

Permanent

Lower teeth

Third molar (wisdom tooth)	17–21
Second molar	11–13
First molar	6–7
Second premolar (second bicuspid)	11–12
First premolar (first bicuspid)	10–12
Canine (cuspid)	9–10
Lateral incisor	7–8
Central incisor	6–7

Figure 6-4. Dentition development sequences. There can be wide variation in the age when teeth shed and erupt. (Reproduced with permission and based on data from McDonald RE, Avery DR, eds. *Dentistry for the Child and Adolescent*, St. Louis, MO: Mosby; 1994.)

and shape of the dental arch itself, and, in the case of the eruption of permanent teeth, the time at which the primary tooth was lost. Radiographs of the maxilla and mandible show whether the teeth are present. Figure 6-4 on page 70 is a guide to the chronology of tooth eruption. Remember that variations may be greater than 1 year in some cases.

Dermatologic Descriptions

The location of some typical skin lesions is shown in Figure 6-5. Following is a list of common terms and findings based on skin, hair, and nail examination. Skin biopsy and other dermatologic diagnostic techniques are discussed in Chapter 19, page 646.

Alopecia Areata: Patchy hair loss on the scalp, face, and sometimes on other areas of the body. Considered an autoimmune skin disease.

Androgenetic Alopecia: Male- or female-pattern baldness. Loss of hair is usually temporal and occipital in men and diffuse thinning in women.

Atrophy: Thinning of the surface of the skin with associated loss of normal markings. Examples: Aging, striae associated with obesity, scleroderma.

Bulla/Bullae: A superficial, well-circumscribed, raised, fluid-filled lesion greater than 1 cm in diameter. Examples: Bullous pemphigoid, pemphigus, dermatitis herpetiformis.

Burrow: A subcutaneous linear track made by a parasite. Example: Scabies.

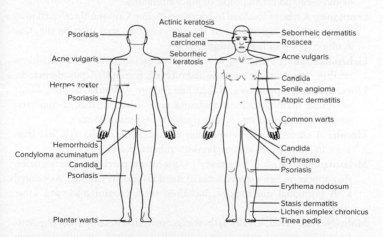

Figure 6-5. Many skin lesions and associated diseases have characteristic anatomic patterns. Some patterns are determined by regional skin features and others by selective exposure to noxious agents. (Reproduced with permission from LeBlond RF, Brown DD, Suneja M, Szot JF. eds. *DeGowin's Diagnostic Examination*, 10e, New York, NY: McGraw-Hill; 2014.)

6

Calluses: A well-circumscribed area of thickened epidermal keratin develops at locations of repeated pressure or friction. Distinguished from verrucae by the preservation of skin lines (dermatoglyphics) in the former.

Crust/Scab: A slightly raised lesion with irregular border and variable color resulting from dried blood, serum, or another exudate. Examples: Scab resulting from an abrasion, impetigo.

Ecchymosis: A flat, nonblanching, initially red-purple-blue lesion that results from extravasation of red blood cells into the skin and turns to a yellow-brown-green after 7 days. Differs from purpura in size; ecchymoses are large purpura lesions. Examples: Trauma, long-term steroid use with minor trauma.

Erosion: A depressed lesion resulting from loss of epidermis due to rupture of vesicles or bullae. Example: Rupture of herpes simplex blister.

Excoriation: A linear superficial lesion, which may be covered with dried blood. Early lesions with surrounding erythema. Often self-induced. Example: Scratching associated with pruritus from any cause.

Fissure: A deep linear lesion into the dermis. Example: Cracks seen in athlete's foot.

Freckles (Ephelides): Small, flat, brown marks most often appear on the face and formed when the skin is exposed to the sun.

Herpetiform: Grouped papules or vesicles arranged like those of a herpes simplex infection.

Keloid: Irregular, raised lesion resulting from hypertrophied scar tissue. Examples: Often seen with burns; African Americans are more prone to keloid formation than people of other ethnicities.

Lentigines: A type of localized hyperpigmentation. Commonly referred to as "liver spots" or "age spots"; are flat, tan to brown, oval spots on the skin. A single spot is called a **lentigo**.

Lichenification: A thickening of the skin with an increase in skin markings resulting from chronic irritation and rubbing. Example: Atopic dermatitis.

Linear Lesions: Appear as a straight line and are suggestive of some forms of contact dermatitis, linear epidermal nevi, lichen striatus, or traumatic lesions (excoriations due to fingernails); are typically linear.

Macule: A circumscribed nonpalpable discoloration of the skin less than 1 cm in diameter. Examples: Freckles, rubella, petechiae.

Melasma: (aka "Mask of pregnancy") Dark brown patches of pigmentation that appear on sun-exposed areas of the skin, usually the face. Associated with hormonal medications, including birth control pills, and other causes.

Mole (Nevus): Small, usually dark, skin growths that develop from pigment-producing melanocytes. They may be flat or raised, smooth, or rough with a wartlike appearance and may have protruding hair. Moles are typically skin-colored but can have other shading (brown, nearly black) and are usually benign (benign nevus). The following changes in a mole may be warning signs of melanoma (known as the **ABCDEs of melanoma**

promoted by the Skin Cancer Foundation: https://www.skincancer.org/skin-cancer-information/melanoma/).

- **A: Asymmetry**. If you draw a line through an asymmetrical mole, the two halves will not match.
- **B: Borders**. The borders of an early melanoma tend to be uneven with scalloped or notched edges.
- **C: Color**. Color changes within the mole; unusual colors; a number of different shades of brown, tan, or black are present. A suspicious mole could have a color significantly different or darker than the person's other moles.
- **D: Diameter**. Suspicious lesions are greater than ¼ in (~6 mm) wide (the size of a pencil eraser).
- **E: Evolving**. Changes in a mole in size, shape, color, elevation, or any new symptom (bleeding, itching, or crusting) are suspicious.

Nail Abnormalities: Nail lesions may suggest an underlying systemic disease.

- **Absent Nails.** Nails may be congenitally absent (ichthyosis) or traumatized nail may prevent regrowth.
- **Beau Lines.** Transverse linear depressions in the nail plate caused by any severe disease that disrupts normal nail growth can be related to trauma and Raynaud disease. (Pearl: Nails normally grow 1 mm every 6–10 days. Measuring from the nail bed to the line allows timing of the illness.)
- **Clubbed Nails and Fingers.** "Clubbing" may be due to the prolonged hypoxemia associated with cardiopulmonary disorders, including congenital cyanotic heart disease, cystic fibrosis, bronchiectasis, severe COPD, lung cancer, and others.
- **Dystrophic Nails.** Include many ill-defined changes (opacities, furrowing, ridging, pitting, splitting, and fraying), all indicating poor nail growth. Associated with chronic nail infections, neuropathy, amyloidosis, and the collagen diseases.
- **Hyperpigmentation.** May be caused by many chemotherapeutic agents, especially the taxanes.
- **Koilonychia/Spoon Nails.** A transverse and longitudinal concavity of the nail, resulting in a "spoon-shaped" nail. Seen in iron deficiency, Raynaud disease, or SLE.
- **Onychogryphosis.** "Ram's horn" configuration with thickened nails that may assume grotesque shape and size. Caused by trauma, vascular disease, neglected nail trimming; most common in elderly.
- **Onycholysis ("Plummer Nails").** The nail plate is separated from the nail bed, results in white discoloration of the affected area. Due to excessive exposure to water, soaps, detergents, alkalis, and industrial cleaning agents; also hyperthyroidism.
- **Onychomycosis.** Also called tinea unguium, a fungal infection of the nail with white or yellow nail discoloration, thickening of the nail, separation of the nail from the nail bed, and nail destruction. May cause nail changes identical to those seen in psoriasis.

6

- **Onychorrhexis.** "Brittle nail" plate where the cut edges of the nail delaminate and have a steplike appearance. Seen with malnutrition, iron deficiency, thyrotoxicosis, or calcium deficiency or cause is unknown.
- **Paronychia.** Inflammation of the lateral or proximal nail folds most commonly due to acute infection secondary to *Staphylococcus aureus*.
- **Pitting.** Punctate depressions in the nail plate. Associated with psoriasis, Reiter syndrome and other connective tissue disorders, sarcoidosis, pemphigus.
- **Splinter Hemorrhages.** Longitudinal lesions associated with endocarditis but can be benign.
- **Subungual Hematoma.** Acute painful bleeding into the closed space between the nail bed and the nail plate usually due to trauma.
- **Subungual Pigmentation.** Manifestation of ungual melanoma.
- **Terry Nails.** Proximal 80% or more of the nail bed is white, associated with hepatic cirrhosis.
- **Yellow Nail Plates:** Yellow-nail syndrome caused by impeded lymphatic circulation.

Nevus: See Mole.

Nodule: A solid, palpable, circumscribed lesion larger than a papule and smaller than a tumor. Examples: Erythema nodosum, gouty tophi.

Nummular lesions: These are circular or coin-shaped. Example: Nummular eczema.

Papule: A solid elevated lesion less than 1 cm in diameter. Examples: Nevi, warts, lichen planus, insect bites, seborrheic keratoses, actinic keratoses, some lesions of acne, and skin cancers.

Patch: A nonpalpable discoloration of the skin with an irregular border, greater than 1 cm in diameter. Example: Vitiligo.

Petechiae: Flat, pinhead-sized, nonblanching, red-purple lesions caused by hemorrhage into the skin. Example: Seen in disseminated intravascular coagulation (DIC), immune thrombocytopenic purpura (ITP), SLE, meningococcemia (*Neisseria meningitidis*)

Plantar Wart (Verruca Pedis or Plantaris): The wart caused by human papilloma virus (HPV) on the foot. Skin lines are disrupted and black spots of hemorrhage may be seen, and weight bearing may cause pain.

Plaque: A solid, flat, elevated lesion greater than 1 cm in diameter. Examples: Psoriasis, discoid lupus erythematosus, actinic keratosis.

Purpura: A condition characterized by flat, nonblanching, red-purple lesions larger than petechiae caused by hemorrhage into the skin. Examples: Henoch–Schönlein purpura, thrombotic thrombocytopenic purpura (TTP).

Pustule: A vesicle filled with purulent fluid. Examples: Acne, impetigo.

Scales: Partial separation of the superficial layer of skin. Examples: Psoriasis, dandruff.

Scar: Replacement of normal skin with fibrous tissue, often resulting from injury. Examples: Surgical scar, burn.

Target (Bull's-Eye or Iris) Lesions: Appear as rings with central duskiness and are classic for erythema multiforme; some cases of Lyme disease.

Telangiectasia: Dilatation of capillaries resulting in red, irregular, clustered lines that blanch. Examples: Seen in scleroderma, Osler–Weber–Rendu disease, cirrhosis.

Tumor: A solid, palpable, circumscribed lesion greater than 2 cm in diameter. Examples include lipomas.

Ulcer: A depressed lesion resulting from loss of epidermis and part of the dermis. Examples: Decubitus ulcers, primary lesion of syphilis, venous stasis ulcer.

Verrucous: These lesions have an irregular, pebbly, or rough surface. Examples: Warts, seborrheic keratoses.

Vesicle: A superficial, well-circumscribed, raised, fluid-filled lesion that is less than 1 cm in diameter. Examples: Herpes simplex, varicella (chickenpox).

Wheal/Hive: Slightly raised, red, irregular, transient lesions secondary to local edema of the skin. Examples: Urticaria (hives), allergic reaction to injections or insect bites.

Xanthomas: Yellowish, waxy lesions, may be idiopathic or may be seen with lipid disorders.

Zosteriform: Lesions clustered in a dermatomal distribution similar to those of herpes zoster.

Neurology Key Elements

The complete neurologic examination, in addition to a complete history and physical exam, includes detailed assessment of:

- Mental status
- Cranial nerves
- Motor function
- Sensory function
- Reflexes
- Coordination and gait

Basic elements of the neurologic exam for both the adult and pediatric populations are reviewed in the basic physical exam section on page 52. Any findings should be compared with the contralateral side, as well as comparing the upper extremity function to the lower extremity function. The clinical data from the neurologic examination coupled with a careful history assist in anatomic localization of the neurologic disease and help guide the diagnostic tests most likely to be informative. See Table 6-4, page 76 for neurologic findings that help identify diagnostic possibilities. Details in the neurologic exam are reviewed here.

Cranial Nerves: There are 12 cranial nerves, the functions of which are noted along with methods of assessing each cranial nerve or groups of cranial nerves.

Table 6-4. Findings Helpful for Localizations within the Nervous System

Region	SIGNS
Cerebrum	Abnormal mental status or cognitive impairment
	Seizures
	Unilateral weakness[a] and sensory abnormalities, including head and limbs
	Visual field abnormalities
	Movement abnormalities (e.g., diffuse incoordination, tremor, chorea)
Brainstem	Isolated cranial nerve abnormalities (single or multiple)
	"Crossed" weakness[a] and sensory abnormalities of head and limbs, e.g., weakness of right face and left arm and leg
Spinal cord	Back pain or tenderness
	Weakness[a] and sensory abnormalities sparing the head
	Mixed upper and lower motor neuron findings
	Sensory level
	Sphincter dysfunction
Spinal roots	Radiating limb pain
	Weakness[b] or sensory abnormalities following root distribution (see Figure 6-6, A and B, pages 80–81)
	Loss of reflexes
Peripheral nerve	Mid- or distal limb pain
	Weakness[b] or sensory abnormalities following nerve distribution (see Figure 6-6, A and B)
	"Stocking or glove" distribution of sensory loss
	Loss of reflexes
Neuromuscular junction	Bilateral weakness, including face (ptosis, diplopia, dysphagia) and proximal limbs
	Increasing weakness with exertion
	Sparing of sensation
Muscle	Bilateral proximal or distal weakness
	Sparing of sensation

[a]Weakness along with other abnormalities having an "upper motor neuron" pattern, i.e., spasticity, weakness of extensors > flexors in the upper extremity and flexors > extensors in the lower extremity, and hyperreflexia.
[b]Weakness along with other abnormalities having a "lower motor neuron" pattern, i.e., flaccidity and hyporeflexia. (Reproduced with permission from Jameson J, Fauci AS, Kasper DL, Hauser SL, Longo DL, Loscalzo J, eds. *Harrison's Manual of Medicine*, 20e, New York, NY: McGraw-Hill; 2018.)

I Olfactory—Smell (consider coffee or toothpaste for the "sniff test"). Often not evaluated unless there is a specific concern. (Note loss of smell [and taste] is a unique characteristic of COVID-19.)

II Optic—Vision acuity, visual fields, and fundi; afferent limb of pupillary response.

III, IV, VI: Oculomotor, trochlear, abducens—Note size, regularity, and shape of pupils; reaction to light, direct and consensual (CN III efferent limb of pupillary response); and convergence (patient follows an object as it moves closer). Check for lid drooping, lag, or retraction. Have patient follow your finger and report any double vision as you move it horizontally to left and right and vertically with each eye first fully adducted, then fully abducted. Identify inability to fully follow the examiner's finger in a particular direction. Note any nystagmus. Test quick voluntary eye movements (saccades) as well as pursuit by "follow the finger." Details of CN associated with the six cardinal positions of gaze can be found in Figure 6-13, page 96. You can isolate the function of CN IV by having the patient look inferiorly and medially and the function of CN VI by lateral gaze.

V Trigeminal—Corneal reflex (afferent), facial sensation V1, V2, and V3; test masseter and temporalis muscle by having patient bite down.

VII Facial—Note any facial asymmetry. Raise eyebrows, close eyes tight, show teeth, smile, or whistle, corneal reflex (efferent).

VIII Acoustic—Hearing; test by finger rub, Weber and Rinne tests (see also page 102); if hearing loss noted based on history or gross bedside testing, obtain more formal audiology testing.

IX, X Glossopharyngeal and vagus—Pharyngeal or "gag" reflex is evaluated by stimulating the posterior pharyngeal wall on each side with a blunt object (e.g., tongue blade); note quality of speech. Palate and uvula should move upward in midline with phonation ("say ahh").

XI Spinal accessory—Shoulder shrug engages trapezius muscle, and head rotation to each side against resistance engages sternocleidomastoid muscle.

XII Hypoglossal—Tongue movement. Test strength by having the patient press tongue against the buccal mucosa on each side while you press a finger against the patient's cheek (exterior). Observe for fasciculations or atrophy/weakness.

Motor: Includes assessment of **muscle bulk, strength, and tone.**

1. **Bulk:** Major muscle groups should appear symmetrically developed when compared with their counterparts on the opposite side. Assess for appropriate development with allowances for the patient's age, gender, and activity level. Palpate the major muscle groups: biceps, triceps, deltoids, quadriceps, and hamstrings. Note any tenderness or tremors. **Parkinson disease** can cause a very characteristic resting tremor that diminishes with voluntarily movement. In contrast, **benign essential tremor** persists

throughout movement and is not associated with any other neurologic findings.

2. **Strength:** This should be tested in upper and lower extremities. Grade strength as follows:

- 5 = active motion against full resistance
- 4 = active motion against some resistance
- 3 = active motion against gravity
- 2 = active motion with gravity eliminated
- 1 = barely detectable motion
- 0 = no motion or muscular contraction detected

  a. **Assess overall upper-limb strength** by checking for **pronator drift** (see Barre sign, page 62).

  b. **Finger flexors**: The patient makes a fist, squeezing their fingers around two of the examiner's fingers.

  c. **Intrinsic hand muscles (C8, T1):** The patient is asked to spread their fingers apart against resistance (abduction) and squeeze them together, with the examiner's fingers placed in between each of their digits (adduction). This assesses the ulnar nerve.

  d. **Wrist flexion (C7, 8, T1):** Patient flexes wrist against resistance and evaluates the median and ulnar nerves.

  e. **Wrist extension (C6, 7, 8):** Have the patient try to extend their wrist against resistance. Evaluates radial nerve.

  f. **Elbow flexion (C5, 6):** With the palm upward and the elbow bent 90 degrees, direct the patient to flex their forearm against resistance.

  g. **Shoulder adduction (C5–T1):** The elbow is flexed and held out from the body at 45 degrees while the patient tries to further adduct the shoulder against resistance.

  h. **Shoulder abduction (C5, 6):** Similar to shoulder adduction, but the resistance is applied by the examiner while the patient tries to further abduct the arm.

  i. **Hip flexion (L2, 3, 4):** The patient is seated, and the examiner places a hand on top of one thigh. The patient is asked to lift the leg up from the table. This assesses the strength of the main hip flexor (iliopsoas muscle, innervated by the femoral nerve).

  j. **Hip extension (L5, S1):** With the patient lying prone, the patient is directed to lift their leg off the table against resistance. This evaluates the main hip extensor (gluteus maximus, innervated by inferior gluteal nerve).

  k. **Hip abduction (L4, 5, S1):** With the patient seated, the examiner places hands on the outside of either thigh and directs the patient to separate their legs against resistance. Several muscle groups are involved.

  l. **Hip adduction (L2, 3, 4):** With the patient seated, the examiner places hands on the inner thighs and asks the patient to push knees together. One major nerve evaluated is the obturator nerve.

 m. Knee extension (L2, 3, 4): With the patient seated, have them push their lower leg against your hand. Keeping your hand on the knee is helpful. Extension is mediated by the quadriceps muscle group (innervated by the femoral nerve).

 n. Knee flexion (L5; S1, 2): The patient should be prone. Have them lift the foot off the table (flexing the knee) against resistance. This assesses the hamstring muscle group (innervated by the sciatic nerve).

 o. Ankle dorsiflexion (L4, 5): With the patient in a seated position, direct them to pull their toes upwards against resistance with your hand on the top of the foot. This assesses the deep peroneal nerve. If this nerve is injured, "foot drop" results with an inability to dorsiflex the foot.

 p. Ankle plantar flexion (S1, 2): With the patient in a seated position, ask them to "step on the gas" against resistance. The gastrocnemius and soleus are tested here and are innervated by a branch of the sciatic nerve.

 q. Ankle plantar flexion and dorsiflexion can be simultaneously assessed by asking the patient to walk on their toes (plantar flexion) and heels (dorsiflexion).

 r. Patterns of paresis are:
- Quadriparesis: Weak in all four limbs
- Hemiparesis: Weak in half of the body
- Paraparesis: Weakness of both upper or both lower extremities
- Monoparesis: Weak in a single limb

3. Tone: For a screening exam, limit this assessment to just the major joints: wrist, elbow, shoulder, hips, and knees. With the muscle group relaxed, the examiner should be able to easily manipulate the joint through its normal ROM in a fluid fashion. **"Cog wheel rigidity"** is a ratchetlike sensation seen in Parkinson disease. **Spasticity** is an increase in tone caused by rapid joint movement and is typically seen with stroke or spinal cord injury.

Sensory: Because most sensory disorders affect distal more than proximal sites, screening should begin distally (i.e., at the toes and fingers) and proceed proximally until the upper border of any deficit is reached. Identify deficits using dermatome and cutaneous innervation diagrams (Figure 6-6 A and B, page 80 and 81).

- Lightly stroking with fingers or a wisp of cotton from the end of a cotton swab across the skin may help elicit dermatomal patterns of sensory loss requiring further evaluation.
- **Pain** (sharp or sharp and dull using two sides of a safety pin) or **temperature** of distal to proximal upper and lower extremities. The loss of pain sensation due to a metabolic or toxic peripheral neuropathy typically follows a stocking-glove pattern, while lesions due to a radiculopathy follow a defined dermatome pattern.

6

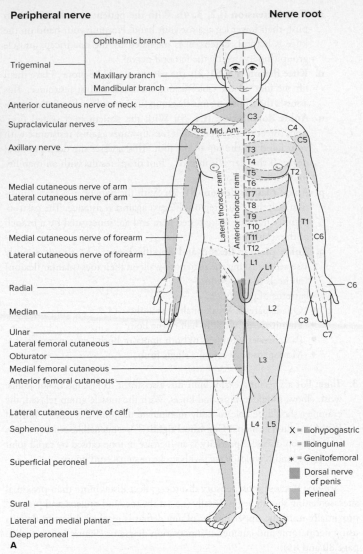

Peripheral nerve

- Trigeminal
  - Ophthalmic branch
  - Maxillary branch
  - Mandibular branch
- Anterior cutaneous nerve of neck
- Supraclavicular nerves
- Axillary nerve
- Medial cutaneous nerve of arm
- Lateral cutaneous nerve of arm
- Medial cutaneous nerve of forearm
- Lateral cutaneous nerve of forearm
- Radial
- Median
- Ulnar
- Lateral femoral cutaneous
- Obturator
- Medial femoral cutaneous
- Anterior femoral cutaneous
- Lateral cutaneous nerve of calf
- Saphenous
- Superficial peroneal
- Sural
- Lateral and medial plantar
- Deep peroneal

Nerve root

C3
C4
Post. Mid. Ant.
C5
T2
T3
T4
T5
T6
T7
T8
T9
T10
T11
T12
T2
T1
C6
L1
L1
C6
L2
C8
C7
L3
L4 L5
S1

Lateral thoracic rami
Anterior thoracic rami

X = Iliohypogastric
† = Ilioinguinal
* = Genitofemoral
▨ Dorsal nerve of penis
▨ Perineal

A

Figure 6-6. A: Dermatomes, nerve roots, and cutaneous innervation patterns, anterior view. (Reproduced with permission from Aminoff MJ, et al., eds. *Clinical Neurology*, 6e, New York, NY: McGraw-Hill; 2005.)

(continued next page)

6

Nerve root

Peripheral nerve

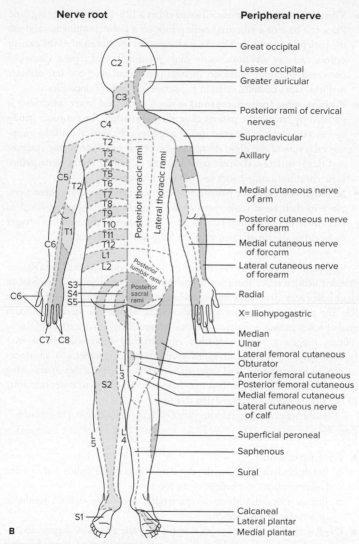

Great occipital

Lesser occipital

Greater auricular

C2

C3

Posterior rami of cervical nerves

C4

Supraclavicular

T2
T3
T4
T5
T6
T7
T8
T9
T10
T11
T12
L1
L2

Axillary

Medial cutaneous nerve of arm

C5

T2

T1

C6

Posterior thoracic rami

Lateral thoracic rami

Posterior cutaneous nerve of forearm

Medial cutaneous nerve of forearm

Lateral cutaneous nerve of forearm

S3
S4
S5

Posterior lumbar rami

Posterior sacral rami

Radial

C6

X= Iliohypogastric

C7 C8

Median

Ulnar

Lateral femoral cutaneous

Obturator

L3

S2

Anterior femoral cutaneous

Posterior femoral cutaneous

Medial femoral cutaneous

Lateral cutaneous nerve of calf

Superficial peroneal

L5

L4

Saphenous

Sural

S1

Calcaneal

Lateral plantar

Medial plantar

B

Figure 6-6.   B: Dermatomes, nerve roots, and cutaneous innervation patterns, posterior view. (Reproduced with permission from Aminoff MJ et al., eds. Clinical Neurology, 6e, New York, NY: McGraw-Hill; 2005.)

6

- **Vibration testing** is conducted using either a 128- or 256-Hz tuning fork. Place the base of a vibrating tuning fork on a bony prominence and ask the patient to say when they can no longer feel the vibration. If the patient cannot feel any vibration, move more proximally and repeat. Causes of decreased vibratory sensation include peripheral neuropathies, diabetes mellitus, tabes dorsalis, vitamin B_{12} deficiency, and myelopathies.
- **Position sense (proprioception)** of distal upper and lower extremities is assessed by having the patient close their eyes while the examiner gently moves a toe (usually the great toe) or a finger in the vertical plane by grasping each side of the digit; do not grasp the toe or finger on the extensor and flexor surfaces. Position sense loss can be caused by the same pathologic conditions noted with loss of vibratory sense.
- **Stereognosis.** Have the patient close their eyes and identify an object you place in their hand (coin, pen) or assess graphesthesia (patient asked to identify letters or numbers traced onto their palm by the examiner's finger or by using the tip of a pen with the ballpoint tip retracted).

Reflexes: "Muscle-stretch reflexes" or "deep tendon reflexes" (DTRs) are assessed using a reflex hammer to test the spinal cord segments involved in their reflex arcs. The reflex testing technique is described in Table 6-5, page 83. The primary nerve root arcs are cervical, lumbar, or sacral. The main goal of reflex testing is to detect absence or asymmetry. Symmetrically absent reflexes suggest a polyneuropathy; symmetrically increased reflexes may indicate bilateral cerebral or spinal cord disease. _Hyporeflexia_ is an absent or diminished response, and _hyperreflexia_ refers to hyperactive or repeating (clonic) reflexes. Elderly patients may have reduced or absent lower extremity DTRs due to normal aging-related changes.

Routine reflex testing and some key DTRs are demonstrated in Figure 6-7, page 84:

- C5–6 nerve root:
  - o Brachioradialis: Striking the distal one-third of the radius with a reflex hammer causes movement of the forearm.
  - o Biceps: Place thumb on biceps tendon and strike thumb; results in movement of the forearm.
- C7–8 nerve root: Triceps reflex is tested with the arm at 90 degrees abduction and the examiner holding the patient's arm with the forearm hanging loosely at a right angle (fingers pointed toward the ground). Tapping the triceps tendon with a reflex hammer should induce an extension in the elbow joint.
- L2–4 nerve root: Striking the tendon just below the patella (leg is slightly bent) induces knee extension through the quadriceps muscle.
- L5 nerve root: Test the posterior tibial reflex by tapping the tibialis posterior muscle either just above or below the medial malleolus. Inversion of the foot occurs with a positive reflex.

Table 6-5. Deep Tendon Reflexes (DTRs) Technique

- The reflex hammer (percussion hammer) is an important tool, and a variety of reflex hammers are available to assess DTRs. The lightweight, triangular-tipped "Taylor" reflex hammer is a common tool used. The heavier, long-handled "Babinski" reflex hammers have weighted heads oriented horizontally or vertically. These heavier hammers are designed so that if you raise them approximately 10 cm from the target and release, they will swing and strike the tendon with adequate force. This allows the examiner to apply the same amount of force to both the left and right side or the same side over time. The smaller hammers should be swung loosely between thumb and forefinger.

- The muscle/tendon group to be tested must be in a neutral position, neither stretched nor contracted, with the target tendon clearly identified. The extremity should be positioned such that the tendon can be easily struck with the reflex hammer.

- If there is difficulty locating the tendon, have the patient contract the muscle to which the tendon is joined. As the muscle contracts, you should be able to see and/or feel the cordlike tendon, confirming the correct location. As an example, if you have difficulty identifying the biceps tendon within the antecubital fossa, have the patient flex their forearm by contracting their biceps muscle while you simultaneously palpate the fossa. The biceps tendon should become taut and easily identified.

- The tendon should be struck with a single brisk stroke. Use the whole length of the reflex hammer; let the hammer fully swing. Don't make small, stabbing thrusts at the tendon. A normal brisk stroke will not cause the patient any pain.

- When testing the biceps tendon, some advocate placing the examiner's thumb on the tendon and striking your thumb.

- The force used to bring out the reflex should be consistent from side to side.

- Eliciting a hyporeflexic DTR requires greater force than a normal or hyperreflexic DTR.

- Routine DTR testing is conducted for the following (see detail in text, pages 82–84): Brachioradialis, biceps, triceps, patella, posterior tibial, Achilles

- **Grade the reflex.** While somewhat subjective, one universal deep tendon reflex grading system is as follows:

    0 = no response; always abnormal
    1+ = a slight but definitely present response; may or may not be normal
    2+ = a brisk response; normal
    3+ = a very brisk response; may or may not be normal
    4+ = a tap elicits a repeating reflex (clonus); always abnormal

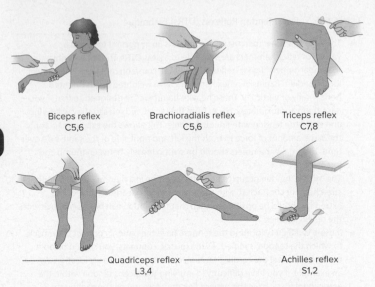

Biceps reflex
C5,6

Brachioradialis reflex
C5,6

Triceps reflex
C7,8

Quadriceps reflex
L3,4

Achilles reflex
S1,2

Figure 6-7. Methods to elicit the deep tendon reflexes showing techniques for eliciting the quadriceps reflex in both seated and supine patients. (Reproduced with permission from LeBlond RF, Brown DD, DeGowin RL. *DeGowin's Diagnostic Examination*. 9e, New York, NY: McGraw-Hill; 2009.)

- S1–2 nerve root: With your non-dominant hand, place slight dorsiflexion pressure on the distal foot while striking the Achilles tendon with a reflex hammer. This will elicit a jerking of the foot toward its plantar surface.
- **Superficial reflexes** can be physiologic or pathologic reflexes. With central motor neuron damage, the superficial reflex response decreases.
  - **T6–12.** The **abdominal reflex** is tested with the patient lying down. Gently stroke the anterior abdominal wall from lateral to medial (bilaterally) in following areas: below the costal arch, around the umbilicus, and above the inguinal ligament. Normal response is a contraction of the abdominal muscles; no contraction is indicative of nerve root damage.
  - **L1–2. Cremasteric reflex** is elicited by stroking the inner thigh with a contraction of the cremaster muscles and upward movement of the ipsilateral testis. With no response suspect nerve root damage.
  - **S3–5.**
    - **Bulbocavernosus reflex:** Squeeze the glans penis or the clitoris. Pelvic floor muscles contract.
    - **Anal reflex:** Stroke the skin around the anus. Normal reflex is contraction of the anal sphincter.

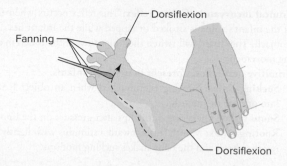

Figure 6-8. An abnormal extensor plantar reflex, the Babinski sign. It is elicited by firmly stroking the lateral border of the sole of the foot. The normal plantar reflex response is flexion of the toes. (Modified from LeBlond RF, Brown DD, DeGowin RL. *DeGowin's Diagnostic Examination*, 9e, New York, NY: McGraw-Hill; 2009.)

- Check for pathologic reflexes. These are sometimes called "primitive reflexes" or "frontal release" signs: a reflex that is **normal in infants and not in adults.** In an adult with a major brain injury these "extinguished" reflexes may reappear.

  o **Plantar reflex:** Use a blunt object (e.g., point of a key or end of reflex hammer) and with a fair amount of pressure (should be a noxious stimulus) stroke the outer border of the sole of the foot from the heel and when you are just proximal to between the fourth and fifth metatarsal, move the object toward the base of the great toe. **Normal plantar reflex** response is plantar flexion of the toes. **Babinski sign** (Figure 6-8) is an abnormal response with extension (dorsiflexion) of the great toe at the metatarsophalangeal joint. May also be associated with abduction (fanning) of other toes and variable degrees of flexion at ankle, knee, and hip.

  o **Palmomental reflex.** This is elicited by scratching the palm of the hand and results in contraction of the ipsilateral chin (mentalis) and perioral (orbicularis oris) muscles.

  o **Glabellar reflex** is elicited by repetitive tapping on the forehead just above the nose; normal subjects blink only in response to the first several taps, whereas persistent blinking is an abnormal response **(Myerson sign).**

  o **Palmar grasp reflex:** Stimulated when an object is placed into the baby's palm. A normally developing neonate responds by grasping the object.

  o **Moro reflex:** With a sudden loud noise, the newborn will throw out the arms and legs and then pull them back towards the body.

o **Truncal incurvation/Galant reflex**: This reflex occurs when the side of the infant's spine is stroked or tapped while the infant lies on their stomach. The infant will twitch their hips toward the touch in a dancing movement

o **Primitive oral reflexes present in newborn infants:**
  - **Sucking reflex:** Sucking is stimulated when an object is inserted into or near the mouth.
  - **Snout reflex:** Puckering of the lips after pressure on the upper lip.
  - **Rooting reflex:** Mouth turns toward a stimulus with lightly touching the cheek and the baby makes sucking motions.

Coordination and Gait:

- **Impaired coordination (ataxia),** which usually results from lesions affecting the cerebellum or its connections, can affect the eye movements, speech, limbs, or trunk. Some tests of coordination:
  o **Heel to shin test**: Ataxia of the lower limbs can be demonstrated by the heel-knee-shin test. The supine patient is asked to run the heel of the foot smoothly up and down the opposite shin from ankle to knee. Ataxia produces jerky and inaccurate movement, making it impossible for the patient to keep the heel in contact with the shin.
  o **Finger to nose**: The patient moves an index finger back and forth between his or her nose and the examiner's finger as the patient moves their finger. The examiner should move the finger far enough away from the patient for the patient's arm to fully or almost fully extend each time.
  o **Rapid alternating movements.** The patient places one hand over the next and asks them to flip one hand back and forth as fast as possible. If abnormal, this is called dysdiadochokinesia. An alternative approach is to have the patient quickly tap their foot on the floor as fast as possible.
- **Gait.** The patient should then be observed walking normally, on the heels, on the toes, and in tandem (one foot placed directly in front of the other), to identify any common gait abnormalities (hemiplegic gait, steppage gait, Parkinsonian gait, others).
- **Romberg test.** A test of stance (i.e., station or no movement) and not gait and provides information related to the function of the cerebellum and vestibular system.
  o Patient stands with feet together, arms at sides with eyes open.
  o The examiner stands facing patient and should be prepared to catch the patient if they fall.
  o Observe the patient for about 20–30 seconds and note any swaying or falling.
  o Next ask the patient to close both eyes for 30 seconds and note if the patient is able to maintain an upright posture.

o Inability to stand with the feet together with the eyes open suggests a cerebellar problem. A positive Romberg sign is a loss of balance requiring the feet to move, swaying, or the patient falling with the eyes closed or unable to keep their eyes closed. This suggests a problem with conscious proprioception and ataxia from dorsal column disease.

o A negative Romberg is minimal swaying.

Obstetrics and Gynecology Key Elements

6

The OB/GYN evaluations are similar to the general adult H&P described on page 43. However, these OB/GYN specialty evaluations are centered on the female reproductive system with the key elements outlined here. Many aspects of this provider–patient interaction can be uncomfortable for both parties. The provider should not be embarrassed or critical and should always be nonjudgmental.

Gynecology History and Physical Key Elements

HPI: Note the patient's age, gravida and parity, and last menstrual period. Age is a critical factor in the approach to the GYN patient, as women have more defined life stages (pubescence, adolescence, childbearing years, premenopausal and postmenopausal years). Gravida refers to the number of pregnancies regardless of outcome. Parity is the number of deliveries over 20 weeks' gestation. Recording the reproductive history commonly uses a four-digit code indicating the number of _T_erm pregnancies, _P_remature deliveries, _A_bortions, and _L_iving children, referred to as **TPAL**. As an example 3-2-1-3 indicates three-term pregnancies, two premature deliveries, one abortion, and three living children.

PMH:

Menstrual history: Age of menarche, characteristics of menses (duration, amount and character of flow, cycle length, any intermenstrual bleeding), menstrual discomfort (dysmenorrhea), climacteric (premenopausal), age at menopause

Gynecologic history: Previous gynecologic surgery, Pap smears, HPV testing, HPV vaccination, breast history (breast disease or biopsy, breastfeeding, last mammogram, use of self-breast exams), infertility (evaluation, treatment, outcome), evidence of DES (diethylstilbestrol) use by patient's mother

Sexual and contraceptive history: Inquire about sexual activities (to include oral or anal sex), including number of partners, sexual orientation, contraceptive methods and satisfaction with current use, concerns about safety or sexual abuse, any prior STIs), may need to specify trichomonas, gonorrhea, syphilis, chlamydia, genital warts, hepatitis B and hepatitis C, human immunodeficiency virus [HIV] or TB exposure)

Other key items: Treatment of PID, salpingitis, endometritis, or tubo-ovarian abscess.

Family History: Due to inheritance patterns, breast, ovarian, and colon cancers are most critical, as this may require genetic evaluation. The time of menopause in the mother or grandmother and any familial history of osteoporosis.

ROS: Vaginal bleeding or discharge, dyspareunia, abdominal or pelvic pain, urinary or fecal incontinence, dysuria, urinary frequency or urgency, hot flashes, night sweats, vaginal dryness.

Physical Examination: Due to the sensitive nature of the female pelvic exam, the following should be considered: having a chaperone present or having a friend or family member in the room for comfort, self-insertion of the speculum, and offering the option to have a mirror so the patient can observe and learn about any issues. Make sure the patient knows they can stop the exam at any time. The American College of Obstetricians and Gynecologists (ACOG) recommends pelvic examinations be performed when indicated by medical history or symptoms and when mutually agreed to by the patient and provider. The pelvic exam is discussed in detail in Chapter 19, page 628.

Vital Signs: Measure height of postmenopausal patients. Height may be lost from osteoporosis and related vertebral fractures.

Breast Exam: The technique for a thorough breast exam is illustrated in Figure 6-1, pages 50–51.

External Genitalia, Speculum, and Bimanual Examination: See Chapter 19, page 628.

Obstetric History and Physical Key Elements

Human pregnancy duration is 280 days or 40 weeks (9 calendar months or 10 lunar months) from the last menstrual period (LMP). The estimated date of delivery (EDD) can be determined by the **Naegele rule**: subtract 3 months from the month of the LMP and add 7 to the first day of the LMP. EDD may also be calculated as 266 days or 38 weeks from the last known ovulation. Gestational age and EDD can also be determined by a pregnancy wheel calculator, and a variety of online and smart phone apps are widely available. Uterine size may provide a general idea of the stage of a singleton pregnancy (Figure 6-9, page 89).

For the obstetric patient, most of the gynecology H&P is similar. Key aspects that should be considered for the OB patient are noted here.

HPI: Note the patient's age, gravida and parity, and LMP (see gynecology H&P). Include any assisted reproductive technologies to achieve pregnancy. Identify any concerns or complications relating to the pregnancy (spotting, contractions, vaginal discharge or rupture of membranes, decreased fetal activity, etc.). Inquire regarding history of gestational diabetes or preeclampsia, perceptions of fetal movement, weight gain, and

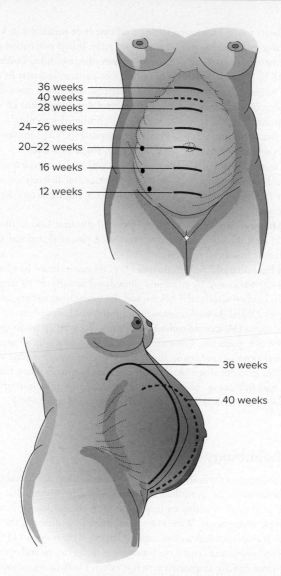

Figure 6-9. Height of fundus at various times during pregnancy. (Reproduced with permission from Bernstein HB. Normal Pregnancy & Prenatal Care. In: DeCherney AH, Nathan L, Laufer N, Roman AS, eds. *Current Diagnosis & Treatment: Obstetrics & Gynecology*, 12e, New York, NY: McGraw-Hill; 2019.)

fetal heart tones. Determine timing and extent of prenatal care and any laboratory or imaging studies performed. The initial perception of fetal movement (the maternal perception of movement is called **quickening**) is at 18 to 20 weeks' gestation in nulliparous patients and may be as early as 14 weeks' gestation in multiparous patients, but this is not a dependable sign of pregnancy. Review any prenatal screening based on current gestational age (first trimester screening ["combined screening"], second trimester screening, chorionic villus sampling [CVS], amniocentesis, other pregnancy screening: see Chapter 10, pages 244–246).

PMH: Obstetric history: Details on past deliveries: dates, type of delivery, sex and weight of the baby, any complications of delivery or anesthesia in mother or baby, including pregnancies ending before 20 weeks' gestation.

Family History: Any known familial/inherited diseases; DM in the family should alert the clinician about an increased risk of gestational diabetes and family history of twinning.

Physical Examination: Fetal heart tones (FHTs) can be heard by a fetoscope at 18–20 weeks and by handheld ultrasound as early as 10 weeks' gestation. Uterine size/fundal height and the gestational age are correlated between 18 and 34 weeks. Measure from the pubic symphysis to the top of the uterus (McDonald technique) at each visit after 20 weeks' gestation (Figure 6-9, page 89). Ultrasound is now used routinely as part of the physical exam to confirm an intrauterine pregnancy, determine viability, estimate gestational age, screen for aneuploidy, and evaluate fetal anatomy and well-being. Near delivery, fetal heart rate monitoring may be employed (see Chapter 20, Specialized Diagnostics, page 698.)

Ophthalmology Key Elements[5]

"Of all the organs of the body, the eye is most accessible to direct examination. Visual function can be quantified by simple subjective testing. The external anatomy of the eye is visible to inspection with the unaided eye and with fairly simple instruments. With more complicated instruments, the interior of the eye is visible through a clear cornea. The eye is the only part of the body where blood vessels and central nervous system tissue (retina and optic nerve) can be viewed directly. Important systemic effects of infectious, autoimmune, neoplastic, and vascular diseases may be identified from ocular examination."[2] The three most common preventable causes of permanent visual loss in developed nations are amblyopia, diabetic retinopathy, and glaucoma.

History

CC and HPI are characterized by the location, duration, frequency, intermittency, and onset of the visual concern. Identify any other ocular and nonocular symptoms that may require specific questioning, as patients may not associate nonocular symptoms with an ocular disease.

PMH should focus on active and past ocular disorders: vascular disorders (diabetes, HTN), use of systemic steroids, glaucoma, any procedures such as laser resurfacing or cataract surgery.

Family History of significant medical diseases such as HTN, CAD, MI, CVA, TIA, PVD, DM, strabismus, amblyopia, glaucoma, or cataracts and retinal problems (detachment, macular degeneration).

ROS should cover common ocular signs and symptoms:

6

- *Symptoms:* Vision loss (unilateral or bilateral, decreased central acuity, peripheral vision deficits), visual aberrations (glare, halos, distortion, flashing or flickering, dimness, wavy or jagged lines, and image magnification or minification, floating spots "floaters" or oscillopsia, a shaking field of vision), photophobia, diplopia. Eye pain may be periocular, ocular, retrobulbar (behind the globe), or poorly localized. Symptoms of dryness, burning, grittiness, and mild foreign body sensation can occur with dry eyes or other types of mild corneal irritation.

- *Signs:* "Red eye" (globe vs. lids vs. periorbital area), conjunctival growth (pterygium is a fleshy growth that covers the cornea; pinguecula is a yellowish, raised growth on the conjunctiva), and asymmetry of pupil size (anisocoria), other color abnormalities such as jaundice. Lids and periocular tissue signs may include edema, redness, focal growths, lesions, and abnormal position or contour, such as ptosis. If secretions are present, classify as severe causing eyes to be fused upon awakening (possible conjunctivitis) to less scant amounts. Evidence of dried matter and crusts on the lashes. Tearing may be of two general types (sudden onset or chronic).

Physical Examination

These basic ophthalmic evaluations should be considered part of a routine general physical examination. A more detailed evaluation may be performed by an ophthalmologist or optometrist and include tonometry (intraocular pressure), indirect ophthalmoscopy, slit lamp examination, and others. Color vision is tested using **Ishihara color plates** that detect red-green color blindness. The test plates contain a hidden number that is visible only to subjects without color blindness and cannot be seen by individuals who are color blind. The test has a very high sensitivity and specificity. This is worth usually screening only male children, since color blindness is almost exclusively X-linked.

External Examination: Skin lesions, growths, and inflammatory signs such as swelling, erythema, warmth, and tenderness. Malposition of the globe, such as proptosis, palpation of the bony orbital rim. Check positions of

6

the eyelids for abnormalities: ptosis (drooping of the upper lid), lid retraction, and symmetry. Enlarged preauricular lymph nodes, sinus tenderness, temporal artery prominence/tenderness may be relevant.

- The upper lid normally covers 1–2 mm of the iris, but this is increased by drooping of the lid (ptosis) due to lesions of the levator palpebrae muscle or to the oculomotor (III) or sympathetic nerve supply and with aging. Can be congenital, myopathic (such as in myasthenia gravis), or due to hypothyroidism or diabetes. Ptosis occurs together with miosis (and sometimes defective sweating, or anhidrosis, of the forehead) in Horner syndrome.
- Abnormal protrusion of the eye from the orbit (exophthalmos or proptosis) is best detected by standing behind the seated patient and looking down at his or her eyes.

Visual Acuity Testing:

- Visual acuity is always tested separately for each eye along with binocular visual acuity and depending on the degree of refractive error with and without corrective lenses/contacts. If 20/20 acuity is not present in each eye, the deficiency in vision must be explained. More extreme degrees of vision loss can be assessed by finger counting, hand movement, or identification of a bright light.
- The **Snellen chart** is the standard wall-mounted eye chart (paper chart or digital screen) used to test acuity at a distance of 6 m (20 ft) (Figure 6-10, below). Patients are asked to read the letters or numbers on successively lower lines (each with smaller images) until you identify the last line that can be read with 100% accuracy. Each line has a fraction written next to it: 20/20 indicates normal vision, and 20/400 means that the patient's vision 20 feet from an object is equivalent to

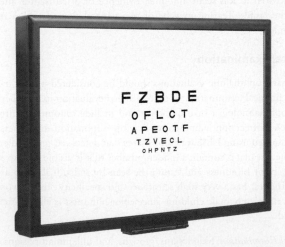

Figure 6-10. Example of a Snellen-style visual acuity chart displayed on an LCD screen. (Reproduced with permission from Riordan-Eva P, Augsburger JJ, eds. *Vaughan & Asbury's General Ophthalmology*, 19e, New York, NY: McGraw-Hill; 2018.)

that of a normal person viewing the same object from 400 feet (the larger the denominator, the worse the vision). All subjects should ideally be able to read the 6/6 m (20/20 ft) line with each eye using their refractive correction lenses if appropriate.

- A smaller-scale version of the Snellen chart is a portable version called the **Rosenbaum card**, which can be held at 36 cm (14 in.) from the patient. Patients who need reading glasses because of presbyopia must wear them for accurate testing with the Rosenbaum card (Figure 6-11, page 94).

- For those who do not understand English or children 3–5 years old, the "Illiterate E" chart is used in a similar fashion to the Snellen chart. (See Figure 6-12, page 95.)

- The **pinhole test** can be used if the patient needs glasses or the glasses/contacts are not available; the corrected acuity can be estimated by testing vision through a "pinhole" disk. Refractive blur due to myopia, hyperopia, or astigmatism is caused by multiple misfocused rays entering through the pupil and reaching the retina, preventing a sharply focused image on the retina. The pinholes help compensate for these refractive errors.

- An **emmetropic eye** is naturally in optimal distance focus, whereas an **ametropic** (**abnormal refractive condition**) eye has **myopia** ("nearsightedness"), **hyperopia** ("farsightedness"), **presbyopia** (loss of near focusing ability after age 40), and **astigmatism** (imperfection in the curvature of cornea or lens). These optical abnormalities collectively are called refractive errors.

Visual Field Testing: This is useful for evaluating peripheral vision that may be affected by diseases such as stroke, glaucoma, retinal detachment, certain brain tumors, and others.

- **Confrontation visual field testing** is a quick way to assess peripheral vision. Visual field testing involves having the examiner standing about an arm's length from the patient. It is useful for the examiner to close one eye so that one can determine if the patient is seeing appropriately in their visual field. The examiner's open eye is serving as a normal control. Ask the patient to cover their left eye with their left hand. The patient should fix their gaze directly on your open eye throughout the test. Close your right eye and maintain fixation on the patient's open right eye with your left eye. Raise your hand to the inferior temporal edge of your peripheral vision halfway between yourself and the patient, while holding up one, two, or five fingers, and ask the patient how many fingers are seen. Repeat for all four visual quadrants of the left eye: inferior temporal, inferior nasal, superior temporal, and superior nasal. Repeat for the patient's right eye (this time your right eye is closed). Note any deficiencies in visual fields. If needed, formal machine measurements (i.e. Humphrey Visual Field Machine) can be used. The size of the patient's central scotoma (blind spot), located in the temporal half of the visual field, can also be measured in relation to the examiner's. The object of confrontation testing is to determine whether the patient's visual field is coextensive with—or more restricted than—the examiner's.

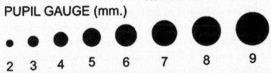

Figure 6-11. The Rosenbaum card is a miniature-scale version of the Snellen chart for testing visual acuity at near distance. This version of the card can be used when held 14 inches from the patient. When the visual acuity is recorded, the Snellen distance equivalent should bear a notation indicating that vision was tested at near, not at 6 m (20 ft), or else the Jaeger number system should be used to report the acuity. (Reproduced with permission from Jameson J, Fauci AS, Kasper DL, et al., eds. *Harrison's Principles of Internal Medicine*, 20e, New York, NY: McGraw-Hill; 2018.)

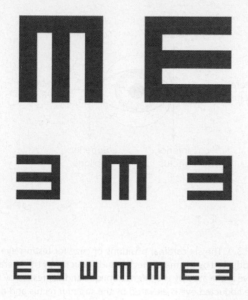

Figure 6-12. "Illiterate E" chart. Used for visual acuity testing in small children (3–5 years of age or older) or if there is a language barrier. The patient is asked to point in the same direction as the three "bars" of the E. (Reproduced with permission from Riordan-Eva P, Augsburger JJ, eds. *Vaughan & Asbury's General Ophthalmology*, 19e, New York, NY: McGraw-Hill; 2018.)

Eye Movements and Alignment.
- **Extraocular movements** are tested by having the patient follow a target (such as a pen light) with both eyes as it is moved in each of the four directions of gaze. Note the speed, smoothness, range, and symmetry of movements and observe for any nystagmus. See Figure 6-13, page 96 for the **six cardinal positions of gaze** as part of the neurologic exam.
- **Alignment** can be tested by several methods. One is the "cover test." The patient is asked to gaze at a distant target with both eyes open. If both eyes are fixating together on the target, covering one eye should not affect the position or continued fixation of the other eye. An abnormal cover test is commonly seen with diplopia.

Pupils: The size of the pupil is dependent on the ambient light and averages 3–4 mm. **Anisocoria** refers to unequal pupils at rest. **Miosis** is

6

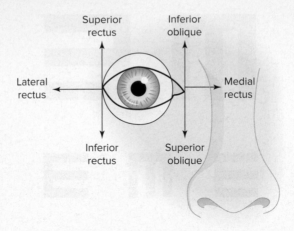

Figure 6-13. The six cardinal positions of gaze for testing eye movement. The eye is adducted by the medial rectus and abducted by the lateral rectus. The adducted eye is elevated by the inferior oblique and depressed by the superior oblique; the abducted eye is elevated by the superior rectus and depressed by the inferior rectus. All extraocular muscles are innervated by the oculomotor (III) nerve except the superior oblique, which is innervated by the trochlear (IV) nerve, and the lateral rectus, which is innervated by the abducens (VI) nerve. (Reproduced with permission from Aminoff MJ, Greenberg DA, Simon RP. *Clinical Neurology*, 6e, New York, NY: McGraw-Hill; 2005.)

<2 mm, and **mydriasis** is considered 5 mm or greater. The Rosenbaum visual testing card (Figure 6-11, page 94) often has a pupil gauge to help estimate pupil diameter. Observe pupils in both bright and dim light. Note abnormalities in the normal round shape of the pupil—any differences should be investigated. Use a penlight to assess the direct pupillary response to light; the **direct response** is constriction of the pupil (graded as brisk or sluggish). The **consensual response** is the normal simultaneous constriction (miosis) of the opposite nonilluminated pupil. The **"swinging flashlight test"** compares the direct and consensual responses in the same eye. Shine the pen light into one eye and note the response. Swing the light into the other eye. If normal optic nerve conduction is present in both eyes, rapid miosis occurs bilaterally as the light is moved back and forth. With impaired nerve conduction in one eye, swinging the light from the normal eye to the impaired eye will produce paradoxical dilatation in the impaired eye, known as an afferent pupillary defect or a "Marcus Gunn pupil." Horner syndrome has a unilateral small pupil and ptosis with normal pupillary response to light. An Adie (tonic) pupil is a unilateral large pupil with sluggish response to illumination.

Table 6-6. Ophthalmoscope Light, Aperture, Filter, and Focus Settings
(see Figure 6-14)

- **Large/medium/small light source:** Allows adjustment of the light source aperture based on the degree of pupil dilation. The large light is best for a dilated pupil (e.g., mydriatic drops). The small light is best when the pupil is very constricted (well-lit room, no dilation). The medium-sized light is used most commonly.
- **Half-circle light:** The half-circle can be used to pass light through only the clear portion of the pupil to avoid light reflecting back if the pupil is partially obstructed by a cataract.
- **Red-free filter:** This setting will make the retina look black and white and is used to visualize the vasculature.
- **Blue light:** Used to look for corneal abrasions or ulcers with fluorescein dye.
- **Slit beam:** Used to examine contour abnormalities of the cornea, lens, and retina.
- **Grid:** Used to approximate distance between retinal lesions.
- **Focusing wheel:** As a baseline focus your ophthalmoscope to the "0" setting. Focusing toward the positive numbers (often marked on the instrument in green or black) focuses on things closer to you, while focusing toward the negative numbers (marked in red) shifts the focus on targets farther away from you. A setting of 0 for a patient with an emmetropic eye and an examiner with an emmetropic eye will be focused sharply on the fundus.

6

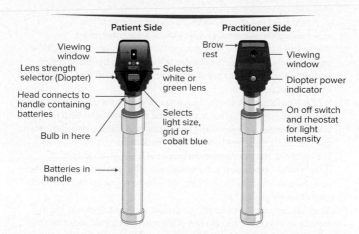

Figure 6-14. Example of a battery-operated ophthalmoscope. Ophthalmoscope features are described in Table 6-6 and how to use in Table 6-7, page 98. The head can be exchanged on many models to function as an otoscope.

Direct Ophthalmoscopy (Fundoscopic Examination): The direct ophthalmo-scope allows examination of inside of the eye to observe the retina, optic nerve, vasculature, and vitreous humor. For step by step instructions on performing the <u>direct ophthalmoscopy exam,</u> see Table 6-7, page 98. This exam produces an upright image of approximately 15 times magnification using a battery-operated ophthalmoscope (Figure 6-14, page 97). The ophthalmoscope settings are reviewed in Table 6-6, page 97. Fundus structures visualized are demonstrated in Figure 6-16, page 100.

Table 6-7. Direct Ophthalmoscopy Exam Technique

1. Position the patient so that the ophthalmoscope is held directly at the level of the patient's eye.
2. Turn on the ophthalmoscope and set the light to the correct aperture. Dim the room lights.
3. Instruct the patient to focus on an object straight ahead on the wall.
4. To examine the patient's RIGHT eye, hold the ophthalmoscope in your RIGHT hand and use your RIGHT eye to look through the instrument (Figure 6-15, page 100).
5. Place your left hand on the patient's head and place your thumb on their eyebrow.
6. Hold the ophthalmoscope about 6 inches from the eye and 15–20 degrees to the right of the patient.
7. Find the red reflex and "drive in on the red reflex."
8. Move in closer to continuously see the red reflex, staying nasally until you see the optic nerve. (See Figure 6-16, page 100.)
9. Start with focusing the diopter dial on 0; move the focus dial back and forth until a retinal vessel is in sharp focus.
   - A farsighted eye requires more plus/green number lenses.
   - A nearsighted eye requires more minus/red number lenses.
10. The normal optic disc is a yellowish, oval structure situated nasally at the posterior pole of the eye. The margins of the disc and the blood vessels that cross it should be sharply demarcated, and the veins should show spontaneous pulsations.
11. Note the disc's outline, shape, color, and size. Assess the papilledema, optic atrophy (pale disc), and glaucoma. It can be seen in patients with multiple sclerosis or other disorders of the optic nerve and is associated with defects in visual acuity, visual fields, or pupillary reactivity.
12. The optic disc has a center portion called the "cup," which is normally quite small in comparison to the entire optic disc. Measure the cup to disc ratio. Normal is usually three-tenths, with a ratio of greater than six-tenths suggestive for glaucoma.
13. Move out temporally to identify the macula and fovea (Figure 6-16); the macula, an area paler than the rest of the retina, is located about two disc diameters temporal to the temporal margin of the optic disc. The macula can also be visualized by having the patient look at the ophthalmoscope light.
    - Examine the macula and fovea, noting the normal foveal reflex (a bright pinpoint of light that moves in response to movement of the ophthalmoscope) centrally and the slight hyperpigmentation. Note any intense pigmentation, scars, or hemorrhages (enhanced by use of the red filter).

(continued)

Table 6-7. Direct Ophthalmoscopy Exam Technique   *(Continued)*

14. Examine the blood vessels as they enter the cup for venous pulsations.

15. Follow each group of vessels out as far as possible and note any arteriolar narrowing. Inspect the retina for hemorrhages and exudates.

    ● Indentation (nicking) of retinal veins by stiff (arteriosclerotic) retinal arteries most often due to chronic hypertension is known as **"A-V nicking."**

    ● In patients with neurologic diseases, the most important abnormality to identify is swelling of the optic disc resulting from increased intracranial pressure (papilledema). In early papilledema the retinal veins appear engorged, and spontaneous venous pulsations are absent. The disc may be hyperemic with linear hemorrhages at its borders. The disc margins become blurred, initially at the nasal edge. In fully developed papilledema, the optic disc is elevated above the plane of the retina, and blood vessels crossing the disc border are obscured. Papilledema is almost always bilateral, does not typically impair vision except for enlargement of the blind spot, and is not painful.

16. Repeat the same technique on the other eye. Refer any suspicious findings to the appropriate specialist. To examine the patient's LFFT eye, hold the ophthalmoscope in your LEFT hand and use your LEFT eye to look through the instrument. Place your right hand on the patient's head and place your thumb on their left eyebrow. Unless you are ambidextrous, it will take a great deal of practice to use your non-dominant eye to look through the ophthalmoscope—this is NOT an option, it is a must if you want to be able to perform a thorough fundoscopic on both eyes.

17. "To dilate or not to dilate" the pupil for the exam is a point of discussion with your supervising attending. Direct ophthalmoscopy is facilitated through the use of mydriatic drops that dilate the pupil. Contraindication to mydriasis is head injury requiring monitoring of the pupils. Rarely acute-angle glaucoma may be precipitated by pupillary dilation (some sources consider this a relative contraindication to dilating the pupil). Some common agents used to dilate the pupil:

    ● Sympathetic agonists include **phenylephrine:** 1 drop of 2.5% or 10% solution, repeat in 10–60 minutes as needed (PRN).

    ● Parasympathetic agents paralyze the circular muscle of the iris, causing mydriasis, and also paralyze the ciliary muscle, causing loss of accommodation. One popular agent is **tropicamide**: 1–2 drops (0.5%) 15–20 minutes before exam, repeat every 30 minutes PRN.

18. The ophthalmoscope can also be used in the evaluation of foreign bodies in the eye and corneal abrasions. Touch the lower lid fornix with a **fluorescein paper strip** (not the cornea) while the patient looks up. Fluorescein is a water-soluble acidic dye that produces green fluorescence in alkaline solution when illuminated with the blue light of the ophthalmoscope. A break in the corneal epithelium (abrasion) permits fluorescein penetration with a bright green appearance of the affected cornea.

6

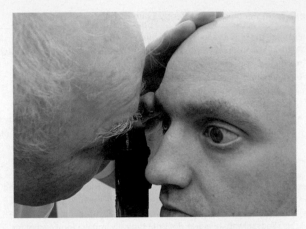

Figure 6-15. Example of direct ophthalmoscopy with the examiner using the right eye to evaluate the patient's right eye. (Reproduced with permission from Riordan-Eva P, Augsburger JJ, eds. *Vaughan & Asbury's General Ophthalmology*, 19e, New York, NY: McGraw-Hill; 2018.)

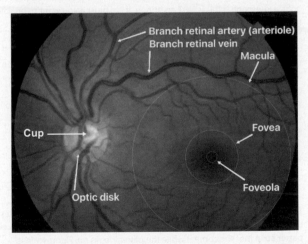

Figure 6-16. Normal fundus and structures seen using the direct ophthalmoscope. The macula is the retinal region responsible for the central, high-resolution color vision. The depression within the macula, the fovea with the foveal center or "foveola," contains the highest density of cone photoreceptors in the retina and provides the greatest visual acuity. Note that the retinal vessels all stop short of and do not cross the fovea. (Reproduced and modified with permission from Riordan-Eva P, Augsburger JJ, eds. *Vaughan & Asbury's General Ophthalmology*, 19e, New York, NY: McGraw-Hill ; 2018; 2018.)

Otolaryngology (ENT) Key Elements

Evaluation of the ears, nose, and throat (ENT) is part of the basic physical exam. Key elements in the ENT evaluation are listed here and are based on guidelines from the American Academy of Otolaryngology (www.entnet.org, accessed May 17, 2020). The ENT evaluation considers the specific ear, nose, or throat concern, but you should also inquire about any associated general symptoms such as fever, weight loss, etc.

History and ROS

- Otologic (tinnitus, otalgia, otorrhea, aural fullness, hearing loss, vertigo); regular exposure to loud music or occupational noise
- Facial (swelling, pain, numbness)
- Nasal (congestion, rhinorrhea, postnasal drip, epistaxis, decreased smell [Note loss of smell is a unique characteristic of COVID-19 infection.])
- Sinus (pressure, pain)
- Mouth (pain, ulcers, masses, bleeding, dental problems, change in or loss of the sense taste [is a unique finding in patients with COVID])
- Throat (pain, odynophagia, dysphagia, globus sensation, throat clearing, ulcers, abnormal growths)
- Larynx (vocal changes or weakness, hoarseness, stridor, dyspnea)
- Neck symptoms (pain, swelling, lymphadenopathy, torticollis, supine dyspnea)

Physical Exam

Ear:

Hearing: In the United States, hearing loss is the third most common chronic health condition (~40 million adults between the ages of 20 and 69 years have hearing loss according to the Centers for Disease Control [CDC], 2017). Guidelines from the American Academy of Pediatrics (AAP) suggest audiology screening for all children at various ages (www.aap.org/en-us/professional-resources/practice-support/Pages/PeriodicitySchedule.aspx, accessed May 25, 2020).

- **Basic bedside hearing screening techniques.** While inferior to formal audiometry, these are quick and easy to perform as part of a routine examination:
  - **Finger rub test:** With the patient's eyes closed in a quiet environment, the examiner stands behind the patient and gently rubs his or her fingers together, testing each ear. With normal hearing, the patient should be able to hear the rubbing of the examiner's fingers approximately 3–4 inches away from each ear. Tests high-frequency hearing.
  - **Whispered speech test:** Examiner whispers a series of numbers or phrases that normally should be heard 2 feet from each ear.
  - **Watch tick:** Noted here for completeness since ticking timepieces are becoming obsolete. Ticking should be heard at 6 inches with normal hearing.

6

o **Rinne and Weber tests**. Sometimes referred to as the Weber and Rinne tests, these tests allow differentiation of conductive vs. sensorineural hearing loss.

- **Weber test.** Tap a 512-Hz tuning fork (conversational sounds are 500–3000 Hz) and place in the midline of the forehead. The tuning fork should be set in motion by striking it on your knee (not the patient's knee or a table). Ask the patient "Where do you hear the sound?"
  - Normal: sound is heard equally in both ears
  - Sensorineural deafness: sound is heard louder on the side of the intact ear
  - Conductive deafness: sound is heard louder on the side of the affected ear

Rinne test. Place a vibrating 512-Hz tuning fork firmly on the mastoid process (apply pressure to the opposite side of the head to make sure the contact is firm). This tests bone conduction.

- Confirm the patient can hear the sound of the tuning fork and then ask them to tell you when they can no longer hear it.
- When the patient can no longer hear the sound, move the tuning fork in front of the external auditory meatus to test air conduction.
- Ask the patient if they can now hear the sound again. If they can hear the sound, it suggests air conduction is better than bone conduction, which is what would be expected in a healthy individual (this is often confusingly referred to as a "Rinne positive" result).
  - o Normal result: Air conduction > Bone conduction (Rinne positive)
  - o Sensorineural deafness: Air conduction > Bone conduction (Rinne positive)—both air and bone conduction are reduced equally
  - o Conductive deafness: Bone conduction > Air conduction (Rinne negative)

- When hearing loss is suspected, **pure-tone audiometry** should be used to evaluate hearing deficits. This measures the patient's hearing across multiple frequencies (measured in hertz) and volumes (measured in decibels).

External ear: Symmetry, piercings, congenital deformities (microtia, preauricular pits), mastoid behind ear. See Figure 6-17, page 103, to identify specific anatomy of the normal ear (pinna).

Otoscopic examination of the external auditory canal, tympanic membrane (see Figure 6-18, page 104), and middle ear. The technique for using an otoscope can be found in Table 6-8, page 103.

External Auditory Canal: S-shaped canal lined with fine hairs, sebaceous and ceruminous glands; normally no evidence of redness, lesions, edema, scaliness, pain, accumulation of cerumen, drainage, or presence of foreign bodies. Common abnormal findings include "swimmer's ear" (otitis externa); malignant otitis externa *Pseudomonas aeruginosa* infection and impacted cerumen.

Middle Ear: Normal tympanic membrane (eardrum) appears as a shallow, circular cone that is shiny and pearl gray in color, semitransparent whitish cord

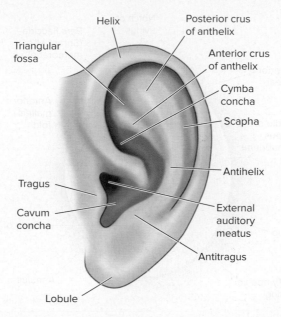

Figure 6-17. Anatomy of the external ear (pinna) with detailed anatomic landmarks. (Reproduced with permission from Lalwani AK, ed. *Current Diagnosis & Treatment Otolaryngology—Head and Neck Surgery*, 4e, New York, NY: McGraw-Hill; 2020.)

6

Table 6-8.   Otoscopy Exam Technique

Using a battery-operated otoscope allows examination of the external auditory canal, tympanic membrane, and indirectly the middle ear. By using a pneumatic attachment, the mobility of the tympanic membrane can also be assessed (common cause of decreased mobility is a middle ear effusion). In children, choose an appropriately sized disposable speculum that allows application of an airtight pneumatic system. The otoscope is held in the hand that correlates with the side of the ear to be examined (patient's right ear, otoscope in the examiner's right hand, etc.). For best viewing with the otoscope in an adult, pull the ear posteriorly, superiorly, and slightly away from the patient to straighten out the external canal. In a child, the ear should be pulled posteriorly. If present remove any debris or cerumen that interferes with visualization of the eardrum. Perform **inflation otoscopy** as noted for the middle ear in the text. Figure 6-18 page 104 demonstrates the detailed anatomy of the ear drum (tympanic membrane).

crossing from front to back just under the upper edge, "cone of light" on the right side at the 4 o'clock position, and normal motion with air inflation. (See Figure 6-18, page 104.) There should be no evidence of bulging, retraction, a lusterless membrane, or obliteration of the "cone of light." Note any fluid level, bubbles, tympanic perforation, otorrhea, bullae, tympanosclerosis, or cholesteatoma. Tympanoplasty tubes may be present in children treated for chronic otitis media. Air inflation otoscopy (pneumatic-otoscope) allows assessment of middle

6

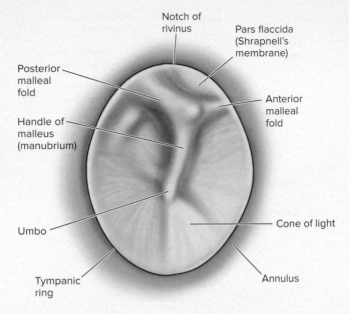

Figure 6-18. Detailed anatomy of the tympanic membrane. The cone of light is a reflection of the light from the otoscope. (Reproduced with permission from Lalwani AK, ed. *Current Diagnosis & Treatment Otolaryngology—Head and Neck Surgery*, 4e, New York, NY: McGraw-Hill; 2020.)

ear disease. The motility of the tympanic membrane is demonstrated by applying positive and negative pressures with the rubber squeeze bulb. Otitis media findings include bulging tympanic membrane, loss of mobility with pneumatic bulb loss of landmarks, and diffuse erythema.

Nose: Anterior rhinoscopy should ideally be performed utilizing a bivalve speculum or otoscope to evaluate the septum and anterior portions of the inferior turbinates.

Throat: Use a light and tongue depressor to systematically inspect all mucosal surfaces, including the gingivobuccal sulci, the gums and alveolar ridge, hard palate, soft palate, tonsils, posterior oropharynx, buccal mucosa, dorsal and ventral tongue, lateral tongue, and floor of mouth. The posterior wall of the oropharynx can be easily visualized via the mouth by depressing the tongue or with a fiber optic scope. Thrush appears as whitish plaques on the mucosal surfaces; atrophic glossitis is the appearance of a shiny tongue with loss of all papilla, causes include iron or vitamin B_{12} deficiency, celiac disease, or others; and black tongue can be due to fungal infection with *Aspergillus*. A geographic tongue is erythematous patches, with atrophy of the filiform papillae of the tongue, with whitish, hyper-keratotic borders.

Neck: Note any masses, palpate the larynx and thyroid, and evaluate for any adenopathy.

Cranial Nerves: A complete head and neck exam includes testing of cranial nerves (see pages 75 and 77).

Pediatric History and Physical Examination

6

Similar to the adult history and physical examination, the details and length of a written H&P can vary with the particular admitting concern, underlying medical conditions, and service to which the patient is admitted. The pediatric H&P has more focus on developmental and social issues than the usual adult version. An example of a complete pediatric H&P write-up is on page 126. The pediatric history should be obtained from the patient when possible, with further details from the parent or appropriate guardian. Age-appropriate language should be used, with detail taken to inquire about the quality of symptoms when speaking with children ("Does it feel like someone is sitting on your belly or someone is poking it with a sharp stick?" "Does the pain stay in one place or does it go to other places?").

History (Pediatric)

Date: XXXX **Time:** XXXX
PCP or Referring Provider: Dr. XXX
History Obtained From: Informant (e.g., patient, relative, old chart), and reliability of the informant
Identification: Name, age, sex, gender identity, referring physician. Identify if an interpreter is needed for the history and what type of interpreter (live in person, telephonic, electronic/computer) with their appropriate identification information.
Chief Concern (CC): State the current problem in the patient's or parent's/guardian's words.
HPI: Define current problem by quality, quantity, anatomic location. Be specific about the time course of illness and how symptoms presented within said time course (progression? regression?). Ask about aggravating, alleviating, and associated factors. History should be organized in chronological order. Related history can be described, including prior treatment and risk factors.
Past Medical History (PMHx): Including diagnoses, accidents, and injuries. Include past hospitalizations.
Pregnancy and Birth Hx: Maternal health during pregnancy (include substance use and infections), gestational age, type of delivery, birth weight, Apgar score if relevant. If patient required neonatal intensive care unit (NICU) stay, identify major elements of hospitalization including

respiratory support, feeding challenges, and hyperbilirubinemia. Results of newborn screening (vision and hearing screening; any other health screening including laboratory tests).

Medications: Dose, formulation (concentration is often important in liquid formulation), route, frequency.

Allergies: If present, indicate the reaction associated with the specific allergy listed.

Immunizations: List received to date or any not received based on guidelines. (See Appendix for immunization recommendations.)

Past Surgical History (PSHx): Prior surgical procedures.

Developmental History: Indicate whether patient obtained milestones within appropriate range, should include gross and fine motor skills, expressive and receptive speech. (See Appendix, page 1065, for some common developmental milestones from the CDC.)

Feeding History: When appropriate, indicate specific feeding plan. This could include an infant feeding plan such as formula or maternal breast milk (may be listed in volume and/or time intervals), dietary restrictions (gluten-free diet in the setting of celiac disease, thickened liquids for a patient with dysphagia), tube feedings for the medically complex child (indicate type of feeding tube: nasogastric [NG] tube, gastrostomy tube, schedule). Inquire about intake of fast food, candy, and sugar drinks.

Family History: Major medical conditions in blood relatives. Can consider use of a family pedigree (see page 61–62) if needed, but also be mindful of relevant conditions as related to HPI.

Psychosocial (Social) History: Identify type of habitat, number of people in home, and relationship to patient. List parental/guardian employment, childcare or grade in school, pets. Identify smoke exposure and if there are firearms in the home and how they are stored.

Note: There should be a separate evaluation of social history for **adolescents**, as the social history can be an essential component to the specific concerns and pathologies seen in adolescent patients. This part of the interview should be conducted with an adolescent without their parent or guardian if possible. The following mnemonic is helpful to remember the components on the adolescent exam:

HEADSS

H—Home: type of home, who lives at home, relationship dynamics, do they feel safe at home

E—Education: school/grade, academic performance with any recent changes, favorite/least favorite subjects, academic struggles, future plans

A—Activities: hobbies/leisure activities, driving/seat belts/texting with driving/driving while intoxicated

D—Drugs: personal use, friend/parental use, type of drug (including tobacco delivery systems, alcohol, prescription drugs) with amount and frequency

S—Sexuality: designated pronouns, sexual orientation/preference, degree and type of sexual experience and acts, number of partners, history of STIs, history of pregnancy/miscarriage/abortion, type of contraception used, safety/consent in encounters

S—Suicide/Depression: sleep issues, feelings of loneliness/hopelessness, history of suicidal ideation or attempts, history of nonsuicidal injurious behssavior, depression, anger/impulsiveness, body dysmorphisms/body image concerns

ROS

Note: Your ability to obtain a pediatric ROS is dependent on patient age. For example, it may be almost impossible to identify whether a 6-month-old infant is experiencing nausea.

General: Weight loss, weight gain, fatigue, weakness, appetite, fever, chills, night sweats

Skin: Rashes, hives, pruritus, bruising, dryness

Head: Trauma, headache, tenderness, dizziness, syncope

Eyes: Vision, changes in visual field, glasses, last prescription change, photophobia, blurring, diplopia, eso/exotropia, redness, discharge, dry eyes, excessive tearing

Ears: Hearing changes, tinnitus, pain, discharge, vertigo, history of ear infections

Nose: Sinus problems, epistaxis, obstruction, polyps, changes in or loss of sense of smell

Throat: Bleeding gums; dental history (last checkup, etc.); ulcerations or other lesions on tongue, gums, buccal mucosa

Respiratory: Ability to keep up with peers, pneumonia, bronchiolitis, wheezing, chronic cough, snoring, sputum, hemoptysis, TB

Cardiovascular: Cyanosis and dyspnea, heart murmurs, exercise tolerance, squatting, chest pain, palpitations, edema

Gastrointestinal: Appetite, abdominal pain/distention, dysphagia, heartburn, nausea, vomiting, diarrhea, constipation, hematemesis, melena (hematochezia), hemorrhoids, change in stool shape and color, jaundice

Gynecologic: Menstrual history when age appropriate (LMP, length of cycle, duration/quality, associated symptoms such as cramping). Age at menarche; LMP (frequency, duration, flow); dysmenorrhea; spotting; history of STIs; vaginal discharge

Genitourinary: Frequency, urgency, hesitancy; dysuria; hematuria; polyuria; nocturia; incontinence; impotence; polyuria; polydipsia; change in urinary stream

Endocrine: Polyuria, polydipsia, polyphagia, temperature intolerance, glycosuria, hormone therapy, changes in hair or skin texture

Musculoskeletal: Arthralgia, arthritis, trauma, joint swelling, redness, tenderness, limitations in ROM, back pain, musculoskeletal trauma

Hematology: Anemia, bleeding tendency, easy bruising, lymphadenopathy

Neuropsychiatric: Syncope; seizures; weakness; ataxia or coordination problems; alterations in sensations, memory, mood, or sleep pattern, anhedonia, loss of energy, decreased ability to concentrate, emotional disturbances; drug and alcohol problems

Physical Examination (Pediatric)

A physical examination of a pediatric patient should be performed in the presence of a parent or guardian. If they are unavailable, a chaperone should be present per policy of the American Academy of Pediatrics (AAP). The order and location of the physical exam may change depending on the age of the patient. Infants under 6 months of age can be examined on an examining table, but from 8 months until 3 or so, it may be more successful to complete this on a parent's lap. Note that for younger children, the cardiac and respiratory exams should be prioritized in the exam before the patient begins crying.

General: Observe patient's general level of comfort, state of well-being (well vs. ill appearing), activity level, physical appearance (neat vs. unkempt), nutritional status. One may also to be able to witness interactions between patient and parent/guardian.

Vital Signs/Physical Assessment: Temperature (note if oral, rectal, axillary or ear), pulse, respirations, BP. Heart rate, respiratory rate, and blood pressure vary by age, and these values should be checked with reference to ensure that they are appropriate.

Growth parameters are essential parts of a pediatric physical exam. The points should be measured and tracked on age-appropriate growth charts. *The CDC recommends that the CDC growth charts be used for children older than 2 years. Under 2 years of age, the World Health Organization (WHO) guidelines should be used.* These parameters include weight, height, and head circumference. Of note, there are specialized growth charts for certain populations such as those with Down syndrome, prematurity, and achondroplasia. Under age 2, it is preferable to measure the patient in the supine position for a length. Head (occipitofrontal) circumferences should be measured until age 3. (Growth charts can be found in the Appendix, pages 1074–1077.)

Skin: Rashes, eruptions, scars, tattoos, birthmarks such as nevi, hemangiomas, Mongolian spots.

Lymph Nodes: Location (head and neck, supraclavicular, epitrochlear, axillary, inguinal), size, tenderness, motility, consistency.

HEENT:

Head: Size and shape, tenderness, trauma, bruits, fontanels, suture lines.

Eyes: Conjunctiva; sclera; lids; position of eyes in orbits; pupil size, shape, reactivity; extraocular muscle movements including muscular control (eso/exotropia); visual acuity (e.g., 20/20 if appropriate for age) (see pages 93–95); visual fields; red reflex, fundi when appropriate.

Ears: Note the position of the ears, hearing test; tenderness, discharge, external canal, tympanic membrane (intact, dull or shiny, bulging, motility, fluid or blood, injected). Otoscopy technique is described in Table 6-8, page 103.

Nose: Symmetry, inspection for obstruction, lesions, exudate, inflammation. Palpation over sinuses if appropriate, though only the maxillary antrum, anterior, and posterior ethmoid cells are present at birth. At 2–4 years the pneumatization of the frontal sinus takes place, but rarely has clinical relevance until age 6 at the earliest. The sphenoid sinus does not assume clinical significance until 5–8 years of age.

Throat: Lips, teeth (count the number and the condition; dentition eruption sequences are reviewed in Figure 6-4, page 70), palate (intact, arch), gums, tongue, pharynx (lesions, erythema, exudate, tonsillar size, presence of crypts).

Neck: ROM, position (torticollis, ability to support head), tenderness, lymph nodes, thyroid examination, location of larynx, position of trachea.

Chest: Shape and symmetry, at rest and with respiration; intercostal retractions; palpation for tenderness, fremitus, and chest wall expansion; percussion (include diaphragmatic movement between tidal breathing and full inspiration); breath sounds; adventitious sounds (rales, rhonchi, wheezes, rubs). If indicated: vocal fremitus, whispered pectoriloquy, egophony (found with consolidation).

Heart: Rate, inspection, and palpation of precordium for point of maximal impulse, apical impulse, and thrills; auscultation at the apex, LLSB, and right and left second intercostal spaces with diaphragm and apex and LLSB. Listen for rate, rhythm, force, quality of sounds, and murmur (location, position in cycle, intensity, pitch, effect of change of position, transmission, effect of exercise).

Breast: Inspection for nipple discharge (can be a normal finding in newborns), inversion, gynecomastia in men and boys, pubertal signs (Tanner staging, Table 6-9, page 110).

Abdomen: Shape (scaphoid, flat, distended, obese); examination for scars; auscultation for bowel sounds; percussion for tympani and masses; liver size (span in midclavicular line); CVA tenderness; palpation for tenderness (if present, check for rebound tenderness); ascites, hepatomegaly, splenomegaly; guarding.

Male Genitalia: Inspection for meatal opening, hypospadias, phimosis, testicles (size, tenderness, masses, varicocele), and hernia; hydrocele; pubertal changes (Tanner staging, Table 6-9, page 110).

Pelvic Exam: If appropriate for adolescent girls; see Chapter 13 for details.

Table 6-9. Tanner Staging System in Males and Females

Males	Testes development	Penis development
I	Prepubertal (<4 mL)	Prepubertal
II	Testes enlarge (≥4 mL), scrotum reddens and changes texture	Slight enlargement
III	Larger	Longer
IV	Scrotum darkens	Larger, wider with development of glans
V	Adult size	Adult size
Female breast development		
I	Prepubertal	
II	Breast and papilla elevated as small mound with palpable subareolar bud, areolar diameter increased	
III	Enlargement and elevation of whole breast	
IV	Areola and papilla form secondary areolar mound	
V	Mature breast contour, nipple projects	
Male and female pubic hair development		
I	None	
II	Sparse, short, straight, at base of penis or medial border of labia	
III	Darker, longer, coarser, and curlier, sparsely over pubic bones	
IV	Coarse, curly, resembles adult hair; but spares thighs	
V	Adult distribution with inverse triangle pattern and spread to medial thighs	

(From Shah SS, Zaoutis LB, Catallozzi M, Frank G. eds. *The Philadelphia Guide: Inpatient Pediatrics*, 2e, New York, NY: McGraw-Hill; 2016. Reproduced with permission.)

6

Rectal: Inspect for fissures, inflammation, lack of tone. A rectal exam is not part of a routine exam but should be considered in a setting of possible abuse, gastrointestinal concerns such as bleeding from rectum, or neurologic concerns involving the spinal cord.

Musculoskeletal: Deformities, visible joint swelling, and ROM; palpation of joints for swelling, tenderness, and warmth. Examine back for sacral dimple, kyphosis, or scoliosis; gait for in-toeing/out-toeing, bowing; hips for developmental dysplasia (Ortolani and Barlow signs; see Physical Signs, Symptoms, and Eponyms, page 60).

Peripheral Vascular: Cyanosis; clubbing; palpation of peripheral pulses; edema.

Neurologic: The pediatric neurologic exam is very observation dependent. Using toys can sometimes help, particularly with extraocular muscles and fine motor control. Aspects such as determining sensation or completing a mental status exam may be challenging in children younger than school-aged.

Mental Status Examination: If appropriate; see Psychiatric History and Physical Examination and Psychiatric Mental Status Examination, page 113.

Cranial Nerves: The functions of the 12 cranial nerves are as follows:

I Olfactory—Smell

II Optic—Vision, visual fields, and fundi; afferent limb of pupillary response

III, IV, VI Oculomotor, trochlear, abducens—Efferent limb pupillary response, ptosis, volitional eye movements, pursuit eye movements

V Trigeminal—Corneal reflex (afferent), facial sensation; test masseter and temporalis muscle by having patient bite

VII Facial—Raise eyebrows, close eyes tight, show teeth, smile, or whistle, corneal reflex (efferent)

VIII Acoustic—Hearing; test by finger rub, Weber and Rinne tests (see also page 102) if hearing loss noted on history or gross testing. (Air conduction lasts longer than bone conduction in a healthy person.)

IX, X Glossopharyngeal and vagus—Gag reflex; speech. Palate should move upward in midline. Ability to swallow and speak clearly.

XI Spinal accessory—Shoulder shrug, push head against resistance.

XII Hypoglossal—Tongue movement. Test strength by having the patient press tongue against the buccal mucosa on each side while you press a finger against the patient's cheek. Observe for fasciculations.

Motor: Test strength in upper and lower extremities proximally and distally. (Grading system: 5, active motion against full resistance; 4, active motion against some resistance; 3, active motion against gravity but not resistance; 2, active motion with gravity eliminated; 1, barely detectable motion; 0, no motion or muscular contraction detected.)

Cerebellum: Romberg test (see page 86). Heel to shin (should not be with assistance from gravity; instruct a patient sitting with legs dangling to drag the heel of one foot up the shin of the other leg **and not down the shin**), finger to nose, heel-and-toe walking, rapid alternating movements of upper and lower extremities

Sensory: Pain (sharp) or temperature of distal and proximal upper and lower extremities, vibration using either a 128- or 256-Hz tuning fork or position sense of distal parts of upper and lower extremities, and stereognosis or graphesthesia. Identify deficits using dermatome and cutaneous innervation diagrams identical to adults (Figure 6-6A and B, pages 80–81).

Reflexes: Brachioradialis and biceps C5–6, triceps C7–8, abdominal (upper T8–10, lower T10–12), quadriceps (knee) L3–5, ankle S1–2. Grading system: 4+, hyperactive with clonus; 3+, brisker than usual; 2+, normal or average; 1+, decreased or less than normal; 0, absent. Reflex technique can be found on page 82.

Neonatal reflexes: Moro reflex (startle), palmar/plantar reflex, suck, walking/step reflex. These should normally extinguish between 4 and 6 months and are described on page 85.

Data

List results of the pertinent laboratory, radiographic, and other studies. You may include the reference ranges for laboratory values if appropriate. If technology allows, you could include a key image from the patient's computed tomography (CT) series or a pathology slide.

Impression and Plan

Impression or assessment should start with a summation sentence similar to the HPI and include the known diagnoses and/or current issues. A thoughtful differential should be included. Then address the patient's problems with a plan for treatment. This can be addressed in a problem-based approach or systems-based if the patient is very complicated. Record the date and time with each entry.

Sign_____
Title_____
Date _____

Tanner Staging (See Table 6-9, page 110)

The Sexual Maturity Rating (SMR), more commonly known as Tanner staging, is an objective classification system to document and track the development and sequence of secondary sex characteristics of children going through puberty from stage 1 (preadolescent) to stage 5 (adult). Significant deviations from these milestones such as precocious puberty or delayed puberty may signal the need for further evaluation for underlying conditions. The onset of puberty ranges from 9–14 years of age in males and from 8–13 years of age in females.

Psychiatric History and Physical Examination

The core elements of the psychiatric history and physical exam are identical to those of the basic H&P and selective use of neurologic elements based on the clinical picture. The main difference involves attention to the past psychiatric history, more behaviorally focused ROS, and a more detailed mental status examination, as described in the following section.

Review of Symptoms

- **Cognitive:** memory or concentration changes
- **Psychosis:** delusions, hallucinations, talking incoherently, and agitation
- **Substance Abuse:** alcohol, drugs of addiction, including prescription drugs
- **Mood:** depression, mania, suicidal ideation, guilt
- **Neurovegetative:** sleep, appetite, libido, interests, energy
- **Anxiety:** anxiety symptoms, panic/agoraphobia, obsessions/compulsions, flashbacks/hypervigilance
- **Eating Disorder:** anorexia, bulimia
- **Violence:** rages, assaults, homicidal ideation
- **Impulse Control:** pathological gambling, trichotillomania, kleptomania, hypersexuality

Psychiatric Mental Status Examination

The mental status examination (MSE) is a component of all medical exams and may be considered the psychological equivalent of the physical exam. The MSE is especially important in neurologic and psychiatric evaluations. The following factors are evaluated as part of the psychiatric mental status examination. A determination of consciousness must be the first step in the MSE. MSEs should not be used as the sole criteria for diagnosing delirium or dementia. (Adapted from Zimmerman M. *Interviewing Guide for Evaluating DSM-IV Psychiatric Disorders and the Mental Status Examination.* Philadelphia, PA: Psychiatric Press Products; 1994:121–122.)

Table 6-10. Basic Elements of the Mental Status Exam

Appearance	Age, gender, race, body build, posture, eye contact, dress, grooming, manner, attentiveness to examiner, distinguishing features, prominent physical abnormalities, emotional facial expression, alertness, gestures, mannerisms
Motor	Slowed movement, agitation, abnormal movements, purposeful movements, gait, catatonia
Speech	Rate, rhythm, volume, amount, articulation, spontaneity, coherence, flight of ideas
Affect	Stability, range, appropriateness, intensity, affect, mood
Thought content	Suicidal ideation, death wishes, homicidal ideation, depressive cognitions, obsessions, ruminations, phobias, ideas of reference, paranoid ideation, magical ideation, delusions, overvalued ideas, worries, hypochondriasis
Thought process	Associations, coherence, logic, stream, clang associations, perseveration, neologism, blocking, attention, evasion
Perception	Hallucinations, illusions, depersonalization, derealization, déjà vu (sensation that a place or event someone is currently experiencing has been experienced before), jamais vu (sensation that everything around him or her is strange and unfamiliar)
Intellect	Global impression: average, above average, below average
Insight	Awareness of illness

1. **Level of consciousness:**
   o **Somnolence:** A state of drowsiness from which a patient can be easily aroused.
   o **Stupor:** Insensitivity bordering on unconsciousness. The patient can only be awoken using a very strong stimulus (e.g., a loud voice) and the patient returns to this state in the absence of further stimuli.
   o **Coma:** Patient cannot be aroused and there is no response to stimuli.
   o **Glasgow Coma Scale** can be used if necessary to evaluate conscious states (see Appendix, pages 1072–1073).
2. **Elements of the mental status exam** are summarized in Table 6-10, above.

   Additional questions can be used to further expand the components of a psychiatric screening exam:

- **Attention:** Ask the patient to count by 2s to 20. This can be used for patients with poor arithmetic skills.

- **Calculation abilities:** Ask the patient to add simple combinations of two-digit numbers. The task can be graded in difficulty.
- **Immediate recall:** Assessed by asking the patient to repeat number sequences up to seven forward and four in reverse order. Best to start with shorter sequences.
- **Memory:** Ask about news events, sports, television shows, or recent meals.
- **Long-term memory:** Use past events confirmed by family members or repeating names of historical figures (e.g., U.S. presidents).
- **Language ability:** Ask patients to explain similarities and differences between common objects (e.g., tree/bush, car/plane, air/water).
- **Thinking processes:** Ask patients to explain common proverbs with which they are familiar (e.g., "People who live in glass houses should not throw stones.")

Folstein Mini-Mental State Examination

Several shortened forms of the MSE have been developed as screening instruments. The Folstein Mini-Mental State Examination (MMSE)[6] is used to check for cognitive impairment (problems with thinking, communication, understanding, and memory) and is useful in assessing for dementia in the elderly and assessing patients with any neurologic or systemic disease affecting the CNS. The MMSE is a quick and simple test, and the results can be followed over time to assess for progression, improvement, or no changes in the underlying process. The MMSE is divided into two sections: one assessing orientation, memory, and attention, and the other testing the patient's ability to write a sentence and copy a diagram (usually two pentagons that intersect to form a four-sided figure). Table 6-11, page 116, shows the Mini-Mental State Exam. Other tests that may be used include the Cognitive Capacity Screening Examination (CCSE) that tests orientation, serial subtraction, memory, and similarities. It is less sensitive for delirium or dementia in the elderly. The Neurobehavioral Cognitive Status Examination (NCSE) is especially good for medically ill patients.

The maximum score for the MMSE is 30; a score of 25 or higher is considered normal. If the score is below 25, the result is considered abnormal (indicating possible cognitive impairment) with the impairment further classified as follows:

- Mild—MMSE score of between 21 and 24
- Moderate—MMSE score of between 10 and 20
- Severe—MMSE score of less than 10

Table 6-11. Folstein Mini-Mental State Examination (MMSE)[6]

Patient	_____	
Examiner	_____	
Date	_____	
	"Mini-Mental State"	
Maximum Score		
	Orientation	
5	What is the (year) (season) (date) (day) (month)?	
5	Where are we? (state) (county) (town) (hospital) (floor)	
	Registration	
3	Name 3 objects: 1 second to say each. Then ask the patient all 3 after you have said them. Give 1 point for each correct answer. Then repeat until he learns all 3. Count trials and record. Trials _____	
	Attention and Calculation	
5	Serial 7s: One point for each correct. Stop after 5 answers. Alternatively, spell "world" backward.	
	Recall	
3	Ask for the 3 objects repeated above. Give 1 point for each correct answer.	
	Language	
9	Point to a pencil, and watch and ask the patient to name it.	(2 point)
	Repeat the following: "No it's, and's, or but's." (1 point)	
	Follow a 3-stage command: "Take a paper in your right hand, fold it in half, and put it on the floor." (3 points)	
	Read and obey the following:	
	Close your eyes	(1 point)
	Write a sentence	(1 point)
	Copy design (two intersecting pentagrams)	(1 point)
	_____ Total Score	
Assess level of consciousness along the following continuum		
Alert	Drowsy	Stupor Coma

Source: Based on Folstein MF, Folstein SE, McHugh PR: *J. Psychiatr Res* 1975;12:189–198. Used with permission.

Patient Health Questionnaire (PHQ)

The Patient Health Questionnaire (PHQ) is a self-administered version of the PRIME-MD diagnostic instrument for common mental disorders. The PHQ-9 is the depression module commonly used to detect depression (Kroenke K, et al. The PHQ-9: Validity of a Brief Depression Severity Measure. *J Gen Intern Med* 2001;16(9):606–613). See Table 6-12.

6

Table 6-12. Patient Health Questionnaire (PHQ-9)

NAME: _____ DATE:_____

Over the last *2 weeks*, how often have you been bothered by any of the following problems? (use "✓" to indicate your answer)

	Not at all	Several days	More than half the days	Nearly every day
1. Little interest or pleasure in doing things	0	1	2	3
2. Feeling down, depressed, or hopeless	0	1	2	3
3. Trouble falling or staying asleep, or sleeping too much	0	1	2	3
4. Feeling tired or having little energy	0	1	2	3
5. Poor appetite or overeating	0	1	2	3
6. Feeling bad about yourself—or that you are a failure or have let yourself or your family down	0	1	2	3
7. Trouble concentrating on things, such as reading the newspaper or watching television	0	1	2	3
8. Moving or speaking so slowly that other people could have noticed. Or the opposite — being so fidgety or restless that you have been moving around a lot more than usual	0	1	2	3

(Continued)

6

9. Thoughts that you would be better off dead, or of hurting yourself

0   1   2   3

add columns 1, 2, and 3

_____ + _____ + _____

(Healthcare professional: For interpretation of TOTAL, please refer to accompanying scoring card.)

Total : _____

10. If you checked off *any problems,* how *difficult* have these problems made it for you to do your work, take care of things at home, or get along with other people?

Somewhat difficult _____
Not difficult at all _____
Very difficult _____
Extremely difficult _____

For initial diagnosis:

1. Patient completes PHQ-9 Quick Depression Assessment.
2. If there are at least 4 ✓s in the shaded section (including Questions #1 and #2), consider a depressive disorder. Add scores to determine severity.

Consider Major Depressive Disorder
- if there are at least 5 ✓s in the shaded section (one of which corresponds to Question #1 or#2)

Consider Other Depressive Disorder
- if there are 2–4 ✓s in the shaded section (one of which corresponds to Question #1 or #2)

Note: Since the questionnaire relies on patient self-report, all responses should be verified by the clinician, and a definitive diagnosis is made on clinical grounds taking into account how well the patient understood the questionnaire, as well as other relevant information from the patient.

Diagnoses of Major Depressive Disorder or Other Depressive Disorder also require impairment of social, occupational, or other important areas of functioning (Question #10) and ruling out normal bereavement, a history of a Manic Episode (Bipolar Disorder), and a physical disorder, medications, or other drugs as the biological cause of the depressive symptoms.

   To monitor severity over time for newly diagnosed patients or patients in current treatment for depression:

1. Patients may complete questionnaires at baseline and at regular intervals (e.g., every 2 weeks) at home and bring them in at their next appointment for scoring or they may complete the questionnaire during each scheduled appointment.
2. Add up ✓s by column. For every ✓: Several days = 1. More than half the days = 2. Nearly every day = 3.
3. Add together column scores to get a TOTAL score.
4. Refer to the accompanying **PHQ-9 Scoring Box** to interpret the TOTAL score.
5. Results may be included in patient files to assist you in setting a treatment goal, guiding treatment, and determining the degree of response to treatment.

Table 6-12. Interpretation of Total Score (*Continued*)

Total Score	Depression Severity
1–4	Minimal depression
5–9	Mild depression
10–14	Moderate depression
15–19	Moderately severe depression
20–27	Severe depression

GENDER TERMINOLOGY IN HEALTHCARE

Table 6-13, page 120 is a guide for healthcare providers when addressing issues in transgender health. This terminology is provided by the World Professional Association for Transgender Health (WPATH) in their Standards of Care (SOC) for the Health of Transsexual, Transgender, and Gender Nonconforming People (https://www.wpath.org/publications/soc; accessed November 8, 2020). This gender terminology is based on the best available science and expert professional consensus.

6

Table 6-13. Terminology Used in Transgender Health (see text for reference)

Transgender: Individuals whose gender identity, expression, and behavior differ to varying degrees from those typically ascribed to their sex at birth

Cisgender: Individuals whose gender identity aligns with their sex at birth

Gender dysphoria: Distress that is caused by a discrepancy between a person's assigned gender at birth and the person's gender identity

Gender identity: An individual's intrinsic sense of being male, female, or an alternative gender (gender variant) that is independent of the gender assigned at birth

Sexual orientation: An individual's attraction to members of the same sex and/or a different sex (i.e., lesbian, gay, bisexual, heterosexual, or asexual)

Gender expression: The manner used by individuals to present themselves socially that may or may not be congruent with their gender identity

Gender variance/gender nonconformity: Expression of gender identity that does not fully adhere to either male or female gender norms

Female-to-male (trans men): Individuals assigned female gender at birth who are changing to a more masculine body/gender role

Male-to-female (trans women): Individuals assigned male gender at birth who are changing to a more feminine body/gender role

EXAMPLE OF A HISTORY AND PHYSICAL EXAMINATION, ADULT

This example is for an adult male admitted to a general medical service.

HISTORY

12/10/20 7:30 PM

Identification: Mr. Robert Jones is a 49-y-old man referred by Dr. Harry Doyle from Whitesburg, Kentucky. The informant is the patient and a photocopy of the EHR records from Whitesburg Hospital accompanies the patient.

CC: "Squeezing chest pain for 10 h, it started yesterday morning"

HPI: Mr. Jones awoke on 12/09 at 6 AM with squeezing substernal chest pain that felt "like a ton of bricks" sitting on his chest. The chest pain was a 9 on a 10-point scale and decreased in intensity shortly after arriving to the Whitesburg emergency department. The pain radiated to the left side of the neck and left elbow and was associated with dyspnea and diaphoresis. The patient denies nausea. The pain got worse with any exertion, and nothing seemed to alleviate it.

Mr. Jones presented to the Whitesburg ER 10 h after the onset of pain and was given 3 NTG tablets SL and 2 mg morphine sulfate.

ECG revealed 3-mm ST depression in leads V_1 through V_4. He was admitted to the ICU at Whitesburg Hospital and had an uneventful course. Troponin on admission was 8 ng/mL and before transfer the next morning was 24 ng/mL. He was given aspirin 325 mg PO, ticagrelor 180 mg oral and a bolus of 4000 units of unfractionated heparin. He was then started on aspirin 81 mg/day, metoprolol and is currently on 50 mg PO q12h, atorvastatin 80 mg/D, ticagrelor 90 mg BID and unfractionated heparin 840 units/hr. His last PTT before transfer was 2.5 X control. He was transferred for possible cardiac catheterization.

Mr. Jones has experienced similar chest pain but less intense occurring intermittently over the last 2 mo. The pain was precipitated by exercise and relieved with rest. He was not seen by a physician since the onset of the chest pain. He attributed the pain to GERD. There is no history of orthopnea, paroxysmal nocturnal dyspnea, dyspnea on exertion, or pedal edema.

Mr. Jones has smoked two packs of cigarettes per day for 35 y, he has a 2-yr history of HTN for which he has been taking chlorthalidone 50 mg/day, and he denies hypercholesterolemia or DM. His BP is 120–130/80-85 at home. The patient's father died of MI at age 54.

PMH:

Medications. Aspirin 325 mg/d PO; metoprolol 50 mg PO q12h; atorvastatin 80 mg/day; ticagrelor 90 mg BID; unfractionated heparin 1,500 units/h; chlorthalidone 50 mg/day; omeprazole 300 mg PO qhs PRN; ibuprofen 200 mg 2–3 tabs PO PRN for back pain; and acetaminophen 500 mg PO for HA. *Vitamins.* One-A-Day OTC. *Herbals.* None.

Allergies. Penicillin, rash entire body at age 20 y

Surgical Procedures. Appendectomy age 20, Dr. Smith, Whitesburg

Hospitalization. See above.

Trauma. Roof fall in mine accident 10 y ago, injured back. Occasional pain, relieved with ibuprofen 200 mg 2–3 tabs

Transfusions. None

Illnesses. No hx of asthma, emphysema, thyroid disease, kidney disease, PUD, cancer, bleeding disorders, TB, or hepatitis. Reports a several-year history of GERD and takes omeprazole PRN

Routine Health Maintenance. Last diphtheria/tetanus immunization 3 yr ago; stools for guaiac were negative X 3 1 yr ago; Refused colonscopy. He has been seen by Dr. Doyle every 3–4 mo for the last 2 yr for HTN and GERD.

Family History:

Mother: age 73, alive and well, cataracts

Father: deceased age 54 from MI; hx of gout and HTN

Sister: age 52, HTN and type 2 DM

Brother: age 55, has not seen in 25 years, unsure of health

Brother: deceased age 51 from pancreatic cancer

Son: age 17, high school senior, no medical problems

Daughter: age 15, high school sophomore, asthma since age 7, well controlled on an inhaler

Psychosocial (Social) History: Mr. Jones has been married for 25 yr and has two children.

He and his family live in a house on 3 acres about 3 miles from Whitesburg. He worked in a coal mine until 10 y ago, when he was injured in a roof fall. He is currently employed in a local chair factory and is a high school graduate. He is Baptist and attends church regularly. Hobbies include woodworking and gardening. He eats breakfast and supper every day and has a soft drink and crackers for lunch. He currently works 8 h/d Monday through Friday. He goes to bed every day by 10:00 PM and awakens at 5:30 AM. He drinks one to two cups of coffee per day and does not drink alcohol and does not use drugs. He has never been exposed to environmental toxins other than when he worked in the coal mine. He has no financial problems but is concerned about how his illness will affect his income. He has health insurance. He has no other stressors in his life. His sources of support are his wife, minister, and a sister who lives near the patient.

ROS: Negative unless otherwise noted.

Eyes: Has worn reading glasses since age 12; blurred vision for 1 year; last eye appointment 2 yr ago. No loss of vision, double vision, or history of cataracts.

Respiratory: Cough every morning for 15-20 years and produces one teaspoon of gray sputum for years. No hemoptysis or pleuritic chest pain. Last CXR before today was 3 years ago.

GI: occ sour taste in his mouth for 10 years, aggravated by tomato sauce, relieved with OTC calcium carbonate or omeprazole.

Musculoskeletal: occ lumbar and lower thoracic pain with heavy lifting; occ wakes him at night, alleviated by change in body position, hx of trauma as per the PMHx.

PHYSICAL EXAMINATION

General: Mr. Jones is a pleasant man lying comfortably supine in bed. He appears to be the stated age.

Vital Signs: Temp 98.6°F orally. Resp 16, HR 64 and regular, BP 110/70 mm Hg left arm supine

Skin: Tattoo left arm, otherwise no lesions

HEENT:

Head. Normocephalic, atraumatic, nontender, no lesions

Eyes. Visual acuity 20/40 left and right corrected. External structures normal, without lesions, PERRLA. EOM intact.

Visual fields intact. Funduscopic examination discs sharp bilaterally, moderate arteriolar narrowing and A–V nicking

Ears. Hearing intact to finger rub at 3 ft bilaterally. Tympanic membranes intact with good cone of light bilaterally

Nose. Symmetrical. No lesions. Maxillary, frontal, and ethmoid sinuses nontender

Mouth. Several dental fillings, otherwise normal dentition. No lesions

Neck. Full ROM, without tenderness. No masses or lymphadenopathy. Carotids +2/4 bilaterally, no bruits. Internal jugular vein visible 2 cm above the sternal angle, patient at 30 degrees

Chest: Symmetrical expansion. Fremitus by palpation bilaterally equal. Diaphragm moves 5.5 cm bilaterally by percussion. Lung fields normal resonance to percussion. Breath sounds normal, except end-inspiratory crackles heard at both bases that do not clear with coughing.

Node: 1 X 1 left axillary node, nontender and mobile. No other palpable lymphadenopathy

Breast: Normal to inspection and palpation

Heart: No cardiac impulse visible. Apical impulse palpable at the sixth intercostal space 2 cm lateral to the midclavicular line. Normal S_1, physio-logically split S_2. S_4 heard at apex. No murmurs, rub, or S_3

Abdomen: Flat, no scars. Bowel sounds present. No bruits. Liver 10 cm midclavicular line. No CVA tenderness. No hepatomegaly or splenomegaly by palpation. No tenderness or guarding. No inguinal lymphadenopathy.

Genital: Normal circumcised man, both testes descended without masses or tenderness.

Rectal: Normal sphincter tone. No external lesions. Prostate smooth without tenderness or nodules. No palpable masses.

Musculoskeletal: Lumbar spine decreased flexion to 75 degrees, extension to 5 degrees, decreased rotary and lateral movement. Otherwise full ROM of all joints, no erythema, tenderness, or swelling. No clubbing cyanosis or edema

Peripheral Vascular: Radial, ulnar, brachial, femoral, dorsalis pedis, and posterior tibial pulses +2/4 bilaterally. Popliteal pulses nonpalpable. No femoral bruits

Neurologic:

Cranial nerves: I through XII intact.

Motor: +5/5 upper and lower extremity, proximally and distally.

Sensory: Intact to pinprick upper and lower extremities proximally and distally. Vibratory sense intact in great toes and thumbs bilaterally. Stereognosis intact.

6

Reflexes: Biceps, triceps, quadriceps, and ankles +2/4 bilaterally. Toes down going bilaterally.

Cerebellum. Romberg sign absent. No pronator drift. Intact finger-to-nose and heel-to-shin bilaterally. Rapid alternating movements intact upper and lower extremities bilaterally

DATABASE

ECG: HR 80, NSR 1-2 mm ST depression and inverted T waves V1 through V5

CXR: Cardiomegaly, otherwise clear

UA: SG 1.020, protein trace otherwise negative PT. 12.1, control 11.7, INR 1.1

Anti-factor Xa activity: 0.65 IU/mL

Chemistry Profile: Na 134, K 4.2 , Cl 108, HCO3 26, Creat 1.0, BUN 16, LFTs normal

Troponin: 16.4 ng/mL

CBC: WBC 9100; HCT 49%; Hbg 16 g/dL; Segs 43, Bands 2, Lymphs 40, Mons 5, Eos10

Date Entered	Date of Onset	Problem	Active	Inactive	Date Inactive
PROBLEM LIST					
12-10-20	12-09-20	1	Coronary artery disease		
12-10-20	12-08-20	1a	Non-ST elevation MI, Type 1		
12-10-20	2017	2	Hypertension		
12-10-20	early 2000s	3	Bronchitis		
12-10-20	2010	4	Heartburn/reflux esophagitis		
12-10-20	2009	5	Back injury		
12-10-20	12-10-20	6	Eosinophilia		
12-10-20	2018	7	Blurred vision		
12-10-20	1990	8		Appendicitis 1990	

ASSESSMENT AND PLAN

Acute Coronary Syndrome (ACS): Mr. Jones presented with a classic history for MI. The troponin and electrocardiogram support the diagnosis. The ST depression without evolving Q waves is consistent with acute non-ST elevation MI Type 1. Mr. Jones is at risk of further myocardial damage and he needs further evaluation before discharge.

- Continue aspirin 81 mg/d PO, metoprolol 50 mg q12h, atorvastatin 80 mg/day, ticagrelor 90 mg q12h and UFH 840 U/hr IV.
- Monitor anti-factor Xa while he is still on UFH. Monitor cardiac rhythm by telemetry.
- Check lipid panel.
- Cardiology team to see Mr. Jones today for risk stratification and possible cardiac cath.
- If no cardiac cath, will consider modified stress test before discharge.
- Continue cardiac rehabilitation and refer for outpatient cardiac rehab.

Hypertension: In view of the patient's age, easily controlled HTN, and there is no evidence of a secondary cause, the HTN is most likely primary in nature. It is important that BP be well controlled with known CAD. Mr. Jones' BP has been well controlled with chlorthalidone, and he is now also taking metoprolol for his ACS. Closely monitor BP.

- Continue chlorthalidone, dietary consult before discharge to instruct patient on low-sodium as well as low-fat diet.

Chronic cough with sputum production: Most likely chronic bronchitis. He is at increased risk for developing bronchogenic carcinoma and when coupled with the palpable axillary LN, will need imaging to R/O lung cancer. CT of the chest before discharge. Encourage smoking cessation.

Eosinophilia: 10% eosinophils, concerned about a parasitic infection possibly from *Strongyloides stercoralis*. Differential includes neoplasia and allergy.

- Obtain *Strongyloides* serology and stool for ova and parasites as an outpatient or before discharge.
- CT of chest as above.

Signature: *Nick Pavona, MD*

Title: *Associate Professor, Blue Medicine Attending*

EXAMPLE OF A HISTORY AND PHYSICAL EXAMINATION, PEDIATRIC

Admission Note
Date: 10/24/2020   **Time:** 4:40 PM
HISTORY

History obtained from: parent (reliable historian), EHR, nursing

CC: Difficulty breathing

HPI: LJ is a 10-month-old previously healthy male with 3 days of congestion and cough and one day of increased work of breathing. Had tactile temperature day prior to admission but no true fever recorded. He has been taking less solids but still drinking formula well, making wet diapers. Older brother also has URI symptoms.

LJ developed worsening rhinorrhea, congestion and cough, and went on have labored breathing at home. Family tried older brother's nebulizer at home without improvement, and brought him in for further evaluation. No evidence of COVID-19 exposure.

In the emergency department, patient was initially febrile and tachypneic. LJ demonstrated hypoxia when he fell asleep and was admitted for further management.

PMHx: No significant PMHx, no hospitalizations

Birth Hx: Born at 7lbs 8 oz at 38 weeks GA via SVD, product of unremarkable pregnancy and without concerns in the newborn period.

Medications: none

Allergies: No known allergies

Immunizations: Up to date excluding flu shot

PCP: Dr. Angela Babidok

PSurg Hx: No prior surgeries

Devel Hx: No current developmental concerns. Pulling to stand, crawling. Babbles and points to things he wants.

Feeds: Regular age appropriate diet, takes stage 1 and stage 2 baby food, some puffs. Also drinks Enfamil Neuropro, 6 ounces every 4 hours along with meals.

Fam Hx: Asthma in father and older brother, COPD and HTN in paternal grandfather, Type II DM in paternal grandmother, osteoarthritis in maternal grandmother.

Social Hx: Lives with parents, 4-year-old older brother. Is in daycare during the day. No smoke exposure, no firearms at home.

ROS: *Constitutional:* Tactile fevers, No weight change, fussiness

Eyes: No redness or discharge

Ears, Nose, Throat: + congestion, + rhinorrhea, no ear tugging

Respiratory: + cough, + SOB

Cardiovascular: No issues

Gastrointestinal: normal appetite, no vomiting, no diarrhea, no constipation

Genitourinary: normal UOP

Skin/Breast: no rashes

Neurological: no seizures

Musculoskeletal: no joint swelling, full range of motion

Lymph: no swollen nodes

PHYSICAL EXAMINATION

General Appearance: Pleasant, no acute distress, cooperative with exam. Nasal cannula in place.

Vital Signs/Physical Assessment:
BP 111/98 | Pulse 171 | Temp 38.4 °C (101.1 °F) | Resp 60 | Wt 11.3 kg (24 lb 14.6 oz) Ht 0.762 m (2' 6") HC 46.7 cm (18.39") Oxygen Saturation (SpO_2) Avg: 96 % Min: 93 % Max: 99 %

    Growth Parameters: Weight: 96 %ile (Z= 1.73) based on WHO (Boys, 0-2 years) weight-for-age data using vitals from 10/24/2020. Height 97%ile based on WHO (Boys, 0-2 years) length-for-age data. HC 92%ile based on WHO (Boys, 0-2 years) HC-for-age data.

Skin: No rashes, no lesions

Head: Atraumatic, normocephalic

Eyes: Eyelids and eyelashes normal, conjunctivae and sclerae clear, pupils equal, round, reactive to light, EOM full and intact

ENT: Tympanic membranes with fluid behind them BL without erythema appreciated, external ears with no lesions or erythema. Lips moist and normal without lesions, buccal mucosa normal, palate normal, soft palate, uvula, and tonsils normal

Neck: Supple without significant adenopathy

Lungs: Very mild supraclavicular retractions, no nasal flaring. Coarse breath sounds bilaterally, intermittent inspiratory expiratory wheezing noted. No focal findings appreciated.

Heart: Tachycardic, but regular rhythm, no murmurs detected

Vascular: Well perfused in the distal extremities, capillary refill <2 seconds

Abdomen: Soft, nondistended, nontender, no masses palpated, no hepatosplenomegaly

GU: normal Tanner 1 male, circumcised, both testes descended, no hernia or hydrocele

Musculoskeletal: No extremity musculoskeletal defects are noted

Neuro: No focal deficits noted, muscle tone normal, muscle strength normal, reflexes 2+ bilaterally

LABS AND STUDIES

RSV/Flu testing negative

ASSESSMENT AND PLAN

10 mo male without significant past medical history who presents with 3 days URI and 1 day of respiratory distress due to acute viral bronchiolitis. Exam findings not consistent with pneumonia or asthma exacerbation.

1. Bronchiolitis: Monitor respiratory status closely, wean oxygen support as tolerated.

    Nasal suction as needed, can use nasal saline spray as needed for congestion.

    Monitor I/Os, continue regular diet and ensure that IVF are not needed.

    No antimicrobials are indicated at this time, but would use contact/droplet precaution.
2. Administer flu vaccine prior to discharge.

Signature: Mac Mulatta, MD

Title: Professor of Pediatrics

References

1. Goddu AP, et al. Do Words Matter? Stigmatizing Language and the Transmission of Bias in the Medical Record. *J Gen Intern Med* 2008;33(5):685-691.
2. Hausmann JS, et al. Using smartphone crowdsourcing to redefine normal and febrile temperatures in adults: Results from the Feverprints Study. *J Gen Intern Med* 2018:33(12):2046–2047.
3. Barnett BJ, et al. Oral and tympanic membrane temperatures are inaccurate to identify fever in emergency department adults. *West J Emerg Med.* 2011 Nov; 12(4):505–511.
4. McGee ZA, Gorby GL. The diagnostic value of fever pattern. *Hospital Practice* 1987;22(10A):103–110.
5. Chang DF. Ophthalmologic examination. In: Riordan-Eva P, Augsburger JJ, eds. *Vaughan & Asbury's General Ophthalmology.* 19th ed. New York, NY: McGraw-Hill, 2018.
6. Folstein M, et al. "Mini-mental state": A practical method for grading the cognitive state of patients for the clinician. *J Psychiatr Res.* 1975;12:189.
7. Jameson J, et al., eds. *Harrison's Manual of Medicine.* 20th ed. New York, NY: McGraw-Hill; 2018.

Chartwork

7

PROMISES AND CHALLENGES OF THE ELECTRONIC HEALTH RECORD (EHR)

The EHR has been a major disruptive change in healthcare over the last 20 years. The adoption of the EHR across the United States was accelerated by the HITECH Act passed by Congress in 2009. EHRs are very expensive, often costing academic medical centers and healthcare systems hundreds of millions of dollars. Besides the actual cost of the EHR, many hours of training staff and physicians are required, often affecting productivity during implementation. Once an EHR is in place, physicians spend many additional hours each week documenting in the EHR compared to before implementation. For many physicians, the EHR in the ambulatory setting, and to a lesser extent in the hospital, is an obstacle to optimal communication with the patient, because physicians will spend a great deal of time during the encounter entering information in the EHR and less "face time" with patients. Additionally, some patients perceive privacy concerns. And lastly, in the past, medical students were excluded from using the EHR. This changed recently when the Centers for Medicare and Medicaid Services (CMS) allowed the use of the student note for the documentation used for billing purposes. Organizations such as the American Medical Association have promoted EHR training for students, and most academic centers now provide that resource to students.

Chapter update by Steven A. Haist, MD, and Leonard G. Gomella, MD

For all of the recognized drawbacks, the EHR appears to be improving the quality of patient care. Vaccination rates increase, as do the use of deep venous thrombosis (DVT) prophylaxis; rates of guideline-based treatment of hypertension increase, and increases in the rate of proper use of antibiotics have all resulted with the implementation of the EHR. There is improved coordination of care between providers in the same healthcare system and across different healthcare systems through health information exchange (HIE) programs. Additionally, patient participation in their own healthcare as a result of HIE is enhanced. Computerized provider order entry (CPOE) was initially intended to address errors that were inherent in handwritten medication orders. Eliminated are medication errors that resulted from illegible handwriting and misspellings, as well as a decrease in errors related to the wrong dose being administered and the ability to send alerts and warnings regarding drug interactions and medication allergies. CPOE for laboratory tests, consultations, and procedures has also provided benefits. When coupled with clinical decision support systems, CPOE can restrict the ordering of expensive laboratory testing except when indicated and can help ensure best practices are followed, such as DVT prophylaxis following certain procedures. Unintended consequences from the CPOE have included alert fatigue, cognitive overload, and increasing demands on physicians to interact with technology, resulting in fewer interactions with patients and some suggestion that EHR documentation contributes to provider burnout.

Another EHR benefit is the ability to improve the health of patient populations through the ability to easily obtain data, such as checking to see if every woman between the ages of 50 and 75 has had a screening mammogram in the last 2 years as per the United States Preventive Services Task Force guidelines. Research related to population health is another benefit. The EHR has the potential to positively affect health disparities through equitable access. The cost of healthcare delivery is potentially lowered through such changes as a reduction in the ordering of redundant laboratory testing. Prescription writing may be enhanced through the use of legible computer-generated prescriptions or by transmission directly to the pharmacy.

Many common tasks included in traditional handwritten chartwork are now available as structured templates in many EHR systems, while other notes must be entered in free-form style. This chapter will outline the basic structure of some commonly used notes. The style and formatting may be unique to each EHR system, but understanding their general structure and utility is essential.

HOW TO WRITE ORDERS

Students are often not allowed to place any orders into the permanent records. Following along with an attending or resident as they use the EHR order entry system is a useful learning activity. There are many electronic templates for admission and inpatient orders, and most include the standard information listed here. Some institutions have preloaded critical pathway admission orders for diagnoses such as acute MI or hip fracture. If given the opportunity in an educational environment, it is best practice to review the orders that have been entered for any patient directly assigned to you. The following conceptual format is useful for the traditional method of writing concise admission, transfer, and postoperative orders and allows you to understand the patient care journey when admitted to the hospital. The one described here (others exist) involves the mnemonic **A.A.D.C. VAAN DISSL**, which stands for **A**dmit/**A**ttending, **D**iagnosis, **C**ondition, **V**itals, **A**ctivity, **A**llergies, **N**ursing procedures, **D**iet, **I**ns and outs, **S**pecific medications, **S**ymptomatic medications, and **L**abs.

A.A.D.C. VAAN DISSL

Admit: Admitting team (i.e., Blue Surgery, General Medicine, Peds ICU, etc.), room number.

Attending: Name of the attending physician (the person legally responsible for the patient's care), as well as the resident, intern, and other providers' names. Case manager if known.

Diagnosis: List admitting diagnosis or procedure if writing postop orders.

Condition: Stable, critical, etc.

Vitals: Determine frequency of vital signs (temperature, pulse, BP, weight, pulse oximetry, other hemodynamic measurements, etc.).

Activity: Bedrest, up ad lib, ambulate QID, bathroom privileges, etc.

Allergies: Drug reactions, food and environmental allergies (e.g., latex, adhesive tape).

Nursing Procedures:
  Bed Position: Elevate head of bed 30 degrees, etc.
  Preps: Enemas, scrubs, showers.
  Respiratory Care: P&PD, TC&DB, etc.
  Dressing Changes, Wound Care: Change dressing BID, wound vac parameters, etc.
  Notify Provider If: Temperature >101°F, BP systolic <90 mm Hg, etc., drain output greater than 20 mL/hr, etc.

Diet: NPO, clear liquid, regular, etc.

Ins and Outs: All "tubes" a patient may have.
  Record Daily I&O
  IV Fluids: Specify type and rate (see Chapter 15, Fluid and Electrolytes).
  Drains (NG Tube, Foley Catheter, ETT, Arterial Lines, Wound Drains, etc.): Specify care desired (e.g., NG to low wall suction, Foley to gravity, suction ETT q2h and PRN).

Specific Medications: Antihypertensive medications, antibiotics, etc. with dosing.

Symptomatic Medications: PRN medications (e.g., pain medications, laxatives, sleep medications).

Table 7-1. Example of Dosing Notation and Timing of Dosing (24-Hour Clock Notation)

Dosing frequency	Administration time
Daily	0900
2 times per day (BID)	0900, 2100
3 times per day (TID)	0900, 1400, 2100
4 times per day (QID)	0900, 1300, 1700, 2100
Every 3 hours	0000, 0300, 0600, 0900, 1200, 1500, 1800, 2100
Every 4 hours	0100, 0500, 0900, 1300, 1700, 2100
Every 6 hours	0600, 1200, 1800, 2400
Every 8 hours	0800, 1600, 2400
Every 12 hours	0900, 2100

Labs: Blood for basic metabolic panel, CBC with differential and platelets, blood cultures, spot urine for electrolytes, and urinalysis. Specific times if applicable. Also include **diagnostic tests** such as ECGs, radiographs, nuclear scans, etc. See end of this chapter for shorthand for common laboratory data.

Consultation Requests: Cardiology, geriatric psychiatry, nutrition, etc.

Standardized Inpatient Medication Dosing Intervals

Most medications to treat specific conditions (infections, hypertension, auto-immune diseases, etc.) are given on a set schedule to ensure appropriate therapeutic levels. Most hospitals have standardized medication administration times based on the individual product labeling. This is one example of these standardized administration times (Table 7-1). Your facility may have alternative administration times that should be reviewed.

SOAP NOTE OR DAILY PROGRESS NOTE

The most commonly used format, **SOAP**, stands for **Subjective, Objective, Assessment, and Plan.** A sample SOAP note is on page 133 (Box 7-1).

S or **subjective** is how the patient says they are feeling. Record their subjective answers to history-related questions in their own words. For example, for a patient admitted with chest pain, record the answers to daily follow-up questions: Any further chest pain? If so, describe it for me. How long did it last? Any shortness of breath? How did you sleep last night?

O or **objective** is the place for recording the physical examination and laboratory data. The physical examination should include, at a minimum, general appearance, vital signs, chest, heart, abdomen, and any other system

Box 7-1.   Example of a SOAP Note

Day 3 of the hospitalization of Mr. Jones whose admission history and physical is noted on page 120.

S) Mr. Jones is day 3 after being transferred here for a non-ST elevation MI. He underwent a cardiac cath yesterday and underwent stenting of a mid-LAD lesion. Mr. Jones does not have any concerns this morning. He denies chest pain and dyspnea. He denies any bleeding from the cath site. He has not had a cigarette since the day before he was admitted to the Whitesburg hospital. He wants to quit smoking and "I will need help once I leave the hospital." His cough is unchanged and he produced two to three spoonfuls of sputum in the last 24 hours. He denies hemoptysis.

O) BP 106/70 mm Hg, HR 64 BPM, Resp 14/min, Temp 98.4°F

Neck: JVP 1 cm above the sternal angle, carotids 2^+ bilaterally w/o bruits.

Chest: percussion bilaterally resonant, end-inspiratory crackles at both bases that do not clear with coughing.

Heart: Nl S_1 and S_2, no S_4 or S_3, no murmur or rub.

Ext: trace edema, pulses $2+$ dorsalis pedis and posterior tibial pulses.

Axilla: Left axillary lymph node 1×1 cm unchanged.

Labs: troponin 1.6 ng/mL, K^+ 4.2, BUN 14 mg/dL, creat 1.1 mg/dL

A & P)

Problem 1. Coronary artery disease with a non-ST elevation MI type 1, S/P LAD stent no further chest pain. Continue his current medical regimen (metoprolol, atorvastatin, aspirin, ticagrelor).

Problem 2. Chronic bronchitis, concerned about lung cancer with axillary node and hx of smoking. Will obtain low-dose CT of the chest before discharge.

Problem 3. Hypertension, well controlled at this time, continue thiazide diuretic.

Problem 4. Eosinophilia, concerned about *Strongyloides stercoralis* or possibly another parasite, will defer complete workup until the cardiac evaluation is complete.

Fluid/Electrolytes/Nutrition: No IV fluids, heparin lock dorsum L hand; K^+ 4.2, all other electrolytes and renal function normal; low-sodium diet

Disposition: Likely discharge to home today pending CT chest. Follow-up with Dr. Doyle to be scheduled in 1 week. Outpatient cardiac rehabilitation to be arranged prior to discharge.

Signature: _____

Title: _____

Date and Time: _____

7

in which there is a new concern or in which there was a finding on admission. Laboratory data may include tests such as radiologic studies performed the previous afternoon or the troponin and CBC drawn in the early morning the day the SOAP note is written.

A is the place for recording the **assessment** of the patient. Evaluate the data and record any conclusions drawn such as presumptive diagnosis.

P is where the **plan** for the day is recorded. Include any new lab tests or medications, changes or additions to previous orders, and discharge or transfer plans. Note that A & P may sometimes be noted together as in the example in Box 7-1.

If the patient has more than one active medical problem, address the **assessment** and **plan** for each problem separately.

1. List each medical, surgical, and psychiatric problem separately: pneumonia, pancreatitis, CHF, etc.
2. Give each problem a number: 1, 2, 3 (as on page 133).
3. Retain the number of each problem throughout the hospitalization.
4. When the problem is resolved, mark it as such and delete it from the daily progress note.

DISCHARGE SUMMARY/NOTE

At most hospitals, a formal discharge summary is required for any admission longer than 24 hours. The framework provided here is a common template that can be used when writing or dictating a discharge summary. The following skeleton includes most of the information needed for a discharge note.

Date of Admission: Specify.
Date of Discharge: Specify.
Admitting Diagnosis: List main reason for initial admission.
Discharge Diagnosis: List primary diagnosis and any secondary diagnoses.
Attending Physician and Service Caring for Patient: Provide attending's name and service or practice group.
Referring Physician: Provide name and contact information (e.g., address, phone number) if available.
Procedures: Include surgery and any invasive diagnostic procedures (e.g., lumbar puncture, arteriogram).
Brief History, Pertinent Physical Findings, and Lab Data: *Briefly* review the main points of the history, physical, and admission lab tests. Do not repeat what is recorded in the admission note; summarize the most important points about the patient's admission.
Hospital Course: Briefly summarize in chronological order the evaluation, treatment, and progress of the patient during the hospitalization. If the patient has more than one active problem during the hospitalization, address each problem separately, and within each problem record the events in chronological order.
Condition at Discharge: Note whether improved, unchanged, or worse.
Disposition: Record the location to which the patient is discharged (e.g., home, another hospital, rehab center, nursing home). Give the specific address, if available, if the patient is transferred to another medical institution, and note who will be assuming responsibility for the care of the patient.
Discharge Medications: List medications, dosing, and refills.

Discharge Instructions and Follow-up: Note clinic return date, appointments for inpatient or outpatient scheduled procedures, labs to be obtained and when, dietary instructions, any restrictions, etc.

Problem List: List active and past medical problems.

ON-SERVICE NOTE

Also known as a "pick-up note," the on-service note is written by a new member of the team who assumes care of a patient. The patient was admitted to the team by another intern, who oftentimes leaves the service, necessitating the handover (handoff). This type of note is more common on internal medicine services. Make the note brief, summarizing the hospital course to date and showing that the patient's care has been reviewed. The following skeleton includes most of the information needed in an on-service note. (The essential elements of a handoff note for cross coverage are reviewed in Chapter 8.)

Date of Admission: Specify.

Admitting Diagnosis: Specify.

Procedures (with Results) Performed to Date: List.

Hospital Course to Date: Summarize briefly.

Brief Physical Examination: Record findings pertinent to the patient's problems.

Pertinent Lab Data: Summarize key lab tests.

Problem List: Use the problem-numbering system as for the SOAP format (page 133).

Assessment: Describe how the patient is progressing and the up-to-date assessment of each problem.

Plan: Outline further testing or therapy planned.

OFF-SERVICE NOTE

If rotating off the service before the patient is discharged, the team member primarily responsible for the patient's care writes an off-service note. The components are identical to those of the on-service note, and these notes will aid the individual taking over the care of the patient.

BEDSIDE PROCEDURE NOTE

Procedure: Lumbar puncture, thoracentesis, etc.

Indications: For example, R/O meningitis, symptomatic pleural effusion.

Permission: Note risks and benefits explained and indicate the consent for the procedure is signed and in the chart.

7

Physicians: Note physicians and others present and responsible for the procedure.

Document "Time Out": This is similar to procedures taking place in the operating room that confirm the patient identity, the procedure, allergies or medical conditions, the specific site, equipment availability and function, and that all present are aware of the proposed procedure and ready to proceed (time out is discussed in Chapter 24 page 809).

Description of Procedure: Indicate type of positioning, prep, anesthesia type and amount (e.g., 2 mL 1% lidocaine). Briefly describe technique and instruments used.

Complications: Note any.

Estimated Blood Loss: If any.

Specimens/Findings Obtained: For example, opening pressure for LP, CSF appearance, and tubes sent to lab, etc.

Disposition: Describe the patient's status after procedure (e.g., Patient alert and oriented with no concerns; BP stable). Note any changes in orders based on the procedure.

PREOPERATIVE NOTE

The specific items in the preoperative note depend on institutional guidelines, the nature of the procedure, and the age and health of the patient. For example, an ECG and blood setup may not be necessary for a 2-year-old being treated for a hernia but are essential for a 70-year-old undergoing aortic valve surgery. The following list includes most of the information needed in a preoperative note.

Preop Diagnosis: Record (e.g., "GSW to the abdomen").

Procedure: Indicate the planned procedure (e.g., "exploratory laparotomy").

Labs: Record results of CBC, electrolytes, PT, PTT, urinalysis, etc.

CXR: Note results.

ECG: Note results.

Blood: Follow institutional blood bank guidelines for recommended quantities (e.g., T&C 2 units PRBC, blood not needed, etc.) (see also Chapter 12).

History and Physical: See chart.

Orders: Note any special preop orders (e.g., preop colon prep, vaginal douche, prophylactic antibiotics).

Permission: If completed, write "consent signed and on chart." If not, indicate plans for obtaining informed consent before the procedure. Note risks and benefits that were discussed.

OPERATIVE NOTE

The operative note is written immediately after a surgical procedure to summarize the operation for those who were not present. The note is meant to complement and not replace the formal operative summary dictated by the surgeon.

The following list includes most of the information needed in an operative note. Hospitals may produce standardized EHR template for this type of note.

Preop Diagnosis: Record the reason for the operation (e.g., "GSW to the abdomen").

Postop Diagnosis: Record the diagnosis based on the operative findings (e.g., "mesenteric lymphadenitis").

Procedure: Specify the operation performed (e.g., "exploratory laparotomy").

Surgeons: List the attending physician, residents, and students who scrubbed on the case, including their titles, for example, MD, CCIV (clinical clerk, fourth year), or MSII (second-year medical student). Identify the dictating surgeon if known.

Findings: Briefly note operative findings (e.g., "perforated duodenum," "subtrochanteric hip fracture," "pyloric stenosis").

Anesthesia: Specify the type of anesthesia (e.g., local, spinal, general, endotracheal).

Fluids: Record the amount and type of fluid administered during the operation (e.g., 1500 mL NS, 2 units PRBC, 500 mL albumin). This information usually is obtained from the anesthesia records.

EBL: Record the estimated blood loss. This information is obtained from the anesthesia or nursing records.

Drains: State location and type of drain (e.g., "Jackson–Pratt drain in LUQ," "T-tube in midline").

Specimens: State any samples sent to pathology and the results of examination of any intraoperative frozen sections.

Complications: Note any complications during or after the operation.

Condition: Note where the patient is taken immediately after the operation and the patient's condition (e.g., "transferred to the recovery room in stable condition").

NIGHT OF SURGERY NOTE (POSTOP NOTE)

This progress note is written several hours after or the night of surgery and may be required on some surgical services.

Procedure: Indicate the operation performed.

Level of Consciousness: Note whether the patient is alert, drowsy, etc.

Vital Signs: Record Temp, BP, and pulse and respiratory rates.

I&O: Calculate amount of IV fluids, blood, urine output, and other drainage and attempt to assess fluid balance.

Physical Examination: Examine the chest, heart, abdomen, extremities, and any other body part pertinent to the surgery and record the findings. Examine the dressing for bleeding or other evidence of saturation.

Labs: Review lab results obtained since the operation.

Assessment: Evaluate the postop course thus far (stable, etc.).

Plan: Note any changes in orders.

DELIVERY NOTE

Fill in # where appropriate. Details noted will vary with the course of the delivery, and requirements for documentation vary by medical center. "G"(gravida) indicates the number of times a woman is/ has been pregnant, regardless of outcome. Current pregnancy is included in this count. Multiple pregnancy is counted as 1. "P" is parity, or "para", and refers to the number of pregnancies reaching viable 20-week gestational age (live births and still-births). The number of fetuses does not determine the parity. A twin pregnancy carried to viable gestational age is counted as 1. "AB" or abortus is the number of pregnancies lost for any reason (induced abortions, miscarriages).

The mother is a ## old (married or single) G ## now para ##, AB ##, notation of whether patient received prenatal clinic care, patient with (estimated date of confinement) EDC ##, and prenatal course (specify uncomplicated, or describe any problems). Labor (describe any unique characteristics (e.g., oxytocin-induced, premature rupture of membranes) draped in the usual sterile manner.

Under controlled conditions delivered a ## lb ## oz (## g) viable (specify male, female or gender unassigned) infant under (specify general, spinal, pudendal, none) anesthesia with delivery date ## and delivery time ##. Delivery was by (specify spontaneous vaginal delivery [SVD]with midline episiotomy, or forceps, or cesarean section, etc.). Apgar scores were ## at 1 min and ## at 5 min (for Apgar scoring, see Appendix, page 1043). Cord blood sent to lab. Placenta expressed intact with trailing membranes. Lacerations and degree (1st, 2nd, 3rd, and 4th) repaired by standard method with good hemostasis and restoration of normal anatomy.

- EBL: ##
- Maternal blood type (MBT): ##
- HCT (predelivery and postdelivery): ##
- Rubella titer: ##
- RPR test, hepatitis B serology, HIV test, and status of other serology or cultures that can affect a mother's or newborn's health: ##
- Condition of mother: ##

OUTPATIENT PRESCRIPTION WRITING

With an EHR system, the formatting of an outpatient prescription is predetermined. This also minimizes prescribing errors due to unclear instructions or illegible handwriting. As you will be prescribing medications at some point in your career, understanding the elements of a prescription, be it computer generated or handwritten, is an essential clinical skill.

The general format for outpatient prescriptions is outlined below and illustrated in Figure 7-1. Today most EHR systems generate automated prescription requests. Controlled substances, such as narcotics, require a DEA number on the prescription. Some states require that the controlled

---

NICK PAVONA, MD
BENJAMIN FRANKLIN UNIVERSITY MEDICAL CENTER
CHADDS FORD, PA 19317

LICENSE <u>MD 685-488-194</u>   **DEA** <u>NP–3612982</u>

                NPI: 2157786991

NAME <u>NICK PAVONA, Sr.</u>   **AGE** <u>65</u>

ADDRESS <u>Box 209</u>   **DATE** <u>10/24/2020</u>

<u>   Cambridge, MD 21613   </u>

            Rx: minoxidil (Rogaine) 2% topical solution
            DISP: 60 mL
            SIG: Apply BID to scalp
                Brand medically necessary

REFILL <u>   X3   </u>

SUBSTITUTION PERMISSIBLE   ☐   *Nick Pavona*   M.D.

TO ENSURE BRAND NAME DISPENSING, PRESCRIBER MUST
SPECIFY "DISPENSE AS WRITTEN" ON THE PRESCRIPTION *

---

*This can vary by state; some require that you write "Brand Medically
Necessary" to specify a brand name and not a generic.

Figure 7-1. Example of an outpatient prescription. As a safety feature, DEA numbers should never be preprinted on a prescription form. The "Dispense as Written" statement can vary by state requirements. This statement requests that the pharmacist fill the prescription as requested and not substitute a generic equivalent.

substance be written or printed out on a special type of prescription pad, with some states also requiring physicians to use an online prescription monitoring system for all controlled substances that link to state agencies for the purpose of combating the opioid epidemic. The database tracks prescribing physicians and dispensing pharmacies of all controlled substances by individual patients. These systems are used to assist physicians in monitoring and treating patients on medications that can be misused. For handwritten prescriptions, the DEA number should never be preprinted on a prescription. The National Provider Identifier (NPI) is a Health Insurance Portability and Accountability Act (HIPAA) Administrative Simplification Standard. The NPI is a unique identification number for covered healthcare providers and must be used by all health plans. The NPI is a ten-digit number that does not carry other information about healthcare providers, such as the state in which they live or their medical specialty. Many prescription stationary papers (handwritten or computer generated) will display a "VOID" pattern if an attempt is made to photocopy or scan it to deter fraud and abuse.

Essential elements of an outpatient prescription include:

Patient's Name, Address, and Age: Print clearly where indicated.
Date: State requirements vary, but most prescriptions must be filled within
    6 months.

License of the Provider: XXX

DEA: If needed for controlled substances.

NPI: Usually required for any prescription to be filled.

Rx: Drug name, strength, and type (usually listed as the generic name). Designate "no substitution" if a specific brand name is preferred. "Rx" is the abbreviation of the Latin word for "recipe." List the strength of the product (usually in milligrams) and the form (e.g., tablet, capsule, suspension, transdermal, and suppository).

Dispense: Amount of drug (e.g., number of capsules) and time period (e.g., 1-month supply, QS [quantity sufficient]). Some insurance companies limit the total amount of a drug that may be dispensed. The maximum is typically 90 days, with some exceptions.

Sig: Short for the Latin "signa," which means "mark through" on patient instructions. Abbreviate the instructions or write them in full. Spelling out directions rather than using abbreviations decreases the likelihood of error. A list of frequently used abbreviations follows. However, the use of abbreviations on prescriptions is becoming less common due to the potential for errors through misinterpretation.

ad lib = as much as wanted

PO = by mouth

PR = by rectum

SL = sublingual

OS = left eye

OD = right eye

OU = both eyes

qd = daily ("qd" **is a dangerous abbreviation and should not be used**; write out "every day" or "Q day"; see "Dangerous Practices," page 141)

PRN = as needed

Write out the number of pills to be taken at each dose "three (3)"

qhs = every night at bedtime

BID = twice per day

TID = three times per day

q6h = every 6 hours

QID = four times a day. Note that QID and q6h are NOT the same orders: QID means the patient takes the medication four times a day while awake (e.g., 8 AM, 12 noon, 6 PM, and 10 PM); q6h means the medication is taken four times a day but by the clock (e.g., 6 AM, 12 noon, 6 PM, 12 midnight).

Refills: How many times this prescription can be refilled.

Substitution: Whether a generic drug can be used instead of the one prescribed.

Tips for Safe Prescribing

1. Verify if the patient has any known drug allergies.
2. Confirm if there are any black box warnings on the medication you are about to prescribe.

3. Determine if any dose modifications are needed based on patient specific factors (renal insufficiency, etc.) or if significant drug interactions exist.
4. For handwritten prescriptions, take time to write legibly.
5. Print if doing so would make the prescription more legible than cursive writing.
6. Computer-generated prescriptions avoid issues with legibility and are becoming the standard in most settings. Direct transmission to the patient's pharmacy of choice is facilitated through the use of the EHR where available.
7. Avoid dangerous abbreviations that should never be used (see later).
8. Carefully print the order to avoid misreading. There are many "look alike and sound-alike" drugs and medications that have similar spellings (e.g., Celexa and Celebrex). See some examples at https://www.ismp.org/recommendations/confused-drug-names-list.
9. The FDA initiated the "Name Differentiation Project" in 2001 to help address the issue of look alike drug names (https://www.fda.gov/drugs/medication-errors-related-cder-regulated-drug-products/fda-name-differentiation-project). Tall man lettering (TML) uses uppercase lettering to help differentiate look-alike drug names. Starting on the left side of a drug name, TML highlights the differences between similar drug names by capitalizing dissimilar letters (e.g., vinBLAStine versus vinCRIStine and CISplatin versus CARBOplatin).

Dangerous Prescription Writing Practices

1. **Never** use a trailing zero.
   Correct: 1 mg; dangerous: 1.0 mg. If the decimal is not seen, a 10-fold overdose can occur.
2. **Never** leave a decimal point "naked." Correct: 0.5 mL; dangerous: .5 mL. If the decimal point is not seen, a 10-fold overdose can occur.
3. **Never** abbreviate a drug name. The abbreviation can be misunderstood and may have multiple meanings.
4. **Never** abbreviate the word "units." The letter U can be read as a zero (e.g., "6 U regular insulin" can be misread as 60 units). Write the order as "6 units regular insulin."
5. **Never** use "qd" (abbreviation for once a day or every day). When poorly written, the tail of the q can make the abbreviation look like "qid," or four times a day. Write out "every day" or "Q day."

SHORTHAND FOR LABORATORY VALUES

The method for manually recording laboratory values is shown in Figure 7-2, page 142. This method is usually limited to reference use when presenting a patient based on the provider's personal handwritten notes.

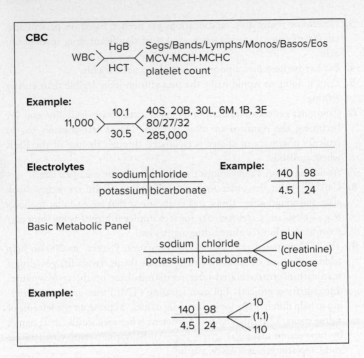

Figure 7-2. Shorthand notation for recording laboratory values.

Oral Presentations and Safe Handovers

8

- ➤ Principles of the Oral Presentation
- ➤ New Patient Presentation on Rounds
- ➤ Follow-up Patient Note and Presentation on Rounds
- ➤ Handovers (Hand-offs)
- ➤ Handovers: The Essential Elements

PRINCIPLES OF THE ORAL PRESENTATION

An essential skill as a medical student and as an intern or resident is being able to provide a concise and organized oral presentation of your patients. Likely outcomes for those who master this essential skill include more efficient rounds and higher ratings on your clerkship evaluations from your attending, residents, and fellows. The one caveat is that the expectations of what information to present and how long you have to present each patient will vary from institution to institution, from service to service, and from attending to attending. On the first day of a new rotation you should inquire about your responsibilities on rounds, including the preferred format of the oral presentation and the maximum length of the presentations, both for the initial presentation and on subsequent days. Additionally, the site of rounds, such as bedside versus a conference room, may influence the amount of time allotted for your presentation. Occasionally, teams will meet in a conference room to review the patients. This may occur before the team goes to the bedside, or the team may not go back to the bedside with the attending if the attending has already seen the patients or if the attending will see the patients in the afternoon after morning clinic.

What you want to avoid is a disorganized presentation that takes 15 or more minutes and is confusing to those who do not know the patient (and, maybe, even to those who do know the patient). The best way to avoid this, especially early on, is to write out the key findings of the history, physical examination, and laboratory data and practice the presentation. Be sure to time yourself!

Obviously, new patient presentations will take more time compared to subsequent hospital days unless the patient after admission has a major complication and/or becomes gravely ill. The various formats for the written

Original chapter by Steven A. Haist, MD, MS, and Andrew R. Hoellein, MD

presentations in Chapter 7 provide you with outlines for your oral presentations on surgical and nonsurgical services, including obstetrics. For the patient in the write-up in Chapter 6 on page 120, below is the information that could be presented on rounds after admission. It is written out as it would be verbalized on rounds. The time of day and format for patient presentations can vary based on the nature of the service (medical vs. surgical vs. psychiatric, for example). This example is typical for medicine services. The new patient presentation as a general rule should be about 3 minutes and not be more than 4 minutes (this may vary for the reasons outlined earlier). Remember, the resident and possibly the attending have already interviewed and examined the patient, so you do not need to, nor should you, report on every piece of history you obtain. While presenting a patient on rounds, focus on the major components of the history and physical examination. After the new patient presentation given here, there is an example of the oral presentation on day 3 in the hospital for the same patient, which coincides with the SOAP note in Chapter 7 on page 133.

NEW PATIENT PRESENTATION ON ROUNDS

- Mr. Jones is a 49-year-old man from Whitesburg, Kentucky, who was transferred yesterday afternoon for further evaluation of a myocardial infarction.
- Two days ago he awoke with substernal chest pain—it felt like a ton of bricks on his chest. The pain radiated to his left neck and arm. There was associated dyspnea and diaphoresis.
- The pain was aggravated by activity, and nothing relieved the pain for 10 hours until treatment at his local hospital.
- He had similar pain but not as intense over the last 3 months, always precipitated by exercise and relieved with rest.
- He has a 2-year history of hypertension for which he takes chlorthalidone, he has a family history for early CAD, and has smoked 2 PPD for 35 years. He is interested in quitting.
- At his local emergency department, he was given 3 NTG, 1 aspirin, and 2 mg of morphine with relief of the pain. ECG showed 3–4 mm of ST depression in V1–V4. Troponin was initially 8 and peaked the next morning at 24. He was admitted to the ICU and started on metoprolol atorvastatin, aspirin, ticagrelor, and unfractionated heparin at 1500 units/hr.

  ROS: Notable for daily cough with gray/white sputum, he denies any hemoptysis, last CXR was 3 years ago; GE reflux for 10 years; back pain with lifting and hx of back injury related to a mining accident.

  Physical examination was notable for a man resting comfortably lying in bed at 30 degrees. BP was 110/70, HR 64.

o Neck: JVP is 2 cm above the sternal angle.

o There is a 1×1 cm mobile axillary node.

o Chest: End-inspiratory crackles at both bases that do not clear with coughing.

o Heart: PMI sixth intercostal space, 2 cm lateral to the midclavicular line, Nl S_1 and S_2, $+S_4$, no murmur, rubs, or S_3.

o ECG: Last evening 1- to 2-mm ST depression and inverted T waves V1–V4. CXR shows cardiomegaly.

o Anti–factor Xa activity 0.70 this morning on 1550 units of unfractionated heparin, troponin 16 last evening, and this morning 6.8.

o CBC: Normal except for 10% eosinophils.

Assessment and Plan: Mr. Jones has four active problems:

o **Problem 1:** Coronary artery disease with a non-ST elevation MI type 1, no further chest pain. The plan is for him to undergo cardiac catheterization later today or tomorrow unless he has further chest pain and, if so, immediate cath. Continue the current medical regimen and titrate heparin to keep the anti–factor Xa activity at 0.5–1.0. Continue the other medications started at his local hospital.

o **Problem 2:** Chronic bronchitis from smoking; axillary node with 70 pack-year hx of smoking. He is at risk for lung cancer. Will obtain low-dose CT of the chest before discharge.

o **Problem 3:** Hypertension, well controlled, continue diuretic. Also now on metoprolol.

o **Problem 4:** Eosinophilia, concerned about *Strongyloides* or possibly another parasite, neoplasia, or allergies; will defer workup until cardiac workup is complete.

FOLLOW-UP PATIENT NOTE AND PRESENTATION ON ROUNDS

After the initial presentation, the student or intern will likely be responsible for presenting the patient on subsequent days. A common and the most straightforward way to present is the SOAP note format. Present the **subjective**, organizing what you say by problem, then the **objective**, and finally, an **assessment** and **plan** for each active problem.

• Mr. Jones is day 3 after being transferred here for a non-ST-elevation MI. He underwent a cardiac catheterization yesterday and underwent stenting of a mid-LAD lesion. Mr. Jones does not have any complaints this morning; he denies chest pain or dyspnea. He denies any bleeding from the cath site. He has not smoked since the day before he was admitted to the Whitesburg Hospital. He wants to quit smoking and "I will need help once I leave the hospital." His cough is unchanged, and he produced two to three spoonfuls of sputum in the last 24 hours. He denies hemoptysis.

o BP 106/70 mm Hg, HR 64 BPM, Resp 14/min, Temp 98.4°F.

o Neck: JVP 1 cm above the sternal angle, carotids 2+ w/o bruits.

o Chest: end-inspiratory crackles at both bases that do not clear with coughing.

o Heart: Nl S_1 and S_2, No S_4 or S_3, no murmur or rub. Ext: trace edema, warm, pulses 2+ dorsalis pedis and posterior tibial pulses.

o **Labs:** troponin 1.6, K^+ 4.2, BUN 14, and creatinine 1.10.

- **There are four active problems:**

  o **Problem 1:** Coronary artery disease with a non-ST-elevation MI, SP LAD stent, no further chest pain. Continue his current medical regimen (metoprolol, atorvastatin, aspirin, ticagrelor).

  o **Problem 2:** Chronic bronchitis, w/axillary node with hx of smoking; rule out lung cancer. Will obtain low-dose CT of the chest before discharge.

  o **Problem 3:** Hypertension, well controlled at this time, continue thiazide diuretic and metoprolol.

  o **Problem 4:** Eosinophilia, concerned about *Strongyloides stercoralis* or possibly another parasite; will complete workup as an outpatient.

- **Disposition:** Discharge to home later today with follow-up within a week with Dr. Pavona.

HANDOVERS (HAND-OFFS)

To Err Is Human: Building a Safer Health System, a book published in 1999, estimated that the number of patient deaths due to medical errors was between 44,000 and 98,000 per year. This Institute of Medicine publication resulted in many changes to how we practice medicine, including the introduction of medication reconciliation, timeouts during surgeries and procedures, and handovers. Discontinuity of care is a necessary evil of medical care. Patient care, either at the end of a shift or when a new day begins, requires that the care be transferred from one nurse to another or from one physician to another. This discontinuity increases the likelihood of medical errors. In academic medical centers, the discontinuity of care increased even more in 2003 with the introduction of duty hour restrictions. How patient care is transitioned from one provider to another can minimize the likelihood of errors occurring.

Handovers that are designed to facilitate the transfer of care have been shown to decrease medical errors. Formally defined by The Joint Commission, which oversees accreditation of healthcare facilities, "A hand-off (handover) is a transfer and acceptance of patient care responsibility achieved through effective communication. It is a real-time process of passing patient-specific information from one caregiver to another or from one team of caregivers to another for the purpose of ensuring the continuity and safety of the patient's care."* Handovers must occur in person and be performed in a standardized

---

*The Joint Commission Center for Transforming Healthcare. Improving transitions of care: Hand-off communications. Oakbrook Terrace, Illinois: The Joint Commission, 2014.

manner. The handover needs to be conducted both verbally **and** in writing without distractions. The communication should be conducted face-to-face and may include others, such as family members or other healthcare professionals when appropriate. Both individuals involved in the handover must be attentive to the communication. Each medical center should continually assess the handover process used at their institution and make changes when appropriate.

There are several standardized handover formats with easy-to-remember mnemonics, including **I-PASS** (**I**llness severity, **P**atient summary, **A**ction list, **S**ituation awareness, and contingency plans, and **S**ynthesis by the receiver) and **ISBAR** (**I**dentification, **S**ituation, **B**ackground, **A**ssessment, and **R**ecommendations). Other mnemonics have been developed for specialized services. The use of electronic health record (EHR) capabilities and other technologies such as apps, patient portals, and telehealth may have a role in enhancing hand-overs between senders and receivers.

8

HANDOVERS: THE ESSENTIAL ELEMENTS

This is based on the following publication: The Joint Commission. Inadequate Hand-off Communication. *Sentinel Alert Event* 2017;58:1–6. Available at https://www.jointcommission.org/assets (accessed November 8, 2020).

- Name of the patient, room number, and nurse caring for the patient
- Illness assessment, including severity
- Patient summary: Briefly outline the events leading to admission, the hospital course, and plans of care
- To-do list: What needs to be done by the receiver (test results to check on, consult notes to review, etc.)
- Contingency plans: What to do if… (who needs to be contacted, what needs to be ordered, what needs to be administered if…)
- Allergies: Should be noted
- Code status: Officially documented in the medical record
- Medications: Routine and PRN
- Laboratory and procedure results: The most current and essential
- Physical examination findings, including vital signs (dated and timed) and any abnormal findings

A sample of a written handover and what would also be communicated verbally to the receiving physician for our patient Mr. Jones on the evening of his third day in the hospital is illustrated here:

- **Robert Jones:** 6E, room 633, and night shift nurse L. Vance, RN.
- **Acute coronary syndrome:** non-ST-elevation MI type 1, 3 days ago, status post cardiac cath with balloon angioplasty for single-lesion mid-LAD 1 day ago; stable.

- **Hypertension:** on chlorthalidone 50 mg/day; BPs 100–108/66–72; excellent control.
- **Chronic bronchitis:** 70 pack-year hx of smoking plus single palpable axillary lymph node, low-dose CT to rule out lung cancer, scheduled for tomorrow morning; stable.
- **Eosinophilia:** unknown cause, rule out parasitic cause; stool for ova and parasites pending, will complete outpatient workup after discharge.
- **Presentation:** Classic history of unstable angina for about 1 month prior to presenting with 10 hr of substernal chest pain, troponin peaked at 24 ng/mL, initially 3–4 mm ST depression V1–V4, upon transfer to UK 1-mm ST depression and inverted T-waves V1–V4. Underwent cath and intervention as noted earlier. No CP since in the ER at his local hospital.
- **Hospital course:** as earlier, uneventful; low-dose CT of chest tomorrow; may discharge to home after CT; follow-up with Dr. Doyle, Whitesburg, Kentucky.
- **To-do list:** only pending test is one stool for ova and parasite, and I will check the results in the morning; please stop by and see if he or his family have any questions about the CT tomorrow; family will be visiting after dinner.
- **Contingency plans:** if any chest pain, immediately contact cardiac cath team.
- **Allergies:** PCN, rash as child.
- **Code status:** full code.
- **Medications:** atorvastatin 80 mg/day, metoprolol 50 mg twice a day, aspirin 81 mg/day, ticagrelor 90 mg twice a day, chlorthalidone 50 mg/day, acetaminophen 500 mg PRN.
- **Laboratory and procedure results:** troponin 1.6 ng/mL this AM; ECG this AM, no ST depression, T-wave changes V1–V4.
- **PE:** BP 106/72 mm Hg, HR 60 BPM, Resp 14/min, Temp 98.8°F; inspiratory crackles both bases, do not clear with coughing; inferiorly and laterally displaced PMI (sixth ICS between anterior axillary line and MCL), S_4 initially, not audible since admission; 1 × 1 cm left axillary LN.

Differential Diagnosis

9

- ➤ Abdominal Distention
- ➤ Abdominal Pain
- ➤ Adrenal Mass
- ➤ Alopecia
- ➤ Amenorrhea
- ➤ Anorexia
- ➤ Anuria
- ➤ Arthritis
- ➤ Ascites
- ➤ Back Pain
- ➤ Breast Lump
- ➤ Chest Pain
- ➤ Chills
- ➤ Clubbing
- ➤ Coma
- ➤ Constipation
- ➤ Cough: Acute and Chronic
- ➤ Cyanosis
- ➤ Delirium
- ➤ Dementia
- ➤ Diaphoresis
- ➤ Diarrhea: Acute and Chronic
- ➤ Diplopia
- ➤ Dizziness
- ➤ Dyspareunia
- ➤ Dysphagia
- ➤ Dyspnea
- ➤ Dysuria
- ➤ Earache
- ➤ Edema

- ➤ Epistaxis
- ➤ Facial Swelling
- ➤ Failure to Thrive
- ➤ Fever
- ➤ Fever of Unknown Origin (FUO)
- ➤ Flank Pain
- ➤ Flatulence
- ➤ Frequency
- ➤ Galactorrhea
- ➤ Genital Sore
- ➤ Gynecomastia
- ➤ Headache
- ➤ Heartburn
- ➤ Hematemesis, Melenemesis, and Melena
- ➤ Hematochezia
- ➤ Hematuria
- ➤ Hemoptysis
- ➤ Hepatomegaly
- ➤ Hiccups (Singultus)
- ➤ Hirsutism
- ➤ Hypersomnia
- ➤ Impotence (Erectile Dysfunction)
- ➤ Incontinence (Urinary)
- ➤ Insomnia
- ➤ Jaundice
- ➤ Loss of Consciousness

- ➤ Low Back Pain
- ➤ Lymphadenopathy and Splenomegaly
- ➤ Melena
- ➤ Nausea and Vomiting
- ➤ Night Sweats
- ➤ Nystagmus
- ➤ Oliguria/Anuria
- ➤ Palpitations
- ➤ Pleural Effusion
- ➤ Pruritis
- ➤ Seizures
- ➤ Sleep Disturbance: Insomnia, Hypersomnia
- ➤ Smell Disorders: Anosmia, Hyposmia, Parosmia, Olfactory hallucination
- ➤ Splenomegaly
- ➤ Syncope
- ➤ Taste Disorders: Dysgeusia, Hypogeusia, Ageusia
- ➤ Tremors
- ➤ Vaginal Bleeding
- ➤ Vaginal Discharge
- ➤ Vertigo
- ➤ Vision Loss, Acute
- ➤ Vomiting
- ➤ Weight loss
- ➤ Wheezing
- ➤ Xerostomia

Chapter update by Brian Calio, MD, and Leonard G. Gomella, MD

This section presents some of the more common presenting symptoms, physical signs, and other conditions that are encountered in daily patient care. It is not an all-inclusive listing but provides a starting point for patient care. This primarily notes common diagnostic possibilities in adults with select pediatric differentials.

ABDOMINAL DISTENTION

Ascites, intestinal obstruction, ovarian/renal cysts, tumors, hepatosplenomegaly, abdominal aortic aneurysm, uterine enlargement (pregnancy), bladder distention/retention, inflammatory mass

ABDOMINAL PAIN (See also Figure 9-1)

Characterized by location of abdominal pain based on Figure 9-1.

Diffuse: Gastroenteritis, intestinal angina, early appendicitis, colitis, diabetic ketoacidosis, hereditary angioedema, mesenteric thrombosis, mesenteric lymphadenitis, peritonitis, porphyria, sickle cell crisis, uremia, renal colic, renal infarct, pancreatitis

Right upper quadrant: Gallbladder disease (cholecystitis, cholangitis, choledocholithiasis), hepatitis, hepatomegaly, pancreatitis, pneumonia, pulmonary embolus, pyelonephritis, renal colic, renal infarct, appendicitis (retroperitoneal)

Left upper quadrant: Esophagitis, hiatal hernia, esophageal rupture, gastritis, pancreatitis, PUD, myocardial infarction, pericarditis, dissecting aneurysm, pneumonia, pulmonary embolus, pyelonephritis, renal colic, renal infarct, splenic abscess, splenic rupture, splenic infarct

Lower abdomen: Aortic aneurysm, colitis including inflammatory bowel disease, diverticulitis including Meckel diverticulum, intestinal obstruction, hernia, perforated viscus, pregnancy, ectopic pregnancy, dysmenorrhea, endometriosis, mittelschmerz (ovulation), ovarian cyst or tumor (especially with torsion), PID, renal colic, UTI, rectal hematoma, bladder distension

Right lower quadrant: Appendicitis, ectopic pregnancy, ovarian cyst or tumor, salpingitis, mittelschmerz, cholecystitis, perforated duodenal ulcer, Crohn's disease

ADRENAL MASS

Adenoma, hyperplasia, metastasis, adrenocortical carcinoma, pheochromocytoma, cyst, varices, hemorrhage, congenital adrenal hyperplasia, ganglioneuroma, micronodular adrenal disease

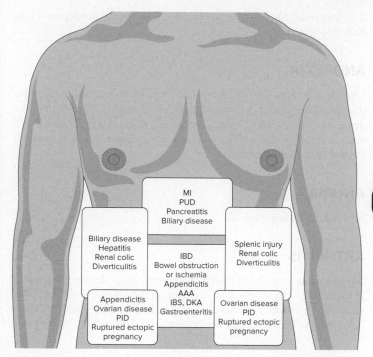

AAA, abdominal aortic aneurysm; DKA, diabetic ketoacidosis; IBD, inflammatory bowel disease; IBS, irritable bowel syndrome; MI, myocardial infarction; PID, pelvic inflammatory disease; PUD, peptic ulcer disease.

Figure 9-1. Abdominal pain differential based on location. (From Stern SC, Cifu AS, Altkorn D. [eds.]. *Symptom to Diagnosis: An Evidence-Based Guide*, 4e, New York, NY: McGraw-Hill; 2006.)

ALOPECIA

Male pattern baldness (androgenic type in both men and women), trauma and trichotillomania, tinea capitis, bacterial folliculitis, telogen arrest, anagen arrest (chemotherapy, radiation therapy), alopecia areata, discoid lupus

AMENORRHEA

Pregnancy, excessive exercise, menopause, severe illness, weight loss, stress, delayed puberty, gonadal dysgenesis (i.e., Turner syndrome), hypothalamic and pituitary tumors, virilizing syndromes (polycystic ovaries), anatomical anomaly (imperforate hymen, uterine agenesis), enzymatic deficiencies (i.e., congenital adrenal hyperplasia), disorders of sexual development (i.e., Kallmann syndrome)

ANOREXIA

Chronic infections, gastritis, duodenitis, esophagitis, hepatitis, carcinomas, digitalis toxicity, uremia, anxiety, depression, alcohol/drug dependence, dementia/delirium, CHF, radiation exposure, chemotherapy, anorexia nervosa, debilitating illness (e.g., end-stage lung disease, terminal cancers), CKD/ESRD, liver cirrhosis

ANURIA

See Oliguria/Anuria, page 163

ARTHRITIS

Bursitis, tendonitis, osteoarthritis, connective tissue disease (rheumatoid arthritis, SLE, scleroderma, gout, psoriatic arthritis, Reiter syndrome, rheumatic fever), infections (bacterial, viral, TB, fungal, Lyme disease), trauma, sarcoidosis, sickle cell anemia, hemochromatosis, amyloidosis, coagulopathy

ASCITES

Use serum albumin to ascetic albumin difference to differentiate cause of ascites. If the difference is >1.1, portal hypertension is present. If the difference is <1.1, the cause is not portal hypertension. CHF, tricuspid insufficiency, constrictive pericarditis, venous occlusion, cirrhosis, pancreatitis, peritonitis, tumor, trauma, myxedema, anasarca (hypoalbuminemia), ovarian fibroma associated with hydrothorax and ascites (Meigs syndrome)

BACK PAIN

Herniated disk, spinal stenosis, ankylosing spondylitis, metastatic tumor, multiple myeloma, mechanical back sprain, vertebral body fracture, osteoporosis-induced fracture, infectious process (osteomyelitis, epidural abscess), referred pain (visceral, vascular) including pyelonephritis and colitis, endometriosis, abdominal aortic aneurysm, psychiatric disorder including malingering, substance abuse, depression

BREAST LUMP

Cancer, fibroadenoma, fibrocystic disease, fat necrosis, gynecomastia (male patients, alcoholic patients)

CHEST PAIN

Deep, dull, poorly localized: Angina, variant angina, unstable angina, AMI, aortic aneurysm, pulmonary embolus, tumor, gallbladder disease, pulmonary hypertension, GERD, anxiety/panic attack

Sharp, well-localized: Pulmonary embolus, pneumothorax, pleurodynia, pericarditis, atypical MI, hyperventilation, hiatal hernia, esophagitis, esophageal spasm, herpes zoster, aortic aneurysm, breast lesions, bony/soft tissue abnormalities (rib fracture, costochondritis, muscle damage), perforated ulcer, pancreatitis, acute cholecystitis

CHILLS

Infection, neoplasm (Hodgkin lymphoma), drug and transfusion reactions, hypothermia

CLUBBING

Clubbing is bulbous enlargement of the ends of one or more fingers or toes. Pulmonary causes (abscess, bronchiectasis, fibrosis, tuberculosis, cancer), AV malformations, cardiac conditions (congenital cyanotic heart diseases, endocarditis), hereditary conditions, thyrotoxicosis, GI (inflammatory bowel disease, cirrhosis)

COMA

Use the mnemonic **AEIOU TIPS: A**lcohol, **E**ncephalitis (other CNS causes such as epilepsy, hemorrhage, mass), **I**nsulin (hypoglycemia, hyperglycemia), **O**piates, **U**remia (and other metabolic conditions such as hyper/hyponatremia, hypercalcemia, hepatic failure, thiamine deficiency), **T**rauma, **I**nfection, **P**sychiatric causes, **S**yncope (including decreased cardiac output from aortic stenosis, arrhythmia)

CONSTIPATION

Dehydration, lack of exercise, bedrest, medications (narcotics, anticholinergics, antidepressants, calcium channel blockers, clonidine, diuretics, aluminum or calcium containing antacids, laxative abuse, megacolon, fecal impaction), neoplasm, intestinal obstruction, vascular occlusion of the bowel, inflammatory process, hemorrhoids, fissures, neurologic disorders (spinal cord lesions/trauma), diabetes mellitus, porphyria, hypothyroidism, hypercalcemia, hypokalemia, hypomagnesemia, irritable bowel syndrome

9

COUGH

Acute: Tracheobronchitis, pneumonia, recently described for SARS-CoV-2 infection, sinusitis, pulmonary edema, foreign body, toxic inhalation, allergy, pharyngitis, asthma, GERD, ACE inhibitors, impacted cerumen or ear foreign body, CHF exacerbation

Chronic: Bronchitis (smoker), chronic sinusitis, emphysema, bronchiectasis, cancer (bronchogenic, head and neck, esophageal), TB, interstitial lung disease, mediastinal lymphadenopathy, GERD, ACE inhibitors

CYANOSIS

Peripheral: Arterial occlusion and insufficiency, vasospasm and Raynaud disease, venous stasis, venous obstruction

Central: Hypoxia, congenital heart disease (right-to-left shunt), pulmonary embolus, pseudo-cyanosis (polycythemia), methemoglobinemia

DELIRIUM

Metabolic: Hypoglycemia, hypoxia, hyponatremia, hypernatremia, hypercalcemia, hypercarbia, uremia, hyperthyroidism

Neurologic: Stroke, subdural and epidural hematoma, subarachnoid hemorrhage, postictal state, traumatic brain injury, meningitis, encephalitis, brain tumor

Drug or toxin induced: Lithium intoxication, ethanol, steroids, anticholinergics, sympathomimetics, poisons (mushrooms, carbon monoxide), drugs of abuse

Other: Sepsis, thiamine deficiency, niacin deficiency. Delirium in the ICU is discussed in Chapter 28, page 886.

DEMENTIA

Chronic CNS disease: Alzheimer disease, Pick disease, Parkinson disease, multiple sclerosis, ALS, brain tumor, normal pressure hydrocephalus, Wilson disease, Huntington disease, Tay–Sachs, Lewy body dementia

Metabolic: Hypoxia, hypoglycemia, hyperammonemia, dialysis, heavy-metal intoxication, pernicious anemia, niacin/thiamine deficiency, medications (barbiturates, phenothiazines, lithium, benzodiazepines)

Infectious: AIDS encephalopathy, brain abscess, chronic meningoencephalitis, encephalitis, Creutzfeldt–Jakob disease

Vascular: Vasculitis, multiple cerebral infarcts (i.e., vascular dementia)

Traumatic: Contusion, hemorrhage, subdural hematoma

Psychiatric: Sensory deprivation, depression (pseudodementia)

DIAPHORESIS

Hypoglycemia, fever, endocarditis, anxiety, MI, heat exhaustion, HIV, hyperhidrosis, hyperthyroidism, malaria, menopause, non-Hodgkin lymphoma and tuberculosis (night sweats), substance abuse

DIARRHEA

Acute: Infection, toxic (food poisoning, chemical), drugs (antibiotics, cholinergic agents, lactulose, magnesium-containing antacids, SSRIs, metformin, acarbose, orlistat, digoxin, sorbitol), appendicitis, diverticular disease, GI bleeding, ischemic colitis, food intolerance, fructose intolerance, fecal impaction (paradoxical diarrhea), serotonin syndrome, recently described with SARS-CoV-2 infection

Chronic: Postoperative state (gastrectomy, vagotomy, bowel resection), Zollinger-Ellison syndrome, ulcerative colitis, Crohn disease, microscopic colitis, irritable bowel syndrome (IBS), malabsorption, diverticular disease, carcinoma, villous adenoma, gastrinoma, lymphoma of the bowel, functional bowel disorder (irritable colon, mucous colitis), pseudomembranous colitis (Clostridioides difficile infection), endocrine disease (carcinoid, hyperthyroidism, Addison disease), radiation enteritis, drugs, Whipple disease, celiac disease, amyloidosis, AIDS-related infection, pellagra

DIPLOPIA

Problems with the third, fourth, or sixth cranial nerve (e.g., from vascular disturbances, meningitis, tumor, demyelination, orbital blow-out fracture); hyperthyroidism; ocular myopathy; strabismus; alcohol intoxication

DIZZINESS

Hyperventilation, depression, hypoglycemia, anemia, volume depletion, hypoxia, trauma, benign paroxysmal positional vertigo, Meniere disease, aminoglycoside toxicity, vestibular neuronitis, multiple sclerosis (MS), brainstem ischemia or stroke, posterior fossa lesions, cerebellar ischemia or stroke, arrhythmia, aortic stenosis, carotid sinus hypersensitivity, postural tachycardia, subclavian steal, vasovagal reaction, medications (vasodilators, benzodiazepines, others), orthostatic hypotension, peripheral neuropathy, primary autonomic failure (multiple sclerosis, multiple system atrophy [Shy–Drager syndrome], Parkinson disease/parkinsonism, Wernicke encephalopathy), secondary autonomic failure (amyloidosis, chronic inflammatory demyelinating polyneuropathy, connective tissue diseases, diabetes mellitus, Lewy body dementia, older age, spinal cord injury, uremia)

DYSPAREUNIA

Atrophic vaginitis, endometriosis, cervicitis, vaginismus, vulvodynia, pelvic inflammatory disease

DYSPHAGIA

Loss of tongue function, pharyngeal dysfunction (myasthenia gravis), Zenker diverticulum, tumors (bronchogenic, head and neck, esophageal), stricture, esophageal web, epiglottitis, eosinophilic esophagitis, esophageal compression (e.g., left atrial dilation from chronic mitral stenosis), laryngeal nerve injury, Schatzki ring, lower esophageal spasm, foreign body, aortic aneurysm, achalasia, scleroderma, diabetic neuropathy, amyloidosis, infection (especially candidiasis), polymyositis, MS, brainstem infarct, Plummer–Vinson syndrome, amyotrophic lateral sclerosis (ALS)

DYSPNEA

Laryngeal and tracheal infections, foreign bodies, and narrowing/stricture; tumors, COPD, asthma, pneumonia, aspiration, interstitial lung disease, lung carcinoma, atelectasis, pneumothorax, pleural effusion, hemothorax, pulmonary embolus, pulmonary infarction, carbon monoxide poisoning, cardiac/noncardiac pulmonary edema, acute coronary syndrome, arrhythmia, aortic stenosis/regurgitation, mitral stenosis/regurgitation, pericardial tamponade, anemia, abdominal distention, myopathies, neuropathies, spinal cord disorders, phrenic nerve and diaphragmatic disorders, GERD, deconditioning, anxiety

DYSURIA

Urethral stricture, stones, blood clot, tumor (bladder, prostate, urethral), prostatic enlargement, infection (urethritis, cystitis, vaginitis, prostatitis), atrophic vaginitis, trauma, bladder spasm, dehydration, urethral syndrome or interstitial cystitis

EARACHE

Otitis media and externa, mastoiditis, serous otitis, otic barotrauma, foreign body, impacted cerumen, referred pain (dental or temporomandibular joint (TMJ)

EDEMA

Right-sided CHF, constrictive pericarditis, liver disease (cirrhosis), nephrotic syndrome, nephritic syndrome, hypoalbuminemia, malnutrition, hypothyroidism/myxedema, hemiplegia, volume overload, obstructive sleep apnea, lymphatic obstruction (malignancy, post-radiation therapy), medications (non-dihydropyridine calcium channel blockers, others), venous insufficiency/stasis, deep vein thrombosis, cellulitis, preeclampsia, eclampsia

EPISTAXIS

Trauma (e.g., nose picking), neoplasm, polyps, foreign body, desiccation, coagulopathy, medications (use of cocaine, nasal spray), infection (sinusitis), uremia, hypertension

FACIAL SWELLING

Allergic reaction, drugs including ACE inhibitors, cellulitis, sinusitis, hypothyroidism, abscess, preeclampsia, eclampsia, angioedema, actinomycosis, trauma, superior vena cava syndrome, C1-inhibitor deficiency

FAILURE TO THRIVE

Environmental: Social deprivation, decreased food intake
Organic: CNS disorder, intestinal malabsorption, cystic fibrosis, parasites, cleft palate, heart failure, endocrine disease, hypercalcemia, Turner syndrome, renal disease, chronic infection, malignant diseases

FEVER

In adults, a morning temperature above 98.8°F or a night temperature above 99.9°F is generally defined as a fever. See Chapter 6, page 53, for details on Temperature Considerations. Infection, neoplasm (lymphoma, leukemia, renal and hepatic carcinoma), hemophagocytic lymphohistiocytosis (HLH) connective tissue disease (SLE, vasculitis, rheumatoid arthritis, adult Still disease, temporal arteritis), heat illness, malignant hyperthermia, neuroleptic malignant syndrome (NMS), serotonin syndrome, thyroid storm, pheochromocytoma, adrenal insufficiency, pulmonary embolus, MI, inflammatory bowel disease, drugs (most commonly antipsychotics, amphotericin, bleomycin, barbiturates, cephalosporins, methyldopa, penicillins, phenytoin, procainamide, sulfonamides, quinidine, cocaine, LSD, phencyclidine, ketamine, 3,4-methylenedioxymethamphetamine [MDMA] [ecstasy] and amphetamines)

FEVER OF UNKNOWN ORIGIN (FUO)

Definition: In adults, defined as a temperature of 101°F or greater for at least 3 weeks and for which a diagnosis is not established after 1 week of hospitalization or three ambulatory visits. In children, the minimum duration is 2 weeks and the temperature is at least 101.3°F.
Causes: TB, fungal infection, endocarditis, abscess (especially hepatic), neoplasm (lymphoma, renal cell, hepatoma, preleukemia), atrial myxoma, connective tissue disease (especially temporal arteritis in the elderly), drugs (see Fever), pulmonary embolus, Crohn disease, ulcerative colitis, hypothalamic injury, factitious disorder

FLANK PAIN

Renal obstruction, renal/ureteral stones, GU malignancy, rib fracture, musculoskeletal, infection/inflammation (pyelonephritis/renal abscess), retroperitoneal fibrosis or other condition causing hydronephrosis, referred pain (thoracic pathologies), dermatologic conditions (shingles)

FLATULENCE

Aerophagia, food intolerance (such as lactose intolerance), bowel motility disorders/disturbances (including diabetes, uremia), gallbladder disease, medications (e.g., acarbose, orlistat), celiac disease, irritable bowel syndrome, certain foods (i.e., beans, dairy)

FREQUENCY

Infection (bladder, prostate), excessive fluid intake, use of diuretics (also coffee, tea, or cola), diabetes mellitus, diabetes insipidus, prostatic obstruction (BPH), bladder stones, bladder tumors, pregnancy, psychogenic bladder syndrome, neurogenic bladder, interstitial cystitis

GALACTORRHEA

Hyperprolactinemia, prolonged breastfeeding, major stress, pituitary tumors, breast lesions (benign, cancer, inflammatory), hypothyroidism, chronic renal failure, cirrhosis, idiopathic with menses, drugs (i.e., oral contraceptives, dopamine antagonists such as first-generation antipsychotics, amitriptyline, SSRIs, opioids, H2 antagonists, verapamil, methydopa, others)

GENITAL SORE

Syphilis (chancre), chancroid, granuloma inguinale, lymphogranuloma venereum, genital herpes, traumatic ulcer, fixed drug eruption, scabies, malignant ulceration (penile cancer), Behçet ulcer

GYNECOMASTIA

Normal (physiologic): Newborn, adolescence, aging
Pathologic: Drugs (cimetidine, spironolactone, estrogens, gonadotropins, marijuana, anti-androgens), decreased testosterone (Klinefelter, testicular failure), increased estrogen production (hermaphroditism, testicular or lung cancer, adrenal and liver diseases)

HEADACHE

Cluster: Severe, sharp, stabbing, usually unilateral clustered every day to every other day, lasting 30 min to 2 hr, classically occur in the early morning (3 AM) over 1–4 mo, relieved with high-flow oxygen

Tension: Steady, nonpulsatile bandlike distribution, stress-related, increases as day progresses

Migraine: Precipitated by a factor such as menses or a food and is classically preceded by an aura, but absence of aura is more common; photophobia, nausea/vomiting, neurologic complaints, unilateral deep, throbbing severe parietal-temporal pain

Other types: Benign exertional, benign cough headache, vascular (menstruation hypertension), ice pick headache, eye strain, acute glaucoma, uveitis, keratitis, sinusitis, dental problems, TMJ disease, trauma, subarachnoid hemorrhage, intracranial mass, carotid or vertebral artery dissection, fever, meningitis, pseudotumor cerebri, trigeminal neuralgia, temporal arteritis, hypoglycemia, toxin exposure (carbon monoxide poisoning), drugs, vasculitis, cerebral abscess

HEARTBURN

GERD, esophagitis, hiatal hernia, peptic ulcer, gallbladder disease, medications (bisphosphonates), tumors, scleroderma, food intolerance. Myocardial ischemia can be mistaken for heartburn.

HEMATEMESIS, MELENEMESIS, AND MELENA

Melena: Black, tarry stools caused by stomach acid or intestinal bacterial conversion of hemoglobin to the black pigment hematin; suggests blood loss of >50–100mL

Hematemesis: Vomiting blood

Melenemesis: Vomiting of material that looks like coffee grounds

Note: These three conditions suggest a bleeding site in the upper GI tract but can be as distal as the right colon with reflux of blood through the pylorus. Swallowed blood (e.g., from epistaxis), esophageal varices, esophagitis, Mallory-Weiss syndrome, hiatal hernia, gastritis, duodenal or gastric ulcer, duodenitis, gastric carcinoma, tumors (small and large bowel), ischemic colitis, and aortoenteric fistula. Bleeding diathesis and anticoagulation can unmask GI tract pathology. Medications (e.g., bismuth-containing medications and iron supplements) can darken stool.

HEMATOCHEZIA

A grossly bloody stool, massive upper GI bleeding, hemorrhoids, anal fissures, diverticular disease, angiodysplasia, polyps, carcinoma, inflammatory bowel disease, ischemic colitis

HEMATURIA

GU neoplasms (malignant and benign), polycystic kidneys, trauma, infection (urethra, bladder, prostate), stones, glomerulonephritis (primary and secondary such as granulomatosis with polyangiitis, anti-glomerular basement membrane disease [Goodpasture synd], SLE, and polyarteritis nodosa), renal infarction, renal vein thrombosis, enterovesical fistula, sickle cell anemia, vigorous exercise ("runner's hematuria"), accelerated hypertension, factitious and vaginal and rectal bleeding. Bleeding diathesis and anticoagulation can unmask GU tract pathology.

False positives: Myoglobinuria, hemoglobinuria, porphyria, foods such as beets, medications that color the urine (phenazopyridine)

HEMOPTYSIS

Infection (pneumonia, bronchitis, fungal, TB), bronchiectasis, cancer (bronchogenic or metastatic), bronchial adenoma, pulmonary embolus, AV malformation, granulomatosis with polyangiitis, anti-glomerular basement membrane disease (Goodpasture synd), SLE, pulmonary hemosiderosis, foreign body, trauma, bleeding diathesis, excessive anticoagulation can unmask underlying pulmonary pathology, cardiogenic pulmonary edema, mitral stenosis

HEPATOMEGALY

Right-sided CHF, tricuspid stenosis, hepatitis, fatty liver, tumors (primary and metastatic), biliary obstruction, hemochromatosis, chronic granulomatous disease, amyloidosis, infection, hepatic vein thrombosis (Budd Chiari synd), Wolman disease. Riedel lobe is a normal-variant, elongated right lobe of the liver with normal total liver volume.

HICCUPS (SINGULTUS)

Uremia, electrolyte disorders, diabetes, medications (benzodiazepines, barbiturates), emotionally induced, gastric distention, CNS disorders, thoracic and diaphragmatic disorders (pneumonia, MI), alcohol ingestion

HIRSUTISM

Idiopathic, familial, adrenal causes (Cushing disease, congenital adrenal hyperplasia, adenoma, and carcinoma), polycystic ovaries, medications, androgen-secreting tumors (i.e., testicular, ovarian)

HYPERSOMNIA

See Sleep Disturbance, page 165

IMPOTENCE (ERECTILE DYSFUNCTION)

Psychogenic, vascular, neurologic (spinal cord injury, radical prostatectomy, rectal surgery, aortic bypass), pelvic radiation, medications (common drugs: antihypertensives, especially thiazide diuretics, beta blockers, methyldopa; antidepressants, especially the SSRIs, anticholinergics; alcohol, narcotics, antipsychotics, H2 blockers, finasteride, spironolactone), history of priapism/Peyronie disease, hyperprolactinemia, testicular failure

9

INCONTINENCE (URINARY)

Cystitis, dementia and delirium, stroke, prostatic hypertrophy, fecal impaction, peripheral or autonomic neuropathy, medications (diuretics, sedatives, alpha-blockers), diabetes, spinal cord trauma or lesions, MS, childbirth, surgery, aging, estrogen deficiency, normal pressure hydrocephalus, seizures

INSOMNIA

See Sleep Disturbance, page 165

JAUNDICE

Hepatitis (alcoholic, viral, autoimmune, medications, toxins), Gilbert disease, Crigler-Najjar syndrome, Dubin-Johnsons syndrome, Wilson disease, drug-induced cholestasis (phenothiazines and estrogen), gallbladder and biliary tract disease (including inflammation, infection, obstruction, and hepatic, primary and metastatic tumors), hemolysis, neonatal jaundice, cholestatic jaundice of pregnancy, total parenteral nutrition (TPN)

LOSS OF CONSCIOUSNESS (See also Syncope)

Seizure, cardiac arrhythmia (bradyarrhythmias, ventricular tachyarrhythmias, supraventricular tachyarrhythmias, pacemaker dysfunction), MI, obstructive cardiomyopathy, acute aortic dissection, cardiac tamponade, carotid sinus syndrome/hypersensitivity syncope, vasovagal (induced by fear, heat exposure, noxious stimuli, pain, stress, other), postural tachycardia syndrome, stroke, pulmonary embolism, substance abuse/overdose, hypoglycemia, malingering, drug-induced hypotension, volume depletion (acute blood loss [e.g., GI bleed, ectopic pregnancy]), diarrhea, inadequate fluid intake, vomiting, primary autonomic failure (multiple sclerosis, multiple system atrophy

[Shy–Drager syndrome], Parkinson disease/parkinsonism, Wernicke encephalopathy), secondary autonomic failure (amyloidosis, chronic inflammatory demyelinating polyneuropathy, connective tissue diseases, diabetes mellitus, Lewy body dementia, older age, spinal cord injury, uremia)

LOW BACK PAIN

Herniated disc, degenerative disc disease, spinal stenosis, spondylolisthesis, lumbar muscle/ligament strain, vertebral compression or traumatic fracture, osteoporosis, scoliosis, kyphosis, tumor in vertebral canal, peripheral vascular disease, malingering, ankylosing spondylitis, Reiter syndrome, sacroiliitis, osteoarthritis, osteomyelitis

LYMPHADENOPATHY AND SPLENOMEGALY

Infection (bacterial, fungal, viral, parasitic), benign neoplasm (histiocytosis), malignant neoplasm (primary lymphoma, metastatic), hemophagocytic lymphohistiocytosis (HLH), sarcoidosis, connective tissue disease (e.g., rheumatoid arthritis, SLE), lipid storage diseases, drugs (e.g., phenytoin), HIV and AIDS, splenomegaly without lymphadenopathy (cirrhosis, hereditary spherocytosis, hemoglobinopathies, hairy cell leukemia, histiocytosis X, amyloidosis, Wolman disease, lysosomal storage disorders)

MELENA

See Hematemesis, Melenemesis, and Melena, page 159

NAUSEA AND VOMITING

Appendicitis, acute cholecystitis, chronic gallbladder disease, PUD, gastritis, pancreatitis, gastric distention, intestinal ischemia, intestinal obstruction, peritonitis, food intolerance, intestinal infection, acute systemic infections, hepatitis, toxins, CNS disorders (tumor, hemorrhagic stroke, hydrocephalus, meningitis; increased intracranial pressure often causes vomiting without nausea), labyrinthitis, Meniere disease, migraine headache, acute coronary syndrome, CHF, endocrine disorders, hypercalcemia, hyperkalemia, hypokalemia, pyelonephritis, nephrolithiasis, uremia, hepatic failure, psychogenic vomiting, pregnancy, PID, drugs, porphyria, radiation therapy

NIGHT SWEATS

Malignancy (lymphoma, leukemia, others), infections (HIV, TB, *Mycobacterium avium* complex, infectious mononucleosis, fungal infections [histoplasmosis, blastomycosis, coccidioidomycosis], lung abscess, endocarditis), endocrine (ovarian failure/menopause, hyperthyroidism, diabetes [nocturnal hypoglycemia], endocrine tumors [pheochromocytoma, carcinoid], orchiectomy/LHRH induced hypogonadism), Takayasu's arteritis, temporal arteritis, obstructive sleep apnea, gastroesophageal reflux disease, chronic fatigue syndrome, illicit drug use or withdrawal (alcohol, heroin)

NYSTAGMUS

Congenital, vision loss early in life, MS, neoplasms, ocular infarct, toxic or metabolic encephalopathy, drugs (phenytoin, lithium, alcohol intoxication), thiamine deficiency (Wernicke encephalopathy), cerebellar degeneration, medications, encephalitis, vascular brainstem lesions, Arnold-Chiari malformation, extreme lateral gaze, gaze fixation on rapidly moving object (train)

OLIGURIA/ANURIA

Definitions: Oliguria is <500 mL urine/24 hr; anuria is <100 mL urine/ 24 hr in adults
Prerenal: Volume depletion, shock, heart failure, intravascular fluid movement to third space (extensive burns, pancreatitis, hypothyroidism, any cause of severe hypoalbuminemia), renal artery compromise
Renal: Glomerular disease, acute tubular necrosis, bilateral cortical necrosis, interstitial disease, transfusion reaction, myoglobinuria, radiographic contrast media (especially with diabetes, dehydration, and elderly patients and those with multiple myeloma), ESRD, drugs (aminoglycosides, amphotericin B, vancomycin, cephalosporins, penicillins, sulfa drugs) malignant hypertension, ischemia, emboli, thrombosis, TTP, HUS, and DIC
Postrenal: Bilateral ureteral obstruction, prostatic obstruction, neurogenic bladder

PALPITATIONS

Anxiety, arrhythmias (sinus tachycardia, atrial fibrillation, paroxysmal supraventricular tachycardia, premature ventricular contractions), cardiac structural problems (mitral valve prolapse), pericarditis, hypoglycemia, hyperthyroidism, stimulants, pheochromocytomas

PLEURAL EFFUSION

(See also Chapter 19, Thoracentesis, page 656.)

Transudate: (Pleural to serum protein ratio <0.5, pleural to serum LDH ratio <0.6, and pleural LDH <2/3 the upper limit of normal for serum LDH), CHF, cirrhosis, nephrotic syndrome, peritoneal dialysis

Exudate: (Pleural to serum protein ratio >0.5, pleural to serum LDH ratio >0.6, or pleural LDH >2/3 the upper limit of normal for serum LDH), bacterial or viral pneumonia, pulmonary infarction, TB, rheumatoid arthritis, SLE, malignancy (most common, breast, lung, lymphoma, leukemia, ovarian, unknown primary, GI, mesothelioma), pancreatitis, pneumothorax, chest trauma, uremia

Chylothorax: Traumatic or postoperative complication

Empyema: Bacteria, fungi, TB, trauma, surgery

Hydrothorax: Usually iatrogenic (central venous catheter complication)

PRURITIS

Dermatologic: Atopic dermatitis, seborrheic dermatitis, contact dermatitis, fiberglass dermatitis, folliculitis, psoriasis, urticaria, infestations (bed bugs, pediculosis, pinworms, scabies), dermatophytosis (tinea corporis/cruris/pedis), psychiatric (anorexia nervosa, depression, delusional parasitosis, obsessive compulsive disorder, stress, neurotic excoriations), fibromyalgia, bullous skin disorders (bullous pemphigoid, dermatitis herpetiformis, drug eruption), lichen planus, lichen sclerosus, neoplasia/paraneoplastic-related, lichen simplex chronicus, cutaneous T-cell lymphoma, advanced age (senile), xerosis, pregnancy-associated, stasis dermatitis (venous eczema), mastocytosis (cutaneous and systemic)

Nondermatologic: Cholestasis (intrahepatic, extrahepatic, drug induced), end-stage renal disease, neurologic (multiple sclerosis, brain neoplasm, cerebrovascular accident, brachioradial pruritus, notalgia paresthetica, postherpetic neuralgia, small fiber neuropathy), hematopoietic diseases (lymphoma, multiple myeloma, myeloproliferative/myelodysplastic disorders [polycythemia vera, essential thrombocytosis, primary myelofibrosis], iron-deficiency anemia), endocrine diseases (diabetes/diabetic neuropathy, thyroid disease, parathyroid disease, gout), connective tissue diseases (dermatomyositis, scleroderma, Sjögren syndrome), medications (most common, opioids, antihypertensives [ACE inhibitors, ARBs, beta-adrenergic blockers, diuretics, calcium channel blockers]), antibiotics, metformin, sulphonyl urea derivatives, chloroquine, hydroxyethyl starch, satins, HIV, senile (age-related) pruritus, post-transplant, intestinal parasites

SEIZURES

Generalized: Grand mal and petit mal (absence), febrile

Partial seizures: Partial motor, partial sensory, partial complex (psychomotor or temporal lobe)

Causes: Primary or metastatic CNS tumors, trauma, metabolic disorders (e.g., hypoglycemia, hypocalcemia, hypomagnesemia, hypophosphatemia, hyponatremia, hypernatremia, acidosis, alkalosis, porphyria, uremia), fever (especially in children), infection (meningitis, encephalitis, abscess), anoxia (arrhythmia, stroke, carbon monoxide poisoning), drugs (bupropion, venlafaxine, TCAs, tramadol, theophylline, antipsychotics, buspirone, fluoroquinolones, cyclosporine, tacrolimus) or substance abuse or withdrawal (cocaine, amphetamines, alcohol, barbiturates), lead, collagen-vascular disease (SLE), chronic renal failure, trauma, hypertensive encephalopathy, toxemia of pregnancy, neurodegenerative disorders (e.g., Alzheimer disease, Down syndrome, neurofibromatosis, tuberous sclerosis, glycogen or lipid storage diseases), Whipple disease, sickle cell disease, psychogenic factors (psychogenic nonepileptic seizures)

SLEEP DISTURBANCE

Insomnia: Alcoholism, altitude sickness, anxiety disorders, bipolar disorder, depression, COPD, thyroid-related (hyperthyroidism, thyrotoxicosis), substance abuse (cocaine, amphetamines, alcohol) or withdrawal (alcohol, opioid), post-traumatic stress disorder, drugs (SSRIs, SNRIs, bupropion, theophylline, beta-agonists, steroids, caffeine, nicotine replacement)
Hypersomnia: Sleep deprivation, obstructive sleep apnea, narcolepsy, depression, multiple sclerosis, metabolic encephalopathy, encephalitis, seizure disorder, chronic fatigue syndrome, fibromyalgia, drugs (antidepressants, antiemetics, antihistamines, benzodiazepines, barbiturates, opioids, seizure medications), systemic lupus erythematous, rheumatoid arthritis

SMELL DISORDERS

Anosmia (loss of ability to smell), *hyposmia* (reduced ability to smell), *parosmia* (distorted odor perception with stimulus), *olfactory hallucination* (occurs without a stimulus)

Nasal and sinus conditions (URI, allergic rhinitis, chronic rhinosinusitis, nasal polyps, COVID-19), head trauma (damage to cribriform plate, intracranial damage; facial trauma), neurodegenerative disorders (Parkinson disease, parkinsonism, Alzheimer disease, mild cognitive impairment, multiple sclerosis), other less common include medications, intoxicants/illicit drugs, toxins, chronic medical conditions, nutritional deficiencies, head and neck radiation, Kallmann syndrome

SPLENOMEGALY

See Lymphadenopathy and Splenomegaly, page 162.

SYNCOPE (See also Loss of Consciousness)

Vasovagal: Simple faint (fear, heat exposure, pain, stress, noxious stimuli)
Orthostatic: Volume depletion from any cause, sympathectomy (either functional or surgical), diabetes, primary autonomic failure (multiple sclerosis, multiple system atrophy [Shy–Drager syndrome], Parkinson disease/parkinsonism,

Wernicke encephalopathy), secondary autonomic failure (amyloidosis, chronic inflammatory demyelinating polyneuropathy, connective tissue diseases, diabetes mellitus, Lewy body dementia, older age, spinal cord injury, uremia), drugs (e.g., TCAs, diuretics, alpha-blockers), postural tachycardia syndrome, postprandial in the elderly

Psychiatric: Anxiety (hyperventilation), depression, conversion disorder

Situational: Micturition, cough, Valsalva, swallowing

Cardiac: Arrhythmia (PAT, AF, VT, and sinoatrial or AV block), pacemaker malfunction, aortic stenosis, hypertrophic cardiomyopathy, primary pulmonary hypertension, large pulmonary embolus, atrial myxoma, cardiac tamponade, aortic dissection, subclavian steal syndrome, acute coronary syndrome, pregnancy

Other: Hypoglycemia, hypoxia, seizure disorder, migraine, subarachnoid hemorrhage, TIA (vertebrobasilar or rarely anterior circulation with simultaneous events on the left and the right or 100% stenosis of the carotid artery with a TIA involving the other side)

TASTE DISORDERS

Dysgeusia (altered taste sensation); *hypogeusia* (reduced ability to taste); *ageusia* (loss of taste)

Upper respiratory and middle ear infections, COVID-19; surgeries to the ear, nose, and throat; head trauma; radiation for head and neck cancers; chemicals (insecticides, pepper gas, ammonia); medications (some common antibiotics and antihistamines); extraction of the third molar (wisdom tooth); poor oral hygiene and dental problems; fungal infections; zinc or copper deficiency

TREMORS

Resting (decreases with movement): Parkinson disease, Wilson disease, brain tumors (rare), drugs (SSRI antidepressants, metoclopramide, phenothiazines)

Action (present with movement): Benign essential tremor (familial and senile), cerebellar diseases, withdrawal syndromes (alcohol, benzodiazepines, opiates), normal or physiologic (induced by anxiety, fatigue)

Ataxic (worse at the end of a voluntary movement): MS, cerebellar diseases

Other: Medication-induced (caffeine, steroids, valproic acid, beta-agonists), febrile, hypoglycemic, hyperthyroidism, pheochromocytoma

VAGINAL BLEEDING

Normal menstruation; dysfunctional uterine bleeding (premenopausal bleeding, oral contraceptives, luteal phase defect); anovulatory abnormal uterine bleeding (hypothalamic and pituitary disorders, stress, thyroid and adrenal disease, endometriosis); pregnancy-related (ectopic pregnancy, threatened or spontaneous abortion, retained products of gestation); neoplasia; uterine fibroids; cervical polyps; endometrial, cervical, ovarian, and vulvar carcinoma; coagulopathy

VAGINAL DISCHARGE

Vaginitis due to *Candida albicans, Trichomonas vaginalis, Gardnerella vaginalis, Neisseria gonorrhoeae, Chlamydia trachomatis, Ureaplasma urealyticum, Mycoplasma genitalium*, herpes simplex I and II, chronic cervicitis, tumors, irritants, foreign bodies, estrogen deficiency

VERTIGO

Peripheral: Benign paroxysmal positional vertigo (BPPV), Meniere disease (vertigo, deafness, tinnitus), labyrinthitis, vestibular neuritis, semicircular canal debris
Central (associated with focal neurologic findings): Brainstem and cerebellum ischemia or infarction, acoustic neuroma
Other: Aminoglycoside toxicity, salicylic acid toxicity, quinine, alcohol

VISION LOSS, ACUTE

Retinal artery occlusion, retinal vein occlusion, acute angle closure glaucoma, retinal detachment, temporal arteritis (giant cell arteritis)

VOMITING

See Nausea and Vomiting, page 162.

WEIGHT LOSS

Normal or increased appetite: Diabetes, hyperthyroidism, anxiety, drugs (thyroid, amphetamines), carcinoid, malabsorption (sprue, pancreatic deficiency), parasites
Decreased appetite: Depression, anorexia nervosa, GI obstruction, assorted malignancies, liver disease, severe infection, severe cardiopulmonary disease including end-stage COPD, uremia, adrenal insufficiency, hypercalcemia, hypokalemia, substance abuse and toxins (alcohol, lead), old age, drugs (amphetamines, digitalis, chemotherapy), HIV and AIDS

WHEEZING

Laryngeal stridor, tracheal stenosis, foreign body, epiglottitis, vocal cord dysfunction, endobronchial tumor, asthma, bronchitis, emphysema, aspiration, pulmonary embolus, anaphylactic reactions, myocardial ischemia with pulmonary edema, carcinoid syndrome

XEROSTOMIA

Numerous medications (antidepressives, antihypertensives, antihistamines, decongestants, muscle relaxants, pain medications), normal aging, cancer therapy (chemotherapy, head and neck radiation), injury or surgery to head or neck area, chronic illness (diabetes, stroke, thrush, Alzheimer disease, autoimmune diseases [Sjögren's syndrome], HIV/AIDS) snoring, tobacco, alcohol use, recreational drug use

Laboratory Diagnosis:
Chemistry, Immunology, Serology

10

- Principles of Laboratory Testing
  - Conventional Units Versus Si Units
  - Stat Testing
  - Critical Lab Values
  - Serum versus Plasma Samples
  - Panel Testing
  - Coding Laboratory Tests
- Acetoacetate (Acetoacetic Acid)
- ACTH (Adrenocorticotropic Hormone, Corticotropin)
- ACTH Stimulation Test (Low and High Dose)
- Acute Phase Reactants (APRs)
- Albumin
- Albumin/Globulin Ratio
- Aldosterone, Serum
- Alkaline Phosphatase

- Alpha-1-Antitrypsin (AAT)
- Alpha-Fetoprotein (AFP), Serum
- ALT (Alanine Aminotransferase) (SGPT)
- Ammonia
- Amylase
- Angiotensin-Converting Enzyme (ACE)
- Anti-CCP (Anti-Cyclic Citrullinated Polypeptide Antibodies)
- Anti-Diuretic Hormone (ADH)
- Antinuclear Antibody (ANA)
- Antistreptolysin (ASO)/Anti-DNASE-B Antibody
- Apolipoprotein (apoB)
- AST (Aspartate Amino-transferase) (SGOT)
- Autoantibodies
  - Antinuclear Antibody (ANA)

- Specific ANA Patterns and Antibodies
  - Rheumatoid Factor (RF)
  - Other Autoantibodies
- Base Excess/Deficit
- Beta-Carotene
- Beta-Hydroxybutyrate (BHB)
- Bicarbonate ("Total CO_2")
- Bilirubin
  - Bilirubin, Neonatal ("Baby Bilirubin")
- Blood Urea Nitrogen (BUN), Urea Nitrogen
- BUN/Creatinine Ratio (BUN/CR)
- B-Type Natriuretic Peptide
- C-Peptide, Insulin ("Connecting Peptide")
- C-Reactive Protein (CRP) and Highly Sensitive CRP (hs-CRP)
- CA 15-3 (Cancer Antigen 15-3)

Chapter update by Steven A. Haist, MD, Benjamin J. Stahr, MD, Morgan H. McCoy, MD, PhD, and Leonard G. Gomella, MD

10

- CA 19-9 (Cancer Antigen 19-9)
- CA 27-29 (Cancer Antigen 27-29)
- CA 125 (Cancer Antigen 125)
- Calcitonin (Thyrocalcitonin)
- Calcium, Serum, and Calcium, Ionized Serum
- Carbon Dioxide, Total ("Total CO_2" or Bicarbonate)
- Carboxyhemoglobin (Carbon Monoxide)
- Carcinoembryonic Antigen (CEA)
- Catecholamines, Fractionated Plasma
- Celiac Disease Serology
- Ceruloplasmin
- Chloride, Serum
- Cholesterol, Total
  - Apolipoprotein B (apoB)
  - High-Density Lipoprotein Cholesterol (HDL, HDL-C)
  - Low-Density Lipoprotein Cholesterol (LDL, LDL-C)
  - Lipoprotein (a) (Lp[a])
  - Triglycerides

- Cholinesterase, Serum and RBC
- Chylomicrons
- Clostridium Difficile Toxin Assay, Fecal
- *Clostridioides* (formerly *Clostridium*) *difficile* Toxin Assay, Fecal
- Cold Agglutinins
- Complement
  - C1 Esterase Inhibitor
  - Complement C3
  - Complement C4
  - Complement CH_{50} (Total Complement)
- Copper
- Coronavirus (COVID-19 or SARS-COV-2) Viral RNA, Antigen and Antibody
- Cortisol, Serum
- Cortisol, Saliva
- Cortodoxone
- Cortrosyn Stimulation Test
- Creatine Kinase/ Creatine Phosphokinase (CK, CPK), Total and Creatine Kinase Isoenzymes
  - Creatine Kinase Isoenzymes
- Creatinine, Serum (SCr)

- Cryoglobulins (Cryocrit)
- Cryptococcal Antigen (Serum and CSF)
- Cystatin C Level
- Cytomegalovirus (CMV) Antibodies
- D-Dimer
- Dehydroepian-drosterone (DHEA)
- Dehydroepian-drosterone Sulfate (DHEAS)
- 11-Deoxycortisol (Cortodoxone, 17-Alpha, 21-Dihydroxyproge-sterone)
- Dexamethasone Suppression Test
- 17-Alpha, 21-Dihydroxyproge-sterone
- Dopamine, Serum
- Drug Levels (Therapeutic Drug Monitoring [TDM])
- Epinephrine, Serum
- Erythropoietin (EPO)
- Estradiol, Serum
- Estrogen/ Progesterone Receptors
- Estriol, Total and Unconjugated
- Estrone
- Ethanol (Blood Alcohol)
- Fatty Acids

➤ Fecal Fat
➤ Fecal Occult Blood Testing (FOBT)
  ➢ Guaiac-based FOBT
  ➢ Fecal immunochemical test (FIT)
  ➢ Multitarget stool DNA testing
➤ Ferritin
➤ Folate (Folic Acid)
➤ Follicle-Stimulating Hormone (FSH)
➤ FTA-ABS (Fluorescent Treponemal Antibody Absorbed
➤ Free Fatty Acids
➤ Fructosamine, Serum
➤ Fungal Serology
➤ Gamma-Glutamyl Transferase (GGT)
➤ Gastrin, Serum
➤ Globulins (Alpha-1, Alpha-2, Beta, and Gamma)
➤ Glucagon
➤ Glucose, Serum
➤ Glucose-6-Phosphate-Dehydrogenase (G6PD)
➤ Glucose Tolerance Test (GTT), Oral (OGTT)
  ➢ Interpretation of GTT
➤ Glycohemoblobin (Glycosylated Hemoglobin, Glycated Hemoglobin, Hemoglobin $A1_c$, HbA_{1c})
➤ Growth Hormone (GH), Somatotropin
➤ Haptoglobin
➤ *Helicobacter pylori* Antigen, Feces
➤ Hepatitis Testing
  ➢ Hepatitis A Virus (HAV)
  ➢ Hepatitis B Virus (HBV)
  ➢ Hepatitis C Virus (HCV)
  ➢ Hepatitis D Virus (HDV)
  ➢ Hepatitis E Virus (HEV)
➤ High-Density Lipoprotein (HDL) Cholesterol
➤ HLA Typing
➤ Homocysteine, Plasma
➤ Human Chorionic Gonadotropin, Serum (HCG)
➤ Human Immunodeficiency Virus (HIV) Testing
  ➢ HIV Antigen/Antibody Assay (Fourth-Generation)
  ➢ HIV-1/HIV-2 Antibody Differentiation Assay
  ➢ HIV Viral Load (Quantitative NAAT)
  ➢ Other HIV Testing
➤ Human Leukocyte Antigen (HLA) Typing
➤ Hydroxypro-gesterone (17-Alpha-Hydroxypro-gesterone)
➤ Beta-Hydroxybutyric Acid (Beta-Hydroxybutyrate [BHB])
➤ Hydroxypro-gesterone (17-Alpha-Hydroxypro-gesterone)
➤ Immunoglobulins, Quantitative
➤ Insulin
➤ Insulin-like Growth Factor-1 (IGF-1) (Somatomedin C)
➤ Iron, Serum
➤ Iron-Binding Capacity, Total (TIBC)
➤ Lactate Dehydrogenase (LD, LDH)
➤ Lactic Acid (Lactate)
➤ Lactose Tolerance Test, Blood
➤ Lactose Tolerance Test, Breath Hydrogen

10

- LAP Score (Leukocyte Alkaline Phosphatase Score/Stain)
- Lead, Blood
- *Legionella* Antigen, Random, Urine
- Lipase
- Lipoprotein Profile/ Lipoprotein Analysis
- Lipoprotein (a)
- Low-Density Lipoprotein-Cholesterol (LDL, LDL-C)
- Luteinizing Hormone, Serum (LH)
- Lyme Disease Serology
- Magnesium
- Manganese
- Methemoglobin
- Methylmalonic acid (MMA)
- β_2-Microglobulin, Serum
- Monospot
- Myoglobin
- Natriuretic Peptide, Brain (BNP)
- Natriuretic Peptide, NT-PRO B-Type Plasma
- Newborn Screening Panel
- Norepinephrine, Serum
- *N*-Telopeptide (NTx) (Urine and Serum)

- 5'-Nucleotidase (5'NT)
- Oligoclonal Banding, CSF
- Osmolality, Serum
- Osteocalcin
- Oxygen
- Parathyroid Hormone (PTH), Intact
- Parathyroid Hormone–Related Peptide (PTHrP)
- Phosphorus (Phosphate)
- Potassium, Serum
- Prealbumin (Transthyretin)
- Pregnancy Screening
  - First-Trimester Screening ("Combined Screening")
  - Second-Trimester Screening
  - Chorionic Villus Sampling (CVS)
  - Amniocentesis
  - Other Pregnancy Screening
- Progesterone
- Prolactin
- Prostate-Specific Antigen (PSA) and PSA Derivatives
  - PSA Velocity/PSA Doubling Time
  - PSA Free and Total
- Protein Electrophoresis, Serum and

Urine (Serum Protein Electrophoresis [SPEP]) (Urine Protein Electrophoresis [UPEP])
- Protein, Serum
- Pyruvate (Pyruvic Acid)
- Rapid Plasma Reagin (RPR) Test and Titers
- Renin, Plasma (Plasma Renin Activity [PRA])
- Renin, Renal Vein
- Retinol-Binding Protein (RBP)
- Rheumatoid Factor (RF, RA Latex Test)
- Rocky Mountain Spotted Fever (RMSF) Antibodies
- Sedimentation Rate
- Semen Analysis
- Sex Hormone–Binding Globin (SHBG)
- Sodium, Serum
- Somatomedin C
- Somatostatin
- Stool for Occult Blood
- Sweat Chloride Test (Quantitative Pilocarpine Iontophoresis Sweat Test)
- *N*-Telopeptide (NTx) (Serum)

- Testosterone, Free and Total
- Thyroglobulin
- Thyroid-Binding Globulin (TBG) (Thyroxine-Binding Globulin)
- Thyroid-Stimulating Hormone (TSH, Thyrotropin)
- Thyroxine, Free (FT$_4$)
- TORCH Battery
- Transferrin
- Transferrin Saturation
- Treponemal Specific Antibody
- Triglycerides
- Triiodothyronine, (T$_3$), Free

- Triiodothyronine (T$_3$), Total
- Troponin I (TI) and Troponin T (TT, Highly Sensitive)
- Urea Nitrogen (Blood)
- Uric Acid (Urate)
- Vasoactive Intestinal Peptide (VIP)
- VDRL Test (Venereal Disease Research Laboratory)
- Vitamin A (Retinol)
- Vitamin B$_1$ (Thiamine)
- Vitamin B$_2$ (Riboflavin)
- Vitamin B$_6$ (Pyridoxine)

- Vitamin B$_{12}$ (Extrinsic Factor, Cyanocobalamin)
- Vitamin C
- Vitamin D 1,25-Dihydroxy-cholecalciferol (Calcitriol)
- Vitamin D 25-Hydroxy-cholecalciferol (Ergocalciferol)
- Zinc

10

PRINCIPLES OF LABORATORY TESTING

This chapter outlines commonly ordered blood chemistry, immunology, and serology tests and other common laboratory investigations. Additional lab tests are described in the following chapters: Hematology, Chapter 11; Urine Studies, Chapter 12; Microbiology, Chapter 13; Blood Gases, Chapter 14; and Fluids and Electrolytes, Chapter 15.

Normal values and a guide to the diagnosis of common abnormalities and some background information on the tests are provided. **It should be noted that each laboratory has its own reference values that may differ from those listed here. The normal values given here should only be used as a guide.** Unless specified, values reflect normal levels in adults. Increased or decreased values that are not clinically useful (e.g., decreased GGT) may not be listed.

Although normal values for laboratory studies may vary between laboratories, normal values for common tests (e.g., potassium, sodium) are generally similar. However, for more specialized tests, normal values may vary considerably, depending upon the measurement method used. These specialized tests may use different units of measurement (mcg/dL vs. pg/dL or mcg/dL vs. mmol/L) from laboratory to laboratory. For specialized tests or tests that you are not familiar with, pay close attention to the units of measurement!

Furthermore, laboratory values that are abnormal are often identified with a different color for the text (red versus black) or by some other method (single asterisk). Also, for critical values (potentially life threatening), the result may be identified by an additional colored font (green versus red versus black) or in some other way (two asterisks versus one versus none) to differentiate a critical value from abnormal but not critical value from normal value. Some institutions have protocols in place where the ordering provider is contacted with any critical laboratory result.

Since it is unusual for phlebotomy to be a routine task for students or residents, this chapter no longer includes the method of collection (i.e., color of tube used) with each laboratory test except when it relates to special procedures such as a lumbar puncture or paracentesis, as described in Chapter 19, Bedside Procedures, page 503. It should be noted that laboratories have standardized collection methods, and the various blood specimen collection tubes are listed on page 666.

10

Conventional Units Versus SI Units

In the United States, most labs are reported using "conventional units," and these are used most frequently and listed in this chapter. The International System of Units (abbreviated SI from the French *le Système international d'unités*) relies on the metric system and is widely used outside of the United States. SI units rely on the meter, the kilogram, and the kelvin. If needed, several online conversion tables are available, such as one from the AMA Manual of Style (https://www.amamanualofstyle.com/page/si-conversion-calculator, accessed February 2, 2020). In this chapter, the first normal reference value uses conventional units, and if there is a second value listed, it uses the SI units. An example of both conventional and SI units for AST:

- Males: 6–34 U/L (0.48–0.55 μkat/L);
- Females: 19–25 U/L (0.32–0.42 μkat/L)

Stat Testing

Tests that are ordered on a "stat" basis (from the Latin *statum*, meaning immediately) receive priority handling in the clinical laboratory. Ordering a test stat should be reserved for situations in which a result is needed for urgent medical care in the judgment of the ordering physician.

Critical Lab Values

Critical lab values are historically defined as "panic" values that are well outside the normal range such that they may constitute an immediate health risk to the patient or require immediate action on the part of the ordering provider. Like all tests, these values may vary by lab. Some common critical values are noted in red in this chapter.

Serum versus Plasma Samples

Serum and plasma are both derived from the liquid portion of the blood that remains once whole blood components are removed. The main difference between plasma and serum is that plasma retains albumin, globulin, and fibrinogen (the main clotting component), which is removed from serum.

Serum is the fluid obtained after whole blood clots; this takes place spontaneously when blood contacts a glass or plastic surface. After phlebotomy, it is common to centrifuge the clotted blood components to the bottom of the tube. The straw-colored liquid above the clot is serum often used for routine chemistry determinations. The disadvantage of serum is that the samples can take time to clot. Serum sample preparation requires at least 30 minutes to 1 hour of waiting time before it can be centrifuged and analyzed.

Plasma is the non-cellular fluid component of blood obtained when a clot-preventing agent (e.g., EDTA [ethylenediaminetetraacetic acid]), heparin, or citrate is added to whole blood and then placed in a centrifuge. This separates the cellular material from the lighter plasma. Plasma specimens can be processed more quickly, shortening the turnaround time for test results. CBC samples are usually collected in an EDTA tube and are not subjected to centrifugation. Sample tubes must be carefully inverted 8–10 times to ensure mixing of the anticoagulant.

Most chemistry reference intervals are based on serum, not plasma. With few exceptions, there is little difference between serum and plasma, except that certain analytes (e.g., LDH, potassium, and phosphate) are higher in serum than plasma due to their cellular release during clotting. Protein and globulins are higher in plasma than serum, because plasma contains fibrinogen. As noted in this chapter, some analytes are preferentially reported on serum or plasma samples. As an example, catecholamines are tested on plasma while aldosterone levels are serum-based.

While lab protocols can vary, stat lab requests for chemistry are often requested in heparin collection tubes, so there is no need for the blood to clot. Anticoagulant tubes with EDTA (lavender) or citrate (blue top) should not be used for chemistry panels, because they chelate minerals (e.g., calcium) and interfere with the results. Details on sample collection tubes used for phlebotomy can be found in Chapter 19, page 666.

Panel Testing

Most laboratories offer "panel" tests, whereby multiple determinations are performed on a single sample, thus reducing the cost to the patient and the healthcare system. These panels were originally endorsed by the American Medical Association (AMA) and now are widely accepted. The downside to panel testing is this: What to do with a laboratory test that is abnormal that you would not have ordered if you ordered each of the tests separately? Is this positive test a false-positive test or is it a true-positive test, indicative of underlying pathology that has yet to display any symptoms or signs? In fact, if you order a panel with 20 tests in someone who is healthy, the odds are high that you have 1 false-positive test rather than 20 normal tests. Remember, normal laboratory tests are defined by 95% of a healthy cohort; thus, for each test, 2.5% of the healthy population will have a value above the reference range and 2.5% will have a value below the reference range.

The traditional "SMA 7" or "Chem 7" and other panels are generally no longer available at most labs. The following panels are endorsed by the AMA and are the most widely recognized:

Basic Metabolic Panel (BMP)

- Total Calcium
- Carbon Dioxide (Bicarbonate)
- Chloride
- Creatinine
- Glucose
- Sodium
- Potassium
- Urea nitrogen (blood) (BUN)

Renal Function Panel

- Albumin
- Calcium
- Carbon Dioxide (Bicarbonate)
- Chloride
- Creatinine
- Glucose
- Inorganic Phosphorus (Phosphate)
- Sodium
- Urea nitrogen (blood) (BUN)

Electrolyte Panel

- Sodium
- Potassium
- Chloride
- Carbon Dioxide (Bicarbonate)

Comprehensive Metabolic Panel (CMP)

- Albumin
- Total Bilirubin
- Total Calcium
- Carbon Dioxide (Bicarbonate)
- Chloride
- Creatinine
- Glucose
- Alkaline Phosphatase
- Potassium
- Total Protein
- Sodium
- Alanine Amino Transferase (ALT) (SGPT)
- Aspartate Amino Transferase (AST) (SGOT)
- Urea nitrogen (blood) (BUN)

10

- **Acute Hepatitis Panel:** Hepatitis A IgM, Antibody, Hepatitis B Core IgM Antibody, Hepatitis B Surface Antigen, Hepatitis C Antibody
- **Hepatic Function Panel:** Total Protein, Albumin, Globulin*, Alb/Globulin Ratio*, Alkaline Phosphatase, Total Bilirubin, Direct Bilirubin, AST/SGOT, ALT/SGPT
- **Lipid Panel:** Cholesterol, Triglycerides, HDL Cholesterol, LDL Cholesterol*, Cardiac Risk Factor*

(*calculated value)

Although laboratories may vary, some other common lab panel tests include the following:

- **CBC (Complete Blood Count)**: WBC (White Blood Cell Count), RBC (Red Blood Cell Count), HGB (Hemoglobin), HCT (Hematocrit), PLT (Platelet Count)
- **H&H**: Hemoglobin/Hematocrit

Coding Laboratory Tests

Every reimbursable laboratory test has an associated CPT code used for billing transactions. The CPT (Current Procedural Terminology) system was developed by and is a registered trademark of the AMA (see Chapter 5). CPT codes have been incorporated as the standard code set for Medicare and Medicaid reimbursement. They also are used in the Health Insurance Portability and Accountability Act (HIPAA) and have been adopted by private insurance carriers and managed care companies.

CPT codes are designated for services that are part of "contemporary medical practice and being performed by many physicians in clinical practice in multiple locations." Each of the codes consists of a five-digit number that is associated with a text descriptor (e.g., 82565, Creatinine; blood).

To comply with government regulations as specified by the Centers for Medicare & Medicaid Services (CMS), clinical pathology laboratories require physicians who order tests to provide the appropriate International Classification of Disease, Tenth Revision (ICD-10) diagnosis and procedure codes that in turn indicate which laboratory tests are reimbursable. (ICD-10 is discussed in Chapter 5.)

ACETOACETATE (ACETOACETIC ACID)

- Normal <1 mg/dL (<0.1 mmol/L)

  Increased: Diabetic ketoacidosis (DKA), alcoholic ketoacidosis, starvation, fasting (β-hydroxybutyric acid >acetoacetate), prolonged exercise

▶ Used to diagnose and monitor ketonemia. Excessive buildup of acetoacetate and other ketones can result in metabolic acidosis, defined as ketoacidosis.

ACTH (ADRENOCORTICOTROPIC HORMONE, CORTICOTROPIN)

- 7–10 AM 9–52 pg/mL (2–11.1 pmol/L); AM values highest levels, PM results are lower

  Increased: Addison disease (primary adrenal hypofunction), ectopic ACTH production (small-cell lung carcinoma, pancreatic islet cell tumors, thymic tumors, renal cell carcinoma, bronchial carcinoid), Cushing disease (pituitary adenoma), congenital adrenal hyperplasia (adrenogenital syndrome with impaired cortisol production)

  Decreased: Adrenal adenoma or carcinoma-producing cortisol, nodular adrenal hyperplasia, pituitary insufficiency, corticosteroid use

▶ Due to diurnal variation and other variables, isolated determination of ACTH is of limited utility. Most useful when using provocative testing (see ACTH stimulation test).

▶ Laboratory value ranges can vary by lab and assay method. Frequently, standards based on the American College of Physicians reference ranges are used (www.acponline.org/sites/default/files/shared/documents/for-meeting-attendees/normal-lab-values.pdf).

ACTH STIMULATION TEST (LOW AND HIGH DOSE)

- Low dose: 1 mcg cosyntropin (Cortrosyn) administered IV for best result
- High dose: 250 mcg cosyntropin (Cortrosyn) IV or IM; basal cortisol at approximately 8 AM before cosyntropin and then cortisol 1 hr after cosyntropin is administered

Normal response: Serum cortisol should increase >20 mcg/dL 60 min after cosyntropin

Subnormal response: Primary or secondary or tertiary adrenal insufficiency; recent injury to the pituitary gland or hypothalamus may have a normal cortisol response to stimulation. Primary can be related to autoimmune, hemorrhagic infarction, adrenoleukodystrophy, fungal, TB, HIV, and drugs; secondary can be related to traumatic brain injury, panhypopituitarism, infection, tumor; also chronic opioid use and chronic high- or moderate-dose glucocorticoid use; primary and secondary can be distinguished by baseline ACTH level.

▶ Cosyntropin (Cortrosyn) exhibits the full corticosteroidogenic activity of natural ACTH. This test's primary use is to diagnose adrenal insufficiency. Low-dose testing is not commonly used in routine practice.

ACUTE PHASE REACTANTS (APRs)

10

(See also individual tests noted.)

- **Increased (APRs that increase with acute inflammation):** C-reactive protein, sedimentation rate, cortisol, α-1-antitrypsin, ceruloplasmin, haptoglobin, ferritin, fibrinogen, plasminogen, complement including C1 esterase inhibitor and C3, mature neutrophils, copper (ceruloplasmin)
- **Decreased (APRs that decrease with acute inflammation):** albumin, prealbumin (transthyretin), transferrin, retinol-binding protein, calcium (albumin), iron (transferrin), zinc (albumin)
- ▶ APR are markers of acute inflammation and they can either increase or decrease as a result of acute inflammation, and many of them change in a matter of hours. Cytokines (IL-6, TNF-α, INF-α, others) produced by macrophages and other cells drive the change in concentration of the acute phase reactants. Sources of acute inflammation include infection, trauma, surgery, collagen vascular diseases (SLE, RA, temporal arteritis, many others), burns, and many cancers including leukemias, lymphomas, multiple myeloma, and metastatic solid cancers. COVID-19 can be associated with a severe inflammatory response from the infection secondary to a "cytokine storm" that can be catastrophic. The changes in the concentrations of copper, calcium, iron, and zinc as a result of acute inflammation is secondary to the change in the protein that binds the element, listed above in the parentheses after the element.

ALBUMIN

- Adult 3.5–5.5 g/dL (35–55 g/L); child 3.8–5.4 g/dL

  Increased: Dehydration

  Decreased: Malnutrition, overhydration, nephrotic syndrome, cystic fibrosis (CF) protein-losing enteropathies, chronic glomerulonephritis, cirrhosis, inflammatory bowel disease, hyperthyroidism, and negative acute phase reactant (decreases with any inflammation such as infection, trauma, surgery, collagen vascular diseases [SLE, RA, temporal arteritis, many others], burns, and cancers including leukemias, lymphomas, multiple myeloma, and metastatic solid cancers)

▶ Assessment of kidney or liver diseases or protein malabsorption. (See also Pre-albumin, page 244, and Chapter 17, page 466.)

ALBUMIN/GLOBULIN RATIO

• 1.0–1.5

Increased: Deficiency or absence of immunoglobulins, leukemia, others

Decreased: Anything that will decrease albumin such as malnutrition, acute illness, cancer, chronic liver disease, protein-losing enteropathies, inflammatory bowel disease, nephrotic syndrome, chronic glomerulonephritis, oral contraceptives, third-trimester pregnancy and/or increase in globulins such as multiple myeloma, Waldenstrom macroglobulinemia, lymphoma, carcinoma, bacterial infections, amyloidosis, myeloproliferative disorders, collagen-vascular diseases

▶ The ratio of albumin present in serum in relation to the amount of globulin; used in the management of some cancers and genetic disorders.

ALDOSTERONE, SERUM

(See also Chapter 11, page 305, Aldosterone, Urine.)

• Serum: salt depleted (10 mEq Na^+/day for 3–4 days), supine 12–36 ng/dL, upright 17–137 ng/dL
• Serum: salt loaded (120 mEq Na^+/day for 3–4 days), supine 3–10 ng/dL, upright 5–30 ng/dL

Increased: Primary hyperaldosteronism, secondary hyperaldosteronism (CHF, sodium depletion, nephrotic syndrome, cirrhosis with ascites, others)

Decreased: Adrenal insufficiency, panhypopituitarism, licorice (with large ingestion aldosterone suppression can last months)

▶ Discontinue antihypertensives and diuretics 2 wk before test. Patients should be salt depleted with upright samples drawn after 2 hr. Primarily used to screen hypertensive patients for possible Conn syndrome (adrenal adenoma producing excess aldosterone with hypertension and hypokalemia). Often determined with plasma renin activity (PRA). Urine aldosterone most sensitive for primary hyperaldosteronism. See Chapter 12, Urine Studies. The Endocrine Society recommends confirmatory testing: captopril challenge test (CCT), fludrocortisone suppression test (FST), oral sodium loading test (SLT), and saline infusion test (SIT).

ALKALINE PHOSPHATASE

- Adult 50–120 U/L (50–120 U/L), child 40–400 U/L (method dependent)

Increased: Highest levels in biliary obstruction and infiltrative liver disease including nonalcoholic fatty liver disease (NAFLD). Increased calcium deposition in bone (hyperparathyroidism), Paget disease, osteoblastic bone tumors (e.g., metastatic prostate, breast, osteogenic sarcoma, others), osteomalacia, rickets, pregnancy, childhood, healing fractures, liver disease (biliary obstruction due to mass effect), hyperthyroidism, drugs (anabolic steroids, estrogens, azathioprine, clopidogrel, tricyclic antidepressants, trimethoprim-sulfamethoxazole, penicillin antibiotics, macrolide antibiotics, chlorpromazine, ACE inhibitors, many others).

Decreased: Malnutrition, excess vitamin D ingestion, pernicious anemia, Wilson disease, hypothyroidism, zinc deficiency

▶ A fractionated alkaline phosphatase was formerly used to differentiate the origin of the enzyme (bone vs. liver). Generally, replaced by GGT (γ-glutamyl transpeptidase).

ALPHA-1-ANTITRYPSIN (AAT)

- 150–350 mg/dL (27.6–64.5 micromol/L)

Increased: Acute phase reactant, any cause of inflammation, carcinoma, acute infection, pregnancy

Decreased: α-1-antitrypsin deficiency, nephrotic syndrome

▶ Used to screen for AAT deficiency (rare genetic disorder) in patients at a young age with COPD or liver disease. AAT is produced by the liver and protects the lungs from immune damage.

ALPHA-FETOPROTEIN (AFP), SERUM

- <10 ng/mL
- Third trimester of pregnancy maximum 550 mg/mL

Increased: Hepatocellular carcinoma, some testicular tumors (embryonal carcinoma, malignant teratoma), ovarian Ca, endometrial Ca, cervical Ca, gastric Ca, colon Ca, neural tube defects (in mother's serum [spina bifida, anencephaly, myelomeningocele]), fetal death, multiple gestations, ataxia–telangiectasia, viral hepatitis, hepatic necrosis, cirrhosis

Decreased: Trisomy 21 (Down syndrome) in maternal serum

Normal: Seminoma

▶ Maternal blood AFP often part of triple (AFP, estriol, and hCG) or quadruple (AFP, estriol, hCG and inhibin A) second-semester screening test for birth defects. AFP is a protein normally produced by the embryonic yolk sac and the fetal liver and can be produced by malignant tumors such as non-seminomatous testicular cancer.

10

ALT (ALANINE AMINOTRANSFERASE) (SGPT)

- Males 7–55 U/L; females 7–45 U/L; higher values in newborns normal

Increased: Liver disease, liver metastasis, biliary obstruction, pancreatitis, liver inflammation (ALT is more elevated than AST in viral hepatitis; AST elevated more than ALT in alcoholic hepatitis), nonalcoholic fatty liver disease (NAFLD), drugs (protease and reverse transcriptase inhibitors, sulfonamides, clindamycin, statins, halothane, acetaminophen, NSAIDs, rifampin, isoniazid, tetracycline, carbamazepine, many others)

▶ ALT previously called serum glutamic-pyruvic transaminase (SGPT). Screens for liver disease. (See also AST.) Generally, parallels changes in AST in liver disease. ALT and AST are sensitive tests for acute hepatocellular injury, as they increase about 1 wk before bilirubin increases. Elevated ALT is more specific for liver injury; alcoholic liver disease is suggested with an AST:ALT ratio greater than 2; in NAFLD ratio is usually <1 and with mild and or early disease, ratio can be > 1 with severe NAFLD.

AMMONIA

- Adult 18–60 mcg/dL (11–35 µmol/L)
- Critical value >110 mcg/dL

Increased: Liver failure, hepatic encephalopathy, Reye syndrome, urea cycle inborn errors of metabolism, organic acidemias, urinary tract infections from urea-splitting bacteria (*Proteus, Klebsiella, Providencia, Morganella,* others), drugs (diuretics, asparaginase), healthy neonate (normalizes within 48 hr of birth).

▶ Normally, ammonia is converted in the liver to urea which is passed in the urine. Elevated levels suggest liver disease, renal failure, and genetic diseases.

AMYLASE

- 40–140 U/L (method dependent)

Increased: Acute pancreatitis, pancreatic duct obstruction (stones, stricture, tumor, sphincter spasm secondary to drugs), pancreatic pseudocyst or abscess, trauma involving pancreas, mumps, parotiditis, renal failure (false elevation), macroamylasemia, cholecystitis, penetrating peptic ulcer, intestinal obstruction, mesenteric thrombosis, postsurgical, drugs (HCTZ, azathioprine)

Decreased: Pancreatic destruction (pancreatitis, cystic fibrosis), healthy infant in first year of life.

▶ Amylase primarily produced by pancreas and salivary glands digests complex carbohydrates (starches). Can also be measured in the urine. After acute pancreatitis, urine amylase may be elevated for weeks after the serum amylase normalizes.

ANGIOTENSIN-CONVERTING ENZYME (ACE)

- 14–82 U/L (adults)

Increased: Sarcoidosis, liver disease, hyperthyroidism, DM, multiple myeloma, amyloidosis, other lung disease (pneumoconiosis, miliary TB, histoplasmosis), leprosy, Gaucher disease
Decreased: Hypothyroidism, COPD, renal disease

▶ Used to follow the activity of sarcoidosis; however, only increased in 60% of patients with sarcoidosis

ANTI-CCP (ANTI-CYCLIC CITRULLINATED POLYPEPTIDE ANTIBODIES)

See Autoantibodies, page 186.

ANTIDIURETIC HORMONE (ADH)

- 1–5 pg/mL (0.9–4.6 pmol/L)

Increased: Syndrome of inappropriate antidiuretic hormone release (SIADH) (CNS [acute thrombosis or hemorrhage, trauma, tumor, infection], cancer especially lung, drugs [SSRIs, opioids, NSAID, carbamazepine])
Decreased relative to a low urine osmolality/increased serum osmolality: Diabetes insipidus, heart failure, drugs including lithium and phenytoin.

▶ Also called vasopressin, ADH is secreted by the posterior pituitary. Used in the diagnosis of hyponatremia, SIADH, diabetes insipidus, and polyuria.

ANTINUCLEAR ANTIBODY (ANA)

See Autoantibodies, page 185.

ANTISTREPTOLYSIN (ASO)/ANTI-DNASE-B ANTIBODY

- ASO: 0–1 year: <200 IU/mL; 2–12 years: <240 IU/mL; 13 years and older: <330 IU/mL

- Anti-DNase-B: 0–6 years: <250 U/mL; 7–17 years: <310 U/mL; 18 years and older: <260 U/mL

Increased: Confirms current/recent infection with *Streptococcus pyogenes* (group A strep) in patients suspected of nonsuppurative complications, e.g., rheumatic fever, poststreptococcal glomerulonephritis

APOLIPOPROTEIN B (apoB)

See Cholesterol, pages 196–197.

AST (ASPARTATE AMINOTRANSFERASE) (SGOT)

- Males: 6–34 U/L (0.48–0.55 μkat/L)
- Females: 19–25 U/L (0.32–0.42 μkat/L)

Increased: AMI, liver disease, nonalcoholic fatty liver disease (NAFLD), Reye syndrome, muscle trauma and injection, pancreatitis, intestinal injury or surgery, factitious increase (erythromycin, opiates), burns, cardiac catheterization, brain damage, renal infarction, drugs (protease inhibitors, reverse transcriptase inhibitors, sulfonamides, clindamycin, statins, halothane, acetaminophen, NSAIDs, rifampin, isoniazid, tetracycline, carbamazepine, many others)

Decreased: Beriberi (vitamin B$_6$ deficiency), diabetic ketoacidosis, liver disease, chronic hemodialysis

▶ Generally parallels changes in ALT in liver disease. Formerly SGOT (serum glutamic oxaloacetic transaminase). ALT and AST are sensitive tests for acute hepatocellular injury, as they increase about 1 wk before bilirubin increases. Mild asymptomatic AST increases are seen in 10% of patients. Elevated ALT is more specific for liver injury; elevated AST can also be caused by extrahepatic diseases (thyroid diseases, celiac sprue, hemolysis, muscle disorders). Alcoholic liver disease is suggested with an AST:ALT ratio greater than 2; in NAFLD ratio is usually <1. (See also ALT.) Besides liver, also found in skeletal and cardiac muscle, RBCs, and brain and kidney tissue.

AUTOANTIBODIES

- Normal: Negative (false positives exist that require further testing)

▶ Autoimmune diseases are pathologic conditions caused by an immune response directed against an antigen within the body of the host, a self-antigen. This autoimmune response may be initiated by a self-antigen or a foreign antigen and usually involves both a T-cell and B-cell response. These activating antigens may be found in all cells (e.g, chromatin or centromeres) or are specific for a cell type in one organ (e.g., thyroglobulin in the thyroid). Most autoantibodies are biomarkers of disease. These disorders include systemic rheumatic diseases (systemic lupus erythematosus [SLE], vasculitis), and tissue/organ-specific, including endocrine and neurologic disorders such as autoimmune thyroiditis and multiple sclerosis.

Antinuclear Antibody (ANA)

▶ Useful screening test in patients with symptoms suggesting autoimmune/collagen–vascular disease, especially if autoantibody titer is >1:160. Up to 30% of healthy people can have a positive test, so a positive test needs to be interpreted based on the clinical setting. If a patient is ANA positive, panels as noted below are used to evaluate for other specific antibodies to help refine the diagnosis. Absence of ANA in a patient with diseases such as suspected SLE makes the diagnosis much less likely. Serologic tests currently used for diagnosis and monitoring in SLE, such as antinuclear antibody (see below), and complement levels, are of limited utility when used in isolation.

Positive: Systemic lupus erythematosis (SLE), drug-induced lupus-like syndromes (e.g., from procainamide, hydralazine, isoniazid), scleroderma, mixed connective tissue disease (MCTD), rheumatoid arthritis (RA), polymyositis, juvenile RA (5–20%). Low titers are also seen in diseases other than collagen–vascular disease.

Specific ANA Patterns and Antibodies

▶ The traditional method for ANA test is microscopic evaluation of indirect immunofluorescence (IIF) slides examining specific laboratory reference cells for patterns that have been treated with the patient's sera. Other, newer methods rely on ELISA testing. It is reported if antibodies are present that react to various parts of the nucleus of cells (hence anti-"nuclear" antibody). Since fluorescence microscopy techniques are often used to detect the autoantibodies in the cells, ANA testing is sometimes called *fluorescent antinuclear antibody test (FANA).*

Homogeneous. Nonspecific, from antibodies to deoxyribonucleoprotein (DNP) and native double-stranded DNA. Seen in SLE and a variety of other diseases. Antihistone is consistent with drug-induced lupus.

Speckled. Pattern seen in many connective tissue disorders.

Centromere pattern. Distinguished from other "speckled" patterns by seeing fluorescent dots along the chromosomes in dividing cells.

Nucleolar pattern. From antibodies to nucleolar RNA. Positive in Sjögren syndrome and scleroderma.

The following are specific antinuclear antibodies for a variety of autoimmune diseases.

Anti-DNA (Anti–double-stranded DNA): SLE (but negative in drug-induced lupus), chronic active hepatitis, mononucleosis

Anticentromere: CREST syndrome, scleroderma, Raynaud disease

Anti-cyclic citrullinated peptide (anti-CCP): Rheumatoid arthritis (often positive early in disease, useful to differentiate RA from other diseases and identify patient who may benefit from specific treatments; specificity >95%, sensitivity 80%, rare false positives with hepatitis C and autoimmune thyroid disease; once a patient develops a positive anti-CCP, it will usually remain positive, despite remission. Normal <20 U; weak positive: 20–39 U; moderate positive: 40–59 U; strong positive: >60 U

Antihistone: Drug-induced lupus

Anti-Jo-1: Polymyositis/dermatomyositis

Anti-Mi-2: Dermatomyositis

Anti-PM-Scl: Overlap syndrome of polymyositis and scleroderma

Anti-RNP: Mixed connective tissue disease (MCTD) and SLE

Anti-Sjögren syndrome antibody (SS-A) (anti-Ro): SLE, cutaneous lupus, SLE/Sjögren overlap syndrome, primary biliary cirrhosis

Anti-Sjögren syndrome antibody (SS-B) (anti-La): Sjögren syndrome

Anti-SCL 70: Scleroderma, at risk for pulmonary fibrosis

Anti-Smith: High specificity for SLE, ~30% of patients with SLE are positive

Antistreptolysin O / anti-DNase-B antibody: See ASO titers, page 183.

Rheumatoid factor (RF)

- Normal: < 40 U/mL (40 kU/L)
- RF is an IgM autoantibody; may be negative early in the disease; a positive/elevated RF suggests more severe disease. Initial workup should include both RF and anti-cyclic citrullinated peptide antibody (anti-CCP) testing. RA (present in 80%); juvenile RA usually negative for RF, false positives can be seen with SLE, scleroderma, Sjögren syndrome, cirrhosis of the liver, lymphomas, and infections (hepatitis, endocarditis, tuberculosis, viral infections, syphilis); 1–2% of healthy persons and >20% of healthy persons >65 yr are positive making measurement of RF of little value as a screening test

Other Autoantibodies

Antiadrenal: Multiple antibodies can cause various diseases, autoimmune adrenalitis, various adrenal steroid deficiencies

Anti–glomerular basement membrane (anti-GBM) antibody disease: Goodpasture syndrome (rapidly progressive GN, pulmonary hemorrhage) or only lung or only renal involvement

Antigranulocyte: Autoimmune neutrophilia and below

Antineutrophil cytoplasmic (ANCA):

o c-ANCA with *proteinase 3 antibodies*: Granulomatosis with polyangiitis (high titer = 1:80, highly predictive)

- o **p-ANCA with *myeloperoxidase antibodies*:** Microscopic polyangiitis, other forms of vasculitis including Churg–Strauss, SLE
- o **x- or atypical ANCA:** Ulcerative colitis

Antimitochondrial: Primary biliary cirrhosis, autoimmune diseases (SLE)

Antiparietal: Autoimmune atrophic gastritis resulting in pernicious anemia

Antiplatelet: Immune thrombocytopenic purpura

Anti-smooth muscle: Low titers in a variety of illnesses; high titers (>1:100) suggestive of chronic active hepatitis

Antithyroid:

- o *Antithyroid peroxidase (antimicrosomal antibodies):* Hashimoto thyroiditis
- o *Antithyroglobulin:* Hashimoto thyroiditis
- o *Thyroid-stimulating hormone receptor:* Graves disease

BASE EXCESS/DEFICIT

- −2 to +2

See Chapter 14, page 400.

BETA-CAROTENE

- 10–85 mcg/dL (0.2–1.6 μmol/L)

   Increased: Vitamin A toxicity (overdose), chronic renal disease, infantile idiopathic hypercalcemia

   Decreased: Malnutrition, malabsorption small bowel (celiac disease), pancreatic insufficiency, carcinoid syndrome, hypothyroidism, abetalipoproteinemia

▶ Also called provitamin A. (See also Vitamin A, page 262.)

BETA-HYDROXYBUTYRATE (BHB)

- 0.2–2.8 mg/dL (<0.27 mmol/L)

   Increased: DKA, starvation, alcoholic ketoacidosis

▶ Produced from fatty acid metabolism in the liver along with acetoacetate. Used in the diagnosis and management of DKA. BHB accounts for about 75% of the ketones in blood; during periods of DKA, BHB increases more than the other two ketoacids (acetoacetate and acetone). BHB assesses the severity of and is used for the management of DKA and to exclude hyperosmolar nonketotic diabetic coma.

BICARBONATE ("TOTAL CO₂")

- 22–28 mEq/L (22–28 mmol/L)
- Critical values: <11 mEq/L

See Carbon Dioxide, page 193, and Chapter 14, page 399.

10

BILIRUBIN

- Adults: Total, 0.1–1.2 mg/dL (2–18 µmol/L)
- Direct, 0.1–0.4 mg/dL (<3.4 µmol/L)
- Indirect, 0.2–0.7 mg/dL; total bilirubin may be lower in African Americans. (See also Bilirubin, Neonatal.)
- Critical values: Newborns, 10.0 mg/dL first 24 hr; 13.0 mg/dL for 1–30 days

Increased total: Hepatic damage (hepatitis, toxins, cirrhosis), congenital liver enzyme defects (Dubin-Johnson, Rotor, Gilbert, Crigler-Najjar), biliary obstruction (stone or tumor), hemolysis, fasting, drugs (any drug causing cholestasis, or hepatocellular injury/hepatitis, or hemolysis).

Increased direct (conjugated): Determination of direct bilirubin is usually unnecessary with total bilirubin levels <1.2 mg/dL; biliary obstruction/cholestasis (gallstone, tumor, stricture), Dubin-Johnson and Rotor syndromes, drug-induced cholestasis.

Increased indirect (unconjugated): Calculated (total minus direct bilirubin). Any type of hemolytic anemia (e.g., transfusion reaction, sickle cell), Gilbert disease, Crigler–Najjar syndrome, physiologic jaundice of the newborn.

Decreased bilirubin: May be due to medications such as penicillin, sulfisoxazole (compete for binding sites on albumin).

▶ Lab assays for total and direct (conjugated) bilirubin, then total minus direct = indirect bilirubin. Most unconjugated bilirubin is from senescent RBC. There is rapid conjugation of indirect bilirubin in the liver, with conjugated bilirubin excreted in the bile and is essentially not in the blood of normal individuals. Due to renal excretion, maximum bilirubin levels are 10–35 mg/dL. However, with renal insufficiency levels may be much higher (up to 75 mg/dL).

Bilirubin, Neonatal ("Baby Bilirubin")

▶ Normal dependent on many factors (e.g., gestational age, postnatal age, birthweight, risk factors, hydration, disease state, breastfeeding, nutritional status of the infant)
- Total bilirubin 0–1 day: 0.0–6.0 mg/dL; 1–2 days 0.0–8 mg/dL; 2–5 days 0.0–12.0 mg/dL; 5 days to 4 months 0.3–1.2 mg/dL; direct bili 0.0–0.4 mg/dL all ages
- Critical values: Total bilirubin 6.0 mg/dL in the first 24 hours of life or >15.0–17.0 mg/dL in term infant

Increased: Erythroblastosis fetalis, physiologic jaundice (may be due to breastfeeding), resorption of hematoma or hemorrhage, obstructive jaundice, hemolytic disease, others.

▶ Bilirubin normally peaks between 3 and 5 days post-delivery. Most infants born between 35 weeks' gestation and full term usually require no treatment for physiologic jaundice as few term newborns with hyperbilirubinemia have serious pathology. Phototherapy (to prevent neurologic toxicity or "kernicterus") should be instituted based on recommendations from the American Academy of Pediatrics. Jaundice is considered pathologic if it presents within the first 24 hours after birth, if total bilirubin increases >5 mg per dL/day or >0.2 mg/dL/h, total serum bilirubin level >95th % for age in hours based on nomograms, or lasts greater than 2 weeks in full-term infants. Breast-fed newborns may be at risk for jaundice and can be classified into two types: breastfeeding jaundice (early onset) and breast milk jaundice (later onset).

10

BLOOD UREA NITROGEN (BUN)

- Birth to 1 yr: 4–16 mg/dL (SI 1.4–5.7 mmol/L)
- Over 1 yr: >10–20 mg/dL (SI 3.6–7.1 mmol/L)
- Slight gradual increase with age
- Critical values: 0–2 yr >65 mg/dL; >2 yr >70 mg/dL

Increased: Renal failure (including drug-induced from aminoglycosides, NSAIDs), prerenal azotemia (renal hypoperfusion secondary to volume depletion, CHF, shock, cirrhosis/ascites, nephrosis), postrenal (obstruction), GI bleeding, drugs (especially aminoglycosides); increased catabolism (high-protein diet, vigorous exercise, burns, etc.)

Decreased: Malnutrition, liver failure, pregnancy, infancy, nephrotic syndrome, overhydration, low-protein diet

▶ Less useful measure of GFR than creatinine because BUN is also related to protein metabolism

BUN/CREATININE RATIO (BUN/CR)

- Mean: 10, range: 6–20; calculation based on serum levels

Increased: Prerenal azotemia (renal hypoperfusion secondary to volume depletion, CHF, shock, cirrhosis/ascites, nephrosis), GI bleed (ratio often >30), increased catabolism (high-protein diet, vigorous exercise, burns, etc.), ileal conduit, drugs (steroids, tetracycline)

Decreased: Malnutrition, pregnancy, low-protein diet, ketoacidosis, hemodialysis, SIADH, drugs, severe diarrhea, vomiting

▶ A rough guide used to differentiate prerenal and postrenal azotemia from renal azotemia

B-TYPE NATRIURETIC PEPTIDE

See Natriuretic peptide, page 240.

C-PEPTIDE, INSULIN ("CONNECTING PEPTIDE")

- Fasting, 0.78–1.89 ng/mL (0.26–0.62 nmol/L); 1 hr after glucose load: 5–12 ng/mL method dependent

    Increased: Insulinoma, sulfonylurea ingestion

    Decreased: Type 1 diabetes mellitus (decreased endogenous insulin), insulin administration (factitious or therapeutic)

▶ A measure of pancreatic beta cell function, half-life is 3–4 times longer than insulin. Used to differentiate endogenous insulin from exogenous insulin; liberated when proinsulin split to insulin; levels reflect endogenous insulin production

C-REACTIVE PROTEIN (CRP) AND HIGH-SENSITIVITY CRP (hs-CRP)

- Normal: CRP: <0–10 mg/dL; hs-CRP: <3 mg/L

    Increased: MI, unstable angina, transplant rejection, pulmonary embolus, last half of pregnancy, oral contraceptives, acute phase reactant (increases with any cause of inflammation including infection, trauma, surgery, collagen vascular diseases [SLE, RA, temporal arteritis, many others], burns, and cancers including leukemias, lymphomas, multiple myeloma, and metastatic solid cancers).

    Decreased (false): Magnesium supplements, NSAIDs, and statins

▶ Classic acute phase reactant, a nonspecific screen for infectious and inflammatory diseases, correlates with ESR. In the first 24 hr ESR may be normal and CRP elevated. CRP returns to normal more quickly than ESR in response to therapy. **High-sensitivity (hs-CRP)** is predictive of cardiovascular risk (<1 mg/dL low risk; 1–3 mg/dL moderate risk; >3 mg/dL high risk); most useful in those who are in the intermediate cardiovascular risk category.

CA 15-3 (CANCER ANTIGEN 15-3)

- <30 U/mL

    Increased: Progressive breast cancer, benign breast disease, and liver disease

    Decreased: Response to therapy (25% change considered significant)

▶ Used to detect breast cancer recurrence and monitor therapy. Levels related to stage of disease. Not FDA approved for screening.

CA 19-9 (CANCER ANTIGEN 19-9)

- <37 U/mL

Increased: GI cancers, e.g., pancreas (elevated in 80%), stomach, liver, colorectal, hepatobiliary; some cases of lung and prostate cancers. Some noncancerous conditions: pancreatitis, nonmalignant GI diseases, cirrhosis, cholangitis, hepatitis.

▶ Utility in determining resectability of pancreatic cancer (i.e., >1000 U/ mL 95% likely unresectable).

CA 27-29 (CANCER ANTIGEN 27-29)

- <38 U/mL

Increased: Early breast cancer recurrence but nonspecific; also ↑ in other cancers (lung, colon, pancreas, renal, ovary, and others) and benign conditions, benign breast disease, early pregnancy, renal and hepatic disease, others

▶ Detects glycoprotein (Muc-1); aid to monitoring breast cancer recurrence similar to CA 15-3

CA-125 (CANCER ANTIGEN 125)

- <35 U/mL

Increased: Ovarian, endometrial, and colon cancer; endometriosis; inflammatory bowel disease; PID; pregnancy; breast lesions; benign abdominal masses (teratomas)

▶ Not useful screening test for ovarian cancer; best used in conjunction with ultrasonography and physical exam. Rising levels after resection predictive of recurrence.

CALCITONIN (THYROCALCITONIN)

- Adolescents and adults: males <12 pg/mL; females <5 pg/mL; higher in infants and young children (method dependent)

Increased: Medullary carcinoma of the thyroid (MCT), C-cell hyperplasia (precursor of medullary carcinoma), small-cell carcinoma of the lung, newborn state, late pregnancy, chronic renal insufficiency, Zollinger–Ellison syndrome, pernicious anemia, leukemia, myeloproliferative disorders, hypercalcemia, thyroiditis, chronic renal failure
Decreased: Surgical resection of medullary thyroid carcinoma

▶ Levels >2000 pg/mL highly likely to be MCT. Values peak at mid-day.

CALCIUM, SERUM, AND CALCIUM, SERUM, IONIZED

See also Chapter 15, page 440, Hypercalcemia, Hypocalcemia, and Chapter 12, page 305, Calcium, Urine.

- Calcium, serum <10 days: 7.6–10.4 mg/dL (1.9–2.6 mmol/L); 10 days to 2 yr: 9–10.6 mg/dL (2.3–2.65 mmol/L); child: 8.8–10.8 mg/dL (2.2–2.7 mmol/L)
- Adult: 8.5–10.5 mg/dL (2.25–2.62 mmol/L); levels decreased in the elderly
- Ionized (free) adult: 4.64–5.28 mg/dL
- Ionized (free) child: 4.8–5.52 mg/dL
- Critical values: Serum calcium: <6.5 mg/dL or >13 mg/dL; Ionized calcium: <2 mg/dL or >7 mg/dL

10

Increased: (*Note:* Critical levels noted may lead to coma and death.) Primary hyperparathyroidism, PTH-related hormone-secreting tumors, vitamin D excess, vitamin A excess, metastatic bone tumors, immobilization, milk-alkali syndrome, Paget disease, thyrotoxicosis, idiopathic hypercalcemia of infants, infantile hypophosphatasia, chronic renal failure, familial hypocalciuria, sarcoidosis, multiple myeloma, ionized Ca^{++} increased in acidosis, drugs (thiazide diuretics, antacids, lithium).

Decreased: (*Note:* Total levels <7 mg/dL may lead to tetany and death.) Hypoparathyroidism (surgical, idiopathic), pseudohypoparathyroidism, insufficient vitamin D, osteomalacia, rickets, hypomagnesemia, RTA, hypoalbuminemia (cachexia, nephrotic syndrome, CF), hyperphosphatemia from any cause (chronic renal failure, ingestion), acute pancreatitis, factitious condition (low protein and albumin), drugs (phenytoin, colchicine), decrease in total calcium secondary to a decrease in the protein-bound calcium without a change in the ionized calcium (any cause of decreased protein or decreased albumin such as starvation, malnutrition, or acute inflammation, calcium is a negative acute phase reactant (decreases because of the decrease in albumin, calcium is bound to albumin; seen with infection, trauma, surgery, collagen vascular diseases [SLE, RA, temporal arteritis, many others], burns, and cancers including leukemias, lymphomas, multiple myeloma, and metastatic solid cancers).

▶ Levels characterized by a high physiological variation (age/sex/season [vit D variation]). Fifty percent of the calcium present in circulation is free (ionized calcium). For interpretation of total calcium, albumin must be known or use ionized calcium. Eighty percent of the bound calcium in the circulation is carried by albumin. If albumin is not normal, corrected calcium is estimated with the following formula. Values for ionized calcium need no corrections.

Corrected total Ca = 0.8 (Normal albumin [4.0] − Measured albumin) + Measured Ca

CARBON DIOXIDE, TOTAL ("TOTAL CO$_2$" OR BICARBONATE)

- Adult 22–28 mEq/l (22–28 mmol/L)
- Child 20–28 mEq/L (20–28 mmol/L)
- See Chapter 14, page 400, for PCO$_2$ values
- Critical values: bicarbonate <10 mEq/L or >40 mEq/L

Increased: Compensation for respiratory acidosis (emphysema) and metabolic alkalosis (severe vomiting, primary aldosteronism, volume contraction, Bartter syndrome), hyperthermia, antacids, thiazide diuretics

Decreased: Compensation for respiratory alkalosis and metabolic acidosis (starvation, DKA, lactic acidosis, alcoholic ketoacidosis, toxins/drugs [salicylates, methanol, ethylene glycol, others], severe diarrhea, renal failure, dehydration, adrenal insufficiency), high altitudes, acetazolamide, aspirin, chlorothiazide diuretics, tetracycline

10

▶ Total carbon dioxide consists of carbon dioxide (CO$_2$) in solution or bound to proteins, bicarbonate (HCO$_3^-$), carbonate and carbonic acid with 80–90% present as HCO$_3^-$. This is reflective of the body's buffering capacity.

CARBOXYHEMOGLOBIN (CARBON MONOXIDE)

- Nonsmoker: <2%
- Smoker 1–2 packs/day: 4–5%
- Smoker, heavy >2 packs/day: 8–9%
- Toxic: >10–15%
- 20–25% recommend hyperbaric oxygen
- Fatal: >40%

Increased: Smokers, smoke inhalation, automobile exhaust inhalation, defective furnaces, smoke from fires and charcoal grills, healthy newborns

▶ pO$_2$ is usually normal in CO poisoning. Studies suggest correlation with CO and atherosclerosis. Percent value refers to saturation of hemoglobin. CO has higher affinity to Hgb than oxygen.

CARCINOEMBRYONIC ANTIGEN (CEA)

- Nonsmoker: <3 ng/mL (3 ug/L)
- Smoker: <5.0 ng/mL (5 ug/L)

Increased: Carcinoma (colon, pancreas, lung, stomach), smokers, non-neoplastic liver disease, Crohn disease, ulcerative colitis

▶ Not a cancer-screening test; used to monitor response to treatment and tumor recurrence in GI tract adenocarcinoma. Usually returns to normal 4–6 wk after resection.

CATECHOLAMINES, FRACTIONATED PLASMA

See also Chapter 12, page 305, Catecholamines, Fractionated, Urine; page 307, Metanephrines, Urine; and page 308, Vanillylmandelic Acid, Urine.

Catecholamine	Plasma (Supine) Levels
Norepinephrine	110–410 pg/mL (SI: 650–2423 pmol/L)
Epinephrine	0–50 pg/mL (SI: 0–273 pmol/L)
Dopamine	<30 pg/mL (SI: <196 pmol/L)
Metanephrine, total free	<200 pg/mL (SI: <1,400 pmol/L)
Normetanephrine	<175 pg/mL (SI: <900 pmol/L
Metanephrine	<25 pg/mL (SI: <500 pmol/L)

Increased: Pheochromocytoma, paraganglioma, neural crest tumors (neuroblastoma); with extraadrenal pheochromocytoma, norepinephrine may be markedly elevated compared with epinephrine; plasma metanephrines have high negative predictive value

▶ Values vary and depend on the lab and method of assay used. Normal levels shown here are based on an HPLC technique. Patient must be supine in a nonstimulating environment with IV access to obtain sample. There are a significant number of false-positive results, making it a poor screening test in a lower-risk population. Metanephrine and normetanephrine are metabolic products of epinephrine and norepinephrine.

CELIAC DISEASE SEROLOGY

• Negative

   Positive: Celiac disease

▶ Celiac disease is also called gluten-sensitive enteropathy or nontropical sprue. Three serum antibodies are used to test for celiac disease: endomysial antibodies (EMAs), deamidated gliadin peptide (DGP) antibodies, and anti-tissue transglutaminase antibodies (tTGs); tTG has a >90% sensitivity and >95% specificity. IgA tTG antibody is the preferred test for screening. Immunoglobulin G (IgG) tests may be used in people with IgA deficiency (frequently seen in celiac disease). Positive test leads to a definitive small bowel biopsy. Test with patient on diet that contains gluten (found in wheat, rye, barley, or oats). HLA variation DQ2 in approximately 95% of celiac patients; if HLADQ2/DQ8 is negative, it virtually excludes celiac disease.

CERULOPLASMIN

- 20–40 mg/dL (200–400 mg/L)

    Increased: Acute phase reactant (any inflammatory diagnosis, infection, and cancers, see page 179), pregnancy, drugs (OCPs, phenytoin)

    Decreased: Wilson disease (low predictive value), other CNS disease, other liver disease, nephrotic syndrome, malnutrition, malabsorption, copper deficiency

▶ Ceruloplasmin stores and carries copper. Test primarily used for the autosomal recessive Wilson disease (copper buildup in the brain and liver).

CHLORIDE, SERUM

- 97–107 mEq/L (96–106 mmol/L)

    Increased: Diarrhea, RTA, renal failure, dehydration, excess saline admin, DI, hyperparathyroidism, respiratory alkalosis, hyperalimentation, medications (thiazide diuretics, acetazolamide, androgens, ammonium chloride), salicylate overdose

    Decreased: Vomiting, diarrhea, upper GI suctioning, DKA, chronic respiratory acidosis, SIADH, mineralocorticoid excess, renal disease with sodium loss

▶ Included with electrolytes in metabolic panels. Chloride is the major extracellular anion and usually reflects changes in serum sodium.

CHOLESTEROL, TOTAL

- See also Lipoprotein Profile/Lipoprotein Analysis, page 236

10

Optimal <200 mg/dL; borderline 200–239 mg/dL; high ≥240 mg/dL; see Table 10-1 and Table 10-2, page 197.

Table 10-1. Cholesterol is included as part of a "Lipid Profile" that includes total cholesterol, HDL cholesterol, LDL cholesterol and Triglycerides. Cholesterol and triglycerides are lipids that are insoluble and are solubilized by attaching to lipoproteins (see page 236). Cholesterol management and guideline recommendations are discussed in the Appendix, page 1054. Some hyperlipidemias are based on inherited factors and are demonstrated in Table 10-2.

Total Cholesterol
- Optimal: <200 mg/dL
- Borderline high: 200–239 mg/dL
- High: ≥240 mg/dL

High density lipoprotein cholesterol (HDL cholesterol aka "good cholesterol")
- Optimal: >60 mg/dL
- Normal: 40–60 mg/dL
- Low: <40 mg/dL

Low density lipoprotein cholesterol (LDL cholesterol aka "bad cholesterol")
- Optimal: <100 mg/dL
- Borderline optimal: 100–129 mg/dL
- Borderline high: 130–159 mg/dL
- High: 160–189 mg/dL
- Very high: ≥190 mg/dL

Triglycerides
- Optimal: <150 mg/dL
- Borderline high: 150–199 mg/dL
- High: 200–499 mg/dL
- Very high: ≥500 mg/dL

THE FOLLOWING LIPOPROTEINS CAN ALSO BE USED TO ASSESS RISK OF HEART DISEASE

Apolipoprotein B (apoB)
- Optimal: <90 mg/dL
- Borderline high: 90–99 mg/dL
- High: 100–130 mg/dL
- Enhancer of ASCVD risk: >130 mg/dL[*]

Lipoprotein (a) [Lp(a)]
- Optimal: <10 mg/dL
- Borderline high: 10–29 mg/dL
- High: 30–49 mg/dL
- Enhancer of ASCVD risk: >50 mg/dL[*]

[*] Apo B >130 mg/dL and/or a Lp(a) >50 mg/dL are both independent risk factors for ASCVD.
Lipid profile date based on: Endocrine Self-assessment Program: Laboratory Reference Ranges. Endocrine Society, Center for Self Learning, Washington, DC, 2015.
LAB update: Apolipoprotein B: A risk factor in the primary prevention of cardiovascular disease. Laboratory Corporation of America, 2019.
Zawacki AW, Dodge A, Woo KM, Ralphe JC, Peterson AL. In pediatric familial hypercholesterolemia, lipoprotein (a) is more predictive than LDL-C for early onset of cardiovascular disease in family members. J Clin Lipidol. 2018;12:1445–1451.

Table 10-2. Classification of Genetic Hyperlipidemias based on the Frederickson Classification. (Adapted from Fitzpatrick's Color Atlas and Synopsis of Clinical Dermatology, 8e. 2017 Reproduced with permission from McGraw-Hill Medical.)

Frederickson Type	Classification	Lipid Profile
I	Familial lipoprotein lipase deficiency (hyperchylomicronemia, hypertriglyceridemia)	TG++, C normal, CM++, HDL-/normal
IIa	Familial cholesterolemia	TG normal, C+, LDL+
IIb	Familial combined hyperlipidemia	TG+, C+, LDL+, VLDL+
III	Familial dysbetalipidemia (remnant particle disease)	TG+, C+, IDL+, CM remnants+
IV	Familial hypertriglyceridemia	TG+C normal/+, LDL++, VLDL++
V	Familial combined hypertriglyceridemia	TG+, C+, VLDL++, CM++

TG, triglycerides; C, cholesterol; CM, chylomicrons; HDL, high-density lipoproteins; LDL, low-density lipoproteins; VLDL, very low-density lipoproteins; IDL, intermediate-density lipoproteins; +, raised; -, lowered

Increased: Familial and polygenic hypercholesterolemia, biliary obstruction, nephrotic syndrome, hypothyroidism, poorly controlled diabetes mellitus, pregnancy, anorexia nervosa, Cushing syndrome drugs (corticosteroids, thiazide diuretics, protease inhibitors, anabolic steroids, others)

Decreased: Liver disease (e.g., hepatitis, cirrhosis), hyperthyroidism, malnutrition (cancer, starvation), malabsorption, chronic anemia, extensive burns, abetalipoproteinemia, familial hypercholesterolemia, AMI

▶ Used to assess risk of heart disease and ASCVD, usually ordered with HDL, LDL, and triglycerides as a lipid profile panel test. Seasonal variation with higher levels (up to 8%) in winter. Positional variation is lower by 5% sitting and 10–15% recumbent as opposed to standing when sample taken.

Apolipoprotein B (apoB)

● Men: 50–123 mg/dL; women: 25–120 mg/dL; see Table 10-1, page 196

Increased: Hyperlipidemia, familial hyperlipidemia, patients with premature CVD, family history of premature CVD.

▶ An LDL receptor ligand found in all four of the ASCVD-promoting lipoproteins LDL, IDL (intermediate density lipoprotein), VLDL, and lipoprotein (a) and also in chylomicrons remnants; elevated levels correlate with CAD risk; a stronger predictor of cardiac risk than LDL cholesterol; levels >130 mg/dL enhancer of ASCVD risk.

High-Density Lipoprotein Cholesterol (HDL, HDL-C)

• Fasting: 40–60 mg/dL, see Table 10-1, page 196

Increased: Estrogen (menstruating women), regular exercise, ethanol intake, medications (gemfibrozil, others)
Decreased: Men, smoking, uremia, obesity, diabetes, liver disease, Tangier disease

▶ HDL-C correlates with the development of CAD; decreased HDL-C leads to increased risk. Levels <40 mg/dL associated with increased risk of CAD. Levels >60 mg/dL associated with decreased risk of CAD.

Low-Density Lipoprotein Cholesterol (LDL, LDL-C)

• Optimal <100 mg/dL, see Table 10-1, page 196

Increased: Excess dietary saturated fats, hyperlipoproteinemia, biliary cirrhosis, endocrine disease (diabetes, hypothyroidism)
Decreased: Malabsorption, severe liver disease, abetalipoproteinemia

▶ Elevated levels correlate with CAD risk; LDL-C is usually a calculated value using the Friedewald formula. The formula estimates the LDL-C level using the following: total cholesterol (TC), triglycerides (TG), and high-density lipoprotein cholesterol (HDL-C). The measurements must be in mg/dL. This formula is not accurate for triglycerides >400 mg/dL.

$$\text{LDL-C (mg/dL)} = \text{TC (mg/dL)} - \text{HDL-C (mg/dL)} - \text{TG (mg/dL)}/5.$$

Lipoprotein (a) (Lp[a])

• 10–30 mg/dL; see Table 10-1, page 196

Increased: Hyperlipidemia, familial hyperlipidemia, patients with premature ASCVD, family history of premature ASCVD; in the absence of hypercholesterolemia, not as strong of a predictor of ASCVD in women than in men

▶ One type of ASCVD-promoting lipoprotein along with LDL, IDL, and VLDL; consisting of LDL particle + specific apolipoprotein A; structurally similar to plasminogen and thought to promote thrombosis; an independent risk factor for ASCVD; levels >50 mg/dL enhancer for ASCVD risk.

Triglycerides

- Optimal: <150 mg/dL; borderline high: 150–199 mg/dL; high 200–499 mg/dL; very high >500 mg/dL. Fasting required for best test results. See Table 10-1, page 196.

   Increased: Nonfasting specimen, hypothyroidism, liver disease (viral hepatitis, cirrhosis, biliary tract obstruction), poorly controlled DM, alcoholism, pancreatitis, AMI, nephrotic syndrome, familial disorders, drugs (OCPs, beta blockers, cholestyramine, corticosteroids)

   Decreased: Malnutrition, malabsorption, hyperthyroidism, Tangier disease, congenital abetalipoproteinemia, drugs (ascorbic acid, nicotinic acid, clofibrate, gemfibrozil)

▶ Triglycerides are carried in the blood by lipoproteins; about 80% of triglycerides are in very low density lipoproteins (VLDL) and 15% in low density lipoproteins (LDL). Lipoproteins are described in detail on page 236. The triglycerides spike in the blood after eating.

10

CHOLINESTERASE SERUM AND RBC

- Serum: 8–18 U/mL (8–18 kU/L)
- RBC: 31.2–61.3 U/g of hemoglobin

   Increased: Hemolytic anemias (in RBC), diabetes, hyperthyroidism

   Decreased: Organophosphate and carbamate poisoning, acute decrease in plasma and a decrease in RBC from chronic exposure; malnutrition, liver disease (cirrhosis, hepatic carcinoma); succinylcholine sensitivity or if prolonged sedation with succinylcholine

▶ Most commonly used to monitor organophosphate poisoning; preop evaluation for succinylcholine sensitivity

CHYLOMICRONS

See Lipoprotein profile/Lipoprotein analysis, page 236.

CLOSTRIDIUM DIFFICILE TOXIN ASSAY, FECAL

See Clostridioides (Formerly Clostidium) Difficile Toxin Assay, Fecal, below.

CLOSTRIDIOIDES (FORMERLY *CLOSTRIDIUM*) *DIFFICILE* TOXIN ASSAY, FECAL

- Normal: Negative

Positive: >90% of cases of pseudomembranous colitis, 50–75% of antibiotic-associated colitis, and 15–25% of antibiotic-associated diarrhea

False positive: Some healthy adults and neonates

▶ Assay only liquid stool in patients with ≥3 loose stools in 24 hr. Two toxins are produced by *C. difficile* (toxin A, an enterotoxin, and toxin B, a cytotoxin) and are usually tested with the assay. Often ordered along with a GDH antigen (GDH enzyme present in all *C. difficile* isolates). *C. difficile* must be distinguished from other causes of diarrhea. Most antibiotic-associated diarrhea is not *C. difficile* related. Antibiotic-associated diarrhea associated with pseudomembranous colitis is nearly always **C. difficile–associated diarrhea (CDAD).** (Note: Based on genetic and ribosomal sequencing, in 2018 the Clinical and Laboratory Standards Institute [CLSI] recognized the taxonomic classification of *Clostridium difficile* should be changed. The name change was from *Clostridium difficile* to *Clostridioides difficile.*)

COLD AGGLUTININS

- <1:32

Increased: Atypical pneumonia (*Mycoplasma pneumoniae*), viral infections, listeriosis, syphilis, parasitic infections, cirrhosis, autoimmune hemolytic anemia, collagen vascular disease, lymphoma and chronic lymphocytic leukemia, multiple myeloma, Waldenström macroglobulinemia

▶ Historically, used to screen for atypical pneumonia. Not commonly ordered for this purpose anymore.

COMPLEMENT

▶ Complement describes a series of sequentially reacting serum proteins that participate in pathogenic processes and cause inflammatory injury, such as autoimmune diseases (SLE, rheumatoid arthritis [RA]). There are nine major classes, but only a few have clinical significance and are noted here.

C1 Esterase Inhibitor

- 20–40 mg/dL

Increased: Acute phase reactant (infection, any inflammatory diagnosis, surgery, traumatic injury, burns, and cancers)

Decreased: C1 esterase inhibitor deficiency, can be genetic (autosomal dominant) or acquired due to autoantibodies or lymphoma mediated

▶ Controls the first step in the classic complement pathway. C1 esterase deficiency leads to activation of C1 and will result in the consumption of C2 and C4. C1 esterase inhibitor also inhibits plasmin, thrombin, and factor X11a. Deficiency causes angioedema.

Complement C3

- 64–200 mg/dL (method dependent)

    Increased: Acute phase reactant (infection, any inflammatory diagnosis, surgery, traumatic injury, burns, and cancers), RA (variable finding), various acute viral hepatitis, MI, pregnancy, amyloidosis, sarcoidosis, thyroiditis

    Decreased: SLE, glomerulonephritis (poststreptococcal and membranoproliferative), RA, Sjögren syndrome, sepsis, SBE, chronic active hepatitis, malnutrition, DIC, gram-negative sepsis, autoimmune hemolytic anemia, paroxysmal nocturnal hemoglobinuria, extensive burns, protein-losing enteropathies

▶ Decreased level suggests activation of the classical or alternative pathway or both

10

Complement C4

- Males: 12–72 mg/dL
- Females: 13–75 mg/dL

    Increased: RA (variable finding), neoplasia (GI, lung, others)
    Decreased: SLE, RA, chronic active hepatitis, cirrhosis, proliferative glomerulonephritis, hereditary angioedema (test of choice), extensive burns, protein-losing enteropathies

Complement CH50 (Total Complement)

- 30–75 U/mL (method dependent)

    Increased: Acute phase reactant (infection, any inflammatory diagnosis, surgery, traumatic injury, burns, and cancers)
    Decreased: Classic complement pathway deficiencies (SLE, glomerulonephritis)

▶ Tests complement deficiency in the classical pathway.

COPPER

- Males: 70–140 ug/dL
- Females: 80–155 ug/dL

    Increased: Wilson disease (autosomal recessive disorder of copper metabolism causing excess copper storage), acute and chronic copper toxicity
    Decreased: Nutritional deficiency

▶ Used in the diagnosis of Wilson disease; assessment primary biliary cirrhosis and primary sclerosing cholangitis.

CORONAVIRUS (COVID-19 OR SARS-COV-2) VIRAL RNA, ANTIGEN AND ANTIBODY

See also Chapter 13, page 380.

SARS-CoV-2 RNA testing:
- Positive: SARS-CoV-2 RNA detected
- Negative: SARS-CoV-2 RNA not detected

SARS-CoV-2 antigen testing
- Positive: antigen detected
- Negative: antigen not detected

Serology:
- IgG antibodies

Positive: Recent or past infection with COVID-19; may signify immunity, but at this time (January 2021) we are unsure how long a positive IgG confers immunity. False-positive results can occur from an infection with another non–SARS-CoV-2 coronavirus.

Negative: No recent infection with SARS-CoV-2; in an epidemic or pandemic, individuals testing negative will be susceptible to infection, or a negative test could be a false-negative

▶ There are two laboratory methods for detecting acute SARS CoV-2 infection: 1) detection of viral RNA, which is the gold standard; initially, results were not available for at least 24 hours and now there is point-of-care (POC) testing for viral RNA and 2) an antigen test that detects specific SARS CoV-2 proteins can be performed in minutes.

▶ RNA detection is by reverse transcriptase polymerase chain reaction (RT-PCR) or other nucleic acid amplification testing (NAAT) methods. POC using PCR is comparable to laboratory-based testing, whereas other NAAT methods have a higher false-negative rate. False-negative rates for RT-PCR are highest on the first day of infection (100%); The false-negative rate decreases to a low on day 8 (day 3 of symptoms). If the test is negative and clinical suspicion is high, the test should be repeated. Improper collection of the specimen increases the false-negative rate.

▶ Nasopharyngeal is the preferred site for specimen collection but swabbing the throat or anterior nares to mid-turbinate is acceptable; however, the yield may not be as high as a nasopharyngeal specimen (see page 328). The nasopharyngeal site may elicit a significant gag reflex. A flocked swab with an aluminum or plastic handle should be used. False-negative results can be caused by foreign substances contaminating the specimen such as wood from a wood-based handle.

▶ When patients become infected with SARS-CoV-2, antibody production and detection varies based on the time lapse since infection and the severity of symptoms. Antibodies are not detected until about 3 days after the onset of symptoms. Sensitivity and specificity of the SARS-CoV-2 IgG assay are 97.6% and 98.8%, respectively, when obtained 14 days after the onset of symptoms (typically ~20 days post-infection). Besides IgG antibodies,

IgM and IgA antibody testing is available. Antibodies to SARS-CoV-2 should not be used for diagnosis except in rare instances, such as very late in the course of the illness and when there are two negative tests for SARS-CoV-2 RNA (usually by PCR) with at least one day between tests. There is often cross-reactivity to other coronaviruses besides SARS-CoV-2.

CORTISOL, SERUM

See also Chapter 12, page 306, Cortisol, Urine.

- 8 AM, 8.7–22.4 μg/dL
- PM, <10 μg/dL (method dependent)

Increased: Adrenal adenoma, adrenal carcinoma, Cushing disease, nonpituitary ACTH-producing tumor, corticosteroid therapy, oral contraceptives, pregnancy, starvation, acute physical stress including from hypoglycemia, hypotension, trauma, surgery, acute bacterial infection from any cause including septic shock, burns, emotional stress including anxiety and major depressive disorder, chronic alcohol use/abuse, false elevation with prednisone methylprednisolone, cortisone, and dexamethasone,

Decreased: Primary adrenal insufficiency (Addison disease), congenital adrenal hyperplasia, Waterhouse–Friderichsen syndrome, ACTH deficiency, decreased corticosteroid binding globulin (nephrotic syndrome)

▶ Discriminates primary and secondary adrenal insufficiency and used in the diagnosis of Cushing syndrome

CORTISOL, SALIVA

- Diurnal variations: 5.6 ng/mL 8:00–9:00 AM, 1 ng/mL at 11:00 PM

    Increased: Evening increased with Cushing syndrome
    Decreased: Morning decreased with adrenal insufficiency

▶ Used to screening for Cushing syndrome serially in ambulatory patients. Useful in the setting of cyclical Cushing syndrome.

CORTODOXONE

See 11-Deoxycortisol, page 207.

CORTROSYN STIMULATION TEST

See ACTH Stimulation Test, page 178.

CREATINE KINASE/CREATINE PHOSPHOKINASE (CK, CPK), TOTAL AND CREATINE KINASE ISOENZYMES

- 50–200 U/L (varies between male and female with a higher normal in a male)
- Critical value: >1500 U/L

Increased: Muscle damage (Acute MI [AMI]), myocarditis, muscular dystrophy, muscle trauma [including injections], postsurgery), brain infarction, defibrillation, cardiac catheterization and surgery, rhabdomyolysis, extensive exercise, polymyositis, hypothyroidism, malignant hyperthermia, generalized seizures, chronic alcohol use, drugs (statins)

▶ Used in suspected MI or muscle diseases. Skeletal and cardiac muscle and brain tissue have high intracellular levels.

Creatine Kinase Isoenzymes

The proportion of CPK isoenzymes is the key to interpretation of the isoenzyme isolated.

CPK 2 (MB): (Normal <6%, heart origin) increased in AMI (begins in 2–12 hr, peaks at 12–40 hr, returns to normal in 24–72 hr); troponin is marker of choice for AMI; also increased in pericarditis with myocarditis, rhabdomyolysis, Duchenne muscular dystrophy, polymyositis, malignant hyperthermia, cardiac surgery

CPK 3 (MM): predominantly skeletal muscle; thus can help distinguish peripheral skeletal muscle disease from cardiac; skeletal muscle diseases include trauma, rhabdomyolysis, adverse reactions to statins, prolonged exercise, muscle inflammatory conditions (e.g., polymyositis), heat injury, muscular dystrophy, and dermatomyositis

CPK 1 (BB): Predominantly elevated in disorders involving brain and central nervous system: stroke, inflammatory CNS disorders, others

▶ Creatine kinase isoenzymes are not as widely used now due to the increased use of troponin to diagnosis AMI (see page 261).

CREATININE, SERUM (SCr)

- 0.7-1.3 mg/dL (61.9-115 µmol/L)
- Children 0.5–0.8 mg/dL; critical values: 0–2 yr >4.2 mg/dL; 2–10 yr >4.8 mg/dL; >10 yr >5 mg/dL
- Critical values: 0 to 2 yr >4.2 mg/dL; 2 to 10 yr >4.8 mg/dL; >10 yr >5 mg/dL

Increased: Renal failure (prerenal, renal, or postrenal obstruction), or medication-induced (aminoglycosides, NSAIDs, others), hypothyroidism, acromegaly, ingestion of red meat, false positive with DKA

Decreased: Pregnancy, decreased muscle mass, severe liver disease, starvation, decreases with aging

▶ A clinically useful estimate of GFR. In general, SCr doubles with each 50% reduction in GFR. Creatinine clearance based on urinary collection is considered the most accurate method (see also Chapter 12, Urine Studies).

CRYOGLOBULINS (CRYOCRIT)

- <0.4% (negative if qualitative)

    Monoclonal: Multiple myeloma, Waldenström macroglobulinemia, B-cell lymphoma, CLL

    Mixed polyclonal or mixed monoclonal: Infectious diseases (viral [hepatitis C, HIV], bacterial, parasitic), infective endocarditis (IE), malaria; SLE, RA, polyarteritis nodosa, essential cryoglobulinemia; hemolytic anemia, lymphoproliferative diseases; sarcoidosis; chronic liver disease (cirrhosis)

- ▶ Cryoglobulins are abnormal proteins that precipitate out of serum at low temperatures. Cryocrit (quantitative) is preferred over qualitative method. Request analysis of positive results for immunoglobulin class and light-chain type.

10

CRYPTOCOCCAL ANTIGEN (SERUM AND CSF)

- Negative (titer is performed on positive specimens)
- ▶ Most *Cryptococcus neoformans* infections involve the lungs in immunocompetent (usually asymptomatic to mild disease) and immunocompromised individuals (more severe disease, may result in respiratory failure). Meningitis can occur, and is commonly seen with HIV/AIDS or other immunocompromised individuals. Serum cryptococcal antigen has a 90% sensitivity for cryptococcal meningitis. There are false positives, most commonly with RA.

CYSTATIN C LEVEL

- 0.5–1.3 mg/L

    Increased: Chronic kidney disease, renal failure

- ▶ Cystatin C is a proteinase that is produced by all nucleated cells and filtered by the kidneys and reabsorbed and metabolized in the proximal tubules. An elevation in cystatin C is seen in any cause of renal dysfunction such as end-stage kidney disease or renal dysfunction from NSAIDs. Useful when you have increased muscle mass (body builders, weightlifters) or decreased muscle mass (malnourishment, cirrhosis, or obesity) in assessing renal function.

CYTOMEGALOVIRUS (CMV) ANTIBODIES

- Both IgG and IgM antibody (Ab) assays are usually reported as either detected or not detected.

    Increased: IgG antibodies suggest previous exposure; IgM antibodies suggest recent or current infection.

▶ May be helpful in determining exposure history or infection status. Most adults have detectable Ab. In neonates, CMV IgG Ab may be present due to passive transfer from mother.

▶ CMV NAAT more useful for diagnosing/screening disease in neonates (saliva and urine commonly collected specimens). CMV infection in adults also commonly diagnosed by CMV NAAT from various specimen types depending on disease process. Quantitative NAAT is commonly performed on plasma specimens for disseminated or systemic disease in certain patient populations, e.g., transplant or other immunosuppressed patients.

D-DIMER

See also Chapter 11, page 286.

- <500 ng/mL

  Increased: DVT/PE, MI, CVA, recent surgery, trauma, malignancy, DIC, sepsis, sickle cell crisis, hypercoagulable states, pregnancy, renal failure

▶ D-Dimers are proteins released with the fibrinolytic breakdown of fibrin; used to rule out suspected DVT and PE; highly negative predictive value in this setting; level returns to normal if clot stabilized (i.e., treated with heparin) and not undergoing any further fibrin deposition or plasmin activation.

DEHYDROEPIANDROSTERONE (DHEA)

- Men: 180–1250 ng/dL
- Premenopausal women: 100–1100 ng/dL
- Postmenopausal: 50–500 ng/dL (peaks age 30 yr, decreases with age)

  Increased: Anovulation, polycystic ovaries, adrenal hyperplasia, adrenal tumors, congenital adrenal hyperplasia (CAH); due to deficiency in 11-hydroxylase, 3-beta-hydroxysteroid dehydrogenase, or 21-hydroxylase.

  Decreased: Menopause, anorexia nervosa, severe illness. Normally decreases with aging.

▶ One of three androgens (DHEA, DHEA-S, androstenedione) produced by the adrenal gland. Abnormal DHEA should only be interpreted in relation to other hormones.

DEHYDROEPIANDROSTERONE SULFATE (DHEAS)

See also, Chapter 12, Urine Studies, page 308, 17-Ketosteroids.

- Men: 40–500 mcg/dL
- Women: 20–320 mcg/dL (peaks age 30 yr, decreases with age)

  Increased: Hyperprolactinemia, adrenal hyperplasia, adrenal tumors, polycystic ovary syndrome (PCOS), ovarian tumors, drugs (metformin, others), smokers, most cases of congenital adrenal hyperplasia (CAH)

Decreased: Menopause, adrenal insufficiency, hypopituitarism, drugs (OCPs, corticosteroids, others)

▶ DHEAS (dehydroepiandrosterone-sulfate) is secreted exclusively by the adrenals, making it a good marker for adrenal androgen production. Sulfated form serves as the circulating storage pool for DHEA. DHEAS is generally preferred over DHEA, as DHEAS has a longer half-life and no circadian variation. Mild elevation in DHEAS is a common feature in women with PCOS, and it is often used in evaluation of females with hirsutism. Values above 700 ng/dL suggest an adrenal neoplasm.

11-DEOXYCORTISOL (CORTODOXONE, 17-ALPHA, 21 DIHYDROXYPROGESTERONE)

10

• <50 ng/dL males; <33 ng/dL females; variable based on age and laboratory

Increased: 11-beta-hydroxylase deficiency (also decrease in cortisol and increase in androgens), metyrapone use

Decreased: 21-hyroxylase deficiency, most common congenital adrenal hyperplasia (CAH) and 17-alpha-hydroxylase deficiency (also decrease in cortisol and increase in androgens for 21-hyroxylase and 17-alpha-hydroxylase deficiency)

▶ Precursor to cortisol. Useful in diagnosis and monitoring of CAH due to 11 β-hydroxylase deficiency.

DEXAMETHASONE SUPPRESSION TEST

Overnight test: The "rapid" screening version. Patient takes 1 mg of dexamethasone PO at 11 PM and fasts overnight; draw red top tube at 8 AM for serum cortisol. If 8 AM cortisol is <5 mcg/dL, the pituitary–adrenal axis suppresses normally, which excludes Cushing syndrome. An 8 AM serum cortisol ≥5 mcg/dL is abnormal. Result should be interpreted cautiously; many false positives (obesity, major anxiety/depression, severe stress, exogenous estrogen or anticonvulsant therapy, pregnancy, alcoholism). Use 24-hr urine collection for urinary free cortisol and creatinine as a screen for Cushing syndrome in these patients (see Chapter 10).

Two-day low-dose dexamethasone suppression test: Day 1, draw a baseline serum cortisol and collect 24-hr urine for free cortisol and creatinine. At 6 AM day 2, give 0.5 mg of dexamethasone PO q6h × 8 doses. On day 3, collect another 24-hr urine for urinary free cortisol excretion and creatinine. On days 3 and 4 draw serum cortisol at 8 AM. Normal: Suppression (cortisol <5 mcg/dL) by day 4 or urinary free cortisol <10% of baseline; this result excludes Cushing syndrome. Failure to suppress serum cortisol and/or urinary free cortisol increases the likelihood of Cushing syndrome; false-positives with rapid metabolizers of dexamethasone, anticonvulsant therapy, severe depression or stress, alcoholism.

High-dose dexamethasone suppression test: Similar to the low-dose test except that 2 mg of dexamethasone is given PO q6h × 8 doses; serum cortisol is not drawn. If urinary free cortisol <10% of baseline, suppressible pituitary adenoma is likely; otherwise, a nonpituitary cause of Cushing syndrome should be ruled out.

▶ Used to confirm or exclude the diagnosis of Cushing syndrome (increased serum cortisol)

17-ALPHA, 21-DIHYDROXYPROGESTERONE

See 11-Deoxycortisol, page 207.

DOPAMINE, SERUM

See Catecholamines, Fractionated, page 194.

DRUG LEVELS (THERAPEUTIC DRUG MONITORING [TDM])

• See Table 10-3, page 209

▶ The goal of TDM is to limit toxicity and determine the optimum dosing for an individual patient. Most commonly used for medications with a narrow therapeutic index or those potentially associated with significant toxicity. Medications such as anticonvulsants, antibiotics, antifungal drugs, antiviral drugs, antidepressants, immunosuppressive drugs, and cardiac drugs are routinely monitored. Timing of the blood collection is important in TDM. Typically, peak concentrations alone are used for toxicity, and trough levels used alone are useful for demonstrating satisfactory dosing. Trough levels are commonly used with medications such as carbamazepine, lithium, theophylline, phenytoin, valproic acid, and others and are usually obtained just before the next dose is scheduled (does not apply to digoxin). Peak and trough levels are routinely used for antibiotics such as gentamicin, tobramycin, and vancomycin to avoid toxicity and ensure antibacterial effect.

EPINEPHRINE, SERUM

See Catecholamines, Fractionated, page 194.

ERYTHROPOIETIN (EPO)

• 5–30 mU/mL

Increased: Pregnancy, secondary polycythemia (e.g., high altitude, COPD), tumors (renal cell carcinoma, cerebellar hemangioblastoma, hepatoma, others), PCKD, anemias with bone marrow unresponsiveness (e.g., aplastic anemia, iron deficiency), hemolytic anemia

Table 10-3. Some Common Drug Levels

Drug Name	Level**
Acetaminophen (for single-dose overdoses use normogram*)	10–30 μg/mL (Toxicity >50 μg/mL)
Alprazolam	10–50 ng/mL
Amikacin (once-daily dosing)	Peak: 20–30 μg/mL (Toxicity >30 μg/mL); trough 1–8 μg/mL (Toxicity >8 μg/mL)
Amiodarone	0.5–2.5 μg/mL
Amitriptyline	80–250 ng/mL
Amobarbital	1–5 μg/mL
Amoxapine	200–600 ng/mL
Atazanavir	150 ng/mL
Bupropion	25–100 ng/ml
Caffeine (infants less than 32 wk postmenstrual age)	5–25 mg/L
Carbamazepine	8–12 μg/mL (Toxicity >14 μg/mL)
Chloramphenicol	10–25 μg/mL
Chlordiazepoxide	0.7–1.0 μg/mL
Chlorpromazine (adult)	50–300 ng/mL
Chlorpromazine (child)	40–80 ng/mL
Chlorpropamide	75–250 mg/L
Clonazepam	15–60 ng/mL
Codeine	10–100 ng/mL
Cyclosporine (Toxicity)	>400 ng/mL
Desipramine	50–200 ng/mL
Diazepam	Diazepam + nordiazepam metabolite: 0.2–2.5 μg/mL (Toxicity: >5.0 μg/mL)
Digoxin	0.5–2.0 ng/mL (Toxicity >2.4 μg/mL)
Disopyramide	2.8–7.0 mg/L
Doxepin	150–250 ng/mL
Efavirenz	1000 ng/mL
Ethosuximide	40–100 μg/mL

*Acetaminophen. In: Nelson LS, Lewin NA, Howland MA, et al. Goldfrank's Toxicology Emergencies, 10e, New York, NY: McGraw-Hill; 2015.
**Ranges vary by lab and can vary by individual patient characteristics.
1 mg/L = 1 μg/mL; 1 μg/mL = 1000 ng/mL; 1 ng/ml = 0.001 μg/mL

Table 10-3. Some Common Drug Levels

Drug Name	Level**
Everolimus	3–15 ng/mL
Fosamprenavir	400 ng/mL (measured as amprenavir)
Gabapentin	2–20 µg/mL
Gentamicin (Conventional dosing q8h)	Trough target @ 24 hr 30 min before dose <1–2 µg/mL (Toxicity >2 µg/mL); Target peak @ 30 min after infusion 6–8 µg/mL; 8–10 µg/mL with serious infections (Toxicity >12 µg/mL)
Haloperidol	5–20 ng/mL
Ibuprofen	10–50 µg/mL
Imipramine	150–250 ng/mL
Isoniazid	1–7 µg/mL
Indinavir	100 ng/mL
Isopropanol (Isopropyl alcohol)	Toxicity >400 mg/L
Lamotrigine	2.5–15 µg/mL
Levetiracetam	12–46 µg/mL
Lidocaine	1.0–6.0 µmL g/mL
Lithium	0.6–1.2 mEq/L (Toxicity >1.5 mEq/L)
Lopinavir	10,000 ng/mL
Lorazepam	50–240 ng/mL
Maprotiline	200–600 ng/mL
Meperidine	0.4–0.7 µg/mL
Methadone	100–400 ng/mL
Methsuximide	10–40 µg/mL
Methyldopa	1–5 µg/mL
Metoprolol	75–200 ng/mL
Methotrexate:	
Toxicity 24 hr after dose	≥10 µmol/L
Toxicity 48 hr after dose	≥1 µmol/L
Toxicity 72 hr after dose	≥0.1 µmol/L

**Ranges vary by lab and can vary by individual patient characteristics.
1 mg/L = 1 µg/mL; 1 µg/mL = 1000 ng/mL; 1 ng/ml = 0.001 µg/mL

(Continued)

Table 10-3.   Some Common Drug Levels (*Continued*)

Drug Name	Level**
Morphine	10–80 ng/mL
Mycophenolic Acid	1.3–3.5 µg/mL
Naproxen	50 µg/mL
Nelfinavir	800 ng/mL
Nevirapine	3000 ng/mL
Nortriptyline	50–150 ng/mL
Oxazepam	0.2–1.4 µg/mL
Oxycodone	10–100 ng/mL
Pentobarbital	1–5 µg/mL
Phenobarbital	15–40 µg/mL (Toxicity >55 µg/mL)
Phenytoin	10–20 µg/mL (Toxicity >30 µg/mL)
	Note: Phenytoin levels are total phenytoin, total = free (~10% of total phenytoin) and phenytoin bound to protein; in protein-deficient states such as malnutrition, cirrhosis, protein-losing nephropathy or enteropathy, etc., a normal phenytoin level may actually be toxic. In this setting consider obtaining a free phenytoin level and assess for symptoms and signs of toxicity such as nausea, confusion, ataxia, and nystagmus.)
Primidone	
In Children	7–10 ug/mL
In Adults	9.0–12.5 ug/mL
Procainamide	10–30 µg/mL
Propoxyphene	0.1–0.4 µg/mL
Propranolol	50–100 ng/mL
Quinidine	2.0–5.0 µg/mL
Salicylates	15–30 mg/dL (Toxicity >40–80 mg/dL)
Saquinavir	100–205 ng/mL
Sertraline	10–50 ng/mL
Sirolimus	4–20 ng/mL

10

**Ranges vary by lab and can vary by individual patient characteristics.
1 mg/L = 1 µg/mL; 1 µg/mL = 1000 ng/mL; 1 ng/ml = 0.001 µg/mL

Table 10-3. Some Common Drug Levels *(Continued)*

Drug Name	Level**
Tacrolimus	3–20 ng/mL
Theophylline	10–20 µg/mL (Toxicity >25 µg/mL)
Thiopental	1–5 µg/mL
Thioridazine	1.0–1.5 µg/mL
Tobramycin (Conventional dosing q8h)	Trough target @ 24 hr 30 min before dose <1–2 µg/mL (Toxicity >2 µg/mL); Target peak @ 30 min after infusion 6–8 µg/mL; 8–10 ug/mL with serious infections (Toxicity >12 µg/mL)
Tocainide	4–10 µg/mL
Topiramate	5–20 µg/mL
Valproic Acid	50–150 µg/mL
Vancomycin	10–20 µg/mL (Toxicity >50 µg/mL)
Verapamil	100–500 ng/mL
Warfarin	1.0–10 µg/mL; maintain an INR of 2.0–3.0
Zidovudine	0.15–0.27 µg/mL

10

Decreased: Bilateral nephrectomy, anemia of chronic disease, renal failure, primary polycythemia, HIV infection treated with AZT.

▶ EPO is a renal hormone that stimulates RBC production. Measuring EPO levels before giving recombinant EPO for renal failure is not usually needed.

ESTRADIOL, SERUM

● Serum levels: See Table 10-4.

Increased: Estrogen-producing cancers (ovarian, adrenal, and testicular); early puberty, girls or late puberty, boys; gynecomastia; cirrhosis; hyperthyroidism; certain antibiotics; herbal or natural remedies; phenothiazines

Decreased: PCOS, Turner syndrome primary ovarian failure, anorexia nervosa

Table 10-4. Serum Estradiol Levels

Female	Normal Value
Follicular phase	20–350 pg/mL
Midcycle Peak	150–750 pg/mL
Luteal Phase	30–450 pg/mL
Pregnancy	
1st trimester	1–5 ng/mL
2nd trimester	5–15 ng/mL
3rd trimester	10–40 ng/mL
Postmenopause	**5–25 pg/mL**
Oral contraceptives	**<50 pg/mL**
Male	
Prepubertal	5–11 pg/mL
Adult	10–50 pg/mL

10

▸ Estradiol and estrone are the two biologically active estrogens in the non-pregnant state. Estradiol is the primary estrogen in premenopausal nonpregnant women. Elevated estrogens have been implicated in depression in young men.

ESTROGEN/PROGESTERONE RECEPTORS

▸ Determined with fresh surgical breast cancer specimens. Presence of the receptors (ER-positive, PR-positive) is associated with improved outcome and increased likelihood of responding to endocrine therapy (e.g., tamoxifen); 50–75% of breast cancers are estrogen receptor positive. "Triple-negative breast cancer" tests negative for estrogen receptors, progesterone receptors, and excess HER2 protein, making them more aggressive and unlikely to respond to hormonal therapy.

ESTRIOL, TOTAL AND UNCONJUGATED

• <2 ng/mL males and nonpregnant women; during pregnancy peaks at about 14 ng/mL

Increased: Pending labor

Decreased (unconjugated): Trisomy 21 (Down syndrome), one of four tests (α-fetoprotein, hCG, and inhibin A) during second trimester used for screening; trisomy 18 (Edwards syndrome); spina bifida; anencephaly

▶ One of three primary estrogens (estrone and estradiol) and the one that is the least biologically active; however, the predominate estrogen during pregnancy. There is a fourth estrogen, estetrol, produced by the fetal liver and only found during pregnancy.

ESTRONE

- Men: 15–65 pg/mL; women: follicular phase 100–250 pg/mL; luteal phase 15–200 pg/mL; postmenopausal 15–55 pg/mL

 Increased: Estrogen-producing cancers (ovarian, adrenal, and testicular); early puberty, girls, or late puberty, boys; gynecomastia; cirrhosis

 Decreased: Polycystic ovary syndrome, Turner syndrome, primary ovarian failure, anorexia nervosa

▶ Estrone and estradiol are the two biologically active estrogens in the nonpregnant state. Estrone is the primary estrogen in postmenopausal women.

ETHANOL (BLOOD ALCOHOL)

- **Normal "0 mg/dL"** (limit of quantification is <10 mg/dL)
- **<50 mg/dL:** Limited muscular incoordination, decreased inhibition
- **80 mg/dL:** Legal limit in all states; 46 United States and District of Columbia have stricter penalties at varying levels above 80 mg/dL that range from 100–250 mg/dL, and five states and District of Columbia have more than one cutoff for stricter penalties (as of February 2020)
- **50–100 mg/dL:** Pronounced incoordination
- **100–150 mg/dL:** Mood and personality changes
- **150–400 mg/dL:** Nausea, vomiting, marked ataxia, amnesia, ysarthria
- **>400 mg/dL:** Coma, respiratory insufficiency, and death risk increase; respiratory failure likely >700 mg/dL

▶ Ethyl alcohol (C_2H_5OH), commonly called ethanol, is in beverages. Physiologic changes can vary with degree of alcohol tolerance of an individual. Serum alcohol levels will read higher than whole blood, which corresponds to breathalyzer; thus, serum may imply intoxication (0.08 mg/dL) where the whole blood or breathalyzer reading would provide a level less than the cutoff for intoxication. The difference is roughly 10–15% higher in the serum [Barnhill MT, Herbert D, Wells Jr, DJ. Comparison of Hospital Laboratory Serum Alcohol Levels Obtained by an Enzymatic Method with Whole Blood Levels Forensically Determined by Gas Chromatography. J Anal Toxicol 2007;31(1):23–30].

FATTY ACIDS

See Free Fatty Acids, page 217.

FECAL FAT

- Quantitative 2–6 g/day on an 80–100 g/day fat diet
- 72-hr collection time (refrigerate sample)
- Random sample Sudan III or IV stain, <60 droplets fat/hpf

Increased: Pancreatic dysfunction (chronic pancreatitis, CF, Shwachman-Diamond syndrome), diarrhea with or without fat malabsorption (any diarrhea state alters fat absorption), regional enteritis (Crohn disease), celiac disease

▶ Aids in diagnosis of malabsorption, steatorrhea. Most fat normally absorbed in small bowel. The qualitative Sudan III stain on a spot sample of stool has 80–99% sensitivity in detecting clinically significant steatorrhea.

10

FECAL OCCULT BLOOD TESTING (FOBT)

- Normal: Negative

Positive: Colon or rectal polyps or cancer, hemorrhoids, anal fissures, esophageal or gastric cancer, peptic ulcers, ulcerative colitis, Crohn disease, GERD, esophageal varices, vascular ectasia, recent dental procedure with bleeding gums

False-positive: False positives noted here limited to guaiac testing: eating red meat within 3 days of test, fish, turnips, horseradish, or drugs such as colchicine and oxidizing drugs (e.g., iodine and boric acid)

False-negative: High doses of vitamin C (guaiac testing)

▶ Used for colorectal cancer (CRC) screening. Annual FOBT reduces colorectal cancer deaths 15–33%. With a positive FOBT, colonoscopy will usually be advised. See Appendix, pages 1051–1052 for recommended CRC screening.

- Guaiac-based FOBT. **Hemocult II, Hemocult SENSA** test card uses guaiac-impregnated paper and developer to detect oxidation of a colorless indicator to a blue color in the presence of hemoglobin pseudoperoxidase in the stool sample. Requires diet free of exogenous peroxidases (fish, horseradish, turnips), no vitamin C or medicines that irritate GI tract (e.g., NSAIDs). Patient typically collects 2–3 consecutive stool specimens and uses a wooden stick to place sample on assay card. Rectal exam sample may also be used. Low-cost FOBT option and is recommended annually.

- Fecal immunochemical test (FIT) for blood. **HemSelect (HS), OC Sensor, FlexSure (FS)** uses anti–human hemoglobin antibodies to detect human hemoglobin in stool. No need to restrict medications or change diet. Requires a special container for collection and should be processed in 24 hr and is recommended annually in the United States.
- Multitarget stool DNA testing. Commercially available in the United States as **Cologuard.** Tests for DNA (KRAS) mutations in shed cancer cells along with FIT testing. Requires special collection kit and is returned by mail. Requires a full stool sample.

FERRITIN

- Men: 30–500 ng/mL
- Women: 12–300 ng/mL
- Child 6 mo–15 yr: 7–142 ng/mL

Increased: Iron excess (hemochromatosis, hemosiderosis, chronic blood transfusions), porphyria, sideroblastic anemia, type 2 DM, postpartum state, hemophagocytic lymphohistiocytosis (HLH), hyperthyroidism, acute or chronic liver disease, chronic alcohol use/abuse, acute phase reactant (infection, [marked elevation with COVID-19 may identify patients with associated cytokine storm], any inflammatory diagnosis, surgery, traumatic injury, burns, and cancers)
- Levels > 1000 seen in HLH, hemochromatosis, adult-onset Still disease, severe COVID-19, sepsis, malignancy.

Decreased: Iron deficiency (earliest and most sensitive test, occurs before RBC morphologic change)

▶ Ferritin is the major storage protein for iron and is most useful in anemia workup; used to differentiate iron deficiency from anemia of chronic disease.

FOLATE (FOLIC ACID)

- Serum 5–25 ng/mL
- RBC folate 166–640 ng/mL

Increased: Folic acid administration
Decreased: Malnutrition/malabsorption (folic acid deficiency), massive cellular growth (cancer) or cell turnover, ongoing hemolysis, medications (trimethoprim, some anticonvulsants, oral contraceptives), vitamin B_{12} deficiency (low RBC and normal serum levels), pregnancy

▶ Serum folate fluctuates with diet; RBC levels are indicative of tissue stores; vitamin B_{12} deficiency can impede the ability of RBCs to take up folate despite normal serum folate level; thus, if RBC folate is low, consider vitamin B_{12} deficiency, while folate replacement in a vitamin B_{12}–deficient patient will correct the anemia, the neurological sequelae will not correct and are irreversible if not treated early.

FOLLICLE-STIMULATING HORMONE (FSH)

- Males (adult): 5–15 mU/mL (5–15 units/L)
- Females: follicular or luteal phase, 5–20 mU/mL (5–20 units/L); midcycle peak, 30–50 mU/mL (30–50 units/L); postmenopausal, greater than 35 mU/mL (>35 units/L)

10

Increased: Postmenopausal, surgical/chemical castration, primary or premature ovarian or testicular failure, gonadotropin-secreting pituitary adenoma, Klinefelter syndrome

Decreased: Prepubertal, hypothalamic and pituitary dysfunction, Kallmann syndrome LHRH analogue treatment, pregnancy, anorexia nervosa, drugs (OCPs, corticosteroids)

▶ Used in workup of impotence, male infertility, and female amenorrhea.

FTA-ABS (FLUORESCENT TREPONEMAL ANTIBODY ABSORBED)

See Rapid Plasma Reagin (RPR) and Titer, page 250.

FREE FATTY ACIDS

- Adults: 8–25 mg/dL (0.28–0.89 mmol/L); children and obese adults <31 mg/dL (<1.0 mmol/L)

Increased: Poorly controlled diabetes, pheochromocytoma, hyperthyroidism, alcoholism,

Decreased: Fatty acid malabsorption (chronic pancreatitis, pancreatic insufficiency, small bowel resection, cystic fibrosis), zinc deficiency

▶ Formed by the breakdown of lipoprotein and triglycerides, may be used to monitor nutritional therapy (malabsorption, starvation, TPN), diabetes management

FRUCTOSAMINE, SERUM

- Normal (nondiabetic): 170–285 μmol/L

Increased: Diabetes mellitus

▶ Fructosamine is a measure of glycosylated protein and provides a measure of glucose control in diabetics over the previous 2–3 wk. Hemoglobin A1c (HbA1c) provides an average over the last 3 mo. Can also be used to monitor DM control in patients with an abnormal hemoglobin.

FUNGAL SEROLOGY

- Negative or no bands identified; various methodologies, e.g., EIA, complement fixation, and immunodiffusion

▶ A screen for fungal antibodies; often used to detect antibodies to *Histoplasma capsulatum, Blastomyces dermatitidis, Aspergillus* species, *Candida* species, and *Coccidioides immitis.* Clinical utility limited due to cross-reactivity; clinical relevance may be greater with CSF specimens.

▶ Serum, plasma, or urinary antigen assays by EIA are available for *H. capsulatum, B. dermatitidis, C. immitis,* and *Aspergillus* spp. Interpretation complicated by cross-reactivity between assays. Fungal culture and fungal stain with morphological identification will be helpful.

GAMMA-GLUTAMYL TRANSFERASE (GGT)

- Men: <50 U/L
- Women: <30 U/L

Increased: Liver disease (acute or chronic hepatitis from any cause, cirrhosis, obstructive jaundice), primary or metastatic liver cancer, pancreatitis, drugs (phenytoin, carbamazepine, others)

▶ Parallels changes in serum alkaline phosphatase and 5′-nucleotidase in liver disease. Sensitive indicator of alcoholic liver disease. Also found in kidney and pancreas.

GASTRIN, SERUM

- Fasting: <100 pg/mL

Increased: Zollinger–Ellison syndrome, pyloric stenosis, pernicious anemia, achlorhydria, atrophic gastritis, ulcerative colitis, renal insufficiency, drugs (calcium [antacids, any source], H2-blockers, proton pump inhibitors [PPIs], glucocorticoids)
Decreased: Vagotomy and antrectomy

▶ Verify patient is not taking H2-blockers or antacids before test.

GLOBULINS (ALPHA-1, ALPHA-2, BETA, AND GAMMA)

See Protein and Protein Electrophoresis, pages 248 and 250.

GLUCAGON

* 20–100 pg/mL

Increased: Hypoglycemia, acute stress, prolonged fasting, exercise, any glucagon-producing tumor

Decreased: Chronic pancreatitis, status post-pancreatectomy, some with type 1 DM with prolonged hypoglycemia have blunted response to hypoglycemia, insulin, zinc

▶ Catabolic peptide hormone produced by the α cells of the pancreas; an insulin counterregulatory hormone along with growth hormone, cortisol, epinephrine, and norepinephrine.

10

GLUCOSE, SERUM

* Fasting, 70–100 mg/dL (3.9–5.6 mmol/L)
* Critical values: Adults <55 mg/dL; >450 mg/dL

Increased: DM (types 1 and 2), Cushing syndrome, acromegaly, increased epinephrine (e.g., injection, pheochromocytoma, stress, burns), acute and chronic pancreatitis, ACTH administration, spurious cause (sample taken from site above IV containing dextrose), advanced age, pancreatic glucagonoma, drugs (glucocorticoids, thiazide diuretics, OCPs, others)

Decreased: Pancreatic islet cell tumors (insulinoma), extrapancreatic tumors (carcinoma of adrenal gland, stomach), celiac disease, Whipple disease, severe hepatic disease (hepatitis, cirrhosis, tumors), endocrine disorders (hypothyroidism, hypopituitarism, cortisol deficiency, GH deficiency), renal diagnosis, pediatric (prematurity, infant of diabetic mother, ketotic hypoglycemia, enzyme diseases), exogenous insulin, oral hypoglycemic agents, malnutrition, sepsis, alcohol, exercise

▶ **American Diabetes Association Diagnostic Criterion for Diabetes:** Normal fasting <100 mg/dL; impaired fasting 100–125 mg/dL; DM 126 mg/dL or higher on more than one occasion or any random level >200 mg/dL with associated symptoms such as polyuria, polydipsia, polyphagia, and weight loss.
▶ Most glucose strips and meters quantify whole blood glucose. Most labs use plasma or serum, which reads 10–15% higher. Samples where the serum is not separated from blood cells have glucose values decreasing at rate of 3–5%/hr at room temperature.

▶ Point-of-care testing (POCT) for glucose is a useful tool for managing diabetes with digital glucometers using a fingerstick drop of blood. The FDA approvals for most glucose POCT include home use by patients and use in the hospital setting. POCT for glucose should be used with caution, if at all, for critically ill patients, who may be affected by hypoxemia, poor perfusion, or severe anemia that could affect device accuracy. While POCT for blood glucose has become the mainstay for serial monitoring and decision-making in the management of diabetes, it cannot replace clinical laboratory testing for precision and accuracy. POCT glucose monitors should not be used to diagnose diabetes mellitus.

GLUCOSE-6-PHOSPHATE-DEHYDROGENASE (G6PD)

10

- Screen: Normal/deficient; quantitative: 7.0–20.5 units/g of Hgb

    Decreased: G6PD deficiency; with hemolysis, qualitative assay may be falsely negative since the G6PD-deficient red cells have been hemolyzed; quantitative method is dependent on the gm/dL of hemoglobin

▶ Used with suspected G6PD deficiency (G6PD deficiency is X-linked inheritance; causes variable forms of hemolytic anemia)

GLUCOSE TOLERANCE TEST (GTT), ORAL (OGTT)

▶ Two fasting glucose levels ≥126 mg/dL or a random glucose >200 mg/dL (11.1 mmol/L) is the threshold for diagnosis of DM. GTT is not necessary for diagnosis of DM and may be useful in gestational DM. Unreliable in the presence of severe infection, prolonged fasting, or after insulin injection. After an 8–12-hr overnight fast (water only), a fasting blood glucose sample is drawn, and the patient ingests a 75-g oral glucose load, usually by drinking Glucola (100 g for gestational DM screening, 1.75 mg/kg ideal body weight in children up to 75 g). For the diagnosis of DM, blood for glucose at baseline, 1 hr, and 2 hr after glucose load. For gestational DM, blood for glucose at baseline, 1 hr, 2 hr, and 3 hr after glucose load.

Interpretation of GTT

Normal glucose tolerance: Glucose <140 mg/dL 2 hr after glucose load

Impaired glucose tolerance: Fasting glucose >110 mg/dL and <126 mg/dL, risk factor for future diabetes. Glucose 140–199 mg/dL 2 hr after glucose load

Diabetes: Glucose >200 mg/dL 2 hr after glucose load

Gestational diabetes: OGTT usually done at about 28 wk with any two of the following glucose levels diagnostic: fasting >105 mg/dL, 1 hr >190 mg/dL, 2 hr >165 mg/dL, or 3 hr >145 mg/dL

GLYCOHEMOGLOBIN (GLYCOSYLATED HEMOGLOBIN, GLYCATED HEMOGLOBIN, HEMOGLOBIN A1$_c$, HbA$_{1c}$)

- Normal nondiabetic: 4.0–5.6%; goal is individualized; generally, the goal for DM is <7%; for the elderly, the goal is 7.5–8.0%

  Increased: DM (uncontrolled), lead intoxication, hemoglobin F
  Decreased: Chronic renal failure, hemolytic anemia, acute or chronic blood loss, hemoglobinopathies

▶ Mean plasma glucose is equal to (HbA1c × 35.6) – 77.3. Useful in long-term monitoring control of blood sugar in diabetic patients; reflects levels over preceding 3–4 mo; not used to diagnose DM (see also Fructosamine).

10

GROWTH HORMONE (GH), SOMATOTROPIN

- 0–7 years: 1–13.6 ng/mL; 7–11 years: 1–16.4 ng/mL; 11–15 years: 1–14.4 ng/mL; 15–19 years: 1–13.4 ng/mL
- Adult males: 0–4.0 ng/mL
- Adult females: 0–18.0 ng/mL

  Increased: Pituitary adenoma (isolated GH or combination GH and prolactin), nonpituitary tumor (rare, lymphoma, pancreatic islet cell), GH insensitivity, malnutrition, drugs (dopamine, L-dopa)
  Decreased: Hypopituitarism (non–GH-secreting adenoma, irradiation, Sheehan syndrome), hypothalamic injury/damage (irradiation), pituitary dwarfism, adrenocortical hyperfunction

▶ Growth hormone (GH) or human growth hormone (HGH) is produced in the anterior pituitary gland, and normal production is controlled by GH-releasing factor. Used to diagnose conditions such as gigantism, acromegaly, and Laron dwarfism (defective GH receptor).

HAPTOGLOBIN

- 50–150 mg/dL (500–1500 mg/L)

  Increased: Acute phase reactant (infection, any inflammatory diagnosis, surgery, traumatic injury, burns, and cancers), obstructive liver disease, MI
  Decreased: Any type of hemolysis (e.g., autoimmune, transfusion reaction, status post-uneventful transfusion), liver disease, oral contraceptives, childhood and infancy

▶ An acute phase reactant synthesized by the liver. Very sensitive test for RBC destruction and useful in the diagnosis and management of an acute transfusion reaction.

HELICOBACTER PYLORI ANTIGEN, FECES

- Normal: Absence of detectable antigen

    Positive: H. *pylori* antigen present in the stool
    Negative: Does not exclude the possibility of *H. pylori* infection.

▶ Collection: 5 g of stool in a screw-capped, plastic container. Submit promptly to lab. Watery, diarrheal specimens or stool in transport media, swabs, or preservatives cannot be tested.

▶ Used to diagnose *H. pylori* infection and monitor *H. pylori* clearing after therapy. Persons without symptoms should not be tested. PPIs and bismuth subsalicylates may cause false-negative results. Sensitivity and specificity are ~95%.

10

HEPATITIS TESTING (HEPATITIS A, HEPATITIS B, HEPATITIS C, HEPATITIS D, HEPATITIS E)

Recommended hepatitis panel tests based on clinical settings are shown in Table 10-5, page 223, and pattern interpretation in Table 10-6, page 225. Profile patterns of hepatitis A and B are shown in Figure 10-1, page 226, and Figure 10-2, page 226.

Hepatitis A Virus (HAV)

(See also Figure 10-1)

Anti-HAV: Total antibody to hepatitis A virus (IgG and IgM); confirms previous exposure to HAV; the IgG component is detectable for life. Positive 8 wk after exposure.

Anti-HAV IgM: IgM antibody to hepatitis A virus; suggests recent HAV infection; declines typically 1–6 mo after symptoms.

Hepatitis B Virus (HBV)

(See also Figure 10-2)

HBsAg: Hepatitis B surface antigen. Earliest marker of HBV infection (excluding NAAT); indicates chronic or acute infection. Also used to screen blood donors for HBV; vaccination does not affect this test.

Anti-HBc-total: IgG and IgM antibodies to HBV core antigen; confirms either previous exposure to HBV or ongoing acute or chronic infection. Used by blood banks to screen donors for HBV.

Anti-HBc IgM: IgM antibody to hepatitis B core antigen. Early and best indicator of acute infection with HBV.

Table 10-5. Hepatitis Panel Testing to Guide the Ordering of Hepatitis Profiles for Given Clinical Settings

Clinical Setting	Test(s)[a]	Purpose
SCREENING TESTS		
Pregnancy	HBsAg	All expectant mothers should be screened during third trimester
High-risk patients on admission (e.g., MSM[b], dialysis patients, IV drug users, etc.)	HBsAg Anti-HBs Anti-HBc	To differentiate chronic from active infection, immunity (prior infection), or vaccination
Percutaneous inoculations		
Donor	HBsAg Anti-HCV	To test patients' blood (esp. dialysis and HIV patients) for potential infectivity if a healthcare worker is exposed
Victim	Anti-HBs Anti-HBc Anti-HCV (known HCV exposure)	To test exposed healthcare worker for immunity of chronic infection For follow-up monitoring after known exposure
Pre-HBV vaccine	Anti-HBc Anti-HBs	To determine if a high-risk individual is infected or has antibodies to HBV
Screening blood donors	HBsAg Anti-HBc Anti-HCV	Used to screen blood donors for HBV and HCV
DIAGNOSTIC TESTS		
Differential diagnosis of acute jaundice, hepatitis, or fulminant liver failure	HBsAg Anti-HBc IgM Anti-HAV IgM Anti-HCV	To differentiate HBV, HAV, and HCV in an acutely jaundiced patient with hepatitis or fulminant liver failure; HCV rarely causes symptomatic acute hepatitis

10

Table 10-5. Hepatitis Panel Testing to Guide the Ordering of Hepatitis Profiles for Given Clinical Settings

Clinical Setting	Test(s)[a]	Purpose
Chronic hepatitis	HBsAg	To help diagnose chronic HBV infection; if positive for HBsAg need to determine infectivity
	HBeAg	Indicates increased infectivity if HBsAg positive; also obtain if HBsAg patient worsens or becomes very ill
	Anti-HBe	Often correlates with loss of HBeAg, i.e., loss of viral production (however, may revert back to HBeAg positive)
	Anti-HDV (total + IgM)	To diagnose concomitant infection with HDV
	Anti-HCV	To diagnose chronic HCV infection. If anti-HCV is +, then order HCV-NAAT to confirm chronic infection (active viral replication)
MONITORING		
Infant follow-up	HBsAg Anti-HBc Anti-HBs	To monitor the success of vaccination and passive immunization for perinatal transmission of HBV 12–15 mo after birth (HBV NAAT also helpful)
Postvaccination screening	Anti-HBs	To ensure immunity has been achieved after vaccination
Sexual contact	HBsAg Anti-HBc Anti-HCV	To monitor sexual partners of a patient with chronic HBV or HCV

[a] See Abbreviations list on pages 222, 225, and 227 for definition of abbreviations;
[b]Men who have sex with men.

Table 10-6. Interpretation of Viral Hepatitis Serologic Testing Patterns

Anti-HAV (IgM)	HBsAg	Anti-HBc (IgM)	Anti-HBc (Total)	Anti-HCV	Interpretation
+	−	−	−	−	Acute HAV
+	+	−	+	−	Acute HAV in HBV carrier
−	+	−	+	−	Chronic HBV[a]
−	−	+	+	−	Acute HBV
−	+	+	+	−	Acute HBV
−	−	−	+	−	Past HBV
−	−	−	−	+	Hepatitis C[b]
−	−	−	−	−	Early HCV or other viral cause or toxin

[a]Patients with chronic hepatitis B (either active hepatitis or carrier state) should have HBeAg and anti-HBe checked to determine activity of infection and relative infectivity. Anti-HBs is used to determine response to hepatitis B vaccination.
[b]Anti-C is often not positive for 3–6 mo. NAAT may allow earlier detection.

10

HBeAg: Hepatitis Be antigen; indicates viral replication/infectivity. Positive in acute or chronic hepatitis B. Order only when evaluating for chronic HBV infection.

HBV NAAT: Most sensitive and specific early evaluation for HBV; may be detectable when all other markers are negative. Positive in acute or chronic hepatitis B, asymptomatic hepatitis B carriers.

Anti-HBe: Antibody to hepatitis Be antigen; associated with loss of viral replication.

Anti-HBs: Antibody to hepatitis B surface antigen; indicates immunity and clinical recovery from infection or previous immunization with hepatitis B vaccine. Use to assess effectiveness of vaccine; request titer. Negative in epatitis B carrier.

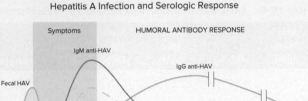

Figure 10-1. Clinical and serological response in a patient with acute hepatitis A virus infection. Fecal HAV = viral shedding in the stool; Viremia = hepatitis A virus in the blood; anti-HAV IgM = IgM antibody to hepatitis A; anti-HAV IgA = IgA antibody to hepatitis A; anti-HAV IgG = IgG antibody to hepatitis A. (Reproduced with permission of Abbott, © 2021. All rights reserved; Scarborough; Adapted from: http://www.benbest.com/health/hepa.html).

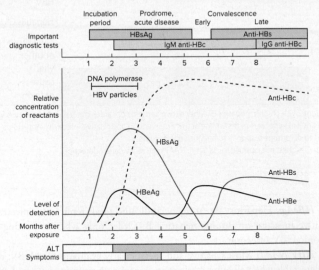

Figure 10-2. Clinical and serologic response in a patient with acute hepatitis B virus infection. ALT = alanine aminotransferase; anti-HBc = antibody to hepatitis B core antigen; anti-HBe = antibody to hepatitis Be antigen; anti-HBs = antibody to hepatitis B surface antigen; HBeAg = hepatitis Be antigen; HBsAg = hepatitis B surface antigen; HBV = hepatitis B virus; IgG = immunoglobulin G; IgM = immunoglobulin M. (Reproduced with permission from Riedel S, Hobden JA, Miller S, Morse SA, Mietzner TA, Detrick B, Mitchell TG, Sakanari JA, Hotez P, Mejia R. Hepatitis Viruses. In: *Jawetz, Melnick, & Adelberg's Medical Microbiology*, 28e; 2019.)

Hepatitis C Virus (HCV)

Anti-HCV: Antibody against HCV. Most commonly used to diagnose chronic infection. Patients who are positive for antibody should have HCV NAAT performed to detect active viral replication (chronic infection). Positive HCV antibody with negative HCV NAAT may indicate cleared infection or false-positive antibody result. The USPSTF recommends one-time screening for all persons ages 18–79 for HCV. Persons who inject drugs should undergo periodic screening, though the interval between screenings has not been determined.

HCV-NAAT: Used to confirm antibody result and to identify chronic infection (active viral replication).

Hepatitis C genotyping: Six genotypes and three additional subtypes (1a, 1b, 2a, 2b, 3a, 3b, 4, 5a, 6a). Genotypes 1, 2, and 3 are the most common genotypes in North America, and genotype 1 is the more difficult genotype to cure.

10

▶ The particular genotype will dicrate the drugs used to treat and the length of treatment.

Hepatitis D Virus (HDV)

Anti-HDV: Total antibody to HDV; confirms previous exposure. Use with known acute or chronic HBV infection.

Anti-HDV IgM: IgM antibody to HDV; indicates recent infection. Use to test in known acute or chronic HBV infection. Positive in 80–90% of chronic HBsAg carriers.

▶ Hepatitis D can only infect HBsAg-positive patients.

Hepatitis E Virus (HEV)

Anti-HEV IgG: Previous infection with HEV
Anti-HEV IgM: Acute infection with HEV
HEV RNA: Detection of virus in blood or stool

▶ HEV is a self-limited disease that does not result in chronic infection. While rare in the United States, HEV is common in many parts of the world and is transmitted through ingestion of fecal matter from contaminated water or food sources. There are four genotypes.

HIGH-DENSITY LIPOPROTEIN (HDL) CHOLESTEROL

See Cholesterol, page 195.

HLA TYPING

See Human Leukocyte Antigens (HLA Typing), page 231.

HOMOCYSTEINE, PLASMA

- Normal fasting: males, 0.54–2.16 mg/L (4–16 μmol/L); females, 0.41–1.89 mg/L (3–14 μmol/L)

Increased: Disorders of methionine metabolism involving methionine synthase or cystathionine beta-synthase and cobalamin metabolism, vitamin B_{12}, B_6, and folate deficiency, renal failure, medications (nicotinic acid, theophylline, methotrexate, levodopa, anticonvulsants), chronic alcohol use, advanced age, hypothyroidism, SLE.

▶ An independent risk factor for CAD and atherosclerosis. Moderate, intermediate, and severe hyperhomocysteinemia refer to concentrations 16–30, 31–100, and >100 μmol/L, respectively. May be useful for screening patients at increased risk for ASCVD and recommendation of strategies for obtaining ideal target of <10 μmol/L (i.e., dietary, lifestyle changes, vitamin supplementation).

HUMAN CHORIONIC GONADOTROPIN, SERUM (HCG)

- Normal <3.0 mIU/mL
- Pregnancy: 10 days after conception, >3 mIU/mL; 30 days, 100–5000 mIU/mL; 10 wk, 50,000–140,000 mIU/mL; >16 wk, 10,000–50,000 mIU/mL. Thereafter levels slowly decline.

Increased: Pregnancy, ectopic pregnancy, hyperemesis gravidarum, testicular tumors (teratoma and seminoma [15%]), trophoblastic disease (hydatidiform mole, choriocarcinoma levels usually >100,000 mIU/mL)

▶ Detection of pregnancy and a tumor marker (choriocarcinoma and some testicular germ cell tumors; mostly non-seminomatous germ cell tumors)

HUMAN IMMUNODEFICIENCY VIRUS (HIV) TESTING

See algorithm in Figure 10-3A and Figure 10-3B, based on CDC guidelines.

▶ HIV testing is recommended by the CDC for all persons between the ages of 13 and 64 years of age one time. Additionally, screen all

Recommended Laboratory HIV Testing Algorithm for Serum or Plasma Specimens

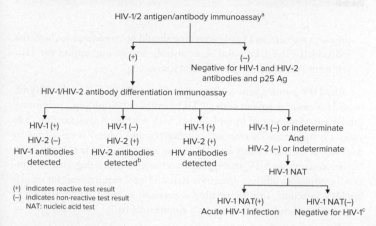

(+) indicates reactive test result
(−) indicates non-reactive test result
    NAT: nucleic acid test

[a]The FDA-approved single-use rapid HIV-1/HIV-2 antigen/antibody immunoassay can be used as the initial assay in the laboratory HIV testing algorithm for serum or plasma. If any instrumented antigen/antibody test is available, it is preferred due to its superior sensitivity for detecting HIV during acute infection.
[b]This includes specimens reported as HIV-2 positive with HIV-1 cross-reactivity.
[c]A negative HIV-1 NAT result and repeatedly HIV-2 indeterminate or HIV indeterminate antibody differentiation immunoassay result should be referred for testing with a different validated supplemental HIV-2 test (antibody test or NAT) or repeat the algorithm in 2–4 weeks, starting with an antigen/antibody immunoassay.

Figure 10-3A. Diagnostic algorithm for HIV infection. (Branson BM, Owen SM, Wesolowski LG. Laboratory Testing for the Diagnosis of HIV Infection: Updated Recommendations. CDC. June 27, 2014, p. 7. https://stacks.cdc.gov/view/cdc/50872. Accessed January 16, 2021.)

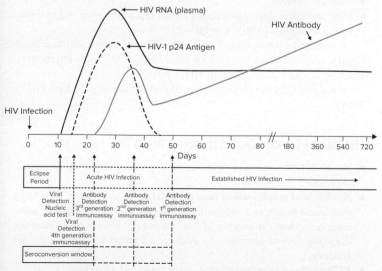

Figure 10-3B. Sequence of appearance of laboratory markers for HIV-1 infection. Units for vertical axis are not noted because the magnitude differs for each marker. (Branson BM, Owen SM, Wesolowski LG. Laboratory Testing for the Diagnosis of HIV Infection: Updated Recommendations. CDC. June 27, 2014, p. 11. https://stacks.cdc.gov/view/cdc/50872. Accessed January 16, 2021.)

pregnant women, and yearly screening should be considered for high-risk individuals. The CDC also recommends an opt-out option for HIV testing as part of preventive laboratory screening.

Any HIV-positive person >6 yr old with a CD4+ T-cell level <200/mL or an HIV-positive patient with a CDC-defined condition (e.g., pulmonary candidiasis, disseminated histoplasmosis, HIV wasting, Kaposi sarcoma, TB, various lymphomas, *Pneumocystis* pneumonia, and others) is considered to have AIDS. Confidentiality in HIV testing is regulated by law. Many states require consent for HIV testing. We recommend contacting your institutional compliance office to determine state and local requirements for reporting HIV infection. This information is normally released only in writing to the ordering attending physician on a confidential basis.

10

HIV Antigen/Antibody Assay (Fourth-Generation)

- Normal: Negative

  Recognize both HIV-1 and HIV-2 antibodies and HIV p24 antigen.
  Uses: Diagnosis of HIV infection. Antibodies develop 1–4 mo after infection, and p24 antigen is detected approximately 2 wk after infection.

HIV-1/HIV-2 Antibody Differentiation Assay

- Normal: Negative
- ▶ Used to confirm HIV Ag/antibody fourth-generation assay and to differentiate antibodies to HIV-1 or HIV-2

  If negative or indeterminate, HIV-1 NAAT may provide clarification; if negative and clinical suspicion is high for recent exposure (early infection) or advanced disease (AIDS), perform HIV-1 NAAT.

  If positive, indicates HIV infection. As part of follow-up, perform HIV-1 NAAT.

HIV Viral Load (Quantitative NAAT)

- Negative: Lower limits of detection are approximately 20–40 copies/mL of plasma.
- ▶ **Nucleic acid amplification tests (NAATs)** are used to detect HIV. Used to evaluate extent and progression of disease and for monitoring treatment (e.g., detect emergence of drug resistance). Should not be used for diagnosis. Several commercially available quantitative RT-PCR tests are available:
- **PCR** most common; results reported as copies/mL of plasma
- **bDNA** (branched-chain DNA assay) reported as units/mL of plasma

- **NASBA** (nucleic acid sequence–based amplification) infrequently used; reported units/mL of plasma

    Increased: Acute HIV infection, AIDS, disease progression, drug resistance

    Decreased: Response to therapy, remission of HIV

▶ In the past, when to initiate antiretroviral treatment was often based on CD4 count and/or the viral load. Now, treatment is almost always instituted when the diagnosis is made or very shortly afterwards. When immune reconstitution inflammatory syndrome is a concern (e.g., cryptococcal meningitis or TB meningitis diagnosed simultaneously with HIV), antiretroviral treatment should **NOT** be instituted until shortly after the treatment of the infection is started. However, initiating early antiretroviral treatment is beneficial in the presence of nonmeningeal TB infections, mild-to-moderate limited Kaposi sarcoma, and non-Hodgkin lymphoma. (https://aidsinfo.nih.gov/guidelines/html/1/adult-and-adolescent-arv/10/initiation-of-antiretroviral-therapy, accessed 3/23/2020).

10

Other HIV Testing

Tropism testing. Used to predict virologic response to CCR5 antagonists (maraviroc, others).

HLA-B*57:01: Screens patients for hypersensitivity to abacavir (occurs in 5–8% of patients).

Oral mucosal transudate test. A pad collects oral mucosal transudate (OMT). This fluid contains HIV antibodies in an HIV-infected person.

Urine HIV antibody test. Detects HIV antibodies, accuracy less than blood and oral tests; confirm positive with Western blot.

Home test kits. These are widely available on the Internet and may use self-pinprick blood, oral pad, or urine testing. The OraQuick In-Home HIV Test, uses an gum swab sample and is the only HIV rapid in-home test approved by the FDA as of 1/2021. All positive home tests require confirmation by formal lab testing.

HUMAN LEUKOCYTE ANTIGEN (HLA) TYPING

▶ Used to identify a group of antigens on the cell surface that are the primary determinants of histocompatibility; useful in assessing transplantation compatibility. Some HLA antigens are associated with specific diseases but are not diagnostic of these diseases.

HLA-A31:01: Carbamazepine sensitivity
HLA-A32:01: Vancomycin sensitivity including eosinophilia
HLA-B15:02: Carbamazepine sensitivity

IRON-BINDING CAPACITY, TOTAL (TIBC)

- Serum: 250–460 µg/dL (45–82 µmol/L)

   Increased: Acute and chronic blood loss, iron-deficiency anemia, acute hepatitis, OCPs, pregnancy

   Decreased: Anemia of chronic disease, cirrhosis, nephrotic syndrome, renal failure, hemochromatosis, iron therapy overload, hemolytic anemia, aplastic anemia, thalassemia, megaloblastic anemia, malnutrition

▶ Used in differential diagnosis of anemia and screen for iron overload disorder

LACTATE DEHYDROGENASE (LD, LDH)

- Adults: 100–190 U/L (1.7–3.2 mkat/L)
- Higher in childhood
- Critical value: >3000 U/L

   Increased: AMI, heart failure, cardiac surgery, prosthetic valve, PE, hepatitis, obstructive liver disease, cirrhosis, malignancy, non-Hodgkin lymphoma, pernicious anemia, hemolysis (anemias or factitious), polycythemia vera, TTP, renal infarction, renal disease, muscle injury, muscle disease, megaloblastic anemia, lung injury, *Pneumocystis jiroveci* infection, hepatotoxic drugs (e.g., acetaminophen overdose, many others)

▶ Tissue breakdown releases LDH. Elevated LDH suggests injury to muscles, liver, red cells, or rapid cell division (e.g., lymphomas).

LACTIC ACID (LACTATE)

- Venous blood: 6–16 mg/dL (0.67–1.8 mmol/L)

   Increased: Lactic acidosis due to hypoxia, hemorrhage, shock, sepsis, cirrhosis, exercise, ethanol intoxication, DKA, regional ischemia (extremity, bowel), generalized seizures, trauma, HIV infection and antiretroviral therapy, spurious factors (prolonged use of a tourniquet), metabolic disease (type 1 glycogen storage disease, pyruvate dehydrogenase deficiency, many others), alcohols and glycols (ethanol, ethylene glycol, methanol, propylene glycol), and drugs (metformin, isoniazid, epinephrine, NRTIs, others)

▶ The most frequent cause of lactic acidosis is poor tissue perfusion (various shock states with tissue hypoxia). Suspect lactic acidosis with elevated anion gap in the absence of other causes (renal failure, ethanol, methanol, ethylene glycol, and salicylate ingestion). Lactic acidosis is a complication of antiretroviral therapy. In the critical care setting, mortality with a serum lactate level >2 mmol/L persisting after 24 hr with acidosis approaches 70%.

LACTOSE TOLERANCE TEST, BLOOD

▶ Lactose load and obtain serum fasting glucose; administer 50 gm lactose load and in 60 and 120 min obtain glucose. Normal is an expected rise of >30 mg/dL in serum glucose after load. Serum glucose <20 mg/dL with GI symptoms suggests lactase deficiency. Diabetes mellitus and delayed gastric emptying can result in false-negative results. Infrequently performed; breath hydrogen test more commonly used.

LACTOSE TOLERACE TEST, BREATH HYDROGEN

▶ Administer lactose after an overnight fast. Expired air samples collected before and at 30-min intervals for 3 hrs to assess hydrogen gas concentration. An increase in breath hydrogen concentration >20 parts per million over the baseline suggests lactase deficiency. Currently the diagnostic test of choice for lactose intolerance.

LAP SCORE (LEUKOCYTE ALKALINE PHOSPHATASE SCORE/STAIN)

• 50–150

Increased: Leukemoid reaction, acute inflammation, Hodgkin disease, pregnancy, liver disease, polycythemia vera
Decreased: CML, PNH, nephrotic syndrome

▶ Differentiates CML from leukemoid reaction; evaluation of polycythemia vera, myelofibrosis with myeloid metaplasia, and paroxysmal nocturnal hemoglobinuria (PNH)

LEAD, BLOOD

See also Chapter 12, Urine Studies, page 306, Heavy metals, Urine.

• Child <6 yr: <10 mcg/dL
• Child 6–18 yr: <25 mcg/dL
• Adult: <40 mcg/dL

Increased: Lead poisoning from ingestion (paint, lead plumbing, moonshine whiskey), occupational exposure (metal smelters, welders, petroleum refinery workers, paint manufactures, others)

▶ Neurologic findings at 15 mg/dL in children and 30 mg/dL in adults; severe symptoms (lethargy, ataxia, coma) >60 mcg/dL

MAGNESIUM

See also Chapter 15, page 444, Hypermagnesemia, Hypomagnesemia.

- Serum: 1.5–2.4 mg/dL (0.62–0.99 mmol/L)
- Critical values: <1.0 and >4.9 mg/dL

Increased: Renal failure, Addison disease, hypothyroidism, trauma, severe dehydration, drugs (magnesium-containing antacids, laxatives, and enemas; lithium, progesterone, diuretics [triamterene, high-dose furosemide])

Decreased: Malabsorption, steatorrhea, acute pancreatitis, alcoholism, uncontrolled hyperglycemia, hyperthyroidism, aldosteronism, hyperparathyroidism, hungry bone syndrome, hyperalimentation without adequate supplementation, NG suctioning, chronic dialysis, renal tubular acidosis, Bartter syndrome, Gitelman syndrome, hypophosphatemia, intracellular shifts with respiratory or metabolic acidosis, drugs (aminoglycosides, cisplatin, cyclosporine, amphotericin B, diuretics, pentamidine, rapamycin, long-term use of PPIs, calcium salts, massive blood transfusion [citrate induced])

▶ Used to monitor preeclampsia patients when using magnesium sulfate, poor nutritional status, malabsorption requiring magnesium monitoring

MANGANESE

- 4–15 mcg/L

Increased: Occupational exposure from welding or contaminated water

▶ Manganese is an essential trace element present in many foods, as a dietary supplement, and is a cofactor for many enzymes. Toxicity from inhalation usually from occupational exposure or contaminated water. Symptoms may be nonspecific (include fatigue, weakness), neurologic (psychosis, Parkinson-like symptoms including tremor and rigidity), respiratory, and reproductive.

METHEMOGLOBIN

- 0.06–0.24 g/dL or <1.5% of hemoglobin

Increased: Hereditary methemoglobinemia (autosomal recessive), oxidant drug induced (local anesthetics [benzocaine, lidocaine, prilocaine], dapsone, sulfa drugs, phenytoin, isoniazid, nitroprusside, nitroglycerin, nitrates, hydralazine, and many others; drugs of abuse [cocaine, amyl nitrite])

▶ Small amounts of methemoglobin normally present in blood. With the conversion of a larger fraction of hemoglobin into methemoglobin, perceptible cyanosis results. Treatment of methemoglobinemia is administration of methylene blue and/or ascorbic acid. (A historic Kentucky note is that one of the most famous discoveries in the treatment of hereditary methemoglobinemia was in a family from the Troublesome Creek and Ball Creek regions near Hazard, Kentucky Cawein M, Behlen CH, Lappat EJ, et al. Hereditary Diaphorase Deficiency and Methemoglobinemia. *Arch Intern Med* 1964;113:578–585.)

METHYLMALONIC ACID (MMA)

- Serum: 150–370 nmol/L

    Increased: Vitamin B_{12} deficiency; CKD (mild increase in levels), genetic (autosomal recessive) may involve multiple genes, methylmalonic CoA mutase (MMUT) is the most common

▶ Used to evaluate megaloblastic anemia (B_{12}/cobalamin deficiency) and methylmalonic academia in children

10

β₂-MICROGLOBULIN, SERUM

See also Chapter 12, page 301, β2-Microglobulin, Spot Urine.

- <2 µg/mL (<170 nmol/L)

    Increased: Inflammatory diseases such as inflammatory bowel disease and autoimmune disease (e.g., SLE), HIV and CMV infection, lymphoid malignant disease (lymphoma, Waldenstrom macroglobulinemia, multiple myeloma), myeloproliferative and myelodysplastic disorders, transplant rejection, renal disease (chronic renal failure, diabetic nephropathy, pyelonephritis, ATN, nephrotoxicity from medications)

▶ A portion of the class I MHC antigen; useful marker for following progression of B-cell malignancies (e.g., multiple myeloma); levels <4 µg/mL good prognosis in multiple myeloma

MONOSPOT

- Normal: Negative

    Positive: Mononucleosis, rarely in leukemia, serum sickness, Burkitt lymphoma, viral hepatitis, rheumatoid arthritis (RA)

▶ The test is not recommended for general use, as the antibodies detected can be due to conditions other than infectious mononucleosis. Moreover, studies have shown that the Monospot produces both false-positive and false-negative results. Epstein–Barr virus (EBV) infection is the most common cause of mononucleosis.

OSMOLALITY, SERUM

- 275–295 mOsm/kg H$_2$O (275–295 mmol/kg H$_2$O)
- Critical value <250 mOsm/kg or >295 mOsm/kg

Increased: Hypernatremia from any cause (severe burns, diarrhea, vomiting, DI, iatrogenic or accidental overdose [excessive NaCl, or NaHCO3]), ethanol, methanol, isopropyl alcohol, or ethylene glycol, acetone ingestion; drugs (corticosteroids, mannitol)

Decreased: Hyponatremia from any cause such as diarrhea, vomiting, SIADH, CHF, cirrhosis, nephrotic syndrome, Addison disease, iatrogenic causes (poor fluid balance usually from too much free water [administration of D5W or ½ NS]), late pregnancy, drugs (diuretics)

▶ The osmolality of a patient is measured using an osmometer or a rough estimation of osmolality is [2(Na$^+$ mEq/L) + BUN mg/dL/2.8 + glucose mg/dL/18]. Measured value is usually less than calculated value. If measured value is 15 mOsm/ kg less than calculated, consider methanol, ethanol, or ethylene glycol ingestion or other unmeasured cations/anions.

OSTEOCALIN

- Adults 10–50 ng/mL; children/adolescents (7–17 yr) 25–300 ng/mL

Increased: Any metabolic bone diagnosis such as osteoporosis, osteomalacia, vitamin D deficiency, Paget disease, bone disease secondary to chronic renal disease, bone metastases, fracture, hyperthyroidism, hyperparathyroidism, acromegaly

Decreased: Hypothyroidism, hypoparathyroidism, growth hormone deficiency, multiple myeloma

▶ Noncollagen protein produced by osteoblasts

OXYGEN

See Chapter 14, Table 14-1, page 400.

PARATHYROID HORMONE (PTH) INTACT

- 10–50 pg/mL (10–50 ng/L) (method dependent)

Increased: Primary hyperparathyroidism, secondary hyperparathyroidism (e.g., hypocalcemia states such as chronic renal failure), vitamin D deficiency, drugs (lithium, furosemide, propofol)

Decreased: Hypoparathyroidism, hypomagnesemia, hypercalcemia not due to hyperparathyroidism, hyperthyroidism

▶ Commonly used for establishing the diagnosis of hyperparathyroidism. The upper limits of the reference range may be lower in different regions of the world with more daily hours of sunshine. If renal function is normal and serum calcium is elevated, an intact PTH concentration of >50 pg/mL strongly suggests primary hyperparathyroidism. PTH fragments (N-terminal and C-terminal remain as research tools)

PARATHYROID HORMONE–RELATED PEPTIDE (PTHrP)

- References ranges vary, serum: 10–65 pg/mL (10–65 ng/L)

  Increased: Hypercalcemia related to malignancy producing PTHrP including lung, breast, head and neck, GU, and gynecologic Ca and myeloma and T-cell lymphoma

▶ PTHrP is a protein secreted by some cancer cells leading to hypercalcemia of malignancy.

10

PHOSPHORUS (PHOSPHATE)

See also Chapter 15, page 446, Hyperphosphatemia and Hypophosphatemia.

- Adults: 3–4.5 mg/dL (0.97–1.45 mmol/L)
- Children: 4.0–6.0 mg/dL
- Critical values: <1.1 or >8.9 mg/dL

  Increased: Hypoparathyroidism (including surgical, pseudohypoparathyroidism), secondary hyperparathyroidism, DKA, lactic acidosis, renal failure, bone disease (healing fractures), osteolytic bony metastases, tumor lysis (especially with heavy tumor burden and responsive to treatment, e.g., lymphomas and leukemias), rhabdomyolysis, Addison disease, acromegaly, drugs (iatrogenic from phosphate-containing medications including enemas, laxative; K^+ containing salts; bisphosphonates, vitamin D, anabolic steroids) childhood, factitious increase (hemolysis of specimen)

  Decreased: Hyperparathyroidism, severe hypercalcemia, vitamin D deficiency, hypothyroidism, GH deficiency, alcoholism, malnutrition, refeeding syndrome, treatment of DKA, acute respiratory alkalosis, hyperalimentation without adequate replacement, dialysis for chronic renal failure, diarrhea, vomiting, acute pancreatitis, gout, salicylate poisoning, hypokalemia, hypomagnesemia, drugs (diuretics, aluminum and magnesium-containing phosphate-binding antacids)

▶ Phosphorus monitoring is used in renal, endocrine, and GI disorders. In ESRD, monitor for renal osteodystrophy (osteomalacia) (obtain serum calcium, phosphorus, and PTH for secondary hyperparathyroidism)

POTASSIUM, SERUM

See also Chapter 15, page 436, Hyperkalemia, Hypokalemia.

- 3.5–5.0 mEq/L (3.5–5.0 mmol/L)
- Critical values: 2.5 mEq/L <1 wk; >1 wk, < 3.0 mEq/L; any age >6.0 mEq/L

Increased: Factitious increase (hemolysis of specimen, thrombocytosis), renal failure, renal tubular acidosis (RTA) (type IV), Addison disease, congenital adrenal hyperplasia, acidosis, dehydration, hemolysis, rhabdomyolysis, massive tissue damage, and drugs (excess intake [oral or IV], potassium-containing medications, spironolactone, triamterene, ACE inhibitors, ARBs, NSAIDs, beta blockers, and TMP-SMX)

Decreased: Diuresis from any cause (e.g., hyperglycemia), decreased intake, vomiting, NG suctioning, villous adenoma, diarrhea, Zollinger–Ellison syndrome, RTA (type I and II), chronic pyelonephritis, metabolic alkalosis, hyperaldosteronism, Cushing syndrome, Gitelman syndrome, drugs (diuretics, beta agonists)

▶ Primarily an intracellular ion (98%) with <2% extracellular. In a patient with hypokalemia, a 1 mmol/L decrease of serum potassium reflects a total body deficit of <100–400 mmol. The deficit depends somewhat on the degree of hypokalemia. With acidemia, potassium moves out of cells and with alkalemia, potassium moves into cells.

PREALBUMIN (TRANSTHYRETIN)

See also Chapter 17, page 466.

- Normal range: 18–40 mg/dL

Increased: Pregnancy, iron-deficiency anemia, ESRD, lymphoma, drugs (anabolic steroids, corticosteroids, and NSAIDs)

Decreased: Malnutrition, starvation, negative acute phase reactant, (decreases with inflammation including from infection, trauma, surgery, collagen vascular diseases [SLE, RA, temporal arteritis, many others], burns, and cancers including leukemias, lymphomas, multiple myeloma, and metastatic solid cancers).

▶ Evaluation of nutritional status and total parenteral nutrition. Useful in nutritional analysis due to short half-life. High concentrations in the CSF make it a key indicator of CSF leakage into the sinus, eyes, and ears with cranial trauma.

PREGNANCY SCREENING

▶ Normal blood values based on gestational age, others based on chromosomal analysis. First-trimester screen offers advantages over second-trimester screen. Negative results reduce maternal anxiety. Positive results allow women to take advantage of first-trimester chorionic villus sampling (CVS) at 10–12 wk or second-trimester amniocentesis (≥15 wk). The American College of Obstetricians and Gynecologists recommends all women >35 yr at delivery be offered CVS or amniocentesis (diagnoses 99.9% of screened chromosomal abnormalities).

First-Trimester Screening ("Combined Screening")

▶ Maternal serum beta-HCG, PAPP-A (pregnancy-associated plasma protein-A, with ultrasound-determined nuchal transparency). Done at 11–13 wk. Screen of low-risk pregnant women (<35 yr) for Down syndrome and trisomy 18 (detects ~85% of cases of Down syndrome and ~97% of trisomy 18). Measures free beta-HCG and PAPP-A in combination with ultrasound assessment of fetal nuchal translucency (measure of fluid in the fetal neck).

Second-Trimester Screening

▶ "Quadruple screening": Maternal serum AFP, HCG, estriol, and inhibin A, done at 15–21 wk of pregnancy to detect open neural tube defects, Down syndrome, and trisomy 18 (detects ~80% of open neural tube defects, ~85% of cases of Down syndrome, and ~60% of cases of trisomy 18).

10

Chorionic Villus Sampling (CVS)

▶ Performed at 10–12 wk of pregnancy; placental tissue removed percutaneously and studied for chromosomal analysis (~1% risk of complications such as miscarriage).

Amniocentesis

▶ Performed at 13–14 wk of pregnancy (early amniocentesis) or at 15 wk and later (traditional amniocentesis). Chromosomal analysis is performed on the fetal skin cells in the amniotic fluid. Risk similar to CVS. (See also Chapter 20, page 677.)

Other Pregnancy Screening

▶ **Initial prenatal visit:** CBC, hepatitis B surface antigen, HIV screening, syphilis and chlamydia screening, antibodies for rubella and varicella, UA for asymptomatic bacteriuria, Rh blood typing and antibody testing of mother. If there is history of gestational DM, then glucose tolerance/challenge test at the initial visit. Screening for gonorrhea is recommended for all women 24 yr and younger, as well as any women considered at high risk. Hepatitis C (HCV) screening is recommended once for all persons 18–79 years of age. For individuals at increased risk, such as individuals who inject drugs, they should be periodically screened for HCV; the interval between screenings has not been determined. Thus, every pregnant patient should be screened for HCV, if not previously tested. For those that have been previously tested, if they are at increased risk, it is reasonable to screen them again. All subsequent visits should include a UA for glucose, ketones, and protein.

Third-trimester 24–28 wk: CBC; if no previous history of gestational DM, then test for gestation diabetes (1-hr glucose tolerance/challenge test with a 50-gm load, if glucose >130–140 mg/dL, then will need 3-hr glucose tolerance/challenge test with 100-gm load); 28–29 wk: if mother Rh neg, repeat antibody testing unless biological father is known to be Rh neg; syphilis at 28–32 wk if at risk; screening for chlamydia and gonorrhea for women at high risk; and HIV before 36 wk if at risk.

Symptomatic pregnant women with COVID-19 are at increased risk of more severe illness compared with nonpregnant peers, with the CDC including pregnant women in its "increased risk" category for COVID-19 illness. Pregnant women admitted with suspected COVID-19 or who develop symptoms suggestive of COVID-19 during admission should be prioritized for testing.

PROGESTERONE

10

See Table 10-7

● Normal values: See Table 10-7

Increased: Luteal phase of menstrual cycle, luteal cysts of ovary; ovarian tumors (e.g., arrhenoblastoma), congenital adrenal hyperplasia, adrenal tumors

Decreased: Gonadal agenesis, fetal death, amenorrhea, toxemia of pregnancy

▶ Used to confirm ovulation and corpus luteum function. Used to monitor patients undergoing ovulation induction.

PROLACTIN

● Men and nonlactating women: 1–25 ng/mL

Increased: Pregnancy, nursing after pregnancy, exercise, prolactinoma, hypothalamic tumors, sarcoidosis or granulomatous disease of the hypothalamus, hypothyroidism, hypoglycemia, renal failure, cirrhosis, CHF, Addison disease, drugs (L-dopa, phenothiazines, haloperidol)

Table 10-7. Progesterone Levels

Sample collection	Normal value (women)
Follicular phase	<1 ng/mL
Luteal phase	5–20 ng/mL
Pregnancy	
1st trimester	10–30 ng/mL
2nd trimester	50–100 ng/mL
3rd trimester	100–400 ng/mL
Postmenopause	<1 ng/mL

▶ Used in workup of infertility, impotence, hirsutism, amenorrhea, and pituitary neoplasm.

PROSTATE-SPECIFIC ANTIGEN (PSA) AND PSA DERIVATIVES

• <4 ng/dL with most experts considering <2.5 ng/dL to be normal. May see slight increases in PSA as men age due to benign prostate hypertrophy.

Increased: Prostate cancer (levels >10 ng/dL increase likelihood of prostate cancer and of spread beyond the prostate), acute prostatitis, benign prostate hypertrophy (BPH), prostatic infarction, prostate surgery (after biopsy, levels are elevated for 4–6 wk), vigorous prostatic massage (routine rectal exam does not clinically elevate levels), rarely after ejaculation (suggest refraining from sexual activity for 24–48 hr before test)

Decreased: Radical prostatectomy (should be "undetectable" or <0.2 ng/dL), response to therapy for prostatic carcinoma (radiation or androgen deprivation therapy that lowers testosterone), response to antibiotics in acute bacterial prostatitis, drugs (5-alpha-reducatse inhibitors finasteride and dutasteride can reduce PSA by up to 50% at 6 months of therapy)

▶ PSA is one of the most reliable tumor markers to assess response to prostate cancer treatment; used for prostate cancer screening (see Appendix, page 1050). Prostate cancer can only be diagnosed by tissue biopsy. There is no PSA level at which you can be sure prostate cancer is present, but levels above 10 are suggestive. Many older men develop forms of non-aggressive prostate cancer that may not require treatment. Some other common lab tests to consider before biopsy in the setting of elevated PSA include 4K score blood test and urine assays MDx Select and ExoDx Prostate test.

PSA Velocity/PSA Doubling Time

A rate of rise in PSA of >0.75 ng/dL/yr (velocity) is suggestive of prostate cancer on the basis of at least three separate assays 6 mo apart. Increased PSA doubling time <3 mo before diagnosis or <10 mo after treatment (radiation or surgery) suggests a poor prognosis.

PSA Free and Total

Prostate cancer tends to be associated with lower free PSA levels in proportion to total PSA; free/total PSA can improve the specificity of PSA in the range of total PSA from 2.0–10.0 ng/mL. Ratio free/total <10% indicates >50% chance of positive biopsy; >25%, 8–10% risk of positive biopsy. Some recommend prostate biopsy only if the free PSA percentage is low; others use the ratio to guide decision for further biopsy after an initial negative biopsy.

PROTEIN ELECTROPHORESIS, SERUM AND URINE (SERUM PROTEIN ELECTROPHORESIS [SPEP]) (URINE PROTEIN ELECTROPHORESIS [UPEP])

▶ Qualitative analysis of serum proteins is used in the workup of hypoglobulinemia, macroglobulinemia, α_1-antitrypsin deficiency, liver disease, and myeloma and occasionally in nutritional assessment. Serum electrophoresis yields five bands (Figure 10-4 and Table 10-8, page 249).

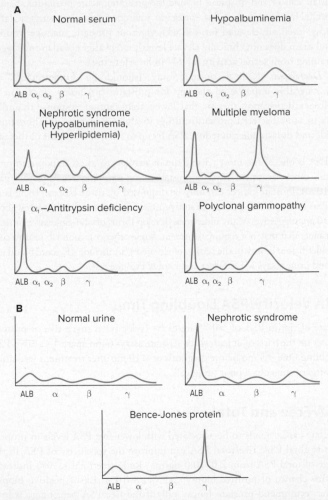

Figure 10-4. Examples of (A) serum (top 6 panels) and (B) urine (bottom 3 panels) electrophoresis patterns. See also Table 10-8, page 249. (Courtesy of Dr. Steven Haist.)

Table 10-8. Normal Serum Protein Components and Fractions as Determined by Electrophoresis, Along with Associated Conditions[a]

Protein fraction	Percentage of total protein	Constituents	Increased	Decreased
Albumin	52–68	Albumin	Dehydration (only known cause)	Nephrosis, malnutrition, chronic liver disease
Alpha-1 (α_1) globulin	2.2–2.4	Thyroxine-binding globulin, antitrypsin, lipoproteins, glycoprotein, transcortin	Inflammation, neoplasia	Nephrosis, α_1-antitrypsin deficiency (emphysema related)
Alpha-2 (α_2) globulin	6.1–10.1	Haptoglobin, glycoprotein, macroglobulin, ceruloplasmin	Inflammation, infection, neoplasia, cirrhosis	Severe liver disease, acute hemolytic anemia
Beta(β) globulin	8.5–14.5	Transferrin, glycoprotein, lipoproteins	Cirrhosis, obstructive jaundice	Nephrosis
Gamma(γ) globulins (Immunoglobulins)	10–21	IgA, IgG, IgM, IgD, IgE	Infections, collagen-vascular diseases, leukemia, myeloma	Agammaglobulinemia, hypogammaglobulinemia, nephrosis

[a]See also Figure 10-4, page 248.

10

If monoclonal gammopathy or a low albumin to globulin fraction (albumin/total protein albumin) is detected, quantitative immunoglobulin tests should be ordered. Urine protein electrophoresis can be used to evaluate proteinuria and to detect Bence Jones protein (light chain), which is associated with myeloma, Waldenström macroglobulinemia, and Fanconi syndrome. Spot urine and 24-hr urine provide the same proportions of the various proteins.

PROTEIN, SERUM

- 6.0–8.0 g/dL
- See also Serum Protein Electrophoresis, above.

Increased: Multiple myeloma, Waldenström macroglobulinemia, benign monoclonal gammopathy, lymphoma, polyclonal gammopathy from any cause (chronic inflammation, HIV, sarcoidosis, viral illnesses), dehydration

Decreased: Malnutrition, nephrotic syndrome, protein-losing enteropathy including Crohn diagnosis and ulcerative colitis, chronic liver disease, acute burns, cancer

PYRUVATE (PYRUVIC ACID)

Increased lactate:pyruvate ratio: >20:1: Mitochondrial respiratory chain diagnosis, pyruvate carboxylase deficiency, and tricarboxylic (TCA) disorders

Decreased lactate:pyruvate ratio: <10:1: Pyruvate dehydrogenase deficiency.

▶ Pyruvate is not a very useful test unless a lactate is obtained simultaneously.

RAPID PLASMA REAGIN (RPR) TEST AND TITERS

See also Treponemal Specific Antibody, page 260, and VDRL Test, page 262.

- Normal: Nonreactive

Positive/reactive RPR: Syphilis (all stages of *Treponema pallidum* infection), false positives: malaria, leprosy, EBV, HIV, *Streptococcus pyogenes* infection, autoimmune disease, pregnancy, intravenous drug use

Negative/nonreactive: Negative treponemal specific antibody suggests infection with *Treponema pallidum* is unlikely unless there is concern for early infection or a poor antibody response, i.e., AIDS or some other cause of severe immune compromise

▶ Figure 10-5A provides a timeline of the percent of patients infected with *Treponema pallidum* who test positive by the various serological tests and at the various stages of syphilis. Screening assay for syphilis uses the "traditional algorithm" (see Figure 10-5B). The RPR assay detects antibody directed against non-treponemal antigens.

  o If RPR is positive, then obtain RPR titer and treponemal specific antibody via automated immunoassay or TP-PA

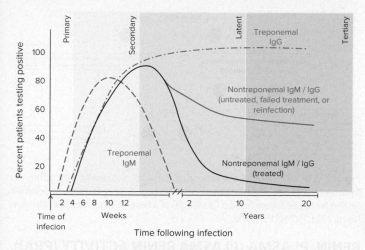

Figure 10-5A. Syphilis staging and serology. FTA-Abs = fluorescent treponemal antibody absorbed; IgM = immunoglobulin M; RPR = rapid plasma reagin; TPHA = T pallidum hemagglutination assay; VDRL = Venereal Disease Research Laboratory. (From Soreng, K, Levy R, Fakile Y. Serologic Testing for Syphilis: Benefits and Challenges of a Reverse Algorithm. *Clin Microbiol Newsl* 2014;36(24):195–202.)

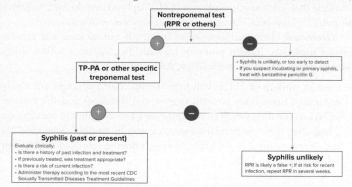

Figure 10-5B. The traditional testing algorithm for *Treponema pallidum*. (Adapted from From Soreng, K, Levy R, Fakile Y. Serologic Testing for Syphilis: Benefits and Challenges of a Reverse Algorithm. *Clin Microbiol Newsl*. 2014;36(24):195–202).

- o A positive treponemal specific assay suggests untreated or undertreated syphilis
- o Serial RPR titers should be used to monitor therapy
  - Positive RPR with positive treponemal specific antibody, likely untreated or undertreated syphilis
  - Positive RPR with negative treponemal specific antibody suggests false-positive RPR unless concern for early infection or poor antibody response, i.e., AIDS or another cause of severe immune compromise
- ▶ RPR has replaced VDRL as the initial test for syphilis. Should **not** be used for testing CSF for neurosyphilis.

10

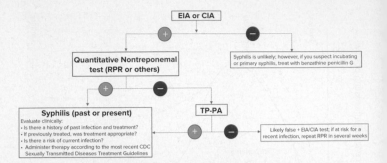

Figure 10-5C. CDC Recommended Reverse Screening Algorithm for *Treponema pallidum*. (Adapted from From Soreng, K, Levy R, Fakile Y. Serologic Testing for Syphilis: Benefits and Challenges of a Reverse Algorithm. *Clin Microbiol Newsl*. 2014;36(24):195–202).

RENIN, PLASMA (PLASMA RENIN ACTIVITY [PRA])

- Adults, normal-sodium diet, upright 1.1–4.1 ng/mL/hr

  Increased: Pregnancy, dehydration, renal artery stenosis, adrenal insufficiency, Bartter syndrome, chronic hypokalemia, upright posture, salt-restricted diet, edematous conditions (CHF, nephrotic syndrome, cirrhosis), drugs (ACE inhibitors, diuretics, oral contraceptives, estrogens)

  Decreased: Primary aldosteronism (renin will not increase with relative volume depletion, upright posture), high-salt diet, supine position, drugs (beta blockers, clonidine, methyldopa, ASA, and NSAIDs)

- ▸ Used in workup of HTN with hypokalemia. Normal ranges are highly dependent upon body position (supine and standing) and the amount of Na^+ in the diet. Going from supine on a low-Na^+ diet to standing on a high-Na^+ diet, the normal ranges may vary by fivefold. Stop diuretics and estrogens for 2–4 wk before testing. Often determined with serum aldosterone (page 180).

RENIN, RENAL VEIN

- Normal L and R should be equal

- ▸ A ratio of >1.5 (affected/unaffected) suggestive of lateralizing renovascular hypertension

RETINOL-BINDING PROTEIN (RBP)

- Adults: 3–6 mg/dL
- Children: 1.5–3.0 mg/dL

  Decreased: Malnutrition, vitamin A deficiency, intestinal malabsorption of fats, chronic liver disease, negative acute phase reactant (decreases with inflammation including from infection, trauma, surgery, collagen vascular diseases [SLE, RA, temporal arteritis, many others], burns, and cancers including leukemias, lymphomas, multiple myeloma, and metastatic solid cancers).

Increased: Advanced chronic renal disease

▶ Used to assess nutritional status

RHEUMATOID FACTOR (RF, RA LATEX TEST)

See Autoantibodies, page 186.

ROCKY MOUNTAIN SPOTTED FEVER (RMSF) ANTIBODIES

- Normal: <4× increase in paired acute and convalescent sera
- IgG <1:64
- IgM <1:8

▶ The diagnosis of RMSF is made with acute and convalescent titers that show a 4× increase or a single convalescent titer >1:64 in the clinical setting of RMSF. Occasional false-positives in late pregnancy.

SEDIMENTATION RATE

See Chapter 11, page 290.

SEMEN ANALYSIS

See Table 10-9 for WHO standards for normal semen analysis.

Alterations in normal parameters: After vasectomy (should be 0 sperm after 3 mo), varicocele, radical prostatectomy, primary testicular failure (i.e., Klinefelter syndrome), secondary testicular failure (chemotherapy, radiation, infections), aftermath of recent illness, congenital obstruction of the vas, retrograde ejaculation, endocrine causes (e.g., hyperprolactinemia, low testosterone)

▶ Collect after 48–72 hr abstinence, analyze within 1–2 hr. May not be valid after a recent illness or high fever. Verify abnormal by serial tests. WHO standards and terminology in Table 10-9, page 254.

SEX HORMONE–BINDING GLOBIN (SHBG)

- Men: 13– 72 nmol/L
- Women: 16–132 nmol/L

Increased: Weight loss, anorexia nervosa, liver disease, hyperthyroidism, HIV, drugs (OCPs [estrogen containing])

Table 10-9. Normal Semen Analysis and Terminology Based on WHO Standards

Characteristic	Reference Standard
Ejaculate volume	>1.5 mL
pH	≥7.2
Sperm concentration	≥15 million/mL
Sperm count	≥39 million/mL
Sperm motility	≥40% total motility and 32% with progressive motility
Sperm morphology	≥4%[1] with normal forms
Term	**Definition**
Normospermia	Normal ejaculate (as defined by reference standards above)
Oligozoospermia	Sperm concentration <15 million/mL
Asthenozoospermia	<32% of spermatozoa with progressive motility
Azoospermia	No spermatozoa in ejaculate
Aspermia	No ejaculate

Based on data from: Cooper TG, Noonan E, von Eckardstein S, et al. World Health Organization reference values for human semen characteristics. *Hum Reprod Update* 2010;16(3):231–245.

Decreased: Weight gain, polycystic ovary syndrome (PCOS), metabolic syndrome, DM type 2, insulin resistance, hypothyroidism, acromegaly, drugs (glucocorticoids, anabolic steroids)

▶ SHBG is a protein made by the liver that binds testosterone, dihydrotestosterone, and estradiol and delivers the sex hormones to various tissues

SODIUM, SERUM

See also Chapter 15, page 430, Hypernatremia, Hyponatremia.

- 136–145 mEq/L (136–145 mmol/L)
- Critical values: <121 mEq/L or >158 mEq/L

Increased: Associated with low total body sodium (drugs [glycosuria, mannitol, diuretics, sorbitol, lactulose], urea, vomiting, diarrhea, excess sweating), normal total body sodium (diabetes insipidus [central and nephrogenic], respiratory losses, and sweating, ethanol, drugs [phenytoin, demeclocycline, amphotericin B, lithium, vinblastine, colchicine]), and increased total body sodium (administration of hypertonic sodium bicarbonate, Cushing syndrome, hyperaldosteronism)

Decreased: Associated with excess total body sodium and water (nephrotic syndrome, CHF, cirrhosis, renal failure), excess body water (SIADH [small-cell lung cancer; pulmonary disease including TB, lung cancer, pneumonia; CNS disease including trauma, tumors, and infections; perioperative stress; acute intermittent porphyria; drugs including SSRIs, ACE inhibitors, carbamazepine, celecoxib, antipsychotics, chemotherapeutic agents; and aftermath of colonoscopy], hypothyroidism, adrenal insufficiency, psychogenic polydipsia, beer potomania), decreased total body water and sodium (drugs [diuretics, mannitol], RTA, urea, mineralocorticoid deficiency, cerebral salt wasting, vomiting, diarrhea, pancreatitis), and pseudohyponatremia (hyperlipidemia, hyperglycemia, multiple myeloma)

▶ Sodium is the major extracellular cation and has a major role in maintaining the normal distribution of water and osmotic pressure. Sodium changes most often reflect changes in water balance rather than sodium balance.

10

SOMATOMEDIN-C

See Insulin-Like Growth Factor-1 (IGF-1), page 233.

SOMATOSTATIN

● <25 pg/mL (<25 ng/L)

Increased: Somatostatinoma located in the pancreas or small bowel, medullary thyroid cancer, pheochromocytoma

▶ Produced by the delta cells of the pancreas and duodenum; inhibitor of multiple GI hormones, insulin, and glucagon; also produced in the hypothalamus, inhibitor of GH and TSH secretion

STOOL FOR OCCULT BLOOD

See Fecal Occult Blood Test (FOBT), page 215.

SWEAT CHLORIDE TEST (QUANTITATIVE PILOCARPINE IONTOPHORESIS SWEAT TEST)

● Normal: <40 mmol/L (>3 mo); <30 mmol/L (<3 mo)

Increased: Cystic fibrosis (not valid on infants <3 wk); Addison disease, meconium ileus, and renal failure can occasionally raise levels.

▶ Collection and quantification of sweat after pilocarpine iontophoresis. Three steps are sweat stimulation, sweat collection, and sweat analysis. Positive test is defined by sweat chloride >60 mmol/L in sweat from both arms.

N-TELOPEPTIDE (NTX) SERUM

See also Chapter 12, page 302, *N*-Telopeptide (NTX), Urine.

- Premenopausal women: 6.2–19.0 nmol bone collagen equivalents (BCE)
- Men >25 yr: 5.4–24.2 nmol BCE

Increased: Osteoporosis, osteomalacia, Paget disease, vitamin D deficiency, primary hyperparathyroidism, bony metastasis, multiple myeloma, hyperthyroidism

Decreased: Response to bisphosphonate therapy (decrease of 30–40% from baseline after 3 mo of therapy is typical of bisphosphonate therapy)

▶ *N*-Telopeptides of type I collagen (NTx) are end products of bone resorption and allow monitoring of bone metabolism. Reported as nanomolar bone collagen equivalents per liter (nM BCE/L). In urine, values are corrected per millimolars of creatinine per liter (mM creatinine/L). Serum NTx provides a quantitative measurement of bone resorption. A baseline NTx level is obtained before antiresorptive therapy (i.e., bisphosphonate) with periodic testing until decrease in NTx achieved.

TESTOSTERONE, FREE AND TOTAL

Normal total ranges (may vary by lab):
- Prepubertal children: 5–20 ng/dL (0.17–0.7 nmol/L)
- Men (≥17 yr): 300–1000 ng/dL (10.4–34.7 nmol/L)
- Women: 20–70 ng/dL (0.7–2.6 nmol/L)
- Free testosterone: adult male range 8.8–27 pg/mL

Increased: Adrenal hyperplasia, adrenocorticoid tumors, testicular feminization, ovarian tumors, ovarian stromal hyperthecosis, polycystic ovary syndrome (POCS), idiopathic hirsutism, menopause, hyperthyroidism

Decreased: Hypogonadism, castration (medical or surgical treatment of prostate cancer), hypopituitarism, Klinefelter syndrome, ethanol, liver disease, chronic renal disease, drugs (spironolactone, digoxin)

- Testosterone is most commonly used as the initial test for hypogonadism in males, less commonly used in the evaluation of virilism and hirsutism in females. Should be obtained from 8 AM to 10 AM, due to higher morning levels. There is not consensus on the lower limits of normal for testosterone. As per the American Association of Clinical Endocrinologists, a decreased testosterone level (free plus protein bound) is <200 ng/dL (or 6.9 nmol/L); The FDA defines decreased as levels <300 ng/dL (or 10 nmol/L), and notes such levels are associated with hypogonadism and warrants further workup in a man.

- Free testosterone useful in males; elevated or decreased SHBG changes the bioavailability of testosterone. It can be used as an adjunct to the patient with low total testosterone levels. For example, obesity is characterized by reduced total testosterone and normal free testosterone due to reduced protein binding. Serum SHBG concentrations increase with age. With increasing age, less of the total testosterone is free or biologically active.

THYROGLOBULIN

- 3–42 ng/mL (3–42 ug/L)

    Increased: Differentiated thyroid carcinoma (papillary, follicular), Graves disease, nontoxic goiter
    Decreased: Hypothyroidism, status post thyroidectomy, autoantibodies to thyroglobulin, drugs (testosterone, steroids, phenytoin, factitious or supratherapeutic dosing of levothyroxine, etc.)

▶ Useful for following nonmedullary thyroid carcinoma. See also Table 10-10.

10

THYROID-BINDING GLOBULIN (TBG) (THYROXINE-BINDING GLOBULIN)

- 10–26 µg/dL (129–335 nmol/L)

    Increased: Genetics, drugs (estrogens)
    Decreased: Euthyroid sick syndrome (acute illness), malnutrition, nephrotic syndrome, liver disease, central hypothyroidism, increase in GH, drugs (anabolic steroids)

▶ One of three thyroid-binding proteins; the other two are albumin and prealbumin (transthyretin). Only the unbound thyroid hormones are active; an increase in TBG will cause an increase in total T_4 and T_3 without an increases in thyroid activity. The opposite is true with a decrease in TBG. See also Table 10-10.

THYROID-STIMULATING HORMONE (TSH, THYROTROPIN)

- 0.4–4.8 uIU/mL (0.4–4.8 mU/L)

    Increased: Primary hypothyroidism, values >5–7 uIU/L suggest borderline or subclinical primary hypothyroidism
    Decreased: Primary hyperthyroidism; in secondary and tertiary hypothyroidism TSH levels can be decreased or normal (these cases make up less than 1% of all cases of hypothyroidism), acute illness, drugs (dopamine, corticosteroids)

▶ Best screening test for thyroid dysfunction; useful for monitoring thyroid replacement therapy and confirming TSH suppression in patients with thyroid cancer taking thyroxine therapy. See also Table 10-10, page 258.

Table 10-10. Overview and Use of Thyroid Tests

Use	Comment	Test
For Screening	Serum thyroid-stimulating hormone (TSH)	Most sensitive test for primary hypothyroidism and hyperthyroidism
	Free thyroxine (FT4)	Excellent test
For hypothyroidism	Serum TSH	High in primary and low in secondary hypothyroidism
	Antithyroperoxidase and antithyroglobulin antibodies	Elevated in Hashimoto thyroiditis
For hyperthyroidism	Serum TSH	Suppressed except in TSH-secreting pituitary tumor or pituitary hyperplasia (rare)
	Triiodothyronine (T3) or free Triiodothyronine (FT3)	Elevated
	^{123}I uptake and scan	Increased uptake, diffuse versus 'hot' foci on scan
	Antithyroperoxidase and antithyroglobulin antibodies	Elevated in Graves disease
	Thyroid-stimulating immunoglobulin (TSI)	Usually (65%) positive in Graves disease
For thyroid nodules	Fine-needle aspiration (FNA) biopsy	Best diagnostic method for thyroid cancer
	^{123}I uptake and scan	Cancer is usually 'cold'; less reliable than FNA biopsy
	^{99m}Tc scan	Vascular or avascular
	Ultrasonography	Useful to assist FNA biopsy and in assessing the risk of malignancy (multinodular goiter or pure cysts are less likely to be malignant). Useful to monitor nodules and patients after thyroid surgery for carinoma

(Reproduced with permission from Papadakis MA, McPhee SJ, Rabow MW. Thyroid Testing. In Current Medical Diagnosis and Treatment. New York, NY: McGraw-Hill Medical; 2020.)

THYROXINE, FREE (FT$_4$)

- Normal: 0.9–2.3 ng/dL (12–30 pmol/L)

Increased: Hyperthyroidism, drugs (exogenous thyroxine administration, amiodarone, iodine, radiographic contrast, interferon, lithium, heparin)

Decreased: Hypothyroidism, drugs (glucocorticoids, dopamine agonists, lithium, iodide, amiodarone, propylthiouracil, methimazole)

▶ Confirms thyroid dysfunction after abnormal TSH. FT$_4$ and TSH provide the best assessment of thyroid function with abnormal serum TBG levels or abnormal binding characteristics (e.g., pregnancy, medications including estrogens, androgens, phenytoin, or salicylates). Total T$_4$ can be misleading due to abnormal binding proteins or major illnesses resulting in "euthyroid sick syndrome." Thus, FT$_4$ is the preferred test over total T$_4$. In euthyroid sick syndrome, reverse T$_3$ will be increased. FT$_4$ can be normal, increased, or decreased in euthyroid sick syndrome. See also Table 10-11, page 258.

10

TORCH BATTERY

- Normal: Not detected
▶ An acronym for a group of infectious diseases (TORCH) that can cause illness in pregnant women and may cause birth defects in their newborns. Traditional acronym for serologic evidence of exposure to **T**oxoplasma gondii, **r**ubella, **C**MV, and **H**SV. Other organisms, including *Treponema pallidum*, parvovirus, varicella zoster and zika virus, are often included with the TORCH infection panel. Reported as detected or not detected for IgG and/or IgM for each infectious agent.

TRANSFERRIN

- 200–380 mg/dL

Increased: Acute and chronic blood loss, iron deficiency, hemolysis, pregnancy, viral hepatitis, drugs (OCPs)

Decreased: Anemia of chronic disease, malnutrition, cirrhosis, nephrotic syndrome, hemochromatosis, negative acute phase reactant (decreases with inflammation including from infection, trauma, surgery, collagen vascular diseases [SLE, RA, temporal arteritis, many others], burns, and cancers including leukemias, lymphomas, multiple myeloma, and metastatic solid cancers).

▶ Used in workup of anemia; transferrin levels can also be assessed by total iron-binding capacity

TRANSFERRIN SATURATION

- Male: 20–50%; female: 15–50%

  Increased: Megaloblastic anemia, sideroblastic anemia, iron overload, malnourishment

  Decreased: Chronic iron deficiency, uremia, nephrotic syndrome inflammation (transferrin is an acute phase reactant and transferrin saturation will decrease along with transferrin from infection, trauma, surgery, collagen vascular diseases [SLE, RA, temporal arteritis, many others], burns, and cancers including leukemias, lymphomas, multiple myeloma, and metastatic solid cancers).

▶ Transferrin saturations <20% indicate iron deficiency. Transferrin saturations >50% suggest iron overload. Total iron-binding capacity is similar to transferrin saturation with parallel increases in iron stores. Transferrin saturation is calculated as (serum iron level × 100)/total iron-binding capacity.

TREPONEMAL SPECIFIC ANTIBODY

- Normal: Negative (screening assay for *Treponema pallidum* using "reverse algorithm," see Figure 10-5A page 251, and 10-5C, on page 252).
▶ Many automated immunoassay platforms are available using enzyme immunoassays (EIA) or chemiluminescent immunoassay (CIA). If treponemal specific antibody is positive, then obtain non-treponemal assay, e.g., RPR and titer. If RPR is negative, then confirm treponemal specific antibody result using an alternative method, e.g. TP-PA.
  - o Positive treponemal specific antibody with positive RPR, likely untreated or undertreated syphilis.
  - o Positive treponemal specific antibody with negative RPR and positive TP-PA suggests previously treated syphilis.
  - o Positive treponemal specific antibody with negative RPR and negative TP-PA suggests false positive.
  - o Negative treponemal specific antibody suggests syphilis is unlikely unless there is concern for early infection or poor antibody response, i.e., AIDS or another cause of severe immune compromise.

TRIGLYCERIDES

See Cholesterol, page 195.

TRIIODOTHYRONINE (T$_3$), FREE

- 250–450 pg/dL

  Increased: Hyperthyroidism, T$_3$ thyrotoxicosis, exogenous T$_4$

  Decreased: Hypothyroidism (should NOT be ordered when evaluating for hypothyroidism)

▶ Like T_4, only a small fraction of T_3 is free or not bound to protein ($<0.5\%$). Rarely patients with hyperthyroidism will have a normal T_4 and an elevated T_3; if hyperthyroidism is suspected but T_4 is normal, obtain a T_3 or free T_3 (T_3 thyrotoxicosis). Free T_3 is helpful if thyroid-binding protein (albumin, TBG) is high (pregnancy) or low (malnutrition, liver disease). See also Table 10-11, page 258.

TRIIODOTHYRONINE (T₃), TOTAL

- 80–200 ng/dL

Increased: Hyperthyroidism, T_3 thyrotoxicosis, pregnancy, exogenous T_4, any cause of increased TBG (oral estrogen or pregnancy)

Decreased: Hypothyroidism and euthyroid sick state, any cause of decreased TBG (liver disease, malnutrition)

▶ Used when hyperthyroidism suspected but T_4 is normal (T_3 thyrotoxicosis); NOT used to diagnose hypothyroidism. See also Table 10-11, page 258.

TROPONIN I (TI) and TROPONIN T (TT, HIGHLY SENSITIVE)

- Troponin I (TI) <0.04 ng/mL (<0.04 µg/L)
- Troponin T (TT) <0.1 ng/mL
- Highly Sensitive Troponin T (TT): Men <22 ng/L; women <14 ng/L (method dependent)

Increased: Myocardial damage from any cause including MI, cardiac surgery, cardiac procedures, CHF, myocarditis; false positives (renal failure, cirrhosis, cardiac contusion, others)

▶ Used to diagnose AMI; increases rapidly 3–12 hr after MI, peak at 24 hr and may stay elevated for several days (TI 5–7 days, TT up to 14 days). Serial testing recommended. The troponins are specific to cardiac muscle and more cardiac-specific than CK-MB.

UREA NITROGEN (BLOOD)

See Blood urea nitrogen (BUN), page 189.

URIC ACID (URATE)

- Men: 2.4–7.4 mg/dL
- Women: 1.4–5.8 mg/dL

Increased: Gout, renal failure, myeloproliferative disorders (leukemia, lymphoma, myeloma, polycythemia vera), tumor lysis, toxemia of pregnancy, lead poisoning, lactic acidosis, hypothyroidism, hyperthyroidism, PCKD with decreased renal function, parathyroid diseases, drugs (diuretics, nicotinic acid)

10

Decreased: SIADH, liver disease, Wilson disease, Fanconi syndrome, uricosuric drugs (salicylates, probenecid, allopurinol)

▶ Increase associated with increased catabolism, nucleoprotein synthesis, or decreased renal clearing of uric acid (i.e., thiazide diuretics, renal failure)

VASOACTIVE INTESTINAL POLYPEPTIDE (VIP)

● 0–70 pg/mL

Increased: Enteropancreatic producing VIP (90% are located in the pancreas); levels >200 pg/mL, VIP-producing tumor highly likely

▶ Used to evaluate patients with chronic watery diarrhea with metabolic acidosis, hypokalemia, and hyperchloremia; VIP-producing tumors are very rare.

VDRL TEST (VENEREAL DISEASE RESEARCH LABORATORY)

Non-treponemal antibody assay commonly used for CSF specimens to help diagnose neurosyphilis. RPR (see page 250) is the standard screening test for serum using traditional algorithm. See also Figure 10-5 A and 10-5B, page 251.

VITAMIN A (RETINOL)

● Normal 30–80 µg/dL (1.05–2.80 µmol/L); lower in children

Increased: Vitamin A toxicity (excess intake), medications (OCP, probucol), chronic kidney disease

Decreased: Abetalipoproteinemia, chronic alcoholism, zinc deficiency, carcinoid syndrome, chronic infections, cystic fibrosis, TB (disseminated), hypothyroidism, liver and pancreatic diseases, protein malnutrition, medications (mineral oil, neomycin, allopurinol, cholestyramine)

▶ One of the fat-soluble vitamins (A, E, D, K); values <0.10 mg/L indicate significant deficiency. Promotes normal vision, skin health, and tissue growth. There are two forms of vitamin A, retinoids (*preformed* vitamin A, found in animal sources, most metabolically active form), and carotenoids, with beta-carotene being the most important one (provitamin A, and plant based).

VITAMIN B₁ (THIAMINE)

● Normal: 2.5–7.5 µg/dL (74–222 nmol/L) whole blood sample

Increased: Excessive intake, leukemia, polycythemia vera, Hodgkin disease

Decreased: Alcoholism (both with and without liver disease), diabetes, severe diarrhea, pellagra, dietary deficiency, carcinoid, drugs (isoniazid, valproic acid)

▶ Water-soluble vitamin. Whole blood best for sample, as most of thiamine found in whole blood. Required for carbohydrate metabolism, brain function, and myelination of peripheral nerves. B_1 deficiency diseases include beriberi and Wernicke-Korsakoff and Leigh syndromes. Cooking reduces food levels.

VITAMIN B₂ (RIBOFLAVIN)

- Normal 4–24 μg/dL (106–638 nmol/L)
- Marginally low: 2 μg/dL
- Diminished: <2 μg/L

10

Increased: Excess vitamin B_2 supplementation.

Decreased: Anorexia nervosa, individuals who avoid dairy (lactose intolerance), malabsorption, celiac disease, long-term use of phenobarbital and barbiturates

▶ Water-soluble vitamin. Ariboflavinosis hallmark (deficiency) is mouth sores.

VITAMIN B₆ (PYRIDOXINE)

- Normal 5–30 ng/mL (20–121 nmol/L)

Increased: Hypophosphatasia

Decreased: Alcoholism, lactation, malabsorption, malnutrition, normal pregnancy, pellagra-like syndrome, dialysis, uremia, drugs (amiodarone, anticonvulsants, cycloserine, disulfiram, ethanol, hydralazine, isoniazid, levodopa, OCP, theophylline).

▶ Water-soluble vitamin. Important in hemoglobin synthesis, a coenzyme in amino acid metabolism and glycogenolysis. Severe deficiency signs and symptoms: Irritability, weakness, depression, dizziness, neuropathy, and seizures. Useful in the evaluation of hypophosphatasia. With doses >2 g/day neurotoxicity (pyridoxine megavitaminosis): tingling, numbness, gait disturbance.

VITAMIN B₁₂ (EXTRINSIC FACTOR, CYANOCOBALAMIN)

- Normal 160–950 pg/mL (118–701 pmol/L)

Increased: Excessive intake, myeloproliferative disorders including leukemia, polycythemia vera

Decreased: Inadequate intake (especially strict vegetarians), malabsorption (celiac disease, inflammatory bowel disease, steatorrhea, bacterial overgrowth), status post gastrectomy, hyperthyroidism, pregnancy, drugs (PPIs, metformin)

▶ Water-soluble vitamin; low-normal levels may cause anemia and neurological findings; thus, levels between 200 and 300 pg/mL may need further evaluation.

VITAMIN C

- 0.4–1.5 mg/dL (23–85 μmol/L)

Decreased: Vitamin C deficiency may occur in up to 5% of the population, but overt scurvy is extremely rare in the United States; initial symptoms are nonspecific such as fatigue, anorexia, and irritability and are followed by more classic findings such as swelling of the gums, petechial rash, perifollicular hemorrhages, "corkscrew" body hair, hemarthroses, splinter hemorrhages (nail beds), flame hemorrhages (fundoscopic exam), and edema; occurs after 8–12 wk of no citrus in the diet; more common in alcoholism, malnutrition, eating disorders, hemodialysis, and type 1 DM.

▶ Water-soluble vitamin

VITAMIN D 1,25,DIHYDROXYCHOLECALCIFEROL (CALCITRIOL)

- 16–65 pg/mL (42–169) pmol/L

Increased: Hyperparathyroidism, vitamin D–resistant rickets, sarcoidosis, lymphomas, vitamin D toxicity

Decreased: Hypoparathyroidism, pseudohypoparathyroidism, chronic renal failure, 1-α-hydroxylase deficiency, osteoporosis

▶ One of the fat-soluble vitamins (A, E, D, K); the most active form of vitamin D_3 is 1-25 dihydroxycholecalciferol (calcitriol or D_3 1,25-OH); vitamins D_3 and D_2 are absorbed through the GI tract and vitamin D_3 is also produced in the skin; both vitamin D_2 and vitamin D_3 are inactive; both are then converted to vitamin D_3 25-OH by the liver and finally converted to vitamin D_3 1,25-OH by the kidneys; vitamin D_3 1,25-OH is not usually measured because of the shorter half-life compared to vitamin D_3 25-OH. Vitamin D_3 1,25-OH can be used to distinguish between vitamin D-resistant rickets and 1-a-hydroxylase deficiency.

VITAMIN D 25-HYDROXYCHOLECALCIFEROL (CALCIFEDIOL)

- 14–60 ng/mL (35–150 nmol/L)

Increased: Vitamin D intoxication, sun exposure, large amount of milk intake

Decreased: Malnutrition, malabsorption, dietary deficiency, no sun exposure, advanced age, renal disease, liver disease, hyperparathyroidism, osteomalacia, drugs (phenytoin, chronic glucocorticoids)

▶ One of the fat-soluble vitamins (A, E, D, K); the most active form of vitamin D_3 is 1,25 dihydroxycholecalciferol (calcitriol or D_3 1,25-OH); vitamins D_3 and D_2 are absorbed through the GI tract and vitamin D_3 is also produced in the skin; both vitamin D_2 and vitamin D_3 are inactive; both are then converted to vitamin D_3 25-OH by the liver and finally converted to vitamin D_3 1,25-OH by the kidneys; vitamin D_3 25-OH is usually measured to detect vitamin D deficiency because of the longer half-life compared to vitamin D_3 1,25-OH.

10

ZINC

- 50–150 µg/dL (7.7–23.0 µmol/L)

Increased: Metal fume fever

Decreased: Pernicious anemia, inadequate dietary intake (parenteral nutrition, alcoholism), malabsorption, increased needs (pregnancy, severe burns, wound healing), acrodermatitis enteropathica, dwarfism, hepatic disease, negative acute phase reactant (decreases because of the decrease in albumin which zinc is bound to; occurs with inflammation including from infection, trauma, surgery, collagen vascular diseases [SLE, RA, temporal arteritis, many others], burns, and cancers including leukemias, lymphomas, multiple myeloma, and metastatic solid cancers).

▶ An essential trace element in over 70 important enzyme systems. Zinc intake is closely related to protein intake. Severe zinc deficiency can cause growth failure, primary hypogonadism, skin disease, impaired taste and smell, and impaired immunity.

FURTHER READING

Caturegli G, et al. Clinical Validity of Serum Antibodies to AARS-CoV-2. *Ann Intern Med.* published online July 6, 2020, doi:10.7326/M20-2889.

Cheng MP, et al. Diagnostic Testing for Severe Acute Respiratory Syndrome-Related Coronavirus 2. *Ann Intern Med.* 2020;172:726–734.

Clinical Laboratory Reference Values. In: Laposata M, eds. *Laposata's Laboratory Medicine: Diagnosis of Disease in the Clinical Laboratory.* 3rd ed. New York, NY: McGraw-Hill.

Crawford MH, eds. *Current Diagnosis & Treatment: Cardiology*. 5th ed. New York, NY: McGraw-Hill; 2017.

Kucirka LM, et al. Variation in False-Negative Rate of Reverse Transcriptase Polymerase Chain Reaction-Based SARS-CoV-2 Tests by Time Since Exposure. *Ann Intern Med*. 2020;173(4):262–267.

Malloy MJ, et al. Disorders of Lipoprotein Metabolism. In: Gardner DG, Shoback D, eds. *Greenspan's Basic & Clinical Endocrinology*. 10th ed. New York, NY: McGraw-Hill; 2017.

Nicoll D, et al. *Guide to Diagnostic Tests*. 7th ed. New York, NY: McGraw-Hill; 2017.

Schuetz P, et al. Procalcitonin to initiate or discontinue antibiotics in acute respiratory tract infections. *Cochrane Database Syst Rev*. 2017;10:CD007498.

Williamson MA, Snyder ML, eds. *Wallach's Interpretation of Diagnostic Tests*. 10th ed. Philadelphia, PA: Lippincott Williams & Wilkins; 2015.

10

Laboratory Diagnosis: Clinical Hematology

11

Chapter update by Amy Gerwitz, MD

BLOOD COLLECTION

Venipuncture is discussed in detail in Chapter 19. The CBC sample is usually venous blood drawn with a 22-gauge or larger needle. Smaller-caliber needles can cause hemolysis. For a routine CBC, venous blood must be placed in a purple top tube, containing an anticoagulant (EDTA), which should be gently mixed with the blood. The CBC should be performed within 24 hours of collection. Most samples for coagulation studies are submitted in a blue top (citrate) tube. (See Chapter 19, Figure 19-14, page 666 for detailed description of blood collection tubes.) If a capillary or heelstick sample (see page 601) is used, the hematocrit may be falsely low or high due to preanalytical collection variables (such as milking the finger to get the sample or sludging of the RBCs).

BLOOD SMEARS: WRIGHT STAIN

When a CBC with differential is ordered, the WBC differential is most commonly performed by an automated CBC instrument (automated differential). Based on the instrumentation and laboratory-specific alerts/flags, a manual differential may be performed. The red cell, white cell, and platelet morphologies are accessed by reviewing a Wright-stained blood smear. Such morphologic assessment can assist in the evaluation of red and white blood cell disorders. The slide is usually available for review by students and house staff upon request. The main benefit is to allow identification of abnormal cells and other subtleties that may not be detected with automated systems (Figure 11-1). Characteristics of some abnormal WBCs are shown in Figure 11-2, page 273.

11

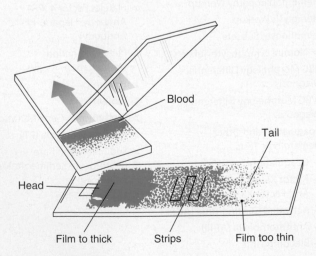

Figure 11-1. Technique of preparing a blood smear for staining and distribution of white and red blood cells on the standard smear.

Table 11-1. Estimate of WBCs Based on Cells Counted in a Blood Smear

WBC/hpf (high dry or 40×)	Estimated WBC (per mm³)
2–4	4,000–7,000
4–6	7,000–10,000
6–10	10,000–13,000
10–20	13,000–18,000

WBC = white blood cells; hpf = high-power field.

Viewing the Film: The Differential WBC

1. Examine the smear in an area where the red cells approximate one another but do not overlap. Acceptable distribution of the white blood cells and red cell morphology occurs in this area, away from the lateral edges of the slide. Morphology should not be accessed in the area of the thinly spread tail or the thick head of the smear. In the thin area of the smear, all red cells look like spherocytes and in the thick areas rouleaux will always be present.

2. In the area where the red cells approximate each other and do not overlap, utilizing the oil immersion objective, count 100–200 cells by running up and down the width or the length of the slide, avoiding the lateral edges.

3. It is best to count in either a vertical or horizontal manner in the ideal area of the smear. In patients receiving chemotherapy, the total white cell count may be so low that only a 25–50-cell sampling for the differential is possible.

4. In smears of blood from patients with very high white counts, such as those with leukemia, count the cells in any well-spread area where the different cell types are easily identifiable. Table 11-1 shows the correlation between the number of cells in a smear and the estimated white cell count. Estimate the platelet count by averaging the number of platelets seen in 10 hpf (under 100× oil immersion) and multiplying by 20,000.

NORMAL CBC VALUES

A CBC panel generally includes WBC count, RBC count, Hgb, HCT, MCH, MCHC, MCV, RDW, and platelets. If a WBC differential is needed, then a CBC with differential should be ordered. Normal CBC, differential, and platelet values can vary by age and patient sex and are outlined in Table 11-2, page 270.

Table 11-2. Normal CBC for Adult Males and Females and Infants to Adolescents of Selected Age Ranges (continued on next page)

Age	WBC count (cells/mm³) [SI: 10⁹/L]	RBC count (10⁶/µL) [SI: 10¹²/L]	Hemoglobin (g/dL) [SI: g/L]	Hematocrit (%)	MCH (pg) [SI: pg]	MCHC (g/dL) [SI: g/L]ᵃ	MCV (µm³) [SI: fL]	RDW
Adult Male	4500–11,000 [4.5–11.0]	4.73–5.49 [4.73–5.49]	14.40–16.60 [144–166]	42.9–49.1	27–31	33–37	76–100	11.5–14.5
Adult Female	As above	4.15–4.87	12.2–14.7	37.9–43.9	As above	As above	As above	As above
11–15 yr	4,500–13,500	4.8	13.4	39	28	34	82	
6–10 yr	5,000–14,500	4.7	12.9	37.5	27	34	80	
4–6 yr	5,500–15,500	4.6	12.6	37.0	27	34	80	
2–4 yr	6,000–17,000	4.5	12.5	35.5	25	32	77	
4 mo–2 yr	6,000–17,500	4.6	11.2	35.0	25	33	77	
1 wk–4 mo	5,500–18,000	4.7±0.9	14.0±3.3	42.0±7.0	30	33	90	
24 hr–1 wk	5,000–21,000	5.1	18.3±4.0	52.5	36	35	103	
First day	9,400–34,000	5.1±1.0	19.5±5.0	54.0±10.0	38	36	106	

ᵃTo convert standard reference value to SI units, multiply by 10.

CBC = complete blood count

WBC = white blood cell; RBC = red blood cell; MCH = mean cell hemoglobin; MCHC = mean cell hemoglobin concentration; MCV = mean cell volume; RDW = red cell distribution width.

Table 11.2. (Continued)

Age	Platelet Count (10³/µL) [SI: 10⁹/L]	Lymphocytes, total (% WBC count)	Neutrophils, band (% WBC count)	Neutrophils, segmented (% WBC count)	Eosinophils (% WBC count)	Basophils (% WBC count)	Monocytes (% WBC count)
Adult Male	238±49	34	3.0	56	2.7	0.5	4.0
Adult Female	270±58	As above	As above	As above	As above	As above	As above
11–15 yr	282±63	38	3.0	51	2.4	0.5	4.3
6–10 yr	351±85	39	3.0	50	2.4	0.6	4.2
4–6 yr	357±70	42	3.0	39	2.8	0.6	5.0
2–4 yr	As above	59	3.0	30	2.6	0.5	5.0
4 mo–2 yr	As above	61	3.1	28	2.6	0.4	4.8
1 wk–4 mo	As above	56	4.5	30	2.8	0.5	6.5
24 hr–1 wk	240–380	24–41	6.8–9.2	39–52	2.4–4.1	0.5	5.8–9.1
First day	As above	24	10.2	58	2.0	0.6	5.8

ᵃTo convert standard reference value to SI units, multiply by 10.
WBC = white blood cell.

NORMAL CBC VARIATIONS

Hbg and HCT are highest at birth (20 g/100 mL and 60%, respectively). The values fall steeply to a minimum at 3 months (9.5 g/100 mL and 32%). Then they slowly rise to near adult levels at puberty; thereafter, both values are higher in men. A normal decrease occurs in pregnancy. The number of WBCs is highest at birth (mean of 25,000/mm³) and slowly falls to adult levels by puberty. Lymphocytes predominate (as much as 60% from the second week of life until age 5–7 years, when neutrophils begin to predominate).

HEMATOCRIT

Because plasma and red cells are lost in equal amounts in acute bleeding, the HCT does not immediately decrease; thus, it does not reflect blood loss during the first few hours. In anemia, the red cell indices and reticulocyte count should be evaluated to guide the differential diagnosis.

11

GRANULOCYTIC MATURATION AND THE LEFT SHIFT

A myeloblast is the most immature cell of granulocytic lineage. As it matures, the round nucleus indents and eventually segments, and the nuclear chromatin simultaneously condenses. The segments (typically 3–4) are connected by thin bands of nuclear chromatin. The cytoplasm, which is light blue, initially demonstrates a small number of primary fuchsia-colored granules, which as the cell matures, are lost and the presence of secondary, salmon-colored granules predominate. A **band cell** is when the nucleus of the neutrophil is indented to more than half the distance to the farthest nuclear margin, but the chromatin is not condensed to a single filament, as in the segmented neutrophil. Figure 11-2 describes the lineage of granulocyte maturation.

The presence of and increased number of immature cells prior to the segmented neutrophil (consisting of myelocytes, metamyelocytes, and a marked increase in bands) constitute a granulocytic **"left shift."** A left shift can be seen in bacterial infection, sepsis, rejuvenating bone marrow, administration of G-CSF, acute stress, acute hemorrhage, and myeloproliferative disorders. (Note the origin of the term "left shift" is historic and debated. It possibly relates to manual cell counters where less mature cell entry keys were on the left side of the counter.)

By convention, **hypersegmented neutrophils** are described as greater than 6 five-lobed neutrophils or 1 six-lobed neutrophil/100 WBCs. While this can be a nonspecific finding, it is often seen in association with megaloblastic anemia, as seen with vitamin B_{12} deficiency. In addition to microscopy, cells can be further identified by cell surface markers.

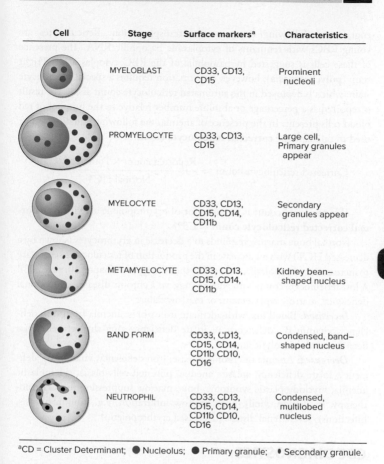

Cell	Stage	Surface markers[a]	Characteristics
	MYELOBLAST	CD33, CD13, CD15	Prominent nucleoli
	PROMYELOCYTE	CD33, CD13, CD15	Large cell, Primary granules appear
	MYELOCYTE	CD33, CD13, CD15, CD14, CD11b	Secondary granules appear
	METAMYELOCYTE	CD33, CD13, CD15, CD14, CD11b	Kidney bean–shaped nucleus
	BAND FORM	CD33, CD13, CD15, CD14, CD11b CD10, CD16	Condensed, band–shaped nucleus
	NEUTROPHIL	CD33, CD13, CD15, CD14, CD11b CD10, CD16	Condensed, multilobed nucleus

[a]CD = Cluster Determinant; ● Nucleolus; ● Primary granule; • Secondary granule.

Figure 11-2. Stages of neutrophil development shown schematically. Granulocyte colony-stimulating factor (G-CSF) and granulocyte–macrophage colony-stimulating factor (GM-CSF) are critical to this process. Identifying cellular characteristics and specific cell-surface markers are listed for each maturational stage. (Reproduced with permission from *Harrison's Principles of Internal Medicine*, 20e, New York, NY: McGraw-Hill Education; 2018.)

RETICULOCYTE COUNT

- Normal: 0.5–2.5% or 20–125 × 10⁹/L

The reticulocyte count is not included in a routine CBC. The reticulocyte count is performed by the CBC instrument and is used in the initial workup of anemia and in monitoring the effect of hematinic or erythropoietin therapy, monitoring recovery from myelosuppression, or monitoring engraftment following bone marrow transplantation. Reticulocytes are young RBCs with remnants of cytoplasmic basophilic RNA. The presence of these cells is suggested by basophilia of the RBC cytoplasm on Wright stain (**polychromasia**); however, confirmation requires a special reticulocyte stain, which is deployed in the automated reticulocyte count assay. The result is reported as a percentage or absolute number relative to the number of red blood cells present. In the presence of anemia, the following equation can be used to calculate the **corrected reticulocyte count**:

$$\text{Corrected reticulocyte count} = \frac{\text{Reported count} \times \text{Patient's HCT}}{\text{Normal HCT}}$$

This corrected count is an indicator of erythropoietic activity. The **normal corrected reticulocyte count $\leq$1.5%**.

Normal bone marrow responds to a decrease in erythrocytes (shown by a decreased HCT) with an increase in the production of reticulocytes secondary to increased erythropoietin produced by the kidneys (see Chapter 10, page 208). A low reticulocyte count with anemia suggests a chronic disease, a nutritional deficiency, marrow replacement, or marrow failure.

Increased: Blood loss with adequate iron stores; anemia from iron deficiency, vitamin B_{12} deficiency, or folate deficiency after the deficiency has been restored; hemolytic anemia

Decreased: Anemia of chronic disease, iron deficiency, vitamin B_{12} deficiency, folate deficiency, aplastic anemia, pure red cell aplasia, sideroblastic anemia, myelodysplastic syndrome, bone marrow suppression (e.g., chemotherapy, irradiation, viral), bone marrow infiltration (e.g., tumor, fibrosis, infections), severe renal disease (decreased erythropoietin)

CBC DIAGNOSTICS

- See Table 11-2, pages 270–271, for age- and sex-specific normal ranges. Beyond the total WBC, RBC, and platelet count, identification of specific CBC alterations may aid in the differential diagnosis of a variety of diseases and conditions. Normal white blood cells consist of a mix of basophils, eosinophils, lymphocytes, monocytes, and polymorphonuclear neutrophils.

White Blood Cells (Leukocytes)

<u>**Total white blood cell counts:**</u> See Figure 11-2, page 273.

Increased: Infection, inflammatory process (rheumatoid arthritis, allergies) leukemia, severe stress (physical or emotional), postoperative state (physiologic stress), severe tissue injury (e.g., burns), corticosteroids

Decreased: Bone marrow failure (aplastic anemia, infection, tumor, fibrosis, radiation damage), medications (e.g., chloramphenicol, linezolid, chemotherapeutics, anticonvulsants, antipsychotics, immunosuppressants, antiinflammatories, other antimicrobials, and others), collagen-vascular disease such as SLE, liver or spleen disease, vitamin B_{12}, or folate deficiency

Basophils: 0–1%
  Increased: Chronic myelogenous leukemia, post-splenectomy, polycythemia, and, rarely, recovery from infection or hypothyroidism
  Decreased: Acute rheumatic fever, pregnancy, postradiation therapy, corticosteroids, thyrotoxicosis, stress

Eosinophils: 1–3%
  Increased: Allergy, parasites, skin disease, malignancy, drugs, asthma, Addison disease, collagen–vascular disease (mnemonic **NAACP: N**eoplasm, **A**llergy/asthma, **A**ddison disease, **C**ollagen–vascular disease, **P**arasites), chronic myelogenous leukemia, and pulmonary diseases such as Loffler syndrome and Churg-Strauss syndrome
  Decreased: Corticosteroids, ACTH, aftermath of stress (infection, trauma, burns), Cushing syndrome

Lymphocytes ("Lymphs"): 24–44% (See also Lymphocyte Subsets, page 278.)
  Increased: Viral infection (HIV, measles, rubella, mumps, smallpox, chickenpox, influenza, hepatitis, infectious mononucleosis), whooping cough, chronic lymphocytic leukemia, and lymphoma with hematogenous spread
  Decreased: Normal in 22% of population; stress, burns, trauma, uremia, some viral infections, HIV and AIDS, bone marrow suppression after chemotherapy, corticosteroids, multiple sclerosis (MS)
  Reactive Lymphocytes: >20%: Infectious mononucleosis, CMV infection, infectious hepatitis, toxoplasmosis; <20%: Viral infections (mumps, rubeola, varicella), rickettsial infections, TB

Monocytes ("Monos"): 3–7%
  Increased: Bacterial infection (TB, SBE, brucellosis, typhoid, recovery from acute infection), protozoan infection, infectious mononucleosis, leukemia, Hodgkin disease, ulcerative colitis, Crohn disease
  Decreased: Aplastic anemia, corticosteroid use, hairy cell leukemia

Polymorphonuclear Neutrophils (PMNs, Segmented Neutrophils, Neutrophils, "Polys"): 40–76%; see also the "Left Shift," page 272.
  Increased:
  Physiologic (Normal): Extensive exercise, last months of pregnancy, labor, surgery, newborn state, corticosteroid therapy
  Pathologic: Bacterial infection, noninfective tissue injury (MI, pulmonary infarction, pancreatitis, crush injury, burn injury), eclampsia, HELLP syndrome, metabolic disorders (DKA, uremia, acute gout), leukemia
  Decreased: Pancytopenia, aplastic anemia, PMN depression (a mild decrease is referred to as **neutropenia**; a severe decrease is called **agranulocytosis**), marrow damage (radiation exposure, toxic chemicals like benzene, antitumor drugs), severe overwhelming infection (disseminated TB,

septicemia), acute malaria, osteomyelitis, infectious mononucleosis, atypical pneumonia, some viral infections, marrow obliteration (osteosclerosis, myelofibrosis, malignant infiltrate), numerous drugs (including chloramphenicol, phenylbutazone, chlorpromazine, quinine, sulfamethoxazole and trimethoprim), vitamin B_{12} and folate deficiencies, hypoadrenalism, hypopituitarism, dialysis, benign ethnic neutropenia most commonly seen in those of African and some Middle Eastern descent.

Red Blood Cells

CBC instruments measure red cell number, mean corpuscular volume (MCV), red cell distribution width (RDW), hemoglobin concentration, and in some cases the hematocrit. The hematocrit and other parameters are usually calculated from those values.

11 Hematocrit

- Men 40–54%; women 37–47%. Calculated from MCV and red cell number; the percentage volume of red cells in a given volume of blood; RBC × MCV

  Increased: Primary polycythemia (polycythemia vera), secondary polycythemia (smoking, COPD, hypoventilation, reduced fluid intake or excess fluid loss, drugs such as EPO or anabolic steroids), congenital or acquired heart and lung disease, high altitude, tumors (renal cell carcinoma, hepatoma)

  Decreased: Megaloblastic anemia (folate or B_{12} deficiencies); iron-deficiency anemia; sickle cell anemia or other hemoglobinopathies; acute or chronic blood loss; sideroblastic anemia, hemolysis; anemia due to chronic disease, dilution, alcohol, or medications

MCH (Mean Cellular [Corpuscular] Hemoglobin)

- 27–31 pg (SI: pg) The amount of hemoglobin in the average red cell. Calculated as:

$$MCH = \frac{\text{Hemoglobin (g/L)}}{\text{RBC} (10^6/\mu L)}$$

  Increased: Macrocytosis (megaloblastic anemia, high reticulocyte count)
  Decreased: Microcytosis (iron deficiency, sideroblastic anemia, thalassemia)

MCHC (Mean Cellular [Corpuscular] Hemoglobin Concentration)

- 33–37 g/dL (SI: 330–370 g/L)

  The average concentration of Hbg in a given volume of red cells. Calculated as:

$$MCHC = \frac{\text{Hemoglobin (g/dL)}}{\text{Hematocrit}}$$

Increased (Hyperchromasia): Very severe prolonged dehydration; spherocytosis

Decreased (Hypochromasia): Iron-deficiency anemia, overhydration, thalassemia, sideroblastic anemia

MCV (Mean Cell [Corpuscular] Volume)
- 78–98 μm^3 (SI: fL)

The average volume of red blood cells; measured directly with the automated cell counter.

Increased (**Macrocytosis**): Megaloblastic anemia (B_{12}, folate deficiency), macrocytic (normoblastic) anemia, reticulocytosis, myelodysplasia, Down syndrome, chronic liver disease, treatment of HIV, chronic alcoholism, cytotoxic chemotherapy, radiation therapy, phenytoin (Dilantin), hypothyroidism, newborn state

Decreased (**Microcytosis**): Iron deficiency, thalassemia, lead poisoning, or polycythemia

Normal: Anemia of chronic disease, acute blood loss, primary bone marrow failure

RDW (Red Cell Distribution Width)
- 11.5–14.5%

RDW is a measure of the degree of **anisocytosis** (variation in RBC size) and is determined with an automated counter.

Increased: Many types of anemia (iron deficiency, B_{12}, folate deficiency, thalassemia), liver disease

Platelets
- 150,000–450,000 μL

Platelet counts may be normal in number but abnormal in function, as occurs in aspirin therapy. Abnormalities of platelet function are assessed by platelet function and platelet aggregation assays.

Increased: Sudden exercise, trauma, fracture, aftermath of asphyxia, postsurgery (especially splenectomy), acute hemorrhage, myeloproliferative neoplasms, post partum, carcinoma, iron deficiency

Decreased: Disseminated intravascular coagulation (DIC), idiopathic thrombocytopenic purpura (ITP), thrombotic thrombocytopenic purpura (TTP), hemolytic uremic syndrome (HUS), congenital disease, marrow suppressants (chemotherapy, alcohol, radiation), burns, snake and insect bites, leukemia, aplastic anemia, hypersplenism, infectious mononucleosis, other viral infections, cirrhosis, massive transfusion, HELLP syndrome (probably a severe form of preeclampsia with microangiopathic hemolysis, elevated liver function tests, and low platelet count), preeclampsia and eclampsia, prosthetic heart valve, numerous drugs (NSAIDs, abciximab, anticonvulsants, thiazides, sulfonamides, linezolid, vancomycin, penicillins, cephalosporins, other antibiotics, heparin, some vaccines, others)

HEMOGLOBINOPATHY WORKUP

- **Normal:** Hemoglobins A, F, and A2 present; normal levels age-dependent

  Hemoglobinopathies are a group of disorders with abnormal production or structure of the hemoglobin molecule and are inherited. Hemoglobinopathy workup consists of analysis of the red cell hemoglobin chains to look for structural abnormalities (i.e., hemoglobins S, C, E) or qualitative production defects as in alpha or beta thalassemias. These results should always be reviewed in conjunction with CBC data. A screening test for hemoglobin S can also be performed, but it is not able to differentiate heterozygous hemoglobin S trait from homozygous hemoglobin S disease. Hemoglobin S trait is clinically silent. Hemoglobin S disease is a serious sickling disorder associated with episodes of marked anemia and painful crisis.

HEMOLYSIS WORKUP

Hemolysis can result in anemia when RBC survival (normal 120 days) is shortened. Destruction of RBC can occur in the bloodstream (intravascular hemolysis) or within the reticuloendothelial system (extravascular hemolysis occurring in the spleen or liver). Factitious hemolysis is from RBC lysis during collection and handling of the blood sample. ↑ lactate dehydrogenase (LDH) and ↓ haptoglobin is 90% specific for hemolysis.

- **Intravascular hemolysis** common causes: mechanical trauma (e.g., micro-angiopathic hemolytic anemia due to mechanical heart valve, DIC, TTP, HUS), autoimmune, ABO incompatibility, snake bites, infectious (e.g., severe malaria, Clostridial sepsis), paroxysmal nocturnal hemoglobinuria.
  - o Labs: Schistocytes **on peripheral smear,** ↑ LDH, ↓ haptoglobin, ↑ free hemoglobin, ↑ urine hemoglobin, hemosiderinuria (stained urine specimen)
- **Extravascular hemolysis** is more common, may be inherited, and usually presents in childhood. Some causes: hemoglobinopathies (e.g., sickle cell disease, thalassemia major) enzyme deficiencies (e.g., deficiencies of G6PD, pyruvate kinase), liver disease, hypersplenism
  - o Labs: Microspherocytes **on peripheral smear,** ↑ LDH, normal to ↓ haptoglobin, ↑ indirect bilirubin, ↑ urine and fecal urobilinogen

LYMPHOCYTE SUBSETS

Specific monoclonal antibodies are used to identify specific T and B cells. Lymphocyte subsets are useful in the diagnosis of AIDS and to guide prophylaxis against certain AIDS-related infections (e.g., CD4 <200 then prophylaxis with TMP-SMX is indicated). Results are most reliably reported as an absolute number of cells/μL rather than as a percentage. A CD4/CD8 ratio of <1 is seen in AIDS. Absolute CD4 count is used to determine when to initiate therapy with antiretroviral agents or to administer prophylaxis for certain infections, e.g., PCP, MAI. The CDC considers an HIV-positive patient to have AIDS if the CD4 count <200. Children with severe combined immunodeficiency (SCID) have a profound deficiency of T and B cells. Used to monitor for B-cell depletion in patients treated with rituximab/anti-CD20 monoclonal antibody for hematologic and autoimmune diseases.

Normal Lymphocyte Subsets

Can vary slightly by lab and age
- Total lymphocytes 660–4600/μL
- T cells (CD3) 644–2201 μL (60–88%)
- B cells (CD19 or CD20) 82–392 μL (3–20%)
- Helper/inducer T cells (CD4) 493–1191 μL (34–67%)
- Suppressor/cytotoxic T cells (CD8) 182–785 μL (10–42%)
- CD4/CD8 ratio >1

11

RBC MORPHOLOGY DIFFERENTIAL DIAGNOSIS

The following are erythrocyte abnormalities and associated conditions normally detected on a Wright stain microscopic exam. See Figure 11-3, page 280. General terms to describe RBC morphology include **poikilocytosis** (irregular RBC shape such as sickle or burr cells) and **anisocytosis** (abnormal RBC size such as microcytes or macrocytes). Normal mature erythrocytes have a uniform, rounded, biconcave shape.

Acanthocytes (spur cells):
- Description: Red blood cells that have circumferential blunt and spiny projections with bulbous tips
- Disease and conditions: Severe liver disease, abetalipoproteinemia

Agglutination:
- Description: Clumping of red cells; can interfere with determination of RBC indices
- Diseases and conditions: Signifies the presence of cold agglutinins (IgM antibodies); mycoplasma pneumonia, cold autoimmune hemolytic anemia, paroxysmal cold hemoglobinuria, IgM-secreting lymphomas

Basophilic stippling:
- Description: Small blue dots seen in red cells (clusters of ribosomes)
- Disease and conditions: Lead or heavy-metal poisoning, thalassemia, severe anemia

11

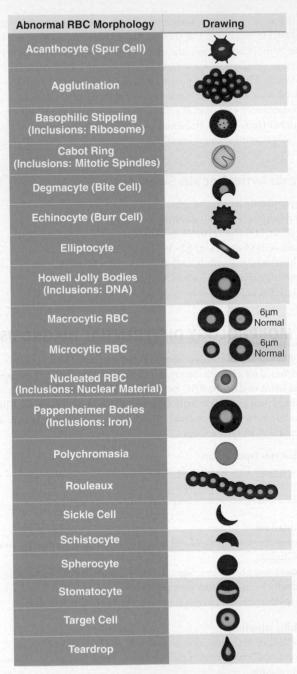

Abnormal RBC Morphology	Drawing
Acanthocyte (Spur Cell)	
Agglutination	
Basophilic Stippling (Inclusions: Ribosome)	
Cabot Ring (Inclusions: Mitotic Spindles)	
Degmacyte (Bite Cell)	
Echinocyte (Burr Cell)	
Elliptocyte	
Howell Jolly Bodies (Inclusions: DNA)	
Macrocytic RBC	6μm Normal
Microcytic RBC	6μm Normal
Nucleated RBC (Inclusions: Nuclear Material)	
Pappenheimer Bodies (Inclusions: Iron)	
Polychromasia	
Rouleaux	
Sickle Cell	
Schistocyte	
Spherocyte	
Stomatocyte	
Target Cell	
Teardrop	

Figure 11-3. Some examples of abnormal RBC morphology.

Cabot rings:
- Description: Ring-shaped, dark purple inclusion body representing residual nuclear material (mitotic spindles), often seen in the presence of polychromasia.
- Diseases and conditions: Asplenia

Degmacytes (Bite cells):
- Description: Red blood cells with an irregular membrane due to splenic macrophage–mediated removal of denatured hemoglobin molecules
- Diseases and conditions: Hemolysis due to oxidative damage, as seen with unstable hemoglobins and red cell enzyme disorders like G6PD deficiency (see Chapter 10) and represent the removal of previously deposited precipitated hemoglobin (Heinz bodies); requires a special stain (not Wright stain) to be visualized.

Echinocytes (Burr cells):
- Description: Circumferential undulations or spiny projections with pointed tips that are uniform in shape and density
- Diseases and conditions: End-stage renal disease, liver disease, starvation, vitamin E deficiency, artifactual

Elliptocytes (ovalocytes):
- Description: RBC cells twice as long as they are wide, pencil shaped
- Diseases and conditions: Iron-deficiency anemia, hereditary elliptocytosis

Howell-Jolly bodies:
- Description: Dotlike, dark purple inclusions representing residual nuclear fragment
- Diseases and conditions: Postsplenectomy, functional asplenia; Howell-Jolly bodies are a useful and sensitive indicator of splenic function

Macrocytosis:
- Description: Enlarged RBC with constant hemoglobin concentration is defined by an MCV of greater than 100 μm^3 (100 fL)
- Diseases and conditions: Vitamin B_{12} or folate deficiency, liver disease, hypothyroidism, myelodysplastic syndrome, drugs (many antineoplastic agents [e.g., methotrexate], some antivirals)

Microcytosis:
- Description: RBC smaller than usual, defined as a MCV of less than 80 μm^3 (80 fL) in adults
- Diseases and conditions: Iron-deficiency anemia, thalassemia, vitamin B_6 (pyridoxine) deficiency, occasionally anemia of chronic disease and sideroblastic anemia (25% of patients with anemia of chronic disease are microcytic, the rest are normocytic/normochromic)

11

Nucleated RBCs:
- Description: Immature RBC that are not normally seen in the peripheral circulation; normal in infants up to 5 days of life
- Diseases and conditions: Severe bone marrow stress (e.g., severe anemia due to hemorrhage, hemolysis, hypoxia), marrow replacement by tumor, extramedullary hematopoiesis, miliary TB

Pappenheimer bodies:
- Description: Similar to basophilic stippling, but larger, more irregular, and grayer than basophilic stippling due to iron-containing mitochondria
- Diseases and conditions: Sideroblastic anemia, asplenia

Polychromasia:
- Description: A bluish red cell on routine Wright stain
- Diseases and conditions: Hemolytic anemia, radiation therapy, certain cancers, paroxysmal nocturnal hemoglobinuria

Rouleaux:
- Description: RBCs are stacked together in long chains caused by an increase in serum proteins
- Diseases and conditions: Plasma cell neoplasms, hypergammaglobulinemia, B-cell lymphomas, acute and chronic infections (acute phase reactants), connective tissue diseases, and chronic liver disease; occasionally artifactual due to poor slide preparation

Sickle cells:
- Description: Under low oxygen tension abnormal sickle cell hemoglobin becomes long and rigid, causing the RBC to become thin and take on the "sickle shape" appearance; causes sludging in tissues
- Diseases and conditions: Sickle cell anemia (SS hemoglobin); with sickle cell trait (AS hemoglobin) less likely to have sickling but sickling can occur at high altitude with exertion

Schistocytes:
- Description: More general term for fragmented RBC; individual cells often referred to by names describing the specific cell shape such as helmet or football; some may resemble commas or triangles
- TTP, HUS, HELLP syndrome, DIC, hemolytic transfusion reaction, burns, mechanical trauma (i.e., mechanical heart valves), medications (cyclosporine, quinine, tacrolimus), transplant rejection; automated cell counters may incorrectly count schistocytes as platelets and if the

number of schistocytes is high, the platelet count may be spuriously increased

Spherocytes:
- Description: Due to loss of part of the cell membrane the RBC are more sphere shaped than biconcave
- Diseases and conditions: Immune-mediated hemolysis and anemia, hereditary spherocytosis, severe burns, ABO transfusion reaction

Stomatocytes:
- Description: RBC with an area of central pallor elongated with a mouth-like shape
- Diseases and conditions: Slide preparation/drying artifact, hereditary stomatocytosis, alcoholic liver disease, Rh null disease, drugs (e.g., dilantin, vinblastine, hydroxyurea, diazepam, phenothiazine)

Target cells (codocytes):
- Description: RBC with a dark circle within the central area of pallor, reflecting redundant membrane
- Diseases and conditions: Thalassemia, hemoglobinopathies, liver disease, post-splenectomy, artifact

Teardrop cells (dacrocytes):
- Description: RBC appearance of a teardrop or pear shape; slightly rounded or blunted ends
- Diseases and conditions: Thalassemia, megaloblastic anemia, marrow infiltration (fibrosis, granulomatous inflammation, hematologic or metastatic malignancy), splenic abnormalities

WBC MORPHOLOGY DIFFERENTIAL DIAGNOSIS

The following are conditions associated with changes in the normal morphology of WBCs. See also Granulocytic Maturation and the Left Shift, page 272.

Auer rods: Acute myeloid leukemia
Döhle inclusion bodies: Severe infection, burns, malignancy, pregnancy, GCSF administration
Hypersegmentation: Megaloblastic anemia (any neutrophils with six or more lobes is diagnostic)
Toxic granulation: Severe illness (sepsis, burns, high fever), GCSF administration

COAGULATION AND OTHER HEMATOLOGIC TESTS

The coagulation cascade is shown in Figure 11-4, page 284. A variety of coagulation-related and other common blood tests follow.

11

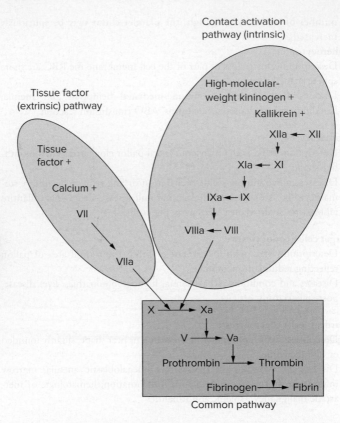

Figure 11-4. Coagulation cascade (Modified and reproduced with permission from Hall JB, Schmidt GA, Kress JP. Bleeding disorders. In *Principles of Critical Care*, 4e, New York, NY: McGraw-Hill; 2015.)

Coagulation Cascade

Activation of the coagulation cascade is organized into pathways that reflect the basic understanding of coagulation events and coagulation function testing. These pathways reflect laboratory techniques used to activate the coagulation cascade. The advantage of these pathway concepts is that they facilitate understanding of common laboratory tests, including PT and PTT. The common pathway describes the final steps in fibrin production from activated factor X to thrombin to fibrin. The tissue factor (extrinsic) pathway is the major and most essential step in the normal initiation of coagulation, beginning with calcium-dependent activation of factor VII by tissue factor. The contact activation (intrinsic) pathway involves activation of factors XII, XI, IX, and VIII. Disorders of coagulation due to primary disturbances of the soluble coagulation factors include congenital deficiencies (e.g., hemophilia A, B), drug-induced coagulopathies (e.g., heparin, warfarin, direct factor Xa inhibitors), depletion of coagulation factors (e.g., vitamin K deficiency, DIC), severe inflammatory states (e.g., sepsis, trauma), and inhibition of activity in autoimmune disease (e.g., antibody inhibitors).

Factor Xa Assay (Anti-Xa Test, Anti-Factor Xa, Heparin Assay)

Used to monitor low molecular weight heparins (LMWHs), unfractionated heparin (UFH), and the direct oral anticoagulants (DOACs) that have anti-Xa activity. Useful when the PTT cannot be used (i.e., a patient with lupus anticoagulant). Only test for monitoring low-molecular-weight heparin (LMWH) (e.g., Lovenox). Monitoring anticoagulant therapy required for IV administration and not essential for subcutaneous use. Elevated in renal failure or when a specimen is contaminated with heparin.

Patients not on heparin: 0 anti-Xa international units/ml (IU/mL)
Therapeutic for DVT treatment: IV administration of UFH (heparin): 0.3–0.7 IU/mL
LMWH: 0.4–1.1 IU/mL for BID dosing or 1–2 IU/mL for once daily
DVT Prophylaxis: measure 3–4 hrs after subcutaneous injection of UFH: 0.1–0.4 IU/mL
LMWH: 0.2–0.5 IU/mL

Activated Clotting Time (ACT)

- 114–186 s

A bedside test used when high levels of unfractionated heparin are needed, such as cardiopulmonary bypass, interventional cardiology, ECMO, and dialysis. Testing is implemented before, during, and shortly after heparin exposure in these settings.

Increased: Heparin, some platelet disorders, severe clotting factor deficiency

Antithrombin III (AT-III)

- 80–120%; used in evaluation of thrombosis; patient must be off heparin for 6 hr

Decreased: Autosomal dominant familial AT-III deficiency, PE, severe liver disease, late pregnancy, oral contraceptives, nephrotic syndrome (lost in urine with resulting increase in factor II and X activity), DIC, heparin therapy
Increased: Warfarin, as an acute phase reactant

Bleeding Time

A test of platelet function of historical interest that measured the amount of time to form a clot from a skin incision. Replaced by platelet aggregation testing (see page 288).

Coombs Test, Direct (Direct Antiglobulin Test)

- Normal = negative
  Tests for the presence of antibody on the patient's **red cells**.

Positive: Autoimmune hemolytic anemia, hemolytic transfusion reaction, some drug sensitizations (methyldopa, levodopa, cephalosporins, penicillins, quinidine), hemolytic disease of the newborn (erythroblastosis fetalis)

Coombs Test, Indirect (Indirect Antiglobulin Test/Autoantibody Test)

- Normal = negative
  Tests for the presence of antibodies against red cell antigens in the patient's serum.

Positive: Isoimmunization from previous transfusion, autoimmune hemolytic anemia, incompatible blood or medication induced (e.g., methyldopa)

Factor V (Leiden) Mutation

- Normal = negative
  Factor V Leiden is the most common hereditary blood coagulation disorder in the United States (5–7%) that increases the risk of thrombosis. Heterozygotes have thrombosis risk **(thrombophilia)** roughly 5 times that of the general population. The risk among homozygotes is 40–80 times that of the general population.

Positive: Factor V mutation; heterozygous or homozygous

Fibrin D-Dimers

(See also Chapter 10, page 206.)

- Negative or <0.25 mcg/mL; Evidence of fibrinolysis following fibrin formation and fibrin cross-linking
  Increased: DIC, thromboembolic disease (PE, arterial or venous thrombosis), post-thrombolytic therapy

Fibrinogen

- 123–370 mg/dL (SI: 1.23–3.7 g/L)
  Most useful in management of DIC and congenital hypofibrinogenemia.

Increased: Acute phase reactant, oral contraceptives, pregnancy, cancer (kidney, stomach, breast)

Decreased: DIC (sepsis, amniotic fluid embolism, abruptio placentae), liver disease (produced in the liver), neoplastic and hematologic conditions, acute severe bleeding, burns, venomous snake bite, severe thrombolysis, post-thrombolytic therapy, congenital hypofibrinogenemia. Depending on the etiology, fibrinogen levels of <100 may require transfusion with cryoglobulin.

Kleihauer–Betke Test

The test is performed to quantitate the number of fetal cells present in the maternal circulation and is commonly used to quantify fetomaternal hemorrhage (the entry of fetal blood into the maternal circulation at the time of delivery). The test measures the amount of fetal hemoglobin transferred from a fetus to a mother's bloodstream, usually performed on Rh-negative mothers. It allows the appropriate RhIG dose to be calculated and administered to prevent the mother from making anti-D antibodies and potentially causing harm during her next pregnancy. Test is based on the principle that red cells containing fetal hemoglobin (HbF) are less susceptible to acid elution than cells containing adult hemoglobin (HbA). After the sample is acid-treated, the slides are stained and examined microscopically. The test should be performed approximately 1 hour after delivery on a maternal sample from all Rh-negative women who deliver an Rh-positive fetus. Results are reported as the percentage of fetal RBCs seen.

11

Mixing Studies (Circulating Anticoagulant Screen)

Used to evaluate prolonged PT or PTT. Normal plasma is mixed with patient plasma, and the abnormal clotting time is measured again in the mix. If the clotting time corrects, a factor deficiency/deficiencies exist. Follow-up testing for levels of factors VIII, IX, XI, and XII if only the PTT is prolonged to identify the specific factor deficiency (note: warfarin may also give this result). If only the PT is prolonged, that is highly suggestive of factor VII deficiency. If both the PT and PTT are prolonged, potential factor deficiencies include factor(s) II, V, VIII, IX, X, XI, and XII and fibrinogen. If the clotting time does not correct, an inhibitor (factor specific or against phospholipid/lupus anticoagulant) is present. Heparin and direct thrombin inhibitors can also result in uncorrected mixing studies. Evaluation of the Russell viper venom time (RVVT), which directly activates factor X, along with testing for antibodies to phospholipids (cardiolipins and B2 glycoprotein), are used to diagnose a lupus anticoagulant (associated with recurrent thrombosis and spontaneous abortions).

MTHFR Mutation

- Normal = negative

   Patients with this mutation have associated severe MTHFR (methylenetetrahydrofolate reductase) deficiency (enzymatic activity 0–20% of normal) and develop hyperhomocysteinuria, which is associated with various conditions, including premature vascular disease and subsequent thromboembolic disorders. MTHFR is an enzyme that breaks down the amino acids, homocysteine, and folate.

Positive: MTHFR mutation; heterozygous of unlikely clinical significance; homozygous may have increased homocysteine levels

Partial Thromboplastin Time (Activated Partial Thromboplastin Time, PTT, aPTT)

- 27–38 s

   Used to evaluate the intrinsic coagulation system (see Figure 11-4, page 284); most often used to monitor heparin therapy

Increased: Heparin, defect in the **intrinsic coagulation system** (fibrinogen and factors II, V, VII, VIII, IX, X, XI, and XII), prolonged application of tourniquet before drawing of sample, hemophilia A and B, von Willebrand disease (sometimes normal), lupus anticoagulant (antiphospholipid antibody), DIC

Platelet Factor 4 (PF4 Antibody, Heparin-PF4 Antibody)

- Heparin-induced thrombocytopenia (HIT) ELISA Optical Density (OD) <0.400 or negative

   Used to evaluate immune-mediated heparin-induced thrombocytopenia (HIT) due to IgG antibodies that bind to a complex of heparin and platelet factor 4

   Positive: HIT should be suspected when the platelet count drops by at least 50% in 5–10 days after the initiation of heparin therapy. The test is sensitive for the presence of immunologically driven HIT; however, the test has poor specificity. HIT is a clinical-pathologic diagnosis, and clinical findings and other laboratory tests should be considered when making the diagnosis.

   If the test findings are indeterminate or negative in a patient with a high clinical suspicion of HIT, utilization of the serotonin release assay (SRA) is recommended.

Platelet Function (Aggregation) Assays

- Collagen/epinephrine ≤175 sec; collagen/ADP ≤120 sec

Commercial assays to evaluate platelet function are available as cartridge-based tests where a citrated whole blood sample travels through a hole in a membrane coated with various platelet agonists to measure platelet adherence, activation, and aggregation. More sophisticated platelet aggregation studies can also be performed exposing the patient's platelets to various platelet agonists. Nonsteroidal medications should be stopped 5–7 days before the test because these agents can affect platelet function. Platelet function (aggregation) assays have essentially replaced bleeding time.

Increased: Thrombocytopenia, von Willebrand disease, defective platelet function, drugs such as aspirin and NSAIDs.

Protein C

- 80–120%
  Used in evaluation of thrombosis; protein C degrades factor Va and VIIIa

Decreased: Inherited protein C deficiency, PE, severe liver disease, vitamin K deficiency, nephrotic syndrome (lost in the urine), DIC, warfarin therapy

Increased (not clinically significant): Heparin therapy, direct thrombin inhibitors

Protein S

- 80–120% of control value
  Used in evaluation of thrombosis; cofactor for protein C

Decreased: Inherited protein S deficiency, PE, severe liver disease, vitamin K deficiency, nephrotic syndrome (lost in the urine), DIC, warfarin therapy

Increased (not clinically significant): Heparin, director thrombin inhibitors

Prothrombin Gene Mutation

- Normal = negative
  Prothrombin gene mutation G20210A results in increased levels of prothrombin and is present in 2–4% in individuals of European ancestry. Carriers are at 3 times the risk of thromboembolic disease.

Positive: Prothrombin gene mutation; heterozygous or homozygous.

Prothrombin Time (PT)

- 11.5–13.5 s (INR, normal = 0.8–1.4)
  Used to evaluate the **extrinsic coagulation system** (see Figure 11-4, page 284), which includes fibrinogen and factors II, V, VII, and X. The use of **INR** instead of the actual PT result in seconds is utilized to guide chronic

11

warfarin therapy, as it resists individual instrument variation and is reproducible across laboratories. **Therapeutic INR** is 2–3 for DVT, PE, TIAs, and atrial fibrillation. Mechanical heart valves require an INR of 2.5–3.5. PT is **NOT** affected by heparin except in doses that greatly exceed therapeutic dosing.

Increased: Drugs (warfarin), vitamin K deficiency, fat malabsorption, liver disease, prolonged application of tourniquet before drawing of sample, DIC, massive transfusion

Sedimentation Rate (Erythrocyte Sedimentation Rate [ESR])

- *Normal*: Adult male: ≤15 mm/hr; adult female: ≤20 mm/hr; child: ≤10 mm/hr; newborn: 0–2 mm/hr

    The "sed rate" is a nonspecific test; high sensitivity and low specificity. Most useful in serial measurement to follow the course of a chronic disease (e.g., polymyalgia rheumatica or temporal arteritis). C-reactive protein is a more sensitive marker of acute inflammation, particularly in the first 24 hours (see Chapter 10).

Increased: Any type of infection, acute or chronic inflammation, rheumatic fever, endocarditis, neoplasm, multiple myeloma

Thrombin Time

- 10–14 s

    Measure of conversion of fibrinogen to fibrin and fibrin polymerization. Used to detect the presence of heparin and hypofibrinogenemia

Increased: Systemic heparin, DIC, fibrinogen deficiency, structurally abnormal fibrinogen molecules

Laboratory Diagnosis: Urine Studies

12

COLLECTING URINE SAMPLES

(See also Urinary Tract Procedures, Chapter 19, page 657.)

- **Random urine samples:** These are collected at any time and are the most common for routine urinalysis.
- **Midstream clean catch urine:** Preferred for routine urine culture and sensitivity. Patients first cleanse the urethral area with a castile soap towelette or other provided wipe. The first portion of the urine stream goes into the toilet, and the midstream sample is captured in a sterile specimen cup. This technique reduces the number of contaminants that enter the sample.
- **First morning specimen:** Considered to be the urine specimen to give the most reliable urinalysis results. Patient voids before bedtime and then provides the morning sample upon awakening. Theoretically, this allows urine to concentrate elements, best for protein determinations and pregnancy testing. Often used to optimize the urinary detection of tuberculosis (TB).
- **Timed sample collection:** Used to collect urine over a specific period (e.g., 8 hr; 24 hr) to measure analytes such as creatinine, calcium, oxalate, catecholamines, and 17-hydroxysteroids that are affected by diurnal variations. Many require sample to be kept on ice.

Chapter update by Rakesh Gulati, MD, and Goni Katz-Greenberg, MD

291

- **Catheter collection:** In patients unable to void, an "in and out" bladder catheter technique can be used (see Urinary Tract Procedures, Chapter 19, page 657). In the setting of a chronic indwelling catheter, the sample must not be obtained from the collection bag and should be directly obtained from the catheter. In patients with urostomy, the stoma should be catheterized to collect the sample and not the collection bag.
- **Suprapubic bladder aspiration** can be performed in infants and children and very selectively in adults. External introduction of a needle through the abdomen into the bladder is sterile under normal conditions when cultured. See Chapter 19, page 662.
- **Pediatric samples** are often collected using a pediatric sterile urine collection bag applied to the skin around the urethra.

HANDLING THE URINE SPECIMEN

- For routine urinalysis (UA), a fresh (less than 2 hr old), clean catch urine sample is preferred. If the analysis cannot be performed immediately, refrigerate the sample (2–8°C) or collect the sample in a preservative-containing tube described below. If refrigerated, rewarm to room temperature just prior to assessment (Note: When urine stands at room temperature for a long time, casts and red cells undergo lysis, and the urine becomes alkalinized with precipitation of salts).
- A variety of urine collection and transfer products are now available to protect healthcare personnel and protect the specimen from contamination. One brand of a closed sterile urine collection cup has a port that allows a vacuum urine collection tube to evacuate the patient-collected sample. This vacuum tube is then submitted to the lab. Alternatively, a special spike can be placed in the specimen and aspirated into a vacuum tube. One company (BD Vacutainer Franklin Lakes, NJ, USA) has several vacuum urine collection tubes that are available: yellow top (no preservative), yellow/cherry red speckled top (preservative) for routine urinalysis, and gray top (boric acid primary preservative, used for culture and sensitivity [C&S], as it reduces the overgrowth of contaminants). These preservatives maintain the specimen in a state identical to refrigeration by suppressing the growth of organisms that could result in bacterial overgrowth or a false-positive culture.

ROUTINE URINALYSIS (UA)

Urinalysis is a noninvasive, widely accessible diagnostic tool. A complete formal test includes three parts: gross appearance, dipstick analysis, and a urine sediment (done with microscopic examination). In many point-of-care clinical settings the microscopic examination is omitted and only the dipstick analysis is performed. The urine dipstick can be visually examined and compared to reference standards on the dipstick container or can be placed into an automated reader if available. Reagent strips should be kept in a sealed air tight container to prevent inaccurate results. An example is nitrite testing; with 1 week of exposure to air, up to one-third of strips give a false-positive result increasing to three-fourths of strips after 2 weeks of air exposure.

1. Pour 5–10 mL of well-mixed urine into a centrifuge tube.
2. **Check for appearance (color, turbidity, and odor).** If a urine sample looks grossly cloudy, it is sometimes advisable to examine an unspun sample.
3. Spin the capped sample at 3000 rpm (450g) for 3–5 min.
4. While the sample is in the centrifuge, perform the **dipstick evaluation** on the remaining sample. Allow 1–2 min before reading the test to avoid false results. Read the results according to the color chart on the test strip container. Tests strips can have some variation, but will usually include: pH, specific gravity, hemoglobin, leukocyte esterase, nitrites, glucose, ketone, urobilinogen, bilirubin, and albumin. Dipstick specific gravity (SG) measurement is possible, but a refractometer also can be used to determine SG.
5. **If a microscopic evaluation of the sediment is to be performed:** Decant and discard the supernatant. Mix the remaining sediment by flicking it with a finger and pouring or pipetting 1 or 2 drops onto a microscope slide. Cover with a coverslip.
   a. First examine ten low-power fields (10× objective) for epithelial cells, casts, crystals, and mucus. Casts are usually reported as number per low-power field (lpf) and tend to collect around the periphery of the coverslip.
   b. Next examine several high-power fields (hpf) (40× objective) for epithelial cells, crystals, red blood cells (RBCs), white blood cells (WBCs), bacteria, and parasites such as trichomonads. RBCs, WBCs, and bacteria are usually reported as number per high-power field. (See Urine Sediment discussion below, page 298, and Figure 12-1, page 294.)

URINALYSIS, NORMAL VALUES

1. *Appearance:* Pale to dark yellow or amber in color and clear.
2. *Specific Gravity (SG):* 1.001–1.035 (typical with normal fluid intake 1.016–1.022). *Note:* Neonates and infants have decreased concentration ability, so their SG will usually be on the low side.
3. *pH*: 4.6–8.0.
4. *Negative for:* Bilirubin, blood, acetone, glucose, protein (*Note:* It should be noted that the UA checks for albuminuria, and not proteinuria), nitrite, leukocyte esterase, and reducing substances.
5. *Trace:* Urobilinogen.
6. *RBC:* Male 0–3/hpf, female 0–5/hpf.
7. *WBC:* 0–4/hpf.

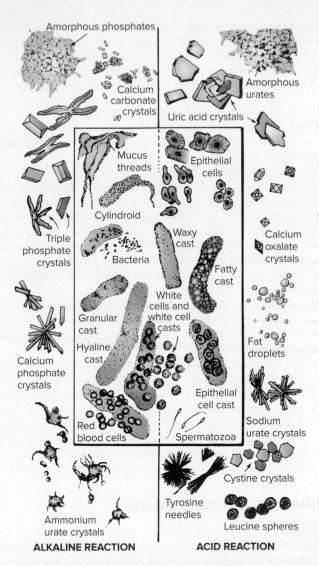

Figure 12-1. Urine sediment as seen with a microscope. (Used with permission from POC Tests/Microscopy, Nicoll D, Mark Lu C, McPhee SJ. *Guide to Diagnostic Tests*, 7e, New York, NY: McGraw-Hill Education; 2017.)

8. ***Epithelial Cells:*** Occasional. Large numbers of squamous epithelial cells in urine suggest contamination of the specimen from the distal urethra in men and the opening of the vagina in women.

9. ***Hyaline Casts:*** Occasional.

10. *Bacteria:* None.
11. *Crystals:* Some limited crystals based on urine pH (see following section).

DIFFERENTIAL DIAGNOSIS FOR ROUTINE URINALYSIS

Appearance

The **normal color** of urine can range from pale to dark yellow; normal color is considered light yellow. Abnormal color can be the result of different pathologies, drugs, or certain foods. Polyuria and diabetes insipidus may contribute to colorless urine.

Gross hematuria, myoglobinuria, or hemoglobinuria all will make urine anywhere from pink to dark red. Bilirubinuria will cause dark yellow to brown-colored urine

Less common pathologies are porphyrinuria or alkaptonuria, which will cause red urine to turn black on standing; urinary tract infections, mainly caused by *Klebsiella* spp., *Escherichia coli, Proteus mirabilis*, or *Enterococcus* spp., can turn urine purple in patients with a permanent Foley catheter ("purple urine bag syndrome"); and chyluria can cause white milky urine.

Cloudy urine can be due to phosphaturia, pyuria, chyluria, lipiduria, hyperoxaluria, or a diet excessively high in purine-rich foods causing hyperuricosuria. Mucus and semen may cause cloudy urine.

12

Drugs that can change urine color:

- Deferoxamine – pink urine
- Indigo carmine dye (renal function, cystoscopy) – blue
- Methocarbamol (muscle relaxant) – green-brown
- Methylene blue (used to identify fistulas)– blue, blue-green urine
- Metronidazole (treatment for *Trichomonas*, amebiasis, *Giardia*) – dark urine, reddish brown
- Nitrofurantoin and chloroquine – brown-black urine
- Phenazopyridine (urinary analgesic), also compounded with sulfonamides – orange-red, acid pH
- Phenytoin – red urine
- Propofol and triamterene – green urine
- Riboflavin (multivitamins) – bright yellow
- Rifampin (TB therapy) – yellow-orange urine
- Food: Beets (red urine), carotene (brown urine), and rhubarb (brown-red urine) are some foods that can change the color of the urine

Bilirubin

Limited utility on dipstick. Early indication of liver disease if positive. Ictotest® Reagent Tablets (Siemens, Malvern PA) are considered more sensitive and can be confirmed by this assay with detection ≥ 0.05 to 0.1 mg bilirubin/dL in urine (0.9–1.7 μmol/L).

Positive (only conjugated bilirubin appears in urine): Obstructive jaundice (intrahepatic and extrahepatic), hepatitis. False-positive with stool contamination of sample.

Blood (Hematuria)

If the dipstick is positive for blood but no red cells are seen, free hemoglobin (Hbg) may be present (transfusion reaction, from lysis of RBCs if pH is <5 or >8) or myoglobin is present (crush injury, burn, or tissue ischemia). Diets high in vitamin C can cause false negative results.

Positive: **Glomerular hematuria**: Familial causes: Fabry disease, hereditary nephritis (Alport syndrome), thin basement membrane disease. Primary glomerulonephritis: Focal segmental glomerulonephritis, Goodpasture disease, Henoch–Schönlein purpura, IgA nephropathy (Berger disease), mesangioproliferative, postinfectious, rapidly progressive glomerulonephritis. Secondary glomerulonephritis: Hemolytic-uremic syndrome, systemic lupus nephritis, thrombotic thrombocytopenic purpura, vasculitis.

Renal causes: Arteriovenous malformation, hypercalciuria, hyperuricosuria, loin pain-hematuria syndrome, malignant hypertension, medullary sponge kidney (MSK), papillary necrosis, polycystic kidney disease, renal artery embolism, renal vein thrombosis, sickle cell disease or trait, tubulointerstitial disease.

Urologic causes: Benign prostatic hyperplasia (BPH), cancer (kidney, ureteral, bladder, prostate, and urethral), infection (cystitis, pyelonephritis, prostatitis), strictures, nephrolithiasis, *Schistosoma* infection, renal TB.

Other: Drugs (e.g., NSAIDs, heparin, LMW heparins, warfarin, cyclophosphamide), trauma (e.g., contact sports, running, Foley catheter), menses, or other causes of vaginal bleeding (contamination).

Glucose

Glucose oxidase technique in most kits is specific for glucose and does not react with lactose, fructose, or galactose; therefore, infant urine should be screened with another assay. Normal threshold: 180 mg/dL.

Positive: Diabetes mellitus, steroids, SGLT2 inhibitors (Empagliflozin (Jardiance), canagliflozin (Invokana), others), RTA. Less commonly in pancreatitis, pancreatic carcinoma, pheochromocytoma, Cushing disease, shock, burns.

Ketones

Utilizes sodium nitroprusside; therefore, detects acetoacetic acid and not acetone or β-hydroxybutyric acid. Trace = 5 mg/dL; moderate = 40 mg/dL; small = 15 mg/dL; large = 80–160 mg/dL.

Positive: Starvation, DKA, vomiting, alcohol, hyperthyroidism, high-fat diet, febrile state (especially in children), aspirin overdose; false-positive:

cystinuria, stimulant laxative (e.g., Ex-Lax), MESNA. Transient positives with strenuous exercise, pregnancy, extended fasting.

Leukocyte Esterase

Used to detect 5 WBCs/hpf or lysed WBCs; detects esterases contained in granulocytic leukocytes. Combined with the nitrite test, leukocyte esterase has a positive predictive value over 90% for UTI if both tests are positive and a negative predictive value of >97% if both tests are negative. Sensitivity is reduced with elevated glucose ($\geq$3 g/dL) or certain medications such as cephalexin, cephalothin, and tetracycline.

Positive: UTI; occasionally with appendicitis, diverticulitis, STI, renal injury false-positive with vaginal/fecal contamination.

Nitrite

Rapid screening test for urinary tract infection; positive for infection when certain bacteria reduce nitrates to nitrites. Includes mainly gram-negative bacteria such as *Escherichia coli, Klebsiella pneumonia,* or *Proteus* spp. (See above, Leukocyte Esterase) False negatives with shortened urine dwell time in bladder (<4 hr) and ingestion of ascorbic acid. Over 10,000 bacteria/mL urine is required for a positive nitrite test. Nitrites may be negative if there is insufficient urinary bladder dwell time for bacteria to convert nitrate to nitrite.

Negative: Negative test does not exclude infection, as some organisms, such as *Streptococcus faecalis* and other gram-positive cocci, do not produce nitrite.

Odor

Limited utility: Normal urine mild ammonia smell. Strong ammonia smell suggests UTI but is not diagnostic and can be due to dehydration or leaving a sample sanding at room temperature for prolonged periods; asparagus consumption gives unique odor often described as sulfur; "sweet-smelling urine" with uncontrolled diabetes; rotten eggs with cystinuria; mousy/musty: phenylketonuria (PKU); sweaty feet: isovaleric/glutaric acidemia; maple syrup: maple syrup urine disease (MSUD). Medications can alter the smell of urine such as chemotherapy, sulfa antibiotics, high dose of vitamin B.

pH

Acidic: High-protein (meat) diet, ammonium chloride, mandelic acid and other medications, acidosis (due to ketoacidosis [starvation, diabetes], chronic obstructive pulmonary disease [COPD]).

Alkaline: UTI, renal tubular acidosis, diet (high vegetarian diet milk, immediately after meals), sodium bicarbonate therapy, vomiting, metabolic alkalosis, diuretic therapy.

Protein

Proteinuria is defined as urinary protein excretion of more than 150 mg per day (10–20 mg per dL) and is the hallmark of renal disease. Proteinuria on dipstick should be quantified with 24-hr urine studies. Normal protein excretion is <150 mg/24 hr or 10 mg/100 mL on a spot specimen (*dipstick approximations are as follows:* negative, 0–50; trace, 50–150; 1+, 150–300; 2+, 300–1000; 3+, 1–3 gm/L; 4+, >3 gm/L). Bence Jones globulins may be missed on dipstick, as it only checks for albumin, and the patient will need urine protein electrophoresis for diagnosis (see Chapter 10, pages 248–250).

Positive: Glomerulonephritis, nephrotic syndrome of different etiologies, pyelonephritis, myeloma, postural causes, preeclampsia, functional causes (fever, stress, heavy exercise), malignant hypertension.

Reducing Substances

These are not normally present in urine or feces. Commonly used in children with failure to thrive who may be lactose intolerant. Does not detect classic galactosaemia.

Positive: Glucose, fructose, galactose, false-positives (e.g., vitamin C, salicylates, antibiotics).

Specific Gravity

Corresponds with osmolarity except with osmotic diuresis (high glucose). Random value 1.003–1.030. Value >1.022 after 12 hr food/fluids fast suggests normal renal concentrating ability. **Isosthenuria** (SG fixed at 1.010 of protein free plasma regardless of fluid intake) suggests renal tubular dysfunction. **Hyposthenuria:** SG <1.010; **hypersthenuria:** SG >1.010.

Increased: Volume depletion, CHF, adrenal insufficiency, DM, SIADH, increased proteins (nephrosis), newborn state; if markedly increased (1.040–1.050), artifact or recent administration of radiographic contrast media.

Decreased: Diabetes insipidus, pyelonephritis, glomerulonephritis, water load with normal renal function (water intoxication).

Urobilinogen

Limited clinical value on dipstick. Normal urine contains small amounts of urobilinogen, the end product of conjugated bilirubin, after it passes into and is metabolized in the intestine. Hemolysis and hepatocellular disease can elevate urobilinogen levels that are usually detected by other means.

URINE SEDIMENT

Many labs no longer do microscopic examinations unless requested or if there is an abnormal dipstick test result. Figure 12-1 is a diagram of materials found in urine sediments.

RBCs: Trauma, pyelonephritis, genitourinary TB, cystitis, prostatitis, stones, tumors (benign or malignant), coagulopathy, and any cause of blood on dipstick test (see Differential Diagnosis for Routine Urinalysis, Blood, page 296).

WBCs: Infection anywhere in the urinary tract, TB, renal tumors, interstitial nephritis, chronic analgesic use, radiation, IgG4-related renal disease.

Renal Tubular Epithelial Cells: Excessive numbers suggests acute tubular necrosis (ATN). More sensitive than granular casts.

Transitional Epithelial Cells: Can be normal in small number. Originate from the bladder, ureters, and renal pelvis.

Squamous Epithelial Cells: 1–5/low power field is normal; >5 may indicate contamination.

Parasites: Trichomonas vaginalis, Schistosoma haematobium infection.

Yeast: Candida albicans infection (especially in diabetic or immunosuppressed patients or if a vaginal yeast infection is present).

Spermatozoa: Normal in men immediately after intercourse or nocturnal emission.

Casts

Localizes some or all of the disease process to the kidney itself.

Hyaline Casts: Acceptable unless "numerous," benign hypertension, nephrotic syndrome, after exercise.

RBC Casts: Acute glomerulonephritis, lupus nephritis, IE, anti-GBM disease, vasculitis, infectious-related glomerulonephritis, and malignant hypertension.

WBC Casts: Pyelonephritis, acute interstitial nephritis, glomerulonephritis.

Granular Casts: Breakdown of cellular casts, leads to waxy casts; **"muddy brown casts"** typical for ATN.

Epithelial (Tubular) Casts: Tubular damage, nephrotoxins.

Waxy Casts: All cellular casts can become waxy casts. Severe chronic kidney disease, amyloidosis.

Fatty Casts: Nephrotic syndrome, DM, damaged renal tubular epithelial cells.

Crystals

- Normal:
  Acidic urine: Calcium oxalate (small, square crystals with a central cross; octahedrons), uric acid (rhomboids, hexagons, squares).
  Alkaline urine: Calcium carbonate/phosphate, triple phosphate (struvite, magnesium ammonium phosphate associated with urea-splitting UTI and possible stone formation [coffin lids]).
- Abnormal:
  Presence of any: Cystine (colorless hexagons), sulfonamide, leucine (bicycle wheels), tyrosine, cholesterol.

12

Excessive: Calcium oxalate (excess vitamin C, spinach or chocolate, ileitis, ethylene glycol poisoning, urolithiasis), uric acid (gout, leukemia, tumor lysis [spontaneous or during chemotherapy]), triple phosphate (urea-splitting UTI and with "infection" stone formation), indinavir (crystals in patients on HIV therapy); acyclovir (bizarre shape).

Contaminants: Cotton threads, amorphous substances (all usually unimportant); "dirty urine" may suggest enterovesical fistula.

Mucus: Large amounts of mucus suggest urethral disease (normal from ileal conduit or continent urinary diversion that uses bowel) or enterovesical fistula.

Glitter Cells: Lysed neutrophils in hypotonic solution.

SPOT OR RANDOM URINE STUDIES

A spot urine, which is often ordered to aid in the diagnosis of various conditions, is done with only a small sample (10–20 mL) of urine.

Spot Urine for Electrolytes

Utility is limited because of variations in daily fluid and salt intake; not useful if a diuretic has been taken.

1. **Sodium <10 mEq/L:** Volume depletion, prerenal azotemia (e.g., CHF, shock), hepatorenal syndrome, some hyponatremia states, glucocorticoid excess.
2. **Sodium >20 mEq/L:** ATN (usually >40 mEq/L), postobstructive diuresis, high salt intake, SIADH, Addison disease, hypothyroidism, interstitial nephritis.
3. **Chloride <10 mEq/L:** Chloride-sensitive metabolic alkalosis (vomiting, excessive diuretic use), volume depletion.
4. **Potassium <10 mEq/L:** Hypokalemia, potassium depletion, extrarenal loss.

Spot Urine for Osmolality

- Normal: 75–300 mOsm/kg, varies with water intake.

Patients with normal renal function should concentrate >800 mOsm/kg after 14-hr fluid restriction; <400 mOsm/kg is a sign of renal impairment.

Increased: Dehydration, SIADH, adrenal insufficiency, glycosuria, high-protein diet.

Decreased: Excessive fluid intake, diabetes insipidus, acute tubular injury, medications (acetohexamide, glyburide, lithium).

Spot Urine for Erythrocyte Morphology

The morphology of red cells in a urine sample positive for blood may indicate the cause of the hematuria. **Isomorphic red cells** are seen in postrenal, nonglomerular bleeding. **Dysmorphic red cells** are associated with glomerular causes of bleeding. Labs vary, but >90% dysmorphic erythrocytes with asymptomatic hematuria indicates a renal glomerular source of bleeding, especially if associated with proteinuria or casts (e.g., IgA nephropathy, poststreptococcal glomerular disease, lupus nephritis). If there are 90% isomorphic erythrocytes or even "mixed" results (10–90% isomorphic erythrocytes), a postrenal cause of hematuria requires urologic evaluation (e.g., urolithiasis, cystitis, trauma, tumors, hemangioma, exercise induced, BPH).

Spot Urine for Microalbumin

- Normal: <30 mcg albumin/mg creatinine
  Used to determine whether a diabetic patient is at risk of nephropathy or cardiovascular disease. Perform two or three separate determinations over 6 mo to confirm; spot urine preferred. Diabetic patients with a level of 30–300 mcg will often benefit from an ACE inhibitor or angiotensin receptor blocker (ARB). Six percent of the healthy population has microalbuminuria.

Spot Urine for Protein

- Normal: <20 mg/dL (0.2 g/L) for a sample taken in midmorning
  See page 298 for the differential diagnosis of protein in the urine.

Spot Urine for Protein Electrophoresis

(See Chapter 10, Protein and Electrophoresis, Serum and Urine, pages 248–250.)

Spot Urine for Myoglobin

(See also Chapter 10, page 240, Myoglobin, Serum.)
- Qualitative negative
  Positive: Drugs (statins, colchicine), skeletal muscle injuries (crush injury, electrical burns, carbon monoxide poisoning, delirium tremens, surgical procedures, malignant hyperthermia), polymyositis.

Spot Urine for β_2-Microglobulin

(See also Chapter 10, page 239, β_2-Microglobulin, Serum.)
- <1 mg/24 hr or 0–160 g/L (keep sample refrigerated)
  Nonspecific marker of renal tubular injury.
  Increased: Diseases of the proximal tubule (ATN, interstitial nephritis, pyelonephritis), viral diseases, drug-induced nephropathy (aminoglycosides),

diabetes, trauma, sepsis, HIV, lymphoproliferative (multiple myeloma, plasmacytoma).

Spot Urine for N-Telopeptide (NTx)

(See also Chapter 10, page 256, N-Telopeptide (NTx), Serum.)

- Healthy women: Premenopausal 19–63 nM BCE/mM creatinine; postmenopausal 26–124 nM BCE/mM creatinine
- Healthy men: 21–83 nM BCE/mM creatinine

Reported as nanomolar bone collagen equivalents per liter (nM BCE/L). In urine, values are corrected per millimolars of creatinine per liter (mM creatinine/L). Serum NTx provides a quantitative measurement of bone resorption. A baseline NTx level is obtained before antiresorptive therapy (i.e., bisphosphonate) with periodic testing until decrease in NTx achieved.

Increased: Osteoporosis, osteomalacia, Paget disease, vitamin D deficiency, primary hyperparathyroidism, bony metastases, multiple myeloma, hyperthyroidism.

Decreased: Response to bisphosphonate therapy (decrease of 30–40% from baseline after 3 mo of therapy is typical of bisphosphonate therapy).

Spot Urine for Cytology

Used as an adjunct in the diagnosis of urothelial cancers (primarily transitional cell carcinoma of the bladder, kidney, and ureter); limited or no role for renal cell carcinoma. Use a 3-hr postvoid and not an a.m. sample. This is often supplemented with a cystoscopic examination and imaging study such as a CT scan of the abdomen and pelvis.

CREATININE CLEARANCE

Normal:

- *Men.* Total creatinine 1–2 g/24 hr; clearance 85–125 mL/min/1.73 m²
- *Women.* Total creatinine 0.8–1.8 g/24 hr; clearance 75–115 mL/min 1.73 m²
- *Children.* Total creatinine (>3 yr) 12–30 mg/kg/24 hr; clearance 70–140 mL/min/1.73 m² (1.17–2.33 mL/s/1.73 m²)

Decreased: Decreased creatinine clearance results in an increase in serum creatinine, usually secondary to kidney injury/disease. See Chapter 10, page 204, for differential diagnosis of increased serum creatinine.

Increased: Early type 1 DM, second trimester of pregnancy.

Methods for Determination of Creatinine Clearance (CrCl)

CrCl is a sensitive indicator of early kidney injury. Clearances are ordered for evaluation of patients with suspected kidney injury or disease and monitoring of patients taking nephrotoxic medications (e.g., gentamicin). CrCl decreases with age; CrCl <20 mL/min indicates severe kidney injury, and when falls <10 mL/min, patient will usually require renal replacement therapy (via dialysis or transplantation). *Of note, CrCl can only be measured when renal function is in a steady state.*

1. **24-hr Urinary Collection for Creatinine Clearance.** Order a concurrent SCr and a 24-hr urine creatinine. A shorter time interval can be used (e.g., 6 or 12 hr), but the formula must be corrected for this change.

    Example: The following are calculations of (a) CrCl from a 24-hr urine sample with a volume of 1000 mL, (b) a urine creatinine of 108 mg/100 mL, and (c) a SCr of 1 mg/100 mL (1 mg/dL).

    $$\text{Clearance} = \frac{\text{Urine creatinine} \times \text{Total urine volume}}{\text{Plasma creatinine} \times \text{Time}}$$

    $$\text{Clearance} = \frac{(108\,\text{mg}/100\,\text{mL})(1000\,\text{mL})}{(1\,\text{mg}/100\,\text{mL})(1440\,\text{min})} = 75\,\text{mL}/\text{min}$$

    To determine whether there is a valid, full 24-hr collection, the sample should contain 20–25 mg/kg/24 hr of creatinine for men or 15–20 mg/kg/24 hr for women. This calculation takes into account an adult of average size, weighing around 150 lb, and with a BSA of 1.73 m². If the values in the previous example are for a 10-year-old boy weighing 70 lb (1.1 m²), the clearance is:

    $$75\,\text{mL}/\text{min} \times \frac{1.73\,\text{m}^2}{1.1\,\text{m}^2} = 118\,\text{mL}/\text{min}$$

2. **Estimated Creatinine Clearance.** Online calculators for adults and children are available at www.niddk.nih.gov/health-information/communication-programs/nkdep/laboratory-evaluation/glomerular-filtration-rate-calculators; accessed January 2, 2020.

    Adults:

- **Modification of Diet in Renal Disease (MDRD) equation** (*Ann Intern Med* 2006;145(4):247–254).

12

$$GFR = 186 \times [SCr]^{-1.154} \times [age]^{-0.203} \times [0.742 \text{ if patient is female or} \times 1.21 \text{ if Black}]$$

- **Chronic Kidney Disease Epidemiology Collaboration (CKD-EPI) equation** (*Ann Intern Med* 2009;150(9):604–612).

$GFR = 141 \times \min(S_{cr}/\kappa, 1)^{\alpha} \times \max(S_{cr}/\kappa, 1)^{-1.209} \times 0.993^{Age} \times 1.018$ [if female] OR $\times 1.159$ [if black]

S_{cr} is in mg/dL

κ is 0.7 for females and 0.9 for males

α is -0.329 for females and -0.411 for males

Of note, neither of the above equations require weight because the results are reported normalized to 1.73 m² body surface area, which is an accepted average adult surface area.

- **Cockcroft-Gault equation:**

$$CrCl \text{ estimate} = \frac{(140 - age) \times wt\,(kg)(\text{if female}, \times 0.85)}{Cr \times 72}$$

Children:

- **Modified Schwartz CKID Formula:**

GFR(mL/min/1.73²) = k (Height)/Serum creatinine

k is the constant = 0.143 for all age groups; height is in centimeters; SCr is in mg/dL.

Staging Chronic Kidney Disease (CKD)

- **Stage 1 CKD:** GFR 90 mL/min/m² or greater
- **Stage 2 CKD:** GFR between 60 and 89 mL/min/m²
- **Stage 3a CKD:** GFR between 30 and 59 mL/min/m²
- **Stage 3b CKD:** GFR between 30 and 59 mL/min/m²
- **Stage 4 CKD:** GFR between 15 and 29 mL/min/m²
- **Stage 5 CKD:** GFR less than 15 mL/min/m²

In stage 1 and 2 CKD there are usually other markers of kidney damage, such as albuminuria (albumin excretion >30 mg/24 hr or albumin:creatinine ratio >30 mg/g [>3 mg/mmol], urine sediment abnormalities, renal histology, imaging abnormalities, and other manifestations.

24-HOUR URINE STUDIES

24-hour urine collections are utilized for the diagnosis and monitoring of a variety of diseases, mostly endocrine based. Each of the following collections requires a special container and storage. Check with the reference lab for specifics.

Aldosterone, Urine

(See also, Chapter 10, page 180, Aldosterone, Serum)
Normal: Urine: Salt-depleted diet (10 mEq Na$^+$/day for 3–4 days) 18–85 mcg/24 hr; Urine: Salt-loaded diet (120 mEq Na$^+$/day for 3–4 days) 1.5–12.5 mcg/24 hr

Increased: Primary hyperaldosteronism, secondary hyperaldosteronism (CHF, sodium depletion, nephrotic syndrome, cirrhosis with ascites, others).

Decreased: Adrenal insufficiency, panhypopituitarism, ingestion of large quantities of licorice (reduction of aldosterone can last months).

Calcium, Urine

(See also Chapter 10, page 192, Calcium, Serum, Including Ionized)
Normal: On a calcium-free diet <150 mg/24 hr, average-calcium diet (600–800 mg/24 hr) 100–250 mg/24 hr.

Increased: Hyperparathyroidism, hyperthyroidism, hypervitaminosis D, distal RTA (type I), sarcoidosis, immobilization, osteolytic lesions (bony metastasis, multiple myeloma), Paget disease, glucocorticoid excess, immobilization, furosemide.

Decreased: Medications (thiazide diuretics, estrogens, oral contraceptives), hypothyroidism, renal failure, fat malabsorption states, rickets, osteomalacia.

Catecholamines, Fractionated

(See also Chapter 10, page 194, Catecholamines, Fractionated, Serum)
Used to evaluate pheochromocytoma and paraganglioma. Avoid drugs that can interfere with the test, leading to falsely high catecholamines: Tricyclics antidepressants, labetalol, levodopa, methyldopa (Aldomet), sotalol, benzodiazepines, amphetamines, decongestants, and most psychoactive agents. All these drugs should be discontinued 2 wk prior to testing.

Normal: Values are variable and depend on the assay method used. Norepinephrine 15–80 mg/24 hr (SI: 89–473 nmol/24 hr), epinephrine 0–20 mg/24 hr (SI: 0–118 nmol/24 hr), dopamine 65–400 mg/24 hr (SI: 384–2364 nmol/24 hr).

Increased: Pheochromocytoma (levels are >twice the upper normal value), paraganglioma, epinephrine administration, presence of drugs (see above).

Cortisol, Free

(See also Chapter 10, page 203, Cortisol, Serum and Chapter 10, page 207, Dexamethasone Suppression Test)
Used to evaluate adrenal cortical hyperfunction; screening test of choice for Cushing syndrome.

Normal: 10–55 μg/24 hr (SI: 27–150 nmol).

Increased: Cushing syndrome (adrenal hyperfunction from a pituitary tumor secreting ACTH or ectopic secretion of ACTH by other tumors such as bronchial carcinoid or adrenal tumor secreting cortisol), stress during collection, pregnancy.

With low-dose dexamethasone suppression test, urinary free cortisol <10% of baseline or <10 mcg/24 hr excludes Cushing syndrome. High-dose dexamethasone test is used to differentiate Cushing disease from ectopic ACTH production.

Creatinine

- See pages 302 and Chapter 10, page 204.

Cysteine

Used to detect cystinuria or homocystinuria and monitor response to medical therapy with agents such as tiopronin (Thiola).

Normal: 40–60 mg/g creatinine.

Increased: Heterozygotes <300 mg/g creatinine; homozygotes >250 mg/g creatinine.

Heavy metals

(See also Chapter 10, page 235, Lead, Serum)
Measures exposure to arsenic (total), arsenic (inorganic), cadmium, lead, and mercury, usually following occupational or environmental exposure.

Normal: Arsenic (total): 0–50 μg/24 hr (<50 μg/L); arsenic (inorganic): <20 μg/L; cadmium:<3.0 μg/24 hr (<2 μg/g creatinine); lead: <80 μg/24 hr (< 50 μg/L); mercury: <20 μg/L.

Increased: Indicative of excess exposure.

5-HIAA (5-Hydroxyindoleacetic Acid)

5-HIAA is a serotonin metabolite useful in the diagnosis of carcinoid syndrome.

Normal: 2–8 mg (SI: 10.4–41.6 mmol)/24-hr urine collection.

Increased: Carcinoid tumors (except rectal), certain foods (banana, pineapple, tomato, walnuts, avocado), phenothiazine derivatives.

Metanephrines

(See also Chapter 10, page 194, Catecholamines, Fractionated, Serum)
Used to detect metabolic products of epinephrine and norepinephrine, primary screening test for pheochromocytoma.

Normal: <1.3 mg/24 hr (7.1 mmol/L) for adults, but variable in children.

Increased: Pheochromocytoma, neuroblastoma (neural crest tumors), false-positive with drugs (phenobarbital, guanethidine, hydrocortisone, MAO inhibitors)

Protein, Urinary

12

Serves as a general guide to the health of the kidneys. Heavy proteinuria on dipstick should be confirmed by a 24-hr collection. See also Urine Protein Electrophoresis Chapter 10, pages 248 and 250. This can help identify the patterns of protein loss: Glomerular, tubular, overflow, or nonselective proteinuria.

Normal: <150 mg/24 hr (<0.15 g/d)

Increased: Nephrotic syndrome (massive proteinuria, hypoalbuminuria, hyperlipidemia, edema, and usually associated with >3.5 g/24 hr; glomerular disease, tubular disease, overflow from elevated plasma proteins (immunoglobulins/immunoglobulin light chains in myeloma), urinary tract inflammation (interstitial nephritis or UTI), trauma, neoplasia.

Protein Electrophoresis, Urine

(See Chapter 10, page 248, Protein Electrophoresis, Serum and Urine)

17-Ketogenic Steroids (17-KGS, Corticosteroids)

Overall adrenal function test, largely replaced by serum or urine cortisol levels.

Normal: Males: 5–24 mg/24 hr (17–83 mmol/24 hr); females: 4–15 mg/24 hr (14–52 mmol/24 hr)

Increased: Adrenal hyperplasia (Cushing syndrome), adrenogenital syndrome.

Decreased: Panhypopituitarism, Addison disease, acute steroid withdrawal.

17-Ketosteroids, Total (17-KS)

(See also Chapter 10, page 206, Dehydroepiandrosterone Sulfate (DHEAS), Serum)
Used to measure DHEA, androstenedione (adrenal androgens); largely replaced by assay of individual elements.

Normal: Men 8–20 mg/24 hr; women 6–15 mg/dL. *Note:* Low values in prepubertal children.

Increased: Adrenal cortex abnormalities (hyperplasia [Cushing disease], adenoma, carcinoma, adrenogenital syndrome), severe stress, ACTH or pituitary tumor, testicular interstitial tumor and arrhenoblastoma (both produce testosterone).

Decreased: Panhypopituitarism, Addison disease, castration in men.

Urea Nitrogen, Urine (Urine Nitrogen, Nitrogen Balance)

12

Measures urine nitrogen concentration as a clinical measure of nutritional replacement ("nitrogen balance"). With sufficient nitrogen intake (hyperalimentation or enteral), normal levels of urea are excreted in the urine. Urea, produced by the liver, generates a metabolite of ammonia (nitrogen) that is excreted in the urine. The nitrogen in ammonia is derived from the deamination of amino acids. Use limited to the evaluation of chronic hyperalimentation or enteral suppelmentation. With kidney disease (<1000 ml urine/day) or dialysis, this test cannot be used. The goal with nutritional support for a depleted person is a positive nitrogen balance of 4 to 6 g nitrogen/24 hours.

Normal: 12 to 20 grams per 24 hours (428.4 to 714 mmol/day) in adults.

Increased: Excess protein breakdown in body (stress, trauma), excess replacement of protein with hyperalimenttion.

Decreased: Renal disease, malnutrition (poor diet or inadequate hyperalimentation replacement).

Vanillylmandelic Acid (VMA)

(See also Chapter 10, page 194, Catecholamines, Fractionated, Serum)
VMA is the urinary product of both epinephrine and norepinephrine; good screening test for pheochromocytoma; also used to diagnose and follow up neuroblastoma and ganglioneuroma.

Normal: <7–9 mg/24 hr (35–45 mmol/L)

Increased: Pheochromocytoma, other neural crest tumors (ganglioneuroma, neuroblastoma), factitious causes (chocolate, coffee, tea, methyldopa).

OTHER URINE STUDIES

Drug Abuse Screen (Urine Drug Screen)

• **Normal** = negative

Several tests can detect common drugs of abuse in the urine. These tests are often used for employment screening for critical jobs. Can be used in the evaluation of conditions such as altered mental status, seizures, vasculitis, and in the setting of chronic pain management. Assays vary by facility and may test for amphetamines, barbiturates, benzodiazepines, marijuana (cannabinoid metabolites), cocaine, methadone, oxycodone, phencyclidine (PCP), tricyclic antidepressants (TCAs), and opiates (codeine, morphine, heroin). Initial screen is often based on immunoassays; with gas chromatography–mass spectrometry (GC/MS) often used to confirm a positive result. Results are qualitative and do not give quantitative results; a single determination cannot differentiate between casual and chronic drug use. (Note: False-positive results can be due to excessive consumption of poppy seeds [false-positive opioid] and common medications such as dextromethorphan, diphenoxylate, pseudoephedrine, diphenhydramine, and others.) Cannabidiol (CBD) products normally do not show up on a blood test but can if trace amounts of delta-9-tetrahydrocannabinol (THC), the active ingredient in marijuana, are present.

12

Xylose Tolerance Test (D-Xylose Absorption Test)

Used to assess proximal bowel function; differentiates malabsorption due to pancreatic insufficiency or due to intestinal problems.

Decreased: Celiac disease (nontropical sprue, gluten-sensitive enteropathy), false decrease with renal disease.

- 5 g xylose in 5-hr urine specimen after 25-g oral dose of D-xylose or 1.2 g after 5-g oral dose
- Collection: Patient is on NPO status after midnight except for water.
- After 8 a.m. void, 25 g of D-xylose (or 5 g if GI irritation is a concern) is dissolved in 250 mL water
- Patient drinks an additional 750 mL water, and urine is collected for the next 5 hr.

URINARY INDICES IN KIDNEY INJURY

Use Table 12-1 to differentiate the causes (renal or prerenal) of oliguria. (See also Oliguria and Anuria, Chapter 9, page 163.)

URINE OUTPUT

Acceptable normal daily urine volume can vary depending on fluid intake and other factors (ranges 750–2000 mL/d). **Polyuria** is usually defined as excessive urine output in a adult of >2.5 L/day. **Oliguria** is typically defined as <0.3 mL/kg per hour or <500 mL/day of urine output), and **anuria** is defined as urine volume of <50–100 mL/d. Normal voiding patterns can

Table 12-1. Urinary Indices Useful in the Differential Diagnosis of Oliguria

Index	Prerenal	Renal (ATN)[a]
Urine osmolality	>500	<350
Urinary sodium	<20	>40
Urine/serum creatinine	>40	<20
Urine/serum osmolarity	>1.2	<1.2
Fractional excreted sodium[b]	<1	>1
Renal failure index (RFI)[c]	<1	>1

[a]Acute tubular necrosis (intrinsic renal failure).

[b]Fractional excreted sodium: $\dfrac{\text{Urine/Serum sodium}}{\text{Urine/Serum creatinine}} \times 100$

[c]Renal failure index: $\dfrac{\text{Urine sodium} \times \text{Serum creatinine}}{\text{Urine creatinine}}$

12

vary but on average an adult voids up to 8 times per day. Pregnancy and older age may increase these numbers.

URINE PROTEIN ELECTROPHORESIS

See Protein Electrophoresis, Serum and Urine, Figure 10-4 and Table 10-8, pages 248–250. The main reason for performing urine protein electrophoresis is to find a light chain myeloma producing an excess of free light chains (Bence Jones protein), an important part of a myeloma screen.

Clinical Microbiology 13

Chapter update by Morgan McCoy, MD, PhD, Vaneet Arora, MD, MPH, D (ABMM), Rose Jung, Pharm D, Steven A. Haist, MD, MS, and Leonard G. Gomella, MD

GENERAL PRINCIPLES OF CLINICAL MICROBIOLOGY

Clinical microbiology has become increasingly complex, requiring interpretive judgment in spite of, and in many cases due to, the advent of laboratory automation and integration of genomics and proteomics. Diagnostic stewardship, which involves appropriate selection of the patient, specimen, and test, is critical in getting results that are accurate, significant, and clinically relevant. Some of the most common tests performed on patients are the procurement of tissue or body fluids for direct detection of pathogenic organisms to prove or disprove the presence of infection. The results of these tests are critical in guiding the selection of antibiotics for targeted therapy.

The three basic questions that need to be answered from the laboratory are: *Is this an infection? If yes, what is the organism? And lastly which antimicrobial agent will likely work against this agent?* The clinical microbiology laboratory provides answers to these questions. Several clinical microbiology principles must be considered when ordering or interpreting the tests:

Severity or Degree of Risk: There is a difference between an otherwise healthy patient with a complaint of dysuria consistent with a urinary tract infection (UTI) versus a patient with neutropenia and a high fever. The first needs a simple urinalysis with a routine bacterial culture. The second needs more extensive testing that may involve specimens from multiple sites and appropriate radiologic studies. The second patient also needs prompt treatment with empiric broad-spectrum antibiotics while waiting on test results because she is at high risk of septicemia and death.

Choice of Antibiotics: Initiation of antibiotics that broadly *cover* a newly recognized infection in a timely and appropriate manner is often lifesaving. Selecting the wrong antibiotic, the wrong dose, an improper route of administration, or delaying treatment can increase morbidity and mortality. While initially a broad-spectrum antibiotic may be employed, de-escalation to a narrow-spectrum antimicrobial or specific therapy is based on information provided by the clinical microbiology laboratory as well as institutional protocols.

Timing: Except for rare instances when not feasible, specimens should always be obtained and cultures performed before antibiotics are started. Negative bacterial cultures should be interpreted in the light of timing of antibiotic administration. However, antibiotics should never be delayed in the face of a possible life-threatening infection, such as meningitis. After the clinical microbiology data such as results of Gram staining, molecular testing (detection of DNA/RNA), and/or culture become available, antibiotic therapy can be narrowed or "de-escalated" to the antibiogram of the recovered organism.

Quality and Choice of Specimen: Proper labeling, collection, and transport of specimens are critical to avoid misleading results, and the clinical laboratory will reject specimens that were not correctly labeled or correctly collected. Each healthcare system must have procedures and policies for appropriate specimen collection and transport in consultation with the clinical laboratory. Actual tissue, aspirates, and fluids are the specimens of choice, especially from surgery, and always superior to a swab of the specimen.

True Infection versus Contamination and Colonization: True infection is almost always accompanied by inflammation with the presence of neutrophils in clinical specimens (but absent in neutropenia) and clinical symptoms and signs. The presence of a large number of epithelial cells in a sample or the growth of normal skin flora of a cultured specimen often signifies contamination and colonization secondary to improper collection of specimens, although there are exceptions. Do NOT demand that a laboratory report and perform susceptibility testing on everything that is growing on culture. Irrelevant information can result in improper treatment.

Capability of the Laboratory: Knowing what the laboratory can and cannot do is always helpful in making the choice of which test to order. Laboratories are required by law to validate the tests and specimen types for in-house tests. This means that not all tests may be available, feasible, or cost-effective to be performed in-house, and some tests may need to be performed at an outside laboratory. Having a conversation with the clinical microbiology laboratory helps manage expectations and avoids delays in care that can have negative outcomes for your patients.

Antimicrobial Resistance: Drug resistance is a serious problem in modern medicine. See Table 13-1 for Centers for Disease Control and Prevention (CDC) recommendations for preventing antibiotic drug resistance. Appropriate use of antimicrobials designated as **"antimicrobial stewardship"** is imperative

13

Table 13-1.   CDC Recommendations to Prevent Antimicrobial Resistance

The CDC has recommended actions for healthcare providers to protect patients and combat antimicrobial resistance:
1. Prevent infections and the spread of germs.
• Follow infection prevention and control recommendations.
• Elicit travel history or treatment at another facility.
• Ensure patients receive recommended vaccinations.
• Alert facilities when transferring patients with resistant organisms.
• Educate patients and stay informed of ongoing outbreaks.
2. Improve antibiotic prescribing
• Follow clinical and treatment guidelines to ensure appropriate antibiotic use.
• Consider other causes in patients not responding to antibiotics; e.g., when treating a patient for a presumed bacterial infection, if the patient is not responding to treatment, consider a nonbacterial cause such as a fungal infection or a rheumatologic etiology. Always be willing to revisit your diagnosis and reorder your differential.
• Use appropriate diagnostic tests to guide therapy.
3. Be alert and take action.
• Be aware of infections and resistance patterns in your community and facility.
• Prompt lab notification for resistant organisms.
• Inform patients if they have an antibiotic-resistant infection.
• Report cases and submit resistance isolates to public health departments as required.

Adapted from: https://www.cdc.gov/drugresistance/pdf/threats-report/Actions-For-Healthcare-508.pdf, accessed 5/7/2020.

to limit the emergence and spread of resistant organisms such as **carbapenem-resistant organisms (CROs)**, which have become a global threat with none to extremely limited choices for treating patients with these infections.

APPROACHES TO LABORATORY ANALYSIS IN CLINICAL MICROBIOLOGY

Laboratory analysis of specimens in the clinical microbiology laboratory involves:

- Gross examination of the specimen (e.g., worms, pus, blood)
- Direct detection: microscopy, staining
- Culture and antimicrobial susceptibility testing
  - o Liquid/solid growth media with manual or automated plating and monitoring for growth
  - o Identification of organism by phenotypic methods (morphology, biochemical reactions—manual or automated); genotypic methods (molecular methods); or mass spectrometry (matrix-assisted laser desorption ionization–time of flight [MALDI-TOF])
  - o Susceptibility testing (manual or automated)
- Serology: Antigen–antibody testing
- Nucleic acid–based tests: e.g., polymerase chain reaction (PCR); microarrays; sequencing

MICROBIOLOGY TECHNIQUES

Acid-Fast Stain (AFB Smear, Kinyoun Stain)

Clinical microbiology labs can perform acid-fast stain for organisms such as *Mycobacterium* species. These **acid-fast bacilli (AFB)** organisms stain pink against a blue background. This stain cannot distinguish between *Mycobacterium tuberculosis* (TB) and non-tuberculous mycobacteria (NTM) such as *M. avium* complex, as they all appear morphologically alike.

- Culture on specialized media or molecular testing is required for confirmation, differentiation of genus of *Mycobacterium* species, and detection of drug resistance such as multidrug-resistant (MDR) TB. Rapid-growing AFB include *Mycobacterium abscessus, Mycobacterium chelonae,* and *Mycobacterium fortuitum* and can usually be cultured in less than 7 days. Most other AFB (*M. tuberculosis, M. avium* complex, *Mycobacterium kansasii, Mycobacterium marinum*) take longer than 7 days to grow. *Mycobacterium gordonae* is thought to be nonpathogenic and may be an environmental or tap water contaminant.
- A "modified" acid-fast stain (Kinyoun stain) can be performed for organisms that are weakly acid-fast staining (e.g., *Nocardia* spp.).

Albert Stain

Helps to distinguish *Corynebacterium diphtheriae* (the cause of diphtheria) from other nonpathogenic diphtheroid that lack the metachromatic granules. Metachromatic granules are a characteristic feature of this bacteria.

Blood Cultures

The microbiologic principles involved in blood cultures are the same as with any culture. A sample of the patient's blood is obtained by aseptic venipuncture and cultured. If growth is detected, the organism(s) are isolated, identified, and tested for antimicrobial susceptibility. In some settings, molecular methods are used to rapidly identify the organism.

- Blood cultures are performed most often when sepsis, endocarditis, osteomyelitis, meningitis, or pneumonia is suspected or to evaluate for fever of unknown origin (see also Chapter 19, page 595). The primary means of establishing a diagnosis of sepsis is by blood culture. Venipuncture is the technique of choice for obtaining blood for culture, as arterial blood cultures are not associated with higher diagnostic yields than venous blood and are not recommended. The number of organisms present in blood is often low, with small blood samples yielding fewer positive cultures than larger volumes of blood. Samples of at least 8–10 mL for each blood culture bottle should be collected from adult patients, but for a child the sample size must be reduced to take account of the smaller blood volume. **A blood culture sample always involves collecting two samples: aerobic and anaerobic.**
- The bacteria most frequently isolated from blood cultures are two gram-positive cocci, *Staphylococcus aureus* and *Streptococcus pneumoniae*, and three gram-negative rods, *Escherichia coli*, *Klebsiella pneumoniae*, and *Pseudomonas aeruginosa*. Viridans streptococci and enterococci may reflect true pathogens or contaminants. Certain pathogenic fungi, including yeast (*Candida* species and *Cryptococcus neoformans*) and molds, can also be isolated from blood cultures.
- A single set of blood cultures positive for coagulase-negative Staphylococci (*Staphylococcus epidermidis* and *Staphylococcus hominis*), viridans-group streptococci, *Corynebacterium* spp., *Propionibacterium* spp., and *Bacillus* spp. other than *B. anthracis*, are usually contaminants.
- While filamentous fungi (e.g., *Aspergilli*, *Mucorales*) often require special media and methods for detection, yeasts such as *Candida* species grow very well in standard blood culture broths unless the patient has been on antifungal therapy.
- Before venipuncture, the skin over the vein must be carefully disinfected to reduce the probability of contamination of the blood sample with skin bacteria. Although it is not possible to "sterilize" the skin, quantitative bacterial skin counts can be markedly reduced with a combination of 70% alcohol and an iodine or hexachlorophene-based antiseptic.

Blood Culture Key Points

- Prior to initiation of antimicrobial therapy, at least two sets of blood cultures taken from separate venipuncture sites should be obtained.
- Blood cultures should not be drawn through an IV catheter at the time of catheter insertion, as this is associated with a higher rate of false-positive cultures.
- In adults, one blood culture set is rarely advisable or sufficient. A positive single culture result may not be interpretable unless an unequivocal pathogen is isolated.
- Most cases of bacteremia are detected by using two or three sets of separately collected blood cultures. More than three sets of blood cultures in a 24-hour period yields little additional information.
- If the volume is adequate, it is rarely necessary to collect more than two or three blood cultures to identify a positive result. In intravascular infections such as infective endocarditis, a single blood culture is positive in greater than 95% of cases. Studies of sequential blood cultures from bacteremic patients without endocarditis have yielded 80–90% positive results on the first culture and 99% in at least one of a series of three cultures.
- Optimum timing of obtaining a blood culture is controversial.
  - The continuous bacteremia of infective endocarditis is usually readily detected, and specimen timing is not critical.
  - Intermittent bacteremia presents the greatest challenge because fever spikes generally occur after, rather than during, the bacteremia.
  - Fever at the time of blood culture collection does not appear to have any relationship with the likelihood of obtaining a positive blood culture.
  - For patients on antibiotic therapy with ongoing concerns for sepsis or endocarditis, blood cultures are ideally drawn just prior to the next dose of antibiotic.
- Blood cultures entered into automated laboratory protocols should routinely be incubated for 5 days. Multiple studies have shown that this incubation time is adequate for the detection of the majority of pathogens, including fastidious gram-negative coccobacillary bacteria that belong to the **Haemophilus, Actinobacillus, Cardiobacterium, Eikenella and Kingella (HACEK) group.** These are oropharyngeal commensals and an infrequent but important cause of infective endocarditis (IE) in non-IV drug abusers. The first four of the HACEK organisms are often encountered with a human bite or when there is a break in the skin after hitting someone in the mouth with a fist. Longer incubation times may be required when fungaemia or bacteriemia caused by *Legionella, Brucella, Bartonella,* or *Nocardia* spp. is suspected. Blood cultures for *Mycobacterium* spp. should be incubated for 4 wk.
- Molecular amplification methods may be needed for detection of bacteria or other organisms that are difficult to detect by culture (e.g., *Tropheryma whippleii,* the causative organism of Whipple disease).

- Some recommended guidelines for obtaining blood cultures are:
  - ○ Acute sepsis: Two or three culture sets from separate sites prior to starting antibiotics.
  - ○ Infective endocarditis: Three blood culture sets with three separate venipunctures over 1–2 hours and begin therapy.
  - ○ Subacute bacterial endocarditis (SBE): Three blood culture sets on day 1. If all negative at 24 hours, obtain three more sets. Blood culture–negative endocarditis is often from *Bartonella* or *Coxiella burnetti* (causes Q fever).
  - ○ The consensus of experts is that, except in very unusual cases, no more than three sets of blood cultures should be collected in one 24-hour period.
- Catheter-related bloodstream infection (CR-BSI). Cultures drawn simultaneously and with the same volume of blood from a central venous catheter (CVC) and from a peripheral blood site can identify a CR-BSI. If the blood culture obtained from the catheter is positive at least 2 hours before the cultures from the peripheral blood site, then the patient likely has a CR-BSI. Also, a CR-BSI is likely when obtaining multiple positive blood cultures (with the same organism and same antibiotic sensitivities) from a central line in the presence of negative peripheral blood cultures. Catheter removal as part of management is strongly encouraged. CRBSI is discussed further on page 352.

Blood Culture Technique

1. See Chapter 19, Venipuncture, page 663, for details on phlebotomy techniques.
2. Gather the materials needed and always use self-shielding needle devices.
   - ○ Aerobic (blue top) and anaerobic (purple top) culture bottles, butterfly, or other self-shielding needle compatible with Vacutainer adaptor, tourniquet, sterile gauze, alcohol pads, chlorhexidine prep pads (2% CHG/70% IPA or 10% povidone iodine), gloves, bandage; optional: syringe with butterfly needed for difficult blood draw).
   - ○ For blood cultures, a common collection system used in the United States is the BD BACTEC Plus Aerobic culture bottle and the BD BACTEC Plus Anerobic culture bottle. The bottles contain necessary growth media, with the "plus" designation indicating resins for antibiotic neutralization. BD BACTEC Lytic Anaerobic contains a lysing agent to increase the detection and recovery of organisms partially phagocytized by white blood cells. BD BACTEC Peds Plus are specialized to accommodate small-volume samples (<3 mL of blood). These BD products (BD, Franklin Lakes, NJ) are designed to fill by vacuum collection using the standard Vacutainer system devices. See Chapter 19, Table 19-14, page 666 for a detailed description of blood sample tubes.

13

3. For infants and individuals with fragile veins, a scalp/butterfly needle and syringe may be more appropriate for the blood sample collection. The sample is then injected into the culture bottles.

4. Wash hands and don gloves.

5. Select the venipuncture site, usually on the arm, then release the tourniquet.

6. Several methods of cleansing the selected venipuncture site have been described, and these cleansing methods may vary from center to center. This is a critical step in minimizing skin bacterial contamination of the culture. Follow your local microbiology lab procedures. One typical skin cleansing procedure is described here:

   o Rub the venipuncture site vigorously with an alcohol prep pad and allow to dry.

   o Apply chlorhexidine gluconate solution (70% alcohol/2% CHG) or 10% povidone-iodine solution over the same area, beginning at the proposed entry site and circling outward to a diameter of approximately 4–5 cm. Let dry 1 minute.

   o If an iodine-based solution is used, cleanse the site a second time with an alcohol prep pad to remove all iodine; otherwise, you can end up with a false-negative blood culture. This step is usually not necessary if chlorhexidine is used.

   o Chlorohexidine should **NOT** be used in infants less than 2 months old. For those pediatric patients, substitute an alcohol pad prep for three applications with 1-minute dry time between each application.

7. Clean rubber caps of blood culture containers with alcohol and allow to dry.

8. Reapply the tourniquet without touching the prepped area, and insert the needle into the vein. When blood flow is established, apply the end of the collecting system to the top of the culture jar and allow the blood to enter the collection device. Keep the collection bottle below the venipuncture site to prevent reflux.

9. Always collect the aerobic sample first, followed by the anaerobic specimen.

10. Additional routine blood work can then be obtained after the cultures are drawn. Special circumstances require more specialized collection devices. Contact your laboratory for specific instructions and special tubes.

    o If there is a request for viral blood cultures, a lavender-top tube containing 8–10 mL of blood (EDTA anticoagulant) may be requested.

    o Special tubes and techniques are required for *Mycobacteria* and filamentous fungi. Centrifugation–lysis (isolator or MGIT-mycobacterial growth indicator tubes) systems are used to culture *Mycobacterium* species and dimorphic fungi such as *Histoplasma capsulatum*.

    o Some labs ask that AFB be cultured using a 10-mL green-top sodium heparin blood collection tube.

11. Repalpation of blood culture collection sites is not recommended. If repalpation of venipuncture site is necessary to locate the vein, disinfect gloved finger with alcohol and iodine (or alcohol and chlorhexidine) and perform venipuncture just above or below the repalpation site. Repeat the procedure for each blood culture set ordered, selecting a different site for each venipuncture. Apply pressure after the needle is removed and apply a bandage. Apply patient identifier to specimens per local protocol.

12. In the evaluation of a potential CR-BSI, follow local protocols for obtaining the blood cultures from a central venous catheter.

Culture Media for Bacterial Pathogens

Microbiology culture media can aid in the isolation and identification of medically important bacteria and fungi. These may be classified as general-purpose nutrient, selective, or indicator media. If you suspect a particular organism, discuss with your laboratory before obtaining the specimen. This will assure the proper medium is used. (see Table 13-2, page 320)

Darkfield Examination

13

Used to identify *Treponema pallidum,* the organism that causes syphilis (see Chapter 10, pages 250 and 260). Rectal and oral lesions cannot be examined with this technique because of the presence of nonpathogenic spirochetes. This technique is rarely used anymore, as it is impractical for most laboratories to maintain control organisms and competency to perform the exam. Additionally, the availability of more sensitive and specific molecular tests is making this technique obsolete.

Giemsa Stain

The standard technique to identify intracellular organisms such as *Plasmodium* (malaria). Also used for other protozoans as well as spirochetes and other organisms (*Chlamydia trachomatis* inclusion bodies, *Borrelia* spp, *Yersinia pestis, Histoplasma* spp., and *Pneumocystis jiroveci* cysts). Unrelated to microbiology, Giemsa is useful for chromosome staining (G-banding) and as a blood film stain for peripheral blood smears and bone marrow specimens.

Gonorrhea Detection

Although *Neisseria gonorrhoeae* (GC or gonococci) can be cultured from many sites, including the female genital tract, male urethra, urine, anorectum, throat, and synovial fluid, and it may be detectable on Gram stain smears, the test of choice for GC is PCR or molecular testing, as these are highly specific, sensitive, and rapid. Because of the high incidence of coinfection with *Chlamydia trachomatis* (CT), combined molecular testing for GC and CT is used most widely for these organisms.

Table 13-2. Some Media Used for Isolation of Bacterial Pathogens (Used with permission from Principles of Laboratory Diagnosis of Infectious Diseases. In: Ryan KJ. eds. Sherris Medical Microbiology, 7e, New York, NY: McGraw-Hill; 2017.)

Medium	Uses
General-purpose Media	
Nutrient broths (e.g., soybean–casein digest broth)	Most bacteria, particularly when used for blood culture
Thioglycolate broth	Anaerobes, facultative bacteria
Blood agar	Most bacteria (demonstrates hemolysis) and fungi
Chocolate agar	Most bacteria, including fastidious species (e.g., *Haemophilus*) and fungi
Selective Media	
MacConkey agar	Nonfastidious gram-negative rods
Hektoen enteric agar	*Salmonella* and *Shigella*
Selenite F broth	*Salmonella* enrichment
Sabouraud agar	Isolation of fungi, particularly dermatophytes
Special-purpose Media	
Löwenstein–Jensen medium, Middlebrook agar	*M tuberculosis* and other mycobacteria (selective)
Martin–Lewis medium	*Neisseria gonorrhoeae* and *Neisseria meningidis* (selective)
Fletcher medium (semisolid)	*Leptospira* (nonselective)
Tinsdale agar	*C diphtheriae* (selective)
Charcoal agar	*Bordetella pertussis* (selective)
Buffered charcoal–yeast extract agar	*Legionella* species (nonselective)
Campylobacter blood agar	*Campylobacter jejuni* (selective)
Thiosulfate-citrate-bile-sucrose agar (TCBS)	*Vibrio cholerae* and *Vibrio parahaemolyticus* (selective)

Gram Stain and Common Pathogens

A Gram stain is essential for differentiating gram-positive from gram-negative bacteria. This is used as an important determinant for selection of antimicrobial therapy. The morphologic features of the organism are also determined by observation of a Gram stain. The procedure can be applied to bacterial cultures and various specimen types such as body fluids such as sputum, bronchoalveolar lavage (BAL), pleural/peritoneal fluid, cerebrospinal fluid, positive blood culture bottles, and others.

1. Smear the specimen onto a glass slide in a thin layer. If time permits, allow it to air-dry. The specimen is fixed under low heat. Heat the slide until it is warm, not hot, when touched to the back of your hand.
2. Timing for the stain is not critical, but allow at least 10 sec for each set of reagents.
3. Apply the crystal violet (Gram stain), rinse with water, apply iodine solution, and rinse with water.
4. Decolorize carefully with acetone–alcohol solution until the blue color is barely visible in the runoff. (Be careful; most Gram stains are ruined in this step.)
5. Counterstain with a few drops of safranin, rinse the slide with water, and blot it dry with lint-free filter paper.
6. Use the high dry and oil immersion lenses on the microscope to examine the slide. On a Gram stain of sputum, an excessive number of epithelial cells (>10/low power field) means the sample contains more oropharyngeal contamination (spit) than sputum. **Gram-positive organisms stain dark blue to purple; gram-negative organisms stain red/pink.**

Common Pathogens: Initial lab reports identify the Gram stain characteristics of the organisms. Gram stain results from sterile body fluids such as blood and cerebrospinal fluid (CSF) are considered critical values at most hospitals and need to have documented communication with the treating physician or pharmacist on call within a specified time (e.g., often within 30 minutes of a positive blood culture bottle), as mortality and morbidity correlate directly with the time to initiation of appropriate therapy. Complete identification requires culture of the organism. The lab algorithms for gram-positive and gram-negative organisms are shown in Figures 13-1 and 13-2, pages 322 and 323. Gram stain characteristics of clinically important bacteria are shown in Table 13-3, page 324.

13

India Ink Preparation

India ink is used primarily on CSF to identify *Cryptococcus* species. Cryptococci appear as blank spaces (round) in a dark background.

KOH Preparation

KOH (potassium hydroxide) preps are used to diagnose fungal infections and are often performed at the bedside. Apply the specimen (vaginal secretion, sputum, hair, skin scrapings) to a slide. Obtain skin scrapings of a lesion by gentle scraping with a no. 15 scalpel blade (see Chapter 19, page 649, for skin biopsy description).

1. Add one or two drops of 10% KOH solution and mix. Gentle heating (optional) may accelerate dissolution of the keratin.

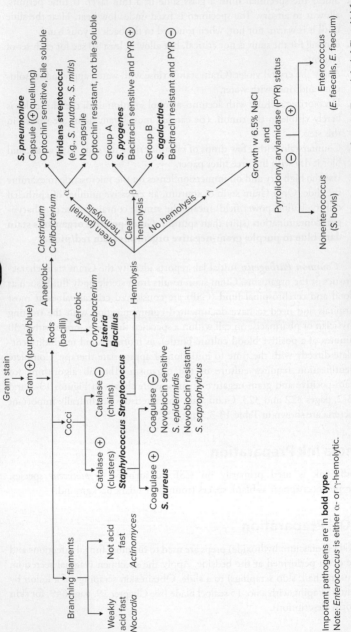

Figure 13-1. Lab algorithm for the identification of gram positive organisms. Modified with permission from Le T, et al. [eds.] First Aid for USMLE Step 1, McGraw-Hill, 2019.

Important pathogens are in **bold type**.

Note: *Enterococcus* is either α- or γ-hemolytic.

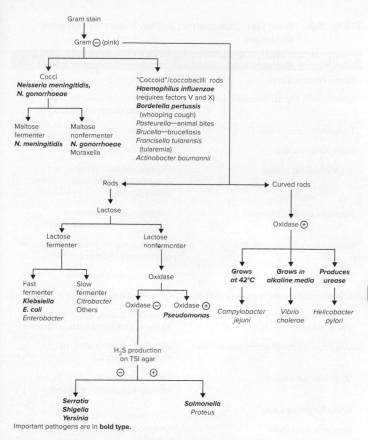

Figure 13-2. Lab algorithm for the identification of gram negative organisms. Modified with permission from Le T, et al. [eds.] First Aid for USMLE Step 1, McGraw-Hill, 2019.

2. Put a coverslip over the specimen, and examine for branching hyphae and blastospores, which indicate the presence of a fungus. KOH should destroy most cellular elements other than fungus. If dense keratin and debris are present, allow the slide to sit for several hours and then repeat the microscopic examination. Lowering the substage condenser provides better contrast between the organisms and the background.

Malaria Smear

Travelers with fever who have recently returned from regions where malaria is endemic need to have malaria ruled out because certain forms can be rapidly fatal. Prophylaxis is never 100%, and breakthrough infections do occur.

The reference standard for malaria diagnosis is examination of multiple sets of thick and thin blood smears. Thin smear is used for speciation and

Table 13-3. Gram Stain Characteristics and Key Features of Common Organisms

Gram Staining Pattern and Organisms	Identifying Key Features
Gram-Positive Cocci	
Enterococcus spp. (*E. faecalis/E. faecium*)	Short chains; catalase-negative; Alpha, beta or gamma hemolysis
Peptostreptococcus spp.	Anaerobic
Staphylococcus spp.	Clusters; catalase-positive
Staphylococcus aureus	Clusters; catalase-positive; coagulase-positive; beta-hemolytic; yellow pigment
Staphylococcus epidermidis	Clusters; catalase-positive; coagulase-negative; skin flora
Staphylococcus saprophyticus	Clusters; catalase-positive; coagulase-negative; novobiocin resistant
Streptococcus spp.	Chains, catalase-negative
Streptococcus agalactiae (group B Strep)	Chains; catalase-negative
Streptococcus pneumoniae (*Pneumococci*)	Diplococci (pairs), lancet-shaped; alpha-hemolytic; optochin-sensitive
Streptococcus pyogenes (group A Strep)	Beta-hemolytic; catalase neg; Bacitracin sensitive
Streptococcus viridans	Chains; catalase-negative; alpha-hemolytic, optochin-resistant
Gram-Negative Cocci	
Moraxella catarrhalis	Diplococci (pairs)
Neisseria gonorrhoeae (gonococcus)	Diplococci (pairs), often intracellular; ferments glucose but not maltose
Neisseria meningitidis (meningococcus)	Diplococci (pairs); ferments glucose and maltose
Gram-Positive Bacilli	
Actinomyces	Branching, rods
Bacilli anthracis (anthrax)	Spore-forming aerobic rods
Clostridium spp. (*C. difficile, C. botulinum, C. tetani*)	Spore forming; anaerobic
Corynebacterium spp. (*C. diphtheriae*)	Small, pleomorphic; (Chinese letter pattern)
Lactobacillus spp.	Common vaginal flora; anaerobic
Listeria monocytogenes	Beta-hemolytic

(Continued)

Table 13-3. Gram Stain Characteristics and Key Features of Common Organisms (*Continued*)

Gram Staining Pattern and Organisms	Identifying Key Features
Mycobacterium spp. (limited staining)	Only rapidly growing species visible on gram stain (*M. abscessus, M. chelonae, M. fortuitum*)
Nocardia	Beaded, branched rods; partially acid-fast-staining
Cutibacterium (formerly Propionibacterium) acnes	Small, pleomorphic diphtheroid; anaerobic
Gram-Negative Bacilli	
Acinetobacter spp.	Coccobacilli
Aeromonas hydrophilia	Lactose-negative (usually) oxidase-positive
Bacteroides fragilis	Anaerobic
Bordetella pertussis	Coccoid rod
Brucella (brucellosis)	Coccobacilli; pleomorphic; variable staining
Citrobacter spp.	Lactose-positive (usually)
Enterobacter spp.	Lactose-positive (usually)
Escherichia coli	Lactose-positive
Fusobacterium spp.	Long, pointed shape; anaerobic
Haemophilus influenzae	Pleomorphic rods; coccobacilli, requires chocolate agar to support growth
Klebsiella spp.	Lactose-positive; mucoid growth
Legionella pneumophila	Stains poorly, use silver stain and special medium
Morganella morganii	Lactose-negative, oxidase-negative
Proteus mirabilis	Lactose-negative, oxidase-negative, indole-negative
Proteus vulgaris	Lactose-negative, oxidase-negative, indole-positive
Pseudomonas aeruginosa	Lactose-negative, oxidase-positive blue-green pigment
Salmonella spp.	Lactose-negative, oxidase-negative
Serratia spp.	Oxidase-negative

13

(*Continued*)

Table 13-3. Gram Stain Characteristics and Key Features of Common
Organisms (*Continued*)

Gram Staining Pattern and Organisms	Identifying Key Features
Serratia marcescens	Lactose-negative, oxidase-negative, red pigment
Shigella spp.	Lactose-negative, oxidase-negative
Stenotrophomonas maltophilia	Lactose-negative, oxidase-negative
Vibrio cholerae (cholera)	Gram-negative curved bacilli
Yersinia enterocolitica	Gram-negative bacilli
Yersinia pestis (plague)	Gram-negative bacilli; safety pin appearance

parasite load. A lateral flow enzyme immunoassay may be used to complement smear examination for improved predictive values.

Molecular Microbiology

Culture-Independent Diagnostic Testing (CIDT) such as molecular techniques are used to identify many pathogens without the need for culturing.
These may involve nonamplification methods like DNA probes or amplification
methods (nucleic acid amplification tests [NAATs] using PCR) with or without the use of additional methods like microarrays and hybridization. Some of
these CIDTs may be for the detection of single organism types such as *C. difficile* by PCR or methicillin-resistant *S. aureus* (MRSA) by PCR, while some may
be for a small number of organisms such as influenza A/B and RSV panel, and
others are multiplex syndromic panels that can identify a large number of organisms from a particular specimen type, e.g., gastrointestinal panel for diarrheal
disease; comprehensive respiratory panel; and meningitis/encephalitis panel
for CSF (see specific disease entities in this chapter). Conventional or next-
generation/whole-genome sequencing is available and increasingly being used
for detection or identification of organisms from specimens or cultures when
other conventional or current methods do not provide answers. (See also
Nucelic acid amplification tests [NAATs].)

Nasopharyngeal Swab

PCR of nasopharyngeal swabs has become the standard for diagnosis of
various respiratory viral infections and is also useful for detection of many
atypical bacterial infections. It has also become the mainstay for the diagnosis
of SARS-Co-V-2, the virus causing COVID-19.

- A common use for the nasopharyngeal swab is in the evaluation of typical
  influenza symptoms: fever, dry or productive cough, runny nose, lethargy,
  and myalgias.

- Panel testing of nasopharyngeal swabs is common, and the specific panel ordered should be based on the specific laboratory's choice of agents. Some of these multiplex panel assays can simultaneously detect up to 20 viruses and several atypical bacteria. In addition to nasal swabs, these panels can be run on bronchoalveolar lavage (BAL) and tracheal aspirates or suction specimens. While nasopharyngeal (NP) swab is the optimal upper respiratory tract specimen collection method for influenza testing, such specimens cannot be collected from infants and many older patients. Alternatively, a combined nasal and throat swab specimen or aspirate specimen can provide good influenza virus yield.

- **It is important to note that these respiratory panels as of September 2020 DO NOT include SARS-CoV-2, which is run as a separate assay.** SARS-CoV-2 testing is reviewed on page 380 and Chapter 10, page 202.

- Panels are not standardized, and nomenclature varies widely by lab: "Respiratory Pathogens Panel," "Respiratory Pathogen Panel by PCR," "Influenza Viruses by PCR," "Respiratory Viruses Panel," "Respiratory Pathogen Molecular Panel Testing," and others. Some illustrative panel examples:

  o **Respiratory Virus Panel:** adenovirus, human metapneumovirus, human parainfluenza virus 1, human parainfluenza virus 2, human parainfluenza virus 3, human RSV A, human RSV B, influenza A, influenza A subtype H1, influenza A subtype H3, influenza B, rhinovirus

  o **Respiratory Pathogen Panel:** adenovirus, human metapneumovirus, rhinovirus/enterovirus, influenza A, influenza A subtype H1, influenza A subtype H3, influenza B, parainfluenza virus (1, 2, 3, 4), RSV-A, RSV-B, bocavirus, coronavirus 229E, coronavirus OC43, coronavirus NL63, coronavirus HKU1, *Chlamydophila pneumoniae, Mycoplasma pneumoniae, Bordetella pertussis* (whooping cough), and *Bordetella parapertussis*

    ▪ **Testing for SARS-CoV-2.** (https://www.cdc.gov/coronavirus/2019-ncov/lab/guidelines-clinical-specimens.html#collecting; accessed July 1, 2020). These tests should be conducted in consultation with a healthcare provider. Specimens should be collected as soon as possible once a decision has been made to pursue testing, regardless of the time of symptom onset. For initial diagnostic testing for SARS-CoV-2, the CDC recommends collecting and testing an upper respiratory specimen. The following are acceptable specimens:

    ▪ NP specimen or an oropharyngeal (OP) specimen collected by a healthcare provider.

    ▪ A nasal mid-turbinate swab collected by a healthcare provider or by supervised onsite self-collection (using a flocked tapered swab).

    ▪ An anterior nares (nasal swab) specimen collected by a healthcare provider or by onsite or home self-collection (using a flocked or spun polyester swab).

- Nasopharyngeal wash/aspirate or nasal wash/aspirate (NW) specimen collected by a healthcare provider.
- Testing lower respiratory tract specimens is also an option. For patients who develop a productive cough, sputum can be collected and tested for SARS-CoV-2. The induction of sputum is not recommended. Under certain clinical circumstances (e.g., those receiving invasive mechanical ventilation), a lower respiratory tract aspirate or BAL sample should be collected and tested.

Nasopharyngeal Swab Technique (Figure 13-3, page 329)

NOTE: If performing nasal swab of a patient under investigation (PUI) for or diagnosed with COVID-19, the healthcare provider should wear appropriate protective equipment (see pages 393–395). A surgical mask, eye protection/face shield, and gloves are recommended at a minimum for all nasopharyngeal testing procedures.

- Collection Method by healthcare worker:
  1. Use sterile flocked swab provided by the reference laboratory. Swab must be sterile Dacron, nylon, or rayon with plastic shafts. Wooden shaft swabs should not be used, as they can be contaminated with nucleic acid residue.
  2. Have patient lie down on their back. If the patient is sitting in a chair, tilt their head back to 70 degrees (head in neutral position is at 90 degrees).
  3. Immobilize patient's head and gently insert sterile flocked swab into one naris while lifting the nostrils.
  4. Continue inserting the swab with a rotating back and forth motion until it reaches the posterior nasopharynx where resistance is met. This will require the swab to bend along the curvature of the nasopharyngeal space. The distance inserted to reach the posterior nasopharynx should be at least a few inches, depending on the age of the patient. Another metric is that the swab should reach a depth equal to the distance from nostrils to outer opening of the ear.
  5. Leave the swab in place for 5–10 seconds. This will likely induce tearing and coughing.
  6. Withdraw the swab slowly with a rotating motion to loosen and collect cellular material while in contact with the mucosal surfaces of the mid-inferior portion of the inferior turbinate.
  7. Immediately place and agitate the swab briskly in a sterile vial containing 2–3 mL of transport media. Viral transport media contains stabilizer, antibiotics to inhibit bacterial and fungal growth, and buffer solutions (e.g., commercial media such as UTM, V-C-M, M4, and others). No medium is necessary if using a test designed to analyze the specimen directly.

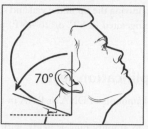

1 Tilt patient's head back 70 to degrees.

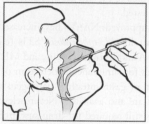

2 Insert swab into nostril. (Swab should reach depth equal to distance from nostrils to outer opening of the ear.) Leave swab in place for several seconds to absorb secretions.

13

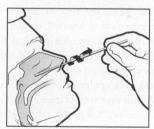

3 Slowly remove swab while rotating it. (Swab both nostrils with same swab.)

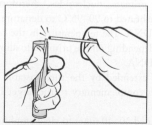

4 Place tip of swab into sterile viral transport media tube and snap/cut off the applicator stick.

Figure 13-3. Technique for nasopharyngeal swab. (From https://www.cdc.gov/flu/pdf/professionals/flu-specimen-collection-poster.pdf. Accessed May 9, 2020.)

8. Cut the swab shaft, leaving the tip in the vial and secure the lid tightly. Keep specimens refrigerated (2-8°C or 26-46°F) prior to shipping to the reference lab.

Nucleic Acid Amplification Tests

NAATs can identify small amounts of DNA or RNA in test samples.

- There are several ways to amplify nucleic acids, with variations of PCR most commonly performed to expand the available nucleic acid specific to the organism(s) being tested.
- The number of FDA-approved NAATs has increased dramatically and includes important tests for *M. tuberculosis*, STIs (e.g., *N. gonorrhoeae*, *C. trachomatis*), groups A and B streptococcus, and MRSA. FDA-approved multiplex NAAT panels for simultaneous detection of several respiratory, central nervous system, or gastrointestinal pathogens and limited antibiotic-resistance markers are also available. Nevertheless, even if NAAT is performed, a culture is still required for drug susceptibility testing of the isolate.

Principles of PCR Amplification

1. At temperatures around 94°C, the two strands of a DNA molecule separate; when the temperature is lowered to around 55°C, the two strands again pair up. By exploiting this physical property of DNA, the core of the PCR technology relies on cycles of repeated heating and cooling for the enzymatic replication of the DNA.
2. PCR uses a thermostable DNA polymerase to produce a twofold amplification of target DNA with each temperature cycle. Conventional PCR, also referred to as end detection PCR, utilizes three sequential reactions—denaturation, annealing, and primer extension.
3. The DNA extracted from the clinical specimen along with sequence-specific oligonucleotide primers, nucleotides, thermostable DNA polymerase, and buffer are heated to 90–95°C to denature (separate) the two strands of the target DNA. The temperature in the reaction is lowered, usually to 45–60°C, depending on the primers, to allow annealing of the primers to the target DNA.
4. Each primer is then extended by the thermostable DNA polymerase by adding nucleotides complementary to the target DNA, yielding the twofold amplification.
5. The cycle is then repeated 30–40 times to yield amplification of the target DNA segment by more than 100-fold.
6. PCR can also be performed on RNA targets, which is called reverse transcriptase PCR. The enzyme reverse transcriptase is used to transcribe the RNA into complementary DNA for subsequent PCR amplification.

Pinworm Preparation (Cellophane Tape Test)

Used to identify infestation with *Enterobius vermicularis*. Wrap a 3-in. piece of *clear* cellophane (e.g., Scotch) tape around a glass slide (sticky side out). Touch the slide to the patient's perianal skin in four quadrants and examine it under a microscope to find pinworm eggs. The best sample is collected either in the early morning before bathing or several hours after retiring.

Sputum Culture

(See Pulmonary Infections, Table 13-4, page 377)

Stool Culture

Routine stool culture is rarely used currently, as it has been replaced by multiplex molecular panels that can detect most of the common diarrheal pathogens, including bacterial, protozoa, fungi, and viruses. Targeted culture for reportable pathogens such as *Salmonella, Shigella, Campylobacter, Listeria,* and Shiga toxin–producing *E. coli* like O157H7 are performed to isolate these organisms so they can be sent to public health laboratories for further studies such as relatedness/fingerprinting for outbreak investigations. (See also Infectious Diarrhea, page 373.)

13

Stool for Ova and Parasites

Routine use of stool for ova and parasites has gone out of favor with the availability of multiplex panels, as described in the Stool Culture and Infectious Diarrhea sections, page 374. Stool for ova and parasites is still used in some populations such as healthy individuals coming through adoption clinics or in cases of persistent diarrhea in international travelers. This involves microscopy looking for the presence of eggs or cysts of various parasites, or in some cases larvae or adult worms.

Syphilis Testing

(See Chapter 10, pages 250–252, 260, and 262.)

Urine Culture

(See page 389)

Vaginal Wet Preparation

(See Chapter 19, page 633)

13

Table 13-4. Organisms Causing Common Infectious Diseases with Recommended Empiric Therapy[1]

Site/Condition	Common / Uncommon but Important	Empiric Antibiotics
BONES AND JOINTS		
Osteomyelitis	*Staphylococcus aureus*, Coagulase negative *Staphylococcus* spp.; if sickle cell disease: *Salmonella* spp.; if nail puncture: *Pseudomonas* spp.; if Peds: *Streptococcus pneumoniae*	Vancomycin + cephalosporin (ceftriaxone, ceftazidime, or cefepime)
Joint, septic arthritis	*S. aureus, Streptococcus pyogenes, Neisseria gonorrhoeae, Kingella* (most common cause <4 yr of age)	Vancomycin, ceftriaxone if gonococci; *Kingella* (NOT covered by vancomycin)
Joint, prosthetic	*S. aureus*, Coagulase negative *Staphylococcus* spp., *Enterococcus* spp., *Streptococcus* spp.	Vancomycin + cephalosporin (ceftriaxone, ceftazidime, or cefepime)
BREAST		
Mastitis, postpartum	*S. aureus*	Mild to moderate:[2] dicloxacillin OR cephalexin Severe[2]: vancomycin (if concerned about MRSA: risk factors for MRSA,[7] local resistance patterns, or poor response to therapy may suggests MRSA[7])
BRONCHITIS	Acute bronchitis: *Mycoplasma pneumoniae*, respiratory viruses Acute exacerbation of chronic bronchitis: *Streptococcus pneumoniae, Haemophilus influenzae, Moraxella catarrhalis, Chlamydia pneumoniae*	Antibiotics are not recommended because most infections are viral. Exacerbation of COPD: azithromycin, clarithromycin, cefuroxime, cefpodoxime, OR cefdinir

CERVICITIS (nongonococcal)	*Chlamydia trachomatis, Trichomonas vaginalis, Mycoplasma genitalium*, Herpes simplex	Azithromycin single dose OR doxycycline (evaluate and treat partner)
CHANCROID	*Haemophilus ducreyi*	Azithromycin OR ceftriaxone as a single dose
CHLAMYDIA		
Urethritis, cervicitis, conjunctivitis, proctitis	*Chlamydia trachomatis*	Azithromycin OR doxycycline (azithromycin if pregnant)
Neonatal ophthalmia, pneumonia	*Chlamydia trachomatis*	Erythromycin (systemic treatment; do NOT use topical alone, may be beneficial as adjunct therapy)
Lymphogranuloma venereum	*Chlamydia trachomatis*	Doxycycline
DIVERTICULITIS		
Mild, no perforation/no peritonitis, outpatient	Enterobacteriaceae, *Bacteroides* spp.	Metronidazole + fluoroquinolone (ciprofloxacin or levofloxacin) OR metronidazole + trimethoprim-sulfamethoxazole (TMP-SMX) OR amoxicillin-clavulanate OR moxifloxacin (if intolerant to metronidazole and beta-lactam agents)
Moderately ill and requires admission	Enterobacteriaceae, *Bacteroides* spp.	Piperacillin/tazobactam, ticarcillin/clavulanic acid, or ertapenem; if immunocompromised: meropenem, imipenem-cilastatin, piperacillin-tazobactam, or doripenem. Multidrug regimens metronidazole with a third-generation cephalosporin or a fluoroquinolone (cefepime + metronidazole, ceftazidime + metronidazole).

13

(Continued)

Table 13-4. Organisms Causing Common Infectious Diseases with Recommended Empiric Therapy[1] (*Continued*)

Site/Condition	Common Uncommon but Important	Empiric Antibiotics
EAR		
Acute mastoiditis: without recurrent acute otitis media or recent antibiotics[3]	*S. pneumoniae, Streptococcus pyogenes, S. aureus*	Vancomycin
Chronic mastoiditis: with history of recurrent acute otitis media or recent antibiotics[3]	Polymicrobial: *P. aeruginosa*, Enterobacteriaceae, anaerobes	Vancomycin + beta-lactam (ceftazidime, cefepime, or piperacillin-tazobactam)
Otitis externa	*Pseudomonas* spp., *Staphylococcus* spp., *anaerobes* Malignant otitis: *Pseudomonas aeruginosa*	Mild:[4] acetic acid-hydrocortisone otic solution Moderate:[4] ciprofloxacin-hydrocortisone otic solution OR neomycin-polymyxin B-hydrocortisone otic solution if the integrity of the tympanic membrane can be confirmed Severe:[4] oral ciprofloxacin for deeper tissue infection
Otitis media	*S. pneumoniae, Haemophilus influenza, Moraxella catarrhalis*, viral, *Streptococcus pyogenes* Nasal intubation: Enterobacteriaceae	Amoxicillin-clavulanate
EMYPEMA		
Community-acquired	*S. pneumoniae; S. aureus*, anaerobes	Metronidazole + cephalosporin (ceftriaxone or cefotaxime) OR ampicillin-sulbactam
Hospital-acquired	*S. aureus*, Enterobacteriaceae, *P. aeruginosa*, anaerobes	Vancomycin + metronidazole + cephalosporin (cefepime or ceftazidime) OR vancomycin + piperacillin-tazobactam

13

ENDOCARDITIS		
Empiric therapy to cover common pathogens		
Native valve	*Streptococcus viridans, Streptococcus pneumoniae, S. aureus, Enterococcus* spp.	Vancomycin
IV drug use	*S. aureus, Streptococcus* spp., *Enterococcus* spp.	Vancomycin
Prosthetic valve	If early (<2 mo after implantation): coagulase-negative *Staphylococcus* (CoNS), *S. aureus, Enterococcus* spp., gram-neg bacilli; If late (>12 month after implantation: more like native valve except CoNS more frequent	Vancomycin + gentamicin + cefepime OR imipenem-cilastatin OR meropenem, OR doripenem
EPIGLOTTITIS	*H. influenza, S. pneumoniae, Streptococcus pyogenes, S. aureus, Neisseria meningitidis, Pasteurella multocida* (immunocompromised host), *Aspergillus*, other fungi (immunocompromised host)	Vancomycin + cephalosporin (ceftriaxone or cefotaxime)
GALL BLADDER		
Cholecystitis: low-risk community-acquired[5]	Acute: *E. coli; Klebsiella; Enterococcus* Chronic obstruction: anaerobes, coliforms, *Clostridium* spp.	Monotherapy: ertapenem Combination therapy: metronidazole + cephalosporin (cefazolin, cefuroxime, ceftriaxone or cefotaxime) OR metronidazole + fluoroquinolones (ciprofloxacin or levofloxacin)
Cholecystitis: high-risk community-acquired[5]		Monotherapy: imipenem-cilastatin, meropenem, doripenem, OR piperacillin-tazobactam Combination therapy: metronidazole + cephalosporin (cefepime or ceftazidime)

13

(Continued)

Table 13-4. Organisms Causing Common Infectious Diseases with Recommended Empiric Therapy[1] (*Continued*)

Site/Condition	Common Uncommon but Important	Empiric Antibiotics
Cholecystitis: hospital-acquired[5]		Metronidazole + cephalosporin (cefepime or ceftazidime) + vancomycin or ampicillin for enterococcus coverage
Cholangitis	*Klebsiella, E. coli, Enterococcus* spp.	See cholecystitis, low-risk community-acquired, high-risk community-acquired, and hospital-acquired
GASTROENTERITIS		
Afebrile, no gross blood or WBC in stool	Virus (norovirus, rotavirus, enteric adenovirus, astrovirus); mild bacterial form	Supportive care only
Febrile, gross blood, WBC in stool	Enteropathogenic *E. coli, Shigella* spp., *Salmonella* spp., *Campylobacter* spp.	Ciprofloxacin OR levofloxacin Fluoroquinolone-resistance or recent travel to Southeast Asia: azithromycin
	Listeria monocytogenes	Pregnant women: amoxicillin, ampicillin, OR TMP-SMX (avoid in the first trimester and last month of pregnancy)
	Vibrio cholerae	Doxycycline, tetracycline, azithromycin, erythromycin, OR ciprofloxacin

13

	Clostridioides difficile	Initial episode: Oral vancomycin OR oral fidaxomicin Fulminant disease:[6] Enteric vancomycin + parenteral metronidazole Recurrent infection: If vancomycin was used for the initial episode: vancomycin pulsed-tapered regimen OR fidaxomicin; If fidaxomicin was used for the initial episode: vancomycin OR vancomycin followed by rifaximin OR fecal microbiota transplantation
GRANULOMA INGUINALE (donovanosis)	*Klebsiella (Calymmatobacterium) granulomatis*	Azithromycin Alternative: Doxycycline, ciprofloxacin, erythromycin, OR TMP-SMX
GONORRHEA (urethra, cervix, rectum, pharynx)	*Neisseria gonorrhoeae*	Single doses of ceftriaxone + azithromycin If ceftriaxone is not available: cefixime + azithromycin
MENINGITIS		
Neonate (<1 mo)	*Streptococcus agalactiae, E. coli, L. monocytogenes*	Ampicillin + cefotaxime OR ampicillin + aminoglycoside (usually gentamicin)
Infant 1–23 mo	*S. pneumoniae, N. meningitidis, S. agalactiae, H. influenza, E. coli*	Vancomycin + third-generation cephalosporin (ceftriaxone or cefotaxime)
Child/adult, community-acquired 2–50 yr	*S. pneumoniae, N. meningitidis*	Vancomycin + third-generation cephalosporin (ceftriaxone or cefotaxime)
Adult >50 yr	*S. pneumoniae, N. meningitidis, L. monocytogenes,* ae·obic gram-negative (*H. influenzae* bacilli)	Vancomycin + ampicillin + third-generation cephalosporin (ceftriaxone or cefotaxime)
HIV infection	*Cryptococcus neoformans*	See Table 13–5

13

(*Continued*)

Table 13-4. Organisms Causing Common Infectious Diseases with Recommended Empiric Therapy[1] (Continued)

Site/Condition	Common Uncommon but Important	Empiric Antibiotics
MENINGITIS, HEAD TRAUMA RELATED		
Basilar skull fracture	S. pneumoniae, H. influenzae, Streptococcus pyogenes	Vancomycin + third-generation cephalosporin (ceftriaxone or cefotaxime)
Penetrating trauma	S. aureus, coagulase-negative Staphylococcus spp. (especially Staphylococcus epidermidis), aerobic gram-negative bacilli (including P. aeruginosa)	Vancomycin + cefepime OR Vancomycin + ceftazidime OR Vancomycin + meropenem
Postneurosurgery	Aerobic gram-negative bacilli (including P. aeruginosa), S. aureus, coagulase-negative Staphylococcus spp. (especially Staphylococcus epidermidis)	Vancomycin + cefepime OR Vancomycin + ceftazidime OR Vancomycin + meropenem
Immunocompromised state	S. pneumoniae, N. meningitidis, L. monocytogenes, aerobic gram-negative bacilli (P. aeruginosa), H. influenzae	Vancomycin + ampicillin + cefepime OR Vancomycin + meropenem
NOCARDIOSIS	Nocardia asteroides	TMP-SMX Severe infection without central nervous system involvement: add amikacin Severe infection with central nervous system involvement: add imipenem-cilastatin
PELVIC INFLAMMATORY DISEASE	N. gonorrhoeae, Enterobacteriaceae, Bacteroides spp., Chlamydia trachomatis, Enterococcus spp., Streptococcus spp., Mycoplasma hominis, Mycoplasma genitalium, Gardnerella vaginalis	Outpatient: doxycycline + cephalosporin (ceftriaxone, cefotaxime, or ceftizoxime) Hospitalized patients: doxycycline + cephalosporin (cefoxitin or cefotetan) OR Clindamycin + gentamicin

13

PERITONITIS

Primary (spontaneous)	*S. pneumoniae* Enterobacteriaceae (*E. coli* most common)	Cefotaxime OR Ceftriaxone
Secondary to bowel perforation, iatrogenic, etc.: mild to moderate community-acquired (e.g., perforated appendix or appendiceal abscess)[5]	*Streptococcus* spp., Enterobacteriaceae (nondrug resistant, including *E. coli*, *K. pneumoniae*), anaerobes (*Clostridium* spp., *Enterococcus* spp., *Bifidobacterium* spp., *Peptostreptococcus* spp.)	Monotherapy: ertapenem OR piperacillin-tazobactam Combination therapy: metronidazole + cephalosporin (cefazolin, cefuroxime, ceftriaxone, or cefotaxime) OR metronidazole + fluoroquinolones (ciprofloxacin or levofloxacin)
Secondary to bowel perforation, iatrogenic, etc.: severe community-acquired[5]	Enterobacteriaceae (drug resistant including *E. coli*, *K. pneumoniae*), *Pseudomonas* spp., *Streptococcus* spp., anaerobes (*Clostridium* spp., *Enterococcus* spp., *Bifidobacterium* spp., *Peptostreptococcus* spp.)	Monotherapy: imipenem-cilastatin, meropenem, doripenem, OR piperacillin-tazobactam Combination therapy: metronidazole + cephalosporin (cefepime or ceftazidime)
Secondary to bowel perforation, iatrogenic, etc.: healthcare-associated[5]	Enterobacteriaceae (multidrug resistant), *Pseudomonas* spp., *Enterococcus* spp. including vancomycin-resistant *Enterococcus*, anaerobes Postbariatric surgery: gram positive cocci, yeast (*Candida* spp.)	Monotherapy: imipenem-cilastatin, meropenem, doripenem, OR piperacillin-tazobactam Combination therapy: metronidazole + cephalosporin (cefepime or ceftazidime) + ampicillin or vancomycin
Tertiary (persistent or recurrent following unsuccessful treatment of secondary)	*Enterococcus* spp. (including vancomycin resistant [VRE]), *Candida* spp., *Pseudomonas aeruginosa*, coagulase-negative *Staphylococcus* spp.	See: Secondary to bowel perforation, iatrogenic, etc.: Healthcare-associated; knowing prior antibiotic Tx influences antibiotics chosen; surgical management is usually required; if VRE, will need linezolid or daptomycin, or other VRE antibiotic
Peritoneal dialysis related	*S. epidermidis*, *S. aureus*, *Streptococcus* spp., *Enterococcus* spp., *Corynebacterium* spp., Enterobacteriaceae, *P. aeruginosa*, *Candida* spp.	Vancomycin + cephalosporin (ceftazidime, cefepime) OR vancomycin + aminoglycoside (gentamicin, tobramycin, or amikacin), or vancomycin + aztreonam

(Continued)

13

Table 13-4. Organisms Causing Common Infectious Diseases with Recommended Empiric Therapy[1] (*Continued*)

Site/Condition	Common Uncommon but Important	Empiric Antibiotics
PHARYNGITIS		
	Respiratory viruses (adenovirus, rhinovirus, coronaviruses) also Epstein-Barr virus, group A Streptococcus (*Streptococcus pyogenes*) Group C and G beta hemolytic streptococci (*S. dysgalactiae, S. equi*) In limited epidemiologic setting: *Arcanobacterium haemolyticum* (teenagers to young adults) *N. gonorrhoeae, Corynebacterium diphtheria; Fusobacterium necrophorum* (prelude to Lemierre syndrome—septic thrombophlebitis of the internal jugular vein)	*S. pyogenes*: penicillin VK or amoxicillin Alternatives: cephalexin, cefuroxime, cefdinir, cefpodoxime, azithromycin, clindamycin
PNEUMONIA		
Neonate: Early onset (age ≤6 days)	Viral: Herpes simplex virus (HSV), CMV Bacterial: *S. agalactiae , L. monocytogenes, E. coli, Klebsiella* spp., *S. aureus, S. pneumoniae* Fungal: *Candida* spp.	Ampicillin + gentamicin HSV: acyclovir
Neonate: Late onset (age >6 days to 1 mo)	*Streptococcus pyogenes, S. aureus, S. pneumoniae,* Enterobacteriaceae, *L. monocytogenes P. aeruginosa, C. trachomatis*	Vancomycin + aminoglycoside (gentamicin)
Infant (1–6 mo)	Viral: (*Respiratory syncytial virus [RSV]*) Bacterial: *S. pneumoniae, S. aureus, S. pyogenes, H. influenzae, M. catarrhalis* Atypicals: *C. trachomatis*	Ceftriaxone or cefotaxime Atypicals: azithromycin

13

Child (6 mo to 5 yr)	*S. pneumoniae, S. aureus, S. pyogenes* Atypicals: *M. pneumoniae or C. pneumoniae*	Outpatient: amoxicillin, amoxicillin-clavulanate, cefdinir, levofloxacin, clindamycin, erythromycin, azithromycin, OR clarithromycin Inpatients: ampicillin, penicillin G, cefotaxime, OR ceftriaxone + Atypicals: azithromycin, erythromycin, levofloxacin
Child (≥5 yr) to 18 yr	Bacterial: *S. pneumoniae, S. aureus, S. pyogenes* Atypicals: *M. pneumoniae, C. pneumoniae*	Outpatients: amoxicillin, cefdinir, cefpodoxime, levofloxacin, clindamycin, erythromycin, azithromycin, OR clarithromycin Atypicals: erythromycin, azithromycin, clarithromycin, OR doxycycline Inpatients: ampicillin, penicillin G, cefotaxime, ceftriaxone + Atypicals: azithromycin, erythromycin OR levofloxacin
Adult community-acquired: otherwise healthy outpatient **without** recent antibiotic use	*S. pneumoniae, H. influenzae* Atypicals: *M. pneumoniae, Legionella pneumophila, C. pneumoniae*	Combination therapy: high-dose amoxicillin + macrolide (azithromycin or clarithromycin) or doxycycline Combination therapy: a third-generation cephalosporin (cefpodoxime) + macrolide (azithromycin or clarithromycin) or doxycycline Monotherapy: respiratory fluoroquinolone (levofloxacin, moxifloxacin, gemifloxacin)
Adult community-acquired: outpatient with major comorbidities (chronic heart, lung, liver, renal disease, DM, alcohol dependence, malignancy, asplenia) smoking, or recent antibiotic use	Bacterial: *S. pneumoniae, H. influenzae, M. catarrhalis* (beta-lactamase-producing); Methicillin-susceptible *S. aureus* (MSSA) Atypicals: *M. pneumoniae, L. pneumophila, C. pneumoniae*	Combination therapy: amoxicillin-clavulanate + macrolide (azithromycin or clarithromycin) or doxycycline Combination therapy: a third-generation cephalosporin (cefpodoxime) + macrolide or doxycycline Monotherapy: respiratory fluoroquinolone (levofloxacin, moxifloxacin, gemifloxacin)

13

(Continued)

13

Table 13-4. Organisms Causing Common Infectious Diseases with Recommended Empiric Therapy[1] (*Continued*)

Site/Condition	Common Uncommon but Important	Empiric Antibiotics
Adult community-acquired: inpatient **without** risk factors for MRSA[7] or *P. aeruginosa*[8]	Respiratory viruses: Influenza, parainfluenza, respiratory syncytial virus, rhinovirus Bacteria: *S. pneumoniae, H. influenzae* Atypicals: *M. pneumoniae, L. pneumoniae, C. pneumoniae*	Combination therapy: cephalosporin (ceftriaxone, cefotaxime, ceftaroline) or ertapenem or ampicillin-sulbactam + macrolide or doxycycline Monotherapy: respiratory fluoroquinolone Influenza therapy discussed in Table 7-3
Adult community-acquired: inpatient **with** risk factors for MRSA[7] or *P. aeruginosa*[8]	*S. pneumoniae, Legionella* spp., gram-negative bacilli including *P. aeruginosa, S. aureus* (MSSA and MRSA), influenza	Combination therapy: Beta-lactam (piperacillin-tazobactam, imipenem-cilastatin, meropenem, cefepime, or ceftazidime) + fluoroquinolone (ciprofloxacin or levofloxacin) For patients with septic shock or respiratory failure: add vancomycin
Adult community-acquired Aspiration	*S. pneumoniae*, oral flora, anaerobes (e.g., *Fusobacterium* spp., *Bacteroides* spp.)	Ampicillin–sulbactam OR amoxicillin–clavulanate
Adult hospital-acquired ventilator-associated: inpatient **without** risk factors for MRSA[7] or *P. aeruginosa*[8]	*S. aureus* (MSSA), Enterobacteriaceae, *S. pneumoniae, Legionella* spp.	Monotherapy: Piperacillin-tazobactam OR cefepime OR levofloxacin
Adult hospital-acquired ventilator-associated: inpatient **with** risk factors for MRSA[7] or *P. aeruginosa*[8]	*S. aureus* (MSSA and MRSA), *S. pneumoniae, P. aeruginosa,* Enterobacteriaceae, *Legionella* spp.	Beta-lactam (piperacillin-tazobactam, cefepime, ceftazidime, imipenem-cilastatin, meropenem, or aztreonam) + aminoglycoside (amikacin, gentamicin, or tobramycin) + MRSA therapy (vancomycin or linezolid) For *Legionella*: replace the aminoglycoside with fluoroquinolone (ciprofloxacin or levofloxacin)

HIV-associated	*Pneumocystis pneumonia, TB, fungi, others*	PCP is discussed in Table 13-6 TB is discussed below Fungi infection is discussed in Table 13-5
SINUSITIS		
Acute sinusitis	*S. pneumoniae, H. influenza, M. catarrhalis, S. pyogenes, S. aureus,*	Acute: amoxicillin, amoxicillin-clavulanate Alternatives: doxycycline, cefixime, cefpodoxime, levofloxacin, OR moxifloxacin
Nosocomial, nasal intubations, etc.	*S. aureus, Pseudomonas* spp., Enterobacteriaceae, *Streptococcus* spp., anaerobes; Fungal: chronic/complicated sinusitis	See adult hospital-acquired ventilator-associated pneumonia above
SKIN/SOFT TISSUE		
Acne	*Cutibacterium acnes*	Topical: benzol peroxide OR retinoids (tretinoin, adapalene, tazarotene, or isotretinoin) OR antibiotic (clindamycin, erythromycin, dapsone, or minocycline) Oral antibiotics: tetracycline, doxycycline, minocycline, sarecycline, erythromycin, trimethoprim-sulfamethoxazole, azithromycin Oral retinoid: isotretinoin
Rosacea	*Possible skin mites*	Metronidazole, azelaic acid, OR ivermectin
Burn wound	*Streptococcus* spp., *Staphylococcus* spp., Enterobacteriaceae, *Pseudomonas* spp., *Providencia* spp., *Acinetobacter baumannii*, herpes simplex virus, *Candida* spp.	Topical: silver sulfadiazine Sepsis: piperacillin-tazobactam or carbapenem (meropenem or imipenem-cilastatin) +/− vancomycin +/− aminoglycoside

(*Continued*)

13

343

Table 13-4. Organisms Causing Common Infectious Diseases with Recommended Empiric Therapy[1] *(Continued)*

Site/Condition	Common Uncommon but Important	Empiric Antibiotics
Bite	**Human:** *Staphylococcus* spp., *Streptococcus* spp., *Clostridium* spp., anaerobic gram-negative rods; *Fusobacterium* spp. **Animal:** *Pasteurella multioculada* (common, classic) or *Capnocytophaga canimorsus* (commonly associated with septic shock and death); *Erysipelothrix* spp., *Actinobacillus*, spp., *Staphylococcus* spp., *Streptococcus* spp., *Moraxella* spp.; often polymicrobial including anaerobes; *Mycobacterium fortuitum, M. kansasii* If rabies/herpes B suspected: contact public health lab for assistance	Ampicillin-sulbactam IV OR amoxicillin-clavulanate
Cellulitis	*Streptococcus* spp. (group A, B, C, G), anaerobes	Cefazolin OR cephalexin Purulent infection: clindamycin, trimethoprim-sulfamethoxazole, OR tetracycline (doxycycline or minocycline)
Diabetic foot infections: mild-moderate[9] **without** risk factors for MRSA[10]	*S. aureus, S. agalactiae, S. pyogenes,* and coagulase-negative *Staphylococcus* spp.	Cephalexin, dicloxacillin, amoxicillin-clavulanate, OR clindamycin
Diabetic foot infections: mild-moderate[9] **with** risk factors for MRSA[10]	*S. aureus* (MSSA, MRSA), *S. agalactiae, S, pyogenes,* and coagulase-negative *Staphylococcus* spp.	Either TMP-SMX or doxycycline + either clindamycin or linezolid or cephalexin or dicloxacillin

13

Infection	Organisms	Treatment
Diabetic foot infections: moderate to severe[9]	Streptococcus spp., S. aureus (MSSA and MRSA), gram-negative bacilli, anaerobes	Monotherapy: ampicillin/sulbactam or piperacillin-tazobactam or carbapenem (imipenem-cilastatin, meropenem, ertapenem) Combination therapy: metronidazole + cephalosporin (ceftriaxone, ceftazidime, cefepime) OR metronidazole + fluoroquinolone (ciprofloxacin, levofloxacin, moxifloxacin) OR metronidazole + aztreonam **With risk factors for MRSA**[10]: ADD vancomycin, linezolid, OR daptomycin
Decubitus: mild-moderate[9]	S. pyogenes, anaerobes, S. aureus, Enterobacteriaceae, often polymicrobial	TMP-SMX + amoxicillin–clavulanate OR clindamycin + fluoroquinolone (ciprofloxacin, levofloxacin, or moxifloxacin)
Decubitus: moderate-severe[9]	S. pyogenes, anaerobes, S. aureus, Enterobacteriaceae, often polymicrobial	Vancomycin + piperacillin-tazobactam, or imipenem-cilastatin, or ceftazidime + metronidazole
Erysipelas	S. pyogenes	Cefazolin, ceftriaxone, OR flucloxacillin
Impetigo	S. pyogenes, S. aureus	Topical: mupirocin, retapamulin Oral: cephalexin or dicloxacillin Alternative: erythromycin or clarithromycin
Tinea capitis (scalp) "ringworm"	Dermatophyte fungus: Trichophyton spp., Microsporum spp.	Griseofulvin, terbinafine
Tinea corporis (body)	Dermatophyte fungus: Trichophyton spp., Epidermophyton spp., Microsporum spp.	Topical: azoles (econazole, ketoconazole, luliconazole, etc.), allylamines (naftifine or terbinafine), butenafine, ciclopirox, tolnaftate Systemic therapy if topical agents fail: terbinafine, itraconazole

13

Table 13-4. Organisms Causing Common Infectious Diseases with Recommended Empiric Therapy[1] (*Continued*)

Site/Condition	Common Uncommon but Important	Empiric Antibiotics
Tinea unguium (nail)/ onychomycosis	Dermatophyte fungus: *Trichophyton rubrum, Candida* spp., nondermatophyte molds, e.g. *Aspergillus* spp.	Oral terbinafine
SYPHILLIS (Less than 1 yr duration)	*Treponema pallidum*	Penicillin G benzathine as single dose Alternative: doxycycline, tetracycline, ceftriaxone
TUBERCULOUS		
Pulmonary (HIV neg)	*Mycobacterium tuberculosis*	Isoniazid (INH) + rifampin (RIF) + ethambutol + pyrazinamide at least 2 mo (+/– pyridoxine); followed by INH + RIF for 4 mo; (combined duration of therapy of 6 mo) Children <5 yr: RIF for 4 mo, retest at 8–12 wk; see below, for >5 yr of age and healthy, repeat TB testing in 8–12 wk
TB exposure (PPD or equivalent neg)		RIF × 3 mo OR INH + RIF × 3 mo OR INH + rifapentine × 3 mo OR INH × 9 mo (INH can be given with or without pyridoxine)
PPD or equivalent positive, or prophylaxis in high-risk patients (immunocompromised, DM, IV drug use)		
ULCER DISEASE (duodenal or gastric; NOT NSAID related)	*Helicobacter pylori*	Clarithromycin + amoxicillin + proton pump inhibitor (PPI) (lansoprazole, omeprazole, pantoprazole, rabeprazole, or esomeprazole) OR clarithromycin + metronidazole + PPI Erythromycin-resistance: bismuth + metronidazole + tetracycline + PPI

URINARY TRACT INFECTION (UTI)

Cystitis	Enterobacteriaceae (E. coli most common) Staphylococcus saprophyticus (nonpregnant premenopausal women without underlying urologic abnormalities), Candida spp., Enterococcus spp.	Nitrofurantoin monohydrate/macrocrystals (Macrobid), TMP-SMX Alternative: amoxicillin-clavulanate, cefpodoxime, cefadroxil, cephalexin, ciprofloxacin, levofloxacin
Urethritis	N. gonorrhoeae, C. trachomatis, Trichomonas, herpes simplex virus, M. genitalium, Ureaplasma urealyticum	Gonococcal: single doses of ceftriaxone + azithromycin Nongonococcal: single dose of azithromycin or 7 days of doxycycline
Prostatitis, acute[11] <35 yr or >35 yr who engage in high-risk sexual behavior (include coverage for N. gonorrhoeae and C. trachomatis)	C. trachomatis, N. gonorrhoeae, Enterobacteriaceae, P. aeruginosa, Cryptococcus (HIV/AIDS)	TMP-SMX, ciprofloxacin, levofloxacin Parenteral: ciprofloxacin or levofloxacin with or without gentamicin or tobramycin
Prostatitis, acute[11] >35 yr	Coliform (E. coli most common)	TMP-SMX, ciprofloxacin, levofloxacin
Prostatitis, chronic bacterial[12]	Coliforms, Enterococcus spp., Pseudomonas	Long-term (at least 6 wk) ciprofloxacin or levofloxacin
Pyelonephritis	Enterobacteriaceae (E. coli most common) Enterococcus spp., Pseudomonas spp., Staphylococcus spp.	No risk for multidrug-resistance: ceftriaxone, piperacillin-tazobactam, ciprofloxacin, levofloxacin Risk for multidrug-resistance[13]: vancomycin + imipenem, meropenem, OR doripenem

13

(Continued)

Table 13-4. Organisms Causing Common Infectious Diseases with Recommended Empiric Therapy[1] *(Continued)*

Site/Condition	Common Uncommon but Important	Empiric Antibiotics
VAGINA		
Candidiasis	Candidiasis: *C. albicans* (most common), *C. glabrata, C. tropicalis,*	Fluconazole
Trichomonas	Protozoan: *T. vaginalis*	Metronidazole or tinidazole (and treat partner)
Vaginosis, bacterial	Polymicrobial: (*Gardnerella vaginalis, Prevotella* spp., *Porphyromonas* spp., *Bacteroides* spp., *Peptostreptococcus* spp., *M. hominis, U. urealyticum, Mobiluncus* spp., *Megasphaera* spp., *Sneathia* spp., *Clostridiales* spp., *Fusobacterium* spp., *Atopobium vaginae*)	Metronidazole (PO or vaginal gel), clindamycin (PO or intravaginally)

[1]All antimicrobial therapy should be based on complete clinical data, including results of gram stains and cultures.

[2]Mild to moderate: persistent symptoms including fever beyond 12–24 hr; severe: hemodynamic instability and progressive erythema on antibiotics.

[3]Recurrent otitis media in children: Three or more episodes in 6 mo or four or more episodes in 12 mo.

[4]Mild: minor discomfort and pruritus, minimal drainage, minimal canal edema; moderate: moderate pain and pruritus, moderate drainage and partially occluded canal; severe: intense pain, erythema and swelling of the outer ear, completely occluded auditory canal, and fever and lymphadenopathy may be present.

[5] Mild to moderate community-acquired: mild to moderate infection in absence of risk factors for antibiotic resistance or treatment failure; severe community-acquired: severe infection with diffuse peritoneal involvement with high risk for antibiotic resistance (e.g., recent travel to areas of the world that have high rates of antibiotic-resistant organisms or known colonization with such organisms) or treatment failure (e.g., delay in initial intervention >24 hr, advanced age (>70 yr), inability to achieve adequate debridement or control of infection with drainage, comorbidities (e.g., renal or liver disease, malignancy), immunodeficiencies (e.g., poorly controlled diabetes mellitus, chronic high-dose corticosteroid use, use of other immunosuppressive agents, neutropenia, advanced HIV infection, B- or T-lymphocyte defects), organ dysfunction, severe peritoneal involvement or diffuse peritonitis, low albumin level, and poor nutritional status); healthcare associated: nosocomial infection, <90 days since hospitalization.

[6]*C. difficile,* fulminant disease: tachycardia, hypotension, oliguria with an increased creatinine, requires mechanical ventilation, leukocytosis with an increase in banded neutrophils; occurs in 3–5% of patients with *C. difficile colitis;* often requires colectomy.

13

[7]Risk factors for MRSA: known MRSA colonization, prior MRSA infection, gram-positive cocci in clusters on a good-quality sputum gram stain, recent hospitalization or antibiotic use in the prior 3 mo, recent influenza-like illness, necrotizing or cavitary pneumonia, empyema, immunosuppression, end-stage kidney disease, crowded living conditions, injection drug use, contact sports participation, men who have sex with men.

[8]Risk factors for P. aeruginosa: known Pseudomonas colonization, prior Pseudomonas infection, detection of gram-negative rods on a good-quality sputum gram stain, hospitalization with receipt of IV antibiotics in the prior 3 mo, recent stay in a long-term care facility, recent antibiotic use of any kind, frequent COPD exacerbation requiring glucocorticoid and/or antibiotic use, other structural lung disease (e.g., bronchiectasis, cystic fibrosis), immunosuppression.

[9]Mild to moderate: limited cellulitis/erythema of surrounding skin and no systemic signs of infection; moderate to severe: deeper soft tissue infection involving fascia and muscle or systemic manifestations of sepsis.

[10]Diabetic foot infection: risk factors for MRSA include purulent infection, prior MRSA infection, known MRSA colonization, prior antibiotic use, previous hospitalization, and currently or previously residing in a long-term care facility.

[11]Acute bacterial prostatitis: severe prostatitis symptoms, systemic infection, and acute bacterial urinary tract infection.

[12]Chronic bacterial prostatitis: chronic bacterial infection of the prostate with or without prostatitis symptoms and usually with recurrent urinary tract infections caused by the same bacterial strain.

[13]A history of any of the following in the prior 3 mo: an MDR gram-negative urinary isolate; inpatient stay at a healthcare facility (e.g., hospital, nursing home, long-term acute care facility); increasing age; obstructive uropathy; use of a fluoroquinolone, TMP-SMX, or broad-spectrum beta-lactam (e.g., third- or later generation cephalosporin); and travel to parts of the world with high rates of multidrug-resistant organisms.

Viral Detection Methods

Viral cultures are used with decreasing frequency, and most clinical laboratories have stopped using viral cultures because rapid and highly sensitive/specific PCR/molecular testing is widely available. In rare occasions, e.g., in some pediatric cases, physicians may request backup viral culture as recommended by guidelines (*Red Book: Report of the Committee on Infectious Diseases.* American Academy of Pediatrics; 2018.) Molecular detection relying on NAAT/PCR is discussed on pages 326 and 330.

- Viral cultures occasionally may include skin lesions for herpes simplex virus (HSV) or varicella zoster virus (VZV), cervical or vaginal cultures for HSV, conjunctival cultures for HSV or adenovirus, and respiratory tract cultures (throat, NP, nasal wash) for HSV, adenovirus, human metapneumovirus, and the respiratory viruses (RSV; influenza A/B; and parainfluenzas 1, 2, 3). Viruses are intracellular pathogens—vigorous swab collections should be obtained to include cellular material.

- Serologic testing for detection of antibodies is used commonly for diagnosis of viral infections, and this may include looking for specific IgM antibodies for recent infection, IgG antibodies for past infections or immunity, or in some cases a fourfold rise in titers between the **acute specimen (titer) obtained** as early as possible in the course of the illness and the **convalescent specimen (titer)** 2–4 wk later. Examples of some serologic tests for viral diseases are below.

- Testing to detect various viruses include:

  o **Cytomegalovirus (CMV)** (see Chapter 10, page 205)
  o **Arthropod-borne viral diseases**
    - **Chikungunya virus** (mosquito borne)
      - Viral culture can be positive in the first 3 days of infection
      - Viral RNA can be detected during the first 8 days of the illness
      - IgM-neutralizing antibodies
    - **Dengue fever** (mosquito borne)
      - rRT-PCR detects viral genomic sequences (collected 7 days or less from symptom onset)
      - Immunoassay for dengue nonstructural protein 1 antigen (may be positive up to 12 days after fever onset)
      - IgM testing most useful 1 week or longer after onset of fever; may cross-react with other flaviviruses
      - IgG, single value is not useful, present for life after infection
    - **Encephalitis** (mosquito borne): Each diagnosed with specific IgM antibodies in the serum or CSF; need confirmatory testing with neutralizing antibodies, often from acute and convalescent serum
      - Eastern equine encephalitis
      - Japanese encephalitis: IgM detected 3–8 days from onset to 30–90 days after infection
      - La Crosse encephalitis
      - St. Louis encephalitis

- West Nile virus: IgM detected 3–8 days from onset to 30–90 days after infection; IgG positive shortly after IgM and may be present for years
- Yellow fever: IgG is also useful; confirmatory testing with plaque-reduction neutralization test; virus RNA can be detected early (3–4 days after onset) but often negative
- **Zika virus** (mosquito borne):
  - NAAT; however, negative test does not exclude Zika virus infection
  - IgM can be used for diagnosis, BUT negative test does not rule out infection; timing of IgM is vital (false negative if test is obtained before antibodies develop or after the antibodies wane); IgM can be a false positive from infection or from a vaccination for another flavivirus
- o **Human immunodeficiency virus-1** (see page 371 and Chapter 10, pages 228–231)
- o **Hepatitis viruses** (see Chapter 10, pages 222–227)
- o **Herpes Simplex Virus (HSV)**
  - PCR to detect HSV DNA from active genital ulcers (more sensitive than culture)
  - Viral culture from genital lesion
  - Glycoprotein G serologic assay, can detect HSV-2 or HSV-1 (sensitivity of 80–98%, false-negatives occur early in the infection)
  - IgM is not useful, not type specific, and can be positive during recurrence of either HSV-1 or HSV-2
- o **Measles**
  - IgM, measles specific
  - RT-PCR of respiratory specimen
  - Urine may contain virus and when coupled with respiratory specimen can increase the likelihood of detecting measles
- o **Mumps**
  - RT-PCR (obtained via buccal swab)
  - Viral culture can also be used for diagnosis
  - Serology: IgM can be used
- o **Rubella**
  - PCR of a throat (best source), nasal, and urine specimens
- o **Varicella-Zoster Virus (VZV)**
  - PCR to detect VZV from vesicles (most sensitive test)
  - Direct fluorescent antibody assay (not recommended because PCR more sensitive)
  - Viral culture (not recommended because it takes longer and PCR more sensitive)
  - Serology: IgM detection is evidence of recent infection (much less sensitive than PCR and poor specificity)
  - Serology: IgG fourfold increase between acute presentation and convalescent, excellent specificity but not as sensitive as PCR

13

COMMON INFECTIONS AND EMPIRIC THERAPY

Tables 13-4 through 13-9 list common infections with common pathogens, with empiric treatment suggestions. These include a variety of infectious diseases, including bacterial and other (Table 13-4), viral (Table 13-5), HIV (Table 13-6), fungal (Table 13-7), parasitic (Table 13-8), and tick-borne diseases (Table 13-9). Additional suggested resources for infectious diseases include the *Sanford Guide to Antimicrobial Therapy* (www.sanfordguide.com), the *Johns Hopkins ABX Guide* (www.hopkins-abxguide.org), and The Medical Letter (www.medicalletter.org). The antimicrobial drug of choice for the management of infection is usually the most active drug against the pathogenic organism or the least toxic alternative. The choice of drug should be based on the site of infection, clinical status (e.g., allergy, renal disease, pregnancy, etc.), and local resistance pattern or antibiogram. Once etiologic pathogens are identified and/or antimicrobial susceptibility results are available, tailored definitive therapy should be prescribed with a narrower antimicrobial spectrum.

COMMON CLINICAL MICROBIOLOGY APPLICATIONS

Catheter-Related Bloodstream Infection

Catheter-related bloodstream infections (CRBSIs) are a common cause of nosocomial infection and can cause significant morbidity, mortality, and increase the length of hospitalization. CRBSIs are commonly associated with IV catheters and central venous catheters (CVCs). Central line–associated bloodstream infections, common in the ICU setting, are referred to as CLABSIs (aka "line sepsis"). Use of full barrier precautions during insertion, shorter duration of catheter use, antibiotic-impregnated catheters, avoidance of femoral venous access, and maintenance care by a central-line team are associated with reduced CLABSI risk. CVCs and IV catheters are discussed in Chapter 19, "Bedside Procedures," pages 533 and 611 (https://www.cdc.gov/infectioncontrol/guidelines/bsi/recommendations.html, accessed May 6, 2020, and Mermel LA, et al. Clinical Infectious Diseases 2009;49:1–4).

Prevention of CRBSI

1. Wear clean gloves for the insertion of peripheral IVs and sterile gloves when inserting of arterial and central catheters. Do not administer systemic antimicrobial prophylaxis routinely before insertion or during use of an intravascular catheter to prevent catheter colonization or CRBSI.
2. Use maximal sterile barrier precautions (cap, mask, sterile gown, sterile gloves, sterile full body drape) for the insertion of CVCs, peripherally inserted central catheters (PICCs), or guidewire exchange.
3. Prepare skin with an antiseptic (70% alcohol, tincture of iodine, or alcoholic chlorhexidine gluconate solution) before peripheral IV insertion.

(Continued on page 363)

Table 13-5. Pathogens and Drugs of Choice for Treating Common Viral Infections

Viral Infection	Drug of Choice	Duration
Cytomegalovirus (CMV)		
Retinitis[1]	Ganciclovir 5 mg/kg IV q12h × 14–21 days, then 5 mg/kg/d IV ganciclovir implant (Vitrasert) no longer manufactured	Retinitis 3–6 mo
	Ganciclovir 5 mg/kg IV q12h × 14–21 days, then valganciclovir 900 mg PO qd	
	Foscarnet 60 mg/kg IV q8h or 90 mg/kg IV q12h × 14–21 days, then 90–120 mg/kg/d IV	
	Cidofovir 5 mg/kg/wk IV × 2 wk, then 5 mg/kg IV q2wk	
Colitis, esophagitis[1]	Ganciclovir 5 mg/kg IV q12h, then valganciclovir 900 mg PO q12h when tolerating PO therapy	Colitis or esophagitis 21–42 days
Epstein-Barr Virus (EBV)	None	
Hepatitis A Virus[2] (HAV)	None, but gamma globulin 0.2 mL/kg/IM × 1 within 2 wk of exposure may limit infection[2]	
Hepatitis B Virus (HBV)		
Chronic hepatitis[3]	**Preferred**	
	Peg-IFN-alpha-2a 180 mcg SC qwk	48 wk
	Entecavir 0.5 mg PO qd	Duration variable
	Tenofovir dipivoxil fumarate 300 mg PO qd	Duration variable

(Continued)

13

353

Table 13-5. Pathogens and Drugs of Choice for Treating Common Viral Infections (*Continued*)

Viral Infection	Drug of Choice	Duration
	Tenofovir alafenamide 25 mg PO qd	Duration variable
	Nonpreferred	
	Lamivudine 100 mg PO qd	Duration variable
	Adefovir 10 mg PO qd	Duration variable
	Telbivudine 600 mg PO qd	Duration variable
Hepatitis C Virus[4] (HCV)		
Genotype	Recommended regimens[4]	Duration[4]
	Treatment-naïve and NOT coinfected with HIV[5]	
Genotype HCV 1a or 1b without cirrhosis or with compensated (Child-Pugh A) cirrhosis	Daily fixed dose of glecaprevir (300 mg)/pibrentasvir (120 mg)[6]	8 wk for patients without cirrhosis 12 wk for patients with compensated cirrhosis
	Daily fixed dose of sofosbuvir (400 mg)/velpatasvir (100 mg)	12 wk
	Daily fixed dose of elbasvir (50 mg)/grazoprevir (100 mg) for patients without baseline NS5A RASs for elbasvir[7]	12 wk
	Daily fixed dose of sofosbuvir (400 mg)/ledipasvir (90 mg)	12 wk
	Daily fixed dose of sofosbuvir (400 mg)/ledipasvir (90 mg) for patients who are nonblack, HIV-**uninfected**, and whose HCV RNA level <6 million IU/mL[8]	8 wk patient without cirrhosis
Genotype HCV 2 or 3 without cirrhosis or with compensated (Child-Pugh A) cirrhosis	Daily fixed dose of glecaprevir (300 mg)/pibrentasvir (120 mg)[5]	8 wk for patients without cirrhosis 12 wk for patients with compensated cirrhosis

	Daily fixed dose of sofosbuvir (400 mg)/velpatasvir (100 mg)	12 wk
Genotype HCV 4 without cirrhosis or with compensated (Child-Pugh A) cirrhosis	Daily fixed dose of glecaprevir (300 mg)/pibrentasvir (120 mg)[5]	8 wk for patients without cirrhosis 12 wk for patients with compensated cirrhosis
	Daily fixed dose of sofosbuvir (400 mg)/velpatasvir (100 mg)	12 wk
	Daily fixed dose of elbasvir (50 mg)/grazoprevir (100 mg)	12 wk
	Daily fixed dose of sofosbuvir (400 mg)/ledipasvir (90 mg)	12 wk
Genotype HCV 5 or 6 without cirrhosis or with compensated (Child-Pugh A) cirrhosis	Daily fixed dose of glecaprevir (300 mg)/pibrentasvir (120 mg)[5]	8 wk for patients without cirrhosis 12 wk for patients with compensated cirrhosis
	Daily fixed dose of sofosbuvir (400 mg)/velpatasvir (100 mg)	12 wk
	Daily fixed dose of sofosbuvir (400 mg)/ledipasvir (90 mg)	12 wk
Human Immunodeficiency Virus (HIV) (See Table 13-6)		
Herpes Simplex Virus (HSV)		
Orolabial herpes ("cold sore," "fever blister") in the immunocompetent with multiple recurrences (usually HSV-1)	Acyclovir (Zovirax) 5% cream applied 5 times per day Penciclovir (Denavir) % cream applied q2h while awake	4 days
	Valacyclovir 1 g PO BID Famciclovir 500 mg PO BID Acyclovir 400 mg PO TID	5–10 days

13

(Continued)

13

Table 13-5. Pathogens and Drugs of Choice for Treating Common Viral Infections (*Continued*)

Viral Infection	Drug of Choice	Duration
Genital herpes (HSV-1 or HSV-2) Initial or recurrent	Valacyclovir 1 g PO BID Famciclovir 500 mg PO BID Acyclovir 400 mg PO TID	5–10 days
Genital herpes (HSV-1 or HSV-2) Chronic suppressive therapy	Valacyclovir 500 mg PO BID Famciclovir 500 mg PO BID Acyclovir 400 mg PO BID	Daily
Mucocutaneous in the immunocompromised	Acyclovir 5 mg/kg IV q8h, then change to oral therapy when lesions regress	Oral therapy until lesions completely heal
Encephalitis	Acyclovir 10–15 mg/kg IV q8h	21 days
Neonatal	Acyclovir 20 mg/kg IV q8h	14–21 days
Acyclovir-resistant	Foscarnet 40 mg/kg IV q8h	Until clinical response
Keratoconjunctivitis	Trifluridine 1% solution, 1 drop topically q2h up to 9 drops/day Ganciclovir 0.15% 1–2 drops 5 × day	10 days
Influenza A and B Virus[9]		
	Oseltamivir 75 mg PO BID (>13 yr of age); <1 yr 3 mg/kg BID; 1–12 yr 30–75 mg BID (based on weight, see package insert or other reference)	5 days
	Zanamivir 10 mg (two 5-mg inhalations) BID by inhaler (>7 yr)	5 days
	Peramivir 600 mg IV over 15–30 min (>13 yr of age); 2–12 yr 12 mg/kg (max 600 mg)	One dose

MEASLES[10]

Baloxavir marboxil >12 yr, <80 kg, 40 mg × 1 dose; ≥80 kg, 80 mg PO × 1 dose

No antiviral helpful in treating measles

MMR vaccine within 72 hr of exposure OR immunoglobulin within 6 days (never simultaneously)

Immunoglobulin IM 0.5 mL/kg (Maximum dose = 15 mL)

Immunoglobulin IV 400 mg/kg

Severe cases in children

Vitamin A

50,000 IU for infants younger than 6 mo of age

100,000 IU for infants 6–11 mo of age

200,000 IU for children 12 mo of age and older

PAPILLOMA VIRUS (HPV)

Anogenital warts11

Imiquimod 3.75% cream applied once at bedtime q night (remove 6–10 hr later)

Imiquimod 5% cream applied once at bedtime 3 times/week (remove 6–10 hr later) for up to 16 wk | Max of 16 wk

Podofilox 0.5% solution or gel applied BID × 3 days followed by 4 days of no therapy and repeat up to 4 total cycles

Sinecatechins 15% ointment (0.5-cm strand of ointment to each wart) applied TID for up to 16 wk

Respiratory Syncytial Virus (RSV)

Ribavirin aerosol treatment 12–18 hr continuously | 3–7 days

Varicella Zoster Virus (VZV)

Exposure prophylaxis in the immunocompromised (HIV, steroids, etc.)

Varicella zoster immune globulin within 10 days of exposure | See package insert

13

(Continued)

13

Table 13-5. Pathogens and Drugs of Choice for Treating Common Viral Infections (*Continued*)

Viral Infection	Drug of Choice	Duration
Varicella (>12 yr old); tx not recommended for age <12 yr	Acyclovir 20 mg/kg (max 800 mg) PO QID Valacyclovir 20 mg/kg (max 1000 mg) PO TID	5 days
Herpes zoster	Valacyclovir 1 g PO TID Famciclovir 500 mg PO TID (for adults only) Acyclovir 800 mg PO 5 × /day	7 days
Varicella or zoster if immunocompromised	Acyclovir 10 mg/kg IV q8h	7 days
Acyclovir-resistant	Foscarnet 40 mg/kg IV q8h	10 days

CMV = cytomegalovirus; EBV = Epstein-Barr virus; HAV = hepatitis A virus; HBV = hepatitis B virus; HCV = hepatitis C virus; HIV = human immunodeficiency virus; HPV = human papilloma virus; HSV = herpes simplex virus; RSV = respiratory syncytial virus; VZV = varicella-zoster virus.

[1]aidsinfo.nih.gov/contentfiles/lvguidelines/adult_oi.pdf (Accessed April 10, 2020).

[2]MMWR May 19, 2006 / Vol. 55 / No. RR-7.

[3]Terrault NA, Lok ASF, McMahon BJ, et al. Update on Prevention, Diagnosis, and Treatment of Chronic Hepatitis B: AASLD 2018 Hepatitis B Guidance. Hepatology. 2018; 67(4): 1560–1599.

[4]American Association for the Study of Liver Disease, HCVGuidelines.org.

[5]For patients in whom prior therapy failed or those coinfected with HIV infection, regimen choice varies based on patient-specific data, including drug interactions and comorbidities.

[6]Three tablets once daily.

[7]For all genotype 1b-infected patients and genotype 1a-infected patients without baseline NS5A resistance-associated substitutions (RASs) at amino acid positions 28, 30, 31, or 93, which confer antiviral resistance.

[8]Only for patients without cirrhosis.

[9]Uyeki TM, Bernstein HH, Bradley JS, et al. Clinical Practice Guidelines by the Infectious Diseases Society of America: 2018 Update on Diagnosis, Treatment, Chemoprophylaxis, and Institutional Outbreak Management of Seasonal Influenza. *Clinical Infectious Diseases*, Volume 68, Issue 6, 15 March 2019, Pages e1– e47.

[10]https://www.cdc.gov/measles/hcp/index.html (Accessed May 5, 2020).

[11]https://www.cdc.gov/std/tg2015/warts.htm (Accessed June 5, 2020).

Table 13-6. Antiretroviral Regimens Recommended for Management of HIV-1 Infection in Antiretroviral-Naïve Patients[1] and Pre-exposure Prophylaxis (PrEP) in High-Risk Adults Who Are HIV Negative

Regimen	Drugs	Daily Pill Burden
Preferred initial regimens		
INSTI + 2 NRTIs	Dolutegravir (Tivicay) 50 mg + one of the following:[2] Tenofovir disoproxil fumerate/emtricitabine (Truvada)[3] Tenofovir alafenamide/emtricitabine (Descovy)[4]	2 tablets PO qd
	Dolutegravir (Tivicay) 50 mg + abacavir[5]/lamivudine (Epzicom) if HLA-B*5701 negative	2 tablets PO qd
	Bictegravir/tenofovir alafenamide/emtricitabine (Biktarvy[6])	1 PO qd
	Darunavir[7]/cobicistat[7] tenofovir alafenamide/emtricitabine (Symtuza[7])	1 PO qd
	Darunavir[7] (Prezista) + booster (ritonavir or cobicistat[7]) + one of the following: Tenofovir alafenamide/emtricitabine (Descovy) Tenofovir disoproxil fumerate/emtricitabine (Truvada) Tenofovir disoproxil fumerate/lamivudine (Cimduo)	2–3 tablets PO qd Darunavir[7]/cobicistat[7] (Prezcobix)
	Raltegravir (Isentress) + one of the following: Tenofovir alafenamide/emtricitabine (Descovy) Tenofovir disoproxil fumerate/emtricitabine (Truvada) Tenofovir disoproxil fumerate/lamivudine (Cimduo)	3 tablets PO qd Raltegravir 1200 mg (two 600-mg tablets) qd

(Continued)

13

Table 13-6. Antiretroviral Regimens Recommended for Management of HIV-1 Infection in Antiretroviral-Naïve Patients[1] and Pre-exposure Prophylaxis (PrEP) in High-Risk Adults Who Are HIV Negative (*Continued*)

Regimen	Drugs	Daily Pill Burden
Alternative	Elvitegravir[7]/cobicistat[7]/ tenofovir alafenamide/emtricitabine (Genvoya)	1 PO qd
	Elvitegravir[8]/cobicistat[8]/tenofovir disoproxil fumerate/emtricitabine (Stribild[8])	1 PO qd
Pre-exposure Prophylaxis (PrEP) (only if neg HIV)	Tenofovir alafenamide/emtricitabine (Descovy)	1 PO qd
	Tenofovir disoproxil fumerate/emtricitabine (Truvada)	1 PO qd

INSTI = integrase strand transfer inhibitor; NRTI = nucleoside reverse transcriptase inhibitor

[1]https://aidsinfo.nih.gov/drugs.

[2]Dolutegravir not recommended for women who are pregnant, wish to become pregnant, or are at risk of becoming pregnant.

[3]Tenofovir disoproxil fumerate associated with lower lipid levels.

[4]Tenofovir alafenamide associated with fewer bone and kidney toxicities. Select based on patient's comorbidities.

[5]Risk of hypersensitivity reaction if HLA-B*5701 positive.

[6]Has not been studied in pregnancy.

[7]Darunavir/cobicistat not recommended for pregnant women.

[8]Elvitegravir/cobicistat not recommended for pregnant women.

13

Table 13-7. Systemic Drugs for Managing Fungal Infections

Infection	Drug of Choice	Alternatives
ASPERGILLOSIS[1]		
Invasive Aspergillus (IA)	Voriconazole or isavuconazole	Liposomal amphotericin B Posaconazole
BLASTOMYCOSIS[2]		
Mild to moderate	Itraconazole	Fluconazole Voriconazole
Moderately severe to severe	Liposomal amphotericin B Step down after clinical response: Itraconazole	Amphotericin B Step down after clinical response: Voriconazole
CANDIDIASIS[3]		
Oropharyngeal	Fluconazole PO	Clotrimazole troches Miconazole mucoadhesive buccal tablet Itraconazole oral solution Posaconazole oral suspension Nystatin suspension
Esophageal	Fluconazole or itraconazole oral solution	Voriconazole Isavuconazole Caspofungin Micafungin Anidulafungin Amphotericin B Lipid formulation of amphotericin B
Vulvovaginal	Fluconazole PO or topical azoles (clotrimazole, butoconazole, miconazole, tioconazole, terconazole)	Itraconazole oral solution
COCCIDIOIDOMYCOSIS		
Mild	Fluconazole PO or Itraconazole PO	Voriconazole PO Posaconazole PO
Bone or joint infections	Itraconazole PO	Fluconazole PO
Severe, nonmeningeal infection	Lipid formulations of amphotericin B Amphotericin B	Addition of fluconazole or itraconazole

13

(Continued)

Table 13-7. Systemic Drugs for Managing Fungal Infections (*Continued*)

Infection	Drug of Choice	Alternatives
Meningeal infections	Fluconazole	Itraconazole Voriconazole Posaconazole
CRYPTOCOCCOSIS		
Meningitis		
Induction	Liposomal amphotericin + flucytosine Amphotericin B + flucytosine	Amphotericin B lipid complex + flucytosine Liposomal amphotericin B + fluconazole Amphotericin B + fluconazole
Consolidation	Fluconazole	Itraconazole
Maintenance	Fluconazole	
Non-CNS	Fluconazole	
HISTOPLASMOSIS		
Primary prophylaxis	Itraconazole	
Moderately severe to severe disseminated disease	Induction: Liposomal amphotericin B Maintenance: Itraconazole	Induction: Amphotericin B lipid complex
Less severe disseminated disease	Induction and maintenance: Itraconazole	Posaconazole Voriconazole Fluconazole
Meningitis	Induction: Liposomal amphotericin B Maintenance: Itraconazole	Voriconazole Posaconazole Fluconazole
MUCORMYCOSIS[4]	Liposomal formulation of amphotericin B	Amphotericin B Isavuconazole Posaconazole
PARACOCCIDIOIDOMYCOSIS[5]		
Mild to moderate	Itraconazole	Trimethoprim/sulfamethoxazole
Severe or disseminated	Amphotericin B, lipid formulations of amphotericin B	
SPOROTRICHOSIS[6]		

Table 13-7. Systemic Drugs for Managing Fungal Infections (*Continued*)

Infection	Drug of Choice	Alternatives
Cutaneous	Itraconazole	Potassium iodide 1–5 mL TID
Systemic	Amphotericin B, lipid formulations of amphotericin B Step down after clinical response: Itraconazole	

[1]Ullmann AJ, Aguado JM,cArikan-Akdagli S, et al. Diagnosis and management of Aspergillus diseases: Executive summary of the 2017 ESCMID-ECMM-ERS guideline. Clin Microbiol Infect. 2018;24(Suppl 1):e1–e38.
[2]Castillo CG, Kauffman CA, Miceli MH. Blastomycosis. Infect Dis Clin North Am. 2016;30(1):247–64.
[3]Pappas PG, Kauffman CA, Andes DR, et al. Clinical Practice Guideline for the Management of Candidiasis: 2016 Update by the Infectious Diseases Society of America. 2016;62(4):e1–e50.
[4]Cornely OA, Alastruey-Izquierdo, Arenz D, et al. Global guideline for the diagnosis and management of mucormycosis: An initiative of the European Confederation of Medical Mycology in Confederation with the Mycoses Study Group Education and Research Consortium. 2019;19(12):e405–421.
[5]Shikanai-Yasuda MA, Mendes RP, Colombo A, et al. Brazilian guidelines for the clinical management of paracoccidioidomycosis. Rev Soc Bras Med Trop. 2017;50(5):715–40.
[6]Kauffman CA, Bustamante B, Chapman SW, et al. Infectious Diseases Society of America; Clinical practice guidelines for the management of sporotrichosis: 2007 update by the Infectious Diseases Society of America. Clin Infect Dis. 2007;45(10):1255–65.

13

(Continued from page 352)

Use >0.5% chlorhexidine preparation with alcohol before CVC and peripheral arterial catheter insertion and during dressing changes.

4. Use sutureless securement devices to reduce the risk of infection from intravascular catheters. The use of antimicrobial-impregnated catheters has significantly reduced the rate of CLABSI.

5. Do not use topical antibiotic ointment or creams on insertion sites, except for dialysis catheters, because of their potential to promote fungal infections and antimicrobial resistance.

6. Replace gauze dressings on short-term CVC sites every 2 days and at least every 7 days for transparent dressings (Note: In pediatric patients, the risk of dislodging the catheter may outweigh the benefit of dressing changes. Transparent, semipermeable polyurethane dressings permit continuous visual inspection of the catheter site and require less frequent changes than do gauze dressings.)

7. Replace transparent dressings used on tunneled or implanted CVC (i.e., Hickman, Broviac catheters) sites no more than once per week unless the dressing is soiled or loose) until the insertion site has healed.

8. There is no need to replace peripheral IVs more frequently than every 72–96 hours to reduce the risk of infection and phlebitis in adults.

Table 13-8. Drugs for Treating Select Parasitic Infections

Infection	Drug
Amebiasis (*Entamoeba histolytica*)	
Asymptomatic	Paromomycin, iodoquinol/diiodohydroxyquin, or diloxanide furoate
Intestinal disease, hepatic abscess	Metronidazole or tinidazole followed by paromomycin, iodoquinol/diiodohydroxyquin, or diloxanide furoate
Ascariasis (*Ascaris lumbricoides*, roundworm)	Albendazole or mebendazole or ivermectin[1]
Cryptosporidiosis (*Cryptosporidium*)	Nitazoxanide
Cutaneous larva migrans (creeping eruption, dog and cat hookworm)	Albendazole or ivermectin
Cyclospora infection	Trimethoprim-sulfamethoxazole
Cystoisosporiasis (*Cystoisospora belli*)[2]	Trimethoprim-sulfamethoxazole
Enterobius vermicularis (pinworm)	Albendazole, mebendazole, pyrantel pamoate
Filariasis (*Wuchereria bancrofti, Brugia malayi, Loa loa*)	Diethylcarbamazine
Giardiasis (*Giardia lamblia*)	Metronidazole or tinidazole or nitazoxanide
Hookworm infection (*Ancylostoma duodenale, Necator americanus*)	Albendazole, mebendazole, pyrantel pamoate
Lice (*Pediculus humanus, P. capitis, Phthirus pubis*)	Topical agents: pyrethrins combined with piperonyl butoxide, permethrin (1%), malathion (0.5%), benzyl alcohol (5%), spinosad (0.9%), ivermectin (0.5%)
Malaria (*Plasmodium falciparum, P. ovale, P. vivax,* and *P. malariae*)	
Chloroquine-resistant *P. falciparum* or *P. vivax*	Artemether-lumefantrine (Coartem) Atovaquone-proguanil (Malarone) Quinine sulfate + doxycycline or tetracycline Quinine sulfate + clindamycin
All *Plasmodium* except chloroquine-resistant *P. falciparum*	Chloroquine phosphate Alternative: hydroxychloroquine
All *Plasmodium* (parenteral)	Artesunate IV
Prevention of relapses: *P. vivax* and *P. ovale* only	Tafenoquine (Krintafel) or primaquine phosphate

13

Table 13-8. Drugs for Treating Select Parasitic Infections

Infection	Drug
Malaria, prevention	
Chloroquine-sensitive areas	Chloroquine phosphate
Chloroquine-resistant areas	Atovaquone-proguanil, mefloquine, doxycycline, tafenoquine
Mites, see Scabies	
Pinworm, see *Enterobius*	
***Pneumocystis jirovecii* pneumonia**	Trimethoprim-sulfamethoxazole Alternative: mild to moderate: dapsone + trimethoprim or primaquine + clindamycin or atovaquone Moderate to severe: pentamidine or primaquine + clindamycin ± corticosteroids
Primary and secondary prophylaxis	Trimethoprim-sulfamethoxazole
Roundworm, see Ascariasis	
Scabies (*Sarcoptes scabiei*)	Permethrin (5%) Alternative: oral ivermectin, topical ivermectin, topical sulfur (5–10%)
Strongyloidiasis (*Strongyloides stercoralis*)	Ivermectin
Tapeworm infection	
Adult (intestinal stage)	Praziquantel Alternative: niclosamide (not available in the United States)
Diphyllobothrium latum (fish)	
Taenia saginata (beef)	
Taenia solium (pork)	
Dipylidium caninum (dog)	
Hymenolepis nana (dwarf tapeworm)	
Larval (tissue stage)	
Echinococcus granulosus (hydatid cyst)	Albendazole
Cysticercus cellulosae (cysticercosis)	Albendazole or praziquantel
Toxoplasmosis (*Toxoplasma gondii*)	Pyrimethamine + sulfadiazine
Trichinosis (*Trichinella spiralis*)	Steroids for severe symptoms + albendazole or mebendazole
Trichomoniasis (*Trichomonas vaginalis*)	Metronidazole or tinidazole

13

(Continued)

Table 13-8. Drugs for Treating Select Parasitic Infections (*Continued*)

Infection	Drug
Trichostrongyliasis (*Trichostrongylus colubriformis*)	Albendazole or mebendazole or pyrantel pamoate
Trypanosomiasis (*Trypanosoma cruzi*, Chagas disease)	Benznidazole or nifurtimox
Trichuriasis (*Trichuris trichiura*, whipworm)	Albendazole or mebendazole
Visceral larva migrans, toxocariasis (*Toxocara canis*)	Albendazole or mebendazole

[1]https://www.cdc.gov/parasites/ascariasis/health_professionals/index.html, accessed May 2, 2020.
[2]https://www.cdc.gov/parasites/cystoisospora/faqs.html, accessed May 2, 2020.

9. CVCs should be removed promptly when no longer needed or when a peripheral IV can be reasonably inserted and serve the same function as the CVC. Maintaining a CVC when it is not necessary increases the risk of bacterial colonization and subsequent CLABSIs over time. Routine catheter changes do not reduce the risk of CLABSIs, and routine guidewire catheter exchanges may increase the rate of infections. Use new sterile gloves before handling the new catheter when guidewire exchanges are performed.

10. Use a guidewire exchange to replace a malfunctioning nontunneled CVC if no evidence of infection is present.

Diagnosis and Management of CRBSI (see Figure 13-4, page 368)

CRBSI should be suspected in patients with vascular catheters who develop fever, chills, or other signs of sepsis, even in the absence of local signs of infection and if no alternative source is recognized. Nasal carriers of *S. aureus* are more likely to experience a CRBSI than noncolonized persons. Catheter replacement at scheduled intervals to reduce CRBSI has not lowered infection rates. The organisms most commonly causing CRBSIs include coagulase-negative staphylococci (31%), *S. aureus* (20%), *Enterococcus* species (9%), *Candida* species (9%), and *E. coli* (6%).

1. Remove peripheral IVs with signs of phlebitis (warmth, tenderness, erythema or palpable venous cord), infection, or malfunction.

2. For suspected CLABSI, paired blood culture samples (aerobic and anaerobic) drawn from the catheter and a peripheral vein should be obtained before initiation of antimicrobial therapy.

Table 13-9. Guide to Common Tick-Borne Diseases[1]

	Rocky Mountain Spotted Fever	Anaplasmosis[2]	Lyme Disease	Babesiosis
Causative Agent	*Rickettsia rickettsii* (bacterium)	*Anaplasma phagocytophilum* (bacterium)	*Borrelia burgdorferi, B. mayonii* (bacterium)	*Babesia microti* and other *Babesia* spp. (protozoan)
Season	Peaks in spring and summer (May–August)	Peaks in summer (June–July), may be seen year-round	Peaks in summer (June–July), may be seen year-round	Mostly spring/summer
Vector habits	American dog tick, Rocky Mountain wood tick, brown dog tick	Blacklegged tick, Western blacklegged tick	Blacklegged tick, Western blacklegged tick	Blacklegged tick
Classical clinical presentation	Sudden onset of fever, headache, maculopapular rash (with plantar/palmar presentation,	Fever, headache, gastrointestinal and constitutional symptoms	Erythema migrans (EM) rash, constitutional symptoms, arthritis, cardiovascular and nervous system involvement	Fever, hemolytic anemia, constitutional symptoms
Incubation period	3–12 days	5–14 days	3–30 days	1–9+ wk
Diagnosis	Clinical serology, PCR assay for bacterium	Clinical serology, PCR assay for bacterium	Clinical serology	Blood smear, PCR assay for protozoan
Treatment	Adults and children—doxycycline Pregnant women—consult specialist	Adults and children—doxycycline Pregnant women—consult specialist	Doxycycline, amoxicillin, cefuroxime	Atovaquone + azithromycin or clindamycin + quinine

[1]https://www.cdc.gov/ticks/tickbornediseases/index.html, accessed May 2, 2020.

[2]Human monocytic ehrlichiosis caused by *Ehrlichia chaffeensis* 1377/yr vs. HGA 5762/yr (Ref: CDC.gov). In 2001, *Ehrlicnia phagocytophilum* was officially renamed *Anaplasma phagocytophilum*. The disease was referred to as human granulocytic anaplasmosis (HGA) or more commonly anaplasmosis. The major species reservoirs are the white-tailed deer and the white-footed mouse. A. phagocytophilum is transmitted by *Ixodes scapularis* (blacklegged tick—East Coast and midwestern regions of US) and *Ixodes pacificus* (Western blacklegged tick—Pacific Coast). It is vectored by *Ixodes ricinus* ticks in Europe and Asia.

13

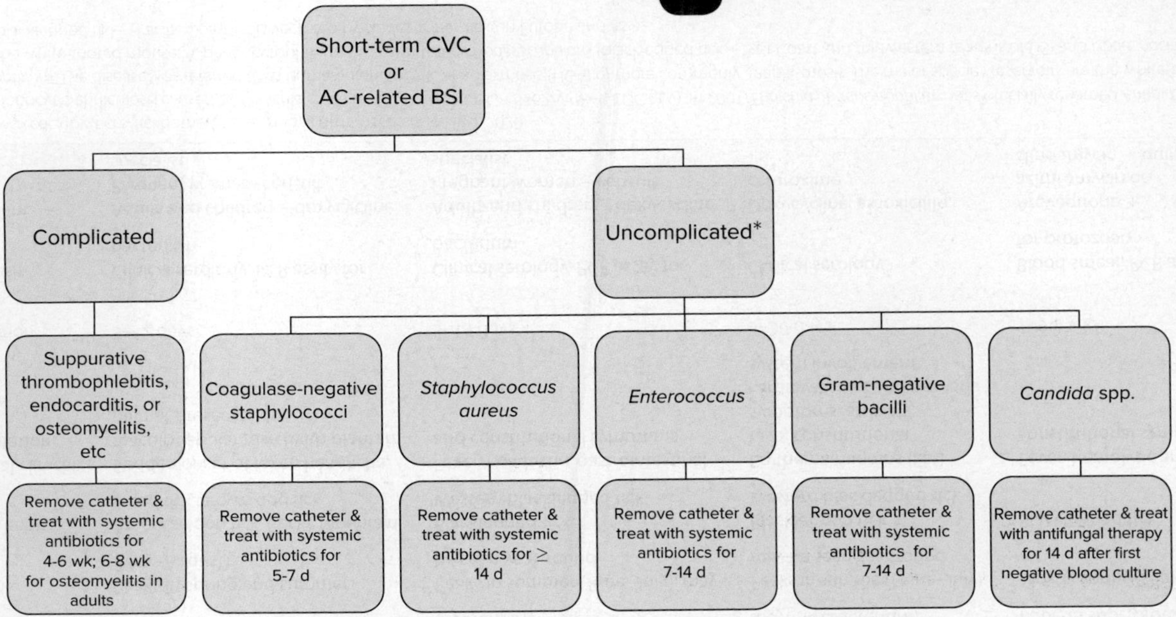

Figure 13-4. Algorithm for management of patients with short-term CVC-related or arterial-catheter-related blood stream infection. AC, arterial catheter; BSI, blood stream infection; CVC, central venous catheter.*Uncomplicated BSI: resolution of BSI within 72 hours; no intravascular hardware; no evidence of endocarditis, suppurative thrombophlebitis, or S. aureus infection; no active malignancy; and no immunosuppression. (From Prevention in the Intensive Care Unit Setting, McKean SC, Ross JJ, Dressler DD, Scheurer DB. Principles and Practice of Hospital Medicine, 2e; 2017, McGraw Hill Medical reproduced with permission)

3. Diagnosis of CLABSI can be by any of the following:

   a. The same organism grown from at least one percutaneous blood culture and from a culture of the catheter tip.

   b. Two blood samples, one from a catheter hub and the other from a peripheral vein; if both cultures are positive, then the criteria for CRBSI are met.

   c. Measurement of the differential time to positivity (the difference in time for blood cultures to become positive when they are drawn simultaneously through a central venous catheter and a peripheral vein) has been shown to be associated with catheter-related infection.

4. When diagnosis of a CLABSI is suspected or confirmed, the catheter should be removed immediately and antibiotics started ASAP. The line should be removed aseptically and 5 cm of the line tip submitted for culture. Isolation of ≥15 CFUs of the catheter tip equals true line-associated infection; <15 CFUs suggest contamination during removal. Do not routinely culture line tips upon removal from asymptomatic patients.

5. When the organism is identified, antibiotics should be tailored to the sensitivity of the organisms grown in culture (Figure 13-4).

13

Central Nervous System Infection

(See also Table 13-4, page 337–338, for specific bacterial pathogens in meningitis and meningitis related to head trauma and Chapter 19, Lumbar Puncture, page 619, for the technique and CSF differential diagnosis.)

1. Obtain a head CT before lumbar puncture (LP) if any of the following is true: focal neurologic signs are present, a seizure has occurred, papilledema is present, the patient's age >60 yr, HIV-1–positive or immunocompromised state is present, or a change in mental status.

2. Details on the LP technique to evaluate CSF can be found in Chapter 19, page 621. Measure opening pressure. A high opening pressure (>25 cm water) suggests a complication of an LP is possible (e.g., brain herniation and risk of death).

3. Order routine tests on the CSF: Cell count with differential, protein, glucose, Gram stain, and bacterial culture.

4. Consider ordering NAAT for the following common viruses: HSV-1/HSV-2 and enterovirus, as well as common bacteria causing CNS infections. May consider viral culture, though yield is often low compared to NAAT. Multiplex panels are able to detect the most common causes of viral and bacterial CNS infections; however, there are significant false negative results

5. Consider ordering CSF cryptococcal antigen test and/or India ink stain for detection of *Cryptococcus* (see Chapter 10, page 205).

6. Because cryptococcal meningitis can be life threatening in HIV/AIDS patients, obtain CSF opening pressure because *Cryptococcus* can impede

the flow of CSF with severe consequences (severe headache, cranial nerve deficits, seizure disorder, and brainstem herniation).

7. Consider ordering fungal culture if a fungal etiology is considered. Fungal culture and stain (KOH/calcofluor white) must be performed since routine bacterial cultures will not effectively identify many pathogenic fungi.

8. Order AFB smear and culture if sufficient clinical suspicion and there are risk factors for CNS mycobacterial infection.

9. Consider ordering syphilis antibody testing, e.g., RPR or treponemal antibody on serum and/or VDRL on CSF if sufficient clinical suspicion and there are risk factors for CNS syphilis infection (see Chapter 10, pages 250–252, 260, and 262).

Hepatitis

(See also Chapter 10, pages 222–227)

Hepatitis is hepatocellular injury that can be from a wide variety of causes. Classically, we think of hepatitis A (HAV) or B (HBV); however, many other processes can cause inflammation of the liver, including other infectious etiologies, toxins, medications, decreased O_2 delivery to the liver (shock, vascular injury, heat stroke), and immune mediated (autoimmune hepatitis). Pathologic processes involving the liver are often classified as obstructive or inflammatory.

- Obstructive processes, such as metastatic carcinoma, will usually have an elevated bilirubin, alkaline phosphatase, and GGT out of proportion to any elevation of AST or ALT.

- In contrast, hepatocellular injury will generally have an elevated AST and ALT (often markedly elevated) out of proportion to elevations of alkaline phosphatase, GGT, and often bilirubin.

- Medications can cause either an obstructive or a hepatocellular injury pattern. Acetaminophen overdose, isoniazid, halothane, and phenytoin are medications that classically cause hepatocellular injury. A number of toxins, including carbon tetrachloride, *Amanita phalloides* (deadly poisonous fungus, often mistaken for an edible mushroom), and alcohol, cause hepatocellular injury. Alcoholic hepatitis is one of the most common causes of hepatitis in the United States.

- Infectious etiologies are predominately viral; however, there are bacterial etiologies (leptospirosis and syphilis), fungal (histoplasmosis), and parasitic etiologies (amebiasis, others). Besides HAV, HBV, HCV, HDV, and HEV, other viruses can cause an acute hepatitis, including CMV, EBV, coxsackievirus, herpes simplex, and others.

1. ***Hepatitis A Testing:*** Acute HAV is diagnosed when anti–HAV IgM antibodies are detected. These antibodies appear soon after the initial infection and persist for approximately 4 mo. Anti–HAV IgG titer

increases slowly, reaching its peak approximately 4 mo after infection, and then persists for many years.

2. *Hepatitis B Testing:* The incubation period of HBV is about 12 wk. HBV surface antigen (HBsAg) usually appears in the first 10 wk after exposure. If HBsAg remains elevated beyond the first 6 mo, then the diagnosis of chronic HBV can be made. Testing for HBeAg and HBV viral DNA should be done to confirm viral replication and infectivity; used to guide treatment.

3. *Hepatitis C Testing:* HCV is screened by detecting anti-HCV antibodies. A positive result does not indicate whether the patient has had a previous infection and cleared the virus (15–30% of patients) or if the patient has a chronic infection. Anti-HCV antibodies do not appear in a naive patient until at least 8–10 wk after exposure. However, since the majority of patients infected with HCV do not present with acute hepatitis, it is those chronically infected that will likely be identified via screening with anti-HCV antibody assay. The U.S. Preventive Services Task Force (USPSTF) recommends offering one-time screening for HCV infection for anyone 18–79 years old. Individuals who inject drugs, they should undergo periodic screening; however, the frequency of screening has not been determined.

13

A. **Confirmatory testing** is performed with HCV NAAT. HCV NAAT testing is divided into two categories:
   - *Qualitative testing,* which may be used to confirm infection.
   - *Quantitative testing* (viral load), which may be used to confirm infection and monitor response to therapy.

B. **Genotyping** of HCV is performed to determine the optimal antiviral regimen. Compared to previous therapies, current direct-acting antiviral therapies cure >95% of patients. Cure is defined as a sustained virologic response (SVR), which is the absence of detectable viral RNA 12 wk following completion of therapy.

HIV TESTING AND SCREENING

(HIV tests are also discussed in Chapter 10, pages 228–231)

Routine HIV testing is done using a fourth-generation screening assay, which detects anti-HIV-1 and anti-HIV-2 antibodies, in addition to HIV P24 antigen. If fourth-generation screening assay is positive, antibodies are differentiated and confirmed using a commercially available supplemental assay. If the supplemental assay fails to confirm antibody, HIV viral RNA NAAT may help for clarification.

1. *Testing for HIV-1 in Acute Retroviral Syndrome:* New infection with HIV often manifests as a protean mononucleosis–like illness that

has been designated **acute retroviral syndrome** (estimated incidence 20–90% in different series). The syndrome occurs 1–6 wk after infection and is marked by fever, lymphadenopathy, myalgia, and pharyngitis (nonexudative, unlike the pharyngitis that occurs with mononucleosis). Maculopapular viral exanthema, usually on the trunk, occurs in about 50% of patients. **The most important factor in the diagnosis of acute retroviral syndrome is to have a high index of clinical suspicion.** Because of its protean nature, the diagnosis is often missed.

Testing for acute retroviral syndrome and newly asymptomatic HIV-1 infection can be problematic. HIV-1 seroconversion (when specific antibodies become detectable in the serum and can be used for diagnostic purposes) usually occurs 4–16 wk after initial infection. HIV-1 P24 antigen appears in the serum usually in the first 2 wk following infection and remains detectable until the host generates sufficient anti-P24 antibody to neutralize the antigen. The fourth-generation HIV screening assays usually detect HIV infection 18–45 days after exposure. Thus, if acute HIV infection is suspected and the initial test is negative, a retest in several weeks may need to be scheduled. Quantitative RT-PCR for HIV-1 RNA is helpful in diagnosing infection and for treatment monitoring.

2. *HIV-1 and Pregnancy:* Decreasing the incidence of vertical transmission of HIV-1 from mother to infant is an issue of paramount importance. The use of **universal prenatal HIV counseling and testing, antiretroviral therapy (ART) for all infected pregnant women,** scheduled cesarean section for women with HIV viral load >1000 copies/mL near delivery, ART for infants, and abstinence from breastfeeding have led to a drop in vertical transmission rates from 25% to <2%. To reduce the risk of perinatal transmission, ART should be administered before, during, and after birth to the woman as well as postpartum to the neonate. ART should be administered to all pregnant women with HIV as early as possible, regardless of their viral load or CD4 count. Drug-resistance genotype assays should be performed before starting ART, but ART should NOT be delayed until results of drug-resistance testing become available.

Maintaining an HIV viral load below the limit of detection during pregnancy and postpartum is critical in reducing the risk of perinatal transmission. Thus, strict adherence to medications is recommended to achieve rapid viral suppression. The decision about which ART to use in a pregnant woman is a complex decision requiring discussion and careful assessment of risk to both mother and fetus. Intravenous zidovudine is recommended to women with HIV if HIV viral load >1000 copies/mL near the time of delivery. All newborns exposed to HIV peripartum should receive ART to minimize the risk of perinatal transmission of HIV.

3. *Baseline Tests after New Diagnosis of HIV and Referral to HIV Specialist:*

ART should be started immediately following the diagnosis except when there is concomitant active infection with *Mycobacterium tuberculosis,* in which case when to start HIV treatment is dependent on the CD4 count. For treatment regimens, see Table 13-6, page 359. The baseline tests used for most of the major clinical decisions regarding HIV-1 therapy are quantitative reverse transcription PCR for HIV-1 RNA (viral load) and CD4 T-cell count. The results are used in decisions on which ART to use, when to change ART in the face of virologic failure (viral load no longer suppressed), and when to give prophylaxis to prevent opportunistic infections such as *P. jiroveci*, cerebral toxoplasmosis, and disseminated *M. avium-intracellulare* infection.

a. Order HIV genotype, including integrase, and HLA-B*5701 to determine which ART regimen is appropriate. The results of these tests are used to modify the initial ART if necessary.

b. Order a series of routine tests such as a comprehensive metabolic panel and a CBC to assess the patient's bone marrow, kidney, and liver function.

c. Order anti-HAV, anti-HBs, anti-HBc, HBsAg, and anti-HCV.

d. Order STD testing: RPR or VDRL, chlamydia and gonorrhea NAAT tests (urine, pharynx, rectum as indicated by sites of exposure).

e. Order TB screening test (e.g., QuantiFERON).

f. Order pregnancy test (if appropriate).

g. Consider a fasting lipid panel because of the risk of adverse lipid effects from treatment with certain classes of ART, such as protease inhibitors.

h. If a patient has an allergy to TMP–SMX and needs prophylaxis to *P. jiroveci*, or develops an allergy during prophylaxis, consider treatment with dapsone; order a G6PD assay to rule out G6PD deficiency, especially if the patient is of Mediterranean or African origin or descent.

i. Consider toxoplasma IgG.

j. Review the initial treatment in this chapter, page 359. Complete up-to-date HIV guidelines are available online at www.aidsinfo.nih.gov/guidelines.

Infectious Diarrhea

(See also Table 13-4, page 336)

Infectious diarrhea can be further classified based on duration.

Acute diarrhea of infectious etiology is passage of a greater number of stools of decreased form from normal lasting <14 days or abrupt onset of 3 or more loose or liquid stools above baseline in a 24 hr. Acute diarrheal infection is also often referred to as gastroenteritis, and some acute gastrointestinal infections may have a vomiting-predominant illness with little or no diarrhea. Infectious diarrhea is usually associated with other clinical features suggesting enteric involvement such as nausea, vomiting, abdominal pain and cramps, bloating, flatulence, fever, passage of bloody stools, tenesmus, and fecal urgency.

Persistent diarrhea is diarrhea lasting between 14 and 30 days, with **chronic diarrhea** generally having diarrheal symptoms lasting for greater than a month. Testing stool for bacterial pathogens is recommended for patients with diarrhea and fever, bloody or mucoid stools, severe abdominal cramping or tenderness, or sepsis (additional testing is recommended in all immunocompromised patients). Blood cultures are recommended for those who are less than 3 months of age, septic, or at risk for enteric fever. Some microbiologic tests used in the evaluation of diarrhea are:

1. **Stool Culture:** NAAT platforms are beginning to replace routine stool culture. Several multiplex panels are able to detect the most common causes of bacterial, parasitic, and viral diarrhea and are commercially available. A fresh stool sample may be cultured for diagnosis of bacterial diarrhea. Most common pathogens, e.g., *Salmonella, Shigella,* and *E. coli* 0.157, can be grown on targeted routine standard media. Less common pathogens, e.g., *Yersinia, Vibrio,* and *Campylobacter,* require special culture media, and their cultures need to be specifically ordered.

2. **Fecal Lactoferrin and Stool Leukocyte Stains (e.g., Fecal Leukocytes, Löffler Methylene Blue Stain):** Both indicate presence of WBCs in stool and signify inflammation of the bowel. Both help differentiate inflammatory from secretory and osmotic diarrhea. Presence of stool leukocytes suggests inflammatory conditions such as bacterial infection, inflammatory bowel disease, TB, and amebic infection.

3. **Clostridoides difficile (formerly Clostridium difficile but still called "C. diff"):** Clinical course can be quite variable, ranging from simple diarrhea of short duration to cases of fulminant pseudomembranous colitis, which can be rapidly fatal. The classic triad of fever, leukocytosis, and diarrhea should suggest the possibility of *C. difficile* colitis. Risk factors for acquisition include antibiotic exposure (clindamycin, second- to fourth-generation cephalosporins, fluoroquinolones, and macrolides are the most common), hospitalization, certain chemotherapeutic regimens (cisplatin, others), advanced age, increasing severity of illness, and anything that disturbs bowel motility, including surgery and medications besides antibiotics such as PPIs and H2-blockers. Immunoassays detecting *C. difficile* antigen and NAAT for toxin gene detection in stool may be used alone or in combination depending on institutional protocol.

4. **Stool for Ova and Parasites:** The Infectious Disease Society of America suggest that patients with persistent diarrhea (>14 days' duration) be tested for parasites, especially if they are immunocompromised or an international traveler. Worldwide *Giardia lamblia* and *Entamoeba histolytica* are the most common intestinal parasites, but the specific parasite can vary based on travel history, exposures, and immune status.

5. **Gastrointestinal Panel Testing.** Some labs may offer fecal PCR panel testing for GI infections caused by the following organisms (individual lab panels may vary): *Campylobacter* species, *Clostridoides (Clostridium) difficile, Plesiomonas shigelloides, Salmonella* species, *Vibrio* species, *V. cholerae, Yersinia* species, *enteroaggregative E. coli, enteropathogenic E.*

coli, enterotoxigenic E. coli, shiga toxin-producing *E. coli, E. coli O157, Shigella, enteroinvasive E. coli, Cryptosporidium* species*, Cyclospora cayetanensis, Entamoeba histolytica, Giardia lamblia,* adenovirus serotypes 40 and 41, astrovirus, norovirus, rotavirus, and sapovirus.

INFECTIVE ENDOCARDITIS PROPHYLAXIS

The most recent guidelines for IE prophylaxis from the American Heart Association was last published in 2007 and endorsed with one modification involving IE prophylaxis for transcatheter prosthetic values in the 2017 American Heart Association/American College of Cardiology (AHA/ACC) Focused Update of the 2014 AHA/ACC Guideline for the Management of Patients with Valvular Heart Disease (Wilson W, et al. Circulation 2009;116:1736–54.; Nishimura RA, et al. Circulation 2017;135:e1159–e1195; Endocarditis Prophylaxis for Dental Procedures. The Medical Letter. 2012; 1399:74–5).

- There is lack of evidence to support aggressive antimicrobial IE prophylaxis. Even with proper antibiotic administration, only a very small number of IE cases can be prevented. Furthermore, no longer is IE prophylaxis recommended based on a patient's lifetime risk, and endocarditis prophylaxis is no longer recommended for GI or GU procedures. The risk of adverse events from the antibiotics used for prophylaxis exceed the benefit from preventing the very rare case of IE as the result of a GI or GU procedure. However, antibiotics for GI or GU procedures may be given for other indications such as acute cystitis. If there is an active GU infection with *Enterococcus* spp. in a patient who needs an elective GU procedure, it is reasonable to eradicate the infection before the procedure.
- For procedures involving dermatologic and musculoskeletal structures, antibiotic prophylaxis is not recommended; however, if there is an infection involving the skin or accompanying structures or musculoskeletal tissue, then antibiotics should be given to treat the known or presumed infection. The antibiotics chosen should cover *Staphylococcus* and beta-hemolytic *Streptococcus*.
- IE prophylaxis is now recommended only for the highest-risk dental procedures for the patients who are at the highest risk. The dental procedures requiring prophylaxis are any procedures involving gingival manipulation or at or around the apex of the teeth or with perforation of the oral mucosa, excluding injections and adjustments or placement of appliances or brackets. See Table 13-10, page 376, for specific regimens.
- Additionally, the highest-risk patients undergoing respiratory tract procedures that involve mucosal biopsy or incision, including tonsillectomy and adenoidectomy, should receive IE prophylaxis. The regimen chosen is the same as for dental procedures (Table 13-10, page 376).

13

Table 13-10. Infective Endocarditis Prophylaxis for Dental and Oral Procedures (and Respiratory Procedures if Incision or Biopsy of the Mucosa)

Prophylaxis	Agent	Regimen (all dosing is 30–60 min before the procedure)
Standard	Amoxicillin	Adults: 2 gm; peds: 50 mg/kg
Unable to take oral meds	Ampicillin	Adults: 2 gm IM^2 or IV; peds^3 50 mg/kg IM^2 or IV
	Cefazolin^1 or ceftriaxone^1	Adults: 1 gm IM^2 or IV; peds 50 mg/kg IM^2 or IV
PCN allergic	Cephalexin	Adults: 2 gm; peds 50 mg/kg
	Clindamycin	Adults: 600 mg; peds 20 mg/kg
	Azithromycin or clarithromycin	Adults: 500 mg; peds: 15 mg/kg
PCN allergic and cannot take PO meds	Cefazolin^1 or ceftriaxone^1	Adults: 1 gm IM^2 or IV; peds 50 mg/kg IM^2 or IV
	Clindamycin	Adults: 600 mg IM^2 or IV; peds 20 mg/kg IM^2 or IV

^{1}DO NOT use if history of severe reaction to PCN (anaphylaxis, angioedema, urticaria).
^{2}DO NOT give IM if on anticoagulation.
^{3}Total peds dose should not exceed adult dose.

- These updated guidelines specify that prophylaxis is reasonable before many dental, oral, or respiratory procedures (with mucosal incision or biopsy) in the following high-risk patients:

   1. Prosthetic cardiac valves, including transcatheter-implanted prostheses and homografts.
   2. Prosthetic material used for cardiac valve repair, such as annuloplasty rings and chords.
   3. Previous IE.
   4. Unrepaired cyanotic congenital heart disease or completely repaired cyanotic congenital heart disease with prosthetic material or implanted device within the first 6 months postop, or status post-repair with residual defects such as valvular regurgitation at the site of or adjacent to the site of prosthetic patch or prosthetic device.
   5. Cardiac transplant with valve regurgitation due to a structurally abnormal valve.

Pulmonary Infections and COVID-19

(See also Table 13-4, page 332, Table 13-5, page 353, and Table 13-7, page 361, for specific bacterial, viral, and fungal pathogens)

Pulmonary infections cover a wide area in medicine, including atypical pneumonia, community-acquired pneumonia, nosocomial pneumonia, bronchitis, influenza, and a variety of other infections due to other viral, fungal and parasitic causes.

Sputum Culture and Stain: An early morning sample is preferred because such samples are more likely from the lower airway. A Gram stain can be used to guide therapy. As with a Gram stain of any clinical specimen, a **high neutrophil to epithelial cell ratio argues against** a contaminated specimen. The presence of >10 epithelial cells/lpf (low power field) suggests the specimen is more likely saliva than sputum and is inadequate for detecting a pulmonary infection. Steps to improve the quality of the sputum collection include:

1. Careful instructions to the patient to produce a sample from the lungs. If the patient cannot mobilize the secretions, P&PD along with nebulizer treatments may help, as may nasotracheal suctioning with a specimen trap.
2. Most labs do not accept anaerobic sputum cultures (critical in the diagnosis of aspiration pneumonia and lung abscesses) unless obtained by transtracheal aspiration or endobronchial endoscopic collection and submitted in special anaerobic transport media.

13

Fungal Culture and Stain: Routine sputum cultures will not effectively identify many pathogenic fungi. If a fungal etiology is suspected, a fungal culture and stain (KOH/calcofluor white) must be performed. *Pneumocystis* pneumonia is difficult to diagnose with expectorated sputum. Therefore, if suspected, an endobronchial lavage or open lung biopsy should be performed. Since *P. jiroveci* cannot be cultured, specialized stains for directly identifying *P. jiroveci*, such as monoclonal immunofluorescence, calcofluor white, methenamine silver, Giemsa, or toluidine blue, must be used. NAAT methods are also frequently used.

Viral Detection: Multiple methods are available to identify specific pathogenic viruses. The collection of most viral samples requires the sample be placed in viral transport medium that contains antimicrobials designed to inhibit overgrowth of bacteria and fungi that may normally contaminate a sample from a nasopharyngeal swab or BAL (see also pages 327–328).

- The role of culture is diminishing as newer tests are developed that provide more rapid results and are able to detect a larger number of viruses. If clinically indicated, viral cultures may still be performed on a variety of respiratory specimens. For viral culture, the specimen should be transported to the microbiology lab without delay, and refrigeration is recommended if a significant delay is anticipated.
- NAAT based on PCR platforms have become commonplace. Several multiplex panels able to detect the most common causes of viral respiratory infection are commercially available. Many single analyte assays are also available when a specific virus is suspected, e.g., influenza or RSV.

- Immunoassays with formation of antigen–antibody through recognition and binding with fluorescent antibody (FA) is widely used in diagnostic virology.
- ***Rapid Viral Testing:*** Rapid antigen, fluorescent antibody, and NAAT platforms for detecting some respiratory viruses, e.g., influenza A and B viruses, in nasopharyngeal swabs are now available as point of care testing.

COVID-19: See also Chapter 10, page 202. See Chapter 28, Critical Care, for specific recommendations on ICU management of the patient with COVID-19, page 938 based on consensus held by the Surviving Sepsis Campaign group (Alhazzani W, et al. Surviving Sepsis Campaign: Guidelines on the Management of Critically Ill Adults with Coronavirus Disease 2019 (COVID-19), Intensive Care Med 2020;48(6):854–887.)

- **Coronavirus and clinical disease.** Coronaviruses are enveloped single stranded RNA viruses that cause upper and lower respiratory tract infections. Coronaviruses have historically been a cause of the "common cold" and over the last 20 years coronaviruses have caused three serious clinical syndromes. Each virus had initially spread amongst animal hosts before jumping to humans. The first of the three viruses, severe acute respiratory syndrome coronavirus (SARS-CoV), was first identified in November 2002. There were approximately 8,000 cases worldwide with a mortality rate of roughly 10%. The second virus, Middle East respiratory syndrome coronavirus (MERS-CoV), was first identified in Saudi Arabia in 2012. A total of approximately 2,500 cases have been identified since 2012 with a mortality rate of about 35%. The third virus, severe acute respiratory syndrome coronavirus-2 (SARS-CoV-2), is the cause of COVID-19, which emerged in mid-November 2019.
- The Coronavirus Study Group of the International Committee on Taxonomy of Viruses has proposed that this virus be designated **severe acute respiratory syndrome coronavirus 2 (SARS-CoV-2),** and the clinical syndrome or disease is referred to as **COVID-19**.
- As of February 7, 2022, worldwide there were approximately 397,400,000 cases of COVID-19 or 50,454 cases/million people and 5,763,000 deaths or 731 deaths/million people. As of January 30, 2022 there are no countries in the world without a case of COVID-19, either active or recovered. In the United States as of February 7, 2022, there were a total of 75,500,000 cases and the number of deaths attributable to COVID-19 was 927,800. These number equte to approximately 227,000 cases/million people and 2,790 deaths/million. There have been five waves of COVID in the United States, April-June 2020, November 2020-January 2021, March-April 2021, July-November 2021 and the fifth wave started in December 2022 and was caused by the omicron variant. While this variant spreads more easily and many people are asymptomatic, the mortality rate is less than with earlier previous variants.
- **Transmission.** While the mortality rate is significantly lower compared to SARS-CoV and MERS-CoV, SARS-CoV-2 spread more rapidly throughout the world in part due to the high prevalence of asymptomatic infections, estimated to be 40–45%, and some experts think this percentage may be

much higher. Asymptomatic infections are more likely to occur in a younger population and more often in women. Even though SARS-CoV-2 infection in children is less severe, children can play a significant role in the spread of the virus. The delta variant is the predominant strain detected in the US in August 2021 (75-80% of new cases). According to the CDC, it is more contagious than chicken pox. In other countries, the delta variant rapidly infected the unvaccinated population, and then the case rate rapidly decreased.

- The incubation period is a median of 5 days and for 97.5% of those infected, the incubation period is <12 days. Transmission is thought to occur between the 3 days prior to symptom onset to approximately 7–10 days after the onset of symptoms for mild to moderate COVID-19. In severe cases of COVID-19, an individual may be infectious up to 20 days after the onset of symptoms. Viral shedding may occur well beyond this infectious period; however, the detection of SAR-CoV-2 RNA does not infer infectivity.

- SARS-CoV-2 is primarily spread via respiratory transmission, and the risk is increased based on proximity to the infected person. This suggests droplet transmission is more likely than aerosol transmission. Increasing ventilation can reduce the risk of secondary household transmission. The risk of direct contact transmission is low. Though rare, there is a risk of vertical transmission. Also, while viral RNA from SARS-CoV-2 is detected in blood, there have been no documented cases of blood-borne transmission.

- **Symptoms and signs.** Though a significant number of infected patients are asymptomatic, flu-like symptoms, including fever, chills, cough, headache, fatigue, and myalgias, are common as well as dyspnea and pleuritic chest pain. Loss of the senses of smell and taste occur in approximately 50% of symptomatic cases and are highly suggestive of SARS-CoV-2 infection. Additionally, patients may have GI symptoms such as nausea, vomiting, and diarrhea. As the disease progresses, many individuals develop dyspnea related to severe lower respiratory involvement that often requires hospitalization and intubation. Some individuals will have a significant inflammatory response from a "cytokine storm." Positive acute phase reactants, such as ferritin, will be markedly increased, and inflammatory markers may identify a subset of patients whose treatment may target the exaggerated cytokine response. Also, there is a high incidence of thromboembolic events in patients with COVID-19. Furthermore, approximately 10% of individuals will continue to have symptoms for months after initially becoming symptomatic. These individuals have been termed "long haulers," and fatigue, myalgias, dyspnea, and cough are common persistent symptoms. Additionally, difficulty concentrating and impaired memory have been referred to as "brain fog" and when associated with marked fatigue resemble chronic fatigue syndrome. There have also been individuals who develop postural orthostatic tachycardia syndrome (POTS) post-COVID-19.

- **Prevention.** In addition to immunization (pages 383 and 1083), social distancing, wearing of masks, and avoiding large gatherings of people slow the spread of SARS-CoV-2. Indoor versus outdoor gatherings are higher risk and if the number of people attending precludes 6 ft of social distancing, the risk is greater. Furthermore, attendees from outside the local

13

community increase the risk. Increasing ventilation within a dwelling can reduce the risk of secondary household transmission. Additionally, in an outpatient study of patients with COVID-19 (Fischer, et al., 2020), having recently gone to a restaurant is reported 2.4–2.8 times more often than in those without an infection. For individuals without a close COVID-19 contact, going to a bar or a coffee shop was reported 3.9 times more often in infected patients compared to uninfected controls.

- **Viral RNA and viral antigen testing for diagnosis of an acute COVID-19 infection**. Viral RNA and viral antigen testing are performed by collecting a nasal, nasopharyngeal, or oropharyngeal sample depending on the test (see Chapter 10, page 202). Point of care testing can now be performed and can provide a positive test in as few as 5 minutes with some manufacturers' tests. Most samples are either tested by hospital clinical laboratories or are sent out to reference laboratories (adding additional time for turnaround). Run time of the assay depends on the specific test performed, but generally ranges from 2–8 hours once the test is initiated. The U.S. Food and Drug Administration authorized the first diagnostic test with a home collection option for COVID-19 in May 2020 under the auspices of the emergency use authorization (EUA). Additionally, an EAU was authorized for at-home testing in November 2020. These tests are available by prescription or can be obtained over the counter.
- **Antibody testing.** The FDA issued an EUA to Cellex Inc., for a SARS-CoV-2 antibody test in early April 2020. Also, in April 2020, the Centers for Disease Control (CDC) developed an antibody test designed for broad-based surveillance. Since April 2020, many other companies have developed and released SARS-CoV-2 antibody assays. Sensitivity of antibody testing <3 days from symptom onset is near 0% and increases to above 90% at 2–3 wk post infection with assays from US based companies. Antibody testing should never be used to diagnosis of COVID-19 except when SARSCoV-2 RNA (usually by PCR) test is negative and a repeat test is also negative and the symptoms have been present for about 2 wk. An antibody test will be beneficial to identify people who were previously infected, recovered, and hopefully immune to reinfection, though there have been many documented cases of patients being infected a second time many months after recovery from the initial infection. Assays for antibodies to the spike protein and nucleocapsid protein are available. Antibodies to the nucleocapsid protein have a higher sensitivity than to the spike protein for SARS-CoV-2 infection. The assay for the spike-protein antibodies can be used to assess for an immune response to vaccination. IgG, IgM, and IgA antibodies can be detected.
- **Immunity.** A full understanding of the immunity conferred following SARS-CoV-2 infection may not be possible for some time. Additional clinical experience with this virus will demonstrate whether infection results in short- or long-term immunity. Long-term immunity would imply that a previously infected person would no longer be at risk for reinfection with SARS-CoV-2; however, this is unlikely (at least for many) since there are more and more cases of someone being infected a second time. Antibody testing will help us better understand the extent to which the virus percolated through the

population via either asymptomatic carriers or mildly symptomatic individuals who did not seek medical attention. Additionally, reliable antibody tests will be useful in assessing immunity conferred during vaccine trials.

- **Treatment.** There are many ongoing research studies on the treatment and prevention of COVID-19. COVID-19 treatment guidelines and recommendations are changing rapidly; and while the treatments below were accurate when they were written, they may have changed. Be sure to review the National Institutes of Health (NIH) or Infectious Disease Society of America (IDSA) recommendations or other references such as the Medical Letter so you can provide the most up-to-date treatment for your patients. The treatments under investigation include many different medications from a wide variety of drug classes. The Food and Drug Administration (FDA) has issued several Emergency Use Authorizations (EUAs) for different treatments, including convalescent plasma, remdesivir, monoclonal antibodies, and a JAK enzyme inhibitor. One problem with issuing a EUA is that patient recruitment for randomized-controlled trails may be hampered and thus delay the completion of trails needed on which to base sound clinical guidelines.

- **Treatment, remdesivir.** Prior to mid-April 2020, the only treatment available was aggressive supportive care, including in some cases, extracorporeal membrane oxygenation (ECMO). Remdesivir, an antiviral active against SARS-CoV-2, received an EUA on May 1, 2020 and full approval by the FDA in October of that year to treat hospitalized patients with COVID-19 who are $\geq$12 years old and weighing $\geq$40 kg. Remdesivir was developed initially to treat Ebola infection and has been shown to shorten time to recovery from COVID-19. The Infectious Disease Society of America (IDSA) recommends a 5-day course of remdesivir in hospitalized patients with severe disease (room air $pO_2 \leq$94% or requiring supplemental oxygen), but NOT for critical disease (mechanical ventilation, or ECMO).

- **Treatment, corticosteroids.** Dexamethasone 6 mg daily for up to 10 days is recommended for patients with increased markers of inflammation and with severe disease (recently hospitalized patients with O_2 sat $\leq$94% on room air, increasing oxygen needs, or requiring high-flow oxygen) or critical disease (use of mechanical ventilation or extracorporeal membrane oxygenation [ECMO]). Besides dexamethazone, recommendations often include remdesivir and/or baricitinib or tocilizumab. If dexamethasone is not available, other corticosteroids can be used such as prednisone 40 mg every day or 20 mg q12 hrs. Corticosteroids should **NOT** be used in patients not requiring supplemental oxygen.

- **Treatment, tocilizumab.** Tocilizumab is a monoclonal antibody that inhibits IL-6. IDSA recommends the combination of tocilizumab with dexamethazone (see above) for hospitalized patients with COVID-19 and who have progressive severe or critical disease and who have elevated markers of inflammation.

- **Treatment, Sotrovimab.** Sotrovimab is another monoclonal antibody that blocks SARS-CoV-2 from entering healthy cells as well as clearing infected cells. The FDA issued an EUA for use in ambulatory patients with mild to moderate disease at risk for progression (overweight, pregnancy, COPD/asthma, hypertension, and other cardiovascular disease). As with the other

13

monoclonal antibodies used to treat COVID-19, **patients receiving monoclonal antibodies who require hospitalization or require oxygen therapy may have worse clinical outcomes compared to patients NOT using the monoclonal antibodies.**

- **Treatment, casirivimab and imdevimab.** On November 21, 2020, the U.S. Food and Drug Administration issued an emergency use authorization (EUA) for casirivimab and imdevimab, two monoclonal antibodies that bind to the spike protein to be administered together for the treatment of mild to moderate COVID-19 in non-hospitalized adults and pediatric patients at risk for disease progression ($\geq$12 years old and weighing $\geq$40 kilograms [about 88 pounds]). Casirivimab and imdevimab reduced medical visits, including in high-risk patients, and in post-hoc analyses reduced the need for hospitalization or emergency room visits. **The use of monoclonal antibodies in hospitalized patients with COVID-19, or patients requiring oxygen therapy, may lead to a worse clinical outcome compared to not using the monoclonal antibodies.**

- **Treatment, baricitinib.** In November, 2020, the FDA issued an EUA for remdesivir in combination with baricitinib, a JAK enzyme inhibitor (FDA approved for rheumatoid arthritis) to treat hospitalized patients with COVID-19 who require supplemental oxygen, invasive mechanical ventilation, or ECMO who are >2 years old. Additionally, for recently hospitalized patients with increased markers of inflammation who require high-flow oxygen or noninvasive ventilation, dexamethasone with or without remdesivir, plus either baricitinib OR tocilizumab, is recommended.

- **Treatment, Favipiravir.** Favipiravir, an antiviral drug, has been approved for use in other countries but is not available in the US as of August 2021. In moderate COVID-19 disease, favipiravir improved time to viral clearance and fewer days to clinical recovery.

- **Treatment, convalescent serum.** There is a EUA for high titer convalescent plasma to treat hospitalized patients early in their disease or in patients with impaired humoral immunity. However, NIH recommends against the use of high titer convalescent serum in hospitalized patients who do not require mechanical ventilation. IDSA recommends to use convalescent serum only for ambulatory patients with mild to moderate disease who are participating in a clinical trial. There is a concern that natural antibody produced secondary to an infection may be diminished and this treatment may affect immunity. As of October, 2020, it is not known whether convalescent serum adversely affects the a patient's natural immune response to SARS-Co-V-2.

- **Treatment, other cytokine mediating drugs.** Drug classes being actively investigated to mitigate the inflammatory response associated with COVID-19 include another monoclonal antibody inhibiting IL-6 receptors (sarilumab), interleukin-1 receptor antagonist (anakinra), interleukin-1-β receptor antagonist (canakinumab), ruxolitinib a JAK enzyme inhibitor (jakafi), several TNF inhibitors, and an anti-CD6 monoclonal antibody (itolizumab). Both interferon beta-1A and interferon beta-1B may have activity as an antiviral as well as mitigate the inflammatory response. Large multi-institutional, well-designed RCTs are essential before these drugs can be recommended to treat COVID-19.

- **Treatment, other drugs or drug classes.** Many drug classes and medications have been or are being considered to treat SARS-Co-V-2 or symptoms of COVID-19. These drugs include: antiviral medications (lopinavir/ritonavir, darunavir/cobicistat, atazanavir, and ribavirin); icatibant (antagonist for bradykinin B2 receptor, FDA approved for treating acute hereditary angioedema) may reduce pulmonary edema associated with COVID-19); ivermectin (used to Tx intestinal strongyloidiasis) may inhibit SARS-Co-V-2; famotidine (an H2-blocker) may inhibit viral replication; colchicine (used to Tx gout) an anti-inflammatory, dipeptidyl-peptidase-4 (DPP-4) inhibitors (FDA approved to treat diabetes mellitus, type 2) may prevent SARS-Co-V-2 infection and/or progression of disease; and fluvoxamine, an SSRI used to treat obsessive compulsive disorder, may decrease cytokine release. To date, (August 2021), much of the research involving these drugs has been retrospective case-controlled trials, cohort trails, or small randomized-controlled trails (often open label) and often the results were mixed. Large multi-institutional RCTs are crucial before these drugs can be recommended to treat COVID-19.

- **Treatment, angiotensin-converting enzyme inhibitors (ACEIs) and angiotensin receptor blockers (ARBs).** ACEIs and ARBs should **NOT be stopped** in patients already on these medications and should **NOT be started** to treat COVID-19. Several studies suggest that patients on ACEIs or ARBs prior to being infected have better outcomes.

- **Treatment, hydroxychloroquine and chloroquine.** Hydroxychloroquine and chloroquine, with or without azithromycin, should **NOT** be used to treat COVID-19 in the hospital and in the ambulatory setting.

- **Treatment, venous thromboembolism prophylaxis (VTE).** Because of the increased risk of MI, DVT/PE, and ischemic stroke, VTE prophylaxis is recommended for critically ill and acutely ill hospitalized patients with COVID-19. Low-molecular weight heparin is the preferred choice.

- **SARS-CoV-2 Vaccines.** In less than a year after the pandemic began, over 100 SARS-CoV-2 vaccines were in various stages of development with over 50 in human trials. At least seven have been approved in at least one country, including three in the United States, Pfizer/BioNtech, Moderna, and Janssen/Johnson&Johnson. Also see Appendix Table A-12, page 1083. Administration of the vaccines began shortly after the Emergency Use Authorizations (EUA) were granted. While vaccine hesitancy and adequate distribution to vulnerable populations must be addressed to adequately respond to the pandemic, as of August 2021, 4.46 billion doses of COVID-19 vaccines have been administered worldwide and over 1.2 billion people are fully vaccinated. In the United States, over 350 million doses have been given and 166 million people are fully vaccinated (just over 50% of the population).

Both the Pfizer and Moderna vaccines utilize messenger-RNA encoding the spike glycoprotein and achieved about 95% efficacy in phase 3 trials. Both of these vaccines require a second dose be administered 21 days (Pfizer) and 28 (Moderna) days after the first dose. The Pfizer vaccine must

13

be kept at $-70°C$ and can be refrigerated only for 5 days at $2–8°C$. The Moderna vaccine requires storage at $-20°C$ and can be refrigerated for up to 4 wks at $2–8°C$. The Johnson&Johnson vaccine utilizes an inactivated adenovirus, as does the Oxford AstraZeneca vaccine in the United Kingdom. The Johnson & Johnson vaccine requires only one dose, whereas the AstraZeneca vaccine requires two doses. Both the Johnson & Johnson and the AstraZeneca vaccines can be refrigerated at $2–8°C$ for up to 3 months. A fifth vaccine by Novovax, utilizes the coronavirus spike protein via nanotechnology and in December 2020 began enrolling volunteers in a phase 3 trial in the United States.

Common side effects include injection site pain, headache, fever, and chills after injection. During phase 3 trails, severe adverse events were no more common than with placebo. However, severe but rare adverse events are often not detected during phase 3 trails because of the number of exposures required to detect rare events. Also, detection of delayed adverse events may not be identified because of the time lag between injection and observation of the event. After EUA of the Johnson & Johnson vaccine, there were numerous cases of thrombosis, including cavernous sinus thrombosis with thromocytopenia. The thrombosis occurred 1-2 wk after vaccination, and cases were predominately in women 18-50 years of age. There were similar reports following administration of the AstraZeneca vaccine. Administration of both vaccines was temporarily stopped and then resumed after review. Furthermore, the FDA added a warning to the Johnson & Johnson vaccine following 100 persons developing Guillain-Barre syndrome (GBS) following vaccination. This complication occurred about 6-8 wk post vaccination. At the time of the warning, over 12 million doses have been administered, equating to approximately 1 case per 120,000 doses of the vaccine.

Pulmonary Tuberculosis (TB)

1. Place all patients with possible pulmonary TB under airborne precautions in a negative pressure room.
2. Evaluate patients with suspected TB with serial **sputum acid-fast bacterial smears and culture.** Obtain three sputa, one per day on separate days. Early morning sputum collection is preferred because the specimen is more likely from the lower airway. Prepare an AFB smear to detect acid-fast bacilli (see page 314). If the smear is positive, continue airborne precautions. TB NAAT platforms are helpful for ruling TB in or out on AFB smear–positive specimens. TB NAAT may have utility on AFB smear–negative specimens for patients with a high clinical suspicion of pulmonary tuberculosis. TB NAAT platforms also provide information on predicted rifampin resistance. Monitor culture results; forward positive cultures to a reference laboratory for antimycobacterial susceptibility testing if not performed in-house.
3. If a patient with possible TB is immunosuppressed and their clinical condition is worsening, consider early bronchoscopy and chest CT to better evaluate the lung parenchyma.

4. Verify the mycobacteria recovered are in the *M. tuberculosis* complex by such techniques as culture on special growth media, nucleic acid probes, and nucleic acid amplification methods.

5. The TB skin test (tuberculin skin test described on page 652) can be difficult to interpret for a variety of reasons. Compared to TB skin testing, interferon-gamma release assays (IGRAs) are more objective and less likely to be affected by BCG vaccination status. Available assays include T-SPOT.*TB*, QuantiFERON-TB Gold, and QuantiFERON-TB Gold Plus. IGRA detect levels of gamma-interferon (cell-mediated immune response) released from patient-derived leukocytes in response to specific TB antigens. An individual is considered positive for *M. tuberculosis* infection if the interferon-gamma (IFN-γ) response to TB antigens is above the test cutoff (after subtracting the background IFN-γ response of the negative control).

6. Promptly report confirmed cases of TB to the local public health authorities. The public health department can also set up direct observed therapy (DOT) to ensure compliance with treatment.

Sepsis

Sepsis (also known as systemic inflammatory response syndrome [SIRS] when the source is suspected to be an infection) is a life threatening clinical syndrome of organ dysfunction caused by the body's response to an infection. In septic shock, there is critical reduction in tissue perfusion; acute multiple organ failure can occur (lungs, kidneys, liver). Common causes in immunocompetent patients include a variety of gram-positive and gram-negative bacteria. Sepsis in immunocompromised patients may be caused by uncommon bacterial or fungal species.

- **Septic shock** is a subset of sepsis with significantly increased mortality due to severe abnormalities of circulation and/or cellular metabolism. Septic shock involves persistent hypotension (defined as the need for vasopressors to maintain mean arterial pressure $\geq$65 mm Hg and a serum lactate level >18 mg/dL [2 mmol/L] despite adequate volume resuscitation.

- **Toxic shock syndrome** is a unique, uncommon form of shock caused by staphylococcal and streptococcal toxins.

Postoperative infection (deep or superficial) should be suspected as the cause of septic shock in patients who have recently had surgery. Signs of sepsis include fever, hypotension, oliguria, and confusion. The diagnosis of sepsis is primarily clinical, combined with culture results demonstrating an infection. Early recognition and treatment is critical. Treatment is aggressive fluid resuscitation, antibiotics, surgical excision of infected or necrotic tissue and drainage of pus, and supportive care.

Clinical practice guides for the management of sepsis have been developed by the **Surviving Sepsis Campaign**, an international collaboration of the Society of Critical Care Medicine and the European Society of Intensive Care Medicine. The **Surviving Sepsis Campaign** partnered with the Institute for Healthcare Improvement (IHI) to create bundles to

Hour One Bundle: Initial resuscitation for sepsis and septic shock

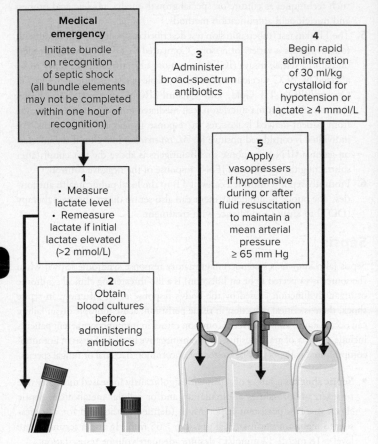

Figure 13-5. Initial treatment of sepsis and septic shock. (Reproduced with permission from Society of Critical Care Medicine and the European Society of Intensive Care Medicine. https://www.sccm.org/SurvivingSepsisCampaign/Guidelines/Adult-Patients; accessed June 4, 2020)

help frontline providers implement the guidelines (Rhoades A, Evans LE, Alhazzani W, et al. Surviving Sepsis Campaign: International Guidelines for Management of Sepsis and Septic Shock: 2016 Intensive Care Med 2017;43:304–377).

The initial management for sepsis is discussed in detail in Chapter 28, "Critical Care," page 944. An infographic is used by the Surviving Sepsis Campaign to increase awareness. The initial resuscitation efforts for sepsis and septic shock (referred to as the "1-hour Bundle") are shown in Figure 13-5. The "1-hour Bundle" encourages clinicians to act as quickly as possible to obtain blood cultures, administer broad-spectrum antibiotics, start appropriate fluid resuscitation, measure lactate, and begin vasopressors if clinically indicated. Ideally these interventions would all begin in the first hour from sepsis recognition but may not necessarily be completed in the first hour. Minimizing the time to treatment acknowledges the urgency that exists for patients with sepsis and septic shock.

Skin and Soft Tissue Infections

(See also Table 13-4, page 343)

The spectrum of skin and soft tissue infections runs the gamut from routine uncomplicated infections such as cellulitis of an extremity to life-threatening emergencies such as necrotizing fasciitis. Two basic questions need to be addressed.

1. Is there a collection (e.g., abscess) in the region of the infection that needs to be drained? If doubt exists, imaging of the infected area can demonstrate abscess formation and provide guidance on drainage. Such drainage procedures yield material for Gram stain, culture, and sensitivity testing. Special fungal and AFB stains and cultures should also be ordered if there is clinical suspicion (e.g., immunocompromised state).
2. Are contiguous structures already involved or at risk if the infection spreads? Examples of contiguous spread are orbital cellulitis leading to meningitis and diabetic foot ulcer or sacral decubitus ulcer leading to osteomyelitis.

13

Streptococcal Pharyngitis

The usual symptoms and signs of streptococcal pharyngitis include sudden onset of sore throat, odynophagia, fever (temperature >100.4°F [38°C]), tonsillar erythema and exudate, and tender cervical adenopathy. Cough, coryza, and diarrhea are more typically associated with viral pharyngitis. For treatment of streptococcal pharyngitis, see Table 13-4, page 340.

- Most "sore throats" are due to viral infection. Only 5–10% of "sore throats" in adults and 15–20% in children are associated with bacterial infections. The finding of a follicular yellowish exudate or a grayish membrane must arouse suspicion that Lancefield group A β-hemolytic streptococcal, diphtherial, gonococcal, fusospirochetal, or candidal infection exists; such signs may also be present in infectious mononucleosis, adenovirus, and other viral infections.
- It is desirable to differentiate bacterial from viral infections and reduce unnecessary antibiotic use. To diagnose bacterial pharyngitis (usually group A beta-hemolytic streptococci–*Streptococcus pyogenes*), an office-based rapid antigen assay or a molecular/PCR test is performed. A positive test does not require a culture, as these tests are very specific, and group A strep is universally susceptible to beta-lactams, but because the sensitivity of the antigen test is about 80%, the culture provides a "backup" in the case of a false-negative result. If a rapid antigen assay is negative but strep throat

is still considered, a throat culture is more definitive, and results will be available in 24–48 hr. Also, if another bacterial cause of pharyngitis, such as group C or G streptococci or *Arcanobacterium,* is suspected, pharyngeal culture may help with the diagnosis. See Pulmonary Infections for sample collection if a virus or *Chlamydia/Mycoplasma* are suspected (page 376).

Throat Culture

1. **Do NOT attempt if epiglottitis (croup) is suspected** (stridor, drooling). May induce laryngeal spasm, creating a life-threatening emergency.
2. Obtain the sample with a tongue blade and a good light source. With the patient's head tilted back and the throat well illuminated, depress the tongue so that the back of the throat can be seen.
3. Use the swab and try to touch only the tonsillar involved area, not the oral mucosa or tongue. If the patient is uncooperative, use an archlike swath that touches both the tonsillar areas and the posterior pharynx. Place the swab in the collection container provided by the lab.
4. If diphtheria (*C. diphtheriae*, which has a characteristic pseudomembrane) is suspected, notify the lab, as special media is required.
5. Normal flora on routine throat culture can include alpha-hemolytic streptococci, nonhemolytic *Staphylococcus,* saprophytic *Neisseria* spp., *Haemophilus* spp., *Klebsiella* spp., *Candida* spp., and diphtheroids.

Urinary Tract Infection (UTI, Non-CAUTI)

See Table 13-4, page 347, for common urinary tract pathogens. UTI signs and symptoms in both women and men include malaise, urinary frequency, urgency, urge incontinence, dysuria, nocturia, suprapubic pain or pressure, cloudy urine, foul-smelling urine, and gross and microscopic hematuria. Catheter-associated UTI (CAUTI) for an infection presenting with an indwelling catheter is discussed in the next section.

1. *Sample collection*
   o A properly collected "midstream" or "clean catch" urine sample, discussed in Chapter 19, page 661, provides accurate results in adults. Improperly collected clean catch and long-term Foley catheter urine specimens are at risk for significant contamination.
   o The best urine is obtained through a recently placed Foley catheter or from a "straight cath" to minimize contamination (see Chapter 19, page 661). Suprapubic needle aspiration is the most accurate method of obtaining urine but is almost never done in adults due to risks associated with the procedure. Any pure-culture (single organism) growth in urine obtained with these in-and-out techniques is considered positive.
   o **Never** collect urine directly from a urostomy bag; it will be grossly contaminated. The presence of a urostomy (i.e., ileal conduit) necessitates that a catheter be placed in the stoma to collect the specimen.

o If a urine specimen cannot be taken to the lab within 60 min, refrigerate it to prevent overgrowth of contaminating bacteria.

o Differentiating a true UTI from contamination or simple colonization can be challenging. Pyuria with bacteriuria usually indicates a UTI. In general, if an infection is present, inflammatory cells (except in neutropenia) should be detected in the urine. UA is used to detect inflammatory WBCs and should be ordered with the culture. The presence of epithelial cells suggests contamination; urinary diversion with a bowel segment is an exception.

2. *Urinalysis*

o (See also Chapter 12, "Laboratory Diagnosis: Urine Studies," pages 292, 297–299.)

o The leukocyte esterase test is used to detect neutrophil granules and is a marker for pyuria. Elevated urine WBCs is a dependable marker for true pyuria. Enterobacteriaceae (gram-negative rods such as *E. coli, Klebsiella,* and *Proteus*) reduce nitrate to nitrite. If the urine nitrite test is positive, a member of the Enterobacteriaceae family is likely present.

o Gram-positive cocci do not convert nitrate to nitrite, so a negative nitrite test does not rule out UTI.

3. *Urine Culture*

o A colony count of <10,000 colony-forming units/mL (cfu/mL) is usually insignificant, as is the presence of mixed organisms. A colony count >100,000 cfu/mL is indicative of true infection. Counts of 10,000–100,000 cfu/mL must be interpreted carefully, usually in conjunction with the UA results and the clinical situation.

o The presence of more than three organisms usually indicates contamination unless the UTI is chronic, a GI fistula is present, or the patient has undergone certain types of urinary diversion.

o Routine urine cultures will not detect *N. gonorrhoeae* and *C. trachomatis.* NAAT methods have largely replaced specialized cultures for detecting these two sexually transmitted organisms.

13

Catheter-Associated Urinary Tract Infection

CAUTI is defined as an infection occurring in a person whose urinary tract is currently catheterized or has been catheterized within the previous 48 hr. CAUTI are the most common type of healthcare-associated infection reported to the National Healthcare Safety Network (NHSN), accounting for 40% of hospital-acquired infections and over 80% of the 900,000 cases of bacteriuria annually. Catheter-associated asymptomatic bacteriuria (CA-ASB) is the presence of bacteria in the urinary tract without signs or symptoms of infection. CAUTI and CA-ASB are often not distinguished from each other in reported cases of catheter-associated bacteriuria and may result in inappropriate antibiotic use.

1. **Prevention**. Strategies include limiting use of urinary catheters, aseptic insertion, early discontinuation of catheter use, use of pre-sealed closed drainage systems, and maintaining the drainage bag below the level of the bladder.

    o The diagnosis of CAUTI is made in patients with signs and symptoms of UTI with current or recent (<48 hr) indwelling urinary catheter or routine intermittent catheter. Symptoms may include chills, rigors, altered mental status, malaise, flank pain, and pelvic discomfort, and signs may include a fever. Patients with a recently removed catheter may report dysuria, urinary urgency, and/or frequency. Spinal cord injury patients may report increased spasticity, autonomic dysreflexia, and/or sense of uneasiness.

    o Definitive CAUTI diagnosis is a positive urine culture growing >10^3 cfu/mL. CA-ASB is defined as cultures growing >10^5 cfu/mL without signs or symptoms of UTI. Urine specimen should be sent for culture prior to initiation of antimicrobials. Catheters should be replaced, if still indicated, and a culture should be obtained from a newly placed catheter.

2. **Treatment.** Optimal duration of antibiotic therapy is unknown, but typically ranges from 3–21 days depending on severity of symptoms (e.g., cystitis, pyelonephritis, associated abscess, or bacteremia). Most literature suggests 7–14 days of therapy for CAUTI. A 3-day regimen has been suggested in younger women (<65 yr) in whom a catheter was recently removed. Catheters placed >2 wk prior should be exchanged at time of diagnosis (prior to cultures being sent) to improve antimicrobial penetration and reduce bacterial concentrations. When possible, antibiotic therapy should be culture driven. Given the incidence of polymicrobial colonization as well as involvement of both gram-positive and gram-negative organisms, no first-line agent can be recommended. Serious infections must be covered with broad-spectrum antibiotics and narrowed based on culture sensitivity patterns. Treatment of minor infections should be delayed until culture sensitivities are available to guide antimicrobial selection.

BIOTERRORISM AND SELECT AGENTS

Recognizing unusual patterns in disease presentation, detecting such events and having a high clinical index of suspicion are critical. Certain situations or patterns should prompt contacting public health officials or the CDC. Select agents or agents of bioterrorism may be detected in naturally occurring zoonotic infections such as anthrax, tularemia, or brucellosis. If any of these are suspected on clinical history and examination, warn the clinical microbiology laboratory so they can take proper precautions to avoid occupational exposure. Any suspected select agent that cannot be ruled out by some basic preliminary tests as defined by the CDC has to be referred to the reference

Public Health Laboratory for confirmation. If confirmed by the reference lab, any and all material (specimens and isolates) must be destroyed by the clinical lab within 7 days, and documentation submitted with evidence of destruction. This is done to ensure such select agents do not end up in the wrong hands. Some examples where select agents may be suspected are any disease or suspected disease in the Category A, B, or C list:

Category A: Anthrax, smallpox, botulism, viral hemorrhagic fevers (e.g., Ebola and Marburg), tularemia, plague

Category B (lower mortality than A): Q fever, typhus, melioidosis (or glanders), psittacosis, brucellosis, toxin related (e.g., ricin)

Category C (emerging pathogens with bioterrorism potential): MDR TB, Nipah virus, others.

- A case of disease or cluster of cases in the wrong season, such as an outbreak of "influenza" that occurs in the summer.
- Appearance of an infectious disease in the wrong region, such as a case of coccidioidomycosis in the northeastern United States.
- Fulminant progression of an usually benign infection in a healthy host.
- An infectious disease occurring without the presence of its mandatory vector. Contact information and additional resources:
  - CDC, www.emergency.cdc.gov
  - CDC Emergency Response Hotline (24/7) (770) 488-7100
  - CDC Botulism Hotline (24/7) (770) 488-7100
  - California Department of Public Health Infant Botulism Consultation (24/7) (510) 231-7600

ISOLATION PROTOCOLS

The combination of standard precautions and disease-specific isolation procedures represents an effective strategy in the fight against healthcare-associated transmission of infectious agents. Current Centers for Disease Control and Prevention-Healthcare Infection Control Practices Advisory Committee (CDC-HICPAC) guidelines describe the methods and indications for these precautions (Siegel JD, et al. 2007 Guideline for Isolation Precautions: Preventing Transmission of Infectious Agents in Healthcare Settings. These guidelines are available at: http://www.cdc.gov/niosh/docket/archive/pdfs/NIOSH-219/0219-010107-siegel.pdf, accessed May 5, 2020) with recent updates summarized by the International Society of Infectious Diseases (/https://isid.org/wp-content/uploads/2018/07/ISID_InfectionGuide_Chapter7.pdf, accessed May 5, 2020). The following category names vary somewhat from institution to institution, but the general principles are generally applicable. Contact your institution's infection control unit with specific questions or if you are unsure of the proper procedure. Specific indications for standard, contact, droplet and

Table 13-11. Indications for Standard and Isolation Precautions*

Standard
All patients interacting with healthcare providers are treated using standard
 precautions (see below)

Contact
Abscess, wound infection: major, draining
Bronchiolitis
Burkholderia cepacia: patient with cystic fibrosis, infection, or colonization
Conjunctivitis: acute viral
Gastroenteritis: *C. difficile*, rotavirus, diapered or incontinent persons for other
 infectious agents
Diphtheria: cutaneous
Hepatitis, type A and E virus: diapered or incontinent persons
Herpes simplex virus: mucocutaneous, disseminated or primary, severe, and
 neonatal
Human metapneumovirus
Impetigo
Lice (pediculosis)
Multidrug-resistant organisms: infection or colonization
Parainfluenza virus
Poliomyelitis
Pressure ulcer: infected
Respiratory infectious disease: acute, infants and young children
Respiratory syncytial virus: in infants, young children, and immunocompromised
 adults
Rubella: congenital
Scabies
Staphylococcal disease: furunculosis, scalded skin syndrome, burns

Droplet
Diphtheria: pharyngeal
Influenza virus: seasonal
Invasive disease: *H. influenzae* type b, *N. meningitidis*, Streptococcus group A
Mumps
Parvovirus B19: erythema infectiosum
Pertussis (whooping cough)
Plague: pneumonic
Pneumonia: Adenovirus, *H. influenzae* type b (infants and children), *Mycoplasma*
Rhinovirus
Rubella
Streptococcus group A disease: pharyngitis and scarlet fever (infants and young
 children)
Viral hemorrhagic fevers due to Lassa, Ebola, Marburg, Crimean- Congo fever
 viruses

(Continued)

airborne precautions are reviewed in Table 13-11 and local isolation protocols
are summarized in Table 13-12.

Standard Precautions: Standard precautions are designed to reduce
the risk of transmission from both recognized and unrecognized sources of

Table 13-11.   Indications for Standard and Isolation Precautions* *(Continued)*

Airborne
COVID-19
Influenza A: avian H7N9, Asian H5N1
Measles
MERS-coronavirus: Middle East acute respiratory syndrome
Mycobacterium tuberculosis: laryngeal and pulmonary disease, extrapulmonary
    draining lesion
Smallpox
Varicella-zoster: disseminated disease, localized disease in immunocompromised
    patient

* Centers for Disease Control and Prevention—Healthcare Infection Control Practices
Advisory Committee guidelines and recommendations of the International Society of
Infectious Diseases (https://isid.org/wp-content/uploads/2018/07/ISID_InfectionGuide_
Chapter7.pdf, accessed May 5, 2020).

Table 13-12.   Summary of Specific Transmission-Based Precautions (consult
                with local infection control unit to confirm local isolation
                protocols)

Precaution	Contact	Droplet	Airborne
Patient room	Private	Private	Private
			Specific ventilation requirements
Gloves	Before entering the room, as in Standard Precautions		
Hand hygiene	Hand antisepsis, as in Standard Precautions		
Gown	If direct contact with patient or environment	As in Standard Precautions	
Mask	Standard	<1 meter of patient	Before entering room Special requirements
Other	Limit patient transport		

Centers for Disease Control and Prevention—Healthcare Infection Control Practices Advisory
Committee guidelines and recommendations of the International Society of Infectious
Diseases (https://isid.org/wp-content/uploads/2018/07/ISID_InfectionGuide_Chapter7.pdf
Accessed May 5, 2020).

infection and are recommended for *all* patients (See Chapter 13, page 392
for details on standard precautions.)

- Wash hands before and after patient care, including before and after using
  gloves in all circumstances!
- Put on gloves before contact with nonintact skin, mucous membranes,
  body secretions, excretions, or fluids, and blood.
- Wear mask and eye protection to protect the mucous membranes of the
  eyes, nose, and mouth, and wear a gown during procedures and activities

that are likely to generate sprays or splashes of either body fluids or blood. Remove a soiled gown immediately and place it in the proper receptacle, then wash your hands.

● Ensure proper handling and disposal of needles and other sharps before, during, and after use.
● Properly clean and disinfect patient care equipment and environment.

Contact Precautions: For numerous conditions that pose a risk for contact transmission. Examples may include lice and scabies, acute diarrhea of a probable infectious cause, *C. difficile* infection, infection with drug-resistant bacteria, or herpes zoster.

● Single occupancy room.
● Use personal protective equipment (PPE), e.g., gown and gloves, during all interactions.
● Don all PPE upon entry into room; doff prior to exit.
● Limit transport of patient within facility and, if required, take steps to contain or cover potentially infectious areas on the patient.
● Use dedicated patient care equipment and adequately clean and disinfect before use on another patient.

Droplet Precautions: For conditions known or suspected to be easily transmitted by respiratory droplets generated during coughing, sneezing, or talking. Examples may include influenza, pertussis, and diphtheria.

● Wear a standard surgical mask upon entry into patient space.
● Limit transport of patient within facility and if transported, mask the patient.

Airborne Precautions: For conditions known or suspected to be easily transmitted by airborne route. Examples may include tuberculosis, chickenpox, and measles.

● Place patient in an airborne infection isolation room (negative pressure).
● Wear N95 mask when entering the patient's room or moulded surgical mask.
● Limit transport of the patient within the facility and if transported, mask the patient.
● Restrict susceptible healthcare personnel from interacting with patient, and provide immunization to any unprotected contacts for vaccine-preventable infections.

Special/Emerging Pathogen Precautions: For special contagious conditions; at least *airborne precautions and contact precautions* in combination with additional institutional protocols for suspected special and emerging pathogens. Examples may include smallpox, viral hemorrhagic fevers, severe acute respiratory syndrome [SARS], and the 2019 pandemic novel coronavirus (2019-nCoV/COVID-19):

- Wear N95 mask/powered air purifying respirators (PAPR), gown, gloves, and other PPE per institutional protocol when involved with direct COVID-19 care or if caring for an individual who is a patient under investigation (PUI) for possible infection from any of those listed above. Place patient in an airborne infection isolation room (negative pressure).
- Seek institutional protocols and procedures on guidance for specimen collection and laboratory testing.
- Limit/restrict transport of the patient within the facility.
- See Chapter 19, "Bedside Procedures," page 508 for a discussion of aerosol-generating procedures that are important to recognize in the care of COVID-19–infected and other high-risk patients.

FURTHER READING

13

Selected References for SARS-CoV-2 and COVID-19
Cases and mortality worldwide and the United States:
https://coronavirus.jhu.edu/map.html (accessed March 18, 2022).
www.worldometers.info/coronavirus/ (accessed March 18, 2022).
www.cdc.gov/coronavirus/2019-ncov/hcp/duration-isolation.html#cecommendations (accessed Match 18, 2022).

Transmission:
Fisher KA, et al. Community and close exposure associated with COVID-19 among symptomatic adults >18 years in 11 outpatient care facilities—United States, July 2020. MMWR 2020 (September 11);69(36):1258–1264.

Lauer SA, et al. The incubation period of Coronavirus Disease 2019 (COVID-19) from publicly reported confirmed cases: Estimation and application. Ann Intern Med 2020;172:577–582.

Meyerowitz EA, et al. Transmission of SARS-CoV-2: A review of viral, host, and enviornmental factors. Ann Intern Med 2021 Jan;174(1):69–79.

Oran AM, Topol EJ. Prevalence of asymptomatic SARS-CoV-2 infection. Ann Intern Med 2020;173:362–367.

Clinical Disease:
Tenforde MW, et al. Characteristics of adult outpatients and inpatients with COVID-19 – 11 academic medical centers, United States, March–May 2020. MMWR 2020 (July 3);69(26):841–846.

Joshee S, et al. Long-Term Effects of COVID-19. Mayo Clin Proc. 2022 Mar;97(3):579–599.

Yang BY, et al. Clinical characteristics of patients with Coronavirus Disease 2019 (COVID) receiving emergency medical services in King County, Washington. JAMA Network Open. 2020;3(7):e2014549. doi: 10.1001/jamanetworkopen.2020.14549.

Wichmann D, et al. Autopsy findings and venous thromboembolism in patients with COVID-19. Ann Intern Med 2020;173:268–277.

Prevention:

Alagoz O, et al. Effect of timing of and adherence to social distancing measures on COVID-19 burden in the United States. Ann Intern Med 2021. doi:10.7326/M20-4096.

Padda IS, Parmar M. COVID (SARS-COV-2) Vaccine. 2022 Feb 22. In: StatPearls [Internet]. Treasure Island (FL): StatPearls Publishing; 2022 Jan. PMID: 33620862

https://www.cdc.gov/coronavirus/2019-ncov/vaccines/index.html (Acessed March 14, 2022)

Molecular, Antigen and antibody testing:

Baldanti F, et al, Choice of SARS-CoV-2 diagnostic test: challenges and key considerations for the future. Crit Rev Clin Lab Sci. 2022 Mar 15:1–15. doi: 10.1080/10408363.2022.2045250. Online ahead of print.

Cheng MP, et al. Diagnostic testing for severe acute respiratory syndrome-related Coronavirus 2. Ann Intern Med. 2020;172:726–734.

Cheng MP, et al. Serodiagnostics for severe acute respiratory syndrome-related Coronavirus 2. Ann Intern Med. 2020 Sep 15;173(11):726–734.

Misra A, Theel ES. Immunity to SARS-CoV-2: What Do We Know and Should We Be Testing for It? J Clin Microbiol. 2022 Mar 7:e0048221. doi: 10.1128/jcm.00482-21. Online ahead of print.

Slev PR. Severe Acute Respiratory Syndrome Coronavirus 2 Serology Testing – A Laboratory Primer. Clin Lab Med. 2022 Mar;42(1):1–13.

Treatment:

For up-to-date information regarding treatment and vaccines refer to the references below:

NIH: https://www.covid19treatmentguidelines.nih.gov/whats-new/

CDC: https://www.cdc.gov/coronavirus/2019-ncov/hcp/clinical-guidance-management-patients.html

IDSA: https://www.idsociety.org/practice-guideline/covid-19-guideline-treatment-and-management/ (also a reference for molecular, antigen, and serologic testing)

The Medical Letter on Drugs and Therapeutics: Treatments considered for COVID-19 (the last update used as a reference, July 23, 2021) Issue 1595e: (https://secure.medicalletter.org/downloads/1595e_table.pdf) and https://secure.medicalletter.org/drugs-for-covid-19

Aghamirza Moghim Aliabadi H, et al. COVID-19: A systematic review and update on prevention, diagnosis, and treatment. MedComm (2020). 2022 Feb 17;3(1):e115. On line ahead of print.

Basu D, et al. Therapeutics for COVID-19 and post COVID-19 complications: An update. Curr Res Pharmacol Drug Discov. 2022;3:100086. doi: 10.1016/j.crphar.2022.100086. Epub 2022 Feb 4. PMID: 35136858. On line ahead of print.

Jorda A, et al. Convalescent Plasma Treatment in Patients with Covid-19: A Systematic Review and Meta-Analysis. Front Immunol. 2022 Feb 7;13:817829. doi: 10.3389/fimmu.2022.817829. eCollection 2022.

Rodriguez-Guerra M, et al. Current treatment in COVID-19 disease: a rapid review. Drugs Context. 2021;10:2020-10-3. eCollection 2021.

13

Blood Gases and Acid-Base Disorders

14

BLOOD GAS BASICS

Blood gases provide information concerning the oxygenation, ventilatory, and acid-base status of the patient. Blood gas results are usually given as pH, PO_2, PCO_2, $[HCO_3^-]$, base excess or deficit (base difference), and O_2 saturation. This test gives information on acid-base homeostasis (pH, PCO_2, HCO_3^-, and base difference) and on blood oxygenation (PO_2, O_2 saturation). Arterial blood gases (ABGs) are most commonly measured; venous, mixed venous, and capillary blood gases are less often measured. Indications for blood gas determinations are as follows:

- To determine a patient's ventilator status ($PaCO_2$), acid-base balance (pH and $PaCO_2$), and oxygenation and O_2-carrying capacity (PaO_2 and O_2Hb)
- To quantitate the response to therapeutic interventions (e.g., supplemental O_2 administration, mechanical ventilation) or diagnostic evaluation (e.g., exercise desaturation)
- Monitoring the severity and progression of documented disease processes (e.g., COPD)

Chapter update by Steven Haist, MD, MS

NORMAL BLOOD GAS VALUES

Normal values for blood gas analysis are given in Table 14-1 below, and capillary blood gases are discussed in a following section. Mixed venous blood gases are reviewed in Chapter 28, pages 895–896 and 898. **The bicarbonate concentration ($[HCO_3^-]$) from the blood gas is a calculated value and should not be used in interpretation of blood gases; the $[HCO_3^-]$ from a concurrent chemistry panel should be used.** *Note:* The HCO_3^- values on the chemistry panel and those calculated from the blood gases should be about the same. A major discrepancy (>10% difference) means one or more of the three values is in error (pH, PCO_2, or $[HCO_3^-]$) or the blood gas and the chemistry panel were not collected at the same time. ABGs and chemistry panels $[HCO_3^-]$ should be obtained at the same time for the most accurate interpretation.

VENOUS BLOOD GASES

There is little difference between arterial and venous pH and $[HCO_3^-]$ (except in severe CHF and shock). Venous blood gas levels may occasionally be used to assess acid-base status, but venous O_2 levels are significantly less than arterial values (see Table 14-1).

CAPILLARY BLOOD GASES

A capillary blood gas (CBG) is obtained from a highly vascularized capillary bed. CBG is often used for pediatric patients because obtaining the sample is

Table 14-1. Normal Blood Gas Values (Adult)

Measurement	Arterial Blood	Mixed Venous Blood[a]	Venous Blood
pH (range)	7.40 (7.37–7.44)	7.36 (7.31–7.41)	7.36 (7.31–7.41)
PO_2 (mm Hg) (decreases with age)	80–100	35–40	30–50
PCO_2 (mm Hg)	36–44	41–51	40–52
O_2 saturation (%) [decreases with age]	>95	60–80	60–85
HCO_3^- (mEq/L)	22–26	22–26	22–28
Base difference (deficit/excess)	−2 to +2	−2 to +2	−2 to +2

[a]Obtained from the right atrium, usually through a pulmonary artery catheter.
See Chapter 28, pages 898, 905, and 955.

easier (through the heel) and less traumatic (no risk of arterial thrombosis or major hemorrhage) compared to obtaining an ABG sample. See Chapter 19, page 601, Heelstick and Fingerstick (Capillary Blood Sampling).

When interpreting a CBG, apply the following rules:

- **pH:** Same as arterial or slightly lower (normal = 7.35–7.40).
- **PCO$_2$:** Same as arterial or slightly higher (normal = 40–45 mm Hg).
- **PO$_2$:** Lower than arterial (normal = 45–60 mm Hg).
- **O$_2$ saturation:** >70% is acceptable. Saturation is probably more useful than PO$_2$ in the interpretation of a CBG.

GENERAL PRINCIPLES OF BLOOD GAS DETERMINATIONS

Interpretation of O$_2$ values is discussed on page 400.

1. The blood gas analyzers in most labs measure pH and PCO$_2$ as well as PO$_2$. The [HCO$_3^-$] and base difference are calculated with the **Henderson–Hasselbalch equation:**

$$pH = pK_a + \frac{\log[HCO_3^-] \text{ in mmol/L}}{0.03 \times PCO_2 \text{ in mm Hg}}$$

or the **Henderson equation:**

$$[H^+] \text{ in nmol/L} = \frac{24 \times PCO_2 \text{ in mm Hg}}{[HCO_3^-] \text{ in mmol/L}}$$

2. For a rough estimate of [H$^+$]
   o [H$^+$] = (7.80 − pH) × 100
   o or add 1 nEq/L to 40 nEq for every 0.01 below 7.40
   o or subtract 1 nEq/L from 40 nEq for every 0.01 above 7.40 (accurate for pH 7.25–7.48)
   At normal pH of 7.40 [H$^+$] = 40 nEq/L. Since pH is a log scale, for every change of 0.3 in pH from 7.40, the [H$^+$] doubles or halves.
   o For pH 7.10, [H$^+$] = 2 × 40, or 80 nmol/L
   o For pH 7.70, [H$^+$] = 1/2 40, or 20 nmol/L
3. The calculated [HCO$_3^-$] should be within 2 mEq/L of the [HCO$_3^-$] of a venous measurement drawn at the same time. If not, an error has been made in collection or in determination of the values, and both samples should be recollected.
4. Two additional relationships derived from the Henderson–Hasselbalch equation should be committed to memory. These two rules are helpful in interpreting blood gas results, particularly in defining a simple versus a mixed blood gas disorder:

14

Rule I: A change in PCO_2 up or down 10 mm Hg is associated with an increase or decrease in pH of 0.08 units. As PCO_2 decreases, pH increases; as the PCO_2 increases, pH decreases.

Rule II: A pH change of 0.15 is equivalent to a base change of 10 mEq/L. A decrease in base (i.e., $[HCO_3^-]$) is termed a **base deficit**, and an increase in base is termed a **base excess**.

ACID-BASE DISORDERS: DEFINITION

1. Acid-base disorders are commonly encountered clinical problems. **Acidemia** is a pH <7.37, and **alkalemia** is a pH >7.44. **Acidosis and alkalosis** are used to describe the process by which pH changes. The primary causes of acid-base disturbances are abnormalities in the respiratory, metabolic, and renal systems. As the Henderson–Hasselbalch equation shows, a respiratory disturbance leading to an abnormal PCO_2 alters the pH, and similarly a metabolic disturbance altering $[HCO_3^-]$ changes the pH.

2. Any primary disturbance in acid-base homeostasis invokes a **normal compensatory response.** A primary metabolic disorder leads to respiratory compensation, and a primary respiratory disorder leads to an acute metabolic response due to the buffering capacity of body fluids *and* chronic compensation (1–2 days) due to alterations in renal function.

3. The degree of compensation can be expressed in terms of the degree of the primary acid-base disturbance. Table 14-2, page 403, lists the major categories of primary acid-base disorders, the primary abnormality, the secondary compensatory response, and the expected compensation based on the primary abnormality. These changes are defined graphically in Figure 14-1, page 404.

MIXED ACID-BASE DISORDERS

1. Most acid-base disorders result from a single primary disturbance of the normal physiologic compensatory response (called **simple acid-base disorders**). In some cases (e.g., serious illness), two or more primary disorders may occur simultaneously, resulting in a **mixed acid-base disorder**. The net effect of mixed disorders can be additive (e.g., metabolic acidosis and respiratory acidosis) and result in extreme alteration of pH. Or the effects can be opposite (e.g., metabolic acidosis and respiratory alkalosis) and nullify somewhat the effect of the other on pH.

2. To determine the presence of a mixed acid-base disorder with a blood gas value, follow the six steps in the Interpretation of Blood Gases (see next section). Alterations in either $[HCO_3^-]$ or PCO_2 that differ from expected

Table 14-2. Simple Acid-Base Disturbances

Acid-Base Disorder	Primary Abnormality	Expected Compensation	Expected Degree of Compensation
Metabolic acidosis	$\downarrow\downarrow\downarrow[HCO_3^-]$	$\downarrow\downarrow PCO_2$	Dec in $PCO_2 = (1.5 \times [HCO_3^-]) + 8 +/- 2$
Metabolic alkalosis	$\uparrow\uparrow\uparrow[HCO_3^-]$	$\uparrow\uparrow PCO_2$	Inc in $PCO_2 = \Delta [HCO_3^-] \times 0.6$
Acute respiratory acidosis	$\uparrow\uparrow\uparrow PCO_2$	$\uparrow[HCO_3^-]$	Inc in $[HCO_3^-] = \Delta PCO_2/10$
Chronic respiratory acidosis	$\uparrow\uparrow\uparrow PCO_2$	$\uparrow\uparrow[HCO_3^-]$	Inc in $[HCO_3^-] = 4 \times \Delta PCO_2/10$
Acute respiratory alkalosis	$\downarrow\downarrow\downarrow PCO_2$	$\downarrow[HCO_3^-]$	Dec in $[HCO_3^-] = 2 \times \Delta PCO_2/10$
Chronic respiratory alkalosis	$\downarrow\downarrow\downarrow PCO_2$	$\downarrow\downarrow[HCO_3^-]$	Dec in $[HCO_3^-] = 5 \times \Delta PCO_2/10$

The number of arrows suggests the degree of change of the value; Inc = increase Dec = decrease.

14

403

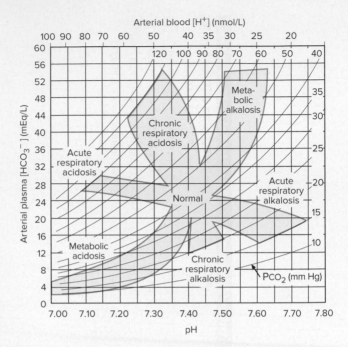

Figure 14-1. Nomogram for acid-base disorders. (Reprinted with permission from Cogan MG: *Fluid and Electrolytes,* Originally published by Appleton & Lange, Copyright © 1991 by the McGraw-Hill Companies, Inc.)

compensation levels indicate a second process. Two of the examples given in the following section illustrate the strategies used in identifying a mixed acid-base disorder.

INTERPRETATION OF BLOOD GASES

Use a consistent, stepwise approach to interpretation of blood gases. (See Figure 14-1, above.)

Step 1: Determine whether the numbers fit.

$$[H^+] = \frac{24 \times PCO_2}{\left[HCO_3^-\right]}$$

The right side of the equation should be within about 10% of the left side. If the numbers do not fit, obtain another ABG and chemistry panel for $[HCO_3^-]$.
Example. pH 7.25, PCO_2 48 mm Hg, $[HCO_3^-]$ 29 mEq/L.

$$56 = 24 \times \frac{48}{29}$$
$$56 \neq 40$$

This blood gas cannot be interpreted, and samples for ABG and $[HCO_3^-]$ must be recollected. The most common reason for the numbers not fitting is that the ABG and the chemistry panel $[HCO_3^-]$ were obtained at different times.

Step 2: Next, determine whether acidemia (pH <7.37) or alkalemia (pH >7.44) is present.

Step 3: Identify the primary disturbance as metabolic or respiratory. For example, if acidemia is present, is the PCO_2 >44 mm Hg (respiratory acidosis), or is the $[HCO_3^-]$ <22 mEq/L (metabolic acidosis)? In other words, identify which component, respiratory or metabolic, is altered in the same direction as the pH abnormality. If both components act in the same direction— e.g., both respiratory (PCO_2 >44 mm Hg) and metabolic $[HCO_3^-]$ <22 mEq/L) acidosis are present—then this is a **mixed acid-base problem** (see Step 4). The primary disturbance is the one that varies the most from normal. That is, with a $[HCO_3^-]$ of 6 mEq/L and PCO_2 of 50 mm Hg, the primary disturbance would be metabolic acidosis; the $[HCO_3^-]$ is only 25% of normal, a change by a factor of 4 (6 = 24/4), whereas the increase in PCO_2 is only 25% above normal (40–50 → 10/40).

Step 4: After identifying the primary disturbance, use the equations in Table 14-2, page 403, to calculate the expected compensatory response. If the difference between the actual value and the calculated value is great, a mixed acid-base disturbance is present.

14

Step 5: Calculate the anion gap:

$$\text{Anion gap} = [Na^+] - ([Cl^-] + [HCO_3^-])$$

A normal anion gap is 8–12 mEq/L. If the anion gap is increased, proceed to Step 6. Be sure to always calculate the anion gap even if there is not an acidemia; you could have a gap metabolic acidosis with a pH >7.44 if the primary disturbance is a respiratory alkalosis or a metabolic alkalosis.

Step 6: If the anion gap is elevated, compare the changes from normal between the anion gap and $[HCO_3^-]$. If the change in anion gap is similar to the change in $[HCO_3^-]$ from normal, a gap acidosis is present and there is **no** metabolic alkalosis **or** nongap metabolic acidosis. If the change in anion gap is greater than the change in $[HCO_3^-]$ from normal, a metabolic alkalosis is also present in addition to gap metabolic acidosis. If the change in the anion gap is less than the change in $[HCO_3^-]$ from normal, a nongap metabolic acidosis is also present in addition to gap metabolic acidosis. (See Examples 5, 6, and 7, starting on pages 416.)

Finally, and most importantly, be sure the interpretation of the blood gas is consistent with the clinical setting.

METABOLIC ACIDOSIS: DIAGNOSIS AND TREATMENT

Metabolic acidosis represents an increase in acid in body fluids reflected by a decrease in $[HCO_3^-]$ and a compensatory decrease in PCO_2.

Differential Diagnosis

The diagnosis of metabolic acidosis (Figure 14-2, page 406) can be classified as anion gap or non–anion gap acidosis. The **anion gap** (normal range, 8–12 mEq/L) is calculated as:

$$Anion\ gap = [Na^+] - ([Cl^-] + [HCO_3^-])$$

Anion Gap Acidosis: Anion gap >12 mEq/L; caused by a decrease in $[HCO_3^-]$ balanced by an increase in an unmeasured acid ion from either endogenous production or exogenous ingestion **(normochloremic acidosis).**

Non–Anion Gap Acidosis: Anion gap = 8–12 mEq/L; caused by a decrease in $[HCO_3^-]$ balanced by an increase in chloride **(hyperchloremic acidosis).** Renal tubular acidosis is a type of nongap acidosis that can be associated with a variety of pathologic conditions (Table 14-3, page 407). A closer look at the anion gap and $[HCO_3^-]$ helps differentiate between (a) pure metabolic gap acidosis, (b) a pure metabolic nongap acidosis, (c) mixed metabolic gap and nongap acidosis, and (d) metabolic gap acidosis and metabolic alkalosis.

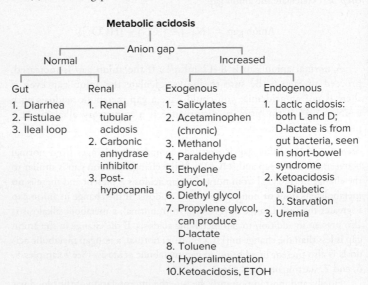

Figure 14-2. Differential diagnosis of metabolic acidosis.

Table 14-3. Renal Tubular Acidosis: Diagnosis and Management

Clinical Condition	Renal Defect	GFR	Serum HCO$_3^-$ mEq/L	Serum K$^+$ mEq/L	Minimal Urine pH	Other Findings	Associated Disease States	Treatment
Normal	None	Nl	24–28	3.5–5.0	4.8–5.2	None	None	None
Classic distal RTA (type I)	Distal H$^+$ secretion	Nl	20–30	↓ (*occ↑)	>5.5	↑ Ca^{++} urine; ↓ citrate urine	Various genetic disorders (*sickle cell, hereditary deafness, medullary kidney dx), autoimmune dx (*lupus nephritis), hyperthyroidism, hyperparathyroidism, liver dx (chronic active hepatitis, cirrhosis, primary biliary cirrhosis), chronic kidney dx (chronic UTIs, *obstructive uropathy, analgesic abuse, nephrocalcinosis, tubulointerstitial dx, rejection of transplanted kidney), toxins/drugs (heavy metals, toluene, *amiloride, amphotericin, foscarnet, lithium, ifosfamide, *pentamidine, *triamterene, *trimethoprim), empty sella syndrome	2–3 mEq HCO$_3^-$/kg/day

(Continued)

* = ↑K$^+$ rather than the usual ↓K$^+$ with other causes of distal renal tubular acidosis; Occ = occasionally.

Table 14-3. Renal Tubular Acidosis: Diagnosis and Management (*Continued*)

Clinical Condition	Renal Defect	GFR	Serum HCO$_3^-$ mEq/L	Serum K$^+$ mEq/L	Minimal Urine pH	Other Findings	Associated Disease States	Treatment
Proximal RTA (type II RTA)	Proximal HCO$_3^-$ reabsorption	Nl	15–18	↓	<5.5	Urine pH >5.5 when HCO$_3^-$ above 18 mEq/L	Fanconi syndrome, various genetic disorders (cystinosis, Wilson dx, fructose intolerance), multiple myeloma, ↓vitamin D, toxins/ drugs (lead, aminoglycosides, acetazolamide, ifosfamide, topiramate, cidofovir), carbonic anhydrase def, chronic rejection of transplanted kidney	Up to 15 mEq HCO$_3^-$/kg/day can use Na$^+$ or K$^+$ HCO$_3^-$ or citrate
Buffer deficiency (type III RTA)	Both proximal HCO$_3^-$ reabsorption & distal H$^+$ secretion	↓	15–18	3.5–5.0	<5.5		Cytosolic carbonic anhydrase gene mutation; drugs (e.g., ifosfamide)	
Generalized distal RTA (type IV RTA)	Hyporeninemic hypoaldosteronism	↓	24–28	↑	<5.5	↑BP; volume overload	Diabetes mellitus and mild CKD (common); renal mineralocorticoid receptor gene mutation (very rare)	Avoid iatrogenic causes of ↑K$^+$

Treatment of Metabolic Acidosis

1. Correct the underlying disorder (e.g., control diarrhea).
2. Bicarbonate therapy is reserved for severe metabolic gap acidosis (pH <7.10 or <7.20 and with renal insufficiency). The total replacement dose of HCO_3^- can be calculated as follows:

$$HCO_3^- \text{ needed in mmol} = \frac{\text{Base deficit (mmol)} \times \text{Patient's weight (kg)}}{4}$$

3. Replace with **one-half the total amount of bicarbonate over 8–12 hr** and reevaluate. Be aware of sodium and volume overload during replacement. The sodium overload produces a hypertonic state resulting in water shifting from the intracellular space to extracellular space.

A normal or isotonic bicarbonate drip is made with 3 amp $NaHCO_3$ (50 mEq $NaHCO_3$/amp) in 1 L D_5W. Sodium or potassium citrate can be an alternative to sodium bicarbonate.

Also, an alternative to sodium bicarbonate therapy is tromethamine (tris-hydroxymethyl aminomethane). The advantages of using tromethamine is that you avoid the hypertonic state from the sodium load and the large volume of fluid associated with sodium bicarbonate drips. Also, tromethamine does not produce CO_2, as is the case with sodium bicarbonate, an advantage when there is a mixed metabolic gap acidosis and a respiratory acidosis.

14

METABOLIC ALKALOSIS: DIAGNOSIS AND TREATMENT

Metabolic alkalosis represents an increase in $[HCO_3^-]$ with a compensatory rise in PCO_2.

Differential Diagnosis

In two basic categories of diseases the kidneys retain HCO_3^- (Figure 14-3). They can be differentiated in terms of response to treatment with sodium chloride and by the urinary $[Cl^-]$, as determined by ordering a "spot" or "random" urine test for chloride (U_{Cl}).

Chloride-Sensitive (Responsive) Metabolic Alkalosis: The initial problem is a sustained loss of chloride out of proportion to the loss of sodium (either by renal or GI losses). This chloride depletion results in renal sodium conservation leading to a corresponding reabsorption of HCO_3^- by the kidneys. In this category of metabolic alkalosis, the urinary $[Cl^-]$ is <10 mEq/L, and the associated disorders respond to treatment with intravenous NaCl.

Chloride-Insensitive (Resistant) Metabolic Alkalosis: The pathogenesis in this category is direct stimulation of the kidneys to retain HCO_3^- irrespective

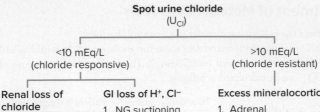

Figure 14-3. Differential diagnosis of metabolic alkalosis. (*Associated with ↑ BP)

of electrolyte intake and losses. The urinary [Cl⁻] >10 mEq/L, and these disorders do not respond to NaCl administration.

Other causes: Milk alkali syndrome, nonreabsorbable anions (penicillins), effective volume depletion (CHF, cirrhosis, nephrotic syndrome).

Treatment of Metabolic Alkalosis

Correct the underlying disorder.

1. **Chloride-responsive**
   a. Replace volume with NaCl if volume depleted.
   b. Correct hypokalemia if present.
   c. NH₄Cl and HCl should be reserved for extreme cases.
2. **Chloride-resistant**
   a. Correct the underlying problem, such as stopping exogenous steroids.

3. Effective volume depletion (edematous states such as CHF, cirrhosis, nephrotic syndrome): if $\downarrow K^+$, replacing K^+ or use of potassium-sharing diuretics may improve metabolic alkalosis.
4. With renal failure, treat with dialysis using a $\downarrow HCO_3^-$ bath concentration.
5. HCl or NH_4Cl can be used in extreme cases but is seldom required; use NH_4Cl with caution with renal or liver disease.

RESPIRATORY ACIDOSIS: DIAGNOSIS AND TREATMENT

Respiratory acidosis is a primary rise in PCO_2 with a compensatory rise in plasma $[HCO_3^-]$. Increased PCO_2 occurs in clinical situations in which decreased alveolar ventilation occurs.

Differential Diagnosis

Neuromuscular Abnormalities with Ventilatory Failure: Muscular dystrophy, myasthenia gravis, Guillain-Barré syndrome, amyotrophic lateral sclerosis, polymyositis, hypophosphatemia, hypomagnesemia

Central Nervous System: Drugs (sedatives, analgesics, tranquilizers, ethanol), CVA, encephalitis, brainstem disorders, central sleep apnea, spinal cord injury (cervical), hypothyroidism, hypothermia

Airway Obstruction: Chronic COPD (severe), acute asthma (severe), upper airway obstruction, obstructive sleep apnea; with severe COPD, administration of O_2 raising the O_2 saturation above 90% may cause acute on chronic retention of CO_2. It is difficult to predict which patients with end-stage COPD will retain CO_2 acutely with O_2 therapy.

Thoracic–Pulmonary Disorders: Bony thoracic cage (flail chest, kyphoscoliosis, pectus excavatum), parenchymal lesions (pneumothorax, severe pulmonary edema, severe pneumonia), large pleural effusions, scleroderma, obesity hypoventilation syndrome (Pickwickian syndrome).

Treatment of Respiratory Acidosis

Improve Ventilation: Intubate patient or may need cricothyrotomy if severe upper airway obstruction and then initiate mechanical ventilation; if already on ventilator increase ventilator rate; may use Ambu bag and mask initially or if the cause is easily reversible; reverse narcotic sedation with naloxone (Narcan), reverse benzodiazepine sedation with flumazenil; suspected anaphylaxis or angioedema administer epinephrine followed by an H1- and H2-blockers and IV steroids (methylprednisolone); continuous positive airway pressure (CPAP) or bilevel positive airway pressure (BiPAP) can be used to treat obstructive sleep apnea.

14

RESPIRATORY ALKALOSIS: DIAGNOSIS AND TREATMENT

Respiratory alkalosis is a primary fall in PCO_2 with a compensatory decrease in plasma $[HCO_3^-]$. Respiratory alkalosis occurs with increased alveolar ventilation.

Differential Diagnosis

Central Stimulation: Anxiety, hyperventilation syndrome, pain, head trauma or CVA with central neurogenic hyperventilation, tumors, salicylate overdose (often mixed metabolic gap acidosis and respiratory alkalosis), fever, early sepsis.

Peripheral Stimulation: PE, CHF (mild), asthma (mild), interstitial lung disease, pneumonia, high altitude, hypoxemia from any cause (see Hypoxia below).

Miscellaneous: Hepatic insufficiency/failure, PRG, progesterone, hyperthyroidism, iatrogenic mechanical overventilation.

Treatment of Respiratory Alkalosis

Correct the underlying disorder.

Hyperventilation Syndrome: Best controlled by having the patient rebreathe into a paper bag to increase PCO_2, decrease ventilator rate, increase amount of dead space with ventilator, or manage underlying cause; if patient is on a ventilator, consider sedation if anxious.

HYPOXIA

The second type of information gained from a blood gas level, in addition to acid-base results, is oxygenation. Results usually are given as PO_2 and O_2 saturation (see Table 14-1, page 400, for normal values). These two parameters are related to each other.

Oxygen saturation at any given PO_2 is influenced by temperature, pH, and the level of 2,3-diphosphoglycerate (2,3-DPG), as shown in Figure 14-4, page 413.

Oxygenation can also be determined noninvasively with pulse oximetry. **Pulse oximetry** is used to measure pulse rate and SaO_2 and can reduce the need for ABG measurements. The transcutaneous technique (detector placed on the finger, toe, top of the ear, earlobe of adults and the foot, palm, great toe, or thumb of children) is sensitive in the detection of arterial desaturation only. The technology is based on the different red and infrared light absorption characteristics of oxygenated and deoxygenated hemoglobin. The technique may be less accurate in cases of poor perfusion, motion, sensor exposure to ambient light, darker skin pigmentation (often inaccurate at saturations <80%), use of IV contrast agents, and

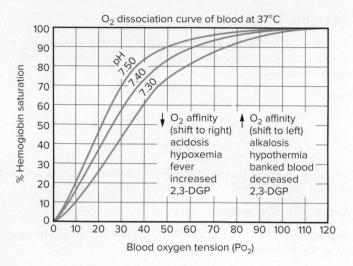

Figure 14-4.   Oxyhemoglobin dissociation curve.

14

the presence of abnormal hemoglobins (carboxy hemoglobin, methemoglobin). **Normal pulse oximetry readings should be 95–99% in a healthy person on room air and can vary slightly according to age, state of fitness, and altitude.** Anemia, elevated bilirubin, and sickle cell disease do not affect readings. (See also Chapter 26, page 838.)

Hypoxia Differential Diagnosis

$\dot{V}/\dot{Q}$ *(Ventilation/Perfusion) Abnormalities:*   COPD (emphysema, chronic bronchitis, asthma), atelectasis, pneumonia, PE, acute respiratory distress syndrome (ARDS), pneumothorax, pneumoconiosis, cystic fibrosis (CF), obstructed airway.

Alveolar Hypoventilation: Skeletal abnormalities, neuromuscular disorders, Pickwickian syndrome, obstructive sleep apnea.

Decreased Pulmonary Diffusing Capacity: Pneumoconiosis, pulmonary edema, drug-induced pulmonary fibrosis (bleomycin), collagen–vascular diseases.

Right-to-Left Shunt: Congenital heart disease (e.g., tetralogy of Fallot, transposition of the great arteries).

SAMPLE ACID-BASE PROBLEMS

In each of these examples, use the technique for blood gas interpretation on page 404 to identify the acid-base disorder.

Example 1

A patient with COPD has a blood gas of pH 7.34, PCO_2 55 mm Hg, and $[HCO_3^-]$ 29 mEq/L. Remember the $[HCO_3^-]$ must be obtained from the serum chemistries.

Step 1:

$$46 = 24 \times \frac{55}{29}$$
$$46 \approx 45$$

The numbers fit because the difference between the calculated and observed values is <10%.

Step 2: pH <7.37, acidemia.

Step 3: PCO_2 >44 mm Hg, and $[HCO_3^-]$ is **not** <22 mEq/L, thus respiratory acidosis is the primary disorder.

Step 4: Normal compensation for chronic (COPD) respiratory acidosis (from Table 14-2, page 403) so there is no secondary disorder.

$$\Delta[HCO_3^-] = 4 \times \Delta(PCO_2/10) = 4 \times \frac{15}{10} = 6$$

Expected $[HCO_3^-]$ is 24 mEq/L + 6 = 30, which is close to the measured $[HCO_3^-]$ of 29 mEq/L, thus simple respiratory acidosis (and no secondary disorder). This patient has chronic respiratory acidosis due to hypoventilation (simple acid-base disorder).

Step 5: Be sure to calculate the anion gap and proceed to Step 6 if there is an elevated anion gap.

Example 2

Immediately after cardiac arrest a patient has pH 7.25, PCO_2 28 mm Hg, and $[HCO_3^-]$ 12 mEq/L.

Step 1:

$$56 = 24 \times \frac{28}{12}$$
$$56 = 56$$

The numbers fit.

Step 2: pH <7.37, acidemia.

Step 3: $[HCO_3^-]$ is <22 mEq/L and PCO_2 is **not** >44 mm Hg; thus, metabolic acidosis is the primary disorder.

Step 4:   (See Table 14-2, page 403.)

$$PCO_2 = (1.5 \times [HCO_3^-] + 8) = (1.5 \times 12) + 8 = 26$$

The expected PCO_2 of 26 mm Hg is similar to the measured value of 28 mm Hg, so this condition is simple metabolic acidosis and there is no secondary disorder. The patient has lactic acidosis following cardiopulmonary arrest (simple acid-base disorder).

Step 5:   Be sure to calculate the anion gap and proceed to Step 6 if there is an elevated anion gap.

Example 3

A young man with a fever of 103.2°F and a fruity odor on his breath has a blood gas of pH 7.36, PCO_2 9 mm Hg, and $[HCO_3^-]$ 5 mEq/L.

Step 1:

$$45 = \frac{24}{5} \times 9$$
$$43 \approx 45$$

The numbers fit.

Step 2:   pH <7.37 indicates acidemia.

Step 3: $[HCO_3^-]$ <22 mEq/L and PCO_2 is **not** >44 mm Hg; thus, a metabolic acidosis is the primary disorder.

Step 4:   The expected compensation in PCO_2 can be calculated as follows (see Table 14-2, page 403):

$$PCO_2 = (1.5 \times [HCO_3^-]) + 8 \pm 2$$
$$= (1.5 \times 5) + 8 \pm 2$$
$$= 17.5 \pm 2$$

The expected PCO_2 is 17.5 mm Hg, but the reading is 9 mm Hg, indicating a secondary disorder, a respiratory alkalosis. This patient has a metabolic acidosis due to DKA and concomitant respiratory alkalosis possibly due to early sepsis and fever (a mixed acid-base disorder).

Step 5:   Be sure to calculate the anion gap and proceed to Step 6 if there is an elevated anion gap.

Example 4

A 30-year-old woman who is 30 wk pregnant presents with nausea and vomiting. Blood gas analysis reveals pH 7.55, PCO_2 25 mm Hg, and $[HCO_3^-]$ 22 mEq/L.

Step 1:

$$28 = 24 \times \frac{25}{22}$$
$$28 \approx 27$$

The numbers fit.

Step 2: pH >7.44 indicates alkalemia.

Step 3: PCO_2 <36 mm Hg and $[HCO_3^-]$ is **not** >26 mEq/L; thus, respiratory alkalosis is the primary disorder.

Step 4: The expected compensation for chronic respiratory alkalosis (i.e., pregnancy) is calculated from Table 14-2, page 403:

$$\Delta[HCO_3^-] = 5 \times \Delta PCO_2/10$$
$$= 5 \times \frac{15}{10} = 7.5$$

The calculated $[HCO_3^-]$ is 24 – 7.5, or 16–17 mEq, but the actual $[HCO_3^-]$ is 22 mEq/L, indicating a relative secondary metabolic alkalosis because the $[HCO_3^-]$ is higher than expected. This patient has respiratory alkalosis due to pregnancy and also has relative secondary metabolic alkalosis due to vomiting.

Step 5: Be sure to calculate the anion gap and proceed to Step 6 if there is an elevated anion gap.

Example 5 (Always Be Sure the Anion Gap Is Appropriate for the Change in [HCO_3^-])

These next two steps should only be done after Steps 1–4 when assessing an acid-base disorder. And Step 5 should always be done regardless of the pH.

A 19-year-old patient with diabetes has an anion gap of 29 mEq/L and a $[HCO_3^-]$ of 6 mEq/L.

Step 5:

> 29 mmol/L actual gap
> –10 mmol/L normal gap
> ──────
> 19 mmol/L expected change in $[HCO_3^-]$

Step 6:

> 24 mmol/L normal $[HCO_3^-]$
> –19 mmol/L expected change in $[HCO_3^-]$
> ──────
> 5 mmol/L expected $[HCO_3^-]$

Actual $[HCO_3^-]$ is 6 mEq/L, close to the expected $[HCO_3^-]$ of 5 mEq/L. Thus, pure metabolic gap acidosis is present, most likely from DKA.

Example 6

A 21-year-old patient with diabetes presents with nausea, vomiting, and abdominal pain. The anion gap is 23 mEq/L, and the $[HCO_3^-]$ is 18 mEq/L.

Step 5:

$$\begin{array}{r} 23 \text{ mmol/L actual gap} \\ \underline{-10 \text{ mmol/L normal gap}} \\ 13 \text{ mmol/L expected change in } [HCO_3^-] \text{ from normal} \end{array}$$

Step 6:

$$\begin{array}{r} 24 \text{ mmol/L normal } [HCO_3^-] \\ \underline{-13 \text{ mmol/L expected change in } [HCO_3]} \\ 11 \text{ mmol/L expected } [HCO_3^-] \end{array}$$

The $[HCO_3^-]$ is 18 mEq/L and not the expected $[HCO_3^-]$ of 11 mEq/L if a pure metabolic gap acidosis was the only metabolic disorder. Because the actual $[HCO_3^-]$ is higher than expected, this condition is mixed metabolic gap acidosis and metabolic alkalosis. The patient has metabolic gap acidosis from DKA and metabolic alkalosis from vomiting.

14

Example 7

A 55-year-old male patient who drinks a fifth of whiskey per day has a 2-wk history of diarrhea. The anion gap is 17 mEq/L, and the $[HCO_3^-]$ is 10 mEq/L.

Step 5:

$$\begin{array}{r} 17 \text{ mmol/L actual gap} \\ \underline{-10 \text{ mmol/L normal gap}} \\ 7 \text{ mmol/L expected change in } [HCO_3^-] \text{ from normal} \end{array}$$

Step 6:

$$\begin{array}{r} 24 \text{ mmol/L normal } [HCO_3^-] \\ \underline{-7 \text{ mmol/L expected change in } [HCO_3^-]} \\ 17 \text{ mmol/L expected } [HCO_3^-] \end{array}$$

Actual $[HCO_3^-]$ is 10 mEq/L and not the expected 17 mEq/L if a pure metabolic gap acidosis was the only metabolic disturbance. Because the actual $[HCO_3^-]$ is lower than expected, a mixed metabolic gap acidosis and metabolic nongap acidosis is present. The patient has metabolic nongap acidosis from diarrhea and metabolic gap acidosis from alcoholic ketoacidosis.

Example 8

One last example to tie it all together: A 35-year-old woman with a history of hypertension and systemic lupus erythematosus has a fever of 103.3°F orally 1 hr ago at home and a cough. Her cough is productive of rusty-colored sputum for the last 12 hr. Prior to today she was afebrile. She is on prednisone 20 mg PO qday and methotrexate 10 mg/wk. She increased her dose of prednisone from 5 mg/day to 20 mg last week when she had a flareup of her joint pain. Her antihypertensive medications include lisinopril 20 mg and chlorthalidone 25 mg every morning. Her BPs at home have been 140–160/90–100 mm Hg. Today her BP is 96/74, HR 120, respiratory rate 20, and temperature 103.8°F. She has crackles in the left lower lung field and has labored breathing. WBC is elevated to 18,600, with 75% segmented neutrophils, 20% banded neutrophils; pH 7.46, $PCO_2 = 20$ mm Hg, $O_2 = 60$ mm Hg; Na^+ 138, K^+ 4.6, Cl^- 98, HCO_3^- 14, glucose 100, BUN 15, and creatinine 1.0.

Step 1:   pH 7.46 = $[H^+]$ 34 nmol/L

$$34 = 24 \times \frac{20}{14}$$
$$34 = 34.3$$

The numbers fit.

Step 2:   Is the pH >7.44 or <7.37? pH = 7.46 indicates an alkalemia.

Step 3:   Is the $[HCO_3^-]$ >26 mEq/L or the PCO_2 <36 mm Hg? The PCO_2 is 20 mm Hg and the (HCO_3^-) <26 mEq/L; thus, the primary disturbance is a respiratory alkalosis, most likely from the pneumonia.

Step 4:   The primary process, the acute respiratory infection (likely a pneumonia), is acute in onset. The expected compensation in HCO_3 can be calculated as follows (see Table 14-2, page 403):

$$\Delta HCO_3^- = 2 \times \frac{40 - 20}{10}$$
$$\Delta HCO_3^- = -4$$

The expected HCO_3^- would be 20 mEq/L (24 − 4) and instead the HCO_3^- is 22, which is likely from measurement error, but there might be a secondary metabolic alkalosis, possibly from the thiazide diuretic.

Remember to always calculate the anion gap, even with a primary respiratory acidosis or alkalosis!

Step 5:

26 mmol/L actual gap
−10 mmol/L normal gap
‾‾‾‾‾‾‾‾‾‾‾‾‾‾‾‾
16 mmol/L expected change in $[HCO_3^-]$ from normal

An anion gap of 26 would necessitate additional laboratory testing, such as lactic acid, ketones, various toxins such as methanol, etc. In this case the lactic acid was markedly elevated, likely from hypoperfusion. Remember, the patient's usual BP was 140–160/90–100 mm Hg and her systolic BP of 96 mm Hg, while "normal," is well below her usual blood pressure, likely leading to hypoperfusion, likely resulting in lactic acidosis.

Step 6:

$$24 \text{ mmol/L normal } [HCO_3^-]$$
$$-16 \text{ mmol/L expected change in } [HCO_3^-]$$
$$\overline{8} \text{ mmol/L expected } [HCO_3^-]$$

The expected $[HCO_3^-]$ is 8 mmol/L; however, the actual $[HCO_3^-]$ is 14, which suggests a metabolic alkalosis in addition to the metabolic gap acidosis.

This patient has a triple acid-base disorder, a respiratory alkalosis secondary to the pneumonia, a metabolic gap acidosis from hypoperfusion, possibly from sepsis, and a metabolic alkalosis, possibly secondary from long-term use of the thiazide diuretic.

14

Fluid and Electrolytes

15

PRINCIPLES OF FLUIDS AND ELECTROLYTES

Physiologic mechanisms regulate volume, electrolytes, osmolality, and acid–base within a narrow homeostatic range. Alterations in homeostasis such as from renal dysfunction and other disease states, deficiency or excess of fluids, and/or electrolytes may lead to perturbations that need correction.

Therapy requires determination and correction of the underlying cause and likely an intervention to correct the resultant fluid and electrolyte disturbances, some of which may be life-threatening and need prompt attention. Therapy needs to be given at the appropriate rate and for the appropriate duration. The assessment and management of various electrolyte disorders are discussed in this chapter.

GOALS OF IV FLUID THERAPY

- Provide maintenance fluids, electrolytes, and nutrition
- Resuscitation in cases of shock
- Correct volume depletion
- Correct electrolyte and/or acid–base disorders
- Correct ongoing loss of fluid and electrolytes

Chapter update by David R. Rudy, MD, and Steven A. Haist, MD, MS

Steps in ordering IVFs

1. Patient assessment: Determine volume status and presence of electrolyte or acid–base disturbances. Assess for underlying medical conditions such as congestive heart failure (CHF), chronic kidney disease, diabetes mellitus (DM), liver disease, etc., and for ongoing losses of fluid and electrolytes such as diarrhea, NG tube drainage, acute pancreatitis, etc.
2. Selection of appropriate IVFs, including additives such as potassium or magnesium.
3. Selection of the rate of administration.
4. Ongoing monitoring and reassessment and adjustments as indicated.

FLUID COMPARTMENTS

Total Body Water (TBW)

TBW varies due to age, gender, and body composition. TBW is approximately 80% in a full-term infant, 60% in a lean male adult, and 40–50% in obese patients and the elderly.

Below are calculations for a 70-kg male with normal body habitus (1 kg = 1 L)

$$TBW = 0.6 \times Body\ wt\ (kg) = 42\ L$$

- 66.6% × TBW = intracellular fluid (ICF) = 28 L
- 33.3% × TBW = extracellular fluid (ECF) = 14 L
  - 25% × ECF = Intravascular fluid (plasma) = 3.5 L
  - 75% × ECF = Interstitial fluid = 10.5 L

Total Blood Volume

Total blood volume = 5600 mL (8% of body water in a 70-kg man)

Red Blood Cell Mass

- Man, 20–36 mL/kg (1.15–1.21 L/m^2)
- Woman, 19–31 mL/kg (0.95–1.0 L/m^2)

The distribution of TBW is important in understanding how to use intravenous fluids (IVFs) appropriately.

Dextrose 5% in water (D5W) is distributed into TBW: 1000 cc of D5W will result in only about an additional 82 cc in the intravascular space. Additionally, slight decreases in serum osmolality (approximately >1%) will lead to a prompt decrease in antidiuretic hormone (ADH), resulting in increased renal elimination of free water. One must be vigilant about the use of hypotonic fluids in patients with increased ADH, such as in the postoperative state, where nonosmotic stimuli for ADH may lead to water retention and hyponatremia. Dextrose-containing fluids should be avoided in patients with diabetes; otherwise, uncontrolled hyperglycemia may result. Likewise, glucose-containing fluids should be avoided in patients with severe hypoglycemia due to the promotion of intracellular shifting of K^+ and resulting in further lowering of plasma K^+.

Normal saline is distributed into the extracellular space: 1000 cc of normal saline will result in an addition of 250 cc into the vascular space. This becomes evident when isotonic fluids, such as normal saline or Ringer's lactate, are used in the resuscitation of critically ill patients where redistribution into the interstitial space may lead to edema. Redistribution may also occur into other extravascular spaces such as the pleural space or the peritoneal cavity, resulting in pleural effusions or ascites, respectively.

Blood, plasma, or albumin will distribute to the intravascular space: 1000 cc of albumin will result in an additional 1000 cc in the vascular space. With the administration of albumin, one must be vigilant of inducing vascular volume overload in susceptible patients, such as in patients with a history of CHF.

Redistribution of body fluids can occur in critical illness with fluids in the circulatory volume moving into the tissues called "third space loss." This can be seen with CHF, renal failure, pancreatitis, or sepsis, all potentially resulting in peripheral edema.

15

Water Balance

- 70-kg man example

The minimum obligate water requirement to maintain homeostasis in adults (if temperature and renal-concentrating ability are normal and solute [urea, salt] excretion is minimal) is about 800 mL/d, which would yield 500 mL of urine. The other losses are from the lungs and skin.

"Normal" Intake: 2500 mL/d (about 35 mL/kg/d baseline)

- Oral liquids: 1500 mL
- Oral solids: 700 mL
- Metabolic (endogenous from oxidation): 300 mL

"Normal" Output: 1400–2300 mL/d

- Urine: 800–1500 mL
- Stool: 250 mL
- Insensible loss: 600–900 mL (lungs and skin). With fever, each degree above 98.6°F (37°C) adds 2.5 mL/kg/d of insensible losses; insensible losses are decreased if a patient is undergoing mechanical ventilation; free water gain can occur from humidified ventilation.

Baseline Fluid Requirements

Afebrile typical 70-kg Adult: 35 mL/kg/24 hr
Children based on body weight: Calculate the water requirement according to the following kg method:

- $\leq$10 kg 100 mL/kg
- >10–20 kg 1000 mL for first 10 kg of body weight plus 50 mL/kg for weight increment above 10 kg
- >20–80 kg 1500 mL for first 20 kg of body weight plus 20 mL/kg for weight increment above 20 kg
- >80 kg 2700 mL/day

Electrolyte Requirements

- 70-kg adult, unless otherwise specified

   Sodium (as NaCl): 80–120 mEq/d (children, 3–4 mEq/kg/24 h)
   Chloride (as NaCl): 80–120 mEq/d
   Potassium: 50–100 mEq/d (children, 2–3 mEq/kg/24 hr). In the absence of hypokalemia and with normal renal function, most of the K^+ is excreted in the urine.
   Calcium: 1–3 g/d, most of which is excreted by the GI tract. Routine administration is not needed in the absence of specific indications.
   Magnesium: 20 mEq/d. Routine administration is not needed in the absence of specific indications, such as parenteral hyperalimentation, massive diuresis, ethanol abuse (frequently needed), or preeclampsia.

Glucose Requirements

- 100–200 g/d (65–75 g/d/m²). During starvation, caloric needs are supplied by body fat and protein; most protein comes from the skeletal muscles. Every gram of nitrogen in the urine represents 6.25 g of metabolized protein. The **protein-sparing effect** is one of the goals of basic IV therapy. Administration of at least 100 g/d of glucose reduces protein loss by more than one half. Almost all IV fluid solutions supply glucose as dextrose (pure dextrorotatory glucose). Pediatric patients need about 100–200 mg/kg/hr of glucose.

COMPOSITION OF PARENTERAL FLUIDS

Parenteral fluids are generally classified according to molecular weight and oncotic pressure.

- **Colloids** are defined as a high molecular weight (MW >8000) substance that largely remains in the intravascular compartment, generating an oncotic pressure. Colloids are rarely used alone and typically used in conjunction with crystalloids.

- **Crystalloids** have a molecular weight <8000 and have low oncotic pressure with limited ability to remain within the circulation and enters the interstitial space. Crystalloids are commonly used as maintenance fluids, for electrolyte replacement, for the administration of intravenous medications, and typically are the first-line choice for fluid resuscitation with hypovolemia, hemorrhage, sepsis, and dehydration.
- In the initial treatment of sepsis/septic shock randomized trials have found no significant difference between using colloid solutions (albumin) solutions vs. crystalloids, and crystalloids can be considered second line therapy for refractory shock. Potential harms from using hydroxyethyl starch in this setting include acute kidney injury and anaphylactic reactions.

Colloids

- Natural colloids
  o Albumin: Normal colloid in plasma (55% of serum proteins, generates 80% of plasma oncotic pressure). Albumin 5% solution is isoosmotic with plasma and 25% is hyperosmotic
  o Blood products (e.g., RBCs, fresh frozen plasma)
  o Plasma protein fraction (Plasmanate) prepared from pools of human plasma; contains 5% albumin, osmotically equivalent to plasma
- Synthetic colloids
  o Gelatins (not used in the United States), dextrans, and hydroxyethyl starch (HES); sometimes used to prime extracorporeal circulation pumps used in cardio-pulmonary bypass

15

Crystalloids

Table 15-1, page 426, describes common crystalloid parenteral fluids.

COMPOSITION OF BODY FLUIDS

Table 15-2, page 427, gives the average daily production and the amount of some of the major electrolytes present in various body fluids.

ORDERING IV FLUIDS

One of the most difficult tasks to master is choosing appropriate IV therapy for a patient. The patient's underlying illness, vital signs, serum electrolytes, and a host of other variables must be considered. The following are general guidelines for IV therapy. Specific requirements for each patient can vary tremendously from these guidelines.

Table 15-1. Composition of Commonly Used Crystalloids

Fluid	Electrolytes (mEq/L)[a]								kcal/L
	Glucose (g/L)	Na$^+$	Cl$^-$	K$^+$	Ca^{2+}	HCO$_3^-$	Mg^{2+}	HPO$_4^{2-}$	
D5W (5% dextrose in water)	50	—	—	—	—	—	—	—	170
D10W (10% dextrose in water)	100	—	—	—	—	—	—	—	340
D20W (20% dextrose in water)	200	—	—	—	—	—	—	—	680
D50W (50% dextrose in water)	500	—	—	—	—	—	—	—	1700
½ NS (0.45% NaCl)	—	77	77	—	—	—	—	—	—
3% NS	—	513	513	—	—	—	—	—	—
NS (0.9% NaCl)	—	154	154	—	—	—	—	—	—
D5 ¼ NS (0.22% NaCl)	50	38	38	—	—	—	—	—	170
D5 ½ NS (0.45% NaCl)	50	77	77	—	—	—	—	—	170
D5NS (0.9% NaCl)	50	154	154	—	—	—	—	—	170
D5LR (5% dextrose in lactated Ringer's)[b]	50	130	110	4	3	27	—	—	180
Lactated Ringer's[b]	—	130	110	4	3	27	—	—	<10
Ionosol MB 5% Dextrose	50	25	22	20	—	23	3	3	170
Normosol M 5% Dextrose	50	40	40	13	—	16	3	—	170

[a]HCO$_3^-$ is administered in these solutions as lactate that is converted to bicarbonate.
[b]Lactated ringers contains calcium and may cause coagulation when mixed with blood transfusions.

Table 15-2.   Composition and Daily Production of Body Fluids

| | Electrolytes (mEq/L) | | | | |
Fluid	Na⁺	Cl⁻	K⁺	HCO₃⁻	Average Daily Production[a] (mL)
Sweat	50	40	5	0	Varies
Saliva	60	15	26	50	1500
Gastric juice	60–100	100	10	0	1500–2500
Duodenal fluid	130	90	5	0–10	300–2000
Bile	145	100	5	15	100–800
Pancreatic juice	140	*75*	5	115	100–800
Ileal fluid	140	100	2–8	30	100–9000
Diarrhea	120	90	25	45	—

[a]In adults.

Maintenance Fluids

The following amounts provide the minimum requirements for routine daily needs:

15

1. **70-kg Man:** 5% dextrose in one-fourth concentration normal saline D5¹/₄NS with 20 mEq/L KCl at 125 mL/hr. (This infusion delivers about 3 L/d of free water.)

2. **Other Adult Patients:** Also use D5¹/₄NS with 20 mEq/L KCl. Determine the 24-hr water requirement with the "kg method" (page 424) and divide by 24 hr to determine the hourly rate.

3. **Pediatric Patients:** In 2018 the American Academy of Pediatrics revised guidelines for prescribing routine maintenance fluids in pediatric patients from 28 days to 18 years of age.[1] The basis of this decision was to limit the development of hyponatremia in this age group. These recommendations do not apply to patients who are neonates, infants less than 28 days, neurosurgical patients, or patients with cardiac or hepatic diseases, cancer, renal dysfunction, severe diarrhea, or extensive burns. Determine the parenteral fluid therapy requirements by either of the following methods (modified from Ref. 2):

Method 1 – Maintenance fluid hourly basis:
- Weight <10 kg – 4 mL/kg/hr
- Weight >10–20 kg – 40 mL/hr for first 10 kg BW plus 2 mL/kg/hr for any increment of BW over 10 kg

- Weight >20–80 kg — 60 mL/hr for first 20 kg of body weight plus 1 mL/ kg/hr for any increment of BW over 20 kg, to a maximum of 100 mL/hr (up to a maximum of 2400 mL daily)

Method 2 – Maintenance fluid 24-hr period:
- Weight <10 kg — 100 mL/kg
- Weight >10–20 kg — 1000 mL for first 10 kg of BW plus 50 mL/kg for any increment of BW over 10 kg
- Weight >20–80 kg – 1500 mL + 20 mL/kg for every kg over 20 (up to a maximum of 2400 mL daily)

Routine maintenance fluid composition in children (see exceptions below)
- **Dextrose 5%**
- **Normal Saline 0.9%**
- **Potassium:** 10 mEq/L weight < 10 kg; ≥10 kg 10–20 mEq/L

Specific Replacement Fluids

Fluids are used to replace excessive, nonphysiologic losses.

Gastric Loss (Nasogastric Tube, Emesis): D5 $^1/_2$ NS with 20 mEq/L KCl

Diarrhea: D5LR with 15 mEq/L KCl. Use body weight as a replacement guide (about 1 L for each 1 kg, or 2.2 lb, lost).

Bile Loss: D5LR with 25 mEq/L of NaHCO$_3$ ($^1/_2$ amp) milliliter for milliliter.

Pancreatic Loss: D5LR D5 with 50 mEq/L of NaHCO$_3$ (1 amp) milliliter for milliliter.

Burn Patients: Use the Rule of Nines formula to determine % body burned. See Appendix, Figure A-11, page 1086. The Parkland (also known as Baxter) formula is commonly used for the fluid replacement.

Rule of Nines. can be used for estimating percentage of body burned. Also, you can use Figure 15-1A and B, pages 429–430, to calculate body burn area in adults and children. This is also useful for determining ongoing fluid losses from a burn until it is healed or grafted.

Parkland Formula.
Adult: Total fluid required during the first 24 hr = (% body burn) × (body weight in kg) × 4 mL

Child: same formula × 3 mL

- Replace with LR over 24 hr as follows:
  o One half of the total over first 8 hr (from time of burn)
  o One half of the total over the next 16 hr

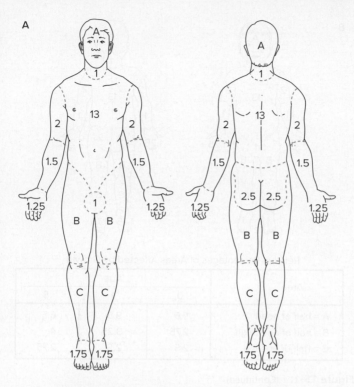

Relative Percentages of Areas Affected by Growth

Area	Age		
	10	15	Adult
A = half of head	5.5	4.5	3.5
B = half of one thigh	4.25	4.5	4.75
C = half of one leg	3	3.25	3.5

Figure 15-1. Tables and graphics for estimating the extent of burns in adults (**A**) and children (**B**). For adults, another way of estimating percentage of the body surface burned is the rule of nines: Each arm is 9%, the front and back of each leg is 9%, the anterior trunk and and posterior trunk are each 18%, the head is 9%, and the perineum is 1%. (Used with permission from Current Surgical Diagnosis and Treatment, 12e, Doherty, GM [editor]. New York, NY: McGraw-Hill; 2006.)

After 24 hr, use $D_5\frac{1}{2}NS$ at a rate to maintain urine output 0.5–1 mL/kg/hr (adults) and 1.0–1.5 mL/kg/hr in children. Consider supplementation of colloid-containing fluid after the first 24 hr postburn. During the second 24-hr period, stop crystalloids and initiate colloids at 20–60% of calculated plasma

B

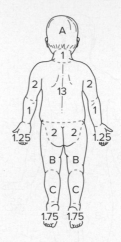

Relative Percentages of Areas Affected by Growth

Area	Age		
	0	1	5
A = half of head	9.5	8.5	6.5
B = half of one thigh	2.75	3.25	4
C = half of one leg	2.5	2.5	2.75

Figure 15-1. (Continued)

volume and dextrose in water. A modified Parkland formula for the second 24 hr uses a 5% albumin colloid infusion of 0.3–1.0/16 mL/kg/%BSA/hr.

ELECTROLYTE ABNORMALITIES: DIAGNOSIS AND TREATMENT

In all of the following situations, the primary goal is to correct the underlying condition. Unless specified, all dosages are for adults.

DISORDERS OF SODIUM AND WATER BALANCE

Disorders of sodium concentration are a reflection of an imbalance between water and sodium, i.e., a disorder of osmolality. Recall that the major determinate of osmolality is sodium concentration. For the most part, these disorders should be treated as problems with water balance. Total body sodium should be thought of as a determinate of volume status. Thus, sodium concentration should be thought of as reflecting osmolality, and total body sodium should be thought of as reflecting volume.

Disorders of sodium concentration, hypernatremia and hyponatremia, are classified according to volume status, and both occur in volume depletion and volume overload, as well as in the euvolemic state.

Disorders of sodium concentration manifest clinically as impaired brain function due to osmotic shifts leading to varying degrees of cerebral edema. In some cases urgent therapy is needed; however, the rate of correction is also critical to prevent neurologic complications both from the initial electrolyte disturbance and potentially from the treatment.

Hypernatremia

- (Na^+ >145 mEq/L)
- Critical value >158 mEq/L

Mechanisms: Most frequent cause is a deficit of total body water.

- **Combined Sodium and Water Losses (Hypovolemic Hypernatremia).** Water loss in excess of Na^+ and anywhere else we have Na, K by itself loss results in low total body Na^+. Due to renal losses (e.g., diuretics, osmotic diuresis from glycosuria or mannitol or increased urea production, postobstructive diuresis) or extrarenal losses (sweating, severe burns, GI [vomiting, NG suction, osmotic-induced diarrhea from sorbitol or lactulose, and respiratory).
- **Excess Water Loss (Isovolemic Hypernatremia).** Total body Na^+ remains normal, but the total body water is decreased. Caused by diabetes insipidus (DI) (central or nephrogenic). Central DI: traumatic brain injury, CNS tumor, CNS surgery, many other causes, including drugs (nephrogenic DI: aminoglycosides, amphotericin B, cisplatin, colchicine, diuretics, penicillins, vinblastine; central DI: ethanol, lithium, phenytoin), and excess skin and/or respiratory losses, and others.
- **Excess Sodium (Hypervolemic Hypernatremia).** Total body Na^+ increased, caused by iatrogenic Na^+ administration (e.g., hypertonic IV fluids, [NaCl, $NaCO_3$], hypertonic dialysis, hypertonic saline enemas, hypertonic feedings, Na-containing medications) and other exogenous sources (seawater ingestion, salt tablets) or adrenal hyperfunction (Cushing syndrome, hyperaldosteronism).

Symptoms: Depend on the absolute level and also how rapidly the Na^+ level increased
- Confusion, irritability, lethargy, stupor, coma, muscle twitching, seizures

Signs: Hyperreflexia, mental status changes

Treatment: Check the serum Na^+ levels frequently while attempting to correct hypernatremia.
- **Hypovolemic Hypernatremia.** Determine whether the patient is volume depleted by determining whether orthostatic changes in BP and HR are present (see Chapter 19, page 627); if volume depleted, rehydrate with NS until patient is hemodynamically stable, then administer hypotonic saline ($^1/_2$ NS).

- **Euvolemic/Isovolemic.** (No orthostatic changes in BP and HR.) Calculate the volume of free water needed to correct the Na$^+$ to normal as follows:

Body water deficit = Normal Total Body Water (TBW) − Current TBW
Normal TBW = 0.6 × Body weight in kg
and

$$\text{Current TBW} = \frac{\text{Normal serum Na}^+ \times \text{TBW}}{\text{Measured serum Na}^+}$$

Give free water as D5W, one half of the volume in the first 24 hr and the full volume in 48 hr. **Caution:** Rapid correction of the Na$^+$ level using free water (D5W) can cause cerebral edema and seizures.

- **Hypervolemic Hypernatremia.** Avoid medications that contain excessive Na$^+$ (e.g., carbenicillin). Use furosemide along with D5W.

Hyponatremia

- (Na$^+$ <136 mEq/L)
- Critical values <121 mEq/L

Mechanisms: Hyponatremia is due to excess body water and is a disorder of osmolality.

The diagnostic approach includes history and physical examination emphasizing assessment of volume status, measurement of serum osmolality, and urinary sodium and osmolality measurements. Symptoms and signs related to cerebral edema include:

Symptoms:
- Mild: Nausea, malaise, forgetfulness, dizzy, irritability
- Moderate: Headache, confusion, lethargy, and muscle cramps
- Severe: Stupor, coma

Signs:
- Mild: Mild cognitive impairment, subtle balance deficits
- Moderate: Gait disturbances
- Severe: Neurologic deficits, seizure, respiratory arrest

The severity of the symptoms and signs depends upon how quickly the sodium decreased to the current level, duration of the hyponatremia, and severity of hyponatremia. Each of these may range from asymptomatic to life-threatening complications, including brain herniation. Too rapid or overcorrection of hyponatremia may lead to catastrophic neurologic consequences: osmotic demyelination syndrome (ODS) (central pontine myelinolysis and extrapontine myelinolysis). For the purposes of therapy, symptoms may be classified as mild to moderate and severe (see below).

Severity of hyponatremia:
Asymptomatic: Patients may not recognize symptoms but they actually are symptomatic with mild cognitive and mild balance issues.

Mild: Nausea, malaise, forgetfulness, dizzy, irritability, subtle cognitive impairment and balance deficits

Moderate: Headache, confusion, lethargy, gait disturbances, muscle cramps, gait disturbances.

Severe: Stupor, seizures, coma, neurologic defects, respiratory arrest

Serum osmolality: The initial test in the evaluation of hyponatremia (normal osm 280–295 mOsm/kg)

Isotonic hyponatremia (osmolality 280–295 mOsm/kg): Pseudohyponatremia, artifactal due to the laboratory method used to measure the serum sodium

Hypertonic hyponatremia (osmolality >295 mOsm/kg): Dilutional, a hyperosmolar solute causes water shifts from intracellular to extracellular compartments and lowers sodium concentration but total body water remains constant.

Hypotonic hyponatremia (osmolality <280 mOsm/kg) (most common form of hyponatremia)

Hyponatremia is further classified by the history, physical, and selected laboratory studies with particular attention to volume status (reflects total body sodium).

History: Inquiry about concurrent medical conditions, medications, vomiting, diarrhea, polyuria, symptoms of hyponatremia.

Physical examination: Focus on volume status; orthostatic vital signs (increase in HR of ≥20 BPM and decrease in systolic BP of ≥10 mm Hg; change in HR occurs before the change in systolic BP), measure JVP, assess skin turgor, look for dry mucous membranes and dry axilla, and review oral and IVF input and urine output measurements, and changes in weight.

Laboratory: Electrolytes, BUN, Cr, serum and urine osmolality, glucose, urine electrolytes. Additional labs are guided by the history and physical exam.

Based upon the clinical assessment of volume status, hypotonic hyponatremia may be further classified as:

Hypervolemic hypotonic hyponatremia: Decreased effective circulating volume leads to increased aldosterone, which leads to renal retention of water in greater proportion than sodium; caused by heart failure, cirrhosis, nephrotic syndrome, or hypoalbuminemia; also seen in advanced kidney disease due to a decreased ability to excrete sodium and water.

Diagnosis: There is evidence of edema, urinary OSM is elevated (>400 mOsm/kg), and urinary sodium is low (<10–20 mEq/L), with the exception being in the presence of diuretic use (a diuretic continues to produce a normal or elevated urine sodium in spite of decreased intravascular volume).

Hypovolemic hypotonic hyponatremia: Causes include extrarenal sodium loss (vomiting, diarrhea, dehydration due to excessive perspiration, and third spacing of fluids [severe burns, pancreatitis, peritonitis, bowel obstruction, or muscle trauma]); renal sodium loss (diuretics [thiazides, mannitol], renal interstitial disease, mineralocorticoid deficiency [Addison disease, hypoaldosteronism], renal tubular disorders, cerebral salt wasting [rare], and ACE inhibitors).

Diagnosis: Evidence of volume depletion such as orthostasis (changes in HR of an increase ≥ 20 BPM and decrease in systolic BP of ≥ 10 mm Hg; change in HR occurs before the change in systolic BP), urinary osm >400 mOsm/kg, and urinary sodium >20 mEq/L.

Isovolemic hypotonic hyponatremia: Five large categories: (1) SIADH, (2) water intoxication, (3) endocrine related, (4) other, and (5) pseudohyponatremia.

1. SIADH: Pain, stress including perioperative stress, nausea, cancer especially lung, pulmonary disease (TB, pneumonia, asthma, CF, ventilator support with PEEP), CNS disease (trauma, tumors, infections, bleed, MS), delirium tremens, acute intermittent porphyria, systemic infections (HIV, RMSF), medications (SSRIs, nicotine, ACE inhibitors, carbamazepine, phenytoin, valproate, many antipsychotics, NSAIDs, celecoxib, tramadol, opioids, 3,4-metthylene-dioxy-methamphetamine [MDMA, ecstasy], and many chemotherapeutic agents (cisplatin, cyclophosphamide, vincristine), osmostat reset.
2. Water intoxication/water intake exceeding excretory capacity: Psychogenic polydipsia, increased water consumption from taking MDMA ("ecstasy"), postoperative, iatrogenic from excess free water intake due to large volumes of sterile water used in procedures (transurethral resection of prostate, multiple tap water enemas), prolonged exercise with hypotonic fluid replacement, beer potomania, tea and toast diet.
3. Endocrine: Hypothyroidism, glucocorticoid deficiency (primary and secondary).
4. Other: Isotonic infusion of glucose or mannitol, severe hyperglycemia (osmotic shifts of fluids from the intracellular space to the extracellular space).
5. Pseudohyponatremia: An artifact due to the laboratory method used to measure the serum sodium, secondary to hyperproteinemia (multiple myeloma, Waldenstrom macroglobulinemia) or severe hyperlipidemia.

Diagnosis:
1. SIADH is a diagnosis by exclusion:
    Urinary osm: less than maximally dilute: >100 mOsm/kg
2. Non-SIADH causes:
    a. Water intoxication: Urinary osmolality <80 mOsm
    b. Endocrine causes: TSH, serum cortisol, ACTH, ACTH stimulation test

Treatment:
    Goals of therapy: To treat symptoms, prevent a further decrease in Na$^+$ concentration, avoid complications (seizures, brain herniation), and avoid overcorrection or too rapid of a correction, which can lead to significant morbidity and mortality.

Treatment of hyponatremia is based upon the duration, severity, and the etiology of the hyponatremia. In addition to treating the underlying cause, some patients may need more rapid correction of the Na$^+$ concentration than would occur by just treating the underlying cause. If acute correction is indicated, the rate of initial sodium correction is 4–6 mEq/L (maximal 8 mEq/L) in the first 24 hr.

The rapidity of correction of hyponatremia and the need for admission to the hospital or intensive care unit depends upon several factors:

Duration of hyponatremia: acute <48 hr or chronic > 48 hr. Inadequate treatment of acute hyponatremia is more likely to lead to complications of cerebral edema, whereas overzealous treatment of chronic hyponatremia is more likely to cause osmotic demylination syndrome (ODS), such as with an initial sodium concentration ≤105 mEq/L with associated hypokalemia from alcoholism, malnutrition, and liver disease. When the duration of hyponatremia is in doubt, assume chronic.

Severity of hyponatremia: Mild (130–134 mEq/L), moderate (120–129 mEq/L), severe (<120 mEq/L).

Severe symptoms: Emergent treatment for acute symptomatic hyponatremia is with hypertonic saline (3%), administered as small boluses (100 mL 3% normal saline over 10 min, checking labs after each bolus for a maximum of three times, if needed) or by infusion to resolve symptoms. The goal is to raise the Na^+ concentration by 4–6 mEq/L/day at a rate of 1–2 mEq/hr over the first 6 hr or a maximum of 8 mEq/day. The serum Na^+ should be checked every hour.

Duration of several hours: Such as from self-induced water intoxication associated with psychosis, marathon running, and taking MDMA. Low risk for ODS, and correction of the Na^+ concentration may proceed more rapidly.

Duration of 1–2 days: Postop hyponatremia, especially in children and women, or secondary to intracranial disease are at higher risk for ODS.

Setting: Preexisting CNS pathology, such as space-occupying lesion, recent intracranial surgery, or recent head trauma requires special attention. These conditions predispose to more complications from hyponatremia-induced cerebral edema and require more aggressive therapy at relatively lesser degrees of hyponatremia compared to other etiologies.

Chronic symptomatic hyponatremia: Apply extreme caution for conditions associated with a high risk of ODS such as chronic symptomatic hyponatremia. Treat with hypertonic saline at a slower rate of correction (≤0.5 mEq/hr). May use boluses of 100 mL 3% saline when chronic symptomatic hyponatremia is complicated by seizures. Once symptoms resolve, the maximal change in 24 hr of Na^+ is 4–6 mEq/L and discontinue the use of 3% saline. Then correct slowly and avoid increasing Na^+ concentration by more than 6 mEq/L in the first day. If a greater degree of correction has occurred, especially in patients at high risk of ODS, consider lowering Na^+ concentration again with ½ normal saline.

Nonemergent treatment of hyponatremia based upon etiology:

Hypervolemic hyponatremia: Treat underlying conditions, such as with loop diuretics or water restriction 1–1.5 L/day. Vasopressin receptor antagonists have a limited role in heart failure and cirrhosis.

15

Hypovolemic hyponatremia: Treat underlying conditions and use isotonic saline.

Isovolemic hyponatremia:

SIADH: Treat underlying cause, restrict fluids (1.5–1 L/day); loop diuretics, demeclocycline, oral salt tablets, and urea have been used in cases of chronic hyponatremia.

Non-SIADH causes: Treat the underlying disorder.

Special considerations:

Concurrent hypokalemia: Treatment of low potassium will raise serum osmolality and serum sodium. Treat hypokalemia first and monitor Na^+ concentration. This will help avoid overcorrection of hyponatremia.

Predisposition to rapid autocorrection of hyponatremia. Treatment of some underlying disorders causing an elevated ADH with water retention, may rapidly decrease ADH secretion and allow a water diuresis with "autocorrection" of hyponatremia. These conditions include the removal of a medication causing SIADH and correction of glucocorticoid insufficiency.

In addition, "autocorrection" may occur with volume restoration in cases of hypovolemic hyponatremia such as postoperative hyponatremia with dehydration. Urinary output and urinary osmolality should be monitored closely during infusion of saline. Once a drop in urine osmolality occurs or if serum sodium corrects too quickly, switch fluids to ½ normal saline.

Do not use isotonic saline in patients with edema (e.g., CHF, cirrhosis, nephrotic syndrome).

Do not use isotonic saline in SIADH. If urine osmolality exceeds 300 mOsm/L, further water retention will occur.

DISORDERS OF POTASSIUM BALANCE

The majority of K^+ (98%) is intracellular (140 mEq/L) and only 2% is extracellular (4–5 mEq/L). The serum K^+ level is normal, about 4.5 mEq/L; the total extracellular pool of $K^+ = 4.5 \times 14\,L = 63$ mEq. K^+ easily interchanges between intracellular and extracellular stores under conditions such as acidemia or alkalemia. K^+ demands increase with diuresis and building of new body tissues (anabolic states).

The clinical manifestations of derangements of potassium concentration are manifested by disturbances of cardiac rhythm, including lethal arrhythmias, and disturbances of neuromuscular conduction in skeletal muscle.

Extreme disorders of potassium concentration require emergent therapy to avoid or treat resultant cardiac arrhythmias. The treatment of hypokalemia needs to be done at an appropriate rate to avoid hyperkalemia and complications thereof.

Hyperkalemia

- $K^+ > 5.0$ mEq/L
- Critical values: any age > 6.0 mEq/L

Since the majority of total body potassium is intracellular, shifts from the intracellular to extracellular compartments may lead to rapid increases in serum K^+ concentration, and extracellular to intracellular shifts can lead to hypokalemia, as discussed in the next section.

The initial response to potassium intake is intracellular uptake of excess K^+. This is facilitated by increased insulin secretion and beta-2-receptor or β_2-receptor stimulation. Renal potassium secretion is regulated by the renin-angiotensin-aldosterone system (RAAS) in response to serum K^+ concentration.

Mechanism: Most commonly due to release from cells, decreased renal excretion, increased intake (iatrogenic is a major cause), or combination of the above.

Release from cells: Pseudohyperkalemia, an artifact from cell lysis with poor phlebotomy technique (excessive tourniquet time or too narrow gauge needle), prolonged storage of specimen, marked thrombocytosis, and severe leukocytosis with CLL due to cell fragility.

Potassium shifts: Increased tissue catabolism from rhabdomyolysis, tumor lysis syndrome, severe burns, hypothermia, reperfusion syndrome; hyperosmolality such as hyperglycemia, decreased insulin with diabetes mellitus; hyperkalemic periodic paralysis; medications including beta blockers, digoxin intoxication, succinylcholine (in the setting of crush injury, burns, or neuromuscular disease), isoflurane.

Decreased renal excretion: Decrease in aldosterone secretion from type IV renal tubular acidosis (RTA), adrenal disorders, medications (ACE inhibitors, NASIDs, calcineurin inhibitors, heparin, beta-blockers [β_1-receptor blockade decreases renin release]); decrease responsiveness to aldosterone (aldosterone resistance), aldosterone antagonists (spironolactone and eplerenone); sodium channel blockade (amiloride, triamterene, trimethoprim); distal RTA (tubulointerstitial disorders from sickle cell disease, cyclosporine toxicity, SLE, others).

Decreased distal Na and water delivery: Pre-renal state, volume depletion.

Hyperkalemia in acute or chronic kidney disease may have one or more of the above causes. Hyperkalemia in the setting of AKI is more severe in the setting of oliguria and/or increased tissue catabolism.

Increased potassium intake: A common iatrogenic cause in hospitalized patents from potassium salts in IVFs, K^+-containing medications such as PCN, dietary salt substitutes, tube feedings, and red blood cell transfusions.

Symptoms: Potassium concentration is a major determinate of neuromuscular resting membrane potential. Both hyperkalemia and hypokalemia may cause muscle paralysis and lethal cardiac arrhythmias. The rate of change of K^+ is more important than the actual serum K^+ concentration.

Hyperkalemia may be asymptomatic or present with weakness or paralysis. Symptoms develop at a K^+ of 6.5–7 mEq/L.

Signs: Physical examination may be normal or may be significant for hypoactive deep tendon reflexes and/or decreased motor strength.

The most important information for the severity of hyperkalemia is an ECG. ECG changes of hyperkalemia necessitate emergent treatment to prevent potentially fatal arrhythmias. All patients with $K^+ \geq 6$ mEq/L and/or with a rapid rise in K^+ should have an emergent ECG performed.

15

ECG changes of hyperkalemia: Follow a progression along the continuum of peaked T waves, shortened QT interval, prolonged PR interval, flattening and then disappearing of P waves, widening of QRS, sine wave, and finally ventricular fibrillation. (See Chapter 27, Figure 27-32, page 872.)

K^+ 7–8 mEq/L ventricular fibrillation risk: 5%

K^+ 10 mEq/L ventricular fibrillation risk: 90%

Treatment:

The underlying etiology of hyperkalemia needs to be addressed, as well as efforts to restore renal function such as correct obstruction or fluids for prerenal azotemia.

If K^+ >6.5 mEq/L and/or ECG changes. Place on cardiac monitoring and discontinue all potassium intake and initiate rapid correction.

Rapid correction:

1. Membrane stabilization: Intravenous calcium gluconate or calcium chloride; onset of action is minutes, and duration of action is 30–60 min; may repeat if ECG changes persists; patients require continuous cardiac monitoring; DO NOT administer with sodium bicarbonate; calcium chloride contains three times the calcium concentration compared to calcium gluconate and can cause irritation at injection site or necrosis with infiltration; calcium chloride 500–1000 mg (5–10 mL of 10% solution) is given over 2–3 min and is the preferred calcium formulation to use in cases of cardiac arrest or cardiac instability, especially when central IV access is available; otherwise, calcium gluconate 10 mL of 10% solution over 10 min is preferred.

2. Shift K^+ intracellularly: Glucose and insulin administration, 10 u regular insulin along with 50 mL dextrose 50% over 5 min; onset of action is 20–30 min, and duration of action is 2–6 hr; monitor glucose every hour for 2–4 hr (6 hr in patients with renal insufficiency); patients with decreased renal function are at increased risk for hypoglycemia and may require an infusion of dextrose 10%; continuous infusion of insulin plus glucose may also be used.

3. Correct metabolic acidosis: Sodium bicarbonate 50 mEq/L (1 amp) over 5 min; onset of action is 30 min, and duration of action is 1–2 hr.

4. Shift K^+ intracellularly: Nebulized albuterol; peak effect in 90 min.

Enhance K^+ excretion is the next step. Membrane stabilization and intracellular shifts are temporizing measures. Definitive therapy is potassium removal from the body via the renal or GI systems and correction of the underlying cause(s).

Strategies to increase K^+ elimination (ongoing careful monitoring in patients with severe hyperkalemia is required until resolved):

1. Diuretics: Loop diuretics in patients with sufficient renal function will enhance renal elimination of K^+. One must be cognizant about inducing volume depletion. Concurrent infusion of normal saline may be

indicated. Loop diuretics in patients with significant renal dysfunction may not be effective.

2. Gastrointestinal cation exchangers: Zirconium cyclosilicate 5- to 10-g pack TID × 48 hr; patiromer 8.5-g, 16.8-g, and 25.2-g doses daily as needed; sodium polystyrene sulfonate (SPS): for decades the primary treatment to enhance GI elimination of K^+; however, it is seldom used now because of adverse GI events including intestinal necrosis. Using the GI tract as the route of elimination takes longer compared to diuretics or hemodialysis.

3. Hemodialysis: Indicated in patients with severe renal dysfunction; there may be rebound hyperkalemia after HD due to re-equilibration from intracellular to extracellular space.

Hypokalemia

- $K^+ <3.5$ mEq/L
- Critical values: 2.5 mEq/L <1 wk old; >1 wk old <3.0 mEq/L

Mechanisms: Due to inadequate intake, loss, or intracellular shifts
- **Inadequate Intake.** Oral or IV.
- **GI Tract Loss.** (Urinary chloride usually <10 mEq/d; chloride-responsive alkalosis) vomiting, diarrhea, excess sweating, villous adenoma, fistula.
- **Renal Loss.** Diuretics and other medications (amphotericin, high-dose penicillins, aminoglycosides, cisplatin), diuresis other than with diuretics (osmotic, e.g., hyperglycemia or ethanol induced), vomiting (from metabolic alkalosis due to volume depletion), renal tubular disease (distal or proximal RTA), Bartter syndrome (due to increased renin and aldosterone levels), hypomagnesemia, ingestion of natural licorice, mineralocorticoid excess (primary and secondary hyperaldosteronism, Cushing syndrome, steroid use), and ureterosigmoidostomy.
- **Redistribution (Intracellular Shifts).** Metabolic alkalosis (each 0.1 increase in pH lowers serum K^+ approximately 0.5–1.0 mEq/L; due to intracellular shift of K^+), insulin administration, beta-adrenergic agents, familial periodic paralysis, and therapy for megaloblastic anemia.

Symptoms:
- Muscle weakness, cramps, tetany
- Polyuria, polydipsia

Signs:
- Decreased motor strength, orthostatic hypotension, ileus
- ECG changes, such as flattening of T waves, U wave becoming obvious (U wave is the upward deflection after the T wave) (see Chapter 27, Figure 27-33, page 872)

Treatment:

- History of HTN, GI symptoms, or use of certain medications may point to the cause.
- Treat the underlying cause.
- A 24-hr urine for K^+ may be helpful if the diagnosis is unclear. Level <20 mEq/d suggests extrarenal loss or redistribution, >20 mEq/d suggests renal losses.
- A serum K^+ level of 2 mEq/L represents a deficit of about 300 mEq in a 70-kg adult. To change K^+ from 3 to 4 mEq/L it takes about 100 mEq of K^+ in a 70-kg adult, and from 2 to 3 mEq/L it may take up to 200 mEq.
- Hypokalemia potentiates the cardiac toxicity of digitalis. In the setting of digoxin use, hypokalemia should be aggressively treated.
- Treat hypomagnesemia if present. It is difficult to correct hypokalemia in the presence of hypomagnesemia.
- **Rapid Correction.** Give KCl IV. Monitor heart rhythm with replacement ≥ 20 mEq/hr. IV K^+ can be painful and sclerose veins.
  Patient <40 kg: 0.25 mEq/kg/hr × 2 hr
  Patient >40 kg: 10–20 mEq/hr × 2 hr
  Severe (<2 mEq/L): Maximum 40 mEq/hr IV in adults. In all cases check a stat K^+ after each 2–4 hr of replacement.
- **Slow Correction.** Give K^+ orally; there are many commercially available supplements; K^+ comes in various salts including KCl; K-gluconate; and combinations of Cl, citrate, bicarbonate, and acetate.
  Adults: 20–40 mEq two to three times a day. Children: 1–2 mEq/kg/d in divided doses.

DISORDERS OF CALCIUM BALANCE

The majority (>98%) of total body calcium is in bone. The serum calcium exists in three forms: ionized (active form) 40%; protein bound chiefly to albumin 45%; and the remainder is complexed to citrate, bicarbonate, and phosphorus (thus acid–base disorders and alterations in phosphorus concentrations will affect calcium concentration). Since a large portion of serum calcium is bound to albumin, the serum calcium should be corrected with hypoalbuminemia:

Corrected total serum calcium mg/dL = measured serum calcium mg/dL + (4 – measured plasma albumin g/dL × 0.8).

Serum calcium concentration is tightly regulated between gut absorption, bone metabolism, and renal elimination through vitamin D and parathyroid hormone.

Disorders of calcium concentration may be reflected in alterations of bone metabolism, nerve conduction, muscle contraction, and CNS symptoms, as well as renal and electrolyte disturbances.

Hypercalcemia

- Serum Ca^{2+} >10.5 mg/dL or ionized Ca^{2+} >5.28 mg/dL.
- Critical serum calcium >13 mg/dL; ionized calcium >7 mg/dL

Mechanisms: Primary hyperparathyroidism and malignancy account for > 90% of cases of hypercalcemia. In hospitalized patients with severe hypercalcemia, malignancy should be suspected.

- Primary hyperparathyroidism with secondary bone reabsorption
- Tertiary hyperparathyroidism (chronic kidney disease)
- Malignancy
  o Humoral hypercalcemia: Mediated by PTHrP; squamous cell carcinoma (lung and head and neck), renal cell carcinoma, breast, prostate, ovary
  o Osteolytic hypercalcemia: Mediated by cytokines; multiple myeloma, metastatic breast, prostate, and non–small-cell lung cancers, some lymphomas, and lymphosarcoma
- Medications (thiazide diuretics, lithium [fairly common], vitamin A intoxication)
- Vitamin D related (vitamin D intoxication; granulomatous diseases such as sarcoidosis, TB, and berylliosis; Hodgkin lymphoma)
- Familial hypocalcuric hypercalcemia
- Other endocrine disorders (hyperthyroidism, acromegaly, pheochromocytoma, adrenal insufficiency)
- Other causes (milk-alkali syndrome, immobilization with Paget disease)

Symptoms: Stones (renal), bones (osteitis fibrosa), moans (abdominal pain), groans (neuropsychiatric symptoms including confusion)

- Renal: Polyuria, polydipsia, flank pain and hematuria from nephrolithiasis
- Neurologic: Memory difficulty, decreased concentration, lethargy, confusion, coma
- Musculoskeletal: Bone pain
- Gastrointestinal: Anorexia, nausea and vomiting, constipation, abdominal pain

Signs:

- Renal: orthostatic changes in HR ($\geq$20 BPM increase) and BP ($\geq$10 mm Hg decrease in systolic BP) with change in position from supine to standing after 2 min; increase in creatinine and BUN from acute and chronic kidney injury
- Neurologic: Mental status changes, decreased concentration, confusion, coma
- Musculoskeletal: Muscle weakness
- Gastrointestinal: Weight loss
- Cardiovascular: Shortening of QT interval, bradycardia, hypertension, arrhythmias

15

Treatment:

The urgency to treat hypercalcemia is based upon the severity of the symptoms and signs, as well as on the level of calcium and the rate of rise.

In addition to the treatment of the underlying etiology, urgent treatment to acutely lower calcium is recommended in patients with albumin-corrected total Ca^{2+} >14 mg/dL or ionized Ca^{2+} >10 mg/dL or in patients with an acute rise in calcium to lesser levels with CNS symptoms of lethargy, stupor, or coma.

Urgent Treatment of Hypercalcemia:

- Volume expansion with isotonic saline. Initial rate 200–300 mL/hr and adjusting rate to maintain urine output of 100–150 mL/hr. Concurrent use of loop diuretics is not recommended in the absence of volume overload due to heart failure of renal insufficiency because of the risk of volume depletion.
- Calcitonin initially at 4 IU/kg subcutaneously or intramuscularly every 12 hr. Due to tachyphylaxis usefulness is usually limited to 48 hr.
- Bisphosphonates are efficacious in treating hypercalcemia due to excessive bone reabsorption.
  - o Zoledronic acid: 4 mg IV over 15 min; do not use in severe renal insufficiency (Cr >4.5 mg/dL); superior to pamidronate.
  - o Pamidronate: 60–90 mg IV over 2 hr; do not use in severe renal insufficiency (Cr >3 mg/dL or GFR <30 mL/min).
- Denosumab, a monoclonal antibody that blocks osteoclast function, may be used in patients refractory to zoledronic acid or in whom bisphosphonates are contraindicated due to severe renal dysfunction; initial dose is 60 mg subcutaneously.
- Hemodialysis or peritoneal dialysis may be used in select patients in which above therapies are contraindicated due to renal failure or heart failure.

Chronic Treatment of Hypercalcemia:

- Treat underlying conditions: Stop offending medications, treat hyperparathyroidism, etc.
- Glucocorticoids may be useful in patients with granulomatous disorders such as sarcoidosis or certain lymphomas.
- Continued bisphosphates may be used in appropriate patients with ongoing increased bone absorption.

Hypocalcemia

- Ca^{2+} <8.5 mg/dL; ionized <4.64 mg/dL
- Critical serum calcium <6.5 mg/dL or ionized calcium <2 mg/dL

Mechanisms: Decreased albumin can result in decreased total Ca^{2+} without a change in the ionized Ca^{2+} (see Chapter 10, page 192).

- **Critical Illness.** Many acute and chronic medical illnesses can cause a decrease in serum Ca^{2+} because of the decrease in albumin that often occurs as a negative acute phase reactant; in this setting check an ionized Ca^{2+}, it is often normal.
- **PTH Deficiency.** Acquired (surgical excision or injury, infiltrative diseases such as amyloidosis and hemochromatosis, irradiation), hereditary hypoparathyroidism (pseudohypoparathyroidism), hypomagnesemia.
- **Vitamin D Deficiency.** Chronic renal failure, liver disease, use of phenytoin or phenobarbital, malnutrition, malabsorption (chronic pancreatitis, aftermath of gastrectomy).
- **Other.** Hyperphosphatemia, acute pancreatitis, osteoblastic metastasis, medullary carcinoma of thyroid, massive transfusion.

Symptoms:
- Peripheral and perioral paresthesia, abdominal pain and cramps, lethargy, irritability in infants

Signs:
- Hypertension
- Hyperactive DTRs, carpopedal spasm (Trousseau sign, see Chapter 6, page 68)
- Presence of Chvostek sign (see Chapter 6, page 63) (facial nerve twitch, present in as many as 25% of healthy adults)
- Generalized seizures, tetany, laryngospasm
- Prolonged QT interval on ECG

Treatment:
- **Acute Symptomatic**
  A total of 100–200 mg of elemental Ca IV over 10 min in 50–100 mL of D5W followed by an infusion containing 1–2 mg/kg/hr over 6–12 hr. 10% Ca gluconate contains 93 mg of elemental Ca. 10% Ca chloride contains 272 mg of elemental Ca. Check magnesium levels and replace if low.
- **Chronic** (vitamin D2-ergocalciferol is used in most cases along with calcium supplements; the dose will vary depending on the indication, for hypoparathyroidism the dose is 50,000–200,000 U/day; vitamin D2-ergocalciferol is useful in cases where more rapid correction via increased absorption is indicated)
  For renal insufficiency/failure, use vitamin D along with oral Ca supplements (see the following lists) and phosphate-binding antacids (e.g., PhosphoGEL, AlternaGEL).
  Oral Ca supplements:
  Ca carbonate (e.g., Os-Cal) 650 mg PO QID (28% Ca^{2+})
  Ca citrate (e.g., Citracal) 950-mg tablets (21% Ca^{2+})
  Ca gluconate 500- or 1000-mg tablets (9% Ca^{2+})

15

Ca glubionate (e.g., Neo-Calglucon) syrup 115 mg/5 mL (6.4% Ca^{2+})

Ca lactate 325- or 650-mg tablets (13% Ca^{2+})

- Monitor calcium and phosphorous to guide adjustments in therapy.

DISORDERS OF MAGNESIUM BALANCE

Magnesium is primarily located intracellularly (99%), primarily in bone, muscle, and soft tissue. Approximately 1% of total body magnesium is located in the plasma, where 65% is ionized, 30% is protein bound, and the remainder is complexed to other ions such as citrate and phosphate. Magnesium homeostasis is primarily regulated by the kidney. Magnesium is involved in a number of metabolic processes, including regulation of ATP, nucleic acids, calcium channels, and membrane stabilization. Alterations in magnesium concentration may result in cardiovascular, neuromuscular, and CNS dysfunction. Alterations in magnesium concentration may also affect serum levels of calcium, potassium, or phosphorus.

Hypermagnesemia

- Mg^{2+} >2.4 mEq/L
- Critical values: >4.9 mg/dL

Mechanisms:

- **Excess Administration.** Used in the management of preeclampsia with magnesium sulfate
- **Renal Insufficiency.** Exacerbated by ingestion of magnesium-containing antacids
- **Others.** Rhabdomyolysis, adrenal insufficiency

Symptoms and Signs:

- 3–5 mEq/L: Nausea, vomiting, hypotension, decreased reflexes
- 7–10 mEq/L: Weakness, drowsiness, hyporeflexia, quadriparesis
- >12 mEq/L: Coma, bradycardia, respiratory failure

Treatment: Clinical hypermagnesemia necessitating therapy is infrequently encountered in patients with normal renal function.

- Ca gluconate: 10 mL of 10% solution (93 mg elemental Ca) over 10–20 min in 50–100 mL of D5W given IV to reverse symptoms (useful in patients being treated for eclampsia)
- Stop magnesium-containing medications (hypermagnesemia is common in patients with renal failure taking magnesium-containing antacids)
- Insulin and glucose as for hyperkalemia (see page 438)
- Furosemide and saline diuresis
- Dialysis

Hypomagnesemia

- Mg^{2+} <1.5 mEq/L
- Critical values: <1.0

Mechanisms:

- **Decreased Intake or Absorption.** Malabsorption, chronic GI losses, deficient intake (alcoholics), TPN without adequate supplementation
- **Increased Loss.** Diuretics, other medications (gentamicin, cisplatin, amphotericin B, others), RTA, DM (especially DKA), alcoholism, hyperaldosteronism, excessive lactation
- **Other.** Acute pancreatitis, hypoalbuminemia, vitamin D therapy

Symptoms:

- Weakness, muscle twitches, vertigo
- Symptoms of hypocalcemia and hypokalemia (hypomagnesemia may cause hypocalcemia and hypokalemia)

Signs:

- Tachycardia, tremor, hyperactive reflexes, asterixis, tetany, seizures
- ECG may show prolongation of PR, QT, and QRS intervals as well as ventricular ectopy and sinus tachycardia

15

Treatment: Underlying causes need to be addressed, i.e., hypomagnesemia associated with PPI use; diuretic-induced magnesium loss may be treated with the addition of potassium-sparing diuretics such as amiloride.

- **Severe: Tetany or Seizures (level is usually <1.0 mEq/L).** Monitor patient with ECG in ICU; 2 g magnesium sulfate in D5W infused over 10–20 min. Follow with magnesium sulfate, 1 g/hr for 3–4 hr; monitor DTRs and monitor Mg^{2+} levels. Repeat replacement if necessary. These patients are often hypokalemic and hypophosphatemic and should be given supplements to correct additional electrolyte abnormalities. Hypocalcemia may also result from hypomagnesemia.
- **Moderate:** Mg^{2+} <1.0 mEq/L but asymptomatic; replace with intravenous magnesium sulfate 1 g/hr for 3–4 hr, monitor levels, and repeat replacement if necessary.
- **Mild:** Mg^{2+} level 1.0–0.5; replace with oral replacement therapy:
  o Magnesium oxide (e.g., Mag-Ox) 240 mg elemental mag per 400 mg tablet (may be associated with diarrhea)
  o Magnesium chloride sustained release (e.g., Slow Mag) 64 mg elemental mag per tab
  o Magnesium L-lactate sustained release (e.g., Mag Tab SR) 64 mg elemental mag per tab

DISORDERS OF PHOSPHOROUS BALANCE

The majority of total body phosphorus (80–85%) is in bone, 14% is intracellular, and 1% is extracellular. Phosphorus homeostasis is maintained via the gut, bones, and the kidneys.

The major complications of severe hypophosphatemia are related to the adverse effects of intracellular phosphate depletion on intracellular ATP. In addition, severe hypophosphatemia via decreased RBC 2,3-diphosphogylcerate (DPG) levels will lead to an increased affinity of hemoglobin for oxygen, leading a decreased oxygen delivery.

Virtually all organ systems—including the CNS, the heart, and smooth and skeletal muscle are affected resulting in decreased diaphragmatic contractility, ileus, dysphagia, myopathy, and rhabdomyolysis. Also, hematologic disturbances including hemolysis, granulocyte and platelet dysfunction, and thrombocytopenia can be caused by hypophosphatemia. Severe hypophosphatemia should be promptly treated to prevent these life-threatening complications. Due to the binding of phosphorus to calcium, the main manifestations of hyperphosphatemia are those of hypocalcemia (see section on hypocalcemia). In addition, there may be soft tissue and vascular deposition of calcium phosphate.

Hyperphosphatemia

- PO_4^{3-} >4.5 mg/dL
- Critical values >8.9 mg/dL

Mechanisms:
- **Increased Intake and Absorption.** Iatrogenic, abuse of laxatives or enemas containing phosphorus, vitamin D intoxication, and granulomatous disease
- **Decreased Excretion** (most common mechanism). Renal failure, hypoparathyroidism, adrenal insufficiency, hyperthyroidism, acromegaly, sickle cell anemia
- **Redistribution and Cellular Release.** Rhabdomyolysis, acidosis, chemotherapy-induced tumor lysis, hemolysis, plasma cell dyscrasia

Symptoms and Signs: Mostly related to tetany as a result of the accompanying hypocalcemia (see page 442) or metastatic calcification (deposition of calcium phosphate in various soft tissues)

Treatment:
- **Acute hyperphosphatemia:** Goal is to increase renal elimination of phosphorus; recovery of renal function usually will result in the correction of acute hypophosphatemia within 12 hr.
  o Phosphate elimination can be further promoted with IV saline +/− the addition of acetazolamide (15 mg/kg q4h) if indicated.

o Hemodialysis may be indicated in cases of acute hyperphosphatemia in AKI or ESRD.
- **Chronic hyperphosphatemia:** Mostly seen in chronic kidney disease.
  o Reduce dietary intake of phosphorus.
  o Phosphate binders such as calcium carbonate, calcium acetate, lanthanum carbonate, or sevelamer carbonate. Due to the risk of aluminum toxicity, aluminum-based phosphate binders are no longer used.

Hypophosphatemia

- PO_4^{3-} <2.5 mg/dL
- Critical values <1.1 mg/dL

Mechanisms:
- **Decreased Dietary Intake.** Starvation, alcoholism, iatrogenic factors (hyperalimentation without adequate supplementation), malabsorption, vitamin D deficiency, phosphate-binding antacids (e.g., AlternaGEL).
- **Redistribution.** Conditions associated with respiratory or metabolic alkalosis (e.g., alcohol withdrawal, salicylate poisoning), endocrine abnormalities (e.g., insulin use, increase in catecholamines), anabolic steroids, hyperthermia or hypothermia, leukemia or lymphoma, hypercalcemia, hypomagnesemia.
- **Renal Losses.** RTA, diuretic phase of acute tubular necrosis (ATN), hyperparathyroidism, hyperthyroidism, hypokalemia, diuretics, hypomagnesemia, alcohol abuse, poorly controlled DM.
- **Other.** Refeeding in the setting of severe protein-calorie malnutrition, severe burns, management of DKA.

Symptoms and Signs: PO_4^{3-} <1 mg/dL weakness, muscle pain and muscle tenderness, paresthesia, cardiac and respiratory failure, CNS dysfunction (confusion and seizures), rhabdomyolysis, hemolysis, impaired leukocyte and platelet function.

Treatment: IV therapy is reserved for severe, potentially life-threatening hypophosphatemia (PO_4^{3-} <1.0–1.5 mg/dL); too rapid correction can lead to severe hypocalcemia. With mild to moderate hypophosphatemia (1.5–2.5 mg/dL), oral replacement is preferred.
- **Severe** (PO_4^{3-} <1.0–1.5 mg/dL). Use potassium or sodium phosphate. 2 mg/kg given IV over 6 hr. **Caution:** Too rapid replacement can lead to hypocalcemic tetany.
- **Mild to Moderate** (PO_4^{3-} >1.5 mg/dL)
  o Sodium–potassium phosphate (Neutra-Phos) or potassium phosphate (K-Phos): 1–2 tablets (250–500 mg PO_4^{3-} per tablet) PO BID or TID
  o Sodium phosphate (Fleet Phospho-soda) 5 mL PO_4^{3-} BID or TID (128 mg PO_4^{3-})

15

References

1. Feld LG, et al. Clinical practice guideline: Maintenance intravenous fluids in children. Pediatrics 2018;142(6).
2. Somers MJ. Maintenance intravenous fluid therapy in children. Up To Date. Accessed February 15, 2020.
3. Schrier RW, ed. Renal and Electrolyte Disorders. Philadelphia, PA, Lippincott, Williams, & Wilkins, 2017.

Transfusion Medicine and the Blood Bank

16

ROUTINE BLOOD DONATION

Voluntary blood donation provides all blood products that are transfused in the United States. Donors usually are >18 yr old, are in good health and afebrile, and weigh >110 lb (50 kg). Donors are usually limited to one unit every 8 wk and six donations per year. A variety of medical conditions and behaviors may temporarily or indefinitely exclude a donor from donating blood; these deferrals are intended to reduce the risk of transfusion-transmitted infections. Donor blood testing includes ABO/Rh type, antibody screen, HIV-1 and -2, HBV, HCV, Zika virus, HTLV-I and -II, and *Treponema pallidum* (syphilis). As of June 2020, the Red Cross began testing donated blood for COVID-19 antibodies. Donors who test positive for COVID-19 antibodies may be invited to donate convalescent plasma.

Chapter update by Alexis Peedin, MD

449

Table 16-1. Blood Groups and Selecting ABO/Rh Types for Transfusion

Type (ABO/Rh)	Population Frequency	Can Receive RBCs From[a]	Can Receive Plasma From
O	45%	O	O, A, B, AB
A	40%	A, O	A, AB
B	11%	B, O	B, AB
AB	4%	AB, A, B, O	AB
Rh-positive	85%	Rh-positive or -negative	
Rh-negative	15%	Rh-negative	

[a]First choice is always the identical blood type; other acceptable combinations are shown. An attempt is also made to match Rh status of donor and recipient; Rh− can be given to an Rh+ recipient safely, but Rh− recipients should receive Rh− only to prevent alloimmunization.

BLOOD GROUPS

Table 16-1 gives information on the major blood groups and their relative occurrences. For RBC units, type O is the **"universal donor,"** and AB is the **"universal recipient."** For plasma units, type AB is the "universal donor" because it lacks both anti-A and anti-B, while type O is the "universal recipient."

BLOOD BANKING PROCEDURES

Type and Screen (T&S): The blood bank tests the patient's ABO and Rh **type** and **screens** for antibodies. If an alloantibody (an antibody formed in response to pregnancy, transfusion, or transplantation targeted against a blood group antigen that is not present on the person's red blood cells) is found that would make crossmatching challenging, the ordering physician usually is notified. If the decision to transfuse is made before the specimen expires (typically 72 hr after collection), the T&S order may be changed to a T&C.

Type and Cross (T&C): The blood bank performs a T&S on the patient's specimen and matches specific donor unit(s) to the patient. The **crossmatch** involves testing the patient's plasma or serum against a small sample from the RBC unit to ensure compatibility. A T&C usually takes approximately 90 min. If the patient does not have alloantibodies, the crossmatch may be performed using an FDA-approved computer system, which takes only a few minutes. For routine requests, the blood is set up at a date and time that you specify and usually held for 24–36 hr.

Stat Requests: The bank sets up blood immediately and usually holds it for 12 hr.

PREOPERATIVE BLOOD SETUP

Most institutions have a "Maximum Surgical Blood Ordering Schedule" (MSBOS) established to simplify blood bank orders before elective surgeries. The MSBOS specifies how many units of PRBCs should be set up before specific surgical procedures or if only a T&S is needed (i.e., intraoperative transfusion is unlikely). Check with the surgeon.

EMERGENCY TRANSFUSIONS

In cases of massive, exsanguinating hemorrhage, the patient may require emergent transfusion and cannot wait for the blood bank to complete the T&C procedure. Uncrossmatched type O PRBC will be issued (Rh-negative usually issued for females <50 yr of age, Rh-positive usually issued for males and females >50 yr) until the patient's ABO/Rh type is established. If uncrossmatched blood is issued, a physician's signature will be required by the blood bank. A specimen should be sent to the blood bank for T&S as soon as possible, but should not delay resuscitation.

BASIC PRINCIPLES OF BLOOD COMPONENT THERAPY

Table 16-2, page 452, shows common indications for and uses of transfusion products. The following outlines the basic transfusion principles for adults.

16

Red Cell Transfusions

Acute Blood Loss: Healthy persons can usually tolerate up to 30% blood loss without transfusion. Patients may manifest tachycardia and mild hypotension without evidence of hypovolemic shock. Start volume replacement (IV fluids, etc.).

- Hgb >10 g/dL: Transfusion rarely indicated.
- Hgb 7–10 g/dL: Transfusion may be indicated if patient is symptomatic of anemia (tachycardia, angina, dyspnea, fatigue, dizziness).
- Hgb <7 g/dL: Transfusion usually indicated.

"Allowable Blood Loss": Often used to guide acute transfusion in the operating room. Losses less than allowable are usually managed with IV fluid replacement.

$$\text{Weight in kg} \times 0.08 = \text{Total blood volume}$$

$$\text{Total volume} \times 0.3 = \text{Allowable blood loss (assumes normal Hbg)}$$

Example: A 70-kg adult

$$\text{Estimated allowable blood loss} = 70 \times 0.08 = 5.6L$$
$$\text{or } (5600 \text{ mL}) \times 0.3 = 1680 \text{ mL}$$

Table 16-2. Blood bank components. All require a specimen to be sent for Type and Screen (T&S).

Product	Description	Common Indications
Whole Blood	No elements removed 1 unit = 450 mL ± 45 mL (HCT ≈ 40%) Contains RBC, plasma, and platelets (may be leukoreduced)	Not routinely transfused Early resuscitation of massively hemorrhaging trauma patients increasingly involves whole blood
Red Blood Cells (RBCs)	1 un t = 250–300 mL (HCT 55–75%) 1 un t should raise Hgb 1 g/dL and HCT 3%	Acute bleeding with hemodynamic instability, symptomatic anemia
Platelets	Prepooled platelet units contain platelets derived from 4 to 6 units of donated whole blood Apheresis-derived platelet units come from 1 donor >3 × 10^{10} platelets/unit 1 unit = 250–300 mL 1 unit should raise platelet count by 30,000–50,000	Threshold to transfuse varies based on clinical scenario: Counts <5000–10,000 (risk of spontaneous hemorrhage), prophylactic transfusion indicated Counts <20,000 if febrile or minor bleeding Counts <50,000 if major bleeding or imminently undergoing invasive procedure or surgery Counts <100,000 if intracranial hemorrhage or undergoing neurosurgery Any count + recent antiplatelet medication + bleeding Usually not indicated in ITP or TTP unless life-threatening bleeding or preoperative status

RBC = red blood cells; WBC = white blood cells; HCT = hematocrit; GI = gastrointestinal; ITP = idiopathic thrombocytopenic purpura; TTP = thrombotic thrombocytopenic purpura; HLA = histocompatibility locus antigen; PT = prothrombin time; PTT = partial thromboplastin time.

16

Plasma (FFP or FP24) FFP = fresh frozen plasma = frozen within 8 hr of collection FP24 = plasma frozen within 24 hr of collection (used interchangeably with FFP)	Contains all clotting factors About 45 min to thaw Weight-based dosing: 10–15 mL/kg. Roughly estimated: <50 kg: 3 units 50–75 kg: 4 units >75 kg: 5 units	Suspected or documented coagulopathy (congenital or acquired) with active bleeding or before surgery Massive transfusion Clotting factor replacement when concentrate unavailable Emergency reversal of warfarin if prothrombin complex concentrate not available Not recommended for volume replacement
Cryoprecipitated Antihemophilic Factor ("Cryo")	Contains fibrinogen, factor VIII, von Willebrand factor, and factor XIII 1 unit = 10 mL Adult dose = 5 or 10 pooled units Expire 4 hr after thawing; only order if you will transfuse it quickly	Fibrinogen deficiency (DIC, obstetrical bleeding) Hemophilia A when factor VIII recombinant or concentrate not available; von Willebrand disease Fibrin surgical glue
Rho Gam (Rho D immune globulin)	Antibody against Rh factor/D antigen (single dose vials = 600 IU (120 mcg), 1,500 IU (300 mcg), 2,500 IU (500 mcg), 5,000 IU (1,000 mcg), and 15,000 IU (3,000 mcg); dosage dependent upon indication)	Give to all Rh− mothers at 28 wk gestation and after vaginal bleeding or trauma If Rh− mother gives birth to Rh+ baby, redose within 72 hr of delivery to prevent hemolytic disease of newborn in future pregnancies
Granulocytes	1 unit = ≈220 mL >1 × 10^{10} PMN/unit, some RBC (must be ABO compatible), lymphocytes, platelets	See page 456

16

RBC = red blood cells; WBC = white blood cells; HCT = hematocrit; GI = gastrointestinal; ITP = idiopathic thrombocytopenic purpura; TTP = thrombotic thrombocytopenic purpura; HLA = histocompatibility locus antigen; PT = prothrombin time; PTT = partial thromboplastin time.

(continued)

Table 16-2. Blood bank components. All require a specimen to be sent for Type and Screen (T&S). *(Continued)*

Product	Description	Common Indications
ALL OF THE AFOREMENTIONED ITEMS REQUIRE A SPECIMEN TO BE SENT FOR TYPE AND SCREEN (T&S). THE FOLLOWING PRODUCTS ARE USUALLY DISPENSED BY MOST HOSPITAL PHARMACIES AND ARE USUALLY ORDERED AS A MEDICATION.		
Factor VIII (Purified Antihemophilic Factor)	Concentrate: From pooled plasma Recombinant factor VIII is synthetic and devoid of infectious risk	Routine for bleeding in hemophilia A (factor VIII deficiency)
Factor IX Concentrate (Prothrombin Complex)	Increased hepatitis risk Factors II, VII, IX, and X Equivalent to 2 units of plasma	Active bleeding in Christmas disease (hemophilia B or factor IX deficiency)
Intravenous Immune Globulin	Precipitate from pooled plasma "gamma globulin"	Immune globulin deficiency Disease prophylaxis (hepatitis A, measles, etc.)
5% Albumin or 5% Plasma Protein Fraction	Precipitate from pooled plasma (see Chapter 15, page 425)	Plasma volume expanders in acute blood loss
25% Albumin	Precipitate from pooled plasma	Hypoalbuminemia, volume expander, burns Draws extravascular fluid into circulation

RBC = red blood cells; WBC = white blood cells; HCT = hematocrit; GI = gastrointestinal; ITP = idiopathic thrombocytopenic purpura; TTP = thrombotic thrombocytopenic purpura; HLA = histocompatibility locus antigen; PT = prothrombin time; PTT = partial thromboplastin time.

Chronic Anemia: Common in certain chronic conditions, such as renal failure, rarely managed with blood transfusion; typically managed with pharmacologic therapy (e.g., erythropoietin, iron replacement). However, transfusion is generally indicated if Hgb <6 g/dL or in the face of symptoms due to low hemoglobin.

Packed Red Blood Cells (PRBC) Transfusion Formula: As a guide, one unit of PRBC raises the HCT 3% (Hgb, 1 g/dL) in the average adult. To estimate the volume of PRBC needed to raise the HCT to a known amount, use the following formula:

$$Volume\ of\ cells = \frac{Total\ blood\ volume\ of\ patient \times (Desired\ HCT - Actual\ HCT)}{HCT\ of\ transfusion\ product}$$

where total blood volume is 70 mL/kg in adults and 80 mL/kg in children. The HCT of PRBC is approximately 60%.

Platelet Transfusions

Indications for using platelet transfusions are in Table 16-2, page 454.

Platelets are usually issued 1 unit at a time. After administration of 1 unit of prepooled or apheresis-derived platelets, the count should rise 30,000–50,000/mm^3 within 1 hr of transfusion. Under normal circumstances, stored platelets that are transfused survive 6–8 days after infusion. Clinical factors (e.g., DIC, splenomegaly, fever) can significantly shorten this time. To standardize the corrected platelet count to an individual patient, use the **corrected count increment (CCI)**. Measure the platelet count immediately before and 1 hr after platelet infusion. If the correction is >5000, the etiology of platelet refractoriness should be determined (e.g., HLA alloantibodies, splenomegaly). Apheresis-derived platelets, in which 1 unit is derived from one donor, may be obtained for patients who require HLA-matched units due to HLA alloantibodies. Providing HLA-matched units also limits exposure to different HLA antigens, reducing the risk of additional antibody production.

$$CCI = \frac{(Posttransfusion\ platelet\ count - Pretransfusion\ count) \times Body\ surface\ area\ (m^2)}{Platelets\ given \times 10^{11}}$$

Plasma Transfusion

Plasma should be dosed based on the patient's weight (10–15 mL/kg). Transfusion of plasma products is indicated in patients with suspected or documented coagulopathy (congenital or acquired) with active bleeding or before surgery. Massive transfusion protocols include plasma in approximately a 1:1 ratio with PRBC units. Warfarin overdose should be treated with prothrombin complex concentrate (PCC), but plasma is an acceptable alternative if PCC is not available.

16

Granulocyte Transfusions

The use of granulocyte transfusions is rarely performed because genetically engineered myeloid growth factors such as GM-CSF are used instead. May be indicated for patients being treated for overwhelming sepsis and severe neutropenia (<500 PMN/μL). The neutropenia should be expected to be reversible (i.e., patient has not yet engrafted after stem cell transplant).

MODIFIED BLOOD COMPONENTS

Irradiation

Patients who are severely immunocompromised, fetuses receiving intrauterine transfusions, and recipients of HLA-matched platelets or directed donations are at risk for transfusion-associated graft-versus-host disease (TA-GVHD). This condition is nearly always fatal, but can be prevented by irradiating blood products that are administered to at-risk patients.

Leukoreduction

Leukoreduced PRBCs and platelets are filtered to remove most WBCs before storage (<5 × 10^6 residual WBCs per unit). Leukoreduced blood should be provided for patients with previous febrile nonhemolytic transfusion reactions and for patients at risk for CMV seroconversion or HLA alloimmunization. Most PRBC/platelet units in the United States are leukoreduced immediately after collection.

Washing

Patients with a prior anaphylactic reaction to a blood transfusion should receive washed PRBCs and platelets, where plasma is washed away and replaced with saline. A significant proportion of the cells in the bag are lost during the washing process (~20% of RBCs and ~40% of platelets). Plasma products cannot be washed (you would be left with a bag of saline!).

TRANSFUSION PROCEDURE

1. Order type and cross in electronic health record system. Identify the patient by referring to the ID bracelet and asking the patient to state, if able, his or her name and date of birth. Draw a pink or purple top tube, label at the bedside, and sign your name on the tube. Send sample and request to the blood bank following institutional protocols.
2. Obtain the patient's informed consent by discussing the reasons for the transfusion and the potential risks and benefits of it. Follow hospital

procedure regarding the need for the patient to sign a specific transfusion consent form.

3. When ready to transfuse, ensure good venous access for the transfusion (18-gauge needle or larger is preferred for adults to prevent mechanical hemolysis of the donor RBCs).

4. Verify the information on each unit of blood with another person, such as a nurse or physician, and with the patient's ID bracelet. Many hospitals have defined protocols for this procedure; check your institutional guidelines.

5. Do not infuse any medications or fluids through the same line as blood products. Isotonic (0.9%) NS may be infused concurrently if absolutely necessary, but using hypotonic products such as D_5W can result in hemolysis of the blood in the tubing. Lactated Ringer's solution should *not* be used because the calcium can chelate citrate, the anticoagulant used in blood products.

6. When transfusing large volumes of PRBC (>10 units) in a short period of time (<24 hr), monitor coagulation tests, platelets, Mg^{2+}, Ca^{2+}, and lactate levels. In massively hemorrhaging patients, it also usually is necessary to transfuse plasma and platelets. If you activate the **massive transfusion protocol (MTP)**, the blood bank will issue PRBC:plasma units in approximately a 1:1 ratio until you discontinue the MTP. Calcium replacement is sometimes needed because the anticoagulant used in the blood (citrate) is a calcium binder, and hypocalcemia can occur after large amounts of blood are rapidly transfused. For massive transfusions, warm the blood to prevent hypothermia and cardiac arrhythmia.

16

TRANSFUSION REACTIONS

Managing Suspected Transfusion Reactions

1. **STOP THE TRANSFUSION!** Monitor the patient. Then, contact the blood bank. Send the bag of blood back to the blood bank.

2. Send new patient specimen to the blood bank. They will repeat ABO/RH type and antibody screen, perform DAT, and check clerical information. Visual inspection of plasma for pink/red color will also be performed (indicative of hemolysis).

3. If hemolysis is a concern, order haptoglobin (becomes undetectable with hemolysis), LDH, and bilirubin. A DIC screen (PT, PTT, fibrinogen, D-dimer) and repeat CBC may be useful as well.

4. If patient experiences respiratory distress, obtain chest x-ray. Transfusion-related acute lung injury (TRALI) is noncardiogenic pulmonary edema that occurs within 6 hr after the transfusion (see below).

Specific Transfusion Reactions

1. **Acute intravascular hemolysis** (1/240,000 to 760,000 units transfused): Fever, chills, flank pain, dark urine, sense of impending doom. Usually caused by ABO-incompatible PRBC transfusion due to clerical errors. Can result in renal failure or death.
   - **Treatment:** Prevent acute renal failure. Place a Foley catheter, monitor urine output closely, and maintain brisk diuresis with plain D_5W, mannitol (1–2 g/kg IV), furosemide (20–40 mg IV), and/or dopamine (2–10 mcg/kg/min IV) as needed. Alkalize the urine with bicarbonate and pressure support (fluids, vasopressors). Monitor for DIC. Initiate renal and hematology consults.
   - **Prevention:** All specimens sent to blood bank for type and screening should be labeled at the bedside immediately after phlebotomy. Two separate specimens should be tested for ABO/Rh type before issuing type-specific blood. Label on blood product should be checked against the patient's wristband immediately before transfusion.

2. **Febrile nonhemolytic reaction** (~2–3/100 units transfused): Usually mild, with fever, chills. Due to cytokines generated from residual WBCs in the unit.
   - **Treatment:** Low-grade fever usually resolves in 15–30 minutes without specific treatment. Oral acetaminophen (325–500 mg) may be used if the episode causes discomfort.
   - **Prevention:** Transfuse leukoreduced PRBC/platelet units can be considered for future transfusions.

3. **Mild allergic reaction** (~1/100 units transfused): Urticaria or pruritus thought to be due to something in the donor's plasma (specific cause usually not identified).
   - **Treatment:** Diphenhydramine (oral or IV) and the dose (25–100 mg) depends on the severity of the reaction and the patient weight.
   - **Prevention:** If prior allergic transfusion reaction, pretreat with diphenhydramine.

4. **Anaphylactic reaction** (1/150,000 units transfused): Acute hypotension, hives, abdominal pain, and respiratory distress. May be seen in IgA-deficient recipients who have anti-IgA antibodies (note: this is *very* rare).
   - **Treatment:** Epinephrine, diphenhydramine, steroids, blood pressure support.
   - **Prevention:** If prior anaphylactic transfusion reaction, pretreat with diphenhydramine, steroids and have crash cart readily available. If IgA-deficient, provide washed PRBC/platelet units or units from IgA-deficient donors (must be specially ordered from blood supplier).

5. **Transfusion-Related Acute Lung Injury (TRALI)** (1/10,000 units transfused): *#1 cause of transfusion-related mortality*. Fever, chills, hypotension, and acute respiratory distress syndrome within 6 hr of

transfusion—essentially ARDS. Bilateral whiteout seen on chest x-ray with hypoxemia (either O_2 saturation <90% on room air or PaO_2/FiO_2 <200 mm Hg). Caused by HLA antibodies in the donor that attack the recipient's lungs.

- **Treatment:** Supportive care only.
- **Prevention:** Blood collection facilities collect plasma and platelet units from male donors or never-pregnant female donors.

6. **Transfusion-associated circulatory overload (TACO)** (1/100 units transfused): Acute dyspnea, tachypnea, rales within 6 hr of transfusion. Volume overload due to rapid infusion of blood product(s) in a patient with CHF, cirrhosis, renal failure, or preexisting volume overload.
- **Treatment:** Diurese with furosemide.
- **Prevention:** Transfuse slowly, taking up to 4 hr if clinical circumstance permits.

7. **Sepsis** (<1/500,000 PRBC units transfused, 1/12,000 platelet units transfused): Usually caused by transfusion of a bacterially contaminated platelet unit (platelets are stored at room temperature). *Staphylococcus epidermidis, Serratia, Pseudomonas,* and *Yersinia enterocolitica* are the more commonly implicated pathogens.
- **Treatment:** Antibiotics, blood pressure support.
- **Prevention:** Thorough cleansing of donor skin at time of phlebotomy, visual inspection for discoloration of units before issuing.

TRANSFUSION-TRANSMITTED INFECTIONS

16

For perspective on interpretation odds of a transfusion transmitting and infectious agent, selected comparative mortality odds ratios are: stroke 1/1,700; pregnancy 1/4,350–1 to 10,000; MVA 1/6,700; anesthesia 1/7,000 to 1/339,450; oral contraceptive use 1/50,000; flood 1/455,000; lightning strike 1/10,000,000.

Hepatitis

One case of transfusion-transmitted hepatitis B occurs for every 205,000–488,000 units transfused; the incidence of hepatitis C is 1/1,800,000 units transfused. Donor screening has greatly reduced hepatitis risk, as has universally collecting blood from unpaid donors.

HIV

The estimated incidence of transfusion-transmitted HIV infection is 1/2,000,000 to 1/3,000,000 units. Nucleic acid and antibody testing is performed on the donor's blood. The window period between HIV exposure and detection of nucleic acid is approximately 9 days.

CMV

The prevalence of CMV infection among donors is very high (approaching 100% in many series). CMV infection represents a major clinical risk mostly for immunocompromised recipients and neonates. Leukoreduction effectively reduces the risk of CMV transmission.

HTLV-I, -II

Very rare (1/514,000 to 1/2,993,000 units transfused). Leukoreduction can further decrease risk of transmission.

COVID-19 (SARS-CoV-2)

Specific viral RNA has been detected in serum from patients with COVID-19. However, the American Association of Blood Banks and the CDC have not recommended any specific SARS-CoV-2-related actions to be taken for blood donations at this time (December 2020). Individuals are not at risk of contracting COVID-19 through the blood donation process or via a blood transfusion, since respiratory viruses are generally not known to be transmitted by donation or transfusion. The U.S. Food and Drug Administration continues to report that there have been no reported or suspected cases of transfusion-transmitted COVID-19 as of January 2021. The FDA does not recommend using COVID-19 laboratory tests to screen blood; however, the Red Cross does screen for COVID-19 antibodies to identify potential plasma donors.

Someone who has symptoms of COVID-19 (fever, cough, shortness of breath) is not healthy enough to donate blood. Standard screening processes already in place will mean that someone with these symptoms will not be allowed to donate. Specific covid-19 related FDA recommendations for donors as of September 2021:

Bacteria, Parasites, and Other Viruses

Sepsis caused by bacteria is rare, but this most often happens due to a contaminated platelet unit rather than PRBC or plasma (see page 459). As of 2019, the FDA is phasing in babesia testing for donors living in babesia-endemic states; other states ask donors if they have ever tested positive for babesia. Donors who test positive are deferred for 2 yr. Careful travel history of blood donors reduces the risk of malaria; there is no testing of donors for malaria.

APHERESIS

Apheresis procedures may be used to collect single-donor platelets (**plateletpheresis**), PRBCs ("double donation" of 2 units at a time), plasma, or

WBC (**leukapheresis**); the remaining components are returned to the donor. **Therapeutic apheresis** is the separation and removal of a particular component to achieve a therapeutic effect (e.g., **erythrocytapheresis** to treat acute stroke or acute chest syndrome in sickle cell disease, or **therapeutic plasma exchange** to treat thrombotic thrombocytopenic purpura). Peripheral IVs should always be the first choice for vascular access, but many patients require an apheresis-compatible catheter placed (same thing as dialysis catheter) if they are vasculopathic or have altered mental status.

- FDA does not recommend using COVID-19 laboratory tests to screen routine blood donors.
- The blood establishment's responsible physician must evaluate prospective donors and determine eligibility. The donor must be in good health and meet all donor eligibility criteria on the day of donation. The responsible physician may wish to consider the following:
  o individuals diagnosed with COVID-19 or who are suspected of having COVID-19, and who had symptomatic disease, refrain from donating blood for at least 14 days after complete resolution of symptoms,
  o individuals who had a positive diagnostic test for SARS-CoV-2 (e.g., nasopharyngeal swab), but never developed symptoms, refrain from donating at least 14 days after the date of the positive test result,
  o individuals who are tested and found positive for SARS-CoV-2 antibodies, but who did not have prior diagnostic testing and never developed symptoms, can donate without a waiting period and without performing a diagnostic test (e.g., nasopharyngeal swab),
  o individuals who received a nonreplicating, inactivated, or mRNAbased COVID-19 vaccine can donate blood without a waiting period,
  o individuals who received a live-attenuated viral COVID-19 vaccine, refrain from donating blood for a short waiting period (e.g., 14 days) after receipt of the vaccine,
  o individuals who are uncertain about which COVID-19 vaccine was administered, refrain from donating for a short waiting period (e.g., 14 days) if it is possible that the individual received a liveattenuated viral vaccine.

COVID-19 CONVALESCENT PLASMA

(https://www.covid19treatmentguidelines.nih.gov/ accessed 11/13/2021)

COVID-19 convalescent plasma is human plasma collected from individuals whose plasma contains anti-SARS-CoV-2 antibodies, and who meet all donor eligibility requirements. It is an investigational product and is not currently approved or licensed for any indication. The NIH sponsored COVID-19 Treatment Guidelines Panel recommends against the use of low-titer COVID-19 convalescent plasma for the treatment of COVID-19. Low-titer COVID-19 convalescent plasma is no longer authorized through the convalescent plasma emergency use authorization (EUA).

- For hospitalized patients with COVID-19 who do not have impaired immunity: The Panel recommends against the use of COVID-19 convalescent plasma for the treatment of COVID-19 in mechanically ventilated patient sand in hospitalized patients who do not require mechanical ventilation, except in a clinical trial.
- For hospitalized patients with COVID-19 who have impaired immunity: There is insufficient evidence to recommend either for or against the use of high-titer COVID-19 convalescent plasma for the treatment of COVID-19.
- For non-hospitalized patients with COVID-19: There is insufficient evidence to recommend either for or against the use of high-titer COVID-19 convalescent plasma for the treatment of COVID-19.

FURTHER READING

1. AABB: Clinical Resources. http://www.aabb.org/programs/clinical/Pages/default.aspx. Accessed January 9, 2021.
2. U.S. Food and Drug Administration: Blood & Blood Products. https://www.fda.gov/vaccines-blood-biologics/blood-blood-products. Accessed June 3, 2019.
3. Busch MP, et al. A New Strategy for Estimating Risks of Transfusion-Transmitted Viral Infections Based on Rates of Detection of Recently Infected Donors. *Transfusion* 2005;45(2):254–264.
4. Padmanabhan A, et al. Guidelines on the Use of Therapeutic Apheresis in Clinical Practice—Evidence-Based Approach from the Writing Committee of the American Society for Apheresis: The Eighth Special Issue. *J Clin Apheresis* 2019;34(3):171–354.
5. Updated Information for Blood Establishments Regarding the COVID-19 Pandemic and Blood Donation. https://www.fda.gov/vaccines-blood-biologics/safety-availability-biologics/updated-information-blood-establishments-regarding-covid-19-pandemic-and-blood-donation?utm_medium=email&utm_source=govdelivery, accessed September 21, 2021.

Nutritional Assessment, Therapeutic Diets, and Infant Feeding

17

INTERPLAY BETWEEN NUTRITION AND ILLNESS

Nutritional factors figure prominently in the pathogenesis of coronary heart disease, cancer, stroke, and type 2 diabetes—diseases that account for more than half of all deaths in the United States. This situation is compounded by the epidemic of obesity in the United States, which is expected to cause sharp increases in the incidence of chronic illness.

However, the link between nutritional status and health risk extends beyond chronic disease to include acute illness. Surveys place the incidence of malnutrition among hospitalized patients between 30% and 55%. Malnutrition increases the risk of adverse clinical outcomes of hospital stays. In short, poor nutrition increases the risk of becoming ill, and when illness does strike, malnutrition complicates treatment and impairs recovery (Table 17-1).

By integrating nutritional assessment into the evaluation of all patients, clinicians not only identify malnutrition but also uncover risk factors for chronic disease and unfavorable clinical outcome, determine nutritional requirements, recognize people likely to benefit from nutritional support, and establish a framework for developing a therapeutic plan. Depending on the clinical setting, nutritional support can be provided through dietary oral intake, enteral tube feedings, or the parenteral route. This chapter focuses on the principles of nutritional assessment and oral therapeutic diets. Chapter 18, Enteral and Parenteral Nutrition, page 485, describes those approaches to nutritional support.

Chapter update by Elizabeth Holt, MD

Table 17-1. Negative Effects of Malnutrition on Clinical Outcome

Greater susceptibility to infectious complications
Reduced immune competence
Poor skin integrity
Delayed wound healing
Higher incidence of surgical complications
Prolonged need for mechanical ventilation
Increased mortality
Extended length of stay, higher healthcare costs

NUTRITIONAL ASSESSMENT

No single assessment technique has the validity to serve as the sole indicator of nutritional status. Nutritional assessment is a comprehensive process that combines objective data with relevant clinical information. Evaluate body composition, anthropometric measurements, and results of laboratory tests, and use the data in the context of the patient's history, physical examination findings, and clinical condition to make decisions concerning nutritional status.

17 ## Body Weight

Body weight is a reliable indicator of nutritional status. Details concerning body weight include deviation of weight from ideal level, change in weight over time, and relation between weight and height. Body weight 20% over or under the ideal level places a patient at nutritional risk. Numerous methods for determining ideal body weight exist, but the Hamwi formula is the most widely used in clinical settings because the calculation is simple and provides a reasonable estimate of ideal body weight (Table 17-2):

Table 17-2. Formula for Determining Ideal Body Weight: Hamwi Formula

Men: 106 lb for 5 ft of height plus 6 lb for every inch of height over 5 ft
Women: 100 lb for 5 ft of height plus 5 lb for every inch of height over 5 ft
Both: ±10% based on frame size

Changes in body weight from baseline carry important prognostic value. Whether or not usual body weight is over or under the ideal, unintentional weight loss is cause for concern. Both the degree of weight loss and the time frame in which it occurs are significant variables. In general, involuntary weight loss of 10% of usual weight over a period of 6 mo represents severe nutritional risk that warrants further investigation. Among children, a downward trend in percentile ranking on growth charts is cause for concern even if the child continues to gain weight. Growth charts can also reveal a tendency toward excessive weight gain, allowing early nutritional intervention and management of obesity.

Body Mass Index

Body mass index (BMI), a ratio of weight to height, is a value that eliminates the influence of frame size. BMI is a reliable indicator of adiposity. An elevated BMI is strongly correlated with the risk of development of cardiovascular disease, diabetes, cancer, hypertension, and osteoarthritis. The formula for calculating BMI is:

$$\text{BMI} = \frac{\text{Weight (kg)}}{\text{Height}^2 \text{ (m)}}$$

Table 17-3 shows the interpretation of BMI values. Each class of obesity represents a higher level of health risk. The BMI formula overestimates body fat in muscular athletes and underestimates fat stores in older persons, limiting the value of the formula in those populations. Detailed BMI tables can be found in the Appendix, page 1047.

Anthropometric Measurements

Anthropometric evaluations are body composition assessments derived through direct measurement. A summary of the techniques used to evaluate body composition appears in Table 17-4. The preferred method of nutritional assessment is a waist circumference measurement to evaluate the distribution of body fat and the health risks associated with abdominal obesity. For men, a waist measurement >40 in (102 cm) indicates a higher risk of cardiovascular

17

Table 17-3. Body Mass Index

BMI	Interpretation
<18.5	Underweight
18.5–24.9	Normal
25–29.9	Overweight
30–34.9	Obesity (class 1)
35–39.9	Obesity (class 2)
>40	Obesity (class 3)

Many BMI calculators are available online; keyword search "BMI." BMI tables can be found in the Appendix, page 1047.

Table 17-4. Techniques for Evaluating Body Composition

Method	Description
Body weight	Actual body weight compared with ideal body weight; used to assess changes over time; results are affected by hydration status
BMI	Used to evaluate weight in relation to height; a reliable indicator of adiposity; higher levels increase health risks
Anthropometric measurements	Measurement of waist circumference and waist to hip ratio, both values linked to health risks; replaces measurement of triceps skinfold thickness and midarm muscle circumference, which lacks validity
Bioelectrical	Assessment of fluid volume and lean body impedance mass by measuring resistance electrical current; assessment used in sports medicine; not fully validated for clinical use
Dual-energy x-ray absorptiometry (DEXA)	Measurement of bone density; may help determine fat and lean body compartments; no clear role in predicting clinical outcome
Neutron activation analysis	Use of shielded counters to measure gamma-ray decay of naturally occurring isotopes; estimate of total body potassium, an indicator of body cell mass; safe for pregnant women and children; used primarily in research

17

disease. Similar risk exists for women with a waist measurement >35 in. (89 cm). Abdominal obesity is one feature of **metabolic syndrome,** a cluster of risk factors, including insulin resistance, dyslipidemia, hypertension, and prothrombotic and proinflammatory states, that increase the risk of cardiovascular disease and type 2 diabetes. Table 17-5 details the identification of metabolic syndrome.

Other body composition testing, such as DEXA, CT, and MRI, provides more direct measurements but is costly. Neutron activation analysis is limited to research at this time.

Laboratory Tests

In primary care, the lipid profile is perhaps the most frequently ordered laboratory test with nutritional implications. Many other routine laboratory tests, such as CBC, blood glucose, electrolyte levels, creatinine, and BUN, also provide information relevant to nutritional status. Although the lipid profile is important during acute illness, nutritional assessment of hospitalized patients also emphasizes evaluation of serum protein concentration.

Visceral protein markers, such as albumin, prealbumin (transthyretin), and transferrin are routinely measured in hospitalized patients (values are discussed

Table 17-5. Diagnostic Criteria for Metabolic Syndrome

Characteristic	Value
Abdominal obesity	Waist circumference
	Men: >40 in (102 cm)
	Women: >35 in (89 cm)
Fasting triglyceride level	>150 mg/dL
HDL cholesterol	Men: <40 mg/dL
	Women: <50 mg/dL
Blood pressure	>130/85 mm/Hg
Fasting blood glucose	>110 mg/dL

The presence of three or more of the risk factors identifies the syndrome.

in Chapter 10, pages 179, 244, and 259). Because of its short half-life, prealbumin is the preferred marker in clinical settings and a key part of the nutritional assessment. These measurements, however, have limited value as nutritional indicators in acutely ill patients. Studies show a strong link between low visceral protein levels and increased risk of morbidity and mortality, but numerous clinical factors other than nutrition can influence visceral protein levels during acute illness. Visceral protein concentrations often reflect hydration status, organ function, or an inflammatory response to injury more than the nutritional state of the patient. In inflammatory states, the liver reprioritizes protein synthesis in favor of acute-phase proteins, causing visceral protein levels to fall. Measuring C-reactive protein in conjunction with visceral protein is a way to differentiate low visceral protein levels caused by nutritional factors from those related to the presence of an inflammatory process.

The assessment of adequate nutritional support must address both energy requirements and protein demands. **Nitrogen balance** is important in assessing nutritional support and is frequently used in injured surgical patients (burn and trauma) requiring long-term nutritional support. Determining urinary urea nitrogen (UUN) and calculating nitrogen balance allows approximation of the trend in nitrogen breakdown and appropriate adjustment of protein goals, particularly when used in conjunction with other clinical monitoring methods. Positive nitrogen balance, a state in which nitrogen intake exceeds losses, implies that the amount of protein being administered is sufficient to promote anabolism and prevent erosion of lean body mass. In general, negative nitrogen balance indicates the need to increase protein intake and possibly energy intake as well. Urinary nitrogen losses of 8–12 g/d indicate a mild stress condition; 14–18 g/d, moderate stress; and 20 g/d, severe stress. The accuracy of nitrogen balance calculations can be improved through measurement over several weeks. When losses of nitrogen are large (e.g., diarrhea, protein-losing enteropathy, fistula, or burns), measurements of nitrogen balance lose accuracy because of the difficulty in collecting secretions for nitrogen measurement. Steps to determine nitrogen balance are as follows:

1. **Measure urine urea nitrogen (UUN)** from a 24-hr urine collection. Because this study shows only nitrogen excretion that occurs as urea, a "fudge factor" of 3 g of nitrogen is added to the urinary loss to account for other nonurea nitrogen losses (skin and feces). Therefore 24-hr UUN + 3 g = 24-hr nitrogen loss.
2. **Determine nitrogen intake.** Calculating nitrogen intake for the 24-hr period of the UUN collection is relatively easy for patients who receive a prescribed amount of protein through parenteral or enteral nutrition, and this is the most common scenario for nitrogen balance testing. To determine 24-hr nitrogen intake, divide protein intake (g/24 hr) by 6.25.
3. **Formula for calculating nitrogen balance:**

$$\text{Nitrogen}_{(balance)} = \text{Nitrogen}_{(intake)} - \text{Nitrogen}_{(output)}$$
$$\text{Nitrogen}_{(intake)} = \text{g protein}_{(intake)} / 6.25$$
$$\text{Nitrogen}_{(output)} = (\text{UUN} \times \text{vol}) + 3$$

UUN, urine urea nitrogen; vol, volume of urine produced over the time of measurement.

Nutritional assessment does not routinely include assays of specific nutrient levels unless clinical circumstances raise concern about potential imbalances. For instance, order iron studies as part of the assessment of a patient with microcytic anemia, but order vitamin B_{12} and folate levels in the evaluation of macrocytosis.

Health History

The health history obtained in the evaluation of every patient is an indispensable source of information regarding nutritional status. The patient interview not only provides an additional opportunity to detect risk factors related to nutrition but also often reveals the mechanisms underlying nutritional problems. The medical history, for example, indicates the impact of disease or previous surgery on nutrient intake, absorption, and metabolism. A review of the patient's current medication profile may reveal drug–nutrient interactions or GI side effects that affect appetite. Symptoms such as nausea, pain, fatigue, dry mouth, and shortness of breath often have negative effects on food intake. Aspects of the patient's social history, such as the presence of substance abuse, financial difficulties, or lack of support systems such as transportation, also are causes of concern about nutritional status. Whenever possible, request a complete nutritional history by a registered dietitian to obtain complete information about nutritional deficits that may exist.

Physical Examination

Use standard physical assessment procedures to evaluate nutritional status. Physical signs of malnutrition are often nonspecific and require correlation with the patient's history, clinical condition, and results of diagnostic studies. As Table 17-6 shows, muscle wasting, poor skin integrity, and loss of subcutaneous fat are typical findings associated with long-standing deficits in protein and energy intake. Patients rarely exhibit the classic signs of vitamin or mineral deficiency that characterize conditions such as scurvy or beriberi. Fortification of the food supply in the United States and widespread use of multivitamin supplements have made physical manifestation of nutrient deficiency an uncommon occurrence.

Assessing GI Function

Although not part of nutritional assessment per se, appraisal of GI function often provides insight into the mechanisms underlying nutritional problems and helps to pinpoint specific nutrient deficiencies that may exist. Any

Table 17-6. Physical Signs of Poor Nutritional Status

Sign	Example	Clinical Implications
Muscle wasting	Loss of muscle mass and tone; concave appearance of the temporal region of the face is evidence of marked muscle wasting, even in the presence of edema	Weakness, reduced stamina and functional status; possible impairment of respiratory effort and ability to cough and clear secretions
Loss of subcutaneous tissue	Loose, elongated skinfolds on the abdomen and in the triceps area; prominent appearance of ribs, scapulae, vertebrae, and pelvic bones	Depletion of fat stores representing marked weight loss and loss of reserves that serve as an energy source during acute illness
Poor skin integrity	Poor turgor, friability, delayed wound healing; edema with severe hypoalbuminemia	Increased risk of pressure ulcers, wound dehiscence, and anastomotic leaks
Obesity	Excess accumulation of body mass and adipose tissue	Serious health risks; truncal obesity more serious risk than fat stores on hips and buttocks

17

alteration in the key GI functions associated with eating—appetite, chewing, swallowing, digestion, absorption, and elimination—can have profound effects on nutritional status. An understanding of GI function is also essential for determining the most appropriate route of nutritional support.

The functional status of the GI tract is a key element in determining when to initiate feeding in postoperative patients. In most cases, patients can safely begin oral intake once they recover consciousness sufficiently to protect their airway. Current studies no longer show that postoperative feeding has to wait for spontaneous resolution of ileus, and the most recent data lean toward early feeding, usually within 24 hr.

ESTABLISHING PROTEIN AND ENERGY REQUIREMENTS

Caloric Expenditure

Establishing target ranges for energy and protein intake helps not only to ensure that the patient receives adequate nutrition but avoids overfeeding. Numerous studies have shown the deleterious effects of overfeeding, including unwanted weight gain, hyperglycemia, hepatic dysfunction, electrolyte imbalances, azotemia, hyperlipidemia, and elevated respiratory quotient. These effects are especially important in patients fed parenterally. Several methods for determining energy expenditure exist, including weight-based calculations, formulas such as the Harris-Benedict equations, and indirect calorimetry techniques. None of these methods is ideal for all situations. Each requires a degree of judgment to account for clinical variables that affect energy needs. The following simple weight-based system is the most practical way to establish goals for caloric intake.

For adults in most clinical settings, a range of 25–30 kcal/kg of body weight is a reasonable estimate of daily energy expenditure. No attempt is made to account for variations in age, sex, body composition, or acuity of illness; hence the need for clinical judgment. Concerns about overfeeding and unfavorable outcome have eliminated the once common practice of providing as much as 35–40 kcal/kg/d to critically ill patients. The weight-based system has a wide margin of error for obese patients. When a patient's BMI falls into an obese category, many clinicians use adjusted body weight (ABW) to determine energy needs. The formula for ABW takes into account that not all of a person's excess weight is adipose tissue but that a portion is metabolically active, lean body mass:

$$\text{Adjusted body weight (ABW)} = [(\text{Actual body weight} - \text{Ideal body weight}) \times 0.25] + \text{Ideal body weight}$$

Consensus does not exist regarding the optimal level of energy intake for obese patients. Studies in which patients received as little as 50% of estimated energy expenditure or 20 kcal/kg of ABW have shown positive outcomes. Further research is needed, however, to establish an accurate prediction of optimal levels of energy intake for obese patients.

Infants and growing children need much higher energy intake per kilogram of body weight than adults. Infants may need as much as 110 kcal/kg/d. Energy intake remains elevated to support growth through the teenage years, but wide variation occurs. Satisfactory growth is the best indication that a child's energy intake is adequate.

Protein Requirements

Healthy persons with normal renal function need 0.8 g of protein per kilogram of body weight per day, but illness and injury can dramatically increase protein needs. For example, postoperative patients need 1.0–1.5 g/kg/d. Sepsis increases protein needs to 1.2–1.5 g/kg/d. Daily protein intake for patients with multiple trauma should fall within 1.3–1.7 g/kg, and burn victims may need 1.8–2.5 g/kg/d. With the exception of patients with burn injuries, guidelines set the upper limit for protein intake at 2.0 g/kg/d. Research suggests that doses of protein above this level exceed the patient's utilization capacity and can lead to azotemia. As with energy intake, protein intake for obese patients should be based on ABW.

Protein needs for children vary with age. The requirement is greatest in the first year of life and then gradually declines. Healthy infants need 2–3 g/kg/d, and children up to age 10 need 1.0–1.2 g/kg/d. The protein requirement of critically ill children is approximately 1.5 g/kg/d.

17

BASIC DIETARY GUIDELINES FOR AMERICANS

Guidance on what comprises basic good nutritional recommendations for adults and children is well established. Several guidelines have been published, and these and other current guidelines emphasize a shift to more plant-based foods (vegetables, fruits, lean protein) and a reduction in saturated fats, sodium, and sugars (see Table 17-7).

THERAPEUTIC DIETS

The term *therapeutic diet* refers to dietary changes that play a role in the management of a medical condition. Some commonly ordered therapeutic diets and their indications appear in Table 17-8. These dietary modifications, which usually require a physician's or other authorized provider's order in the hospital, typically call for a change in the consistency of the food served or an adjustment in the quantity of one or more nutrients in the diet. Most hospitals have diet manuals available for reference, and registered dietitians are usually on staff for consultation in clinical situations that necessitate a therapeutic diet.

Table 17-7. Key Dietary Recommendations for Americans from the U.S. Department of Health. (Based on data from Dietary Guidelines for Americans 2015-2020, 8th ed.; U.S. Department of Health and Human Services and US Department of Agriculture; www. health.gov, accessed April 20, 2020 and reproduced with permission from *Contemp Pediatr* 2020;37[1]).

Healthy eating patterns include:	• Variety of vegetables from all subgroups (dark greens, red and orange, legumes, starchy, and other) • Fruits, especially whole • Grains, half of which are whole • Fat-free or low-fat dairy products • Variety of proteins, including seafood, lean meats and poultry, eggs, legumes, nuts/seeds, and soy • Oils
Healthy eating patterns limit:	• Saturated fats (consume <10% of calories/d) and trans fats • Added sugars (consume <10% of calories/d) • Sodium (consume <2300 mg/d)

Modifying the Consistency of Food

Changing the consistency or texture of the diet is a simple way to make food easier to chew, swallow, and digest. For instance, patients with poor dentition may benefit from a pureed diet. Other patients may benefit from thickening agents added to some foods. Patients with dysphagia frequently need a change in texture or consistency of food to enhance the safety of eating and avoid aspiration. An evaluation of swallowing function by a speech-language pathologist is essential in determining the appropriate diet for patients with impaired swallowing. Dysphagia occurs most often as a result of neurologic conditions, but many medical and surgical problems can compromise swallowing. A swallowing evaluation is warranted before the start of oral intake in any situation that increases the risk of dysphagia, including cognitive or functional decline, surgery or radiation of structures involved in swallowing, prolonged intubation, and recent tracheostomy.

Modifying Nutrient Content of the Diet

Because illness frequently alters nutrient requirements or nutrient tolerance, diet modification is a common therapeutic intervention in the management of many chronic diseases. In some cases, the therapeutic diet may simply limit a single nutrient, such as sodium. At other times diet prescription may require broad changes in eating habits. The dietary changes recommended for prevention and treatment of cardiovascular disease fall

Table 17-8. Commonly Prescribed Therapeutic Diets Used in the Hospital Setting (refer to local hospital dietary listings that may vary from the diets listed here)

Diet	Guidelines	Indications
House/regular	Adequate in all essential nutrients All foods are permitted Can be modified according to patient's food preferences	No diet restrictions or modifications
Mechanical soft	Includes soft-textured or ground foods that are easily masticated and swallowed	Decreased ability to chew or swallow Presence of oral mucositis or esophagitis May be appropriate for some patients with dysphagia
Pureed	Includes liquids as well as strained and pureed foods	Inability to chew or swallow solid foods Presence of oral mucositis or esophagitis May be appropriate for some patients with dysphagia
Full liquid	Includes foods that are liquid at body temperature Includes milk/milk products Can provide approximately: 2500–3000 mL fluid 1500–2000 cal 60–80 g high quality protein <10 g dietary fiber 60–80 g fat/d	May be appropriate for patients with severely limited chewing ability Not appropriate for lactase-deficient patients unless commercially available lactase enzyme tablets provided

(Continued)

17

Table 17-8. Commonly Prescribed Therapeutic Diets Used in the Hospital Setting (refer to local hospital dietary listings that may vary from the diets listed here) (*Continued*)

Diet	Guidelines	Indications
Clear liquid	Includes foods that are liquid at body temperature Foods are Very low in fiber Lactose-free Virtually fat-free Can provide approximately: ≥2000 mL fluid 400–600 cal <7 g low-quality protein 1 g dietary fiber <1 g fat/d This diet is inadequate in all nutrients and should not be used >3 d without supplementation	Ordered as initial diet in the transition from NPO to solids Used for bowel preparation before certain medical or surgical procedures For management of acute medical conditions warranting minimized biliary contractions or pancreatic exocrine secretion
Low-fiber	Foods that are low in indigestible carbohydrates Decreases stool volume, transit time, and frequency	Management of acute radiation enteritis and inflammatory bowel disease when narrowing or stenosis of the intestinal lumen is present
Carbohydrate controlled diet (ADA)	Calorie level should be adequate to maintain or achieve desirable body weight (DBW) Total carbohydrates are limited to 50–60% of total calories Ideally fat should be limited to ≈30% of total calories	Diabetes mellitus

Acute renal failure	Protein (g/kg DBW) Calories (per kilogram) Sodium (g/d) Potassium (g/d) Fluid (mL/d)	0.6 35–50 1–3 Variable Urine output +500 cc	For patients in renal failure who are not undergoing dialysis
Renal failure hemodialysis	Protein (g/kg DBW) Calories (per kilogram DBW) Sodium (g/d) Potassium (g/d) Fluid (mL/d)	1.0–1.2 30–35 1–2 1.5–3 Urine output +500 cc	For patients in renal failure on hemodialysis
Peritoneal dialysis	Protein (g/kg DBW) Calories (per kilogram DBW) Sodium (g/d) Potassium (g/d) Fluid (mL/d)	1.2–1.6 25–35 3–4 3–4 Urine output +500 cc	For patients in renal failure on peritoneal dialysis
Hepatic	In the absence of encephalopathy do not restrict protein In the presence of encephalopathy initially restrict protein to 40–60 g/d, then liberalize in increments of 10 g/day as tolerated Specify sodium and fluid restriction according to severity of ascites and edema		Management of chronic liver disorders

17

(Continued)

17

Table 17-8. Commonly Prescribed Therapeutic Diets Used in the Hospital Setting (refer to local hospital dietary listings that may vary from the diets listed here) *(Continued)*

Diet	Guidelines	Indications
Low lactose/lactose-free	Limit or restrict milk products Commercially available lactase enzyme tablets can be used	Lactase deficiency
Low-fat	<50 g total fat per day	Pancreatitis Fat malabsorption
Fat/cholesterol restricted	Total fat <30% total calories Saturated fat limited to 10% of calories <300 mg cholesterol <50% calories from complex carbohydrates	Hypercholesterolemia
Low-sodium	Sodium allowance should be as liberal as possible to maximize nutritional intake yet control symptoms "No added salt" is 4 g/d; no added salt, no cooking with salt, and no highly salted food and avoids processed foods (i.e. meats) is 2 g/d <1 g/d is unpalatable and thus compromises adequate intake	Indicated for patients with hypertension, ascites, and edema associated with the underlying disease

into the latter category. Any diet that restricts one or more nutrients poses nutritional risks. One concern is that in adhering to a dietary restriction, patients may unintentionally omit other essential nutrients. In addition, patients frequently find restrictive diets unpalatable, a problem that leads to poor intake or noncompliance. A patient who has been given a prescription for a medically indicated therapeutic or modified diet needs instruction by a clinical dietitian before discharge or as an outpatient. Table 17-9 lists some common medically prescribed diets that patients may use on a long-term basis. While beneficial, potential complications can be encountered; therefore, nutritional counseling is important to minimize some of these problems.

There are several other special dietary considerations to consider in nutritional assessment and counseling. Because of family preferences or religious beliefs or due to limited resources, individuals may choose to alter their diet. One common diet choice primarily limits intake of animal proteins. Table 17-10 reviews some of the frequently encountered variations on **vegetarian diets**. When performing nutritional assessment, patients may describe a "plant-based diet." Further questioning is usually warranted, such as "do you eat dairy, eggs, etc.?"

Oral Nutritional Supplements

For patients unable to tolerate sufficient food to maintain adequate nutritional status, oral nutritional supplements can halt or reverse nutritional decline and improve clinical outcome. For elderly patients, for example, the use of oral supplements improves nutritional status and reduces mortality. The nutritional products, which are available without a prescription, come in a variety of forms, including high-protein, high-calorie beverages; puddings; snack bars; and soups. Ensure (Ross Laboratories) and Boost (Novartis) are two common examples of liquid oral supplements. These products are flavored for oral consumption, but they are also appropriate for administration through a feeding tube. Depending on the circumstances, patients can consume these products in addition to regular meals or as a meal replacement. Most oral supplements on the market are lactose-free, an important consideration for persons who cannot tolerate milk-based supplements. Unlike most snack foods, commercially prepared oral supplements provide a balanced mix of nutrients, including vitamins and minerals. Encourage patients to try a variety of supplements to avoid taste fatigue, a common problem among patients who consume only one supplement over an extended period. Adding flavoring such as chocolate or coffee syrup to oral supplements can improve palatability. Sustained success with oral supplements frequently requires the creative support of the entire healthcare team and family.

17

Table 17-9. Some Medically Prescribed Diets to Address a Variety of Conditions with Potential Complications

Prescribed Diet	Medical Indication	Potential Complications
Gluten-free	Celiac disease; nonceliac gluten sensitivity	Poor growth; constipation; deficiencies in iron, calcium, fiber, thiamin, riboflavin, niacin, folate
Lactose-free	Lactose intolerance; galactosemia	Deficiencies in calcium and vitamin D; poor weight gain if hypocaloric
Dairy-free	Milk protein allergy	Possibly low in protein, calories, and calcium
Elimination	Allergy/intolerance; eosinophilic esophagitis	Deficiencies in calcium, iron, zinc, vitamins D, E, folate, and B_{12}; poor growth and weight gain. Risks will be based on the specific food
Specific carbohydrate diet	Inflammatory bowel disease	Potential decreased caloric intake with subsequent poor growth, vitamin D deficiency, and other micronutrient deficiency if not monitored
High-fiber	Constipation; irritable bowel disease	Diarrhea, abdominal pain, gas
Low-fiber	Intestinal strictures	Constipation
Sorbitol- or fructose-free	Sorbitol and fructose intolerance	Constipation; poor weight gain if hypocaloric
Ketogenic	Intractable seizures; metabolic disorder	Poor growth/weight gain; gastrointestinal (vomiting, diarrhea, constipation); anorexia; dehydration; lethargy; irritability; renal stones; acidosis; hyperlipidemia; hypoglycemia; hypertriglyceridemia; bone demineralization; vitamin, mineral, and nutrient deficiencies (vitamins D and E, magnesium, potassium, calcium, selenium, and carnitine)

		Deficiencies in micronutrients; poor growth and weight gain
Metabolic	Metabolic diseases	Deficiencies in micronutrients; poor growth and weight gain
High-caloric diet	Poor weight gain	Hyperlipidemia, excessive protein/fat consumption; refeeding syndrome; obesity if not monitored
Low FODMP**	Irritable bowel disease, high ileostomy output, short bowel syndrome	Weight loss, micronutrient deficiency if not monitored
Specific carbohydrate diet	Irritable bowel disease	Potential decreased caloric intake with subsequent poor growth, vitamin D deficiency, and diarrhea

These represent a starting suggestion, and each patient's diet should be individualized with nutritional consultation to optimize outcomes and minimize complications. Many patients can have more than one issue, such as Crohn disease and irritable bowel syndrome, which may have opposing dietary recommendations.

** FODMP (fermentable oligo-, di- mon-osaccharides and polyols) are found in a wide variety of foods, including fruits and vegetables, grains and cereals, nuts, legumes, lentils, dairy foods, and manufactured foods.

(Modified and reproduced with permission from Contemp Pediatr 2020;37[1]).

17

Table 17-10. Various Types of Vegetarian Diets

Diet	Inclusion/Exclusion	Potential Nutrient Deficiencies
Lactovegetarian	Plant-based (grains, legumes, nuts, fruits, vegetables) including milk and milk products. Excludes eggs, meat, seafood/fish, poultry.	• Vitamin B_{12} • Zinc • Iron
Lacto-ovo-vegetarian	Plant-based (grains, legumes, nuts, fruits, vegetables) including eggs and dairy. Excluding meat, seafood/fish, poultry.	• Vitamin B_{12} • Zinc • Iron • n-3 fatty acids
Ovo-vegetarian	Plant-based (grains, legumes, nuts, fruits, vegetables). Excludes milk, dairy products, meats, poultry, and seafood.	• Vitamin B_{12} • Vitamin D • Calcium • Zinc • Iron
Vegan	Excludes all animal products.	• Energy deficit • Protein • Vitamin B_{12} • Vitamin D • Zinc • Calcium • n-3 fatty acids • Iron

(Modified and reproduced with permission from Contemp Pediatr 2020;37[1]).

INFANT FEEDING

Breastfeeding

Clinical practice guidelines consistently endorse breastfeeding as the sole source of infant nutrition for the first 6 mo of life. Breast milk is uniquely suited to the nutritional needs of growing infants, supporting optimal nutrition and reducing the risk of childhood obesity. Research findings suggest that the presence of long-chain polyunsaturated fatty acids in human milk may also enhance neurocognitive development. Breastfed infants gain protection against infectious disease early in life from maternal immunoglobulins present in breast milk and may have fewer infantile allergies than their formula-fed counterparts. In addition to these physiologic advantages, breastfeeding offers psychological benefits to both mother and infant and reduces the cost of infant feeding.

Commercial Infant Formulas

Despite compelling evidence of the benefits of breastfeeding to both infant and mother, commercial infant formulas continue to play a prominent role as a source of infant nutrition in the United States. Commercial infant formulas serve as an appropriate substitute for breast milk in the presence of medical contraindications to breastfeeding, when the mother decides against breast-feeding, or if maternal milk production is inadequate. Because manufacturers have refined the nutrient profile of commercial infant formulas to more closely resemble the composition of breast milk, homemade infant formulas are no longer considered an acceptable substitute. Most commercial infant formulas have a cow's milk base, but soy-based formulas are also available. Soy formula does not prevent colic or allergy, as once thought, and has no role as a primary method of infant feeding.

Commonly used formulas are outlined in Table 17-11. Most infant formulas are iso-osmolar (e.g., Similac 20, Enfamil 20, and SMA 20 with and without iron). These formulas are used most often for healthy infants.

If possible, preterm infants should receive human milk (breast milk can be fortified to meet the elevated requirements of a rapidly growing infant). Commercial formulas for premature infants contain 24 kcal/oz (e.g., Similac 24, Enfamil 24, "preemie" SMA 24). Many other specialty formulas are available for infants with medical conditions such as inborn errors of metabolism, malabsorption syndromes, and milk and protein sensitivity.

Commercial formulas are available with and without iron, but current guidelines call for use of an iron-fortified formula for most infants. Many pediatricians recommend vitamin supplements with some formulas if the infant is taking <32 oz/day. However, at this point most infants are beginning solid food that serves as an additional source of vitamins and minerals.

Oral Rehydration Solutions

Infants with mild or moderate dehydration, often due to diarrhea or vomiting, may benefit from oral rehydration formulas. These solutions typically include glucose, sodium, potassium, and bicarbonate or citrate. Common formulations include **Pedialyte, Lytren, Infalyte, Resol,** and **Hydrolyte.**

Initiating Infant Feeding

Most healthy term infants can begin breastfeeding immediately after birth. The initial feeding for bottle-fed infants generally takes place within the first 4 or 5 hr of life as long as the infant displays signs of readiness for feeding, such as alertness, active bowel sounds, and rooting and sucking behavior. For preterm and sick infants, conduct a detailed assessment before introducing feeding. In this setting, feedings should begin only if the infant has hemodynamic stability; no excessive oral secretions; no vomiting; no bile-stained

17

Table 17-11. Infant Enteral Feedings: Types and Indications

Formula	Indications
Human milk	All infants: supplement with Vitamin D 400 IU/d; iron at 4 months
Breast milk fortifiers	Preterm infant (<1800 g and <34 weeks): supplement with Vitamin D 400 IU/d; iron; and MV[a]
Cow milk–based formulas: MV[a] if <32 oz./d (~1 L/d)	
Enfamil Infant Similac Advance Similac Organic	Full-term infants: as supplement to breast milk
Enfamil Gentlease/Similac Sensitive	Term infants: to reduce fussiness or gas
Gerber Good Start	Term infants: whey protein; moderate mineral content; may be more palatable
Enfamil Added Rice	Rice starch added for thickening after ingestion (pH sensitive). Used for simple reflux. Not indicated for preterm infants
Preterm formulas	
Enfamil Premature 20, 24, and 30 Similac Special Care 20, 24, and 30	Preterm infants: for infants on fluid restriction or who cannot handle required volumes of 20-calorie formula to grow 24 and 27 formulas are higher osmolality than the 20 formulas which are iso-osmolar. Calcium and phosphorus content to mimic intrauterine accretion rates
Enfamil Premature 24 High Protein Similac Special Care 24 High Protein	Approximately 10% more protein than above formulas at same caloric density
Enfamil EnfaCare Similac NeoSure	Preterm infants preparing for discharge; increased protein, calcium, phosphorous, vitamins A and D; promotes better mineralization. Use up to 6–9 months corrected age
Soy formulas: MV[a] if <32 oz./d (~1 L/d) MV (*Note*: Soy formulas not recommended in infants <1800 g)	
Enfamil ProSobee (lactose and sucrose free) Gerber Good Start Soy Similac Soy Isomil (lactose free)	Term infants: milk sensitivity, galactosemia, carbohydrate intolerance, desire for vegetarian diet. Term infants; hydrolyzed soy proteins *Do not use soy formulas in preterm infants. Phytates can bind calcium and cause rickets*
Protein hydrolysate formulas (casein predominant): MV[a] if <32 oz./d (~1 L/d)	
Nutramigen with Enflora LGG (Probiotic LGG)	Term infants: hypoallergenic, hydrolyzed casein with lactose, galactose, and sucrose free for gut sensitivity to proteins, galactosemia, multiple food allergies, persistent diarrhea, colic due to cow milk allergy

(Continued)

Table 17-11. Infant Enteral Feedings: Types and Indications (*Continued*)

Formula	Indications
Pregestimil	Preterm and term infants: disaccharides deficiency, fat malabsorption, diarrhea, GI defects, cystic fibrosis, food allergy, celiac disease, transition from TPN to oral feeding
Similac Alimentum	Term infants: lactose-free formula; protein sensitivity, pancreatic insufficiency, diarrhea, severe food allergies, colic, carbohydrate, and fat malabsorption
Free amino acid elemental formulas	
Neocate	Term infants: severe cow milk protein allergies; contains 100% free amino acids (elemental formula)
EleCare for Infants	Elemental formula containing amino acids indicated for malabsorption, protein malabsorption, short bowel syndromes
Special formulas: MV[a] and Fe if standard formula weight >1500 g	
Similac PM 60/40	Preterm and term infants: problem feeders on standard formula; infants with renal, cardiovascular, or digestive diseases that require decreased protein and mineral levels; breast-feeding supplement; initial feeding
Enfaport	For infants with chylothorax and LCHAD deficiency
Metabolic formulas	Special metabolic formulas are available for infants with inherited metabolic disorders www.meadjohnson.com www.abottnutrition.com

Fe, iron; GI, gastrointestinal; LCHAD, long-chain 3-hydroxyacyl-CoA dehydrogenase; MV, multivitamin; TPN, total parenteral nutrition.
[a]Such as Poly-Vi-Sol (Mead Johnson). Modified and reproduced with permission from Gomella TL, ed. Neonatology, 8e, New York, NY: McGraw-Hill; 2020.

17

gastric aspirate, normal bowel sounds; and a nondistended and soft abdomen and can coordinate breathing, sucking, and swallowing. Because tachypnea increases the risk of aspiration, verify that the infant's respiratory rate is within normal limits before offering a bottle for the first time. Infants who have been weaned from a ventilator should exhibit no evidence of respiratory distress for at least 6 hr after extubation before feeding.

Infant Feeding Progression

The initial feeding for bottle-fed infants is usually sterile water or D5W. Do not use hypertonic solutions such as D10W.

Controversy exists regarding the optimal way to introduce commercial infant formula after the initial feeding with water or D5W. Some clinicians advocate diluting infant formula with sterile water and advancing the concentration as tolerated (e.g., start with 1/4 strength, increase to 1/2 strength, and then progress to 3/4 strength before giving full-strength formula). Others believe this gradual progression is unnecessary and start with full-strength formula after the infant tolerates the initial feeding with water or D5W without difficulty. Breastfed infants typically begin feeding without first receiving a water feeding, and **breast milk is never diluted.**

Considerations for Preterm Infants

Many preterm infants lack the coordination to take oral feedings safely. In this situation, provide nutrients through a feeding tube. Considerable controversy remains concerning the timing of initial enteral feeding of preterm infants. For larger (>1500 g) premature infants in stable condition, give the first feeding within the first 24 hr of life. Early feeding may allow the release of enteric hormones that exert a trophic effect on the intestinal tract. On the other hand, apprehension about necrotizing enterocolitis (mostly in very low-birthweight infants) precludes initiation of enteral feeding in the following circumstances: perinatal asphyxia, mechanical ventilation, presence of umbilical vessel catheters, patent ductus arteriosus, indomethacin treatment, sepsis, and frequent episodes of apnea and bradycardia. Consensus does not exist regarding the optimal timing and method of introducing feeding to preterm infants with those conditions. In general, preterm infants begin enteral feeding in the first 3 days of life. The objective is to reach full enteral feeding by 2–3 wk of life. Start parenteral nutrition, including amino acids and lipids, at the same time as enteral feeding to provide adequate caloric intake.

CANDIDATES FOR NUTRITIONAL SUPPORT

When nutritional assessment reveals evidence of poor or declining nutritional status, investigate the causes and develop a plan for intervention. This process includes management of underlying medical problems, management of symptoms that interfere with appetite and eating, and efforts to increase intake with dietary modification and oral supplements. Consider enteral or parenteral nutrition when nutritional deficits persist despite efforts to improve oral intake or when the patient's clinical condition precludes safe or adequate intake by mouth (see Chapter 18, Enteral and Parenteral Nutrition, page 485).

Enteral and Parenteral Nutrition   18

DEFINITIONS

Nutritional support is the provision of nutrients with therapeutic intent by either the enteral or the parenteral route. Technically, the term **enteral nutrition** includes oral supplements as well as tube feeding, but in practice, clinicians usually use the term to refer strictly to tube feeding. **Parenteral nutrition (PN)** refers to the intravenous administration of nutrition that may include protein, carbohydrate, fat, minerals and electrolytes, vitamins, and other trace elements. Parenteral nutrition is sometimes referred to as **total parenteral nutrition (TPN)**. PN is reserved for patients who are unable to eat or absorb enough food through tube feeding or by mouth to maintain a good nutrition status.

Enteral and parenteral nutrition are important in the management of many medical conditions. Safe and effective nutritional therapy depends on careful selection for the individualized patient and a thorough understanding of the complications that can occur. Principles of nutritional assessment and oral diets are presented in Chapter 17, Nutritional Assessment, Therapeutic Diets, and Infant Feeding, page 463.

ENTERAL NUTRITION

"If the gut works, use it." This simple adage is the guiding principle of nutritional support. Clinical practice guidelines consistently endorse the use

Chapter update by Elizabeth Holt, MD

Table 18-1. Advantages of Enteral Nutrition

Maintains normal metabolic pathways
Allows delivery of a full range of nutrients
Triggers the release of cholecystokinin
Preserves hepatic lipid metabolism
Maintains normal intestinal pH and flora
Supports the GI tracts as an organ of the immune system
Promotes wound healing
Lowers cost
Reduces infectious complications

of enteral nutrition for patients who have a functional GI tract but cannot take enough nutrients orally to maintain adequate nutritional goals. Enteral nutrition has physiologic and practical benefits that make tube feeding superior to parenteral nutrition (Table 18-1).

Technological advances in enteral access techniques have increased the numbers of patients who can safely receive tube feeding. The indications for enteral nutrition are summarized in Table 18-2.

Principles of Enteral Tube Feeding

Timing: The optimal time for initiating enteral nutrition depends on the patient's baseline nutritional status and clinical condition. Well-nourished patients in stable condition can tolerate suboptimal nutritional intake for 7–14 days without harmful effects. On the other hand, a convincing body of evidence has shown that early enteral feeding improves clinical outcomes among critically ill patients. Many ICUs have established protocols calling for the initiation of tube feeding within 24–36 hr of admission to the intensive care unit.

Delivery Site: The fundamental decision in planning tube feeding is to determine whether nutrients should be delivered to the stomach (gastric) or the small intestine (postpyloric). For most patients, including critically ill patients, gastric feeding is recommended, as there is insufficient data to suggest postpyloric feeding is superior or has fewer complications. Postpyloric feeding should be used in patients intolerant of gastric feeding or if gastric feeding is contraindicated, for example, delayed gastric emptying due to medications, underlying disease process, or carcinoma.

Enteral Access Devices: Tubes inserted through the nose or the mouth are most appropriate for short-term use or in situations in which unstable clinical status prevents more invasive placement procedures. In patients with

Table 18-2. Indications for Enteral Nutrition

Poor Oral Intake (Won't Eat)
Anorexia
Depression
Disabilities
Eating disorders
Early satiety
Nausea
Painful swallowing
Unsafe Oral Intake (Can't Eat)
Altered level of consciousness
Dysphagia
Endotracheal intubation
Gastroparesis
Impaired sucking and swallowing
Proximal intestinal obstruction
Elevated Needs (Can't Eat Enough)
Burns
Open wounds
Pressure ulcers
Sepsis
Trauma

18

head or facial injuries, insert tubes orally to avoid potential injury. Nasogastric tube placement is discussed in Chapter 19, Bedside Procedures, page 597.

The two categories of nasogastric tubes are small-bore and large-bore. Each type has benefits and drawbacks. **Small-bore** feeding tubes are soft and flexible; a guidewire or stylet provides the rigidity needed for insertion. **Large-bore** tubes are usually made of polyvinyl chloride (PVC), a stiff material that allows placement without a stylet. PVC becomes more rigid during use, and this characteristic increases the risk of otitis media, sinusitis, and nasal irritation but allows the tube to be used for suction. Small-bore tubes improve patient comfort and are less likely to cause ear and sinus problems, but small tubes are prone to clogging and become displaced more easily. The presence of a tube of any size across the lower esophageal sphincter increases the risk of reflux and aspiration.

When enteral feeding is expected to last >30 days, a **feeding enterostomy** is superior to nasally placed tubes. The most common sites for placement are the stomach and the jejunum, although a feeding enterostomy can be placed in the pharynx or esophagus. A percutaneous endoscopic gastrostomy (PEG) tube is one of the most widely used feeding enterostomies. Other placement options include radiologic, laparoscopic, and open surgical techniques. Less invasive placement methods are preferred, but not all patients are candidates for these procedures. Morbidly obese patients and those with tumors, GI obstruction, adhesions, or abnormal anatomy may need open surgical placement. Techniques for placing percutaneous jejunostomy tubes have replaced older methods that involved threading a small-bore feeding tube through an existing gastrostomy or using a needle–catheter device to achieve access to the jejunum.

Dual-lumen, or combination, feeding tubes are safe and effective conduits for enteral nutrition. With combination tubes, one lumen terminates in the stomach and the second extends into the small intestine, allowing simultaneous gastric decompression and intestinal feeding. These tubes, which are inserted through the nose or through an enterostomy, are especially beneficial for postoperative patients and other patients with impaired gastric emptying.

Enteral Formulas: A vast number of enteral formulas are available, and many formulas are quite similar in composition. Most hospitals maintain an enteral formulary that contains representative examples of each formula category. With the exception of infant formulas and blenderized adult formulas, enteral formulas are gluten-free and contain no lactose. Characteristics to consider in selecting an appropriate enteral formula include nutrient composition, caloric density, free water content, osmolality, and the presence of fiber. Table 18-3 lists types of enteral formulas and their composition.

Ordering and Advancing Tube Feedings

Depending on institutional policies and professional licensure laws, responsibility for ordering tube feeding falls to physicians, dietitians, clinical nurse specialists, or pharmacists. As with medication prescriptions, orders for enteral nutrition must specify the name of the enteral formula and the route of delivery. The order must also include the target rate for tube feeding as well as a schedule for advancing the feedings to the goal. Start tube feedings slowly and increase them as the patient tolerates. In hospitalized patients, tube feedings are frequently administered continuously with the aid of an infusion pump. In particular, patients with a jejunal tube usually need a pump to avoid feeding intolerance. Rapid infusion of enteral formula into the jejunum can produce diarrhea and distention. Pump-controlled feedings typically begin at 10–40 mL/hr and increase in increments of 10–25 mL/hr every 4–6 hr as tolerated. For patients who are eating but are not meeting their nutritional needs, an enteral feeding pump can be used to administer nutrients during the night to supplement oral intake.

Table 18-3. Enteral Formulas

Category	Description	Clinical Considerations	Examples (Common Brand Names)
Standard low-residue or fiber enriched: 1.0–1.2 kcal/mL, 270–490 mOsm/L	Contains intact protein, fat, and carbohydrate; free water ~84%	For routine tube feeding; not for use in hypermetabolic illness; unflavored products not for oral use.	Ensure, FiberSource, Isocal, Isosource, Jevity, Nutren 1.0, Osmolite, Ultracal
Concentrated low-residue: 1.5–2.0 kcal/mL, 430–525 mOsm/L	Nutrients similar to standard low-residue formulas; contain less free water and more fat; free water ~74%	Used to restrict fluid, relieve symptoms from high-volume feeding, and to meet elevated nutrient needs. Closely monitor hydration status.	Comply, Ensure Plus, Deliver 2.0, TwoCal HN, Isosource 1.5, Nutren 1.5, 2.0
Elemental/semielemental: 1.0–1.5 kcal/mL, 270–650 mOsm/L	Nutrients in easily digested form; many contain MCT oil or little long-chain fat, no fiber	For patients with impaired digestion and absorption; appropriate for patients with fat intolerance.	Alitraq, Criticare, Isotein, Intensical, Peptamin, Subdue, Vital, Vivonex
Renal failure: 2.0 kcal/mL, 600 mOsm/L	Low protein with emphasis on essential amino acids; may not provide vitamins or electrolytes; free water ~70%	Intended to improve nitrogen retention with minimal effect on uremia.	Renalcal, Suplena
Renal failure with dialysis: 2.0 kcal/mL, 570–665 mOsm/L	Provides moderate protein; vitamin and mineral content modified for renal failure; free water ~70%	Provides moderate protein for patients with losses from dialysis; vitamin and electrolyte profile adjusted for altered renal metabolism.	Magnacal Renal, Nepro

(Continued)

18

489

Table 18-3. Enteral Formulas (Continued)

Category	Description	Clinical Considerations	Examples (Common Brand Names)
Respiratory failure: 1.5 kcal/mL, 330–650 mOsm/L	Contains low levels of carbohydrate, high fat; no fiber; free water ~78%	Developed to reduce CO_2, produced by carbohydrate metabolism; some contain omega-3 fatty acids and antioxidants.	Novasource Pulmonary, Nutrivent, Pulmocare, Respelor, Oxepa
Wound healing: 1.0–1.5 kcal/mL, 340–560 mOsm/L	Very high protein content; some have enhanced vitamin profile; free water ~78–83%	Designed to support healing of surgical wounds and pressure ulcers.	Isosource VHN, Promote, Protain XL, Resource, Replete, Traumacal
Immune modulation: 1.0–1.5 kcal/mL, 375–630 mOsm/L	Designed for patients with hypermetabolic illness; usually high in protein; many are enriched with specific nutrients, e.g., arginine, glutamine, and omega-3 fatty acids; some contain fiber	Designed for use during hypermetabolic illness; theoretical benefits for immune function. Use with caution in critically ill, septic patients.	Alitraq, Crucial, Impact, Immunaid
Diabetes: 1.0–1.06 kcal/mL, 300–380 mOsm/L	Low carbohydrate and high ratio of monosaturated fatty acids; contains fiber	Used for patients with abnormal glucose tolerance; nutrient profile meets American Diabetes Association guidelines; many can be consumed orally.	Diabetisource, Choice DM, Glytrol, Glucerna

Under certain circumstances, tube feeding can be administered without a pump. This method, called bolus feeding, is most appropriate for patients with a gastrostomy tube as the sole source of nutrition. With bolus feeding, patients receive 200–400 mL four to six times a day. The entire food bolus flows into the stomach through the barrel of a 50- or 60-mL syringe attached to the feeding tube. Bolus feeding is widely used in subacute and home care settings.

Complications of Enteral Nutrition

Aspiration: Aspiration pneumonia is a common and life-threatening complication of enteral nutrition by tube feeding. Table 18-4 lists risk factors for aspiration.

The single most effective measure for preventing aspiration with enteral tube feeding is to elevate the head of the bed 30–45 degrees during feeding. Multiple other interventions to decrease aspiration risk such as post-pyloric feeding tubes, motility drugs, and checking gastric residual volumes (GRV) have not been shown to significantly decrease the risk. However, these options can be considered on a case-by-case basis. GRVs do not correlate well with aspiration risks and should not be routinely checked. Enteral feeding should not be held for a GRV <500 mL unless there is evidence of intolerance, such as distention, nausea, or vomiting.

Diarrhea: Occurs in 10–60% of patients receiving enteral feedings. Many factors contribute to the incidence of diarrhea among tube-fed patients, including underlying illness, the presence of bacteria, medications, and feeding intolerance. Each of these must be systematically ruled out as the cause of the problem. As a starting point, rule out *Clostridioides* (formerly *Clostridium*) *difficile* colitis by ordering toxigenic culture and cell cytotoxicity neutralization assay for patients with diarrhea who have received antibiotics. The protocol for diagnosing *C. difficile* colitis may vary by institution. If this test result is negative, administer antidiarrheal agents to control symptoms. Administering a probiotic such as lactobacillus acidophilus (Lactinex) can help restore normal flora and decrease diarrhea. Medications frequently cause

18

Table 18-4. Risk Factors for Aspiration

- Advanced age
- Impaired consciousness
- Neuromuscular disease
- Impaired gag and cough reflex
- Endotracheal intubation
- Mechanical ventilation
- Tracheostomy
- Gastroesophageal reflux (presence of tube)
- Delayed gastric emptying, elevated gastric residual volume

diarrhea in patients receiving tube feeding. Electrolytes, particularly magnesium, phosphorus, and potassium, are notorious offenders, as are drugs that contain sorbitol. Changing the enteral formula or adjusting the feeding regimen may provide relief.

Constipation: Although less common than diarrhea, constipation can occur in patients receiving enteral nutrition, especially those in long-term care facilities. Switching to a fiber-enriched enteral formula may alleviate the problem. Adequate hydration is important in promoting regular bowel movements. Provide additional free water as periodic water boluses or as a separate enteral infusion.

Dehydration: One of the most common metabolic disorders among tube-fed patients. Numerous factors contribute to the problem, including the use of concentrated, high-protein formulas, poor oral intake of liquids, hyperglycemia, fever, diarrhea, and failure to administer the prescribed volume of formula. Weight loss and elevations in sodium, chloride, and BUN are characteristic of dehydration related to enteral nutrition. Keep in mind that the percentage of free water in enteral formulas ranges from 70–84% of the volume administered. On average, patients should receive 30 mL/kg/d of free water. Patients in whom dehydration develops may need a less concentrated enteral formula or additional free water.

PARENTERAL NUTRITION

Indications

In circumstances in which lack of function of the GI tract prevents oral or enteral nutrition, parenteral nutrition (PN) is used. PN is expensive and carries a high risk of complications. IV nutrition therefore is reserved for situations in which there are no other options for providing nutritional support. Examples of situations in which PN is indicated appear in Table 18-5. **Although well-nourished patients with GI dysfunction can receive conventional IV fluids for 7–10 days without harmful effects, patients with existing nutritional deficits or metabolic stress and those not expected to resume oral intake for 5–10 days need PN within 3–5 days.** The decision to initiate PN is not an emergency. Adverse effects of PN are less likely to occur in patients who have good glycemic control, stable hemodynamic status, and electrolyte levels within normal limits. Issues such as prognosis, possibility of benefit, and the patient's views regarding artificial feeding also are factors to consider before beginning PN.

Composition of Parenteral Nutrition Formulas

PN formulas are highly complex IV fluids containing the nutrients essential for metabolism and growth: protein, carbohydrates, lipids, electrolytes, vitamins, trace elements, and water. The composition of PN formulas can be

Table 18-5.   Indications for Parenteral Nutrition (PN)

Category	Examples
Conditions that impair absorption of nutrients	Short-bowel syndrome Enterocutaneous fistula Infectious colitis Radiation or chemotherapy effects Small-bowel obstruction
Need for bowel rest	Inflammatory bowel disease Ischemic bowel Severe pancreatitis Chylous fistula Preoperative status
Motility disorders	Prolonged ileus Scleroderma Pseudo-obstruction Visceral organ myopathy
Inability to achieve or maintain enteral access	Unstable clinical condition Hyperemesis gravidarum Eating disorders

tailored to meet the demands of hypermetabolic illness and to accommodate limitations in organ function.

Depending on hospital policy, PN formulas can be compounded in two ways. All of the ingredients can be mixed in a single container, a method called **total nutrient admixture** (TNA), or the lipid emulsion can be excluded from the primary solution and administered separately. Lipid emulsions are isotonic and can be given safely by peripheral vein. Although TNA offers many advantages over conventional dextrose/amino acid formulas, numerous factors affect the stability of the formula. The integrity of the PN formula is a critical consideration that demands the expertise of a pharmacist familiar with stability and compatibility data.

Protein: Supplied as crystalline amino acids in a mix of essential and nonessential amino acids. Standard amino acid solutions are available in concentrations ranging from 3–15%, with the upper range being used most frequently in adults. In general, 1 g of amino acids is equivalent to 1 g of protein. As with dietary protein, IV amino acids yield 4 kcal/g.

Manufacturers offer modified amino acids to meet disease- and age-specific requirements; however, current studies do not support routine use of these specialty formulations.

Carbohydrate: Dextrose monohydrate is the principal energy substrate in PN formulas. This form of carbohydrate provides 3.4 kcal in concentrations ranging from 3–70%. Studies have shown that dextrose dosing of 4–7 mg/kg/min provides optimal protein sparing, although hyperglycemia occurs less often when the dextrose infusion is limited to 4 mg/kg/min.

18

Fat: IV fat emulsions contain soybean oil or a mixture of safflower and soybean oils with egg phospholipid added as an emulsifier. Patients allergic to eggs or soybeans may have reactions to lipid emulsions, including hives, back pain, shortness of breath, and anaphylactic shock. Lipid emulsions are available in concentrations of 10%, 20%, and 30%, providing 1.1, 2.0, and 3.0 kcal/mL, respectively. More efficient lipid clearance occurs with 20% fat emulsions than with 10% products, making the 20% form preferable, especially for pediatric patients. Provision of 1–4% of the patient's daily energy requirements as lipid emulsion prevents essential fatty acid deficiency, a condition that causes dry skin, hair loss, poor wound healing, and diarrhea after weeks to months of fat-free parenteral feedings. **Current guidelines for adults set the daily limit for lipid dose at 2.5 g/kg, but a growing body of evidence suggests that 1 g/ kg may be a safer limit.** Monitor triglyceride levels to determine whether lipid emulsion can safely be used or continued.

Electrolytes: PN formulas must contain sufficient electrolytes for critical metabolic activities. The usual electrolyte profile of PN formulas is sodium, potassium, calcium, magnesium, chloride, acetate, and phosphorus. Unlike conventional IV fluids, electrolyte PN formulas contain the acetate or chloride salt of the electrolyte to help maintain acid–base balance. Sodium bicarbonate is used in PN but may precipitate additives, particularly calcium and magnesium. In most cases, hospital pharmacies offer a standard electrolyte product that provides typical maintenance doses of electrolytes. Table 18-6 lists daily electrolyte requirements for adult patients in stable condition. Patients with diarrhea, fistula output, and gastric losses often have altered electrolyte homeostasis and need higher levels of certain electrolytes. On the other hand, the electrolyte content of the PN formula may have to be restricted if a patient has impaired renal function.

Vitamins: All PN formulas must contain the vitamins needed to support normal metabolism. Life-threatening vitamin deficiencies can develop within 2–3 wk in patients who receive PN without vitamins. Table 18-7 lists the composition of a typical parenteral vitamin product for adults. Individual vitamins, such as A, C, and folic acid, are used to supplement the standard multivitamin combination when a disease-specific or treatment-related deficiency exists.

Trace Minerals: Trace minerals are essential for efficient substrate utilization and other supportive functions. Typical PN solutions contain zinc, chromium, copper, and manganese according to established guidelines. Table 18-8 shows dosing recommendations for trace minerals. Patients receiving long-term PN also need selenium to prevent potentially fatal cardiomyopathy. Commercial trace mineral products do not contain iron. Current guidelines call for administering iron as a separate infusion as needed. Clinical conditions that impair trace mineral excretion may necessitate restricting certain trace minerals in PN formulas. For example, in patients with biliary disease, copper and manganese must be restricted from PN formulas to avoid toxicity.

Table 18-6. Electrolytes for Parenteral Nutrition

Electrolyte	Form	Recommended Daily Requirement
Sodium	Sodium chloride Sodium acetate Sodium phosphate	1–2 mEq/kg
Potassium	Potassium chloride Potassium acetate Potassium phosphate	1–2 mEq/kg
Chloride	Sodium chloride Potassium chloride	As needed for acid–base balance
Acetate	Sodium acetate Potassium acetate	As needed for acid–base balance
Phosphate	Sodium phosphate Potassium phosphate	20–40 mmol
Magnesium	Magnesium sulfate	8–20 mEq
Calcium	Calcium gluconate	10–15 mEq

Table 18-7. Parenteral Vitamin Formulas

Vitamin	Recommended Daily Dose
A (retinol)	1 mg (3300 IU)
B_1 (thiamin)	6 mg
B_2 (riboflavin)	3.6 mg
B_3 (niacin)	40 mg
B_6 (pyridoxine)	6 mg
B_{12} (cobalamin)	5 mcg
Biotin	60 mcg
C (ascorbic acid)	200 mg
D (ergocalciferol)	5 mcg (200 IU)
E (tocopherol)	10 IU
Folic acid	600 mcg
K^+	150 mcg

18

Table 18-8. Trace Element Requirements for Parenteral Nutrition

Element	Recommended Daily Dose
Zinc	2.5–5.0 mg[a]
Copper	0.3–0.5 mg
Selenium	20–60 mcg
Chromium	10–15 mcg
Manganese	60–100 mcg

[a]Requirements may be as high as 15 mg/day in stress states (e.g., burns) or in patients with high-output fistulas.

Central Versus Peripheral Administration

PN formulas that rely on glucose as a primary energy source frequently have an osmolarity that approaches 1800 mOsm/L, more than twice the limit for administration through peripheral veins. Safe infusion of such hypertonic fluids requires placement of an IV line in the central venous circulation, as described in Chapter 19, Bedside Procedures, page 533. However, the osmolarity of PN formulas that contain lipid emulsion and low concentrations of dextrose may fall below 900 mOsm/L, making these formulas suitable for peripheral administration. **Peripheral parenteral nutrition (PPN)** is appropriate for patients with adequate peripheral venous access who need PN for a brief time, usually less than 2 wk. Because peripheral PN formulas contain relatively low concentrations of nutrients, this form of nutritional support is more helpful in preventing malnutrition than in correcting existing deficits. For similar reasons, patients with elevated requirements due to hypermetabolism or those who need fluid restriction are not candidates for PPN.

Initiating and Managing Parenteral Nutrition

Beginning Parenteral Nutrition: Because PN can induce metabolic disturbances or worsen existing problems, do not start PN until a patient has a stable fluid and electrolyte profile. It is usually unwise to begin PN in a patient who needs large amounts of fluid, who may need resuscitation after trauma, or who is in a septic state. Recommended baseline laboratory tests are serum electrolytes (ionized calcium, magnesium, and phosphorus), glucose, prealbumin, triglycerides, creatinine, BUN, and liver function tests. These measurements help identify whether the patient is at risk of metabolic complications and help guide the design of the initial PN formula.

Begin PN at a reduced level and advance to goal according to the patient's response. Because carbohydrate is the substrate most likely to induce metabolic disturbances, initial formulas frequently have a limited dextrose load, usually 200–250 g for the first day. Many institutional protocols allow patients to receive the target level of protein and lipid emulsion initially and increase dextrose to goal over 2 days. Some situations call for a more cautious introduction of PN. For example, a patient with a baseline serum glucose level of 120–150 mg/dL should only receive 100–150 g of dextrose in an initial PN formula. Increase the dextrose in the PN formula over several days while closely observing serum glucose level and insulin requirements.

Refeeding Syndrome: Beginning PN at a reduced level is prudent for patients at risk of refeeding syndrome, a life-threatening metabolic complication that occurs in the setting of severe weight loss or long-standing malnutrition. Risk factors for this problem include anorexia nervosa, chronic alcoholism, cancer cachexia, and other wasting syndromes. In refeeding syndrome, severe fluid and electrolyte disturbances occur in the first few days of therapy. The hallmark of refeeding syndrome is hypophosphatemia, which can be fatal if not recognized and corrected promptly. To avoid refeeding syndrome for patients at risk, current guidelines call for correcting phosphate levels ≤2.0 mEq/dL before beginning PN. In this setting, the initial PN formula should limit dextrose to 150 g and begin with only 50% of the patient's caloric requirements. Vigilant electrolyte replacement is essential and may take several days to achieve full repletion. Calorie and protein intake should progress to goal only when fluid and electrolyte status stabilizes.

Ordering PN: Writing orders for PN is a step-by-step process that takes into account energy needs, nutrient requirements, and electrolyte status. The first step is to set goals for energy intake and to distribute the calories among the protein, carbohydrate, and fat in the PN formula. The following example illustrates these steps for a 70-kg man. The formula produced in this process is a reasonable estimated goal. This PN can then be adjusted to account for clinical circumstances that affect nutrient needs, such as severity of illness and organ function.

18

1. **Establish goals for energy and protein intake.**
   a. Provide 25–30 kcal/kg. For a 70-kg man, the range is 1750–2100 kcal/day. (See Chapter 17, page 470, regarding use of adjusted body weight.) Start at the low end of the range to avoid overfeeding.
   b. Give protein 1.0–1.5 g/kg, a range of 70–105 g/day, for a 70-kg man. Round the goal to 100 g to meet the patient's needs and to simplify compounding.
2. **Determine nonprotein calories.** Subtract protein calories from total calories (100×4 kcal/g = 400 protein calories). **Example:** $1750 - 400 = 1350$ nonprotein calories.
3. **Determine carbohydrate dose.** The standard lipid dose for most adult patients is 50 g or 500 kcal. Subtract lipid calories from nonprotein calories to determine the amount of dextrose needed to meet the patient's energy needs. **Example:** $1350 - 500 = 850$ carbohydrate calories. Divide the calorie goal for carbohydrate by 3.4 cal/g. Example: $850 \div 3.4 = 250$ g.

Table 18-9. Adjusting the Volume of Parenteral Nutrition (PN) Formulas[a]

Example Formula	Standard PN	Fluid Restriction	High Volume
Goal: 1750 kcal			
Protein:	10% AA	15% AA	10% AA
100 g	1000 mL	500 mL	1000 mL
Dextrose:	D_{50} W	D_{70} W	D_{25} W
250 g	500 mL	357 mL	1000 mL
Lipid:	20% fat	30% fat	10% fat
50 g	250 mL	204 mL	500 mL
Volume	1750 mL	1265 mL	2500 mL

[a]Highly concentrated or dilute formulas may affect stability of total nutrient admixture.
AA = amino acids.

4. **Order the PN formula.** Total energy, 1750 kcal; protein, 100 g; carbohydrate, 250 g; fat, 50 g. Safety guidelines for PN call for ordering substrates in grams to avoid confusion. (Some hospitals require that these values be converted to percent solutions in the PN order.) Consult with a pharmacist. As Table 18-9 shows, the identical PN formula can be adjusted to meet the patient's hydration requirements by use of different concentrations of amino acids, dextrose, and fat.

5. **Make appropriate additions to PN formula.** Individualize the electrolyte content of the PN formula according to the patient's laboratory tests and organ function. Sodium and potassium are available as both chloride and acetate salts (acetate is converted to bicarbonate on an equimolar basis). Using higher or lower amounts of these salts can help maintain acid–base balance. Stability and compatibility limits exist for calcium, phosphorus, and magnesium. Many hospitals use standard formulations for vitamins and trace minerals to avoid the need to order each entity individually.

Monitoring Response to Therapy

Carefully monitor patients receiving PN to identify problems and to assess progress toward the therapeutic goal. Measure electrolytes, including calcium, magnesium, and phosphorus, daily until the levels are stable, and order weekly liver function tests and prealbumin and triglyceride levels. Measure blood glucose level by fingerstick every 6 hr until the level is stable. Patients receiving insulin or tapering doses of steroids and those with changing clinical status may need closer blood glucose monitoring. Typical PN protocols call for weighing the patient daily and keeping accurate intake and output records.

No single criterion is a reliable indicator of the effectiveness of PN. Because indicators of protein status are affected by illness, albumin and prealbumin levels are not reliable markers of response to therapy. Nitrogen balance studies do shed light on the adequacy of protein intake, particularly when long-term serial studies are performed (see Chapter 17, page 467). Finally, clinical status is evidence that the nutritional regimen is appropriate. Adequate wound healing, increased stamina, and improved functional status all suggest the nutritional regimen is meeting the patient's needs.

Preventing and Managing PN Complications

Hyperglycemia: The most common metabolic complication of PN. Severe hyperglycemia causes osmotic diuresis that depletes electrolytes, especially potassium, sodium, and phosphorus. If left uncorrected, severe hyperglycemia can progress to **hyperglycemic hyperosmolar nonketotic (HHNK) syndrome**, a rare but potentially fatal condition. Advances in monitoring and delivery techniques have made HHNK an uncommon occurrence. Evidence that tight glucose control during PN greatly improves clinical outcome has made glycemic control a priority during PN therapy.

The goal is to maintain blood glucose level no higher than 120 mg/dL for critically ill patients and no higher than 150 mg/dL for patients in stable condition receiving PN. Keeping dextrose infusion rates ≤ 4 mg/kg/min decreases the incidence of hyperglycemia. Patients with diabetes mellitus and those who are critically ill often need insulin to control blood glucose level during PN. Insulin is stable and is compatible with PN formulas, although a portion of the insulin dose adheres to the administration bags and tubing. Guidelines typically call for 0.05–0.1 units of regular insulin for each gram of dextrose in the PN formula. For example, for an initial dextrose dose of 200 g, 10–20 units of insulin would be added to the PN formula. Closely monitor blood glucose level, and provide additional subcutaneous insulin coverage as needed. The insulin in the PN formula should be increased in increments of 0.05 units per gram of dextrose or by adding two-thirds of the subcutaneous insulin coverage for the previous 24 hr to the next PN formula until blood glucose level stays within target range. In cases of extreme hyperglycemia or insulin resistance, a separate continuous insulin drip allows greater flexibility in controlling glucose levels. After glycemic control is achieved, increase the dextrose dose 50 g/d and maintain the same insulin to dextrose ratio.

Hypoglycemia can develop in patients receiving PN formulas containing insulin. If the blood glucose level stays consistently <80–100 mg/dL, reassess the insulin dose. This step is particularly necessary for patients with renal insufficiency, which delays insulin clearance, and for patients who are receiving tapering steroid doses. Table 18-10 contains guidelines for maintaining tight glucose control in patients receiving PN.

Fluid and Electrolyte Disturbances: Candidates for PN often have pre-existing nutritional deficits and nutrient losses due to GI disorders, which

18

Table 18-10. Blood Glucose Management with PN

Goal: Aim for glucose level of 80–120 mg/dL in critically ill patients. Goal for blood glucose for stable patients ranges from 100–150 mg/dL.

1. **Order fingerstick blood glucose measurement q6h,** with standing sliding scale regular insulin orders.
2. **Use regular insulin.** Do not use NPH or long-acting insulin to avoid fluctuation in blood glucose levels due to variation in drug action.
3. **For patients with a history of diabetes or baseline blood glucose 120-150 mg/dL,** limit initial dextrose dose to 150 g in PN.
4. **For patients with baseline blood glucose 150–200 mg/dL,** limit initial dextrose dose to 150 g and add insulin 0.1 units/g dextrose (15 units).
5. **Review 24-hr insulin coverage.** Add two-thirds of the insulin coverage to the next PN *or* increase insulin in PN by 0.05 units/g dextrose to a goal of 0.2 units/g dextrose.
6. **Consider using an insulin drip** for blood glucose levels persistently >200 mg/dL (e.g., 250 units of regular human insulin in 250 mL of normal saline [1 U/mL]); follow local nursing protocol for infusion and monitoring.
7. **Maintain the insulin/dextrose ratio** when increasing or decreasing dextrose in PN.
8. **Reassess insulin needs daily.** Reduce insulin in PN 30–50% for blood glucose levels that drop below desired level.

make fluid and electrolyte shifts especially common in this population. The principles of fluid and electrolyte management for patients receiving PN are similar to those for any patient. In cases in which fluid restriction is called for, PN formulas can contain the most concentrated form of the nutrients to reduce the volume of the solution.

Hepatobiliary Complications: Abnormalities of hepatic function occur frequently in patients receiving PN. Early in therapy adults may have mild, transient elevations in liver enzymes that resolve when PN stops. However, neonates and patients receiving long-term PN may experience progressive, irreversible hepatic failure. Research findings show a strong association between excessive carbohydrate administration and liver dysfunction during PN. A number of additional risk factors have emerged, suggesting a multifactorial cause of PN-related hepatic dysfunction. PN also places recipients at risk of cholelithiasis, particularly patients who cannot tolerate any oral or enteral nutrition.

Strategies for preventing and managing hepatic complications of PN include avoiding overfeeding, limiting dextrose dose to 30–50% of calories, providing 10–30% of calories as lipid, infusing PN over 12–16 hr thus giving "time off" to mimic a postabsorptive state, and avoiding complete bowel rest if possible. Treatment with ursodeoxycholic acid may help patients with cholestasis.

Pulmonary Complications: The CO_2 produced by carbohydrate metabolism can place added stress on patients with CO_2 retention and those who are being weaned from mechanical ventilation. To avoid problems related to CO_2 production, the formula must meet, not exceed, the patient's requirements. In addition to avoiding overfeeding, reducing the carbohydrate dose and increasing the proportion of calories provided as fat can help prevent adverse pulmonary effects of PN.

Catheter-Related Bloodstream Infection: PN increases the risk of catheter-related bloodstream infection (CR-BSI). Meticulous protocols for the insertion and maintenance of central venous catheters can greatly reduce the risk of this serious complication. CR-BSI may necessitate removal of the vascular access device or treatment with antibiotics, depending on the type of catheter, clinical status of the patient, and type of organism isolated from the patient's blood. Unexplained fever or elevated WBC count in a patient receiving PN should raise suspicion concerning CR-BSI. CR-BSI is also discussed in Chapter 13, pages 352, 363, 366, 368–369.

Terminating PN Therapy

When oral or enteral intake resumes, patients should gradually receive fewer nutrients parenterally. Some clinicians infuse PN only at night in an effort to minimize the risk of rebound hypoglycemia, but no results of controlled trials exist to support this practice. There is rarely a need for a formal schedule of weaning from PN. If concerns about rebound hypoglycemia exist, a 5% dextrose solution can be infused after PN is discontinued.

18

Bedside Procedures

19

Chapter update by Michael J. Pucci, MD, Joon Yau (JY) Leong, MD, Seth Teplitsky, MD, and Leonard G. Gomella, MD; Endotracheal Intubation and Other Airway Management Procedures Update by Eric S. Schwenk, MD, and Eugene Viscusi, MD

503

- ➤ Peripheral Insertion of Central Catheter (PICC)
- ➤ Peritoneal Lavage
- ➤ Peritoneal (Abdominal) Paracentesis
- ➤ Pulmonary Artery Catheterization

- ➤ Pulsus Paradoxus Measurement (Paradoxical Pulse)
- ➤ Skin Biopsy and Other Techniques for Dermatologic Diagnosis
- ➤ Skin Testing
- ➤ Thoracentesis

- ➤ Urinary Tract Procedures
- ➤ Venipuncture
- ➤ Venous Access: Intraosseous (IO) Infusion

PROCEDURE BASICS

Universal* and Standard Precautions

The Centers for Disease Control (CDC) published guidelines in 1983, "Blood and Body Fluid Precautions," for healthcare workers. These precautions were to be used when a patient was known to be infected or suspected to be infected with a bloodborne pathogen such as HIV or hepatitis B. In 1987 the CDC published "Recommendations for Prevention of HIV Transmission in Health-Care Settings." These stated that blood and body fluid precautions be used for all patients regardless of their infection status. Since pathogens transmitted by blood and body fluids pose a hazard to healthcare personnel, particularly during invasive procedures, special precautions are required with all patients whether they are infected or not. **The CDC has called this approach "Universal Precautions" where blood and body fluids of all patients are considered potentially infectious.** The "Bloodborne Pathogens Standard" of the Universal Precautions guidelines lists other potentially infectious materials (OPIMs) beyond blood. These OPIMs include semen, vaginal secretions, cerebrospinal fluid, synovial fluid, pleural fluid, pericardial fluid, peritoneal fluid, amniotic fluid, saliva in dental procedures, any body fluid that is visibly contaminated with blood, all body fluids in situations where it is difficult or impossible to differentiate between body fluids, and any unfixed tissue or organ (other than intact skin) from a human (living or dead) and also in some research lab settings.

Common infections that can be transmitted through contact with blood or body fluids include HIV; hepatitis A, B, and C; staphylococcal and streptococcal infections; gastroenteritis (*Salmonella, Shigella, C. difficile,* norovirus, rotavirus); pneumonia; syphilis; TB; malaria; measles; chickenpox; herpes simplex virus; urinary tract infections; and bloodstream infections. The greatest transmission risks are from HIV and hepatitis B and C. Many other diseases such as Ebola virus, avian flu, West Nile virus, SARS, MERS,

*https://www.osha.gov/SLTC/etools/hospital/hazards/univprec/univ.html and https://www.cdc.gov/infectioncontrol/basics/standard-precautions.html Accessed April 24, 2020.

COVID-19, H1N1, Zika virus, and seasonal influenza are increasingly recognized as transmittable agents that may be spread by aerosolization. Simply protecting healthcare providers from blood and body fluids with gloves and gowns is no longer considered sufficient. Since airborne and bloodborne transmission represented a risk to both patients and providers in 1996, the CDC expanded beyond the concept of universal precautions and established the term and principles of **"Standard Precautions."**

Standard Precautions are the minimum infection prevention practices that apply to all patient care, regardless of suspected or confirmed infection status of the patient, in any setting where healthcare is delivered. These practices are designed to protect healthcare providers and prevent providers from spreading infections among patients. Standard Precautions include the following major components: hand hygiene, use of personal protective equipment (PPE) (e.g., gloves, masks, eyewear), respiratory hygiene/cough etiquette, sharps safety (engineering and work practice controls), safe injection practices (i.e., aseptic technique for parenteral medications), sterile instruments and devices, and the cleaning and disinfection of environmental surfaces. These precautions should be used whenever an invasive procedure or patient care encounter exposes the healthcare provider to potentially infectious agents.

A. Standard Precautions: Key Components
Assess the risk of exposure to body fluids (e.g., blood, urine, feces, sputum), aerosol-generating procedures, or contaminated surfaces before any healthcare activity.

1. *Standard Precautions:* **Hand hygiene** before and after patient contact.
    a. **Hand washing** (40–60 sec): Wet hands and apply soap; rub all surfaces; rinse hands and dry thoroughly with a single-use towel; use towel to turn off faucet.
    b. **Hand rubbing** (20–30 sec): Apply enough product (alcohol-based products gels, rinses, foams) to cover all areas of the hands; rub hands until dry.
    c. **Wearing gloves** without correct hand hygiene can contaminate the gloves. Studies show that less direct patient contact also occurs when clinicians wear gloves. Do not wear the same pair of gloves to perform tasks on two different patients or to perform two different tasks at different sites on the same patient.
    d. **Clean vs. sterile gloves:** The World Health Organization (WHO) recommends wearing clean gloves prior to insertion of peripheral intravascular catheterization, and sterile gloves are to be worn for insertion of arterial, central, and midline catheters when guidewire exchanges are performed. Wear either clean or sterile gloves when changing the dressing on intravascular catheters. Nonlatex gloves are recommended for contact with blood, body fluids, secretion, contaminated items, mucous membranes, and nonintact skin.

19

e. **Coronavirus (COVID-19) hand hygiene (CDC 2020 Guidelines **)**
    i. Alcohol-based hand rub (ABHR) with greater than 60% ethanol or 70% isopropanol in healthcare settings.
    ii. Hands should be washed with soap and water for at least 20 sec when visibly soiled, before eating, and after using the restroom.
    iii. Benzalkonium chloride, along with both ethanol and isopropanol, is deemed eligible by the FDA for use in healthcare personnel hand rubs. However, evidence indicates benzalkonium chloride has less reliable activity against certain bacteria and viruses than either of the alcohols.

2. *Standard Precautions:* **Personal Protective Equipment (PPE).** Specialized clothing or equipment worn to protect the respiratory tract, mucous membranes, skin, and clothing from infectious agents or other hazards. Examples of PPE include gloves, goggles, facemasks, surgical masks, respirators, face shields, foot covering, and gowns. The 2020 COVID-19 pandemic has focused interest on PPE and in particular the use of facemasks and respirators. One important distinction that must be made when discussing respirator use in healthcare settings is the **difference between respirators and facemasks.** **Facemasks** include **surgical masks**, which are fluid resistant, and **procedure or isolation masks**, which are not fluid resistant. A **respirator** is a device worn over the nose and mouth to protect the wearer from hazardous materials in the breathing zone. Respirators include N95 masks and powered air-purifying respirators (PAPRs).

Check your institutional PPE guidelines for specific requirements for procedures or various clinical settings. For facial protection (eyes, nose, and mouth) wear (1) a surgical or procedure mask and eye protection (eye visor, goggles) or (2) a full-face shield to protect mucous membranes of the eyes, nose, and mouth during activities that likely generate splashes or aerosolized sprays of blood, body fluids, secretions, and excretions.

a. **Face masks** are loose-fitting, disposable devices that create a physical barrier between the mouth and nose of the wearer and potential contaminants in the immediate environment. There are two general categories: procedural masks and surgical masks.
    o **Procedural or isolation masks** are not designed to be as fluid resistant as surgical masks and are used for performing patient procedures or when patients are in isolation to protect them from potential contaminants. Procedure/isolation masks are commonly used to protect both patients and staff from the transfer of respiratory secretions, fluids, or other debris. Procedure/isolation masks are used for general "respiratory etiquette" to prevent clinicians, patients, and visitors from spreading germs by talking, coughing, or sneezing. Procedure masks

have ear loops for quick donning, and since they do not slide on the hair, they can be worn without a surgical cap.

- **Surgical masks** are specifically designed to be fluid resistant. The degree of fluid resistance is determined by standards. If worn properly, a surgical mask is meant to help block large-particle droplets, splashes, sprays, or splatter that may contain viruses and bacteria, keeping them from reaching the mouth and nose, and provide protection from splashes, sprays, and splatter. Surgical masks do not seal tightly to the wearer's face and can reduce exposure of the wearer's saliva and respiratory secretions to others. They are normally tied behind the head. These masks may not filter or block all very small particles in the air that may be transmitted by coughs, sneezes, or certain medical procedures. Some may come with an attached clear face shield.

b. A **respirator** is a respiratory protective device designed to achieve a very close facial fit with very efficient filtration of airborne particles. **The designation "N95 respirator" means that the respirator blocks at least 95% of very small (0.3 micron) particles.** For proper functioning, the N95 respirator must be carefully "fitted" to the face of the wearer, and beards should not be worn with an N95, as facial hair interferes with the close fit. They are usually secured tightly to the face by elastic bands and are not tied. The N95 respirator can make it more difficult for the wearer to breathe. Some models have exhalation valves that can make exhalation easier and help reduce heat buildup. However, N95 respirators with exhalation valves should not be used when sterile conditions are needed such as in the operating room.***

c. **Surgical masks vs. N95 respirators.** The Center for Evidence Based Medicine (CEBM (www.cebm.net, Accessed April 22, 2020) has concluded:

- o "Standard surgical masks are as effective as respirator masks (e.g., N95) for preventing infection of healthcare workers in outbreaks of viral respiratory illnesses such as influenza. No head to head trial of these masks in COVID-19 has yet been published, and neither type of mask prevents all infection. Both types of masks need to be used in combination with other PPE measures. **Respirator masks are recommended for protection during aerosol generating procedures (AGPs).**"

d. A **powered air-purifying respirator (PAPR)** is a respirator that protects the user by filtering out contaminants in the air and uses a battery-operated blower and filter to provide the user with clean air through a tight-fitting respirator, a loose-fitting hood, or a helmet. Their use is usually limited to only the most high-risk patient care settings with high potential for aerosolized pathogens (severe acute respiratory syndrome [SARS], Middle Eastern respiratory syndrome [MERS], COVID-19, etc.).

19

***http://www.cdc.gov/niosh/npptl/pdfs/UnderstandDifferenceInfographic-508.pdf and www.cdc.gov/niosh/npptl/pdfs/UnderstandDifferenceInfographic-508.pdf. Accessed April 22, 2020.

e. **Aerosol-generating procedures** result in the release of airborne particles (aerosols/droplets) that can lead to the spread of respiratory infections such as coronavirus (COVID-19) and are listed here:

o Endotracheal intubation and extubation
o Bag mask ventilation
o ENT, oral surgery, and other airway manipulation cases
o Care of the intubated patient outside the operating room setting (in case of inadvertent disruption of closed ventilator circuit)
o Tracheostomy care or suctioning
o Sputum induction, chest physiotherapy
o Bronchoscopy, upper respiratory endoscopy
o Open airway suctioning
o High-flow oxygen therapy
o Noninvasive ventilation (Bi-PAP, CPAP)
o High-frequency oscillatory ventilation
o Nebulizer treatment
o Active obstetrical labor (second stage)
o CPR

f. **Gowns** should be used for blood or body fluid contact and to prevent soiling of clothing. Remove soiled gown as soon as possible and perform immediate hand hygiene.

g. **Specific recommendations for PPE use.**

i. Use additional barrier precautions for invasive procedures in which considerable splatter or aerosol generation is likely. Such splatter does not occur during most routine patient care bedside activities listed in this chapter but can occur in the operating room, ER, and ICU; during invasive bedside procedures; and during CPR. Always wear a mask when goggles are called for, and consider wearing goggles when a mask is called for. Eye protection along with masks is the standard in most operating room environments.

ii. When caring for patients with known or suspected COVID-19 infection (patient under investigation [PUI]), it is generally recommended that healthcare providers adhere to **Standard, Contact, and Droplet Precautions**, including the use of the following PPE: facemask (i.e., surgical mask or N95 based on local protocol), eye protection (i.e., goggles, disposable face shield, or mask with face shield attached), gown, and gloves. **Standard, Contact, and Droplet Precautions** are noted on Chapter 13, Clinical Microbiology, page 391.

3. *Standard Precautions:* **Respiratory hygiene and cough etiquette.** Persons with respiratory symptoms should apply source control

measures: Cover their nose and mouth when coughing/sneezing with tissue or mask, dispose of used tissues and masks, and perform hand hygiene after contact with respiratory secretions.

4. *Standard Precautions:* **Sharps precautions.** Avoid recapping used needles; avoid bending, breaking, or manipulating used needles by hand; and place used sharps in designated puncture-resistant containers. Use self-shielding safety needle devices whenever possible (see Figures 19-1A-F and Figure 19-38, pages 511–513 and page 602, for examples).

5. *Standard Precautions:* **Safe injection practices** (i.e., aseptic technique for parenteral medications). Never administer medications from the same syringe to more than one patient, even if the needle is changed, and do not enter a vial with a used syringe or needle. Hepatitis C virus, hepatitis B virus, and HIV can be spread from patient to patient when these simple precautions are not followed. Medications packaged as single-use vials should never be used for more than one patient.

6. *Standard Precautions:* **Sterile instruments and devices.** Before use on each patient, sterilize critical medical and surgical devices and instruments that enter normally sterile tissue or the vascular system or through which a sterile body fluid flows (e.g., blood).

7. *Standard Precautions:* **Cleaning and disinfecting environmental surfaces.** Emphasis for cleaning and disinfection should be placed on surfaces that are most likely to become contaminated with pathogens, including clinical contact surfaces (e.g., frequently touched surfaces such as door handles, light switches, trays, switches on devices, computer equipment, patient bed controls, etc.) in the patient-care areas. (See page 509 for specific cleaning agents.) Useful terminology to understand in the world of medical care cleaning and disinfection includes the following terms:

   a. **Decontamination:** The use of physical or chemical means to remove, inactivate, or destroy bloodborne pathogens on a surface or item to the point where there is no longer any risk of transmitting infectious particles and the surface or item is rendered safe for handling, use, or disposal.

   b. **Disinfection**: The destruction of pathogens, but not spores, using a chemical or physical means of disinfection.

   c. **Sterilization:** The process by which all pathogens, including spores, are destroyed. Sterilization can be done with moist heat, a combination of heat and pressure, gas, radiation, and boiling water.

   d. **Antiseptic**: A germicidal solution that inhibits the growth of some microorganisms. Some examples include hexachlorophene, iodine, and others. Many can be used directly on the skin.

19

Needlesticks*

The FDA has recommended safer needle devices, including devices that place a barrier between hands and needle after use. Needlestick injury is an occupational injury among healthcare workers in the United States. OSHA estimates that 5.6 million workers in the healthcare industry and related occupations are at risk of occupational exposure to bloodborne pathogens and estimates that 600,000–800,000 needlestick injuries occur each year. Healthcare workers are at risk of transmission of more than 20 known bloodborne pathogens (e.g., HIV, hepatitis B and C viruses). Although it is not possible to eliminate the risk of needlestick injury, it has been estimated that 62% to 88% of sharps injuries can be reduced with devices and procedures designed to protect healthcare workers from exposed needles. A variety of self-shielding or manual shielding needle devices are on the market for procedures such as heelstick and fingerstick (capillary blood sampling), IV techniques, and venipuncture. **Figure 19-1 Panels A–F.** Examples of styles of safety needles and needless IV tubing systems designed to reduce the risk of accidental needlesticks in healthcare providers.

Informed Consent

Before any procedure, counsel the patient about the reasons for the procedure, alternative treatment, and the risks and benefits. Explaining the various steps is likely to help gain the patient's cooperation and make the procedure easier on both parties. In general, procedures such as bladder catheterization, NG intubation, and venipuncture do not require written informed consent beyond normal hospital sign-in protocols. More invasive procedures, such as thoracentesis or lumbar puncture, typically require written consent, which must be obtained by a licensed physician or other authorized licensed provider. Consult local institutional guidelines concerning which procedures require a specific consent.

Preprocedure Patient Assessment

Invasive procedures that may require sedation. Conduct a complete preprocedure assessment with every patient undergoing an invasive procedure that may require sedation. Assess the patient's airway (i.e., difficulty to intubate the patient in an emergency), past medical history including previous complications with anesthetics, history of bleeding problems, and a complete history of allergies to medications such as anesthetics or latex. Be aware of the patient's current medications, with an emphasis on anticoagulants (e.g., heparin, low-molecular-weight [LMW] heparins, warfarin, direct oral anticoagulants) and be aware of the most recent lab coagulation parameters. Additionally, pay particular attention to cardiovascular, drugs which

(continued on page 513)

---

*https://www.osha.gov/SLTC/etools/hospital/hazards/sharps/sharps.html#safer Accessed May 13, 2020.

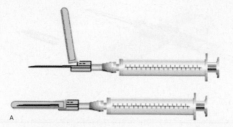

Figure 19-1A **Add on "Safety Feature."** Hinged or sliding shields can be attached to phlebotomy needles, winged steel needles, and blood gas needles, acting as an "add-on" safety feature.

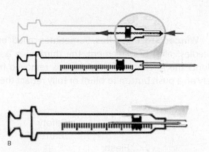

Figure 19-1B **Syringe with Retractable Needles.** After the needle is used, an extra push on the plunger retracts the needle into the syringe, removing the hazard of needle exposure.

19

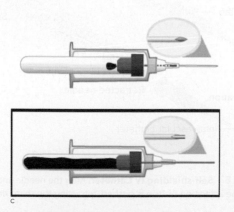

Figure 19-1C **Blunt-Tipped Blood Drawing Needles.** After blood is drawn, a push on the collection tube moves the blunt tip needle forward through the needle and past the sharp needle point. The blunt point tip of this needle can be activated before it is removed from the vein or artery.

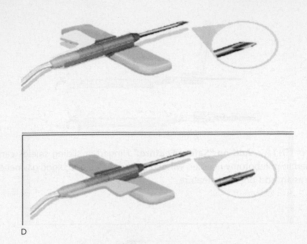

D

Figure 19-1D Winged Steel Needles. Sometimes called "butterfly needles" or "scalp vein needles," after IV placement, the third wing is rotated to a flat position. This blunts the needle point before it is removed from the patient. Other systems rely on a push button to blunt or fully retract the needle.

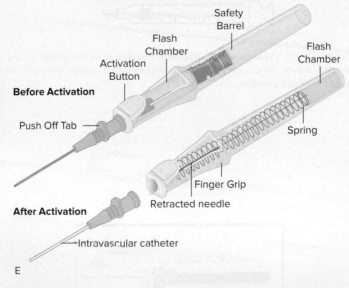

E

Figure 19-1E Self-shielding IV Catheter. After the needle and catheter are in the vein, the activation button is pushed, retracting the sharp needle into the barrel.

Before connection

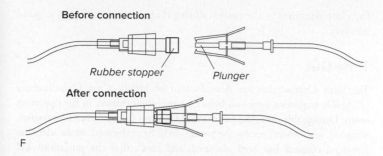

Rubber stopper

Plunger

After connection

F

Figure 19-1F IV connector systems reduce needle sticks by using needleless connector systems with IV setups to minimize occupational exposure to needles and bloodborne pathogens. Avoid using needles where safe and effective alternatives are available.

Figure 19-1 Panels A–F. Examples of styles of safety needles and needless IV tubing systems designed to reduce the risk of accidental needlesticks in healthcare providers. (https://www.osha.gov/SLTC/etools/hospital/hazards/sharps/sharps.html#safer. Accessed January 21, 2020.)

Preprocedure Patient Assessment (continued from page 510)

may contribute to hemodynamic instability perioperative or postoperatively. Review any relevant recent studies directly associated with the anticipated procedure.

Beside procedures that may not require sedation. Review important medications, bleeding, and allergy history as noted above. It is critical to have your patient's cooperation and understanding of the proposed procedure. Even the most "routine" medical procedure such as obtaining a blood sample or placing a bladder catheter can generate patient anxiety. Explain the procedure to the typical nonmedical professional patient in simple terms. Explain what you are doing and why you are performing the procedure. Some patients may be squeamish about medical procedures and may not want to know the details of what you are doing. Be sensitive to your patient's unique needs and try to appropriately address any concerns before, during, and after the procedure. Make the patient as comfortable as possible before the procedure by adjusting the bed, room lighting, and temperature. Some patients may prefer the TV or radio on to provide a distraction. Patients may become upset if a "routine" procedure takes an unacceptably long time. Try to be as efficient as possible; be sure all supplies are readily available. Where appropriate and based on the complexity of the intervention, have an assistant or chaperone present for the start of the procedure to maximize efficiency.

19

Pay close attention to the patient during the procedure by being a "good listener."

Time Out

The Joint Commission on Accreditation of Health Care Organizations (JCAHO) requires a time out before surgical intervention in the operating room. During this time, the members of the team (nurses, anesthesiologists, surgeons, and others) review the procedure to be performed, make sure that informed consent has been obtained, and check that the procedure will be performed on the correct patient and on the correct part of the body (e.g., right or left side of the chest). JCAHO has produced a universal protocol for "The Prevention of Wrong Site, Wrong Procedure, Wrong Person Surgery." The three principal components of this universal protocol include a preprocedure verification, site marking, and a time out. Originally developed for the operating room (see Chapter 24, Introduction to the Operating Room, page 801), many facilities use "time outs" before bedside invasive procedures such as thoracentesis, chest tube placement, lumbar puncture, and others. During a time out, all activity ceases, and a "time out" moment will be taken, with the following verified verbally by each member of the team for bedside procedures:

A. **Correct patient identity**
B. **Correct side and site**
C. **Agreement on the procedure to be done**
D. **Correct patient position**
E. **Availability of correct equipment and/or special requirements**

Bedside Procedure Note

More invasive bedside procedures such as lumbar puncture, thoracentesis, and central line placement (and others) should be carefully documented in the patient's record. An example of the structure of a typical bedside procedure can be found in Chapter 7, Chartwork, page 135.

Latex Allergy

People with certain medical conditions or in occupations that are heavily exposed to products containing natural rubber latex (NRL) may become sensitized and develop allergic reactions to NRL. It is estimated that 7% of healthcare workers have this type of allergic reaction. Any group of patients frequently and intensely exposed to latex, such as those undergoing repeated surgical procedures and treatments such as intermittent catheterization, are at increased risk. Classic examples include children with spinal bifida who are exposed to medical devices such as bladder catheters from a young age. Local and systemic allergic reactions can often be dramatic and occasionally are life-threatening. The treatment is the same as for any acute allergic reaction (remove exposure, administer epinephrine and steroids for anaphylactic-like reactions; see Chapter 29, Common Emergencies, page 996).

If a patient has a known latex allergy, it should be noted on prominently displayed signs in the patient's room and in the patient's chart, and the patient should wear an alert bracelet. Latex is found in medical equipment in addition to gloves (e.g., anesthesia masks, catheters, hemodialysis components, NG tubes, drains, and syringes) and in consumer products (e.g., balloons, rubber bands, scuba diving equipment, underwear). Most hospitals have an inventory of latex-free products, and operating rooms have latex allergy procedures in place. Some hospitals have completely banned latex products in the operating room. Nitrile gloves are becoming common in hospitals because of this growing problem.

Basic Bedside Procedure Equipment

Table 19-1 lists useful instruments and supplies that aid in completion of many of the bedside procedures described in this chapter. Complete kits are commercially available for many of these specific procedures. Local anesthesia is discussed in Chapter 25, Suturing Techniques and Wound Care, page 818.

The size of various catheters, tubes, and needles is often designated by the **French unit** (1 Fr = ⅓ mm in diameter) or by **needle gauge**. Reference listings for these designations are shown in Figure 19-2, page 517. Chapter 29, Common Emergencies, page 1016, contains a useful table that summarizes the sizes of a wide variety of tubes and devices used on pediatric and adult patient care.

Designs of standard surgical scalpels used in the performance of many basic bedside procedures and in the operating room are shown in Figure 19-3, page 518. Scalpels with self-retracting blades are also available and are more commonly used for bedside procedures rather than in the operating room.

19

Antiseptic Solutions, Disinfection, and Sterilization

1. Antiseptic Solutions
The use of topical antiseptic agents for skin disinfection is important in reducing and preventing healthcare-associated infections (HAIs) and surgical site infections (SSIs). Additional information can be found in Chapter 24, Introduction to the Operating Room, page 803, which discusses preoperative surgical scrubs. The most common skin pathogens implicated are *Staphylococcus aureus,* other gram-positives (coagulase-negative *Staphylococcus, Enterococcus,* and group A streptococci), and gram-negative rods (*Escherichia*

Table 19-1. Some of the Instruments and Supplies Used in the Completion of Common Bedside Procedures

MINOR PROCEDURE TRAY
Sterile gloves
Sterile towels/drapes
4×4 gauze sponges
Prep solution: Povidone-iodine (Betadine), chlorhexidine-based preparation with alcohol
Syringes: 5, 10, 20 mL
Needles: 18, 20, 22, 25 gauge. Self-shielding devices always preferred.
Local anesthesia such as 1% lidocaine (with or without epinephrine) or topical agents (See Chapter 25, page 818, for details.)
Adhesive tape, dressings, topical antibiotic products as appropriate

BASIC PROCEDURE INSTRUMENT TRAY
Scissors
Needle holder
Hemostat
Scalpel and blade (no. 10 for adult, no. 15 for children or delicate work)
Suture of choice (2-0 or 3-0 silk or nylon on cutting needle; cutting needle is best for suturing tubes to skin)

coli and *Pseudomonas* are common). General rules for procedure site preparation are noted in adults.

a. **Thirty-second cleansing is more effective than 5- to 10-second cleansings in decreasing bacterial colony counts.**

b. **Always allow antiseptics to dry on the site** (at least 30 sec is recommended). Read manufacturer's recommendations on time to dry.

c. **Remove iodophor solutions off the wider area at the end of the procedure** except right at the procedure insertion site.

d. **Verify that antiseptic is not pooling** under the patient when prepping, as it can cause skin irritation/damage.

2. **Commonly used topical antiseptics.**

a. **Alcohol** (70% to 90% ethyl or isopropyl) is effective against gram-positive and gram-negative bacteria, including MRSA and VRE, as well as mycobacteria and fungi, and is rapid acting. It is commonly used for skin prep of minor procedures (e.g., phlebotomy), but it is not used on mucous membranes. It can be used alone or in combination with chlorhexidine gluconate (CHG). Apply three times in a circle starting at the center of the site of insertion or incision site and going outward. Ethyl and isopropyl alcohol and CHG are NOT for major

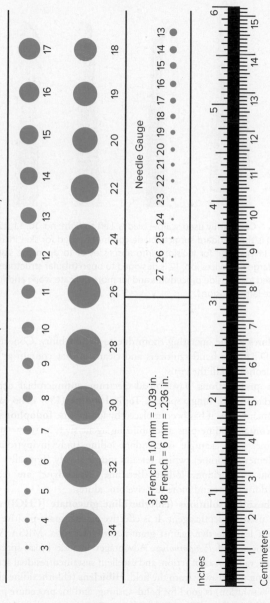

Figure 19-2. French catheter guide and needle gauge reference. A complete table of relative French sizes for a variety of tubes and other devices can be found in Chapter 29, Common Emergencies, page 1016. (Courtesy Cook Medical, Bloomington IN.)

French Catheter Scale
in French units (1 French = 1/3 mm diameter)

Needle Gauge

3 French = 1.0 mm = .039 in.
18 French = 6 mm = .236 in.

Inches

Centimeters

19

517

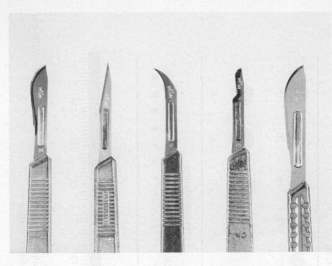

Figure 19-3. Commonly used scalpel blades. Left to right: no. 10, 11, 12, 15, and 20. No. 10 is the standard surgical blade commonly used for skin incisions in adults; no. 11 is useful for incisions into abscesses or to open the skin for placement of large IV devices; no. 12 is designed to open tubular structures; no. 15 is widely used for bedside procedures and for more delicate work; and no. 20 is used to make large incisions.

procedures in the operating room due to flammability. Concerning COVID-19, use hand sanitizers and cleansers that contain at least 60% alcohol to kill the virus.

b. **Iodine preparations** have broad-spectrum antimicrobial activity (bacteria, viruses, fungi, spores). **Topical iodine** (1%) is no longer recommended, as it has been replaced by iodophors. **Iodophor solutions** contain iodine plus a solubilizing agent such as surfactant or povidone. One example is povidone-iodine (polyvinylpyrrolidone plus elemental iodine), which releases iodine slowly. Typically, 10% solutions of povidone iodine (Betadine, Wescodyne) are recommended for major and more invasive procedures.

c. **Chlorhexidine solutions (chlorhexidine gluconate [CHG])** are a widely used antiseptic agent. It is effective against gram-positive bacteria but less effective against gram-negative bacteria, MRSA, VRE, streptococci, and *Pseudomonas*. Advantages include broad-spectrum coverage, rapid onset of action, and excellent sustained/residual activity after being wiped away from the field. **Hibiclens** (chlorhexidine gluconate 4% solution) is good for hand washing, and for procedure preparation **Chlora-Prep** (2% chlorhexidine in 70% isopropyl alcohol).

d. **Hexachlorophene (pHisoHex)** is effective against gram-positive bacteria (especially *Staphylococcus* strains) but is less effective against gram-negative bacteria, fungi, and mycobacteria. It has residual activity for several hours after use and reduces bacterial counts after multiple uses by a cumulative effect. Newer agents, with better antimicrobial coverage and fewer side effects, have replaced hexachlorophene as a common surgical scrub.

e. **Benzalkonium chloride (BZK)** is the main ingredient in alcohol-free popular hand sanitizer brands, including Germ-X and Purell. Benzalkonium chloride is bactericidal against many gram-positive and gram-negative bacteria but is inconsistent in covering fungi, viruses, and mycobacteria. These products may reduce the growth of the germs but not kill them. It has a low incidence of irritant contact dermatitis, but like hexachlorophene, it has been replaced by antiseptics with better antimicrobial coverage as a medically intensive skin procedure prep. BZK towelettes are used for periurethral cleansing for catheter insertion. BZK sanitizers combined with at least 60% alcohol are most effective against viral strains such as the coronavirus.

3. **Disinfection and Sterilization**
   o **Disinfection** involves reduction of pathogenic organisms to safe levels.
   o **Sterilization** inactivates all microbes, including spores. These are important for instruments and surfaces. Bacterial spores are among the most resistant of all living cells. The most important spore formers are members of the genera *Bacillus* and *Clostridium*.

   a. **Autoclave:** Pressurized steam >120°C. Sporicidal but may not reliably inactivate prions. Prions are abnormal, transmittable pathogenic protein agents found most abundantly in the brain. Prion proteins lead to brain damage with prion diseases usually always fatal (e.g., Creutzfeldt-Jakob Disease).

   b. **Alcohols.** Denatures proteins and disrupts cell membranes but are not sporicidal.

   c. **Chlorhexidine.** Denatures proteins and disrupts cell membranes but are not sporicidal.

   d. **Chlorine** (sodium hypochlorite, the active ingredient in bleach). Oxidizes and denatures proteins. Kills enveloped and nonenveloped viruses and fungi and is sporicidal.

   e. **Ethylene oxide (EtO).** Low-temperature gas sterilization. Alkylating agent and is sporicidal.

   f. **Hydrogen peroxide.** Free radical oxidation and is sporicidal.

   g. **Iodine and iodophors.** Halogenation of DNA, RNA, and proteins and sometimes sporicidal.

   h. **Quaternary amines** (benzalkonium chloride, others). Impair permeability of cell membranes and are not sporicidal. Effective against gram-negative and gram-positive bacteria and enveloped viruses and less effective against nonenveloped viruses, such as norovirus, and are rarely effective against TB.

4. **Coronavirus (COVID-19) surface cleaning summary (CDC 2020 Guidelines):**

19

a. Bleach 1/3 cup/gallon water or 4 teaspoons bleach/quart of water.
b. Hydrogen peroxide 3%; allow contact time at least 1 min.
c. Alcohol 70%: Isopropyl and ethanol (ethyl alcohol).
d. Other commercial products may be effective surface cleaners. Check if the product has been certified by the EPA. The registration number can be crosschecked on the EPA.gov website under **List N: Disinfectants for Use against SARS-CoV-2 (Coronavirus).**

Learning Bedside Procedures

Previously, traditional medical education had often used the apprenticeship concept of "see one, do one, teach one." While that approach allowed the newcomer to gain clinical experience, the inconsistency of the learning environment and the risk that this may pose to patients has made this approach of historical interest only. The development and widespread deployment of medical simulation allows the acquisition of clinical skills through deliberate practice rather than this traditional "apprentice style" of clinical learning. Simulation tools serve as an alternative to real patients, allowing a trainee to make mistakes and learn from them without harming any patient.

There are increasing concerns for the quality of patient care and increased attention to error reduction in healthcare, making improvements in patient safety a high priority. Today most medical centers have some type of simulation center for all their trainees in various disciplines to allow experience in simulated "real-life" clinical scenarios. Acquisition of clinical skills has many components such as developing skills in communication, physical examination, laboratory interpretation, differential diagnosis, procedural skills, and recognizing and responding to common emergencies, to name just a few. The bedside procedures reviewed in this chapter are provided as an introduction of these common elements of daily patient care. These descriptions will not make you a procedural expert but provide an overview on how these procedures are used clinically and will enhance your understanding on your journey to becoming a clinically proficient healthcare provider. We encourage you to take advantage of your local simulation center to practice many of these bedside procedures as part of your regularly prescribed core curriculum.

A broad spectrum of medical simulators and task trainers are available today at most academic centers. These range from basic task trainers through so-called "high-fidelity simulators" that are mannequins that replicate many human characteristics. This chapter encompasses many of the clinical procedures that are in the category of basic tasks such as venous and arterial vascular access, lumbar puncture, pelvic exam trainers, endotracheal intubation, and airway management simulators. We encourage you to "see one, do one, teach one" many times in the simulation lab before your resident or attending gives you the ultimate privilege of applying your new procedural knowledge on a real patient in need of one of these bedside interventions.

AMNIOTIC FLUID FERN TEST

Indication

• Assessment for rupture of membranes

Contraindications

• Active labor (relative)

Materials

• Sterile speculum and swab
• Glass slide and microscope
• Phenaphthazine (Nitrazine) paper (optional)

Background

The fern test is used to aid in the diagnosis of ruptured membranes by detecting the presence of amniotic fluid. This fluid, when placed on a glass slide, is allowed to dry. The sodium chloride crystals will form on the protein in the amniotic fluid, causing the resultant ferning (arborized) pattern in confirmation of membrane rupture. **Commercial** amniotic fluid-specific biomarker tests for rupture of membranes ae available but not widely used.

19

Procedure

1. Using a sterile speculum, swab a sample of fluid "pooled" in the vaginal vault onto a glass slide and let it air dry.
2. Amniotic fluid yields an arborization, or "fern," pattern seen under $10\times$ magnification. False-positive: Cervical mucus collection; however, the ferning pattern of mucus is coarser. The test is unaffected by meconium, vaginal pH, and blood–to–amniotic fluid ratios >1:10. Samples heavily contaminated with blood may not fern.
3. Another test for ruptured membranes is performed with Nitrazine paper, which has a pH turning point of 6.0. Normal vaginal pH in pregnancy is 4.5–6.0; amniotic fluid pH is 7.0–7.5. Positive Nitrazine test: color change in the paper from yellow to blue. False-positive: more common with the Nitrazine test; blood, meconium, semen, alkalotic urine, cervical mucus, and vaginal infections can raise the pH.

Complication

- Infection

ARTERIAL LINE PLACEMENT

Indications

- Continuous BP readings (e.g., critically ill patient or intraoperative monitoring)
- Facilitation of frequent ABG measurements (e.g., patients who need ventilatory support)
- Assessment of response to therapeutic interventions (e.g., insulin in patients with diabetic ketoacidosis)
- Procurement of blood sample in an acute emergency setting when venous sampling is not available (unusual)

Contraindications

- Arterial insufficiency with poor collateral circulation (see Allen test, page 526)
- Local infection, thrombus, or distorted anatomy at the puncture site
- Severe peripheral vascular disease of the artery or active Raynaud syndrome
- Thrombolytic therapy or coagulopathy (relative)
- Planned cardiac surgery if the radial artery must be preserved for harvest for CABG (relative)

Materials

- Minor procedure and instrument tray
- Heparin flush solution (1:1000 dilution)
- Arterial line setup according to local ICU routine (transducer, tubing, and pressure bag with pre-heparinized saline, monitor)
- Arterial line catheter kit *or* 20-gauge catheter over a needle, 1½–2 in (4–5 cm). (Insyte Autoguard™ Shielded IV catheter, Angiocath-N™ Autoguard Shielded IV catheter) with 0.025-in (0.6-mm) guidewire (optional)

Procedure

1. The radial artery is most frequently used and is described here. Other sites, in decreasing preference: ulnar, dorsalis pedis, femoral, brachial, and axillary arteries. **Never puncture the radial and ulnar arteries in the same hand;** doing so can compromise the blood supply to the hand and fingers.

2. Using the Allen test (page 526) or Doppler ultrasonography, verify collateral circulation between the radial and ulnar arteries. Prepare the flush bag, tubing, and transducer, paying particular attention to removing air bubbles.

3. Place the forearm on an arm board with a roll of gauze behind the wrist to hyperextend the joint. Prep with povidone-iodine and drape with sterile towels. Wear gloves and a mask.

4. Palpate the artery, and choose the puncture site where the artery appears most superficial. Using a 25-gauge needle and 1% lidocaine, raise a very small skin wheal at the predetermined puncture site. Draw back on the syringe before injecting lidocaine so as not to inadvertently inject into the artery.

5. **a. Standard technique:** (See Figure 19-4) While palpating the path of the artery with your nondominant hand, advance the 20-gauge (preferably 1½-in [4-cm] long) catheter-over-needle assembly into the artery at a low (30–45 degrees) angle. Once a "flash" of blood is seen in the hub, advance the entire unit 1–2 mm so that the needle and catheter are in the artery. If blood flow in the hub stops, carefully pull the entire unit back until flow is reestablished. When flow is established, position the hub of the catheter downward (decreasing the angle between catheter and skin), allowing catheter advancement in less of an acute angle direction. Hold the needle steady and advance the catheter over the needle into the artery. The catheter should slide smoothly into the artery. Activate the safety button on the catheter to automatically shield the needle. Withdraw the shielded needle completely and check for arterial blood flow from the catheter. A catheter that does not "spurt" blood is not in position. Briefly occlude the artery with manual pressure while the pressure tubing is being connected. *Note:* The pressure tubing system must be pre-flushed to clear all air bubbles before connection.

   b. Prepackaged kit technique: Kits, sometimes called "quick catheters," with a needle and guidewire (floppy J-tip is preferred to reduce the risk of endovascular injury) can be used for the **Seldinger technique** (described in step 8). Place the entry needle at a 30- to 45-degree angle to the skin site and insert until a flash of blood appears in the catheter. The catheter does not have to be advanced, but advance both the guidewire (orange handle in some kits) and the catheter into the vessel. Remove the wire and connect the catheter to the pressure tubing.

6. If placement is not successful, apply pressure to the site for 5 min and reattempt one or two more times. If still not successful, move to another site. The artery may spasm, making cannulation more difficult with repeated punctures.

7. Suture the catheter in place with 3-0 silk, and apply a sterile dressing. Splint the dorsum of the wrist to limit mobility and stabilize the catheter.

8. For larger vessels, such as the femoral artery, use the **Seldinger technique** (see Figure 19-9, page 537) of cannulation: Locate the vessel lumen

19

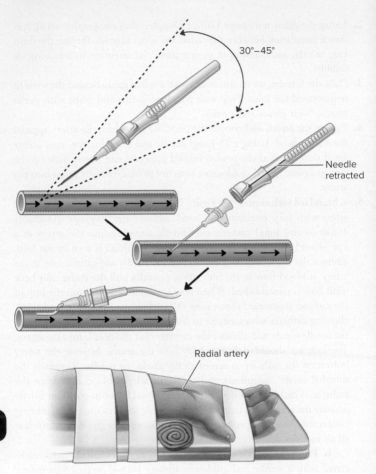

Figure 19-4. Technique of arterial line placement. The self shielding needle assembly needle assembly should be directed at a 30- to 45-degree angle (Reprinted with permission from Gomella TL, ed. Gomella's Neonatology: Basic Management, On-Call Problems, Diseases, Drugs, 8e, New York, NY: McGraw-Hill; 2020.)

with a small-gauge, thin-walled needle; pass a 0.035 floppy-tipped J ("J" describes the configuration of the end of the floppy wire) guidewire into the lumen; a floppy J-tip is preferred to reduce the risk of endovascular injury; and use the guidewire to pass a larger catheter into the vessel. Use a 16-gauge catheter assembly at least 6 in (15 cm) long for the femoral artery. *Note:* If a dilator is used with the kit, take care to dilate only skin and subcutaneous tissue; inadvertent dilation of an artery causes excessive bleeding.

9. Any amount of heparin can make coagulation studies (PTT) inaccurate. If an arterial line sample is obtained and unexpectedly high results are seen, repeat the test and consider conventional venipuncture. Even after discarding a 5- to 10-mL sample from the line, some heparin may remain and can contaminate the line.

10. Always compare the arterial line pressure with a standard cuff pressure. An occasional difference of 10–20 mm Hg is normal and should be considered when monitoring the BP.

Complications

Thrombosis, hematoma, arterial embolism, arterial spasm, arterial insufficiency with tissue loss, infection, hemorrhage, and pseudoaneurysm formation.

ARTERIAL PUNCTURE

Indications

- Blood gas determinations and acquisition of arterial blood for certain chemistry determinations (e.g., ammonia levels)
- To obtain blood samples when venipuncture is unsuccessful

Contraindications

- Overlying skin infection at arterial puncture sites

Materials

19

- Cup of ice
- Blood gas sampling kit
  or
- 3- to 5-mL syringe
- 23- to 25-gauge needle (radial artery); 20- to 22-gauge (femoral artery)
- Heparin (1000 U/mL), 1 mL
- Alcohol or povidone-iodine swabs

Procedure

1. Use a heparinized syringe for blood gas and nonheparinized syringe for chemistry determinations. If a blood gas kit is not available, heparinize a 3- to 5-mL syringe by drawing up 1 mL of 1:1000 solution of heparin through a small-gauge needle (23–25 gauge) into the syringe, pulling the plunger back. The heparin is then expelled, leaving only a small coating.

2. In order of preference, use the radial, femoral, or brachial artery. For the radial artery (Figure 19-5), perform an **Allen test** to verify patency of the ulnar artery. You do not want to damage the radial artery if there is no collateral flow from the ulnar artery. **To perform the Allen test**, have the patient make a tight fist. Occlude both the radial and

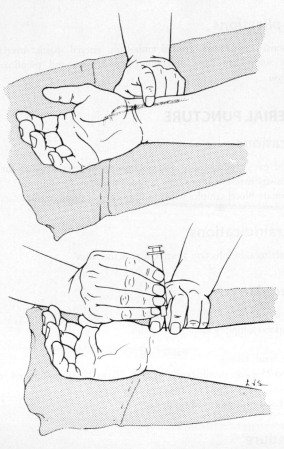

Figure 19-5. Radial artery puncture technique. After performing the Allen test, identify the point of maximum pulsation of the radial artery. After prepping the site index and middle fingers of the nondominant hand, identify again the point of maximal pulsation and path of the artery to identify the radial artery puncture site. Non-gloved hands shown for illustrative purposes. (Reproduced with permission from Stone CK and Humphries RL, eds. CURRENT Diagnosis & Treatment: Emergency Medicine, 8e. Copyright © 2017 by McGraw-Hill Education, Inc.).

ulnar arteries at the wrist and have the patient open the hand. While maintaining pressure on the radial artery, release the ulnar artery. If there is collateral flow from the ulnar artery, the entire hand flushes red within 6 sec, and radial puncture can be safely performed. If flushing is delayed or part of the hand remains pale, do **not** perform the radial puncture because collateral flow is inadequate. Choose an alternative site. Doppler ultrasonography can also be used to determine the patency of the ulnar artery.

3. For the femoral artery, use the mnemonic **NAVEL** to locate groin structures. Palpate the femoral artery just below the inguinal ligament. From lateral to medial, the structures are **N**erve, **A**rtery, **V**ein, (**E**mpty space, **L**ymphatic). (See Figure 19-13, page 548, for anatomy of the groin structures.)

4. Prep the area with either chlorhexidine solution or alcohol swab.

5. With sterile gloves, palpate the chosen artery carefully; lidocaine SQ can be used (small needle such as a 25–27 gauge), but this often turns a "one-stick procedure" into a "two-stick procedure." Palpate the artery proximally and distally with two fingers, or trap the artery between two fingers placed on either side of the vessel. Hyperextension of the joint brings the radial and brachial arteries closer to the surface.

6. See Figure 19-5, page 526. Hold the syringe as shown in Figure 19-5 with the needle bevel up and enter the skin at a 60- to a 90-degree angle. Often you can feel the arterial pulsations as you approach the artery.

7. Maintaining a slight negative pressure on the syringe, obtain blood on the downstroke or on slow withdrawal (after both sides of the artery have been punctured). Aspirate very slowly. A good arterial sample requires only minimal back pressure. If a glass syringe or special blood gas syringe is used, the barrel usually fills spontaneously, and it is not necessary to pull on the plunger.

8. If the vessel is not encountered, withdraw the needle without coming out of the skin, and redirect.

9. After obtaining the sample, withdraw the needle quickly and apply **firm pressure** at the site for **at least 5 min** (longer if the patient is receiving anticoagulants). To prevent compartment syndrome from extravasated blood, apply pressure even if a sample was not obtained. Activate the needle shielding mechanism.

10. If the sample is for a **blood gas determination**, expel any air from the syringe, mix the contents thoroughly by twirling the syringe between your fingers, remove and dispose of the needle assembly, and make the syringe airtight with a cap. Place the syringe in an ice bath if more than a few minutes will elapse before the sample is processed. Note the inspired oxygen concentration and time of day the sample was obtained on the lab slip.

19

ARTHROCENTESIS (DIAGNOSTIC AND THERAPEUTIC)

Indications

- **Diagnostic.** Evaluation of new-onset arthritis; ruling out infection in acute or chronic, unremitting joint effusion
- **Therapeutic.** Instillation of steroids, drainage of septic arthritis; relief of tense hemarthrosis or effusion

Contraindications

Cellulitis at injection site. Relative contraindication: Bleeding disorder; caution if coagulopathy or thrombocytopenia is present or if the patient is receiving anticoagulants.

Materials

- Minor procedure tray; 18- or 20-gauge needle (smaller for finger or toe)
- Ethyl chloride spray can be substituted for lidocaine.
- Two heparinized tubes for cell count and crystal examination
- Microbiology lab's preferred transport fluid/medium for bacterial, fungal, AFB culture, and Gram stain; Thayer-Martin plate for *Neisseria gonorrhoeae* (GC)
- Optional: A 5-mL syringe containing the medication of choice such as long-acting corticosteroid such as methylprednisolone (Depo-Medrol) or triamcinolone when performing a "therapeutic" arthrocentesis

General Arthrocentesis Procedures

1. Obtain consent after describing the procedure and complications.
2. Determine the optimal site for aspiration—knee, wrist, or ankle (see below); identify landmarks and mark site with an indentation or sterile marking pen. Avoid injecting into tendons.
3. If aspiration is followed by corticosteroid injection, maintain a sterile field with sterile implements to minimize the risk of infection.
4. Clean the area with chlorhexidine. Let the area dry and wipe the aspiration site with alcohol because chlorhexidine can render cultures negative. Let the alcohol dry before beginning the procedure.
5. Using a 25-gauge needle, anesthetize the puncture site with lidocaine; **do not inject into the joint space** because lidocaine is bactericidal. Avoid lidocaine preparations with epinephrine, especially in a digit. Alternatively, spray the area with **ethyl chloride ("freeze spray")** just before needle aspiration.
6. Insert the aspirating needle (18- or 20-gauge, smaller for finger or toe), applying a small amount of vacuum to the syringe (5-mL syringe is often

the ideal size to create enough vacuum). When the capsule is entered, fluid usually flows easily. Remove as much fluid as possible, repositioning the syringe if necessary.

7. If corticosteroid is to be injected, remove the aspirating syringe from the needle (using a hemostat to hold the needle in place may aid when exchanging syringes), which is still in the joint space. (*Note:* Ensure that the syringe can easily be removed from the needle before step 6). Attach the syringe containing corticosteroids, pull back on the plunger to ensure the needle is not in a vein, and inject contents. Never inject steroids when there is any possibility that the joint is infected. Remove the needle and apply pressure to the area (leakage of SQ steroids can cause localized atrophy of the skin). In general, the equivalent of 40 mg of methylprednisolone is injected into large joints such as the knee and 20 mg into medium-size joints such as the ankle and wrist. Warn the patient that a postinjection "flare" (pain several hours later) can occur and, if so, it is treated with ice and NSAIDs.

8. Note volume aspirated from the joint. The knee typically contains 3.5 mL of synovial fluid; in inflammatory, septic, or hemorrhagic arthritis, volumes are usually higher. A bedside test for viscosity is to allow a drop of fluid to fall from the tip of the needle. Normal synovial fluid is highly viscous and forms a several-inch-long string; viscosity is decreased in infection. A **mucin clot test** (clot normally forms in <1 min; delayed result suggests inflammation), once a standard test for RA, is no longer routinely performed.

9. Joint fluid is usually sent for the following:
   o Cell count and diff (purple or green top tube)
   o Microscopic crystal exam with polarized light microscopy (purple or green top tube); **normally** no debris, crystals, or bacteria; urate crystals are present with gout; calcium pyrophosphate crystals are seen in pseudogout.
   o Glucose (red top tube) Gram stain and cultures for bacteria, fungi, and AFB as indicated (check with your lab or deliver immediately in a sterile tube with no additives)
   o Cytology if malignant effusion is suspected

Arthrocentesis of the Knee

1. Fully extend the knee with the patient supine. Wait until the patient has a relaxed quadriceps muscle because its contraction approximates the patella against the femur, making aspiration painful.

2. Insert the needle posterior to the *lateral* portion of the patella into the patellar-femoral groove. Direct the advancing needle slightly posteriorly and inferiorly (Figure 19-6, page 530).

19

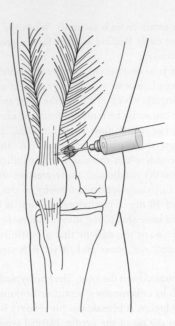

Figure 19-6. Arthrocentesis of the knee. (Reprinted with permission from Haist SA, Robbins JB, eds. Internal Medicine on Call, 4e, New York, NY: McGraw Hill; 2005.)

3. To inject the knee joint, have the patient sitting down with the leg flexed and enter the knee anteriorly over the medial joint line. Follow General Arthocentesis guidelines (page 528).

Arthrocentesis of the Wrist

1. The easiest site for aspiration is between the navicular bone and radius on the dorsal wrist. Locate the distal radius between the tendons of the extensor pollicis longus and the extensor carpi radialis longus to the second finger. This site is just ulnar to the anatomic snuff box. Direct the needle perpendicular to the mark (Figure 19-7, page 531). The wrist space also can be approached from the ulnar side by placement of the needle just distal to the ulnar bone. Follow General Arthocentesis guidelines (page 528).

Arthrocentesis of the Ankle

1. The most accessible site is between the tibia and the talus. Position the angle of the foot to leg at 90 degrees. Make a mark lateral and anterior to the medial malleolus and medial and posterior to the tibialis anterior tendon. Direct the advancing needle posteriorly toward the heel (Figure 19-8, page 531).

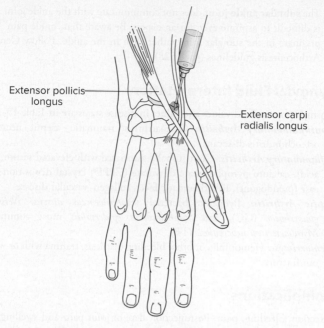

Extensor pollicis
longus

Extensor carpi
radialis longus

Figure 19-7. Arthrocentesis of the wrist. (Reprinted with permission from Haist SA, Robbins JB, eds. Internal Medicine on Call, 4e, New York, NY: McGraw-Hill; 2005.)

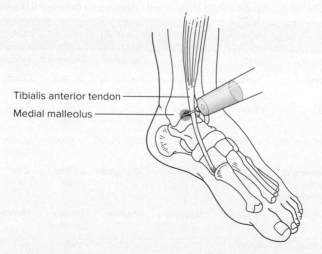

Tibialis anterior tendon
Medial malleolus

Figure 19-8. Arthrocentesis of the ankle. (Reprinted with permission from Haist SA, Robbins JB, eds. Internal Medicine on Call, 4e, New York, NY: McGraw-Hill; 2005.)

2. The **subtalar ankle joint** does not communicate with the ankle joint and is difficult to aspirate even for an expert. Be aware that "ankle pain" can originate in the subtalar joint rather than in the ankle. Follow General Arthocentesis guidelines (page 528).

Synovial Fluid Interpretation

Normal synovial fluid values and values in disease states are in Table 19-2.

Noninflammatory Arthritis: Osteoarthritis, traumatic, aseptic necrosis, osteochondritis dissecans

Inflammatory Arthritis: Gout (usually associated with elevated serum uric acid), calcium pyrophosphate dihydrate (CPPD) crystal deposition disease (pseudogout), RA, rheumatic fever, collagen–vascular disease

Septic Arthritis: Pyogenic bacterial (*Staphylococcus aureus*, *Neisseria gonorrhoeae* (GC), and *Staphylococcus epidermidis* most common), *Mycobacterium tuberculosis* (TB)

Hemorrhagic: Hemophilia or other bleeding diathesis, trauma with or without fracture

Complications

Infection, bleeding, pain. Postinjection flare of joint pain and swelling can occur after steroid injections and persist for as long as 24 hr. This complication

Table 19-2. Synovial Fluid Analysis and Categories for Differential Diagnosis[a]

Parameter	Normal	Noninflam-matory	Inflam-matory	Septic	Hemorr-hagic
Viscosity	High	High	Decreased	Decreased	Variable
Clarity	Transparent	Transparent	Translucent-opaque	Opaque	Cloudy
Color	Clear	Yellow	Yellow to opalescent	Yellow to green	Pink to red
WBC (per mL)	<200	<3000	3000–50,000	>50,000[b]	Usually <2000
Polymorpho-nuclear leukocytes (%)	<25%	<25%	50% or more	75% or more	30%
Culture	Negative	Negative	Negative	Usually positive	Negative
Glucose (mg/dL)	Approx. serum	Approx. serum	>25, but <serum	<25, <serum	>25

[a]See above and page 528 for additional information.
[b]May be lower if antibiotics initiated.
WBC = white blood cells.

is believed to be crystal-induced synovitis caused by the crystalline suspension used in long-acting steroids.

CENTRAL VENOUS CATHETERIZATION

Indications

- Resuscitation/CPR allows rapid infusion and high volume of fluids
- Insertion of pulmonary artery catheter or transvenous pacemaker (see Chapter 28, Critical Care, page 895)
- Measurement of central venous pressure (see Chapter 28, Critical Care, page 893)
- Administration of phlebitic or vasoactive medications (chemotherapy, calcium chloride, vasopressors)
- Hemodialysis, ultrafiltration, plasmapheresis, other blood filtering processes (Shiley or Quinton catheter for dialysis)
- Administration of hyperalimentation solutions (TPN)
- Long-term IV therapy
- Recurrent and/or difficult phlebotomy
- Access for extracorporeal therapy (ECMO)

Contraindications

- No absolute contraindication if the need for immediate venous access outweighs the risks
- Venous thrombosis in target vein; infection at insertion site.
- Coagulopathy dictates the use of the femoral or median basilic vein approach to minimize complications.

19

Background

A central venous catheter, often referred to as a **"deep line"** or **"central line,"** is a catheter with a tip that lies within the proximal superior vena cava, the right atrium, or the inferior vena cava. Central lines can be inserted through a peripheral vein (peripherally inserted central catheters or PICC) or a proximal central vein, most commonly the internal jugular, subclavian, or femoral veins. Central lines are used instead of peripheral IVs, as they provide higher flow rates for injections and are indicated for specific medications or treatments that cannot be given through a peripheral vein. They are also useful for long-term venous access. These catheters are indispensable in various settings, such as the intensive care unit, emergency room, and operating room. Their use can be associated with significant complications, so the decision to place a central venous catheter requires careful consideration. An overview of the various attributes of central venous catheters can be found in Table 19-3, page 534.

Table 19-3. Central Venous Catheters Overview

Subclavian Vein: Tip termination in superior vena cava (ideally at the cavoatrial junction corresponding to the right mainstem bronchus on CXR).

Advantages: Lowest-risk clot; bony landmarks easily palpated (even in obese patients); least uncomfortable.

Disadvantages: ↑ risk of pneumothorax relative to other sites, greatest risk in patients with COPD, asthma, high PEEP, upper thoracic trauma; unable to compress vessel puncture site if bleeding; might consider other sites in patients with coagulopathy; not recommended for chronic hemodialysis (higher risk of thrombosis).

Internal Jugular Vein: Tip termination in superior vena cava (ideally at the cavoatrial junction).

Advantages: Complication risk similar to subclavian but lower risk of pneumothorax; easier to control bleeding.

Disadvantages: ↑ risk of carotid puncture; technically difficult if intubated, presence of tracheostomy, excessive pulmonary secretions, and marked obesity; avoid if postoperative cervical spine procedure.

Femoral Vein: Tip termination in inferior vena cava (ideally at the cavoatrial junction).

Advantages: Easiest during cardiopulmonary arrest, no risk of pneumothorax.

Disadvantages: Medication delays during code; highest risk of infection, clot; requires immobilization after insertion; avoid if known vena cava clot, extrinsic compression of IVC.

PICC (pronounced "pick") (For full discussion see page 636) **P**eripherally **i**nserted **c**entral **c**atheters (PICC) are placed via the mid-arm through basilic or cephalic vein; a PICC line catheter tip should be located at the inferior aspect of the SVC (the arch of the azygous vein). PICC lines are smaller in diameter than central lines since they are inserted in smaller peripheral veins, and they are much longer than central venous catheters (50–70 cm vs. 15–30 cm). Therefore, the rate of fluid flow through PICC lines is considerably slower than central lines, rendering them unsuitable for rapid, large-volume fluid resuscitation. Multilumen PICCs include the **PowerPICC Catheter** and **Groshong Catheter.**

Advantages: Lower risk of infection than non-tunneled central lines and can be used for extended periods of time. They avoid the complications of central line placement (e.g., pneumothorax, accidental arterial cannulation), and they are relatively easy to place under ultrasound guidance and cause less discomfort than central lines.

Non-tunneled Central Venous Catheters are fixed in place at the site of insertion and are used for short-term therapy and in emergent situations at the bedside, in the ER or ICU.

(Continued)

Table 19-3. Central Venous Catheters Overview *(Continued)*

Tunneled Central Lines: Tunneled central lines are typically indicated for long-term use, typically greater than 2 wk. Often these are placed under fluoroscopic guidance in the interventional radiology suite or in the OR. These are NOT placed emergently. Tunneled catheters are passed under the skin away from the vessel insertion site to a separate exit site with the subcutaneous tunnel ~8-10 cm long on chest wall. A subcutaneous cuff is usually present at the exit site that fibroses and seals and secures the catheter in place. Outpatient hemodialysis most common indication. Hemodialysis catheters tend to be larger (16 Fr) and capable of high flow rates (200-300 mL/min necessary for hemodialysis). Types include Power Hickman, Multi-Lumen Hickman, Broviac, and Groshong Tunneled Central Venous Catheter.

Advantages: Lower risk of infection because all elements buried beneath the skin, no dressing is required when not in use.

Disadvantage: More frequent vascular access may ↑ risk of infection at skin over the port; limited in its ability to tolerate repeated use while retaining its ability to function as a barrier to infection.

Implanted Port: Similar to a tunneled catheter but it is entirely under the skin. Cannisters implanted in a subcutaneous pocket (chest: Port-a-Cath, arm: PAS-port). These surgically implanted infusion ports are commonly placed below the clavicle (infraclavicular fossa), with the catheter threaded into the right atrium through a large vein. Once implanted, the port is accessed via a "gripper" noncoring, Huber-tipped needle. Ports can be used for medications, chemotherapy, and blood sampling. Since ports are located completely under the skin, they are easier to maintain and have a lower risk of infection than central venous or PICC catheters. An implanted port is less obtrusive than a tunneled catheter or PICC line, requires little daily care, and has less impact on the patient's day-to-day activities. Port access requires specialized equipment and training and needs to be flushed regularly.

Advantages: Indicated for patients who require intermittent, repeated, >3-mo vascular access for infusion and/or phlebotomy.

Triple-lumen catheter: While central venous catheters are available in single- or double-lumen varieties, triple lumens are frequently used in the ICU for short-term central venous access. However, guidelines from the CDC suggest using the minimum number of infusion channels to reduce infection risk. The three infusion channels allow for multiple therapies to be administered simultaneously. The 7 Fr size is commonly used in adults, and they have one 16-gauge channel and two 18-gauge channels. In distinction to the French scale (Fr), the larger the gauge number, the smaller the catheter diameter.

Introducer sheaths: These sheaths are larger than the catheters (8–9 Fr) and facilitate the passage of temporary devices such as pulmonary artery catheters or pacemakers. The introducer sheath is placed first, and then the device is passed through the sheath and into the vessel (See Pulmonary Artery Catheter, Chapter 28, page 895). These sheaths can also serve as stand-alone devices for rapid infusion given their large diameter.

19

Based on data from McKean SC, Ross JJ, Dressler DD, Scheurer DB., eds. Principles and Practice of Hospital Medicine, 2e, 2017, New York, NY: McGraw-Hill.

Seldinger Technique

A technique used in the placement of devices such as central venous catheters is known as the **Seldinger technique.** Developed by a Swedish radiologist in the 1950s, the principle is to use over-wire catheter insertion to obtain safe percutaneous access to vessels and a variety of hollow spaces/organs (e.g., pleural space, trachea). A needle is used to puncture the structure and a floppy-tipped J guidewire is threaded through the needle; when the needle is withdrawn and removed from the wire, a catheter is threaded over the wire. The wire is then withdrawn, leaving the catheter in place in the vessel or organ. It is commonly used in vascular access procedures, including entry into veins and arteries. Other applications include placement of devices in hollow organs such as gastrostomy tubes, nephrostomy tubes, chest tubes, and suprapubic catheters, to name a few. The basic principles of the Seldinger technique are illustrated in Figure 19-9, page 537.

Central Venous Catheter Techniques

Verify the need for this type of invasive venous catheter placement and the plan for its use, including planned duration and specific device requirements. Before inserting any central venous catheters, obtain a thorough history, asking about any bleeding diathesis, anticoagulant use, previous catheter placement, history of DVT, and presence of a transvenous pacemaker. Note any abnormal laboratory values, especially elevated PT/PTT or low platelets. Correction of any such abnormalities with platelet transfusions, fresh frozen plasma transfusions, vitamin K, or discontinuation of anticoagulation may be required before placement of nonurgent central venous catheters.

For the placement of a central venous catheter, use the Seldinger technique (Figure 19-9, page 537). A less common central vein technique involves puncturing the vein with a larger-bore needle. These devices are known as **intracatheters** (brand name Intracath) and consist of a large-bore needle surrounded by a catheter. They are inserted into the vein as a unit, and the needle is withdrawn, leaving the catheter in the vessel. This section focuses on the commonly used Seldinger technique and placement of either a triple-lumen catheter or a sheath through which a smaller catheter (e.g., pulmonary artery catheter) can be placed. The internal jugular and subclavian approaches are commonly used. The femoral approach, although infrequently used due to increased infection risk, offers several advantages (see Femoral Vein Approach, page 547).

A PICC line is a thin catheter inserted into an upper arm vein and then guided into the superior vena cava on the right side of the heart. PICC placement is discussed in detail on page 636. Insertion of the sheaths needed for items such as a pulmonary artery/Swan-Ganz catheter device and related techniques are discussed in Chapter 28, page 895.

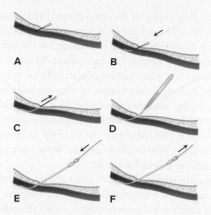

Figure 19-9. Description of the **Seldinger technique** used for safe percutaneous access to vessels and other structures such as central venous catheterization, arterial lines, chest tubes, and other procedural applications. **A.** Needle is inserted through skin and vessel wall until blood is aspirated. **B.** Guidewire is inserted gently through the needle and advanced. **C.** Needle is removed over guidewire. **D.** The skin is incised. **E.** Dilator or catheter is inserted over the guidewire. **F.** The guidewire is removed. (Reproduced with permission from Tintinalli JE, Ma O, Yealy DM, et al. Tintinalli's Emergency Medicine: A Comprehensive Study Guide, 9e, New York. NW; McGraw Hill; 2020.)

Many of the central catheters placed for long-term elective use such as tunneled or dialysis catheters, **Multi-Lumen Hickman, Broviac**, etc., are placed with fluoroscopic guidance. Increasingly, routine bedside central line placement is performed using point-of-care ultrasound. Studies have suggested lower failure rates, reduced complications, lower costs, and faster access compared with the standard physical "landmark" placement techniques. Point-of-care ultrasound imaging of the internal jugular and femoral veins is much easier than imaging of the subclavian vein because the view is hampered by the clavicle. Ultrasound-guided catheter placement in the subclavian vein is possible with the use of a slightly more lateral approach into the infraclavicular axillary vein.

Central Venous Catheter General Complications

Immediate Complications. Complications can be specific to the site of insertion and are noted following each technique. If expertise and equipment are available, point-of-care ultrasound can reduce the immediate complication rate. Immediate complications can include failure to successfully place the catheter, bleeding, inadvertent arterial puncture or puncture of another organ, pneumothorax, hemothorax, arrhythmia, malposition of the catheter, injury to the thoracic duct (with the left-sided unternal jugular approach), and venous air embolism. **Air embolism** is a serious and unique complication to this bedside procedure when air enters the vascular space when a needle or catheter is left open to the atmosphere. Fatal volumes of air measuring as little as 50–200 mL have been reported to be lethal. However, the minimum volume of air that is lethal to humans has not been clearly established. When inserting a central venous catheter, be aware of these symptoms: arrhythmias, chest pain, cardiovascular collapse, gasping, coughing, dyspnea, hypoxia, and respiratory distress. These signs and symptoms in association with central line insertion or manipulation are suspicious for venous air embolism. Trendelenburg with left lateral decubitus positioning (**Durant maneuver**) has been advocated to trap the air in the atrium along with supportive care including 100% inspired oxygen. **Never** leave an open end of a central venous catheter exposed to the air.

Delayed Complications: Common to all devices are delayed complications like development of a fibrin sheath, catheter fracture, malfunction or migration of the catheter, pulmonary emboli, vessel thrombosis or stenosis, or infection. Fibrin sheaths encase the outer wall and the catheter tip, leading to dysfunction in terms of difficult aspiration and/or high resistance to the injection of fluids. Catheter-related bloodstream infections (CRBSIs) have been associated with central venous catheters, and CRBSI is an active area of hospital quality improvement initiatives. The CDC (https://www.cdc.gov/hai/pdfs/bsi-guidelines-2011.pdf, accessed April 25, 2020) recommendations to reduce catheter-related infections include the following:

- When adherence to aseptic technique cannot be ensured (i.e., catheters inserted during a medical emergency), replace the catheter as soon as possible within 48 hr.
- **Do not** administer systemic antimicrobial prophylaxis routinely before insertion or during use of an intravascular catheter to prevent catheter colonization or CRBSI.
- Evaluate the catheter insertion site daily by palpation through the dressing to discern tenderness and by inspection if a transparent dressing is in use. Gauze and opaque dressings should not be removed if the patient has no clinical signs of infection. If the patient has local tenderness or other signs of possible CRBSI, an opaque dressing should be removed and the site inspected visually.
- Replace dressings used on short-term CVC sites every 2 days for gauze dressings and at least every 7 days for transparent dressing.
- **Do not** use topical antibiotic ointment or creams on insertion sites, except for dialysis catheters, because of their potential to promote fungal infections and antimicrobial resistance.
- **Do not** routinely replace CVCs, PICCs, hemodialysis catheters, or pulmonary artery catheters to prevent catheter-related infections.
- **Do not** remove CVCs or PICCs on the basis of fever alone. Use clinical judgment regarding the appropriateness of removing the catheter if there is evidence of an infection elsewhere or if a noninfectious cause of fever is suspected.

- **Do not** use guidewire exchanges routinely for non-tunneled catheters to prevent infection.
- **Do not** use guidewire exchanges to replace a non-tunneled catheter suspected of infection.
- Use a guidewire exchange to replace a malfunctioning non-tunneled catheter if no evidence of infection is present.
- Use new sterile gloves before handling the new catheter when guidewire exchanges are performed.

Materials

Prepackaged trays contain all the necessary drapes, needles, wires, sheaths, dilators, suture materials, and anesthetics needed. If needles, guidewires, and sheaths are collected from different places, make sure that the needle will accept the guidewire, that the sheath and dilator will pass over the guidewire, and that the appliance to be passed through the sheath will fit the inside lumen of the sheath because sizes are not standard. Basic supplies should include the following:

- Minor procedure and instrument tray (Table 19-1, page 516); 1% lidocaine (mixed 1:1 with sodium bicarbonate 1 mEq/L to reduce the sting of the injection).
- The CDC recommends maximal sterile barrier precautions, including the use of a cap, mask, sterile gown, sterile gloves, and a sterile full body drape, for the insertion of CVCs, PICCs, or guidewire exchanges.
- Prepare clean skin with a >0.5% chlorhexidine preparation with alcohol before central venous catheter and peripheral arterial catheter insertion and during dressing changes. If there is a contraindication to chlorhexidine, tincture of iodine, an iodophor, or 70% alcohol can be used as alternatives.
- Sutureless securement devices may be available to reduce the risk of intravascular catheter infections.
- Sterile gauze or sterile, transparent, semipermeable dressing is used to cover the catheter site.
- Guidewire (usually 0.035 floppy-tipped J wire).
- Vessel dilator.
- Intravascular device.
  o **Intravenous central catheter.** Choices include single, double, or triple lumen. Triple-lumen catheter (size varies from 4 to 9 Fr with 7 Fr a common size in adults); includes a 16-gauge and two smaller 18-gauge infusion channels. Central venous catheters used in the internal jugular and subclavian veins are typically 15–30 cm (approximately 6–12 in) long.
  o **Sheath introducer.** Commonly referred to as a "Cordis," "Swann sheath," and "angio sheath," and some introducer brand names are Cordis and Arrow. Sheath introducers are long, wide-bore (4–11 Fr;

19

average 8 Fr), single-lumen catheters with a wide plastic hub on the proximal end, which has a central smaller hole (one-way-valve prevents backflow of blood), through which various other catheters can be inserted, including triple-lumen central lines, Swann-Ganz catheters, temporary external pacing wires, and coronary angiography catheters. These introducers provide a "sheath" around the other catheters noted and provide a clean protected portal for these special catheters to enter a vessel and be carefully manipulated if necessary. The proximal port allows simultaneous administration of fluids (see Chapter 28, page 897 for additional information on sheaths used for Swan-Ganz placement).

- Heparinized flush solution 1 mL of 1:100 units heparin in 10 mL of NS (to fill catheter lumens before placement to prevent clotting during placement).
- IV infusion setup with fluid of choice and connecting tubing.
- ECG monitoring should be considered, as the guidewire may enter the heart and induce an arrhythmia (uncommon).
- Point-of-care ultrasound with appropriate probes and sterile covers should be available along with expertise of the operator. Ultrasound guidance should only be used by those fully trained in its technique.

Subclavian Vein Approach (Left or Right)

The left subclavian approach affords a gentle, sweeping curve to the apex of the right ventricle and is a preferred site for temporary transvenous pacemaker without fluoroscopy. Hemodynamic measurements are easier from the left subclavian approach; catheters do not have to negotiate an acute angle, as is the case at the junction of the right subclavian vein with the right brachiocephalic vein en route to the superior vena cava. This site is commonly complicated by kinking of the line, but it also has the lowest risk of infection. Thus, the CDC recommends this site if not contraindicated for insertion of non-tunneled central venous catheters in adults. The CDC also suggests avoiding the subclavian site in hemodialysis patients and patients with advanced kidney disease to avoid subclavian vein stenosis/thrombosis. The subclavian vein can be cannulated via supraclavicular, infraclavicular, or axillary approaches. *Caution:* The thoracic duct is on the left side, and the dome of the pleura rises higher on the left than the right.

Procedure

1. Use sterile technique (chlorhexidine prep, gloves, mask, gown, and a sterile field).
2. Place the patient flat or with head slightly down (Trendelenburg position) in the center or turned to the opposite side. (*Note:* The "ideal" position is controversial and based on operator preference.) Placing a towel roll along the patient's spine may help.

3. Administer 1% lidocaine and use a 25-gauge needle to make a small skin wheal 1 in (2 cm) below the mid clavicle. Then use a larger needle (e.g., 22-gauge) to anesthetize the deeper tissues and locate the vein.

4. Attach a large-bore, deep-line needle (a 14-gauge needle with a 16-gauge catheter at least 8–12 in [20–30 cm] long) to a 10–20 mL syringe and introduce it into the site of the skin wheal.

5. Advance the needle under the clavicle, aiming for a location halfway between the suprasternal notch and the base of the thyroid cartilage. Place your index or middle finger in the sternal notch and aim for just above your finger (Figure 19-10). The vein is encountered under the clavicle, just medial to the lateral border of the clavicular head of the sternocleido-mastoid muscle. In most patients, the site is roughly two fingerbreadths lateral to the sternal notch. Apply gentle pressure on the needle at the skin entrance site to assist in lowering the needle under the clavicle, aiming the tip of the needle toward the sternal notch. Do not aim the needle toward the floor; that is how the pleura can be hit, resulting in a pneumothorax.

6. Apply back pressure while advancing the needle deep to the clavicle, but above the first rib, and watch for a "flash" of blood.

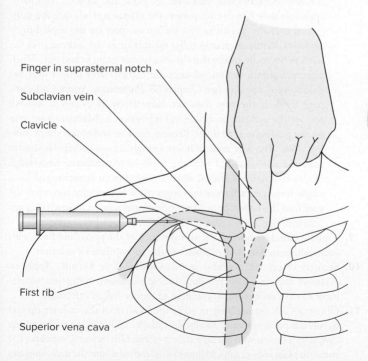

Finger in suprasternal notch

Subclavian vein

Clavicle

First rib

Superior vena cava

Figure 19-10.   Technique for the catheterization of the subclavian vein.

19

7. Free return of blood indicates entry into the subclavian vein. Remember that occasionally the vein is punctured through *both* walls, and a flash of blood may not appear as the needle is advanced. Therefore, if free return of blood does not occur on needle advancement, withdraw the needle slowly with intermittent pressure. Free return of blood heralds entry of the end of the needle into the lumen. Bright red blood that forcibly enters the syringe indicates that the subclavian artery has been entered. If arterial entry occurs, remove the needle. In most patients, the surrounding tissue will tamponade any bleeding from the arterial puncture. *Note:* The artery is under the clavicle; holding pressure has little effect on bleeding.

8. a. If you are using an intracatheter-style device, remove the syringe, place a finger over the needle hub, and advance the catheter an appropriate distance through the needle. Withdraw the needle to just outside the skin and snap the protective cap over the tip of the needle.

   b. For the Seldinger wire technique (see page 536 and Figure 19-9 page 537), pulse or ECG should be monitored during wire passage because the wire can induce ventricular arrhythmias if it enters the heart. Arrhythmias usually resolve when the wire is pulled out several centimeters. Nick the skin with a no. 11 blade and advance the dilator approximately 2 in (5 cm); remove the dilator and advance the catheter in over the guidewire (use the brown port on the triple-lumen catheter). While advancing either the dilator or the catheter over the wire, periodically ensure that the wire moves freely in and out. When placing a sheath system, advance the catheter and dilator over the guidewire as one unit (see Chapter 28, Pulmonary Artery Catheters, page 899). If the wire does not move freely, it usually is kinked; remove the catheter or dilator and reposition it. Maintain your grip on the guidewire at all times. Remove the wire and attach the IV tubing. *Note:* The wire used to insert a single-lumen catheter is shorter than the wire supplied with the triple-lumen catheter. Knowledge of this difference is critical when a triple-lumen is exchanged for a single-lumen catheter; use the longer triple-lumen wire and insert the wire into the brown port. Use the Seldinger wire technique (see page 536 and Figure 19-9 page 537) to place hemodialysis catheters.

9. Aspirate blood, remove all the air from each of the ports, and flush with saline solution. Attach the catheter to the appropriate IV solution.

10. Securely suture the assembly in place with 2-0 or 3-0 silk. Apply an occlusive dressing with povidone-iodine ointment. Sutureless securement devices are becoming common to reduce risk of infection.

11. Obtain a CXR immediately to verify the location of the catheter tip and to rule out pneumothorax. Ideally, the catheter tip lies in the superior vena cava at its junction with the right atrium (about fifth thoracic vertebra (T5) based on plain radiograph). Malpositioned catheters into the neck veins can be used only for saline infusion and not for monitoring or TPN infusion.

12. Catheters that cannot be manipulated into the chest at the bedside can usually be positioned properly during an interventional radiology procedure with fluoroscopy.

13. Point-of-care ultrasound may reduce the mechanical complications associated with CVC insertion. See an example in Figure 19-12, page 545.

Right Internal Jugular Vein Approach

There are three sites of access to the right internal jugular vein: anterior (medial to the sternocleidomastoid muscle belly), middle (between the two heads of the sternocleidomastoid muscle belly), and posterior (lateral to the sternocleidomastoid muscle belly). The middle approach is most commonly used and has well-defined landmarks. The major disadvantage of the internal jugular site is patient discomfort (difficult to dress, uncomfortable when turning the head). Most larger hospitals are equipped with portable ultrasound scanners and needle guides (such as Site-Rite Ultrasound by Bard) to facilitate accurate internal jugular cannulation, minimizing the incidence of inadvertent carotid artery puncture.

Procedure

1. Sterilize the site with chlorhexidine and drape the area with sterile towels. Administer local anesthesia with lidocaine in the area to be explored, as noted in the previous section.

2. Place the patient in the **Trendelenburg** (head-down) position.

3. If using a portable ultrasound scanner, pass the head of the scanner through the sterile sheath, and after applying ultrasound gel locate the internal jugular vein (it is larger and more compressible than the carotid artery). Advance the large-bore, deep-line needle through the needle guide and watch it enter the vein on the ultrasound monitor. If not using ultrasonography, use a small-bore (21-gauge) needle with a syringe to locate the internal jugular vein. It may help to have a small amount of anesthetic in the syringe to inject during exploration if the patient feels discomfort. Some clinicians prefer to leave this needle and syringe in the vein and place the large-bore needle directly over the smaller needle, into the vein. This method is commonly called the "seeker needle" technique.

4. Make sure the internal diameter of the needle used to locate the internal jugular vein is large enough to accommodate the passage of the floppy-tipped guidewire (typically 22-gauge or larger).

5. Make the percutaneous entry at the apex of the triangle formed by the two heads of the sternocleidomastoid muscle and the clavicle (Figure 19-11, page 544).

19

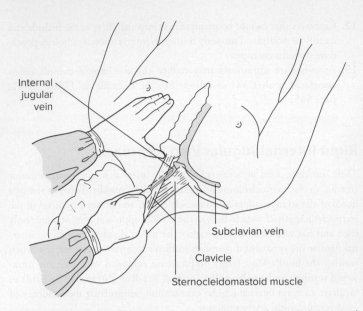

Figure 19-11. Technique for the catheterization of the right internal jugular vein using the "middle approach" (between the two heads of the sternocleidomastoid muscle).

6. Direct the needle slightly lateral toward the ipsilateral nipple and enter at a 45-degree angle to the skin.

7. A notch can sometimes be palpated on the posterior surface of the clavicle; this step can help locate the vein in the mediolateral plane because the vein lies deep to this shallow notch.

8. Vein puncture often is accomplished at an unnerving depth of needle insertion and is heralded by sudden aspiration of nonpulsatile venous blood. Bedside point-of-care ultrasonography is available in most ORs or ICUs and can aid in localization of the internal jugular vein if the standard techniques fail. An example of using a point-of-care ultrasound to localize the key structures is shown in Figure 19-12, page 545. The figure shows the critical structures and the appearance of the guidewire in the internal jugular vein.

9. Inadvertent carotid artery puncture is common if the needle is inserted medial to where it should be on the middle approach and is common with the anterior approach. With arterial puncture, the syringe fills without negative pressure because of arterial pressure, and bright red blood pulsates from the needle after the syringe is removed. In this case, remove the needle and apply manual pressure for 10–15 min. Use of POC ultrasound helps avoid inadvertent arterial puncture. See POC ultrasound images in Fgiure 19-12, page 545.

10. Follow steps 8–12 as for subclavian line (page 542) to confirm position and end procedure.

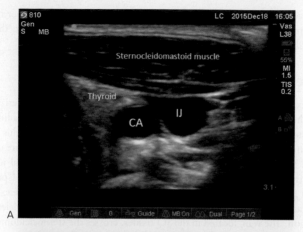

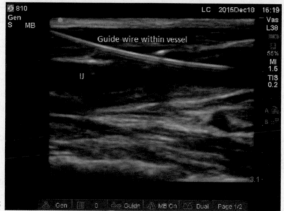

Figure 19-12. Point-of-care ultrasound imaging of internal jugular vein catheterization. **A.** Ultrasound image of critical structures including the internal jugular vein (IJ) and carotid artery (CA). **B.** Ultrasound image of guidewire in internal jugular vein (IJ) after cannulation. (Reproduced with permission from Oropello JM, Pastores SM, Kvetan V, eds. Critical Care, New York, NY: McGraw-Hill; 2020.)

19

Left Internal Jugular Vein Approach

The left internal jugular vein approach is not commonly used for central lines. Try one of the better options before using this approach. The procedure is similar to the right internal jugular vein approach. In addition to the usual complications, the left internal jugular vein approach has unique complications, including inadvertent left brachiocephalic vein and superior vena cava puncture with intravascular wires, catheters, and sheaths and laceration of the thoracic duct causing chylothorax, and higher risk of pneumothorax because of the dome of the pleura rises higher on the left than the right.

External Jugular Vein Approach

The external jugular vein is a safe approach to central venous catheterization, but the method is technically demanding owing to difficulty threading the catheter into the central venous system and is infrequently used. This site is uncomfortable for the patient because the dressing and IV tubing are on the neck. If the central venous system cannot be entered, the external jugular vein is also a site of last resort for placing a standard IV catheter ("peripheral") for the administration of routine nonsclerosing IV fluids. The external jugular vein is usually visible with the patient in a 30-degree Trendelenburg position. The vein, located in the SQ tissues, crosses the sternocleidomastoid muscle arising from just behind the angle of the jaw inferiorly where it drains into the subclavian vein just lateral to the inferior aspect of the sternocleidomastoid muscle.

Procedure

1. Place the patient in the Trendelenburg position with the head turned away from the side of insertion. Prep and drape the neck from the ear to the subclavicular area.
2. Have the patient perform the Valsalva maneuver or gently occlude the vein near its insertion into the subclavian vein to help engorge the vein.
3. At the midpoint of the vein, make a skin wheal with a 25-gauge needle and lidocaine solution. Use a 21-gauge needle to anesthetize the deeper SQ tissue and to locate the vein.
4. Remove the syringe from the needle and insert a floppy-tipped J wire into the needle. Use the guidewire with gentle pressure to negotiate the turns into the intrathoracic portion of the venous system. With difficult wire passage, have the patient turn his or her head slightly to help direct the wire. **Never forcibly push the wire.** As a last resort, use fluoroscopy to direct the wire into the superior vena cava.
5. Once a sufficient length of the guidewire is passed, remove the needle.
6. Nick the skin with a no. 11 blade to accommodate the catheter; advance the catheter over the guidewire, and remove the guidewire. Aspirate blood from the end of the catheter to confirm venous placement.
7. Follow steps 8–12 as for placement through the subclavian vein (page 542).

Complications: Internal Jugular Vein Catheterization

- Overall, a safe procedure when the small-bore needle is used to identify the vein. Safety can be further enhanced through the use of localizing ultrasound techniques. (See also General Complications of Central Vein Catherization page 537.)
- Pneumothorax may be detected when a sudden gush of air is aspirated instead of blood. Always obtain a postprocedure CXR to rule out pneumothorax and check line placement. Pneumothorax necessitates chest tube placement in almost all cases, especially when the patient is receiving mechanical ventilation or is a trauma patient. The left-sided approach is associated with higher pneumothorax risk (higher dome of the left pleura).
- Perforation of endotracheal tube cuffs.
- Hemothorax (vascular injury) or hydrothorax (administration of IV fluids into the pleural space).
- **Deep venous thrombosis:** The greatest risk factor for upper extremity DVT is a history of or the presence of a subclavian or an internal jugular deep line.
- **Catheter tip embolus: Never** withdraw the catheter through the needle (can shear off the tip).
- **Air embolus: Always** keep the open end of a deep line covered with a finger. As little as 50–100 mL of air in a vein can be fatal. For suspected **air embolization, place the patient's head down and turn the patient to his or her left side to keep the air in the right atrium.** A stat portable CXR will show whether air is present in the heart.

Femoral Vein Approach

The femoral vein approach is safe (arterial and venous sites are easily compressible with excessive bleeding), and pneumothorax is not possible. Placement can be accomplished without interrupting CPR. This site can be used to place a variety of intravascular appliances, including temporary pacemakers, pulmonary artery catheters (expertise with fluoroscopy may be needed), and triple-lumen catheters. The main disadvantages are the high risk of sepsis, the immobilization it causes, and the need for fluoroscopy to ensure proper placement of pulmonary artery catheters and transvenous pacemakers. There is also a higher reported incidence of catheter-related deep vein thrombosis compared with jugular or subclavian access. However, compared to subclavian and jugular access sites, the femoral veins may be preferred in a patient with a coagulopathy or thrombocytopenia due to the ability to provide direct pressure at this access site.

19

Procedure

1. Place the patient in the supine position.
2. Use sterile preparation and appropriate draping. Administer local anesthesia in the area to be explored.
3. Palpate the femoral artery. From lateral to medial use the mnemonic NAVEL to locate the vein (nerve/artery/vein/empty space/lymphatic) (Figure 19-13). If the arterial pulse is difficult to palpate, point-of-care ultrasonography may aid in locating the artery.
4. Guard the artery with the fingers of one hand.
5. Explore for the vein just medial to your fingers with a needle and syringe as described previously.
6. It may be helpful to have a small amount of anesthetic in the syringe to inject with exploration.
7. Direct the needle cephalad at about a 30-degree angle and insert it below the femoral crease.
8. Puncture is heralded by the return of venous, nonpulsatile blood upon the application of negative pressure to the syringe.
9. Advance the guidewire through the needle.

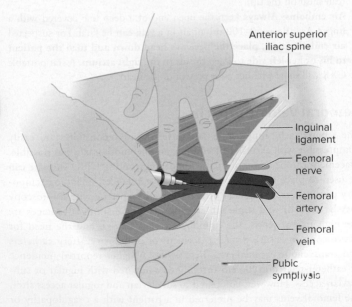

Figure 19-13. Technique for femoral vein access. "NAVEL" helps identifying the structures from lateral to medial (**n**erve/**a**rtery/**v**ein/**l**ymphatic). (In Vascular Access, Tintinalli JE, Ma O, Yealy DM, Meckler GD, Stapczynski J, Cline DM, Thomas SH. Tintinalli's Emergency Medicine: A Comprehensive Study Guide, 9e, New York, NY: McGraw Hill; 2020.)

10. The guidewire should pass with ease into the vein to a depth at which the distal tip of the guidewire is always under your control, even when the sheath–dilator or catheter is placed over the guidewire.
11. Remove the needle once the guidewire has advanced into the femoral vein.
12. For catheter size >6 Fr, make a skin incision with a no. 11 scalpel blade and use a vessel dilator. Advance the catheter along with the guidewire into the femoral vein. Maintain control on the distal end of the guidewire.
13. Follow steps 8–12 as for the subclavian line.

Complications: Femoral Vein Catheterization

The femoral site has the highest risk of contamination and sepsis. If an occlusive dressing can remain in place and free from contamination, this option is safe.

DVT has occurred after femoral vein catheterization. The risk of DVT increases if the catheter remains in place for a prolonged period.

Uncontrolled retroperitoneal bleeding can occur if the iliac or common femoral artery is inadvertently punctured above the inguinal ligament.

Other potential complications include catheter migration, nerve injury, and catheter embolization. (See also General Complications of Central Vein Catherization page 537.)

Removal of a Central Venous Catheter (Any Site)

1. Turn off the IV flow.
2. For subclavian and jugular approaches, place the patient lying down in a slight Trendelenburg (supine position with bed on 15- to 30-degree incline). Cut the retention sutures and gently withdraw the catheter. Visually inspect the catheter to ensure it is intact.
3. Apply pressure for at least 2–3 min and apply a sterile dressing. Undo the Trendelenburg positioning and place the patient in reverse Trendelenburg to decrease venous engorgement for catheters placed in the internal jugular or subclavian veins.

Removal of Tunneled Catheters

Hickman or Broviac tunneled catheters usually have been placed in the OR or interventional radiology suite. These catheters pass through from the internal jugular or the subclavian vein and are then tunneled subcutaneously and emerge from the chest wall. They also have an antibiotic-impregnated cuff near the skin exit site to prevent infection and promote tissue growth.

1. Wearing sterile gloves, gown, and mask, prep the patient as if placing a central line. Be sure to prep the catheter outside of the skin as well.
2. Cut skin sutures while holding the catheter in place.
3. Infiltrate field with 1% lidocaine using a 25-gauge needle. Use caution to not inject directly into the catheter (infiltrate only surrounding tissue).

19

Palpate the antibiotic cuff through the skin. It should be a few centimeters from the skin exit site, although this distance varies by catheter type and length of the catheter outside the skin.

4. If it has been placed within the past 2–4 wk, the catheter may slide out with gentle traction, much like other central lines. More commonly, however, the antibiotic disk causes an inflammatory response that creates a tissue cuff around the cuff and catheter track. Begin by using a hemostat or scissors placed through the exit site to bluntly separate the surrounding connective tissue from the cuff. You may have to use scissors to sharply cut some of this soft tissue. Take great care not to cut the catheter itself.

5. Once the cuff is free, gently attempt to pull out the catheter. If it does not release from underlying adhered tissue with gentle traction, do not pull harder because the catheter tip can snap off, leaving part of it in the right atrium.

6. If the catheter is still not free, continue to cut tissue immediately surrounding it down to the catheter itself. Once you see the white color of the catheter, gently pull again and slide it out.

7. Once the catheter is removed, hold pressure for at least 5 min both at the site of entry into the vein (the internal jugular or subclavian) and at the exit site from the skin. Undo the Trendelenburg positioning.

8. If the cuff is far from the skin exit site of the catheter, make a counterincision through the skin higher on the chest wall to aid in freeing the cuff from surrounding tissue at that location.

CHEST TUBE PLACEMENT (CLOSED THORACOSTOMY, TUBE THORACOSTOMY)

Indications

- Pneumothorax (simple or tension)
- Hemothorax, pleural effusion, hydrothorax, chylothorax, or empyema evacuation
- Pleurodesis for chronic recurring pneumothorax or effusion refractory to standard management (e.g., malignant effusion)

Contraindications

- Anticoagulation, overlying infection or a bleeding diathesis may be a relative contraindication (needle thoracostomy may be a preferred initial option in such patients)

Materials

- Chest tube (adult, 16–24 Fr for pneumothorax, 28–36 Fr for hemothorax or pleural effusion; newborn, 12–18 Fr; 1–2 yr, 14–24 Fr; 5 yr, 20–32; >5 yr, as for adult)

- Water-seal drainage system (e.g., Pleur-evac) with connecting tubing to wall suction (see Figure 19-14.2, Panel B, page 555)
- Minor procedure tray and instrument tray (see Table 19-1 page 516)
- Silk or nylon suture (0 to 2-0) on cutting needle
- Petrolatum gauze (Vaseline) (optional)
- 4 × 4 gauze dressing and cloth tape
- Pulse oximeter monitoring (recommended)

Background

A chest tube is usually placed to manage an ongoing intrathoracic process that cannot be managed with simple thoracentesis (page 653). The traditional methods of chest tube placement are described. Percutaneous tube thoracostomy kits for the Seldinger technique (see page 536) are used for small pneumothoraces when there is no risk of ongoing air leak and are contraindicated in end-stage severe COPD, major pneumothorax >20%, tension pneumothorax, and chronic effusion. This procedure can be painful and may require conscious sedation.

Critical to the safe performance is the suction collection apparatus that creates a water seal to prevent air or fluid form re-entering the pleural space. Originally designed as a "three-bottle apparatus" (collection/air seal/pressure regulator), a popular commercial system is the Pleur-evac self-contained system. The operating principles of this device are demonstrated in Figure 19-14.2, Panel B, page 555.

Procedure

1. Before placing the tube, review the CXR unless the emergency situation does not allow time. For pneumothorax, choose a high anterior site (second or third ICS, midclavicular line, or subaxillary position). Subaxillary placement leaves the best appearance from a scar standpoint. Place a low lateral chest tube in the fifth or sixth ICS in the midaxillary line and direct it posteriorly for fluid removal (usually corresponds to the inframammary crease). In traumatic pneumothorax, use a low lateral site because it is usually associated with bleeding. In rare instances, loculated apical pneumothorax or effusion may necessitate placement of an anterior tube in the second ICS at the midclavicular line. When a tube is placed on the right side, the right hemidiaphragm may be slightly elevated because of the anatomic position of the liver. Insert the tube above the diaphragm in the pleural space.

2. Choose the appropriate chest tube. Use a 16- to 24-Fr tube for pneumothorax and 28–36 Fr for fluid removal. A **"thoracic catheter"** has multiple holes and works best for nearly all purposes and is considered essential for removal of fluid.

19

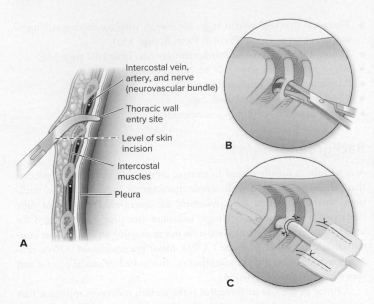

Intercostal vein,
artery, and nerve
(neurovascular bundle)

Thoracic wall
entry site

Level of skin
incision

Intercostal
muscles

Pleura

A

B

C

Figure 19-14.1 Chest tube insertion technique. **Step A**. A subcutaneous tunnel is created with the skin incision lower than the thoracic wall entry site over the top of the rib. **Step B**. The pleura is punctured. **Step C**. The skin site is closed and the tube is secured here using suture and tape on the chest tube technique. **NOTE:** If a patient has signs of tension pneumothorax (acute shortness of breath, hypotension, distended neck veins, tachypnea, tracheal deviation) before a chest tube is placed, urgent treatment is needed. Insert a 14-gauge needle into the chest in the second ICS in the midclavicular line, which will rapidly decompress the tension pneumothorax, and then you can proceed with chest tube insertion. Do not wait for chest X-ray confirmation before inserting a needle into the chest if the diagnosis of tension pneumothorax is suspected. (Reprinted with permission from Gomella TL, ed. Neonatology: Basic Management, On-Call Problems, Diseases, Drugs, 8e, New York, NY: McGraw-Hill; 2020.)

19

3. Position the patient in an appropriate manner. If the patient is supine, have him or her raise the ipsilateral arm over the head to expose the rib space. If the patient is in the lateral decubitus position, have him or her place the ipsilateral arm on a bedside tray table.

4. Wear a mask, eye protection, hat, gown, and sterile gloves. Prep the area with chlorhexidine solution and drape it with sterile towels. Use lidocaine (with or without epinephrine) to anesthetize the skin, intercostal muscle, and anterior periosteum of the rib; start at the center of the rib and gently work over the top. Remember, the neurovascular bundle runs under the rib (Figure 19-14.1, Step A), and these structures are to be avoided. The needle then can be gently "popped" through the pleura, and the aspiration of air or fluid confirms the correct location for the

chest tube. Back out the needle slowly until no fluid or air is aspirated just outside the parietal pleura, and inject lidocaine. There is no benefit in injecting lidocaine inside the pleural space. If the procedure is elective, the patient is extremely anxious, and the patient's respiratory status is not compromised, **occasionally** sedation is helpful. When the procedure is performed under conscious sedation with anxiolytics and IV narcotics, place the patient in a monitored setting.

5. Make a 2-3 cm transverse incision over the center of the rib with a no. 15 or no. 11 scalpel blade. Use a blunt-tipped clamp to dissect over the top of the rib and make a subcutaneous (SQ) tunnel (see Figure 19-14.1, Step A, page 552).

6. Puncture the parietal pleura with the hemostat and spread the opening (see Figure 19-14.1, Step B, page 552). **Be careful not to injure the lung parenchyma with the hemostat tips.** If the tube is inserted for a pneumothorax, a rush of air usually is heard on entry into the pleural cavity. If the tube is placed for effusion, fluid under pressure may be released at this time. Insert a gloved finger into the pleural cavity to gently clear any clots or adhesions so as to avoid accidentally puncturing the lung by the tube.

7. Carefully insert the tube into the desired position with a hemostat or gloved finger as a guide. Make sure all the holes in the tube are inside the chest cavity. Attach the end of the tube to a water-seal or Pleur-evac suction system. One indication of proper placement in the pleural place is fogging on the inner tubing of the chest tube that varies with respiration. To guarantee an intrapleural position, make sure you observe respiratory variation within the tube or suction system to guarantee an intrapleural position. Some chest tubes have sharp trocars that are used to pierce the chest wall and place the chest tube simultaneously with minimal amounts of dissection. These instruments are extremely dangerous and are usually placed in the anterior high position (i.e., second, third, or fourth ICS).

8. Secure the tube in place. Several methods are available. Place a heavy silk or polypropylene (0 or 2-0) suture through the incision next to the tube. Tie the incision together, then tie the ends around the chest tube. Make sure to wrap the suture around the tube several times. Tie the suture around the tube tightly enough that the tubing dimples slightly but not so tightly as to occlude the lumen. This step prevents the tube from slipping through the suture. As an alternative, place a purse-string suture (or "U stitch") around the insertion site or suture the securing tape to the skin as shown in Figure 19-14.1, Step C, page 552. Make sure all of the suction holes are in the chest cavity before the tube is secured.

9. Cover the insertion site with plain gauze. Make the dressing as airtight as possible with tape, and secure all connections in the tubing to prevent accidental loss of the water seal. Some physicians wrap the insertion site with petrolatum (Vaseline or Xeroform) gauze, but these materials

19

can be troublesome (i.e., they are not water soluble and act as a foreign body), inhibit wound healing, and may not seal the site.

10. Connect the tube to the suction apparatus. Start Pleur-evac suction (usually –20 cm water in adults, –16 cm in children) and obtain a portable CXR immediately to check the placement of the tube and to evaluate for residual pneumothorax or fluid. See Figure 19-14.2.

Chest Tube Placement Using Seldinger Technique

Kits for chest tube insertion by the Seldinger technique (see page 536 and Figure 19-9, page 537) are good for nonemergency chest tube placement, make the tube easier to insert, and cause less patient discomfort than other equipment.

1. After sterile prepping and draping, anesthetize the skin over the desired ICS (see details above). Insert the needle over the rib space to avoid injury to the intercostal bundle.

2. Once air (from pneumothorax) or fluid (from effusion) is aspirated, use the Seldinger technique (page 536 and Figure 19-9, page 537) to introduce a floppy J-tip guidewire, serial dilators, and finally the desired chest tube using the guidewire. Remove the wire. Secure the chest tube to the skin and connect it to the Pleur-evac system as described earlier.

Chest Tube Removal

1. Verify that the pneumothorax or fluid is cleared. Check for air leak by having the patient cough; observe the water-seal system for bubbling that indicates either a system (tubing) leak or persistent pleural air leak.

2. Take the tube off suction **but not off water seal** and cut the retention suture. Have the patient inspire deeply and perform the Valsalva maneuver while you apply pressure with petrolatum gauze or with a sufficient amount of antibiotic ointment on 4 × 4 gauze with an additional 4 × 4 gauze squares. Pull the tube rapidly while the patient performs the Valsalva maneuver, and make an airtight seal with tape with the petrolatum or antibiotic ointment saturated gauze. Check an "upright" exhalation CXR for pneumothorax.

Pleurodesis

1. Used for recurrent pneumothorax or in recurrent malignant effusion to obliterate pleural space. This is an uncomfortable procedure, and sedation with a short-acting narcotic is recommended. Sclerosing agents used include doxycycline (500–1000 mg in 100 mL NS), talc (2 g/100 mL NS), and bleomycin (60 units/100 mL NS).

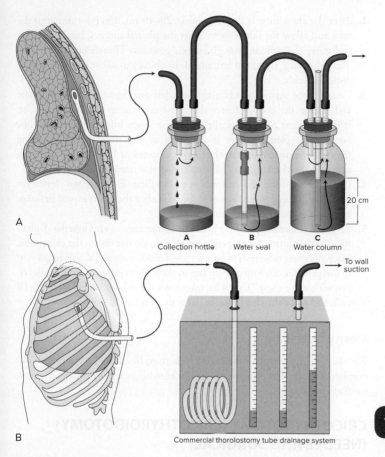

A

A
Collection bottle

B
Water seal

C
Water column

20 cm

To wall
suction

B

19

Commercial thorolostomy tube drainage system

Figure 19-14.2 **Panel A.** Diagram of tube thoracostomy and three-bottle suction apparatus. Bottle A is connected to the thoracostomy tube and collects pleural drainage for inspection and measurement of volume. Bottle B acts as a simple valve to prevent collapse of the lung if tubing distal to this point is opened to atmospheric pressure. Pulmonary air leak can be detected by the escape of bubbles from the submerged tube. Bottle C is a system for regulating the negative pressure delivered to the pleural space. Wall suction should be regulated to maintain continuous vigorous bubbling from the middle open tube in bottle C. The resulting negative pressure (in cm H_2O) is equal to the difference in the height of the fluid levels in bottles B and C. **Panel B.** The Pleur-evac system works in a similar manner graphically demonstrated in the lower panel). One end is attached to the chest tube and the other end is attached to suction. Each chamber of the Pleur-evac is filled with sterile water to the level noted in the manufacturer's instructions. (Reproduced with permission from Dunphy JE, Way LW. Current Surgical Diagnosis & Treatment, 5e, New York, NY: Lange; 1981.)

2. After the chest tube is in place, inject 20–40 mL 1% lidocaine into the tube and allow the lidocaine to enter the pleural space. Clamp the tube, and move the patient through various positions (Trendelenburg, reverse Trendelenburg, right and left lateral decubitus) to allow the lidocaine to disperse evenly.
3. Connect the syringe containing the sclerosing agent to the chest tube and release the clamp. Inject the agent and clamp the tube for 4 hr. It is important to use a sterile technique when injecting into the tube because the pleural cavity is sterile. If at any time during clamping the tube the patient experiences severe dyspnea or hypoxia, unclamp the tube because the lung may have collapsed and needs to be re-expanded.
4. Unclamp the tube and connect it to the Pleur-Evac suction device for 24–48 additional hours. Remove the tube after there is minimal drainage and a CXR shows no pneumothorax.
5. To prevent tension pneumothorax or subcutaneous emphysema if pleurodesis is performed for a persistent air leak, do not clamp the chest tube. Place the chest tube system on water-seal mode over an IV pole to prevent drainage of the sclerosing agent but to allow air to escape if pressure develops within the chest. After 4 hr, take down the tubing system from the IV pole and place the chest tube back on suction for 24–48 hr.

Complications

For chest tube placement in general: infection, bleeding, lung damage, SQ emphysema, persistent pneumothorax or hemothorax, poor tube placement, cardiac arrhythmia

CRICOTHYROTOMY (CRICOTHYROIDOTOMY) (NEEDLE AND SURGICAL)

Indications

- Immediate mechanical ventilation when an endotracheal or orotracheal tube cannot be placed (e.g., severe maxillofacial trauma, excessive oropharyngeal hemorrhage or swelling)

Contraindications

- There are no absolute contraindications to emergency cricothyroidotomy in adults.
- Relative contraindications include transection of the trachea, laryngotracheal disruption with retraction of the distal trachea into the mediastinum, or a fractured larynx.
- Child <12 yr (increased risk for developing subglottic stenosis); use needle approach instead.

Basic Materials

- Oxygen connecting tubing, high-flow oxygen source (tank or wall). Ventilation is most effective for the needle techniques if the cannula is attached to a high pressure (45 psi) jet ventilator
- Bag valve mask ventilator

Needle Cricothyroidotomy

- 12- to 14-gauge catheter-over-needle assembly (Angiocath or other)
- 6–12-mL syringe
- 3-mm pediatric ET adapter
- Prepackaged emergency "Cric" kits are available. Contents may vary, and some include a cuffed cricothyroidotomy cannula kit and others a needle cricothyrotomy, cannula kit which includes a special oxygen flow modulator. One kit is based on the Seldinger technique (Melker Cuffed Emergency Cricothyrotomy Catheter Set, Cook Medical) that includes a 6-mL syringe, an 18-gauge needle with overlying catheter, a guidewire, a tissue dilator, a modified cricothyroidotomy airway catheter, and tracheostomy tape.

Surgical Cricothyroidotomy (Minimum Requirements)

- Minor procedure and instrument tray (page 516) plus tracheal spreader if available
- No. 5–7 tracheostomy tube (6- to 8-Fr ET can be substituted)
- Tracheostomy tube adapter to connect to bag valve mask ventilator and oxygen source

19

Background

Cricothyrotomy (also called cricothyroidotomy) involves an incision in the cricothyroid membrane to establish an emergency airway. Cricothyrotomy is rarely performed (less than 0.3% of all emergency intubations) but serves as a lifesaving procedure of last resort in the patient when you cannot establish an airway by less aggressive means. Critical in performing the procedure is localization of the cricothyroid membrane, located about 2 cm caudal to the laryngeal prominence and can be identified by a slight depression in this area. Obesity can make this landmark difficult to identify. For those providers who are most likely to perform this rare procedure, reviewing the anatomy on a variety of patients and equipment on a recurring basis will help in the performance of this time-sensitive and stressful procedure. While formal "cric" kits are available, something as simple as a large-bore IV catheter to puncture the membrane can be lifesaving. Several different approaches to the procedure have been described with a few common variations presented here. The common procedures involve the use of a simple needle technique, a prepared cricothyroidotomy kit, and a surgical incision. Needle cricothyroidotomy techniques are arguably simpler and quicker to perform than the surgical approach.

Procedure

Needle Cricothyroidotomy

1. With the patient supine, place a roll behind the shoulders to gently hyperextend the neck if possible.
2. Palpate the cricothyroid membrane, which resembles a notch between the caudal end of the thyroid cartilage and the cricoid cartilage (see Figure 19-15A, page 559). Prep the area with povidone-iodine solution. Local anesthesia can be used if the patient is awake.
3. Mount the syringe on the 12- or 14-gauge catheter-over-needle assembly, and advance the syringe through the cricothyroid membrane at a 45-degree angle with the needle pointed inferiorly (toward the feet), applying back pressure on the syringe until air is aspirated.
4. Advance the catheter and remove the needle. Attach the hub to a 3-mm ET adapter that is connected to the oxygen tubing. Use a Y-connector or a hole in the side of the tubing to turn the flow on and off, allowing oxygen to flow at 15 L/min for 1–2 sec on, then 4 sec off.
5. The needle technique is only useful for up to 45 min because the exhalation of CO_2 is suboptimal if the upper airway is obstructed.

Needle Cricothyroidotomy Seldinger Technique

1. Follow steps 1 and 2 as for needle cricothyroidotomy. Open the prepared kit.
2. Follow the procedure outlined in Figure 19-15B, page 559.
3. Secure the airway catheter to the neck using the tape provided. Ventilate the patient with the Ambu bag and adapter.

Surgical Cricothyroidotomy

1. Surgical cricothyroidotomy should not be performed in prepubescent children because of the risk of damaging the cricoid cartilage. Follow steps 1 and 2 as for needle cricothyroidotomy.
2. Make a 2- to 3-cm transverse skin incision through the cervical fascia and strap muscles in the midline over the cricothyroid membrane (see Figure 19-15C, page 560.) Expose the cricothyroid membrane and make a horizontal incision. Insert the knife handle and rotate it 90 degrees to open the hole in the membrane. Use a hemostat or tracheal spreader to dilate the opening.

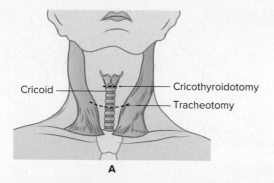

Figure 19-15A Neck anatomy indicating location of cricothyroidotomy (needle and surgical). The location where a formal non-emergent surgical tracheotomy incision would be placed is also shown. (Reproduced with permission from Troob S, Long S. Airway Management and Tracheostomy. In Lalwani AK, ed. Current Diagnosis & Treatment Otolaryngology—Head and Neck Surgery, 4e, New York, NY: McGraw-Hill; 2020.)

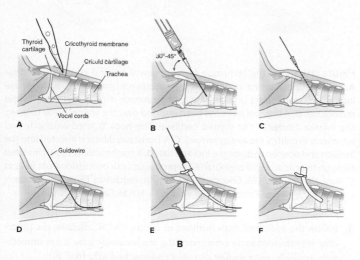

Figure 19-15B The percutaneous cricothyroidotomy using a cricothyroidotomy kit. **A.** A stab incision is made in the midline over the cricothyroid membrane. **B.** A catheter-over-the-needle is inserted at a 30- to 45-degree angle to the skin and advanced inferiorly. Negative pressure is applied to a saline-containing syringe during catheter insertion. Air bubbles in the saline confirm intratracheal placement of the catheter. **C.** The catheter has been advanced until the hub is against the skin. The needle and syringe have been removed. A guidewire is inserted through the catheter. **D.** The catheter has been removed, leaving the guidewire in place. **E.** The dilator/airway catheter unit is advanced over the guidewire and into the trachea. **F.** The guidewire and dilator have been removed, leaving the airway catheter in place. (Reproduced with permission from Boland C, Nasr NF, Voronov GG. Cricothyroidotomy. In: Reichman EF. eds. Reichman's Emergency Medicine Procedures, 3e, New York, NY: McGraw-Hill; 2018.)

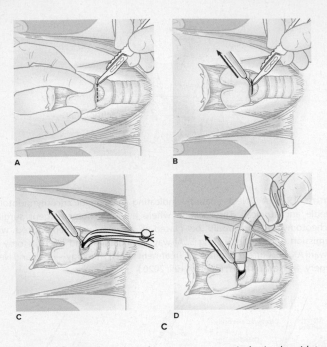

C

Figure 19-15C The technique for emergency surgical cricothyroidotomy. **A.** The nondominant hand stabilizes the cricothyroid membrane. A transverse incision is made through the skin, subcutaneous tissue, and cricothyroid membrane. **B.** A tracheal hook has been inserted over the scalpel blade to grasp the inferior border of the thyroid cartilage. The hook is lifted anteriorly and superiorly to control the airway (arrow). **C.** A Trousseau dilator is inserted into the incision and opened to dilate the incision site. **D.** A tracheostomy tube is inserted through the cricothyroid membrane. (Reproduced with permission from Boland C, Nasr NF, Voronov GG. Cricothyroidotomy. In: Reichman EF. eds. Reichman's Emergency Medicine Procedures, 3e, New York, NY: McGraw-Hill; 2018.)

3. Follow the additional steps outlined in Figure 19-15C. Because the procedure is performed in an emergency, if a tracheostomy tube is not immediately available, use a smaller diameter endotracheal tube (6–7 Fr).
4. Attach to an oxygen source and ventilate. Listen to the chest for symmetrical breath sounds.
5. A surgical cricothyroidotomy should be replaced with a formal tracheostomy after the patient's condition has stabilized, generally within 24–36 hr.

Complications

Bleeding, infection, esophageal perforation, tracheal bleeding, SQ emphysema, pneumomediastinum and pneumothorax, CO_2 retention (especially with the pure needle procedure).

CULDOCENTESIS

Indications

- Diagnostic technique for acute abdominal pain in women
- Evaluation of a female patient with signs of hypovolemia and possible intraabdominal bleeding
- Evaluation of ascites, especially if gynecologic malignant disease is suspected

Contraindications

- Cysts, masses, or other structures that might contaminate the peritoneal cavity if perforated
- A fixed retroverted uterus or a bleeding diathesis

Materials

- Vaginal Speculum
- Antiseptic swabs
- Chlorhexidine
- 1% lidocaine
- 18- to 21-gauge spinal needle
- Two (10 mL) syringes
- Tenaculum (a slender ring handle forecps with teeth at the tip fro grasping structures such as the cervix)

Procedure

1. Follow the basic principles of the pelvic exam (page 628). Perform a careful pelvic exam to document uterine position and rule out a pelvic mass at risk of perforation by the culdocentesis.
2. Obtain informed consent and prep the vagina with an antiseptic (e.g., chlorhexidine).
3. Using the long needle, inject 1% lidocaine submucosally in the posterior cervical fornix before applying the tenaculum.
4. Improve traction by applying the tenaculum to the posterior cervical lip.
5. Connect an 18- to 21-gauge spinal needle to a 10-mL syringe filled with 1 mL of air.
6. Moving the needle forward through the posterior cervical fornix, apply light pressure to the syringe until the air passes. Maintain traction on the tenaculum while advancing the spinal needle to maximize the surface area of the cul-de-sac for needle entry.
7. After the abdomen has been entered, ask the patient to elevate herself on her elbows to allow gravity drainage into the area of needle entry. Apply negative pressure to the syringe. Slowly rotating the needle and slowly removing it may aid in the detection and aspiration of a pocket of fluid.

19

8. If the first culdocentesis attempt is not successful, repeat the procedure with a different angle of approach.
9. Although perforation of a viscus is a possibility, the complication rate of culdocentesis is low. Fresh blood that clots rapidly is probably the result of a traumatic tap, and the procedure can be repeated.
10. If blood is aspirated, spin it for HCT, and place it in an empty glass test tube to determine the presence or absence of a clot. Failure of blood to clot suggests old hemorrhage.
11. If pus is aspirated, send specimens for aerobic and anaerobic bacteria and include cultures for *Neisseria gonorrhoeae* (GC), *Chlamydia, Mycoplasma,* and *Ureaplasma*.
12. If a malignant tumor is suspected, send fluid for cytologic evaluation.

Complications

Infection, hemorrhage, nerve injury, perforated viscus

DOPPLER PRESSURES

Indications

- Evaluation of peripheral vascular disease (ankle/brachial [A/B] or ankle/arm [A/I] index) (See also Chapter 20, page 678, Ankle Brachial Index)
- Routine BP measurement in infants or critically ill adults

Materials

- Doppler flow monitor
- Conductive gel (lubricant jelly can also be used)
- BP cuff

Procedure (A/B or A/I Index)

1. Determine the BP in each arm.
2. Measure the pressures in the popliteal arteries by placing a BP cuff on the thigh. The pressures in the dorsalis pedis arteries (on the top of the foot) and the posterior tibial arteries (behind the medial malleolus) are determined with a BP cuff on the calf. Ideally, measure these pressures with the patient in the supine position.
3. Apply conductive jelly and place the Doppler transducer over the artery. Inflate the BP cuff until the pulsatile flow is no longer heard. Deflate the cuff until the flow returns. This is the systolic, or Doppler, pressure. *Note:* The Doppler examination does not give the diastolic pressure, and a palpable pulse need not be present to perform Doppler studies.
4. The **A/B** or **A/I** index is often computed from Doppler pressure. It is equal to the best systolic pressure in the ankle (usually from the posterior tibial artery) divided by the systolic pressure in the arm. An A/B index

>0.9 is usually normal, and an index <0.7 is usually associated with significant symptomatic peripheral vascular disease and individuals might develop ulcers and gangrene. In patients with long-standing diabetes, the foot arteries can be severely calcified, and thus ankle systolic pressures may be falsely elevated because of the pressure needed to compress the calcified arteries while the patient may have severe small vessel disease putting the patient at risk for foot ulcers.

ELECTROCARDIOGRAM

Basic ECG interpretation is described in Chapter 27, starting on page 851.

Indications

- Evaluation of chest pain and other cardiac conditions

Materials

- ECG machine with paper and lead electrodes
- Adhesive electrode pads

Procedure

Most hospitals have fully automated ECG machines. Become acquainted with the machine at your hospital before using it. The following is a general outline.

1. Start with the patient in a comfortable, recumbent position. Explain the steps of the procedure to the patient. Instruct the patient to lie as still as possible to decrease tracing artifact.
2. Plug in the ECG machine and turn it on.
3. Attach the electrodes as follows:
   a. **Patient Cables.** A standard ECG machine has five lead wires, one for each limb and one for the chest leads. Newer machines have six precordial electrodes, all of which are placed in the proper positions before the procedure. The leads may be color-coded in the following manner:
      - RA (right arm): White
      - LA (left arm): Black
      - RL (right leg): Green
      - LL (left leg): Red
      - C (chest): Brown
   b. **Limb Electrodes.** Machines have disposable self-adhering electrode pads. Place each electrode on the limb indicated at the wrist or ankle, usually on the ventral surface. In case of amputation or presence of a cast, placing the lead on the shoulder or groin has minimal effect on the tracing.

19

c. **Chest (Precordial) Electrodes.** With newer machines, all leads can
   be placed before the ECG is run with all pads applied at the same
   time. This makes locating the proper positions quick and easy (Figure
   19-16). It is attached in sequence to each of the positions on the precordium. Precordial leads are placed as follows:
   - V_1 = fourth ICS just to the **right** of the sternal border
   - V_2 = fourth ICS just to the **left** of the sternal border
   - V_3 = midway between leads V_2 and V_4
   - V_4 = midclavicular line in the 5th ICS
   - V_5 = anterior axillary line at the same level as V_4
   - V_6 = midaxillary line at the same level as leads V_4 and V_5

4. When everything is ready, follow the directions for your particular
   machine to obtain the ECG tracing. It should include 12 leads: I, II, III,
   AVR, AVL, and V_1–V_6. Standard paper speed is 25 mm/s.

5. If the machine does not automatically label the tracing with the patient's
   name, date, and time be sure to do so manually and include any other
   useful information, such as medications, and your name. A routine
   12-lead ECG should take 4–8 min.

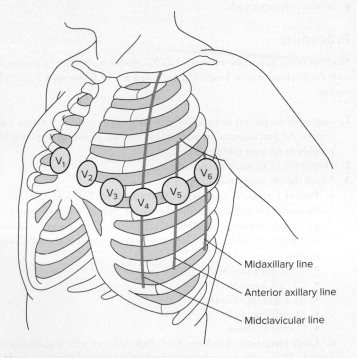

Figure 19-16. Location of the precordial chest leads used in obtaining a
routine 12 lead ECG.

Helpful Hints

1. The second rib inserts at the sternal angle, and therefore the second ICS is directly inferior to the sternal angle. Palpate two ICS inferiorly to identify the fourth ICS to position V_1 and V_2.
2. Learn the commonly used color scheme for the leads; doing so can be very useful in an emergency. Some memory aids for unmarked leads include:
   a. Red and green go to the legs: "Christmas on the bottom" or "When driving your car you use your left leg to brake (red light) and your right leg to go (green light)."
   b. Black (left) and white (right) go to the arms: "Remember white is right and black is left."
   c. Brown is for the chest.

ENDOTRACHEAL INTUBATION AND OTHER AIRWAY MANAGEMENT PROCEDURES*

(See also Chapter 28, page 914: Guidelines for Airway Management)

Indications

- Airway management during CPR.
- Anticipated clinical deterioration.
- Anatomic airway compromise: Neck trauma, angioedema/anaphylaxis, thermal or caustic exposures, mouth and neck infections, tumor, oral bleeding.
- Hypoxic or hypercarbic respiratory failure.
- Neurologic failure to protect the airway (disability): Intracranial catastrophes (stroke, trauma), profound central nervous system (CNS) depression, status epilepticus.
- Neuromuscular weakness syndromes (myasthenia gravis, amyotrophic lateral sclerosis [ALS], Guillain-Barré syndrome) may cause critical airway or breathing embarrassment, depending on whether they primarily insult airway reflexes or the muscles of respiration.
- Difficult fighting patient—especially with high concern for an associated dangerous condition—too agitated to properly manage without aggressive sedation. There is no role for the gag reflex in determining the need for endotracheal intubation or the patient's ability to protect their airway. A more reliable sign of the patient's capacity for airway protection is the ability for the patient to swallow secretions.

19

---

*Sections adapted from Oropello JM, Pastores SM, Kvetan V. eds. Critical Care, New York, NY: McGraw-Hill; 2020 and Tintinalli JE, Ma O, Yealy DM, Meckler GD, Stapczynski J, Cline DM, Thomas SH. Tintinalli's Emergency Medicine: A Comprehensive Study Guide, 9e, New York, NY: McGraw-Hill; 2020.

Special Considerations

The following are only relative contraindications to endotracheal intubation:
- Severe airway trauma or obstruction that does not permit safe passage of an endotracheal tube. Emergency surgical airway management (cricothyrotomy or tracheostomy) is indicated.
- Cervical spine injury can present challenges to endotracheal intubation. Minimizing cervical spine motion during intubation is critical. The induction must balance the concerns of cervical spine stability and preventing aspiration of gastric contents. Careful maintenance of in-line cervical immobilization has not been shown to lead to iatrogenic cervical spinal cord injury.

Background

Understanding safe and effective airway management is an essential skill for physicians and other providers who work in both the inpatient and outpatient environment. Knowledge and understanding of the indications for emergency airway intervention such as endotracheal intubation and other devices and techniques available for airway management are important to understand. While anesthesiologists, critical care, and emergency room providers are most likely to be called upon to address emergency airway issues, all healthcare providers may be called upon to assist in an emergency patient care situation with respiratory compromise ranging anywhere from an allergic reaction through major trauma or a resuscitation code event.

Immediate, definitive airway management is needed when the patient cannot protect his or her airway or is unable to adequately oxygenate or ventilate. Urgent airway management is indicated when a patient develops respiratory distress or when symptoms are progressing rapidly. In addition, airway management often is indicated when the patient appears clinically stable but the clinician anticipates clinical decline such as in the ICU setting or if an unprotected airway presents a risk to the patient who requires transport to another facility or to radiology for extensive diagnostic studies.

Materials (See Figure 19-17, page 568 and Table 19-4, page 567)

Note: Endotracheal intubation is considered an aerosolizing procedure as defined on page 508. If a patient is COVID-19 positive or under investigation for the coronavirus or other significant respiratory pathogen, maximum PPE (N95 mask plus a face shield or a powered air-purifying respirator [PAPR]) should be available to the team members in proximity or participating in the intubation. See page 508 for details on specific PPE. Table 19-4, page 567 is a list of the equipment that can be used for endotracheal intubation.

Table 19-4. Listing of Recommended Equipment for Endotracheal Intubation

- Appropriate Personal Protective Equipment (PPE)
- Essential equipment (see Figure 19-17, page 568)
- Oxygen source and tubing
- Endotracheal tubes (ETT)—various sizes based on anticipated needs (Figure 19-18A and Table 19-5, pages 569 and 578.)
- Stylets, assorted: To stiffen or angulate the ETT to facilitate placement (see Figure 19-18B, page 569)
- Laryngoscope (rigid) handle with batteries and a working backup (Figure 19-19, page 570)
- Laryngoscope blades (straight [Miller] or curved [Macintosh or "MAC"]); size no. 3 for adults, no. 1–1.5 for small children) (Figure 19-20, page 570)
- Bag valve mask; masks with various sizes and shapes should be available (Figure 19-21, page 571)
- Oropharyngeal airways—small, medium, large (Figure 19-22 A, page 572)
- Nasopharyngeal airways—small, medium, large (Figure 19-22 B, page 572)
- Suction catheters and suction source: Yankauer, tracheal suction catheters, nasogastric suction connection tubing for particulate matter and large amounts of vomitus
- Pulse oximetry monitoring system
- Carbon dioxide detector (end tidal CO_2/$EtCO_2$ monitor) (Figure 19-23, page 573)
- Syringes: 10 mL for endotracheal tube cuff inflation
- Magill forceps: A right-handed instrument angled in two planes, which allows for it to be used in the oropharynx and hypopharynx under direct vision during laryngoscopy to assist in ETT placement and to remove foreign bodies.
- Tongue blade
- Intubating stylet (gum elastic bougie): Also called an "introducer," is a device that allows a Seldinger-like technique of intubating a patient's airway. The device is inserted into the airway first, then an endotracheal tube is placed over the bougie into the airway, after which the device is removed. (See example in Figure 19-17, page 568.)
- Water-soluble lubricant or anesthetic jelly
- Rescue devices: Video laryngoscopes, supraglottic airways (e.g., laryngeal mask airway, King LT [King Systems, Noblesville, IN]) (Figure 19-24, page 574)
- Surgical cricothyroidotomy commercial kit (e.g., *Cook Melker Cricothyrotomy Catheter Set* that uses Seldinger wire placement technique, Figure 19-15B, page 559)
- Medications for topical airway anesthesia, sedation, and rapid-sequence intubation (RSI) (Table 19-6, page 583)

See Figure 19-17, page 568, for a graphical representation of the most essential equipment for endotracheal intubation. (ETT: endotracheal tube) (Adapted from Tintinalli JE, Ma O, Yealy DM, et al. Tintinalli's Emergency Medicine: A Comprehensive Study Guide, 9e, New York, NY: McGraw Hill; 2020.)

19

Procedure

1. Endotracheal intubation is sometimes referred to as **tracheal intubation.** **Orotracheal intubation** is most commonly used and is described here. **Nasotracheal intubation** is used with severe angioedema with resultant

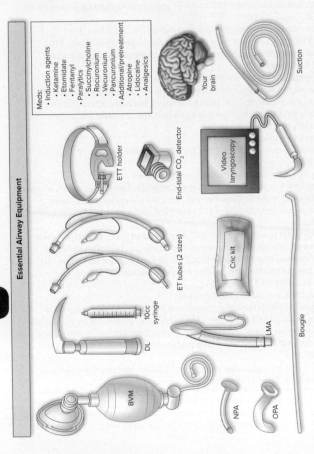

Essential Airway Equipment

Meds:
- Induction agents
  - Ketamine
  - Etomidate
  - Fentanyl
- Paralytics
  - Succinylcholine
  - Rocuronium
  - Vecuronium
  - Pancuronium
- Additional/pretreatment
  - Atropine
  - Lidocaine
  - Analgesics

Your brain

ET holder

End-tidal CO_2 detector

Video laryngoscopy

Suction

DL

10cc syringe

ET tubes (2 sizes)

Cric kit

LMA

NPA

OPA

BVM

Bougie

Figure 19-17. Graphical representation of some essential equipment for endotracheal intubation with a more complete listing in Table 19-4, page 567. Endotracheal tube selection should be based on Table 19-5, page 578. Medications noted are some agents that may be used if rapid sequence intubation (RSI) is planned. BVM: bag valve mask; DL: direct laryngoscope; ET: endotracheal; NPA: nasopharyngeal airway; OPA: oropharyngeal airway; Cric kit: cricothyrotomy kit; LMA: laryngeal mask airway. (Reproduced with permission from Stone CK, Humphries RL. Compromised Airway in CURRENT Diagnosis & Treatment: Emergency Medicine, 8e, New York, NY: McGraw-Hill 2020.)

19

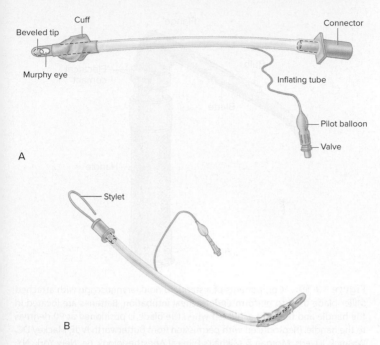

Figure 19-18   A. Endotracheal tubes (ETTs) are most commonly made from polyvinyl chloride. The patient end of the tube is beveled to aid visualization and insertion through the vocal cords. Murphy ETT have a hole (the "Murphy eye") to decrease the risk of occlusion, should the distal tube opening abut the carina or trachea. **B.** The shape and rigidity of ETTs can be altered by inserting a malleable stylet to facilitate passage through the vocal cords. (Reproduced with permission from Butterworth IV JF, Mackey DC, Wasnick JD, eds. Morgan & Mikhail's Clinical Anesthesiology, 6e, New York, NY: McGraw-Hill; 2018.)

19

tongue or lip swelling, severe trismus, or oral cancer, severe oral facial trauma or with fiber-optic intubation. As noted, nasotracheal intubation was once advocated in suspected cervical spine injury, but recent studies suggest properly performed orotracheal intubation is preferred over nasotracheal intubation.

2. **If endotracheal intubation is being considered in the emergency care setting, first assess the patient and their airway.**
   a. Determine the patient's level of consciousness and note the presence of respirations and grade respiratory effort. In patients with known or suspected cervical spine (C-spine) injury, all assessments and maneuvers should be undertaken with the C-spine immobilized in a neutral position to prevent spinal cord injury. The use of flexible fiber-optic bronchoscopy or video laryngoscopy to perform intubation can be considered, although no clear difference in outcome has been demonstrated

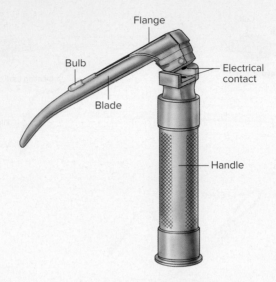

Flange

Bulb

Blade

Electrical contact

Handle

Figure 19-19. Components of a standard rigid laryngoscope with attached Miller blade used to perform endotracheal intubation. Batteries are located in the handle and the light activated when the blade is positioned at 90 degrees to the handle. (Reproduced with permission from Butterworth IV JF, Mackey DC, Wasnick JD, eds. Morgan & Mikhail's Clinical Anesthesiology, 6e, New York, NY: McGraw-Hill; 2018.)

19

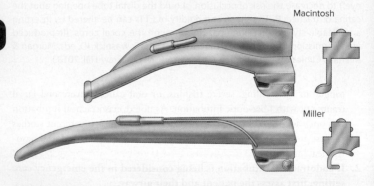

Macintosh

Miller

Figure 19-20. Laryngoscope blades commonly used in endotracheal intubation. Curved or Macintosh blade and the straight or Miller blade are connected to a standard rigid laryngoscope (Figure 19-19). To visualize the vocal cords the curved Macintosh blade is placed anterior to the epiglottis into the vallecula, while the straight Miller blade is passed under the epiglottis. See Figure 19-28, page 579, for further details on blade insertion. (Reproduced with permission from Butterworth IV JF, Mackey DC, Wasnick JD, eds. Morgan & Mikhail's Clinical Anesthesiology, 6e, New York, NY: McGraw-Hill; 2018.).

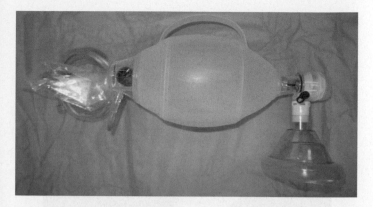

Figure 19-21. Example of a bag valve mask also known by a common manufacturer's name as an "Ambu bag" used to ventilate patients. Bag valve masks contain a self-inflating insufflation device coupled with a facemask and a valve to prevent reinhalation of exhaled air. Typically used with supplemental oxygen, the mask can be removed and the device placed on the end of the endotracheal tube for manual ventilation. (Reproduced with permission from Tintinalli JE, Ma O, Yealy DM, Meckler GD, Stapczynski J, Cline DM, Thomas SH. Tintinalli's Emergency Medicine: A Comprehensive Study Guide, 9e, New York, NY: McGraw Hill; 2020.)

compared to direct laryngoscopy with cervical in-line stabilization. In the setting of complete cardiopulmonary arrest, CPR and resuscitation protocols are discussed in Chapter 29, Common Emergencies, page 965.

b. In the apneic, unconscious patient without C-spine injury use the **chin-lift maneuver** to open the airway (Figure 19-25A, page 575). For patients with potential C-spine injuries, some advocate that the **jaw-thrust maneuver** should be used, with some studies suggesting the chin lift is also acceptable. Jaw-thrust involves placing the index and middle fingers to physically push the posterior aspects of the lower jaw upwards while the thumbs push down on the chin to open the mouth (Figure 19-25B, page 575). With forward displacement of the mandible, the tongue is pulled forward and prevents it from obstructing the trachea. Clear the airway of obstructions, including dentures, and use a rigid suction catheter to remove any blood, vomitus, or secretions from the oropharynx. Remove any large visible obstructing foreign bodies from the oropharynx manually or, if available, with Magill forceps. A "blind finger sweep" of the oropharynx if foreign body is suspected is discouraged.

c. If the patient remains apneic, begin ventilation using a bag-valve-mask device with supplemental oxygen. Place the head in the **"sniffing position"** in preparation for endotracheal intubation (Figure 19-26,

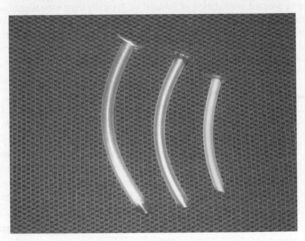

A

B

Figure 19-22. Basic airway devices to relieve upper airway obstruction from collapsed pharyngeal tissues. **A.** Oral (oropharyngeal) airways. **B.** Nasal (nasopharyngeal) airways. (Reproduced with permission from Stone CK and Humphries RL, eds. CURRENT Diagnosis & Treatment: Emergency Medicine, 8e. Copyright © 2017 by McGraw-Hill Education, Inc.)

page 576). In the **sniffing position**, the head is slightly extended, and the neck is flexed on the shoulders. This aligns the axis of the airway with the mouth and pharynx, facilitating direct visualization of the vocal cords during intubation. It is particularly important in young children and infants, in whom the larynx is considerably more

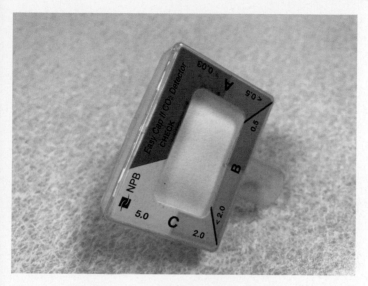

Figure 19-23. Carbon dioxide colormetric detector (end tidal CO_2/EtCO$_2$ monitor) helps rapidly verify correct endotracheal tube placement. This device attaches directly to the endotracheal tube and responds to exhaled CO_2 by changing from purple to yellow suggesting proper tracheal placement. (Reproduced with permission from Tintinalli JE, Ma O, Yealy DM, Meckler GD, Stapczynski J, Cline DM, Thomas SH. Tintinalli's Emergency Medicine: A Comprehensive Study Guide, 9e, New York, NY: McGraw Hill; 2020.)

anterior. Placing a pad underneath the occiput will lift the head and align the ear with the sternal notch, facilitating optimal positioning for intubation. This position cannot be used when there is cervical spine injury. The various bag-valve-mask techniques using one hand or two hands to maintain the airway are demonstrated in Figure 19-27, page 577.

3. **The basic techniques for endotracheal intubation are similar in the emergency and controlled settings.** Specific considerations for intubation in the ICU setting are discussed in Chapter 28, page 914. In the Emergency Department rapid sequence intubation (RSI) may be employed and is discussed below. For the student learning endotracheal intubation, the best opportunity is to practice on the many simulators available and consider an elective anesthesia rotation in the operating room, which provides the most optimum and controlled experience for working with patients.

4. **Before attempting endotracheal intubation, oxygen should be supplied, either with a mask like a nonrebreather in spontaneously breathing patients or with small tidal volumes using positive pressure**

19

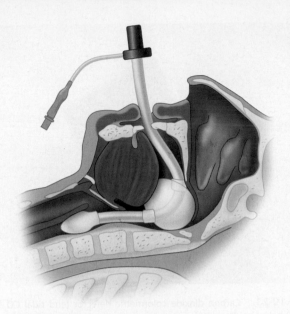

Figure 19-24. King Systems Airway (King-LT) (Ambu US Columbia, MD). The tube has ventilation ports between two inflatable cuffs. The distal cuff seals the esophagus and the prominal cuff seals the oropharynx. (Reproduced with permission from Butterworth IV JF, Mackey DC, Wasnick JD, eds. Morgan & Mikhail's Clinical Anesthesiology, 6e, New York, NY: McGraw-Hill; 2018.)

19

with a bag-valve-mask until expert help arrives. Begin preoxygenation as soon as possible before intubation, even for patients with no apparent hypoxia or hypoxemia. The technique for bag-valve-mask ventilation is demonstrated in Figure 19-27, page 577. Administer 100% oxygen for at least 3 min using a mask supplied with at least 15 L/min of oxygen. The American Society of Anesthesiologists' difficult airway algorithm should be followed, and both facemask and a supraglottic airway device, such as a laryngeal mask airway, should be immediately available.

5. Extend the laryngoscope blade to 90 degrees to verify the light is working. The light intensity should remain constant with a blinking light suggesting a poor electrical contact, and a fading light indicates depleted batteries. Confirm all necessary items are readily available. A backup laryngoscope and several different size and style blades should be available. The appropriately sized endotracheal tube should be available based on Table 19-5, page 578.

6. Place the patient's head in the "sniffing position" (neck extended anteriorly and the head extended posteriorly) (Figure 19-26, page 576). This brings the oral axis and the pharyngeal axes into better alignment, facilitating visualization of the vocal cords as demonstrated in Figure 19-28, page 579.

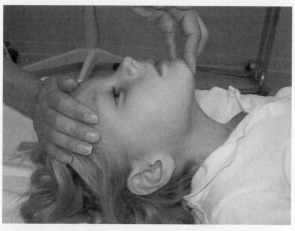

A

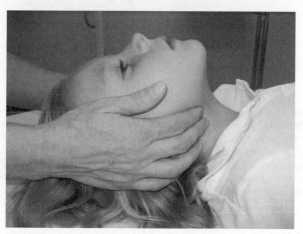

B

Figure 19-25   A. Opening the airway with the head tilt and chin lift in patients without concern for spinal trauma: gently lift the chin with one hand and push down on the forehead with the other hand. **B.** Opening the airway with jaw thrust in patients with concern for spinal trauma: lift the angles of the mandible moving the lower incisors superiorly compared to the inferior incisors; this moves the jaw and tongue forward and opens the airway without bending the neck. (Reproduced with permission from Hay Jr. WW, Levin MJ, Abzug MJ, Bunik M, eds. Current Diagnosis & Treatment: Pediatrics, 25e, New York, NY: McGraw-Hill; 2020.)

19

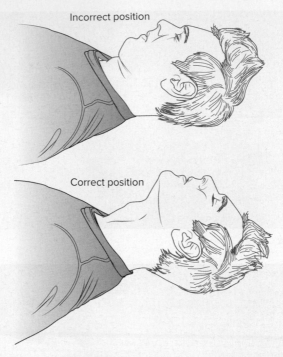

Incorrect position

Correct position

Figure 19-26. The sniffing position (designated as the "correct position"), a combination of flexion of the neck and extension of the head, helps to open the airway and is considered to be the optimum position for direct laryngoscopy and endotracheal intubation. In the "incorrect position," the airway is likely obstructed. (Reproduced with permission from Stone CK, Humphries RL. Compromised Airway in CURRENT Diagnosis & Treatment: Emergency Medicine, 8e, New York, NY: McGraw-Hill; 2020.)

19

7. Hold the laryngoscope in your left hand. Hold the mouth open with your right hand with a scissor motion to open the mouth and facilitate laryngoscope passage. The **"scissor maneuver"** is best done by pressing caudally on the patient's lower incisors with the operator's thumb and cranially on the patient's upper incisors with the operator's index or middle finger (see Figure 19-29, page 580). The right hand can also be used to manipulate the larynx to enhance visualization and to insert the ETT.

8. Use the blade to push the tongue to the patient's left while keeping it anterior to the blade (Figure 19-30, page 581). Advance the blade carefully toward the midline until the epiglottis is visualized. Use suction if needed to clear the airway.

9. At this point the procedure varies based on the style of blade used, curved or straight (Figure 19-20, page 570). If a **straight laryngoscope blade**

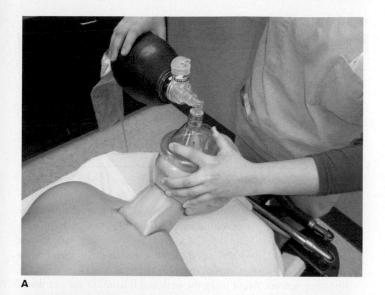

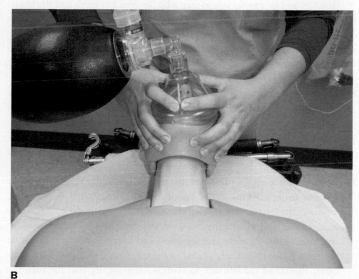

Figure 19-27. **A.** One-person bag-valve-mask ventilation. **B.** Two-handed mask seal. Note the proper hand position to maintain the airway. (Reproduced with permission from Tracheal Intubation in Tintinalli JE, Ma O, Yealy DM, Meckler GD, Stapczynski J, Cline DM, Thomas SH. Tintinalli's Emergency Medicine: A Comprehensive Study Guide, 9e, New York, NY: McGraw Hill; 2020.)

19

Table 19-5. Recommended Endotracheal Tube Sizes Based on Age

Patient	Internal Diameter (mm)	
Premature infant	2.5-3.0	(uncuffed)
Newborn infant	3.5	(uncuffed)
3-12 mo	4.0	(uncuffed)
1-8 y	4.0-6.0	(uncuffed)[a]
8-16 y	6.0-7.0	(cuffed)
Adult	7.0-9.0	(cuffed)

[a]Rough estimate is to measure the little finger.

(Miller) is used, pass it under the epiglottis and **lift** upward to visualize the vocal cords. If the **curved blade (Macintosh)** is used, place it anterior to the epiglottis (into the vallecula) and gently lift anteriorly (Figure 19-30, page 581). In either case, **do not use the handle to displace the epiglottis,** but rather gently lift to expose the vocal cords (i.e., minimize torqueing action). Avoid using the teeth as a fulcrum to prevent dental damage, and be careful not to trap a lip between the teeth and the blade.

10. To decrease the risk of aspiration, have an assistant place firm pressure over the cricoid cartilage to occlude the esophagus and help prevent aspiration during intubation (**Sellick maneuver**). This cricoid pressure can also facilitate visualization of the vocal cords in patients whose larynx is situated more anteriorly than usual, such as in children.

11. While maintaining visualization of the cords, pass the ETT through the vocal cords. The critical anatomy is demonstrated in Figure 19-30, page 581. With more difficult intubations, a malleable stylet may be used to direct the endotracheal tube (Figure 19-18B, page 569). Correct ETT placement in the adult is a minimum of 2 cm above the carina (approximately 23 cm at the incisors in men and 21 cm in women).

12. When using a cuffed tube (adults and older children), gently inflate with air using a 10-mL syringe until the seal is adequate (about 5 mL). Connect the circuit to the end of the ETT and ventilate the patient while auscultating and visualizing both sides of the chest to verify positioning. Auscultate the right and left chest and over the stomach to ensure the tube is not mistakenly placed in the esophagus. (Figure 19-31, page 584). Failure of the left side to ventilate may signify that the tube has been advanced down the right mainstem bronchus. If this is a concern, withdraw the tube 1–2 cm, and recheck the breath sounds. Use an end tidal CO_2 ($EtCO_2$) monitor colorimetric device to confirm the placement of the tube by connecting the device to the ETT between the adapter and the ventilating device (Figure 19-23, page 573). Point-of-care ultrasonography has been used for confirmation of ETT placement by imaging the trachea and/or lungs after intubation.

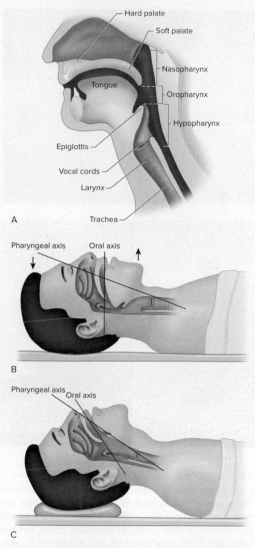

Figure 19-28. **A.** Anatomy of the airway and key structures to identify in endotracheal intubation. **B.** In preparation for endotracheal intubation the **sniffing position** with the head extended and the neck flexed in the direction of the arrows. C (bold C). This aligns the axis of the airway with the mouth and pharynx, facilitating direct visualization of the cords during intubation. (Panel A reproduced with permission from Butterworth IV JF, Mackey DC, Wasnick JD, eds. Morgan & Mikhail's Clinical Anesthesiology, 6e, New York, NY: McGraw-Hill; 2018; Panel B/C reproduced with permission from Oropello JM, Pastores SM, Kvetan V, eds. Critical Care, New York, NY: McGraw-Hill; 2020.)

19

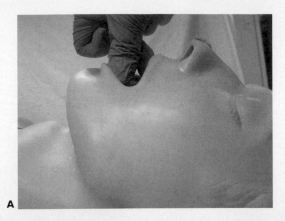

A

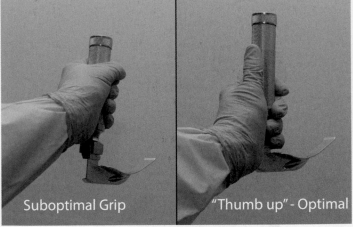

Suboptimal Grip   "Thumb up"- Optimal

B

Figure 19-29. **A.** The "scissor maneuver" is used to hold the mouth open to facilitate passage of the laryngoscope. It is usually performed using the right hand while the laryngoscope is held in the left hand. **B.** The laryngoscope should be gripped as low as possible in the left hand with the thumb extended for optimal control. This makes a natural extension of the forearm. (Panel A reproduced with permission from Stone CK and Humphries RL, eds. CURRENT Diagnosis & Treatment: Emergency Medicine, 8e, Copyright © 2017 by McGraw-Hill Education, Inc.; Panel B reproduced with permission from Knoop KJ, Stack LB, Storrow AB, Thurman R, eds. The Atlas of Emergency Medicine, 4e, New York, NY: McGraw-Hill; 2018.)

13. Use commercial EET tube holder (shown in Figure 19-17, page 568), adhesive tape, or umbilical tape to secure the tube. Do not tape to the vermillion border of the lip, as this will create trauma. Tape only to intact skin. Note the position of the properly inserted ETT at the lips in case

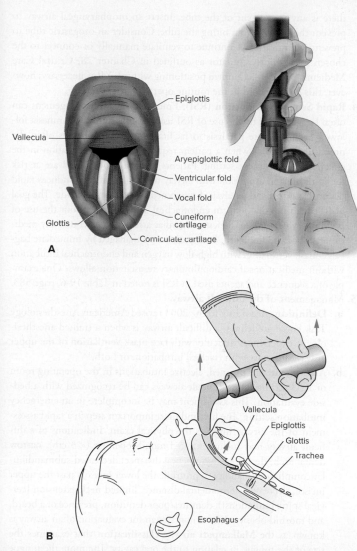

Figure 19-30.   A. Typical view of the glottis during laryngoscopy. The blade pushes the tongue to patient's left while keeping it anterior to the blade before the endotracheal tube is passed through the vocal cords. **B.** The curved Macintosh laryngoscope blade is passed into the mouth trough the pharynx with the tip of a curved blade is usually inserted into the vallecula. If the straight Miller blade tip is used, it would cover the epiglottis. With either blade, the handle is raised up and away from the patient in a plane perpendicular to the patient's mandible to expose the vocal cords. (Panel A reproduced with permission from Butterworth IV JF, Mackey DC, Wasnick JD, eds. Morgan & Mikhail's Clinical Anesthesiology, 6e, New York, NY: McGraw-Hill; 2018.)

there is any movement of the tube. Insert an oropharyngeal airway to prevent the patient from biting the tube. Consider an orogastric tube to prevent regurgitation. Continue to ventilate manually or connect to the chosen mechanical ventilator as outlined in Chapter 28, Critical Care Medicine, page 914. Confirm positioning with a CXR if necessary; however, this not standard in the routine operating room setting.

14. **Rapid Sequence Induction (RSI).** Emergency airway management can often be facilitated by the use of RSI using agents to induce amnesia followed by immediate paralysis to facilitate intubation. This is often the procedure of choice when a patient requires emergent intubation in the emergency department setting. Patients who have not fasted are at risk for vomiting and aspiration with airway manipulation. RSI induces rapid unconsciousness and paralysis through neuromuscular blockade. The goal of RSI is to rapidly perform endotracheal intubation without the use of preliminary ventilation. Patients in cardiac arrest do not require any medications prior to intubation. Such patients are managed by immediate bag-valve-mask ventilation with high-flow oxygen and endotracheal intubation without medications if cardiopulmonary resuscitation allows. One example of a sequence and agents used in RSI is noted in Table 19-6, page 583.

15. **Management of the difficult airway.**
    a. **Definition.** According to the 2003 revised American Anesthesiology Task Force guidelines, a difficult airway is when a trained anesthesiologist experiences difficulty with face mask ventilation of the upper airway, difficulty with tracheal intubation, or both.**
    b. **Assessment.** For planned, elective intubations in the operating room or ICU setting, most difficult airways can be recognized with a bedside evaluation. This assessment may be incomplete in an emergency intubation setting. The first and most important step in a rapid assessment of the airway involves the physical exam. Indications of a difficult airway may include limited mouth opening (<3 cm), narrow dental arch, decreased thyromental distance, decreased submandibular compliance (inability to protrude the lower incisors past the upper incisor, decreased sternomental distance, limited neck extension [cervical spine limitations]), dentures/poor dentition, presence of a beard, and morbid obesity. A common system for evaluation of an airway is known as the **Mallampati airway classification** that examines the size of the tongue in relation to the oral cavity. The more the tongue obstructs the view of the pharyngeal structures, the more difficult intubation may be (Figure 19-32, page 585). Class 1 suggests an easy intubation, while Class 4 predicts a more difficult intubation.
    c. **Management options.** The following are some options for emergency endotracheal intubation in the setting of a difficult airway. It is recommended that these devices be readily available during any attempt at intubation.

**Apfelbaum JL, et al. Practice guidelines for management of the difficult airway: An updated report by the American Society of Anesthesiologists Task Force on Management of the Difficult Airway. Anesthesiology. 2013;118(2):251–270.

Table 19-6. Rapid Sequence Induction (RSI) and Endotracheal Intubation

1. **Preparation**
   a. Obtain IV access; monitor EKG, blood pressure, and pulse oximetry.
   b. Prepare equipment
      i. Make sure to prepare a rescue/backup airway device or technique
   c. Place patient in the best position for success (supine, head in sniffing position if no cervical spine injury suspected)
2. **Preoxygenation**
   a. With spontaneous breathing: provide high concentration O_2 with a non-rebreather mask
   b. Apnea or profound hypoventilation: provide cautious or no ventilations with bag valve mask attached to 100% O_2 (use cricoid pressure to reduce abdominal distension)
3. **Pretreatment**
   a. **LOAD**
      i. **L**idocaine: 1–1.5 mg/kg IV (blunt sympathetic response to intubation)
      ii. **O**pioids- Fentanyl: 1–1.5 mcg/kg IV (blunt sympathetic response to intubation)
      iii. **A**tropine: 0.01 mg/kg IV – use in children and in those receiving more than one succinylcholine dose
      iv. **D**efasciculating agent – provide a fraction of paralyzing dose a few minutes prior to induction
4. **Paralysis with induction**
   a. Choose an induction agent (etomidate, ketamine, or propofol)
      i. Etomidate: 0.1–0.3 mg/kg IV (preserves cardiovascular function; causes adrenal suppression)
      ii. Ketamine: 1–2 mg/kg IV (sympathomimetic; bronchodilator; mostly preserves cardiovascular function; can cause hallucinations and nightmares)
      iii. Propofol: 1.5–2 mg/kg IV (causes cardiovascular depression and hypotension; only use if not concerned about hypotension or in patients with good cardiovascular function)
   b. Choose a neuromuscular blocking agent
      i. Depolarizing – Succinylcholine: 1–2 mg/kg IV
      ii. Nondepolarizing
         1. Rocuronium: 1.2 mg/kg IV
         2. Vecuronium: 0.2 mg/kg IV
5. **Protection**
   a. Apply cricoid pressure to prevent aspiration of gastric contents
6. **Placement of the endotracheal tube and confirmation**
   a. Intubate using direct laryngoscopy, video laryngoscopy, or flexible fiberoptic bronchoscopy
   b. Confirm placement with $EtCO_2$ monitoring
7. **Post-intubation management**
   a. Note tube depth and secure tube with tape or a commercial device
   b. Inform treating team of need for ongoing sedation
   c. Patient disposition as appropriate

19

i. **Noninvasive positive-pressure ventilation (NIPPV)** provides positive-pressure airway support through a face or nasal mask without the use of an endotracheal tube or other airway device. In adults, NIPPV includes **continuous positive airway pressure**

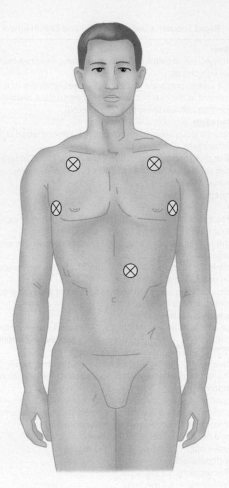

Figure 19-31. Auscultation points to confirm proper endotracheal tube placement. The epigastric ascultation point helps identify incorrect esophageal intubation. (Reproduced with permission from Butterworth IV JF, Mackey DC, Wasnick JD, eds. Morgan & Mikhail's Clinical Anesthesiology, 6e, New York, NY: McGraw-Hill; 2018.)

(CPAP) and **bilevel positive airway pressure (BiPAP)**. NIPPV helps to augment spontaneous respirations. Ideal patients for NIPPV are cooperative, have protective airway reflexes, and have intact ventilatory efforts. NIPPV is not appropriate in patients who have absent or agonal respiratory effort, impaired or absent gag reflex, altered mental status, severe maxillofacial trauma, potential basilar skull fracture, life-threatening epistaxis, or bullous lung

Class I   Class II   Class III   Class IV

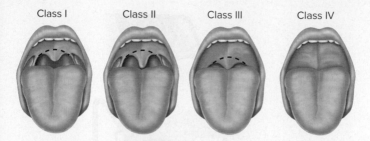

Figure 19-32. The Mallampati scoring system for determining a difficult airway for endotracheal intubation. Class I: The entire palatal arch, including the bilateral faucial pillars, is visible down to the bases of the pillars. Class II: The upper part of the faucial pillars and most of the uvula are visible. Class III: Only the soft and hard palates are visible. Class IV: Only the hard palate is visible. (Reproduced with permission from Tracheal Intubation, Tintinalli JE, Ma O, Yealy DM, et al. Tintinalli's Emergency Medicine: A Comprehensive Study Guide, 9e, New York, NY: McGraw Hill Educational; 2020.)

disease. CPAP delivers a constant positive pressure throughout the respiratory cycle. BiPAP provides different levels of positive airway pressure during inspiration (inspiratory positive airway pressure [IPAP]) and expiration (expiratory positive airway pressure). Occasionally, patients develop anxiety and agitation during NIPPV treatment due to the claustrophobic feeling of the mask or the discomfort of positive-pressure ventilation. Anxiety and agitation can increase the work of breathing and result in NIPPV asynchrony. Although often relieved with encouragement and verbal support, this may require sedatives or anxiolytics.

ii. **Video laryngoscopes (VLs)** use an integrated high-resolution camera and video monitor to facilitate indirect glottic visualization and ETT placement. VLs create a magnified view of the airway with many commercial devices being available (Figure 19-33, page 586). The GlideScope Video Laryngoscope (Verathon, Inc., Bothell, WA) has a one-piece rigid plastic handle and curved blade with a bedside video screen connected by a cable. The McGrath MAC Video Laryngoscope (Medtronic, Minneapolis, MN) also has a curved blade and attached video monitor. While initially used for the difficult airway intubation, many providers use these as a primary laryngoscope for intubation.

iii. **The flexible fiber-optic bronchoscope (FFB)** uses fiber-optic technology embedded in a flexible tube to facilitate visualization of and access to the airway. Newer flexible scopes use video technology, not fiber-optics, and interface directly with VL monitors. FFB is often easiest through the nasal route, allowing easier midline

19

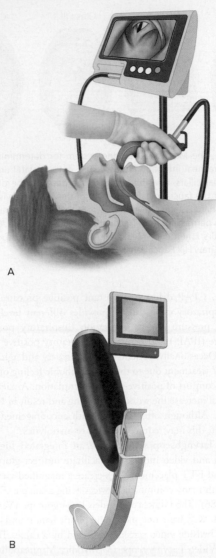

A

B

Figure 19-33. Video laryngoscope examples. **A.** The GlideScope Video Laryngoscope (Verathon, Inc., Bothell, WA) has a one-piece rigid plastic handle and curved blade with the light and camera eye at the tip. The image is transmitted to a screen at bedside. **B.** McGrath MAC Video Laryngoscope (Medtronic, Minneapolis, MN) features a curved blade and intrinsic video monitor. (Reproduced with permission from Butterworth IV JF, Mackey DC, Wasnick JD, eds. Morgan & Mikhail's Clinical Anesthesiology, 6e, New York, NY: McGraw-Hill; 2018.)

airway positioning and entry of the glottis at a less acute angle. Once the scope is through the vocal cords, pass the ETT over the scope in Seldinger fashion and remove the scope.

 iv. **Use of a supraglottic airways** such as a laryngeal mask airway or LMA. Supraglottic airways are discussed below.

 v. **Invasive surgical airway including needle or surgical cricothyrotomy or tracheostomy as a last resort.** See Cricothyrotomy (Cricothyroidotomy) (Needle and Surgical), pages 559–560.

16. **Additional airway management devices and techniques**

 a. **Bag-Valve-Mask.** Bag-valve-masks (Figure 19-21, page 571) contain a self-inflating bag coupled with a facemask and a valve to prevent rebreathing. The device can be connected to an endotracheal tube or supraglottic airway to mechanically ventilate a patient. Although typically used with supplemental oxygen, the bag-valve-mask can be life-saving even when used with room air. Most bag-valve-mask systems deliver approximately 75% oxygen with optimal use.

 b. **Oropharyngeal (Oral) Airway.** An oropharyngeal or oral airway (Figure 19-22A, page 572, and Figure 19-34A, page 588) is a curved, rigid device used to prevent the base of the tongue from occluding the hypopharynx. Use only in a comatose or deeply obtunded patient without a gag reflex. May be used along with an endotracheal tube in an intubated patient to prevent tube occlusion from biting. To determine the appropriate size of the oropharyngeal airway, hold the airway beside the patient's cheek with the flange at the corner of the mouth. The tip of an appropriately sized airway should just reach the angle of the mandibular ramus.

 c. **Nasopharyngeal (Nasal) Airway.** A nasopharyngeal or nasal airway (Figure 19-22B, page 572, and Figure 19-34B, page 588) is pliable and inserted into the nostril, displacing the soft palate and posterior tongue. Nasal airways are helpful in patients with an intact gag reflex. Nasopharyngeal airways can be used in some settings where oropharyngeal airways cannot be visualized, such as oral trauma or trismus (restriction of mouth opening including spasm of muscles of mastication). Nasopharyngeal airways may also help facilitate bag-valve-mask ventilation. To determine the appropriate size of the airway, when held against the side of the face, a correctly sized airway will extend from the tip of the nose to the tragus of the ear. Lubrication of the nasopharyngeal airway prior to insertion is helpful.

 d. **Supraglottic airway devices (SGAs),** sometimes called extraglottic airway devices, are devices placed in the oropharynx that sit above the trachea, allowing for oxygenation and ventilation without the visualized insertion of a tube into the trachea. SGAs can be a bridge to endotracheal intubation, a rescue device after unsuccessful intubation efforts, or a method of facilitating ventilation during general anesthesia. Although SGAs provide adequate oxygenation and ventilation

19

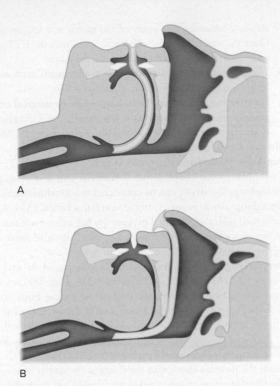

A

B

Figure 19-34. **A.** The oropharyngeal airway in place. The airway follows the curvature of the tongue, pulling it and the epiglottis away from the posterior pharyngeal wall and providing a channel for air passage. **B.** The nasopharyngeal airway in place. The airway passes through the nose and extends to just above the epiglottis. (Reproduced with permission from Butterworth IV JF, Mackey DC, Wasnick JD, eds. Morgan & Mikhail's Clinical Anesthesiology, 6e, New York, NY: McGraw-Hill; 2018.)

for short periods of time, they are not usually used for prolonged ventilation. A SGA may be used during general anesthesia for shorter-duration cases. SGAs should not be used in any patient needing high inspiratory pressures (e.g., adult respiratory distress syndrome), morbidly obese patients, and in patients with a full stomach. SGAs are most often placed in apneic, unconscious patients, as their large cuffs can cause gagging and discomfort in awake patients. In general, SGAs have a higher risk of aspiration than cuffed endotracheal tubes, and the large cuffs may cause hypopharyngeal mucosal damage. Thus, endotracheal tubes are better suited for long-term ventilation. There are many different designs and manufacturers of these devices. A few common devices are listed here.

i. ***Laryngeal Mask Airway (LMA™):*** Was the first laryngeal airway and LMA is a registered trademark. It consists of an inflatable silicone mask and rubber connecting tube (Figure 19-35, page 590). Many design modifications of the classic LMA are now available, such as the LMA ProSeal, LMA FasTrach, or the LMA Supreme. Inserted blindly into the pharynx, a cuff is inflated that forms a low-pressure seal around the laryngeal inlet, allowing gentle positive-pressure ventilation. *Note:* The black line on the airway tube must be oriented toward the upper lip, and a bite block must be in place. Aspiration may be less common with an LMA than with a bag mask.

ii. ***Esophagotracheal Airway (Combitube or ETC):*** A multilumen airway that consists of a single, dual-lumen tube (esophageal/tracheal) with two cuffs designed for blind placement. After placement, port 1 (blue pilot balloon) is inflated with 100 mL of air, then port 2 (white pilot balloon) is inflated with 15 mL of air. Ventilate through the longer blue tube 1; if breath sounds are heard, and auscultation of gastric insufflation is negative, continue ventilation. If auscultation of breath sounds is negative and auscultation of gastric insufflation positive, ventilate through the shorter clear tube 2. It is used in emergency medicine and prehospital settings since placing it does therefore not require laryngoscopy or additional equipment. The Combitube is also used as a rescue device in difficult airway algorithms (Figure 19-36, page 593).

iii. ***King Systems Airway (King-LT):*** A single-lumen supraglottic airway designed to be blindly inserted into the pharynx. Choose correct size (sized based on patient height: yellow 4–5 ft, red 5–6 ft), and using a lateral approach with your dominant hand holding the tube at the connector. Open airway with chin lift and advance tube behind tongue while rotating tube back to midline so the blue orientation line faces patient's chin. Advance tube until connector is aligned with teeth or gums and inflate balloon with 60 cm H_2O. Attach bag-valve-mask and while gently bagging patient, withdraw King LT until ventilation is easy. Add more air to balloon if needed to maximize seal (Figure 19-24, page 574).

19

Complications

See Table 19-7, page 591, for common complications, prevention, and management of endotracheal intubation. Key concepts in airway management include:

- While the persistent detection of CO_2 is the best confirmation of tracheal placement of an ETT, it cannot exclude endobronchial intubation. In addition to asymmetric ventilation and unilateral breath sounds, other early signs of endobronchial intubation may include an increase in peak

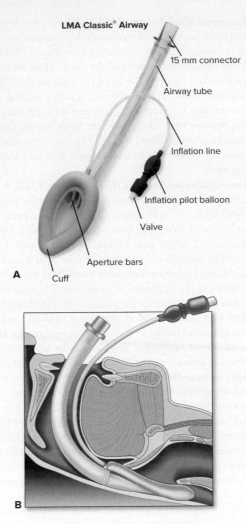

Figure 19-35. **A.** Classic laryngeal mask airway (LMA) is available in eight sizes (1, 1½, 2, 2½, 3, 4, 5, and 6) that can be used in patients ranging from neonates to large adults. Typical adults are treated with a size 3–4 for average females and 4–5 for average males. Its role in difficult or failed facemask ventilation is well established. More advanced modifications of the classic LMA allow for higher pressure ventilation and passage of nasogastric tubes and other features. **B.** Proper positioning of the LMA around the laryngeal inlet. (A. reproduced with permission from Hall, JB, Schmidt GA, Kress JP. Principles of Critical Care, 4e, New York, NY: McGraw Hill; 2018; B. reproduced with permission from Gomella TL, ed. Neonatology: Basic Management, On-Call Problems, Diseases, Drugs, 8e, New York, NY: McGraw-Hill; 2020.)

Table 19-7. Complications of Endotracheal Intubation, Preventive Strategies, and Potential Corrective Actions (Reproduced with permission from Wang HE, Carlson JN. Tracheal Intubation. In: Tintinalli JE, Ma O, Yealy DM, Meckler GD, Stapczynski J, Cline DM, Thomas SH, eds. Tintinalli's Emergency Medicine: A Comprehensive Study Guide, 9e, New York, NY: McGraw-Hill; 2018.)

Complication	Preventive Strategies	Correction Action
ETT misplacement	View ETT entry through glottis	Quick recognition. Remove and replace ETT.
ETT dislodgement	Secure ETT, minimize patient movement, use continuous capnography	Quick recognition. Remove and replace ETT.
Mainstem intubation	View ETT entry through glottis, know appropriate ETT depth	Quick recognition. Adjust ETT position.
Oxygen desaturation	Preoxygenate patient prior to intubation	Verify ETT position. Clear ETT. Hyperventilate.
Hypotension	Ensure adequate blood pressure before intubation efforts, minimize use of medications known to induce hypotension	Place patient in Trendelenburg position. Give IV fluids. Give pressors. Avoid hyperventilation.
Bradycardia	Ensure adequate heart rate before intubation efforts	Hyperventilate. Give atropine or epinephrine.
Cardiac arrest	Ensure adequate heart rate, blood pressure, oxygen saturation before intubation efforts.	Initiate CPR.
Aspiration	Avoid aggressive BVM ventilation, keep patient upright before intubation.	Large-bore suction or oropharynx and ETT.
Injury to oropharynx or hypopharynx	Careful laryngoscopy	
Pneumothorax	Careful laryngoscopy, avoid aggressive BVM ventilation	Insert chest tube or pigtail.

(Continued)

19

Table 19-7. Complications of Endotracheal Intubation, Preventive Strategies, and Potential Corrective Actions (Reproduced with permission from Wang HE, Carlson JN. Tracheal Intubation. In: Tintinalli JE, Ma O, Yealy DM, Meckler GD, Stapczynski J, Cline DM, Thomas SH, eds. Tintinalli's Emergency Medicine: A Comprehensive Study Guide, 9e, New York, NY: McGraw-Hill; 2018.)

Complication	Preventive Strategies	Correction Action
Gastric/visceral perforation	Careful laryngoscopy, avoid aggressive BVM ventilation	
Vocal cord injury	Careful laryngoscopy, careful ETT placement	
ETT cuff leak	Check cuff before intubation, avoid rubbing cuff against teeth	Remove and replace ETT.
ETT obstruction (secretions, vomitus, foreign body)	Suction oropharynx before intubation efforts	Suction ETT. Clear obstruction.
Hyperventilation	Judicious control of manual ventilations	
Interruptions in CPR chest compressions	Minimize CPR interruptions during intubation, use a supraglottic airway instead of ETT	
Failed intubation/inability to intubate	Anticipate and plan for intubation difficulty	Immediate rescue with supraglottic or other airway.

Abbreviations: BVM = bag-value mask; EFF = endotracheal tube.

19

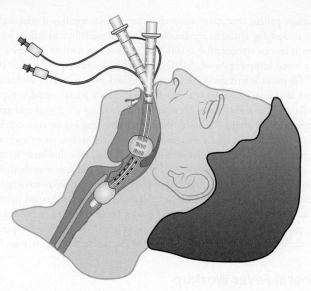

Figure 19-36. Esophagotracheal airway (Combitube or ETC). The diagram depicts the Combitube (Covidien/Medtronic, Minneapolis, MN) in the esophagus with ventilation accomplished by the proximal side ports. (Reproduced with permission from Lalwani AK, ed. Current Diagnosis & Treatment Otolaryngology—Head and Neck Surgery, 4e, New York, NY: McGraw-Hill; 2020.)

inspiratory pressure and a decrease in $EtCO_2$, although none of these is reliable. Confirmation of proper ETT placement can be accomplished with point-of-care ultrasound showing bilateral lung sliding during mechanical ventilation or with a flexible fiber-optic bronchoscope showing the tip of the ETT above the carina.

- If esophageal intubation goes unrecognized, it can produce catastrophic results. To prevent this complication, direct visualization of the tip of the ETT passing through the vocal cords, careful auscultation for the presence of bilateral breath sounds, absence of gastric gurgling while ventilating through the ETT, chest radiography, point-of-care ultrasound, or use of fiber-optic bronchoscopy are all potentially useful techniques. However, the gold standard that combines simplicity, speed, and availability is the confirmation of sustained $EtCO_2$, which can be measured with a single-use calorimetric CO_2 detector.

FEVER WORKUP

Although not considered a standard "bedside procedure," fever workup involves judicious use of the physical examination, laboratory, and diagnostic procedures and is a common "on-call" problem encountered in daily patient care. The true definition of a *fever* varies from service to service and may depend

19

on certain patient characteristics such as immunocompromised state secondary to underlying illness or medications. General guidelines to follow are that a fever is an oral temperature >100.4°F (38°) on a medical or surgical service and a rectal temperature of ≥101°F (38.3°C) or oral temperature ≥100°F (37.7°C) in an infant or immunocompromised patient. When evaluating a patient for a fever, consider whether the temperature is oral, rectal, tympanic, or axillary (rectal and tympanic temperatures are about 1°F higher and axillary temperatures are about 1°F lower than oral); drinking hot or cold liquids or smoking recently can falsely increase or decrease the temperature; and taking antipyretics can lower an elevated temperature. Also, note that body temperature is highest at about 8 P.M. (+0.5°F from 98.6°F) and lowest at about 4 A.M (−1 to 1.5°F). Differential diagnosis of fever and fever of unknown origin are discussed in Chapter 9, page 157. Note that specific fever evaluation pathways may be specified by your institution or by certain services (i.e., "febrile neutropenia protocol" on a bone marrow transplant unit) (also refer to Temperature Considerations considerations are discussed in detail in Chapter 6, page 53).

General Fever Workup

1. Quickly review the chart and medication record if the patient is not familiar to you.
2. Question and examine the patient to locate any obvious sources of fever.
   a. **Ears, nose, sinuses, and throat:** Especially in children.
   b. **Neck:** Pain with flexion suggesting meningitis.
   c. **Nodes:** Adenopathy in the neck or groin.
   d. **Lungs:** Rales (crackles), rhonchi (wheezes), decreased breath sounds, or dullness to percussion. Can the patient generate an effective cough?
   e. **Heart:** A new or changing heart murmur suggesting endocarditis.
   f. **Abdomen:** Presence or absence of bowel sounds, guarding, rigidity, tenderness, bladder fullness, or costovertebral angle tenderness.
   g. **Genitourinary:** If a Foley catheter is in place, note appearance of the urine both grossly and microscopically.
   h. **Rectal exam:** Tenderness or fluctuance suggests an abscess or acute prostatitis.
   i. **Pelvic exam:** Especially in the postpartum patient or sexually active woman with multiple partners.
   j. **Wounds:** Erythema, tenderness, swelling, or drainage from surgical sites.
   k. **Extremities:** Signs of inflammation at IV sites. Look for thigh or calf tenderness and swelling, which suggest a localized infection or deep vein thrombosis.
   l. **Miscellaneous:** Consider the possibility of a drug fever (eosinophil count on the CBC may be elevated) or NG tube fever (sinusitis). Look at all IV sites, looking for erythema suggesting cellulitis, check patency of IV, and look for a "cord" in the vein suggesting thrombophlebitis;

and also remember central lines and PICC lines as potential sources of fever. Do all of the above before beginning to investigate the less common or less obvious causes of a fever.

3. **Laboratory Studies**
   a. **Basic:** CBC with diff, UA, cultures, and Gram stains: urine, blood, sputum, wound, and may include spinal fluid (**strongly consider** in children <4–6 mo old)
   b. **Other:** Order based on clinical findings:
      i **Radiographic:** Chest or abdominal films, CT, or ultrasound exam
      ii **Invasive:** LP, thoracentesis, paracentesis are more aggressive procedures that may be indicated.

Fever of Unknown Origin (FUO)

Before launching into an expensive and time-consuming workup, the clinician should know and apply the accepted definition of "fever of unknown origin." This typically has specific criteria and requires that the patient have

1. An illness that has lasted at least 3 wk
2. Fever of more than 38.3°C on several occasions
3. No diagnosis after routine workup for 3 days in hospital or after three or more outpatient visits

A duration of 3 wk or longer was chosen to eliminate self-limiting viral illnesses that are generally difficult to diagnose and that resolve within that time period. A temperature of more than 38°C was chosen to eliminate those individuals at the far right of the normal temperature distribution curve who normally may have a slightly higher core temperature set point and/or an exaggerated diurnal temperature variation. Recognizing that, presently, most patients with FUO are now diagnosed and managed as outpatients, the third criterion has been modified to include outpatient diagnostic testing, as well as tests conducted in the hospital. The diagnosis of FUO should not be applied to patients who have prolonged hospitalizations and have undergone multiple procedures. The approach to these patients should be similar to that described for the new onset of fever as noted above. Table 19-8 is a suggested approach to the patient with an FUO.

Miscellaneous Fever Facts

1. **Causes of Fever in the Postop Patient:** Think of the "Six Ws":
   a. **Wind:** Atelectasis secondary to intubation and anesthesia is the most common cause of immediate postop fever. To treat, have the patient sitting up and ambulating, using incentive spirometry, P&PD, etc.
   b. **Water:** UTI; may be secondary to a bladder catheter
   c. **Wound:** Infection; a very high fever in the immediate postoperative period can be indicative of a clostridial or group A streptococcal

a catheter-tipped syringe in the air vent will often clear the tube. Both the Salem sump and Levin tubes have radiopaque markings. In general, for suspected obstruction place an 18-Fr tube; smaller-diameter tubes are less effective at suctioning and become clogged more easily than wider tubes. Most adults require a 16–18 Fr sump tube.

2. **Intestinal Decompression Tubes** (also called "long intestinal tubes"). These tubes have largely fallen out of favor because of a lack of data supporting their use in intestinal obstruction.

   a. **Cantor Tube:** A long single-lumen tube with a rubber balloon at the tip. The balloon is partially filled with mercury (5–7 mL through a tangentially directed 21-gauge needle, then the air is aspirated), which allows it to gravitate into the small bowel with the aid of peristalsis. Used for decompression of distal bowel obstruction.

   b. **Miller–Abbott Tube:** A long double-lumen tube with a rubber balloon at the tip. One lumen is used for aspiration; the other connects to the balloon. After the tube is in the stomach, inflate the balloon with 5–10 mL of air, inject 2–3 mL of mercury into the balloon and then aspirate the air. Functioning and indications are essentially the same as for the Cantor tube. **Do not** tape these intestinal tubes to the patient's nose, or the tube will not descend. The progress of the tube can be followed on radiographs.

3. **Feeding Tubes.** Although any NG tube can be used as a feeding tube, it is preferable to place a specially designed nasoduodenal feeding tube. These tubes are of smaller diameter (usually 8 Fr) and are more pliable and comfortable for the patient. Weighted tips tend to travel into the duodenum, which may help prevent regurgitation and aspiration. Most feeding tubes are supplied with stylets that facilitate positioning, especially if fluoroscopic guidance is needed. Always verify the position of the feeding tube with a radiograph before starting tube feeding. Commonly used tubes include mercury-weighted varieties (**Keogh tube, Duo-Tube, Dobbhoff**), tungsten-weighted (**Vivonex tube**), and unweighted pediatric feeding tubes. Take great care with these tubes because complications such as tracheobronchial intubation can easily occur and can be catastrophic if feeding is instituted before tube placement is verified.

4. **Miscellaneous Gastrointestinal Tubes**

   a. **Esophageal-gastric balloon devices:** (See Figure 19-37) These are triple-lumen tubes used exclusively for the control of bleeding esophageal varices by tamponade. One lumen is for gastric aspiration, one is for the gastric balloon, and the third is for the esophageal balloon. Types include the **Sengstaken–Blakemore Tube, Linton,** and **Minnesota Tubes**. These tubes are not routinely used unless there is quick access to endoscopy allowing for more efficient treatment under direct visualization.

   b. **Ewald Tube:** An orogastric tube used almost exclusively for gastric evacuation of blood or drug overdose. The tube is usually double lumen and large diameter (18–36 Fr).

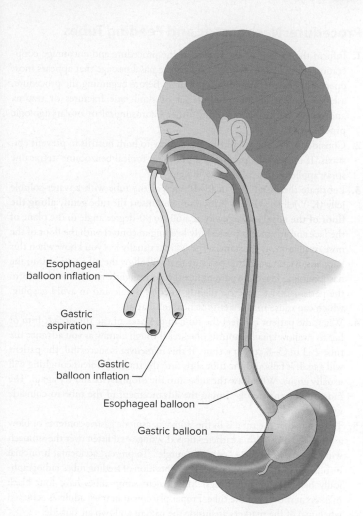

Esophageal
balloon inflation

Gastric
aspiration

Gastric
balloon inflation

Esophageal balloon

Gastric balloon

19

Figure 19-37. Correct insertion of the esophageal-gastric balloon device will result in the large gastric balloon in the relatively free space of the stomach with traction in order to place compression at the gastroesophageal (GE) junction to control variceal bleeding. (Reproduced with permission from Tintinalli JE, Stapczynski J, Ma O, et al. Tintinalli's Emergency Medicine: A Comprehensive Study Guide, 8e, New York, NY: McGraw-Hill Education; 2016.)

    c. **Dennis, Baker, Leonard Tubes:** Used for intraoperative decompression of the bowel and are manually passed into the bowel at the time of laparotomy.

Procedure: Nasogastric and Feeding Tubes

1. Inform the patient of the nature of the procedure and encourage cooperation if the patient is able. Choose the nasal passage that appears most open. The patient should sit up if able. Before beginning the procedure, ask the patient about recent facial or skull base fractures or trauma and recent transsphenoidal and other neurosurgical or otolaryngologic procedures.

2. Consider 0.5% phenylephrine nasal spray to both nostrils to prevent epistaxis. If intractable gagging is a problem, topical benzocaine–tetracaine spray applied to the pharynx will help

3. Lubricate the distal 3–4 in (8–10 cm) of the tube with a water-soluble jelly (K-Y Jelly or viscous lidocaine), and insert the tube gently **along the floor of the nasal passageway** at a 60- to 90-degree angle to the plane of the face and advance it posteriorly keeping in contact with the floor of the nose until it meets resistance. The patient usually lets you know when this happens. Maintain gentle pressure that will allow the tube to pass into the nasopharynx. Have the patient flex the neck slightly from neutral. Inform the patient that it may be slightly uncomfortable and to avoid gasping, which can cause inadvertent tracheal intubation.

4. When the patient can feel the tube in the back of the throat, ask him or her to swallow small amounts of water through a straw as you advance the tube 2–3 in (5–8 cm) at a time. If this maneuver is successful, the patient will gag. If it fails and the tube slips into the trachea, violent coughing will usually ensue. Withdraw the tube into the oropharynx and try again. The most important step is timing the advancement of the tube to coincide with the swallow.

5. To be sure that the tube is in the stomach, aspirate gastric contents or blow air into the tube with a catheter-tipped syringe and listen over the stomach with a stethoscope for a "pop" or "gurgle." To prevent accidental bronchial instillation of tube feedings, **verify** the position of feeding tubes radiographically before starting feedings. Most Salem sump tubes have four black markers at the end of the tube. Proper placement in most adults is achieved when two of the markers are inside the patient and two are outside.

6. NG tubes are attached either to low continuous wall suction (Salem sump tubes with a vent) or to intermittent suction (Levin tubes); the latter allows the tube to fall away from the gastric wall between suction cycles.

7. Pediatric feeding and feeding tubes in adults are more difficult to insert because they are more flexible. Many are provided with stylets that make passage easier. Feeding tubes are best placed in the duodenum or jejunum to decrease the risk of aspiration. Administer 10 mg of metoclopramide IV 10 min before insertion to aid in propagation of the tube into the duodenum. Once the feeding tube is in the stomach, place the bell of the stethoscope on the right side of the middle portion of the patient's abdomen. While advancing the tube, inject air to confirm progression of the

tube to the right, toward the duodenum. If the sound of the air becomes fainter, the tube is probably curling in the stomach. Pass the tube until a slight resistance is felt, heralding the presence of the tip of the tube at the pylorus. Holding constant pressure and slowly injecting water through the tube is often rewarded with a "give," which signifies passage through the pylorus. The tube often can be advanced far into the duodenum with this method. The duodenum usually provides constant resistance that will give with slow injection of water. Placing the patient in the right lateral decubitus position may help the tube enter the duodenum. Always confirm the location of the tube with an abdominal radiograph.

8. Tape the tube securely in place, but do not allow it to apply pressure to the ala of the nose. (*Note:* Intestinal decompression tubes should not be taped because they are allowed to pass through the intestine.) Patients have been disfigured because of ischemic necrosis of the nose caused by a poorly positioned NG tube or tape causing undue pressure to the tip of the nose.

9. Be extremely careful with sedated and intubated patients because it is possible to introduce small feeding tubes past the ET into the trachea and furthermore into the distal bronchial tree, causing pneumothorax. If you meet any resistance, stop immediately and obtain a CXR to assess placement.

Complications

- Inadvertent passage into the trachea can provoke coughing or gagging in the patient.
- Aspiration
- If the patient is unable to cooperate, the tube often becomes coiled in the oral cavity.
- The tube is irritating and may cause a small amount of bleeding in the mucosa of the nose, pharynx, or stomach. The drying and irritation can be lessened with throat lozenges or antiseptic spray.
- Intracranial passage in a patient with a basilar skull fracture.
- Esophageal perforation.
- Esophageal reflux caused by tube-induced incompetence of the distal esophageal sphincter.
- Sinusitis from edema of the nasal passages that blocks drainage from the nasal sinuses.

19

HEELSTICK AND FINGERSTICK (CAPILLARY BLOOD SAMPLING)

Indications: Heelstick

- **Blood collection in infants,** when only a small sample (one drop to <1 cc) is needed or when there is difficulty obtaining samples by venipuncture or other sources.

1. **Common capillary blood studies:** Complete blood count (CBC), general chemistry labs, glucose estimation, liver function tests, thyroid levels, bilirubin levels, toxicology/therapeutic drug levels, newborn metabolic screening panel.
2. Capillary blood gas: Satisfactory for pH and PCO_2, but not PO_2.
3. These cannot usually be done by capillary blood sampling: Coagulation studies, chromosomal analyses, ESR, immunoglobulin titers, others

Contraindications

- Local infection, poor perfusion, significant edema, injury of the foot, or any congenital anomaly of the foot.

Materials: Infant Heelstick

- Automated self-shielding lancets (see Figure 19-38) are preferred in neonates (some devices include BD QuikHeel lancet, Tenderfoot)
  - Full-term neonate: incision depth 1 mm, length of 2.5 mm; preterm neonate incision depth of 0.85 mm and length of 1.75 mm)
- Sterile manual lancets are not recommended but may be used in some facilities (infant sizes based on weight: 2 mm for <1500 g and 4 mm for >1500 g)
- Collection containers for low-volume samples:
  - Glass capillary tube, pre-heparinized capillary tubes for blood gas analysis, Caraway tubes (larger volume 0.3 mL blood); clay or caps to seal the glass capillary tube
  - Designed for low-volume skin puncture blood collection with or without additives such as heparin or coagulating gel (e.g., BD Microtainer tube [with Micro-Guard closure], Multivette 600µl)

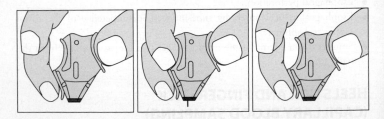

Figure 19-38. Retracting lancets are used for both fingerprick and heelstick. This single-use lancet fires and retracts automatically after use, removing the sharps hazard. Other styles of automated lancets activate only when positioned and pressed against the skin and then retract. (Adapted from https://www.osha.gov/SLTC/etools/hospital/hazards/sharps/sharps.html#safer, accessed January 21, 2020.)

- Filter paper card for newborn screening based on specific state requirements (if appropriate)
- Warm washcloth with a diaper or heel warming device (e.g., a chemically activated packet)
- Antiseptic solution/ swabs (alcohol/chlorhexidine swabs)
- Nonsterile or sterile gloves

Background

Capillary blood sampling, also called "skin puncture" "heelstick," and "fingerstick," involves the collection of a sample from any highly vascularized capillary bed. The heel in newborns, finger pad, earlobe, and great toe are all potential sites. To avoid the risk of repeated venous punctures, especially in infants, assays have been developed that rely on very small volumes of blood. Fingerstick also can be used for small samples in older children and adults (e.g., point-of-care glucose monitoring).

Capillary blood sampling is considered the most common painful form of blood collection, but the least invasive and safest of those done on neonates. Most sources confirm that venipuncture, not capillary blood sampling, by a skilled operator is the method of choice for blood sampling in term neonates. Lower pain scores are seen with venipuncture in infants. Capillary blood sampling is done by puncturing the dermis layer of the skin to access capillaries running through the subcutaneous layer. The sample is a mixture of arterial and venous blood (from arterioles, venules, and capillaries) plus interstitial and intracellular fluids. The proportion of arterial blood is greater than that of venous, due to increased pressure in the arterioles leading into the capillaries. The areas on the bottom surface of the heel contain the best capillary bed, and warming of the puncture site further arterializes the blood. Infant heels are appropriate for blood collection until approximately 6-12 mo. Labs can analyze small samples from pediatric patients. While glass capillary and Caraway tubes are still used for small-volume sample collections, they have been replaced in many settings with specialized low-volume collection tubes (e.g., Multivette 600 Capillary Collection Device and BD Microtainer tubes with color coding indicating the additives in the tube). For a capillary blood gas, the blood is usually transferred to a 1-mL heparinized syringe and placed on ice.

Newborn screening is a public health service managed by each state to identify and treat early a variety of inherited metabolic disorders (organic acidemias, fatty acid oxidation and amino acid disorders) and other conditions. The screening is done a few days after birth by a capillary blood sample on a state by state specific blood sample card. (https://www.hrsa.gov/advisory-committees/heritable-disorders/rusp/index.html, accessed April 25, 2020).

19

Procedure: Heelstick

1. Infant should be supine. Some advocate for the infant to be on their stomach with the limb lower than the level of the heart to increase blood flow.

2. Warm the heel to increase arterial inflow (this is controversial). Apply a heel warmer (special designed heel pack for single use that is temperature controlled and safe) or use a warm washcloth with a diaper wrapped around it or warm water submersion (need to control the temperature). This prewarming may increase the local blood flow in the capillaries (hyperemia) and reduce the difference between the arterial and venous gas pressures.

3. Consider pain management strategies, as heelsticks are very painful. The American Academy of Pediatrics (AAP) recommends nonpharmacologic pain prevention such as oral sucrose/glucose, breastfeeding, kangaroo care, swaddling, rocking, non-nutritive sucking, facilitated tucking, gentle human touch, or other methods (but no analgesics on very premature infants). Automated devices vs. manual lancets reduce the duration of the collection of blood, thereby indirectly reducing the pain.

4. Choose the area of puncture (Figure 19-39, page 605). Always avoid the end (crown) of the heel (the posterior curvature where the calcaneus bone is close to the skin), as this area is associated with an increased incidence of osteomyelitis and the key nerves and blood vessels are more centrally located. Vary the sites to prevent bruising, tissue injury and inflammation. Fingertips and toes are not recommended in infants and are only recommended in children >1 yr.

5. Wash hands and wear gloves prior to procedure. Wipe the proposed heelstick area with povidone-iodine, followed by a saline wipe and let dry for approximately 30 sec. Some sources advocate only a 70% alcohol prep pad and let dry. Do not use cotton balls. (Note: Povidone-iodine can interfere with potassium, bilirubin, phosphorus, and uric acid analyses. If the area is wet with alcohol hemolysis may occur, altering the results.)

6. As noted, two general devices are available: automated and manual. Automated devices (spring loaded) are recommended.

   a. Using an automated lancet (preferred method). Prepare the unit and hold the device either perpendicularly to the skin, or at 90 degrees to the long axis of the foot (Figure 19-39, page 605). Depress the trigger to activate the device and automatically make the puncture. Immediately discard the device. Other style automated lancets activate only when positioned and pressed against the skin, facilitating a consistent puncture depth.

   b. Using a standard (not automated) lancet. Encircle the heel with the palm of your hand and index finger (Figure 19-39B, page 605). Make a quick puncture. Never puncture >2.4 mm to avoid complications in infants.

19

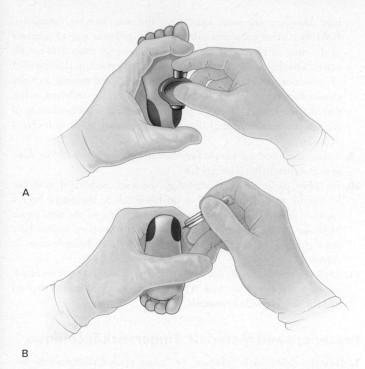

A

B

Figure 19-39. Preferred sites and technique for a heelstick in an infant demonstrated by the red-shaded area. Using these areas limits injury to plantar nerves and arteries. **A.** Use of a self-shielding lancet is recommended. The device is held 90 degrees to the axis of the foot and activated. **B.** Standard lancet device. (Reprinted with permission from Gomella TL, ed. Neonatology: Basic Management, On-Call Problems, Diseases, Drugs, 8e, New York, NY: McGraw-Hill; 2020.)

19

7. Wipe off the first drop of blood with gauze, as it is often contaminated with tissue fluid that may result in a high potassium, specimen dilution, hemolysis, and clotting. Wiping off the first drop also permits the sample to flow better as platelets may otherwise aggregate at the site. DO NOT puncture the skin more than once with the same lancet, and do not use a single puncture site more than once because this can lead to bacterial contamination and infection.

8. Gently apply pressure to the heel ("tennis racket grip"), hold heel in a dependent position, and place the collection tube at the site of the puncture. Fill the capillary tube by touching the open tip of the tube to a blood drop, which is drawn into the tube by capillary action. Gently "pump" the heel to continue the blood flow to collect drops in a larger

tube (controversial; some sources say this may increase hemolysis). Hold specialized collection tubes with the collector end of reservoir to the drop of blood. Fill plasma and hematology tubes between fill marks. Overfilling or underfilling of a tube may result in clotting and/ or erroneous test results. Fill serum tubes to required volume. Samples should flow freely enough that the specimen can be collected in less than 2 min. Longer collection periods may result in microclotting of the sample. Seal the end of the capillary/Carraway tubes with clay if necessary.

9. Collect the blood gas sample first, hematology studies should be done next and chemistry/toxicology last.

10. For filter paper newborn screening, the state authorized card can be directly applied to the heel or the blood can be transferred from a capillary tube that does not contain anticoagulants to the filter paper. Methods of collecting filter paper samples for newborn screens have strict guidelines and vary between laboratories and different states in America.

11. Maintain pressure on the site with a dry sterile gauze pad until the bleeding stops and elevate the foot. A gauze can be wrapped around the heel and left on to provide hemostasis.

Procedure and Materials: Fingerstick Technique

1. Formally called "skin puncture" or "finger prick technique," the finger is usually the preferred site for capillary testing in an adult patient. Frequently used for point-of-care glucose determinations using reagent strips and a detection device such as the Accu-Chek.

2. In an adult the depth of the puncture should not go beyond 2.4 mm, so a 2.2-mm lancet is the longest length typically used. The recommended depth for a fingerstick for a child up to 8 yr is 1.5 mm and 2.4 mm for a child over 8 yr. Fingersticks are not recommended for children less than 1 yr of age.

3. When available, always use automated self-shielding lancets. Devices such as the BD Contact Activated Lancets are available for fingersticks in different sizes; the blue device has a depth of 2.0 mm, and is suitable for fingersticks on most children. The Accu-Check Safe-T-Pro Plus are available for as a single use lancet and has three adjustable depth settings: 1.3, 1.8, and 2.3 mm for specific patient conditions (poor circulation, calloused fingers).

4. Wash hands, put on gloves. Clean the puncture site with alcohol, and allow to air dry. The best digits to use for fingersticks are the middle and ring fingers. The incision should be made off center and perpendicular to the fingerprint lines over the pad of finger. This region (slightly lateral of the ball of the finger) is generally less calloused, improving the ease of puncture, and may be a slightly less painful puncture location.

5. Remove the protective cap from the safety lancet. Depending on the specific manufacturer press the white activation button with your thumb or apply pressure to the end of the device; the lance advances and then retracts. Discard device into sharps container.

6. Gently massage from base of the finger towards the puncture site to collect the sample. Holding the patient's hand below the level of the elbow will enhance blood flow. For glucose determinations with a device such as the BD Genie needle lancet, only a drop of blood is needed to apply to the reagent strip for glucose determination. A lancet-style device is not necessary because of the small amount of blood needed.

7. The puncture site should face downward (fingernail facing up) to facilitate collection. Wipe away the first drop of blood because it may be contaminated with tissue fluid or debris (sloughing skin). Avoid squeezing the finger too tightly because this dilutes the specimen with tissue fluid (plasma) and increases the probability of hemolysis.

8. Follow the steps for heelsrick to collect larger volumes of blood by capillary action. When the blood collection procedure is complete, apply firm pressure to the site to stop the bleeding

Complications: Heelstick

1. Infectious
   a. Cellulitis. Risk can be minimized with sterile technique. If present, a culture from the affected area should be obtained and the use of broad-spectrum antibiotics considered.
   b. Osteomyelitis. Usually occurs in the calcaneus bone. Avoid the posterior curvature of the heel, and do not puncture too deep. If osteomyelitis occurs, tissue should be obtained for culture, and broad-spectrum antibiotics should be started until a specific organism is identified. Infectious disease and orthopedic consultation is usually obtained.
   c. Other infections. Abscess and perichondritis have been reported.

2. Scarring of the heel. Occurs when there have been multiple punctures in the same area. If extensive scarring is present, consider another technique or site for blood collection.

3. Pain and hypoxemia. Heelstick-related pain can cause declines in hemoglobin oxygen saturation as measured by pulse oximetry.

4. Calcified heel nodules. These can occur because of repetitive punctures but usually disappear by 30 mo of age.

5. Other complications. Nerve damage, tibial artery laceration (medial aspect of heel), burning of the skin with too hot of water while warming the heel, bleeding, bruising, hematoma, and bone calcification.

Complications: Fingerstick

1. Pain and soreness at the insertion site. Infectious complications are rare.

19

INJECTION TECHNIQUES

Indications

- **Intradermal:** Most commonly used for skin testing (e.g., PPD allergy testing)
- **Subcutaneous:** Useful for low-volume medications such as insulin, heparin, and some vaccines
- **Intramuscular:** Administration of parenteral medications that cannot be absorbed from the SQ layer or of high volume (≤10 mL) (e.g., penicillin, vaccines such as Gardasil, d Hepatitis A and B., LHRH agonists such as leuprolide)

Contraindications

- Allergy to any components of the injectate
- Active infection or dermatitis at the injection site
- Coagulopathy/anticoagulation (IM injections)

Materials

- Appropriate needle and syringe for medication to be administered. Needle gauge suggested for route of administration is shown below. Many medications today come in single-use packaging (syringe and needle assembly).
- Always use self-shielding needles if none is supplied with the product (page 511).
- Gloves, alcohol swabs.

Procedure

Before any injection, always verify patient identity and determine any allergies or any medications such as blood thinners that may cause bleeding especially with IM injections. The different standard injection techniques, intramuscular, subcutaneous, and intradermal, are demonstrated in Figure 19-40, page 609.

Intradermal: (See Skin Testing, page 650)

Subcutaneous

1. The goal is to deposit the drug within the fat but above the muscle. With careful placement of the injection, nerve injury is rarely a danger.
2. Choose a site free of scarring and active infection. Injection sites include the outer surface of the upper arm, anterior surface of the thigh, and lower abdominal wall. For repeated injections (e.g., for diabetic patients), rotate the sites.

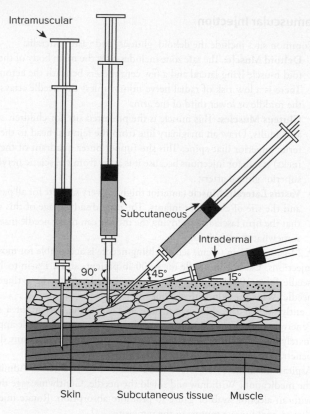

Figure 19-40. Demonstration of the different types of injection, intramuscular, subcutaneous, and intradermal, noting the ideal angle of insertion of the needle.

19

3. 25–27 gauge 3/4–1 in (2–2.5 cm) needles are most commonly used; volume of medication must not exceed 5 mL. Draw up the medication if appropriate. Hold the needle upright to expel any air bubbles.
4. Clean the site with an alcohol swab. Bunch up the skin with your thumb and forefinger so that the SQ tissue is off the underlying muscle.
5. Warn the patient that there will be "pinch" or "sting" and insert the needle firmly and rapidly at a 45-degree angle until a sudden release signifies penetration of the dermis.
6. Release the skin, aspirate to make certain a blood vessel has not been entered, and inject slowly.
7. Withdraw the needle and apply gentle pressure. Activate the automatic needle shield (e.g., BD SafetyGlide shielding hypodermic needle) and discard the needle in a sharps box. A dressing is not usually necessary. Apply pressure longer if there is bleeding from the site.

Intramuscular Injection

1. Common sites include the deltoid, gluteus, and vastus lateralis.
   - **Deltoid Muscle:** The safe zone includes only the main body of the deltoid muscle lying lateral and a few centimeters beneath the acromion. There is a low risk of radial nerve injury unless the needle strays into the middle or lower third of the arm.
   - **Gluteus Muscles:** This muscle is the preferred site for children >2 yr and adults. Draw an imaginary line from the femoral head to the posterior superior iliac spine. This site (upper outer quadrant of the buttocks) is safe for injections because it is away from the sciatic nerve and superior gluteal artery.
   - **Vastus Lateralis Muscle** (anterior thigh): A very safe site for all patients and the site of choice for infants. The only disadvantage of this site is that the firm fascia lata overlying the muscle can make needle insertion somewhat more painful.
2. A 22-gauge, 1½ in (4 cm) self-shielding needle is acceptable for most IM injections. Use a 2-in needle for a 200-lb patient, and a 1¼-in to 1½-in needle for a 100-lb patient. Remove air bubbles from the syringe and needle. Wipe the skin with alcohol.
3. Gently stretch the skin to one side and warn the patient of a sting. Penetrate the skin at a 90-degree angle, and advance the needle approximately 1 in (2.5 cm) into the muscle. (Obese patients may require deeper penetration with a longer needle.)
4. Aspirate to make sure a blood vessel has not been entered. Administer the medication. Withdraw and shield the needle. Gently massage the site with an alcohol swab or gauze to promote absorption. Rotate injection sites to avoid tissue trauma to the same site.

19

Intramuscular Z-track technique

1. This is a modification of the IM injection (Figure 19-41, page 611). The goal is to minimize leakage of irritating or discoloring medications such as iron dextran into the subcutaneous tissue. In elderly patients who have decreased muscle mass, this may help with retention of medication in the muscle. Some practitioners advocate that all IM medication be given this way.
2. Prepare the medication and cleanse site as for IM injection above. No more than 5 mL should be placed IM. The gluteal site is common for this technique.
3. Displace the skin and subcutaneous tissue by pulling the skin laterally or downward from the injection site with your nondominant hand at least 1 in. While holding the skin taut quickly insert the needle into the muscle at a 90-degree angle.
4. Aspirate to verify you are not in a vessel. Inject the medication slowly (10 sec/mL).

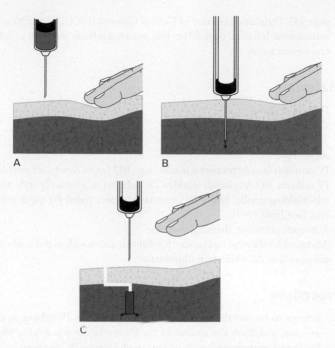

Figure 19-41. "Z-track" technique for IM injections. **A.** The skin is pulled to one side by 1–2 in. **B.** While holding the skin, the needle is inserted into the muscle at a 90-degree angle and the medication administered. **C.** While withdrawing the needle the tension on the skin is released and the needle track shifts, helping to retain the medication in the muscle.

19

5. Slowly withdraw needle while releasing skin to create a "zig-zag" pattern for the needle track. Apply pressure to the site with a clean gauze and do not massage site. Apply bandage is appropriate.

Complications

- Nerve and arterial injury.
- Abscesses (sterile or septic). Use good technique and rotate injection sites.
- Bleeding can usually be controlled with pressure.

IV TECHNIQUES

Indication

- Intravenous (IV) access for administration of fluids, blood products, or medications (other techniques include Central Venous Catheterization, page 533, Peripheral Insertion of Central Catheter [PICC], page 636, and Intraosseous Infusion, page 671). This section addresses common peripheral venous access.

Materials

- IV fluid of choice
- Connecting tubing
- Tourniquet
- Alcohol swab
- IV cannulas (a catheter over a needle [e.g., BD Insyte Autoguard shielded IV catheter, BD Angiocath shielded IV catheter] or a butterfly-style with self-shielding needle. Many IV cannulas are color coded for quick reference (see Table 19-9).
- Antiseptic ointment, dressing, and tape
- Advanced localization equipment for difficult access such as point-of-care ultrasound or AccuVein vein illuminator.

Procedure

1. It helps to lay out the necessary supplies, attach the IV tubing to the solution, and flush the air out of the tubing before you begin. Wash hands and wear gloves (sterile or non-sterile) for the IV insertion.
2. The upper, nondominant extremity is the site of choice for an IV unless the patient is being considered for placement of permanent hemodialysis access. In this instance, the upper nondominant extremity should be "saved" as the access site for hemodialysis. If the patient has previously undergone axillary lymph node dissection (e.g., some breast cancer

Table 19-9. Sizes and Suggested Uses of Peripheral IV Catheters (Some Manufacturers Color Code Hubs)

IV Catheter Size	Hub Color	Suggested Use
14G	Orange	Major trauma where large volumes of fluid or blood need to be infused.
16G	Gray	Used in major surgery where multiple large-volume infusions are likely.
18G	Green	Commonly used for blood transfusions or large-volume infusions.
20G	Pink	Considered a general-purpose IV in adults.
22G	Blue	Frequently used for chemotherapy; patients with small veins; elderly or pediatric patients.
24G	Yellow	Best for elderly or pediatric patients with fragile veins.

operations), start the IV on the side opposite the surgical site. Choose a distal vein (dorsum of the hand) so that if the vein is lost, you can reposition the IV more proximally. Figure 19-42, page 613, shows common upper extremity veins; avoid veins that cross a joint space when placing an IV. Also, avoid the leg because of the increased risk of thrombophlebitis.

3. Apply a tourniquet above the proposed IV site. Use the techniques described in Venipuncture (page 663) to help expose the vein. Carefully clean the site with an alcohol or povidone-iodine swab. If a large-bore IV

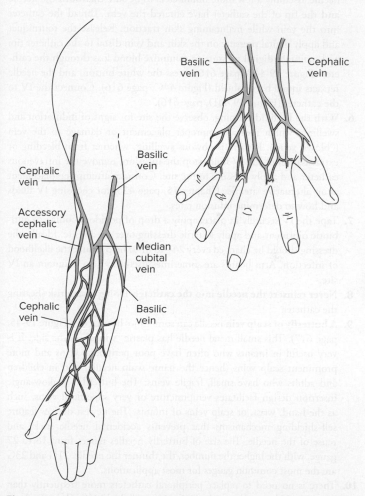

Figure 19-42. Principal veins of the arm used for IV access and in venipuncture in the child and adult. The pattern can be highly variable. (Reprinted with permission from Stillman RM, ed. *Surgery, Diagnosis, and Therapy,* Norwalk, CT: Appleton & Lange; 1989.)

needle is to be used (16- or 14-gauge), local anesthesia (lidocaine injected with a 25-gauge needle) is helpful.

4. Stabilize the vein distally with the thumb of your free hand (Figure 19-43A, page 615). Using the catheter-over-needle assembly, there are several approaches to inserting the needle into a vein (Figure 19-43B and C, page 615).
5. Once the vein is punctured, blood should appear in the "flash chamber" (Figure 19-44A, page 616). Lower the needle assembly and advance the needle assembly a few more millimeters to be sure that **both** the needle **and** the tip of the catheter have entered the vein. Thread the catheter into the vein while maintaining skin traction. Release the tourniquet and apply digital pressure on the skin and vein distal to the catheter tip, and maintain digital pressure to minimize blood loss through the catheter (Figure 19-44B, page 616). Press the white button, and the needle retracts into a barrel shield (Figure 44C, page 616). Connect the IV to the catheter (Figure 19-44D, page 616).
6. With the IV fluid running, observe the site for signs of induration and swelling, which indicate improper placement or damage to the vein ("blown vein"). If there is obvious swelling, whether from bleeding or extravasation of the IV fluid, stop the infusion, remove the intravenous catheter and apply pressure to the site. Consider attempting placement at an alternative site. See Chapter 15, page 425, for choosing IV fluids and how to determine infusion rates.
7. Tape the IV securely in place; apply a drop of povidone-iodine or antibiotic ointment and apply a sterile dressing over the IV site. Ideally, the dressing should be changed every 24–48 hr to help reduce the likelihood of infection. Arm boards are sometimes useful to help maintain an IV site.
8. **Never reinsert the needle into the catheter.** Doing so can risk shearing the catheter.
9. **A butterfly** or **scalp vein** needle can sometimes be used (see Figure 19-45, page 617). This small metal needle has plastic "wings" on the side. It is very useful in infants who often have poor peripheral veins and more prominent scalp veins (hence the name scalp needle) and in children and adults who have small, fragile veins. The butterfly's shallow-angle insertion design facilitates venipuncture of very superficial veins, such as the hand, wrist, or scalp veins of infants. The newest devices feature self-shielding mechanisms that prevents accidental needle sticks and reuse of the needle. The size of butterfly needles ranges from 18 to 27 gauge, with the higher the number, the thinner the needle. 21G and 23G are the most common gauges for most applications.
10. There is no need to replace peripheral catheters more frequently than every 72–96 hr to reduce risk of infection and phlebitis in adults. Evaluate the catheter insertion site daily by palpation through the dressing to discern tenderness and by inspection if a transparent dressing is in use.

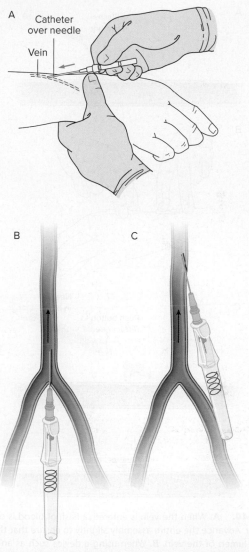

Figure 19-43. Technique for insertion of a standard catheter-over-needle device for IV access. **A.** Stabilize the vein with gentle traction. There are two common approaches to inserting the needle into a vein. **B.** The entry point can be in the "Y" or "crotch" region where two branches of the vein come together. **C.** Another entry point can be on the side of the vein where the needle is inserted into the skin and then advanced 0.5–1 cm before puncturing the side of the vein. Another method is to enter the vein directly through the skin. However, there is an increased risk of "blowing" the vein by perforating the posterior wall if the angle of insertion is too steep.

19

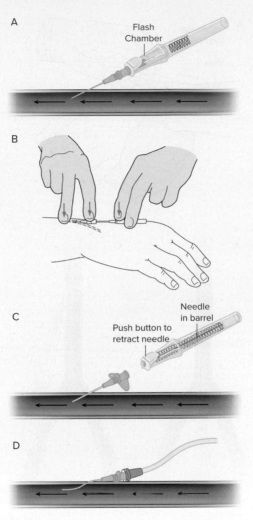

Figure 19-44. **A.** When the vein is entered, a flash of blood is observed in the chamber. Advance the entire assembly slightly to ensure that the catheter tip is in the lumen of the vein. **B.** When using a device such as an Angiocath Autoguard (BD Biosciences), before pressing the autoshield button, apply digital pressure as shown to stabilize the catheter and to prevent blood from escaping after the needle is removed. **C.** Advance the catheter off the end of the needle and push the button to retract the needle. Remove the tourniquet. **D.** Connect the IV fluid and dress the site.

Gauze and opaque dressings should not be removed if the patient has no clinical signs of infection. If the patient has local tenderness or other signs of possible CRBSI, an opaque dressing should be removed and the

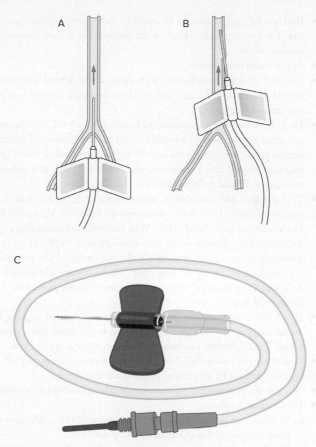

Figure 19-45.   Example of a butterfly needle ("scalp needle") assembly and the two different techniques of entering a vein for IV access. **A.** Direct puncture. **B.** Side entry. **C.** This needle design can also be used for phlebotomy when connected to a vacuum blood collection tube. This butterfly needle features a retractable needle design. (Reprinted with permission from Gomella TL, ed. Neonatology: Basic Management, On-Call Problems, Diseases, Drugs, 5e, New York, NY: McGraw-Hill; 2004.)

19

   site inspected visually. Remove peripheral venous catheters if the patient develops signs of phlebitis (warmth, tenderness, erythema or palpable venous cord), infection, or a malfunctioning catheter

11. **Troubleshooting difficult IV placement**
   - Tapping or gently flicking the vein may result in engorgement.
   - Place the extremity in a position lower than the heart to allow gravity to engorge the veins.

- Inflate a BP cuff to around 30 mm Hg above the proposed insertion site. Do not go much higher on the pressure, as it may compromise arterial inflow.
- Apply warm compresses.
- Try the multiple tourniquet technique using several tourniquets spaced apart above the site; collateral veins should appear; a third if needed can be applied.
- Deep veins are deep and difficult to locate; a 3- to 5-mL syringe can be mounted on the catheter assembly to aid in identification. Determine proper positioning inside the vein by aspirating blood. If blood specimens are needed for a patient who also needs an IV, use this technique to start the IV and collect samples at the same time.
- Technologies are available at many facilities to assist with localization of veins. One device is known as AccuVein that provides a visual map of peripheral veins. Vein visualization technology (also known as vein illumination) uses near-infrared (NIR) imaging for detecting veins. Lasers provide a real-time image of the subcutaneous vasculature up to 10 mm deep. Point-of-care ultrasound can help localize peripheral veins and may significantly reduce the need for central access.
- If no extremity vein can be found, consider external jugular vein access (see page 546). Placing the patient in the head-down position (deep Trendelenburg) can help distend the external jugular vein.
- If all these maneuvers fail, insert a central venous line (page 533).

12. Considerations for IV placement in infants and children.
   - The general principles of IV insertion in adults are similar (see above).
   - IV site considerations
     o In newborns and infants, scalp veins can be used in addition to the usual peripheral veins (Figure 19-46, page 619).
     o Hand and foot veins can be used in children. Foot veins are best in children who are not walking yet. Avoid a dorsal hand vein in a child's dominant hand.
     o Forearm and upper arm sites are suitable for all children. Infants and toddlers may have difficult to locate veins under their more substantial subcutaneous fat.
     o Cephalic, basilic, or median cubital veins are suitable for all children and are easy to locate in infants. Because these antecubital sites are also used for phlebotomy and peripherally inserted central catheter placement, it should not be a first choice. These sites are uncomfortable and require immobilizing the elbow.
   - Use a tourniquet appropriate for the age and size of the child. For scalp vein placement use a rubber band placed above the eyes and ears.
   - Use smaller-gauge catheters than in adults. Use at least a 24-gauge for blood transfusion; 22- to 24-gauge catheters are often used in children.

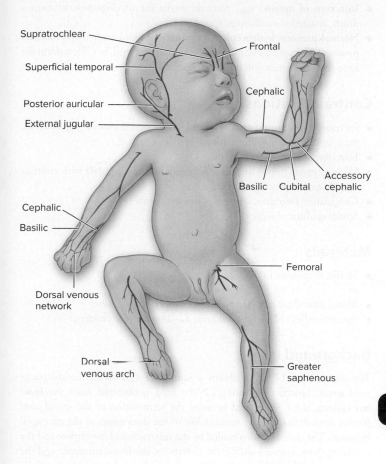

Supratrochlear

Frontal

Superficial temporal

Cephalic

Posterior auricular

External jugular

Accessory
cephalic

Basilic   Cubital

Cephalic

Basilic

Femoral

Dorsal venous
network

Dorsal
venous arch

Greater
saphenous

19

Figure 19-46. Frequently used veins in the newborn for venous access.
(Reprinted with permission from Gomella TL, ed. Neonatology: Basic
Management, On-Call Problems, Diseases, Drugs, 8e, New York, NY: McGraw-Hill;
2020.)

LUMBAR PUNCTURE

Indications

- **Diagnosis:** Analysis of CSF for conditions such as meningitis, encephalitis, subarachnoid hemorrhage, Guillain–Barré syndrome, carcinomatous meningitis, and lymphoma staging
- **Measurement of CSF pressure** or its changes with various maneuvers (e.g., Valsalva)

- **Injection of agents,** e.g., contrast media for myelography, antitumor drugs, analgesics, antibiotics, spinal anesthesia
- **Normal-pressure hydrocephalus evaluation:** Fluid analysis and measure pressure; if symptoms improve after removal of 50 mL of CSF, a shunt for long-term treatment will likely be successful

Contraindications

- Increased intracranial pressure when a mass lesion is present (papilledema, mass lesion, Chiari malformation)
- Infection near the puncture site
- Planned myelography or pneumoencephalography or MRI with contrast to evaluate for meningeal enhancement
- Coagulation disorders, severe thrombocytopenia
- Spinal epidural abscess

Materials

- Sterile, disposable LP kit
  or
- Minor procedure tray (see page 516) with collection tubes
- Spinal needles (22-gauge for adults, 22–24-gauge for children)

Background

The objective of LP is to obtain a sample of CSF from the subarachnoid space. Specifically, during LP the fluid is obtained from the **lumbar cistern,** the CSF located between the termination of the spinal cord (conus medullaris) and the termination of the dura mater at the coccygeal ligament. The cistern is surrounded by the subarachnoid membrane and the overlying dura. Located within the cistern are the filum terminale and the nerve roots of the cauda equina. When LP is done, the main body of the spinal cord is avoided, and the nerve roots of the cauda are simply pushed out of the way by the needle. The termination of the spinal cord in adults is usually between T12 and L1, and in pediatric patients between L2 and L3. The safest site for LP is the interspace between L4 and L5. An imaginary line drawn between the iliac crests (the **supracristal plane**) intersects the spine at either the L4 spinous process or the L4–L5 interspace. A spinal needle introduced between the spinous processes of L4 and L5 penetrates the layers in the following order: skin, supraspinous ligament, interspinous ligament, ligamentum flavum, epidural space (contains loose areolar tissue, fat, and blood vessels), dura, "potential space," subarachnoid membrane, and subarachnoid space (lumbar cistern) (Figures 19-47 and 19-48, pages 621 and 622).

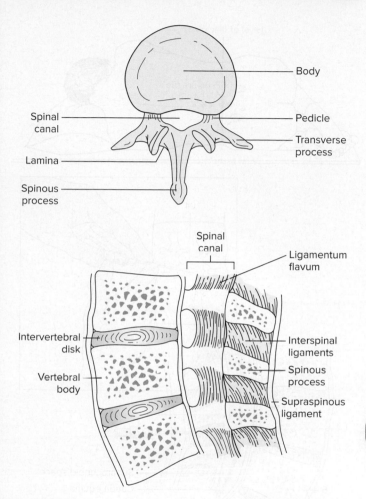

Figure 19-47. Basic anatomy for lumbar puncture. The spinal cord and cerberospinal fluid are located within the spinal canal.

Procedure

1. Examine the fundus for evidence of papilledema, and review the CT or MRI of the head if available. Discuss the relative safety and lack of discomfort to the patient to dispel any myths. Some clinicians prefer to call the procedure "subarachnoid analysis" rather than a spinal tap. As long as the procedure and the risks are outlined, most patients agree to the procedure. Have the patient sign an informed consent form.

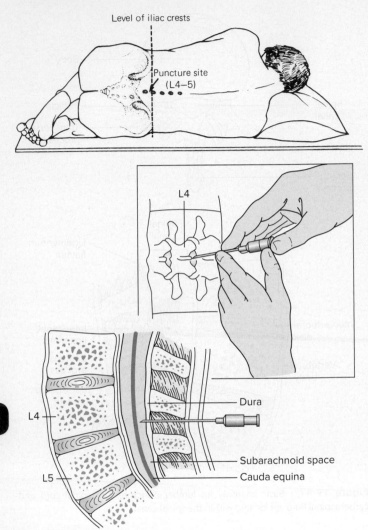

Figure 19-48. For lumbar puncture, place the patient in the lateral decubitus position, and locate the L4–L5 interspace usually defined by the imaginary line between the two iliac cresrs referred to as the supracristal line or plane. Control the spinal needle with two hands, and enter the subarachnoid space.

2. Place the patient in the lateral decubitus position close to the edge of the bed or table. The patient (held by an assistant, if possible) should be positioned with knees pulled up toward the stomach and head flexed onto the chest (Figure 19-48). This position enhances flexion of the vertebral spine

and widens the interspaces between the spinous processes. Place a pillow beneath the patient's side to prevent sagging and ensure alignment of the spinal column. Alternatively, LPs may be performed with patients sitting up and bent forward if measurement of CSF pressure is not necessary; additionally this position may be preferred with patients who are obese or have arthritis or scoliosis.

3. Palpate the supracristal plane (see Background, page 620) and carefully determine the location of the L4–L5 interspace.

4. Open the kit, put on sterile gloves, and prep the area with povidone-iodine solution in a circular manner and covering several interspaces. Drape the patient.

5. With a 25-gauge needle and lidocaine, raise a skin wheal over the L4–L5 interspace. Anesthetize the deeper structures using a 22-gauge needle. Some practitioners wear a mask as well to potentially further reduce risk of infection, but this has not been studied in a controlled way.

6. Examine the spinal needle (20- or 22-gauge) with a stylet for defects and then insert it into the skin wheal and the spinous ligament, with the bevel placed upward to minimize cutting the fibers of the spinous ligament and dura. Hold the needle between your index and middle fingers with your thumb holding the stylet in place. Direct the needle cephalad at a 30- to a 45-degree angle in the midline and parallel to the bed (see Figure 19-48, page 622).

7. Advance the needle through the major structures and "pop" into the subarachnoid space through the dura. An experienced operator can feel these layers, but an inexperienced one may need to periodically remove the stylet to look for return of fluid. It is important to always replace the stylet before advancing the spinal needle. The needle may be withdrawn, however, with the stylet removed. This technique may be useful if the needle has passed through the back wall of the canal. Slowly remove the needle without the stylet and see if CSF fluid returns.

8. If no fluid returns, it is sometimes helpful to rotate the needle slightly. If still no fluid appears and you believe the needle is within the subarachnoid space, inject 1 mL of air; it is not uncommon for a piece of tissue to clog the needle. **Never** inject saline solution or distilled water. If no air returns and if spinal fluid cannot be aspirated, the bevel of the needle is probably in the epidural space; advance it with the stylet in place.

9. When fluid returns, attach a manometer and stopcock and measure the pressure, ensuring that the patient is relaxed and not straining (which can elevate the pressure reading). The normal opening pressure is 70–180 mm H_2O in the lateral position. Increased pressure may be due to a tense patient, CHF, ascites, subarachnoid hemorrhage, infection, or a space-occupying lesion in the cranial cavity. Decreased pressure may be due to CSF leak, needle position, or obstructed flow (you may need to leave the needle in for a myelogram because if it is moved, the subarachnoid space may be lost).

19

10. Collect 0.5- to 2.0-mL samples in serial, labeled containers. Send them to the lab in this order:
    - **First tube for bacteriology:** Gram stain, routine C&S, AFB, and fungal cultures and stains.
    - **Second tube for glucose and protein:** Also, if MS is suspected, order oligoclonal bands and assay for myelin basic protein.
    - **Third tube for cell count:** CBC with diff.
    - **Fourth tube for special studies as clinically indicated:** VDRL (neurosyphilis), polymerase chain reaction (PCR) for *Haemophilus influenzae, Streptococcus pneumoniae, Neisseria meningitidis*, Mycobacterium tuberculous, and herpes simplex encephalitis, and cytology if meningeal carcinomatosis is suspected. If *Cryptococcus neoformans* is suspected (most common cause of meningitis in AIDS patients), India ink preparation and cryptococcal antigen (latex agglutination test) can be ordered.
    - *Note:* Some clinicians prefer to send the first and last tubes for CBC because this procedure allows better differentiation between **subarachnoid hemorrhage and a traumatic tap.** In a traumatic tap, the number of RBCs in the first tube should be much higher than in the last tube. In subarachnoid hemorrhage, the cell counts should be equal, and **xanthochromia** of the fluid be present, indicating the presence of old blood.
11. Withdraw the needle and place a dry, sterile dressing over the site.
12. The patient may ambulate immediately, as studies have not demonstrated any benefit associated with bed rest in prevention of post-LP headache. Previous recommendations for bed rest no longer apply. Similarly, studies have not found any benefit associated with fluid intake with regard to treating spinal headache.
13. Interpret the results using Table 19-10, page 625.

Complications

- **Spinal headache:** The most common complication (about 20%) appears within the first 24 hr after LP. It is usually relieved when the patient lies down and is aggravated when the patient sits up. Sometimes positioning helps, and the prone position may alleviate pain more than the supine position. Spinal headache is characterized by a severe throbbing pain in the occipital region and usually abates within 1–3 days, though it can last up to a week. It is thought to result from intracranial traction caused by acute volume loss of CSF and by persistent leakage from the puncture site. To help prevent spinal headache, encourage intake of fluids (especially caffeinated drinks such as coffee, tea, and soft drinks), use the smallest needle possible, and keep the bevel of the needle parallel to the long axis of the body to help prevent persistent CSF leak. If the headache persists, a blood patch (peripheral blood injected into the epidural space, usually performed by anesthesia service) usually seals the leak though this is rarely done before 4–5 days have elapsed since the LP.

Table 19-10. Differential Diagnosis of Cerebrospinal Fluid

Condition	Color	Opening Pressure (mm H$_2$O)	Protein (mL/100mL)	Glucose (mg/l00mL)	Cells #/mm³
NORMAL					
Adult	Clear	70–180	15–45	45–80	0–5 lymphocytes
Newborn	Clear	70–180	20–120	2/3 serum	40–60 lymphocytes
INFECTIOUS					
Viral infection ("aseptic meningitis")	Clear or opalescent	Normal or slightly increased	Normal or slightly increased	Normal	10–500 lymphocytes (PMN early)
Bacterial infection	Opalescent yellow, may clot	Increased	50–10,000	Decreased, usually <20	25–10,000 PMN
Granulomatous infection (TB, fungal)	Clear or opalescent	Often increased	Increased, usually >100, in TB >1000	Decreased, usually <20	50–500 lymphocytes (early or with acute presentation PMNs may predominate)

(Continued)

19

Table 19-10. Differential Diagnosis of Cerebrospinal Fluid *(Continued)*

Condition	Color	Opening Pressure (mm H$_2$O)	Protein (mL/100mL)	Glucose (mg/l00mL)	Cells #/mm^3
NEUROLOGIC					
Guillain-Barré syndrome	Clear or cloudy	Normal	Increased, typically <100	Normal	Normal or increased lymphocytes
Multiple sclerosis	Clear	Normal	Normal or mildly increased, oligoclonal bands, intrathecal IgG synthesis	Normal	0–20 lymphocytes
Pseudotumor cerebri	Clear	Increased	Normal	Normal	Normal
MISCELLANEOUS					
Neoplasm	Clear or xanthochromic	Increased	Normal or increased	Normal or decreased	Normal or increased lymphocytes
Traumatic tap	Bloody, no xanthochromia	Normal	Normal or increased depending upon degree of contamination	Increased	RBC = peripheral blood; fewer RBC in tube 4 than in tube 1
Subarachnoid hemorrhage	Bloody or xanthochromic after 2–8 hr	Usually increased	Increased	Normal	WBC/RBC ratio same as blood, RBC in tube 1 = tube 4

WBC = white blood cells; RBC = red blood cells; PMN = polymorphonuclear neutrophils.

19

o **Back pain:** This develops at the site of the puncture and usually resolves within a few days. This is quite common, and in one large series, is more common than headache
o **Sixth nerve (abducens) palsy:** This occurs in fewer than 1% of individuals and is typically transient.
- **Trauma to nerve roots or the conus medullaris:** Much less frequent (some anatomic variation does exist, but it is very rare for the cord to end below L3). **If the patient suddenly complains of paresthesia** (numbness or shooting pain in the legs), **stop the procedure**.
- **Herniation of either the cerebellum or the medulla:** Occurs rarely during or after a spinal tap, usually occurs in a patient with increased intracranial pressure. This complication may be reversed medically if it is recognized early.
- **Meningitis**
- **Bleeding** in the subarachnoid or subdural space can occur with resulting paralysis, especially if the patient is receiving anticoagulants, has severe liver disease with coagulopathy, or has severe thrombocytopenia. Either spinal or cerebral subdural hematoma can occur. Antiplatelet therapy is not associated with increased risk of major bleeding.

ORTHOSTATIC BLOOD PRESSURE MEASUREMENT

Indication

- Assessment of volume depletion

Materials

- BP cuff and stethoscope

Procedure

1. Changes in BP and pulse when a patient moves from supine to the upright position are very sensitive bedside tests for detecting volume depletion. Even before a person becomes overtly tachycardic or hypotensive because of volume loss, the demonstration of orthostatic hypotension aids in the diagnosis.
2. Have the patient assume a supine position for 5–10 min. Determine the BP and pulse.
3. Have the patient stand up. If the patient is unable to stand, have the patient sit at the bedside with legs dangling.
4. After about 2–3 min, measure BP and pulse again.
5. A drop in systolic BP greater than 10 mm Hg or an increase in pulse rate greater than 20 beats/min (16 beats/min in the elderly) indicates **volume**

depletion. A change in heart rate is more sensitive and occurs with a lesser degree of volume depletion. Other causes of a drop in BP with body position change (usually without an increase in heart rate) include peripheral neuropathy, surgical sympathectomy, diabetes, and some medications (prazosin, hydralazine, or reserpine).

PARACENTESIS: SEE PERITONEAL (ABDOMINAL) PARACENTESIS, page 642

PELVIC EXAMINATION

Indications

- Pelvic examinations should be performed only when indicated by medical history or symptoms (see also Chapter 6, Gyencologic History and Physical Key Elements, page 87.)
- Screening exam for malignancy (cervical, ovarian, uterine, vaginal, or vulvar).
- Evaluation of certain infections (*Chlamydia, Gonorrhea*, condyloma [warts], candidiasis, bacterial vaginosis). The USPSTF, the CDC, and other professional organizations recommend routing periodic screening for *Chlamydia* for all sexually active women under 25 yr of age and older women at high-risk since screening decreases the incidence of PID. The use of self-collected vaginal swabs for *Chlamydia* screening or the use of urine PCR testing is replacing the routine pelvic exam for this screening.
- Evaluation of other pathology: Atrophic vaginitis, cervical polyps, uterine prolapse, cystocele, fibroids, etc.
- Prior to the provision of an intrauterine device but not for routine hormonal contraception.

Materials

- Sterile gloves
- Vaginal speculum and lubricant
- Thin prep liquid-based Pap smear, cotton swabs, endocervical brush, and cervical spatula prepared for a Pap smear

Materials for Other Diagnostic Tests

- Culture media to test for gonorrhea, *Chlamydia,* herpes
- Sterile cotton swabs
- Plain glass slides
- KOH
- Normal saline solutions, as needed

Background

The utility of the routine pelvic examination has recently been called into question. Traditionally, a pelvic examination is performed for asymptomatic women as a screening tool for gynecologic cancer and infections. The ability to screen for sexually transmitted infections using less invasive methods and the role of the pelvic examination for asymptomatic, nonpregnant women has been evaluated by the American College of Obstetricians and Gynecologists (ACOG).**

Data from recent studies do not support a recommendation for or against performing a routine screening pelvic examination among asymptomatic, nonpregnant women who are not at increased risk of any specific condition. ACOG recommends that that pelvic examinations be performed when indicated by medical history or symptoms. With a current or a history of cervical dysplasia, gynecologic malignancy, or in utero diethylstilbestrol exposure women should be screened and managed according to guidelines specific to those gynecologic conditions. The decision to perform a pelvic examination should be a shared decision between the patient and her care provider. After reviewing risks and benefits, the pelvic examination also may be performed if a woman expresses a preference for the examination. Note that United States Preventive Services Task Force 2018 guidelines have differing recommendations concerning cancer screening (see PAP Smear, Appendix, page 1049).

Procedure

1. In most situations involving sensitive exams such as this, a chaperone is often present for the examination along with the provider. Follow local policy for the role of medical chaperones. If present, the individual should be identified in the procedure note.
2. Perform the pelvic exam in conditions that are as comfortable as possible for both patient and physician. Drape the patient appropriately and help her place her feet in the stirrups on the examining table. Prepare a low stool for the examiner, a good light source, and all needed supplies before starting the exam. In unusual situations, examinations are conducted on a gurney or bed; if so, raise the patient's buttocks on one or two pillows to elevate the perineum off the mattress.
3. Inform the patient of each step in advance. Glove hands before proceeding.
4. **General inspection**
   a. Observe the skin of the perineum for swelling, ulcers, condylomas (venereal warts), and color changes.
   b. Separate the labia to examine the clitoris and vestibule. Multiple clear vesicles on an erythematous base on the labia suggest herpes.

19

**Committee on Gynecologic Practice. The Utility of and Indications for Routine Pelvic Examination. *Obstet Gynecol.* Oct 2018; 132.

    c. Observe the urethral meatus for developmental abnormalities, discharge, neoplasm, and abscess of Bartholin glands at the 4 and 8 o'clock positions.

    d. Inspect the vaginal orifice for discharge and protrusion of the walls (cystocele, rectocele, urethral prolapse).

5. Speculum examination.

    a. Use a speculum moistened with warm water or lubricant. Touch the speculum to the patient's leg to assess whether the temperature is comfortable. There are two general types of vaginal specula: the **Graves speculum**, which is wide billed (vaginal canal may be wider in parous women) and used in most adults, and the **Pedersen speculum**, which is narrow billed speculum and used in teenage girls who've been sexually active or in women with a narrow introitus (Figure 19-49A, page 631). Many specula used today are disposible and clear plastic.

    b. Because the anterior wall of the vagina is close to the urethra and bladder, do not exert pressure in this area. Place pressure on the posterior surface of the vagina. With the speculum directed at a 45-degree angle to the floor, spread the labia and insert the speculum fully, with pressure directed posteriorly. The cervix should come into view with some manipulation as the speculum is opened. If the cervix is not visualized, you might be behind the cervix; slowly remove the speculum about 1–3 in and see if the cervix appears.

    c. Inspect the cervix and vagina for color, lacerations, growths, Nabothian cysts, and evidence of atrophy.

    d. Inspect the cervical os for size, shape, color, and discharge. See Figure 19-49B, page 631.

    e. Inspect the vagina for secretions and obtain specimens for Pap smear, and other smears and culture (see tests for vaginal infections and Pap smear in step 8).

    f. Inspect the vaginal wall; rotate the speculum as you draw it out to see the entire canal. Have the patient perform a Valsalva maneuver that may indicate the presence of relaxation/laxity of the pelvic floor and demonstrate cystocele, urethrocele, rectocele, or vaginal prolapse. This laxity often due to multiple pregnancies with vaginal deliveries.

    g. Use caution when removing the speculum (especially if it is metal) because it can close quickly if not held open while being withdrawn and can trap vaginal mucosa.

6. Bimanual examination.

    a. Stand up for this part of the exam. Use whichever hand is comfortable to do the internal vaginal exam. Replace a clean glove on the hand used to examine the abdomen.

    b. Place lubricant on the first and second gloved fingers used for the internal portion of the examination, and keeping the pressure on the posterior fornix, introduce the fingers into the vagina.

    c. Palpate the tissue at the 5 and 7 o'clock positions between the first and second fingers and the thumb to rule out any abnormality of

19

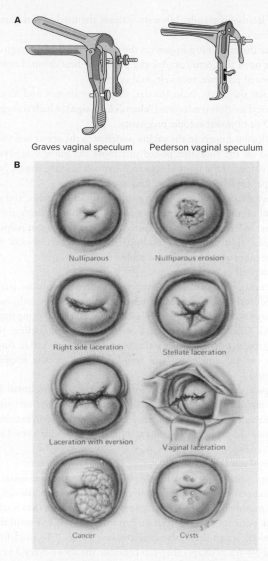

Graves vaginal speculum   Pederson vaginal speculum

Nulliparous   Nulliparous erosion

Right side laceration   Stellate laceration

Laceration with eversion   Vaginal laceration

Cancer   Cysts

Figure 19-49. **A.** Examples of the larger-billed Graves speculum and the narrow-billed Pedersen speculum used for pelvic examinations. Many devices today are made of clear plastic and disposable. **B.** Normal and pathologic appearance of the uterine cervix. (Panel A used with permission from Pernoll ML. Benson & Pernoll's Handbook of Obstetrics and Gynecology, 10e, New York, NY: McGraw-Hill; 2001 and Panel B used with permission from Bernstein HB. Normal Pregnancy & Prenatal Care. In: DeCherney AH, Nathan L, Laufer N, Roman AS, eds. CURRENT Diagnosis & Treatment: Obstetrics & Gynecology, 12e, New York, NY: McGraw-Hill; 2019.)

19

the Bartholin glands. Likewise, palpate the urethra and paraurethral (Skene) glands.

d. Place the examining fingers on the posterior wall of the vagina to further open the introitus. Ask the patient to bear down. Look for evidence of prolapse, rectocele, and cystocele.

e. Palpate the cervix. Note the size, shape, consistency, and motility and cervical motion tenderness (**"chandelier" sign**), which is suggestive of PID or ruptured ectopic pregnancy.

f. With your fingers in the vagina posterior to the cervix and your other hand on the abdomen placed just above the pubic symphysis, force the corpus of the uterus between the two examining hands. Note size, shape, consistency, position, and motility.

g. Move the fingers in the vagina to one or the other fornix, and place the hand on the abdomen in a more lateral position to bring the adnexal areas under examination. Palpate the ovaries (often not palpable), for masses, consistency, and motility. Unless they are diseased, the fallopian tubes usually are not palpable.

7. Rectovaginal examination.

a. Rectovaginal exam is no longer considered a routine part of the pelvic exam and should be performed only when indicated (e.g., to assess for pelvic pain, endometriosis, rectal symptoms, or a pelvic mass). Communicate with the patient before performing rectal portion of examination. Insert your index finger into the vagina, and place the well-lubricated middle finger in the rectum.

b. Palpate the posterior surface of the uterus and the broad ligament for nodularity, tenderness, and masses. Examine the uterosacral and rectovaginal septum. Nodularity may represent endometriosis.

c. It may also be helpful to do a test for occult blood if a stool specimen is available.

8. Papanicolaou (Pap) smear

The Pap smear is helpful in early detection of cervical intraepithelial neoplasia and carcinoma. Endometrial carcinoma is occasionally identified on routine Pap smears. It is recommended that once they reach age 21, low-risk patients undergo routine Pap smears every 3 yr until the age of 30 (United States Preventive Services Task Force 2018 guidelines). For women 30–65 yr of age, they can continue the above every 3 yr or begin high-risk HPV testing alone every 5 yr or co-testing with high-risk HPV testing and cytology every 5 yr. High-risk patients such as those exposed in utero to DES; patients with HPV infection or history of HIV infection; and those with a history of cervical cancer or cervical intraepithelial neoplasia may require more frequent testing. (See also American Cancer Society Guidelines, Appendix Table A-3, page 1049).

a. With a lubricated speculum in place, use a plastic cervical spatula to obtain a scraping from the squamocolumnar junction. Rotate the spatula 360 degrees around the external os. Place spatula into liquid Pap smear solution, which is identified with patient's name and date of birth.

b. Obtain a specimen from the endocervical canal using an endocervical brush and place into liquid medium.

c. Complete the appropriate order. Forewarn the patient that she may experience spotty vaginal bleeding after the Pap smear.

9. **Tests for cervical and vaginal infections.**

   a. **GC and** *Chlamydia* for nucleic acid amplification via a cervical swab, vaginal swab or urine specimen with higher sensitivity than cultures. Culture for GC and Chlamydia may need to be obtained if antibiotic resistance is a concern.

   b. **Vaginal saline (wet) prep:** Helpful in the diagnosis of *Trichomonas vaginalis* and bacterial vaginosis. Mix a drop of discharge with a drop of NS on a glass slide and cover it with a coverslip. Observe the slide while it is still warm to see the flagellated, motile trichomonads. If *Trichomonas vaginalis* is suspected and the wet prep is negative, nucleic amplification testing can be used. Bacterial vaginosis is most often caused by *Gardnerella vaginalis* and can be diagnosed by the presence of "clue cells," which represent PMNs dotted with the *G. vaginalis* bacteria; vaginal pH >4.5; and a fishy amine odor with the addition of KOH to the secretions. It is also possible to see these cells by using a hanging drop of saline and a concave slide. DNA probe-based test and other FDA approved tests are available. *Lactobacillus* organisms are normally the predominant bacteria in the vagina in the absence of specific infection, and the normal pH is usually <4.5.

   c. **Potassium hydroxide prep:** If a thick, white, curdy discharge is present, the patient may have *Candida albicans* (monilial) yeast infection. Prepare a slide with one drop of discharge and one drop of aqueous 10% KOH solution. The KOH dissolves the epithelial cells and debris and facilitates viewing of the hyphae and mycelia of the fungus that causes the infection. There are other commercially available tests for *Candida*.

   d. **Gram stain:** Material can easily be stained in the usual manner (Chapter 13, Clinical Microbiology, page 320). Gram-negative intracellular diplococci (so-called "GNIDs") are pathognomonic of *N. gonorrhoeae* infection. The bacteria most commonly found in Gram stains are large gram-positive rods (lactobacilli), which are normal vaginal flora.

   e. **Herpes cultures:** A routine Pap smear of the cervix or a Pap smear of the herpetic lesion (multiple, clear vesicles on a painful, erythematous base) may show herpes inclusion bodies. Swab the suspicious lesion or the endocervix to obtain a specimen for herpes viral culture. PCR can also be used for the diagnosis of genital herpes.

19

PERICARDIOCENTESIS

Indications

- Emergency treatment of cardiac tamponade
- Diagnosis of the cause of pericardial effusion

Contraindications

- Minimal pericardial effusion (<200 mL)
- Aftermath of CABG because of risk of injury to grafts
- Uncorrected coagulopathy
- When the effusion is associated with aortic dissection or myocardial rupture (potential risk of rapid pericardial decompression and restoration of systemic arterial pressure)

Materials

- ECG machine
- Prepackaged pericardiocentesis kit or procedure and instrument tray (page 516) with pericardiocentesis needle or 16- to 18-gauge needle 10 cm long

Background

Cardiac tamponade results in decreased cardiac output, increased right atrial filling pressure, and pronounced pulsus paradoxus. Acute cardiac tamponade is associated with **Beck triad. The three signs are hypotension, decreased heart sounds, and increased jugular venous pressure**. Some causes of pericardial effusion with or without tamponade include malignancy, uremia, iatrogenic, post-acute MI, infection, acute pericarditis, rheumatologic diseases (SLE, others), idiopathic and other unknown causes.

Procedure

1. If time permits, use sterile prep and draping with gown, mask, and gloves. If available, ultrasound is useful at identifying the location of the effusion and is useful needle placement.
2. Use a left para xiphoid or left parasternal approach through the fourth ICS. The para xiphoid approach is safer, more commonly used, and described here (Figure 19-50, page 635, see below).
3. Anesthetize the insertion site with lidocaine. Connect the needle with an alligator clip to the chest lead (brown) on the ECG machine. Attach the limb leads and monitor the ECG monitor.
4. Insert the pericardiocentesis needle just to the left of the xiphoid process and directed 45 degrees upwards toward the left shoulder.

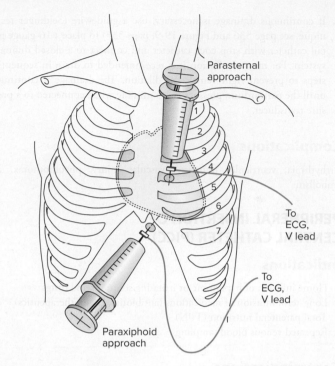

Parasternal
approach

To
ECG,
V lead

To
ECG,
V lead

Paraxiphoid
approach

Figure 19-50. Techniques for pericardiocentesis. The paraxiphoid inferior approach is the most frequently used.

19

5. Aspirate while advancing the needle until the pericardium is punctured and the effusion is tapped. If you feel the ventricular wall, withdraw the needle slightly. If the needle contacts the myocardium, pronounced ST segment elevation will be recorded on the ECG.
6. If pericardiocentesis is performed for cardiac tamponade, removal of as little as 50 mL of fluid dramatically improves BP and decreases right atrial pressure.
7. Blood from a bloody pericardial effusion is usually defibrinated and does not clot, whereas blood from the ventricle does clot.
8. Send fluid for HCT, cell count, or cytology if indicated.
   Differential diagnosis of pericardiocentesis fluid:
   • **Serous fluid:** Consistent with CHF, bacterial infection, TB, hypoalbuminemia, or viral pericarditis
   • **Bloody fluid (HCT >10%):** May result from trauma; iatrogenic; or due to MI, uremia, coagulopathy, or malignant disease (lymphoma, leukemia, breast, lung most common)

9. If continuous drainage is necessary, use a guidewire (Seldinger technique, see page 536 and Figure 19-9, page 537) to place a 16-gauge pig tail catheter with stop cock catheter and connect to a closed drainage system. For massive effusion it is recommended to drain in sequential steps to prevent right ventricular dilation. The drainage is continued until the pericardium pressure is <5 mm Hg when connected to a pressure transducer.

Complications

Arrhythmia, ventricular puncture, vascular injury, pneumothorax, air embolism

PERIPHERAL INSERTION OF CENTRAL CATHETER (PICC)

Indications

- Home infusion of hypertonic or irritating solutions and drugs
- Long-term infusion of medications (antibiotics, chemotherapeutics)
- Total parenteral nutrition (TPN)
- Repeated venous blood sampling

Contraindications

- Infection over placement site
- Inability to identify veins in an arm with a tourniquet in place

Materials

- PICC catheter kit (contains most items necessary, including the Silastic long arm line, such as the Introsyte™ Autoguard system)
- Tourniquet, sterile gloves, mask, sterile gown, heparin flush, 10-mL syringes

Background

Placement of a PICC allows for central venous access through a peripheral vein. See Central Venous Catheterization, this chapter, page 533, for a full discussion and comparison of all central venous catheterization approaches, including PICC. Typically, a long arm catheter is placed into the basilic or cephalic vein, usually with bedside portable ultrasound guidance (see Figure 19-42, page 613) and is threaded into the subclavian vein and superior vena cava. PICCs are useful for long-term home infusion therapy. The design of PICC catheters vary, and the operator should be familiar with the features of the device being used (attached hub or detachable hub designs). Typically, these catheters are placed by specialized PICC nurses at the bedside or by interventional radiologists under fluoroscopic guidance, but it is prudent to be aware of the technique because any trained medical personnel can be called on to place these catheters. The CDC recommends a PICC if an intravenous therapy is to last longer than 6 days.

Procedure

1. Explain the procedure to the patient and obtain informed consent. Have the patient sit or lie down with the elbow extended and the arm in a dependent position. The arm should be externally rotated.
2. Using a measuring tape, determine the length of the catheter required. Measure from the extremity vein insertion site to the subclavian vein.
3. Wear a mask, gown, protective eyewear, and sterile gloves. Set up an adjacent sterile working area. Anyone within about 3 ft of the bedside should have a cap and mask on and observe maximal sterile barrier precautions. Prep and drape the skin in the standard manner. Prepare the area of insertion utilizing an institutional-approved bactericidal agent and allow the solution to dry. Avoid alcohol, as it can cause degradation of some catheters. Tourniquet proximal to the insertion site.
4. Anesthetize the skin at the proposed area of insertion.
5. Trim the catheter to the appropriate length. Most PICC lines have an attached hub, and the distal end of the catheter is cut to the proper length based on previous measurement. Flush with heparinized saline.
6. Insert the catheter and introducer needle (usually 14-gauge in adults) into the chosen arm vein, as detailed on page 611 discussing IV techniques (Figure 19-51A, page 638). A flash of blood will be observed near the activation button when the vein has been entered. Decrease the insertion angle, and advance the catheter and needle assembly farther into the vein.
7. Once the catheter is in the vein, release the tourniquet. Apply pressure to the vein beyond the tip of the catheter and needle assembly to limit blood loss (Figure 19-51B, page 638). Push the white activation button on the Introsyte device to shield the needle by retracting into the sheath and discard the needle assembly (Figure 19-51C, page 639).
8. Place the PICC line in the catheter and advance it using forceps if provided by the manufacturer of the kit or a separate sterile instrument (Figure 19-51D, page 639). Gradually advance the catheter the requisite length. If present, remove the inner stiffening wire slowly once the catheter has been adequately advanced.
9. Split the introducer wings and peel away the introducer catheter as shown in Figure 19-52, page 640). Attach the Luer-Lock and flush the catheter with heparin solution. Attempt to aspirate blood to verify patency.

19

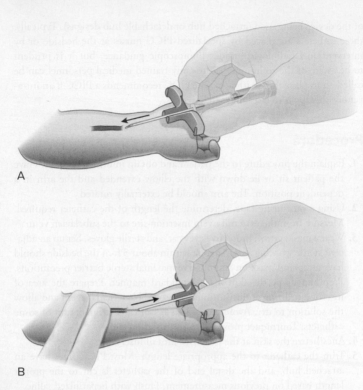

A

B

19

Figure 19-51. Demonstration of the PICC line placement **A.** The specially designed PICC introducer needle is passed into the vein, demonstrated here in a child but usually in the upper extremity in an adult. Once in the vein, a flash back of blood can be seen when the needle is in the vein. Thread introducer sheath at least about 1/4 in off the end of the needle into the vessel. Release the tourniquet and apply pressure to the vein just beyond the tip of the catheter. **B.** The catheter is stabilized. Push the white button on the introducer device and the needle retracts into the sheath as shown in Panel C. (continued on next page)

10. Attach the provided securing wings in the kit and suture them in place. Apply a sterile dressing over the insertion site.
11. Confirm placement in the central circulation with a CXR. Always document the type of PICC, the length inserted, and the site by radiologically confirmation.
12. If vein cannulation is difficult, a surgical cutdown may be necessary to cannulate the vein. If the catheter does not advance, fluoroscopy may be helpful.

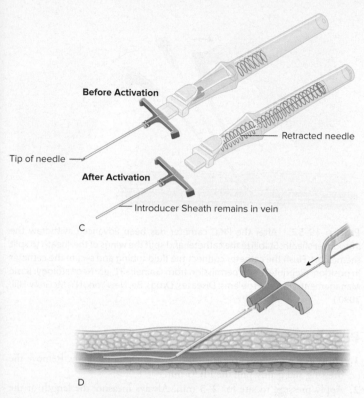

Figure 19-51. (continued from previous page) **C**. The device is activated to withdraw the needle safely into the sheath, leaving the introducer catheter in place. **D.** Place the PICC line catheter with its stiffening wire in the catheter and advance it using a forceps through the introducer sheath. (Reprinted with permission from Gomella TL, ed. Neonatology: Basic Management, On-Call Problems, Diseases, Drugs, 8e, New York, NY: McGraw-Hill; 2020.)

19

13. Instruct the patient and their caretaker on the maintenance of the PICC. The PICC should be flushed with heparinized saline solution after each use. Dressing changes should be performed at least every 7 d under sterile conditions. Instruct the patient to evaluate the PICC site for signs and symptoms of infection. Also, instruct the patient to come to the ER for evaluation if a fever develops.

14. For venous samples, withdraw a specimen of at least the catheter volume (1–3 mL) and discard it. The PICC must always be flushed with heparinized saline solution after each blood draw to avoid clotting.

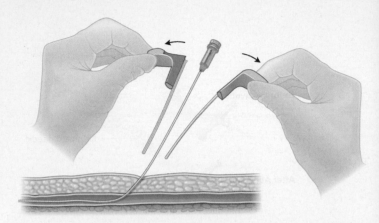

Figure 19-52. After the PICC catheter has been advanced, withdraw the introducer sheath. Stabilize the catheter and split the wings of the sheath to split them apart. Flush the catheter connect the fluid tubing and secure the catheter in position. (Reprinted with permission from Gomella TL, ed. Neonatology: Basic Management, On-Call Problems, Diseases, Drugs, 8e, New York, NY: McGraw-Hill; 2020.)

PICC Removal

1. Position the patient's arm at a 90-degree angle to the body. Remove the dressing and gently pull the PICC out.
2. Apply pressure to site for 2–3 min. Always measure the length of the catheter and check previous documented length to ensure that the PICC line has been removed in its entirety. If a piece of a catheter is left behind, an emergency interventional radiology or cardiology consult is in order.

Complications

Site bleeding, clotted catheter, subclavian thrombosis, infection, broken catheter (leakage or embolization), arrhythmia (catheter inserted too far)

PERITONEAL LAVAGE

Indications

- Peritoneal lavage, formally known as **diagnostic peritoneal lavage (DPL)** is used in the evaluation of intraabdominal trauma (bleeding, perforation) (*Note:* Spiral CT of the abdomen has largely replaced DPL as an initial screening tool for intraabdominal trauma in the emergency setting.)

- Acute peritoneal dialysis and management of severe pancreatitis.
- Aid in the diagnosis of diaphragmatic injury in select patients

Contraindications

- No absolute complications (except in the presence of a clear indication for immediate laparotomy). Relative contraindications: Multiple abdominal procedures, pregnancy, known retroperitoneal injury (high false-positive rate), cirrhosis, morbid obesity, coagulopathy.

Materials

- Prepackaged DPL or peritoneal dialysis tray

Procedure

1. A Foley catheter and an NG or orogastric tube **must** be in place to decompress the bladder and viscera. Prep the abdomen from above the umbilicus to the pubis.
2. The site of choice is in the midline 1–2 cm below the umbilicus. Avoid the sites of old surgical scars (danger of adherent bowel). If a subumbilical scar or pelvic fracture is present, use a supraumbilical approach.
3. Infiltrate the skin with lidocaine with epinephrine. Incise the skin in the midline vertically and expose the fascia.
4. Either pick up the fascia and incise it or puncture it with the trocar and peritoneal catheter. Exercise caution to avoid puncturing any organs. Use one hand to hold the catheter near the skin and to control the insertion while using the other hand to apply pressure to the end of the catheter. After the peritoneal cavity is entered, remove the trocar and direct the catheter inferiorly into the pelvis.
5. During a diagnostic lavage, gross blood indicates a positive tap. If no blood is encountered, instill 10 mL/kg (about 1 L in adults) of Ringer's lactate or normal saline into the abdominal cavity.
6. Gently agitate the abdomen to distribute the fluid; after 5 min drain off as much fluid as possible into a bag on the floor. (Minimum fluid for a valid analysis is 200 mL in an adult.) If the drainage is slow, try instilling additional fluid, carefully repositioning the catheter.
7. Send the fluid for analysis (amylase, bile, bacteria, hematocrit, cell count). Interpret the findings using Table 19-11, page 642.
8. Remove the catheter and suture the skin. If the catheter is inserted because of pancreatitis or for peritoneal dialysis, suture the catheter in place.
9. Negative DPL does not exclude retroperitoneal trauma. False-positive DPL can be caused by a pelvic fracture or bleeding induced by the procedure (e.g., laceration of an omental vessel).

19

Table 19-11. Criteria for Evaluation of Peritoneal Lavage Fluid

Positive	>20 mL gross blood on free aspiration (10 mL in children)
	≥100,000 RBC/mL
	≥500 WBC/mL (if obtained >3 hr after the injury)
	≥175 units amylase/dL
	Bacteria on Gram stain
	Bile (by inspection or chemical determination of bilirubin content)
	Food particles (microscopic analysis of strained or spun specimen)
Intermediate	Pink fluid on free aspiration
	50,000–100,000 RBC/mL in blunt trauma
	100–500 WBC/mL
	75–175 units amylase/dL
Negative	Clear aspirate
	≤100 WBC/μL
	≤75 units amylase/dL

Source: Reprinted with permission from Way, L., Doherty GM (eds). Current Surgical Diagnosis and Treatment, 11e, New York, NY: McGraw-Hill; 2003.
RBC = red blood cells; WBC = white blood cells.

Complications

Infection, peritonitis, superficial wound infection, bleeding, perforated viscus (bladder, bowel)

PERITONEAL (ABDOMINAL) PARACENTESIS

Indications

- Determining the cause of ascites
- Determining whether intraabdominal bleeding is present or whether a viscus has ruptured (Note that diagnostic peritoneal lavage or CT based imaging is considered a more accurate test, see preceding procedure, page 640)
- Therapeutic removal of fluid when distention is pronounced, or respiratory distress is present (acute treatment only)

Contraindications

- Abnormal coagulation factors
- Bowel obstruction, bowel distension, pregnancy
- Uncertainty whether distention is caused by peritoneal fluid or due to a cystic structure (usually can be differentiated with ultrasonography)

Materials

- Minor procedure tray (see page 516)
- Catheter-over-needle assembly (Angiocath™ Autoguard, Insyte™ Autoguard 18- to 20-gauge with 1½-in [4 cm] needle)
- 20–60-mL syringe
- Sterile specimen containers

Procedure

Peritoneal paracentesis is surgical puncture of the peritoneal cavity for aspiration of fluid. Ascites is indicated by abdominal distention, shifting dullness, and a palpable fluid wave; generally ultrasonography is used to confirm ascites.

1. Explain the procedure and have the patient sign an informed consent form. Have the patient empty the bladder or place a Foley catheter if voiding is impossible or if marked changes in mental status are present.
2. The entry site is usually the midline 1–1½ in (3–4 cm) below the umbilicus. Avoid old surgical scars because the bowel may be adherent to the abdominal wall. An alternative entry site is the left or right lower quadrant midway between the umbilicus and the anterior superior iliac spine or the patient's flank, depending on the percussion of the fluid wave (Figure 19-53, page 644). Avoid the rectus abdominus because of bleeding potential.
3. Prep and drape the area and raise a skin wheal with the lidocaine over the entry site.
4. A "Z track" technique helps limit persistent leakage of peritoneal fluid after the procedure (Figure 19-41, page 611). Manually retract the skin caudally and release traction on the skin when the peritoneum is entered. With the catheter mounted on the syringe, go through the anesthetized area while aspirating. There is resistance as the fascia is entered. When there is free return of fluid, leave the catheter in place, and remove the needle or activate the self-shielding mechanism. Begin to aspirate; reposition the catheter as needed because of abutting bowel.
5. Aspirate the amount of fluid needed for laboratory testing (20–30 mL). If the tap is therapeutic, 10–15 L can be safely removed. The removal of a large volume can be facilitated by the use of vacuum container bottles (500 mL–1 L) supplied at most hospitals. Tubing is first connected to the catheter and then to the vacuum container bottles.
6. Apply a sterile 4 × 4 gauze square, and apply pressure with tape. In patients with chronic ascites, a purse-string suture may be placed at the puncture site to minimize ongoing leakage of ascitic fluid from the tap.
7. Depending on the patient's clinical condition, send samples for cell count, including differential, total protein, albumin, amylase, LDH, glucose, cytology, and C&S.

19

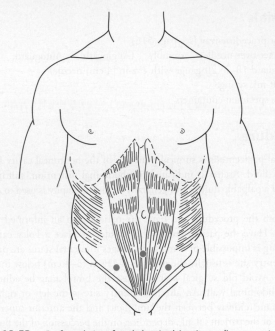

Figure 19-53. Preferred sites for abdominal (peritoneal) paracentesis in an adult. Be sure to avoid old surgical scars.

Complications

Peritonitis, perforated viscus (bowel, bladder), hemorrhage, precipitation of hepatic coma if the patient has severe liver disease, oliguria, or hypotension

Diagnosis of Ascitic Fluid

A differential diagnosis of ascitic fluid can be found in Chapter 9, page 152. The older classification of ascitic fluid as either transudative or exudative is no longer used. The cause of ascites is more likely to be found by determining the serum-to-ascites albumin gradient. See Table 19-12, page 645, to interpret the results of the ascitic fluid analysis.

PULMONARY ARTERY CATHETERIZATION

Details on the applications and insertion of the pulmonary artery catheter can be found in Chapter 28, Critical Care, page 895.

Table 19-12. Differential Diagnosis of Ascitic Fluid

Albumin Gradient:
Serum Albumin – Ascites Albumin = X
if X >1.1 g/dL, then portal hypertension
if X <1.1 g/dL, etiology other than portal hypertension
Cell Count: Absolute neutrophil count >250/μL, presume infected; absolute neutrophil count should be corrected for RBCs (subtract 1 PMN for every 250/μL RBCs
Bacterial Culture: Blood culture bottles 85% sensitivity
Routine cultures 50% sensitivity
Bacterial Peritonitis: Spontaneous versus secondary
Secondary: (1) polymicrobial; (2) total protein >1.0 g/dL; (3) LDH >normal serum value; (4) glucose <50 mg/dL
Food Fibers: Found in most cases of perforated viscus
Cytology: Bizarre cells with large nuclei may represent reactive mesothelial cells and not malignancy. Malignant cells suggest a tumor.

Source: Modified from from Haist SA, Robbins JB, eds. Internal Medicine on Call, 4e, New York, NY: McGraw-Hill; 2005.

PULSUS PARADOXUS MEASUREMENT (PARADOXICAL PULSE)

Indication

- Used in the evaluation of cardiac tamponade and other diseases (e.g., severity of asthma)

Materials

- BP cuff and stethoscope

Background

(See also Chapter 28, Page 891)
Pulsus paradoxus is an exaggeration of the normal inspiratory drop in arterial pressure. Inspiration decreases intrathoracic pressure. The result is increased right atrial and right ventricular filling with an increase in right ventricular output. Because the pulmonary vascular bed also distends, these changes lead to a delay in left ventricular filling and subsequently decreased left ventricular output. This drop in systolic BP is usually <10 mm Hg. In the case of cardiac

19

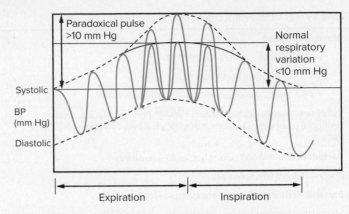

Figure 19-54. Graphical representation of paradoxical pulse.

compression (e.g., acute asthma or pericardial tamponade), the right side of the heart fills more with inspiration and decreases the left ventricular volume to an even greater degree as a result of compression of the pericardial sac. This exaggerated decrease in left ventricular output decreases systolic pressure >10 mm Hg. See Figure 19-54, for a graphic representation of a paradoxical pulse.

Procedure

1. For a simple, **qualitative method**, palpate the radial pulse, which "disappears" on normal inspiration.
2. For a more precise **quantitative method**, measure systolic BP at end exhalation during tidal breathing.
   a. Determine systolic BP at end-inspiration during tidal breathing.
   b. The difference in systolic pressure between end exhalation and end inspiration should be <10 mm Hg. If >10 mm Hg, a so-called "paradoxical pulse" exists.
3. Differential diagnosis includes pericardial effusion, cardiac tamponade, pericarditis, COPD, bronchial asthma, restrictive cardiomyopathy, hemorrhagic shock, massive PE, tricuspid stenosis, and mitral stenosis.

SKIN BIOPSY AND OTHER TECHNIQUES FOR DERMATOLOGIC DIAGNOSIS

Indications

- Any skin lesion or eruption with an unclear diagnosis
- Any refractory skin condition

Contraindications

- Any skin lesion suspected of being malignant (e.g., melanoma) should be referred to a plastic surgeon or dermatologist for a formal excisional biopsy rather than punch or shave biopsy; a full-thickness biopsy is critical for diagnosis and accurate staging of lesions such as melanoma.

Background

Skin biopsy is an easily performed bedside procedure. Techniques include skin punch, shaving with a scalpel or razor blade, and sharp excision. Selection of the technique appropriate for each lesion and for technical performance of the biopsy is based on the experience of the operator.

Punch biopsies yield full-thickness samples and can be used for rashes or blistering lesions involving the dermis that require dermal or subcutaneous tissue for diagnosis (e.g., drug reaction, cutaneous lymphoma, erythema multiforme, Kaposi sarcoma, SLE, pemphigoid, pemphigus, vasculitis). Punch biopsies can be excisional or incisional, based on the size of the lesion and the type of tissue that needs to be obtained.

A superficial shave biopsy can be used for raised lesions that are predominantly epidermal without extension into the dermis, such as warts, papillomas, skin tags, superficial basal or squamous cell carcinomas, and seborrheic or actinic keratoses. Shave skin biopsy is not considered appropriate for suspicious pigmented lesions (e.g., melanoma). Indications for biopsy of suspected melanoma are not usually considered a bedside procedure. The skin punch and shave biopsy techniques are described here.

Materials

- For shave and punch biopsy:
  - Antiseptic skin prep (e.g., povidone/iodine, chlorhexidine)
  - Topical anesthetic (e.g., lidocaine 1% or 2%, with or without 1:100,000 epinephrine with needle (21G) and syringe (see page 516)
  - Specimen container with formalin or preservative requested by the lab
  - Drape, clean towels, gauze pads, forceps, scissors
  - Bandage and topical antibiotic of choice
  - Useful to have hemostatic agents such as silver nitrate sticks or pencil electrocautery available
- For shave biopsy:
  - Double-sided flexible razor blades, no. 15 scalpel blade or commercial flexible shave biopsy instrument (DermaBlade™)
- For punch biopsy
  - 2-, 3-, 4-, or 5-mm skin punch
  - Curved iris scissors and fine-toothed forceps (ordinary forceps may distort a small biopsy specimen and should not be used)
  - Needle driver with suture material (3-0 or 4-0 nylon)

19

Procedure: Punch Biopsy

1. Obtain informed consent.
2. If more than one lesion is present, choose one that is well developed and representative of the dermatosis. For patients with vesiculobullous disease, choose an early edematous lesion rather than a vesicle. Avoid lesions that are excoriated or infected.
3. Mark the biopsy area with a skin-marking pen. Inject lidocaine to form a skin wheal over the site of the biopsy.
4. After putting on sterile gloves and preparing a sterile field, obtain the punch biopsy specimen. Immobilize the skin with the fingers of one hand, applying pressure perpendicular to the skin wrinkle lines with the skin punch. Core out a cylinder of skin by twirling the punch between the fingers of the other hand (Figure 19-55, page 649). As the punch enters into the SQ fat, resistance lessens. At this point, remove the punch. The core of tissue usually pops up slightly and can be cut at the level of the SQ fat with a curved iris scissors without forceps. If the tissue core does not pop up, elevate the core gently using a hypodermic needle or fine-toothed forceps. Be sure to include a portion of the SQ fat in the specimen.
5. Place the specimen in the specimen container.
6. Apply pressure with the gauze pad to achieve hemostasis.
7. Defects from 1.5- and 2-mm punches usually do not require suturing and heal with minimal scarring. Punch defects measuring 2–4 mm can generally be closed with a single 3-0 or 4-0 nylon suture.
8. Apply a dry dressing with or without antibiotic ointment and remove it the following day.
9. Sutures can be removed as early as 3 days from the face and 7–10 days from other areas (see Chapter 25, page 821, for additional information on Suturing and Wound Care).

Procedure: Shave Biopsy

1. and **2.** as above
3. Hold the blade of choice parallel to the skin and slowly remove the lesion or a disk of skin. The specimen is typically less than 1 mm and includes epidermis and upper dermis.
4. Apply a dry dressing with or without antibiotic ointment and remove it the following day.

Other Dermatologic Diagnostic Techniques

Skin scrapings. Used most commonly to diagnose fungal dermatoses or skin infestations. Gently scrape the edge of the skin lesion with a no. 15 scalpel blade. Keep blade perpendicular to skin surface to prevent laceration.

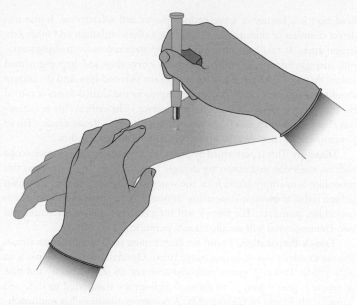

Figure 19-55. Demonstration of skin biopsy using the punch biopsy technique.

- For skin infestations such as scabies (infestation of the skin with the mite *Sarcoptes scabiei* is suspected because of the appearance of 5- to 10-mm-long tracks or burrows on finger-webs, wrists, or genitalia), place glycerol or mineral oil over a burrow or papule (prevents dispersion of mites during scraping), which is then unroofed with the edge of a scalpel. Scrapings are placed directly under a coverslip with mineral oil to identify mites, feces, or eggs to confirm the diagnosis.
- If fungal infection is suspected obtain a skin specimen by using a scalpel blade to scrape scales from the skin lesion onto a glass slide or to transfer the top of a vesicle to the microscope slide. Then a drop of 10% to 20% potassium hydroxide is added. The alkaline KOH solution separates and eventually destroys cells of the stratum corneum, permitting the hyphae and spores of dermatophytes to become more clearly visible. Allow the KOH prep to sit at room temperature until the material has been cleared. The slide may be warmed. Examine the smear under low-power (10×) and high-dry (40×) lenses for mycelial forms. Hyphae, budding yeast, or both confirm the diagnosis of fungal infection (candidiasis, tinea versicolor, trichophyton others).

Wood Light Examination. A 360-mm "black light" (long-wave ultraviolet light) is useful for detecting bacterial or fungal infection or accentuating features of some skin lesions. Fluorescence in skin and hair (scabies and

19

head lice) is a feature of some dermatophytes and infestations. It also can detect disorders of skin pigment including vitiligo, melasma, and other skin irregularities. It can help distinguish hypopigmentation from depigmentation (depigmentation of vitiligo fluoresces ivory-white and hypopigmented lesions do not). The light is not harmful to the skin and eyes, and the patient should be reassured. (*Note:* Most tinea capitis in the United States is caused by *Trichophyton* species, which do not fluoresce.) The earliest clue to cutaneous *Pseudomonas* infection (e.g., in burns) may be green fluorescence. (Trivia: Systemic tetracycline therapy causes the urine to fluoresce yellow.)

Diascopy. This is performed by pressing a magnifying lens or microscope slide on the lesion and observing changes in vascularity. The purpose of this procedure is to empty blood from the superficial vessels to determine if skin redness is due to blood within vessels (erythema) or extravasated into the skin (petechiae, purpura). The former will blanch with pressure; the latter will not. Hemangiomas will usually blanch; purpuric lesions will not.

Tzanck Preparation. Useful for determining presence of herpes viruses (herpes simplex virus or herpes zoster virus). Optimal lesion to sample is an early vesicle. Lesion is gently unroofed with no. 15 scalpel blade, and base of vesicle is gently scraped as above. Scrapings are transferred to slide and stained with Wright or Giemsa stain. A positive preparation has multinucleated giant cells. Culture or immunofluorescence testing must be performed to identify the specific virus. Testing (direct fluorescent antibody [DFA]) testing or PCR are preferred to the Tzanck smear. DFA testing of vesicular fluid or a corneal lesion can identify the varicella-zoster virus antigen. DFA and PCR have far greater sensitivity and specificity than the Tzanck smear and can differentiate between herpes simplex virus and varicella-zoster infections.

Complications

Skin biopsy infections are unusual; hemorrhage (usually controlled by simple application of pressure); keloid formation, especially in a patient with a history of keloid formation

SKIN TESTING

Indications

- Screening for current or past infection delayed-type hypersensitivity (e.g., TB, coccidioidomycosis).
- Screening for immune competency (so-called anergy screen) in debilitated patients.
- Skin testing is considered the gold standard for the detection of IgE-mediated reactions by exposing the mast cells of the skin to the suspected allergen. **Allergy testing** is conducted by close monitoring after injection of allergen extracts.

Materials

- Appropriate antigen (usually 0.1 mL) (e.g., 5 TU PPD)
- A small, short needle (25-, 26-, or 27-gauge)
- 1-mL syringe
- Alcohol swab

Background

Skin tests for **delayed-type hypersensitivity (type IV, tuberculin)** are the most commonly administered and interpreted. Delayed hypersensitivity (so-called due to a lag time of 24–48 hr required for a reaction) is caused by the activation of previously sensitized lymphocytes after contact with an antigen (cell-mediated arm of the immune system). A positive tuberculin skin test (TST) does not distinguish between prior and current infection. The inflammatory reaction results from direct cytotoxicity and the release of lymphokines. Allergy tests (immediate wheal and flare) are rarely performed by students or house officers and require specialized training and monitoring and are not discussed here.

The effects of Bacille Calmette-Guérin (BCG) vaccination on the results of the tuberculin skin test (TST) depend on the age at time of vaccination. When BCG is given in infancy, as is now recommended by the World Health Organization, its effect on the TST is negligible after 10 yr. Therefore, a TST with 10 mm or more of induration in an adolescent or adult with risk factors for infection who received BCG in infancy is indicative of tuberculosis infection. Individuals who received BCG as older children or adults are more prone to false-positive tuberculin skin test results, although this risk also diminishes with time. Use of an interferon-gamma release assay, which does not contain antigens present in BCG, may be useful to clarify the results of TST in these patients and to exclude false-positive TST results. Guidelines from the Centers for Disease Control and Prevention (CDC) in May 2019 stated that, following baseline screening, healthcare workers should no longer undergo routine annual screening for latent TB. Continuing annual screening is reasonable for workers at increased risk for occupational TB exposure (pulmonologists, respiratory therapists, emergency department physicians, nurses, etc.). Institutional policies should be individualized to incorporate these factors.

19

Procedure

1. The most commonly used site is the flexor surface of the forearm, approximately 4 in (10 cm) below the elbow crease.
2. Prep the area with alcohol. With the bevel of the 27-gauge needle up, introduce the needle into the upper layers of skin, but **not** into the subcutis (about a 15-degree angle). Inject 0.1 mL of antigen, such as PPD. The

goal is to inject the antigen intradermally (see Figure 19-40, page 609). If the injection has been done properly, a discrete white bleb approximately 10 mm in diameter (known as the **Mantoux test**) rises. The bleb should disappear soon, and no dressing is needed. If a bleb is not raised, move to another area and repeat the injection. Do not inject too superficially (in the epidermis); doing so causes epidermal–dermal separation resulting in blister formation and an inaccurate test result.

3. Mark the test site with a pen; if multiple tests are being administered, identify each one. Document the site or sites in the patient's chart.

4. To interpret the skin test, examine the site 48–72 hr after injection. If nonreactive, at 48 hr, recheck at 72 hr. **Measure the area of induration (the firm raised area), not the erythematous area.** Use a ballpoint pen held at approximately a 30-degree angle and bring it lightly toward the raised area. Where the pen touches the area of induration, mark the skin and repeat at 180 degrees on the other side of the induration. Do this again at 60–90 degrees from the previous marks. Measure the two diameters and take the average.

5. It is important to check the PPD and other tests at intervals. If the patient develops a severe reaction to the skin test, apply hydrocortisone cream to prevent skin sloughing.

Specific Skin Tests

TST (Tuberculin Skin Testing): Routine TST on persons at low risk is not recommended. Persons at high risk should undergo periodic TST, including those with CXR findings suspicious for TB or recent contact with known or suspected TB cases (includes healthcare workers); immigrants from high-risk areas (Asia, Africa, Middle East, Latin America), the medically underserved (IV drug users, persons with alcoholism, homeless persons); persons undergoing long-term institutionalization; and persons with HIV infection and others who are immunosuppressed.

The **Mantoux test** is the standard technique for TST and relies on the intradermal injection of **PPD**. The **tine test** for TB is no longer recommended by the CDC. The PPD comes in three tuberculin unit strengths: 1 TU (first), 5 TU (intermediate), and 250 TU (second). One TU is used if the patient is expected to be hypersensitive (history of a positive skin test); 5 TU is the standard initial screening test. A patient who has a negative response to a 5-TU test dose may react to the 250-TU solution. A patient who does not respond to 250-TU is considered nonreactive to PPD. A patient may not react if he or she has not been exposed to the antigen or is anergic and unable to respond to any antigen challenge. A positive TST indicates the presence of *Mycobacterium tuberculosis* infection, either active or past (dormant), and intact cell-mediated immunity.

Interpretation of a positive PPD test is based on the clinical scenario. **Patients who have been previously immunized with percutaneous BCG may have a false-positive PPD, usually 10 mm or less.** Interferon gamma release assays (IGRAs) carry a 70% to 90% concordance with PPD testing and are used in all circumstances in which TST is currently used. The IGRA is more specific than TST but more expensive and requires whole blood testing.

- 0–5 mm induration: Negative response
- ≥5 mm: Considered positive in contacts of known TB cases, CXR findings consistent with TB infection or HIV infection or in patients who are immunosuppressed, occasionally in non-TB mycobacterial infection due to cross-reactivity
- ≥10 mm induration: Considered positive in patients with chronic disease (diabetes, alcoholism, IV drug abuse, other chronic diseases), homeless persons, immigrants from known TB regions, and children <4 yr
- >15 mm induration: Positive in persons who are healthy and otherwise do not meet the preceding risk categories

Anergy Screen (Anergy Battery): An anergy screen is based on the assumption that a patient has been exposed in the past to certain common antigens and that a healthy person is able to mount a reaction to them. In anergy screening, an antigen such as mumps or *Candida* is applied, and the results are interpreted similar to PPD testing (a reaction of >5 mm induration is considered a positive test and indicates intact cellular immunity). Anergy screens are sometimes used to evaluate a patient's immunologic status. This test is not commonly used today as the reagents are increasingly costly and becoming unavailable.

THORACENTESIS

Indications

- Determining the cause of a pleural effusion
- Therapeutic removal of pleural fluid in the event of respiratory distress
- Aspirating small pneumothoraces when the risk of recurrence is small (e.g., postoperative without lung injury)
- Instilling sclerosing compounds (e.g., tetracycline) to obliterate the pleural space

Contraindications

- No absolute contraindications. Relative: Pneumothorax, hemothorax, any major respiratory impairment on the contralateral side; coagulopathy

Materials

- Prepackaged thoracentesis kit with either needle or catheter (preferred) *or*
- Minor procedure tray (page 516)

19

- 20- to 60-mL syringe, 20- or 22-gauge needle 1½-in (4 cm) needle, three-way stopcock
- Specimen containers

Background

Thoracentesis is a surgical puncture on the chest wall for aspiration of fluid or air from the pleural cavity. The area of pleural effusion is dull to percussion with decreased breath sounds. Pleural fluid causes blunting of the costophrenic angles on CXR. Blunting usually indicates that at least 300 mL of fluid is present. If you suspect that less than 300 mL of fluid is present or that the fluid is loculated (trapped and not free-flowing), obtain a lateral decubitus film. Loculated effusions do not layer out. Thoracentesis can be done safely on fluid visualized on a lateral decubitus film if at least 10 mm of fluid is measurable on the decubitus X-ray. Ultrasonography may also be used to localize a small or loculated effusion. The pleural fluid may be classified as a transudate or an exudate. Transudates occur secondary to an increase in the pulmonary capillary hydrostatic pressure or a decrease in the capillary oncotic pressure. This results in an accumulation of protein-poor pleural fluid. Common causes: CHF, nephrotic syndrome, cirrhosis, hypoalbuminemia, pulmonary embolism. Exudates are due to conditions that cause inflammation or increased pleural vascular permeability that results in an accumulation of protein rich pleural fluid and cells. Common causes: pneumonia, cancer, tuberculosis.

Procedure

1. Explain the procedure and have the patient sign an informed consent form. Have the patient sit up comfortably, preferably leaning forward slightly on a bedside tray table. A pillow on the bedside tray table can help with comfort. Ask the patient to practice increasing intrathoracic pressure using the Valsalva maneuver or by humming.
2. The usual site for thoracentesis is the posterior lateral aspect of the back superior to the diaphragm but inferior to the top of the fluid level. Confirm the site by counting the ribs based on the CXR and percussing out the fluid level. Avoid going below the eighth ICS because of the risk of peritoneal perforation. A good frame of reference is the inferior angle of the scapula, which is located horizontally at the seventh rib or seventh intercostal space.
3. Use sterile technique, including gloves, chlorhexidine, and drapes. Thoracentesis kits come with an adherent drape with a hole in it.
4. Make a skin wheal over the proposed site with a 25-gauge needle and lidocaine. Change to a 22-gauge, 1½-in (4 cm) needle and infiltrate up and over the rib (Figure 19-56, page 655); try to anesthetize the deeper structures and the pleura. During this time, aspirate back for pleural fluid. Once fluid returns, note the depth of the needle and mark it with a hemostat. This maneuver gives you an approximate depth. Remove the needle.
5. Use a hemostat to measure the 14- to 18-gauge thoracentesis needle to the same depth as the first needle. Penetrate through the anesthetized area with the thoracentesis needle. **Make sure that you "march" over**

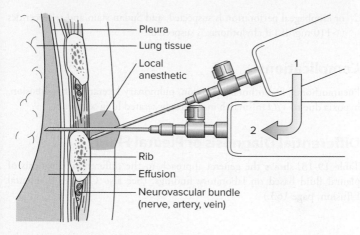

Pleura
Lung tissue
Local anesthetic

1

2

Rib
Effusion
Neurovascular bundle (nerve, artery, vein)

Figure 19-56. In thoracentesis, the needle is passed over the top of the rib to avoid the neurovascular bundle.

the top of the rib to avoid the neurovascular bundle that runs below the rib (see Figure 19-56). With the three-way stopcock attached, advance the thoracentesis catheter through the needle, withdraw the needle from the chest and the catheter, and place the protective needle cover over the end of the needle to prevent injury to the catheter. Next, aspirate the amount of pleural fluid needed. Turn the stopcock and evacuate the fluid through the tubing. **Never remove more than 1000–1500 mL per tap in patients with chronic effusions (e.g., malignant effusions).** Doing so can cause hypotension or development of pulmonary edema due to re-expansion of compressed alveoli. In acute effusions (e.g., traumatic hemothorax or postoperative pleural effusions after cardiac surgery) >1000 mL can be removed at one time without major side effects. In the event of re-expansion pulmonary edema, treat the patient with aggressive diuresis, supplemental oxygenation, potential endotracheal intubation, and continuous hemodynamic and oxygen saturation monitoring.

6. Have the patient hum or do the Valsalva maneuver as you withdraw the catheter. This maneuver increases intrathoracic pressure and decreases the risk of pneumothorax. Place a sterile dressing over the site.

7. Obtain a CXR to evaluate the fluid level and to rule out pneumothorax. An expiratory film is preferred because it is superior in identification of a small pneumothorax.

8. Distribute fluid into specimen containers, attach label slips, and send containers to the lab. Always order pH (collect in an ABG syringe), specific gravity, protein, LDH, cell count and differential, glucose, Gram stain and cultures, acid-fast cultures and smears, and fungal cultures and smears. Optional lab studies can include cytology if malignancy is suspected, amylase if effusion secondary to pancreatitis (usually on the left)

19

or esophageal perforation is suspected, and Sudan stain and triglycerides (>110 mg/dL) if chylothorax is suspected.

Complications

Pneumothorax, hemothorax, infection, pulmonary laceration, hypotension, hypoxia due to $\dot{V}/\dot{Q}$ mismatch in the newly aerated lung segment

Differential Diagnosis of Pleural Fluid

Table 19-13, shows the general approach to the differential diagnosis of pleural fluid based on laboratory findings. (See also Chapter 9, Pleural Effusion, page 163.)

Table 19-13. Differential Diagnosis of Pleural Fluid

Lab Value	Transudate	Exudate
Appearance	Clear yellow	Clear or turbid
Specific gravity	<1.016	>1.016
Absolute protein	<3 g/100 mL	>3 g/100 mL
Protein (pleural to serum ratio)	<0.5	>0.5
LDH (pleural to serum ratio)	<0.6	>0.6
Absolute LDH	<200 IU	>200 IU
Glucose (serum to pleural ratio)	<1	>1
Fibrinogen (clot)	No	Yes
WBC (pleural)	Very low	>2500/mm³
Differential (pleural)		PMN early, monocytes later

OTHER SELECTED TESTS

Cytology: Bizarre cells with large nuclei may represent reactive mesothelial cells and not malignancy. Malignant cells suggest a tumor.

pH: Generally >7.3. If between 7.2 and 7.3, suspect TB or malignancy or both. If <7.2, suspect empyema.

Glucose: Normal pleural fluid glucose is 2/3 serum glucose. Pleural fluid glucose is much lower than serum glucose in effusions due to rheumatoid arthritis (0–16 mg/100 mL); and low, <40 mg/100 mL in empyema.

Triglycerides and positive Sudan stain: Chylothorax

Eosinophilia >10%: drug-induced pleural disease (eosinophilia >10%)

LDH = lactate dehydrogenase; WBC = white blood cells; RBC = red blood cells; PMN = polymorphonuclear neutrophils; TB = tuberculosis.

Transudate: Cirrhosis with hepatic hydrothorax, congestive heart failure (CHF most common), CSF leak to the pleural space (rare), glomerulonephritis, hypoproteinemia, nephrotic syndrome, peritoneal dialysis/continuous ambulatory peritoneal dialysis, superior vena cava obstruction, urinothorax

Exudate: Acute respiratory distress syndrome, asbestos induced pleural effusion, CABG (s/p), chylothorax, drug-induced pleural disease (eosinophilia >10%), fungal infection, hypothyroidism, intra-abdominal abscess, SLE, malignancy (malignant mesothelioma, others), Meig syndrome, ovarian hyperstimulation syndrome, pancreatic pseudocyst, pericardial disease, pneumonia, pseudochylothorax, pulmonary embolism (major), rheumatoid pleuritis, TB

URINARY TRACT PROCEDURES

Bladder Catheterization

Indications

- Relief of urinary retention with or without bladder outlet obstruction
- Collection of an uncontaminated urine specimen for diagnostic purposes
- Monitoring of urinary output in critically ill patients or during prolonged surgical procedures
- Bladder tests (cystogram, cystometrogram)
- During and following specific surgeries of the genitourinary tract or adjacent structures
- Management of hematuria associated with clots. Can be used to irrigate the clots or rinse the bladder with continuous bladder irrigation (CBI) usually with a three-way catheter.
- Management of patients with neurogenic bladder
- Intravesical pharmacologic therapy such as BCG, mitomycin, others for bladder cancer

Contraindications

- Urethral disruption, often associated with pelvic fracture (presence of blood at the meatus or gross hematuria associated with trauma should be first evaluated with retrograde urethrogram)
- Acute prostatitis (relative contraindication)

Materials

- Prepackaged bladder catheter tray (may or may not include a catheter or appropriate drainage bag)
- Catheter (several examples are shown in Figure 19-57, page 658). Latex catheters are usually yellow or red colored. Many catheters are available

19

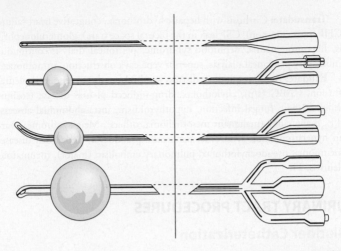

Figure 19-57. Bladder catheters, top to bottom: straight Robinson or red rubber catheter, Foley catheter with standard 5-mL balloon, Coudé catheter, and three-way irrigating catheter with 30-mL balloon. All catheters with a distal balloon have an inflation valve shown. Catheters have been shortened for illustrative purposes.

in silicone (clear- or blue-colored) if there is latex sensitivity. The catheter size is indicated by the color of the plastic hub on the balloon port. Catheters are designated by their diameters in French units where 1 French unit = ⅓ mm (see page 517)

Catheter size (French Units)	10 Fr	12 Fr	14 Fr	16 Fr	18Fr	20 Fr	22 Fr	24 Fr
Hub color	Black	White	Green	Orange	Red	Yellow	Purple	Blue

Foley: Describes a straight catheter with a retention balloon at the tip to keep it in the bladder. Use a 14–18 Fr for adults (the higher the number, the larger the diameter). Irrigation catheters (three-way Foley) should be larger (22–24 Fr) to allow the evacuation of clots. These so called "hematuria catheters" will usually have a larger retention balloon (30 mL) to allow for tamponade against the prostate when placed on traction. A typical Foley catheter size for an adult patient is 14–18 Fr with a 5 or 10 cc retention balloon to be filled with only with sterile water. Smaller sizes (6–10F) are available for children. See Chapter 29, Table 29-7 for description of recommended urethral catheter sizes for all ages.

Coudé (pronounced "coo-DAY"): Refers to elbow-tipped catheter useful in men with prostatic hypertrophy. The catheter is passed with the tip pointing to the 12 o'clock position. An indicator nub is at the 12 o'clock position near the inflation hub to assist with orientation.

Council catheter: Has a reinforced hole at the tip of the catheter that allows the catheter to be passed into the bladder over a wire or catheter stylet.

Red rubber catheter (Robinson): Plain rubber or latex catheter without a balloon, usually used for in-and-out catheterization, in which urine is removed, but the catheter is then removed.

Procedure

1. Use sterile technique.
2. Explain the procedure to the patient. Have the patient lie supine in a well-lighted area; female patients should lie with knees flexed wide and heels together to get adequate exposure of the meatus.
3. Get all the materials ready before attempting to insert the catheter. Open the kit and put on the gloves. Open the prep solution and soak the cotton balls. Apply the sterile drapes.
4. Inflate and deflate the balloon of the Foley catheter to ensure proper functioning. Coat the end of the catheter with lubricant jelly.
5. In **female patients**, use one gloved hand to prep the urethral meatus in a pubis-toward-anus direction; hold the labia apart with the other gloved hand. For uncircumcised male patients, retract the foreskin to prep the glans; use a gloved hand to hold the penis still.
6. Do not let the hand used to hold the penis or labia touch the catheter; use the disposable forceps in the kit insert the catheter or use the forceps to prep and then use the gloved hand to insert the catheter.
7. For **male patients**, stretch the penis upward perpendicular to the body to eliminate any internal folds in the urethra that might lead to a false passage. Use **steady, gentle** pressure to advance the catheter. The bulbous urethra is the most likely part to tear. Any significant resistance encountered may represent a stricture and requires urologic consultation. In men with BPH, a Coudé tip catheter may facilitate passage. Tricks used to get a catheter to pass in a male patient are to make sure that the penis is well stretched and to instill 30–50 mL of sterile water-based surgical lubricant (K-Y jelly) into the urethra with a catheter-tipped syringe before passing the catheter. Viscous lidocaine jelly for urologic use can help lubricate and relieve the discomfort of difficult catheter placement. Allow at least 5 min after instillation of the lidocaine jelly for the anesthetic effect to take place.
8. For both male and female patients, insert the catheter to the hilt of the drainage end. In male patients, compress the penis toward the pubis. These maneuvers help ensure that the balloon inflates in the bladder and not in the urethra. Inflate the balloon with 5–10 mL of sterile water. The catheter valve balloon will specify the volume to inflate the retention balloon. After inflation, pull the catheter back so that the balloon comes

19

to rest on the bladder neck. There should be good urine return when the catheter is in place. If a large amount of lubricant jelly was placed into the urethra, you may have to flush the catheter with sterile saline to clear the excess lubricant. A catheter that will not irrigate is probably **in the urethra, not the bladder**.

9. In uncircumcised male patients, reposition the foreskin to prevent massive edema of the glans (paraphimosis) after the catheter is inserted.

10. Catheters in female patients can be taped to the leg. In male patients, the catheter should be taped to the abdominal wall to decrease stress on the posterior urethra and help prevent stricture formation. The catheter is usually attached to a gravity drainage bag or a device for measuring the amount of urine. Many new kits come with the catheter already secured to the drainage bag. These systems are considered closed; do not open them if at all possible. The catheter may drain into a leg bag (capacity 300–900 mL) or an "overnight or nighttime" bag that cannot be worn but has a capacity up to 2 L.

11. Catheterization in children is similar except that in young infants catheter retention balloons are not used. In neonates feeding tubes or umbilical catheters are often used and taped in place.

Troubleshooting Difficult Catheter Placement

- **Adult males.** With a very tight phimosis a small catheter may be able to be passed blindly into the meatus. If unsuccessful a dorsal slit with anesthesia may be performed at the bedside usually by a urologist to open the phimosis. In obese males or those with massive edema, the meatus may be difficult to locate. Have an assistant use downward pressure around the base of the penis to depress the fat. With significant penile edema, manual pressure or an elastic compression wrap around the penis for no more than 15–20 min may reduce the edema to allow visualization of the meatus. If a catheter does not pass proximally in a male it may be due to stricture or prostatic enlargement. Injecting 20 mL of sterile lidocaine jelly may facilitate passage. A Coude tipped catheter may bypass an enlarged prostate. Urologic consultants have additional tools such as guide wires, flexible cystoscopes, and emergency suprapubic catheters that may be necessary if a catheter is needed but cannot be placed.

- **Adult female.** The urethral meatus in a female may be difficult to identify due to obesity, vaginal atrophy, or a tight introitus. In female adults the normal position of the urethra is 2.5 cm inferior to the glans clitoris. The use of stirrups, enhanced lighting, Tendelenberg positioning and an assistant retracting the labia may help. A vaginal speculum or gentle digital retraction on the posterior vaginal fornix may bring the meatus into direct vision.

"In-and-Out" Catheterized Urine

1. If urine is needed for analysis or C&S, especially for a female patient, a so-called in-and-out catheterization can be done. This procedure is also useful for measuring residual urine in male or female patients. The incidence of inducing infection with this procedure is about 3%.
2. The procedure is identical to that described for bladder catheterization. The main difference is that a red rubber catheter (no balloon) is often used and is removed immediately after the specimen is collected.
3. In children, the American Academy of Pediatrics recommends straight in and out catheter urine samples in young children with risk factors, including female sex, persistent fever above 102°F, and absence of an alternative cause for the fever.

Complications: Bladder catheterization

1. Catheter-associated urinary tract infection (CAUTI) is a catheter-associated complication. The duration of catheterization generally determines the development of bacteriuria. (See Chapter 13, page 389.) An indwelling catheter should be placed using aseptic technique and sterile equipment. The drainage bag along with its connecting tube must be kept below the level of the bladder and disconnecting the end of the catheter to the drainage tubing should be minimized. The urethral catheter should be removed as soon as possible when it is no longer needed.
2. Urethral, prostate or bladder trauma (perforation). Usually associated with forceful catheter placement in the setting of abnormal anatomy (stricture, prostate enlargement).
3. Paraphimosis in uncircumcised males due to failure of repositioning the foreskin in an uncircumcised male.

19

Clean-Catch Urine Specimen

1. Clean-catch urine is useful for routine urinalysis, is usually good for culturing urine from male patients, but is only fair for culturing urine from female patients because of the potential for contamination.
2. For male patients:
   a. Expose the glans, clean with povidone-iodine solution and dry the area with a sterile pad.
   b. Collect midstream urine in a sterile container after the initial flow has escaped.
3. For female patients:
   a. Separate the labia widely to expose the urethral meatus; keep the labia spread throughout the procedure.
   b. Cleanse the urethral meatus with povidone-iodine solution from front to back, and rinse with sterile water.
   c. Catch the midstream portion of the urine in a sterile container.

Urine Collection Techniques in Children

The most common clinical need for a urine collection in a child is the evaluation of a urinary tract infection. Options include a clean voided sample, bagged collection, catheterized sample, or a suprapubic bladder aspiration (described in the next section).

1. Bladder catheterization in infants and children is generally similar to the technique described previously in adults. The main issue is the use of an appropriately sized urethral catheter. (See Chapter 29, Table 29-7.) Use latex-free catheters whenever possible.

2. Clean voided urine samples are best in children who are toilet trained. In females the labia should be spread and the perineum cleansed two to three times with mild antiseptic solution or mild soap. In boys the foreskin if present retracted and the penis and the perineum should be cleansed. Obtain a midstream urine sample in a sterile cup for both boys and girls. A technique used in infants less than 6 mo involves having the infant suspended in a parent's or assistant's arm after feeding for a period of time. The genitalia are cleansed and an attentive assistant holds the sterile cup ready to obtain the sample. Tapping over the bladder with paravertebral massage may encourage spontaneous urination in the infant.

3. Bag specimens are not ideal but sometimes necessary in children who are not toilet trained. The genitalia and perineum are cleaned with an antiseptic solution. A specifically designed urine collection bag is used. The adhesive backing is removed and the bag is applied over the vulva in females and over the penis and scrotum in boys. It is left in place until an adequate sample is collected and removed.

Percutaneous Suprapubic Bladder Aspiration

Indications

Used most frequently in infants and young children (<2 yr).
- Inability to obtain urine with a less invasive method
- Urethral abnormalities
- Refractory UTI

Contraindications

- Voiding within the last hour (children)
- Inability to percuss the bladder
- Abdominal distension, organomegaly, volume depletion, or congenital anomalies of the GI or GU systems.

Procedure

1. This procedure is almost exclusively limited to infants younger than 6 mo.
2. Immobilize the child. Do not attempt this procedure if the child has voided within the last hour.

3. Palpate the bladder above the pubic symphysis (the bladder sticks out high above the pubis in a young child when it is full). Some clinicians suggest occluding the urethra in boys by holding the penis and in girls by inserting a finger in the rectum to exert pressure. Percuss out the limits of the bladder. Point-of-care ultrasound can help identify the bladder and direct the needle placement procedure

4. Obtain a 20-mL syringe with a 23- or 25-gauge, 1½-in (4 cm) needle. Prep with povidone-iodine and alcohol ½–1½ in (1.5–4 cm) above the pubis. Anesthesia is not routinely used.

5. Insert the needle perpendicular to the skin in the midline; maintain negative pressure on the downstroke and on withdrawal until urine is obtained (Figure 19-58, page 664).

6. If no urine is obtained, wait at least 1 hr before reattempting the procedure.

7. Point-of-care ultrasound is considered essential at some centers if suprapubic aspiration is to be performed to verify an acceptable volume of urine is present.

Complications: Percutaneous Suprapubic Bladder Aspiration

Major complications may include gross hematuria, abdominal wall abscess, and intestinal perforation.

VENIPUNCTURE

Indications

- Venipuncture (**phlebotomy**) is the puncture of a vein to obtain a sample of venous blood for analysis.
- Occasionally, medications are given intravenously.

Contraindications

- With evidence of cellulitis or abscess at the site; presence of a hematoma; presence of a vascular shunt, graft or access device; above the level of an IV site

Materials

- Tourniquet (acceptable replacements for a standard tourniquet 1½-in [4 cm] Penrose drain, or BP cuff is an acceptable replacement)
- Alcohol prep pad, gauze pad, and adhesive bandage. For blood culture sample chlorhexidine is recommended to be used. (Note: Samples contaminated with povidone-iodine may interfere with test results of potassium, phosphorus, and uric acid.)

19

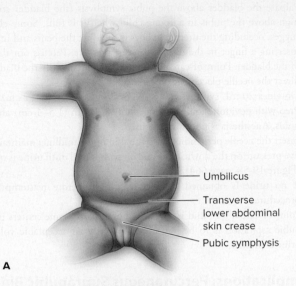

Umbilicus

Transverse lower abdominal skin crease

Pubic symphysis

A

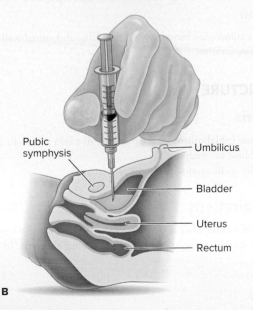

Pubic symphysis

Umbilicus

Bladder

Uterus

Rectum

B

Figure 19-58. Technique and anatomic structures in suprapubic bladder aspiration. Point-of-care ultrasound is recommended to visualize adequate urine in the bladder. (Reprinted with permission from Gomella TL, ed. Neonatology: Basic Management, On-Call Problems, Diseases, Drugs, 8e, New York, NY: McGraw-Hill; 2020.)

- Proper specimen tubes for desired studies (red top, purple top, etc.) (Table 19-14, page 666).
- Appropriate-sized syringe for the volume of blood needed (5 mL, 10 mL, etc.). For routine sample collection, a vacuum collection tube system is most commonly employed (e.g., Vacutainer tube, appropriate needle, and Vacutainer holder. The BD Eclipse blood collection system includes a manually activated needle shield).
- A 20- to 22-gauge needle in adults; 23- to 25-gauge needle in infants and children. (Larger needles are uncomfortable, and smaller ones can cause hemolysis or clotting; the higher the gauge number, the smaller the needle, see Figure 19-2, page 517.) In the setting of infants and fragile elderly veins, a scalp needle connected to a vacuum tube collection system can be used.

Procedure

Blood cultures, IV techniques, and arterial punctures are discussed elsewhere in this book.

1. Collect the necessary materials before you begin, including extras in case there is a problem. Confirm the identity of the patient from whom the sample is to be taken.
2. The common sites for routine venipuncture are the veins of the antecubital fossa (see Figure 19-42, page 613). Use caution in the antecubital fossa, as major arteries and nerve trunks are very superficial and can be easily damaged in this area. Alternative sites include the dorsum of the hand, the forearm, the saphenous vein near the medial malleolus ernal jugular vein. If peripheral sites are unacceptable, use the femoral vein. **Never draw a blood sample proximal to an IV site** because of the high concentration of IV fluid in the veins. If you are obtaining blood from the same area as an IV, puncture the vein 3–4 in below the site of the IV.
3. Apply the tourniquet at least 2–3 in (5–8 cm) above the venipuncture site. Have the patient make a fist to help engorge the vein. Do not have the patient clench and unclench the fist repeatedly (pumping). To facilitate vein locating, the patient may be asked to hold a rubber ball, or a thick wad of gauze, etc. Also, never leave a tourniquet on the arm for more than 1 min without releasing it. If veins are difficult to locate, try gently slapping or flicking the vein to cause reflex dilation, hanging the extremity in a dependent position, wrapping the extremity in a warm wet towel, substituting a BP cuff for the standard tourniquet, or applying nitroglycerin paste below and over the area to help dilate the veins.
4. Swab the site with the alcohol prep pad (70%) and allow the alcohol to evaporate. Do not do this if a blood alcohol level is being determined.
5. The vacuum blood tube systems (e.g., **Vacutainer system BD, Franklin Lakes, NJ)** have become the standard means of collecting blood for

19

Table 19-14.   Identification of Commonly Used Blood Collection Tubes (BD Vacutainer)

BD Vacutainer Tubes with BD Hemogard™ Closure	BD Vacutainer® Tubes with Conventional Stopper	Additive	Number of Inversions* at Blood Collection	Laboratory use
Gold	Red/Gray	• Clot activator and gel for serum separation	5	For serum determinations in chemistry. May be used for routine blood donor screening and diagnostic testing of serum for infectious diseases. Tube inversions ensure mixing of clot activator with blood. Blood clotting time: 30 minutes.
Light Green	Green/Gray	• Lithium heparin and gel for plasma separation	8	For plasma determinations in chemistry. Tube inversions prevent clotting.
Red	Red	• Silicone coated (glass) • Clot activator, Silicone coated (plastic)	0 5	For serum determinations in chemistry. May be used for routine blood donor screening and diagnostic testing of serum for infectious disease. Tube inversions ensure mixing of clot activator with blood. Blood clotting time: 60 minutes.
Orange		• Thrombin-based clot activator with gel for serum separation	5 to 6	For stat serum determinations in chemistry. Tube inversions ensure mixing of clot activator with blood. Blood clotting time: 5 minutes.

Tube	Additive	Inversions	Use
Orange	• Thrombin-based clot activator	8	For stat serum determinations in chemistry. Tube inversions ensure mixing of clot activator with blood. Blood clotting time: 5 minutes.
Royal Blue	• Clot activator (plastic serum) • K₂EDTA (plastic)	8 8	For trace-element, toxicology, and nutritional-chemistry determinations. Special stopper formulation provides low levels of trace elements (see package insert). Tube inversions ensure mixing of either clot activator or anticoagulant (EDTA) with blood.
Green	• Sodium heparin • Lithium heparin	8 8	For plasma determinations in chemistry. Tube inversions ensure mixing of anticoagulant (heparin) with blood to prevent clotting.
Gray	• Poasium oxalate/ sodium fluoride • Sodium fluoride/ Na₂ EDTA • Sodium flurodie (serum tube)	8 8 8	For glucose determinations. Oxalate and EDTA anticoagulants will give plasma samples. Sodium fluoride is the antiglycolytic agent. Tube inversions ensure proper mixing of additive with blood.
Tan	• K₂EDTA (plastic)	8	For lead determinations. This tube is certified to contain less than .01 mcg/mL(ppm) lead. Tube inversions prevent clotting.

(*Continued*)

19

Table 19-14. Identification of Commonly Used Blood Collection Tubes (BD Vacutainer) *(Continued)*

BD Vacutainer® Tubes with BD Hemogard™ Closure	BD Vacutainer® Tubes with Conventional Stopper	Additive	Number of Inversions* at Blood Collection	Laboratory use
	Yellow	• Sodium polyanethol sulfonate (SPS)	8	SPS for blood culture specimen collections in microbiology.
		• Acid citrate dextrose additives (ACD): **Solution A—** 22.0 g/L trisodium citrate, 8.0 g/L citric acid, 24.5 g/L dextrose	8	ACD for use in blood bank studies, HLA phenotyping, and DNA and paternity testing.
		Solution B— 13.2 g/L trisodium citrate, 4.8 g/L citric acid, 14.7 g/L dextrose	8	Tube inversions ensure mixing of anticoagulant with blood to prevent clotting.
Lavender	Lavender	• Liquid K_3EDTA (glass)	8	K_2EDTA and K_3EDTA for whole blood hematology determinations. K_2EDTA may also be used for routine immunohematology testing, and blood donor screening.
		• Spray-coated K_2EDTA (plastic)	8	Tube inversions ensure mixing of anticoagulant (EDTA) with blood to prevent clotting.

19

Tube color	Additive	Number of inversions	Use
White	• K_2EDTA and gel for plasma separation	8	For use in molecular diagnostic test methods (such as, but not limited to, polymerase chain reaction [PCR] and/or branched DNA [bDNA] application techniques.) Tube inversions ensure mixing of anticoagulant (EDTA) with blood to prevent clotting.
Pink	• Spray-coated K_2EDTA (plastic)	8	For whole blood hematology determinations. May be used for routine immunohematology testing and blood donor screening.* Designed with special cross-match label for patient information required by the AABB. Tube inversions prevent clotting.
Light Blue	• Buffered sodium citrate 0.105M Na citrate (approx 3.2%)	3–4	For coagulation determinations. CTAD for selected platelet function assays and routine coagulation determination. Tube inversions ensure mixing of anticoagulant (citrate) to prevent clotting. Certain tests may require chilled specimens.
Clear	• 0.129M Na citrate (3.8%)	3–4	
	• Citrate, theophylline, adenosine, dipyridamole (CTAD)	3–4	
Red/Light Gray			
Clear	• None (plastic)	0	For use as a discard tube or secondary specimen tube.

Note: Tubes for pediatric and partial draw applications can be found on the company website: www.bd.com/vacutainer.

Source: Reproduced with permission from BD Diagnostics, Franklin Lakes, NJ.

*Invert gently, do NOT shake

19

669

analysis. Screw an appropriate sided needle (adult 20–22 gauge) on the BD Vacutainer single use cup, and rotate the safety shield back. In the Eclipse needle system (BD Biosciences), a shield covering the end of the needle is manually activated after the sample is collected. Remove the protective needle cap.

6. Keep the needle bevel up, and puncture the skin alongside the vein. After the needle is through the skin, use the thumb of your free hand to stabilize the vein and prevent it from rolling. Enter the vein on the side at about a 30-degree angle. An alternative technique is to enter both the skin and vein in one stick at an angle of 15–30 degrees. (Figure 19-59). This maneuver requires practice because the vein is often punctured through and through.

7. Advance the appropriate collection tube (see Table 19-14, page 666) onto the needle inside the Vacutainer cup to puncture the diaphragm of the stopper by pushing the tube forward and initiating vacuum suction. The vacuum inside the tube automatically collects the sample. If only a single collection tube is required, when the vacuum is tube is completely filled, release the tourniquet, and remove the tube from the needle assembly. Place a piece of dry gauze over the needle and withdraw the needle carefully. If serial specimens are to be obtained (see tube sequence below), hold the Vacutainer cup steady and remove the tube you just collected and insert an empty tube and repeat. Serial tubes can be collected in this manner.

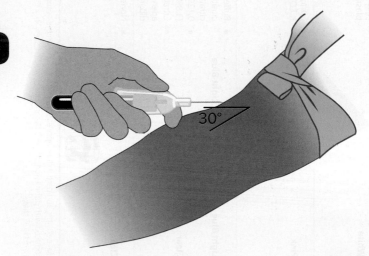

Figure 19-59. Technique of venipuncture in the antecubital fossa. The skin entry is approximately a 30-degree angle. Note the vacuum collections system with the safety needle that will cover the needle after the sample is obtained.

8. Tubes should be filled until the vacuum and blood flow is exhausted. Tubes containing additives (EDTA, citrate, heparin, etc.) should be filled until the volumes are complete. These additive-containing tubes should be mixed gently by inverting several times to mix well.

9. After the blood is collected, remove the tourniquet, withdraw the needle, and apply firm pressure with the alcohol swab or sterile gauze for 2–3 min. The BD Eclipse needle allows rapid one-handed reshielding of the needle tip. Elevation of the extremity helps limit hematoma formation. Bending the arm and heavy lifting immediately after phlebotomy increases the size of the venipuncture site and should be discouraged. Excessive bleeding (longer than 5 min) should be further evaluated.

10. If no peripheral veins can be located, point-of-care ultrasound can be used to locate a vein or the **femoral vein can be utilized**. Locate the femoral vein using the **NAVEL** mnemonic from lateral to medial (see Figure 19-13, page 548). The femoral vein should be just medial to the femoral artery. After prepping the skin, insert the needle perpendicular to the skin, and gently aspirate. The vein should be about 1–1½ in (2.5–4 cm) below the skin. Apply firm pressure after collecting the sample; hematomas are frequent complications of femoral venipuncture. If the femoral artery is accidentally entered, it is acceptable to collect the sample. Apply pressure for at least 5 min if the artery is entered.

11. In children and elderly persons with fragile veins, a butterfly (21–25 gauge) can be used to obtain a sample (see Figure 19-45, page 617). Attach a syringe or use a needleless Vacutainer like system with a push button that retracts the needle.

12. If preprinted labels are not available, all specimens must be labeled with both the patient's first and last name as well as a second identifier such as the patient's birth date or medical record number.

13. When multiple specimens are drawn from a single venipuncture site, the following order is recommended: (1) sterile blood culture tubes, (2) nonadditive clotting tubes (red), (3) coagulation tubes and tubes containing citrate (blue), (4) gel-barrier tubes and tubes with additives (red), (5) tubes containing heparin (green), (6) tubes containing EDTA (lavender, royal blue), (7) tubes containing acid citrate dextrose (yellow), and (8) tubes containing sodium fluoride and potassium oxalate (gray).

VENOUS ACCESS: INTRAOSSEOUS (IO) INFUSION

Indications

- Emergency vascular access when standard techniques cannot be used
- When rapid high-volume fluid infusion is needed (hypovolemic shock, burns)
- Difficult vascular access in the setting of seizures, extensive burns, obesity, massive edema

Contraindications

- Cutaneous infection or burn overlying the insertion site.
- Previous attempt at IO placement at the same site or same extremity.
- Fracture in the target bone or major injury to the extremity proximal to the insertion site.
- Osteopetrosis, osteopenia
- For sternum insertion, previous sternotomy or fracture or vascular injury near the sternum

Materials

- Materials for skin sterilization
- Lidocaine, 1%, with 5-mL syringe and 25-gauge needle
- Short, large-bore bone marrow needle or 13- to 18-gauge IO infusion needles of choice from various manufacturers:
  o Sur-Fast intraosseous needle (Cook, Bloomington, IN)
  o Jamshidi needle and Jamshidi disposable Illinois sternal/iliac needle (Baxter Healthcare, McGaw Park, IL)
  o Sussmane-Raszynski needle (Cook, Bloomington, IN)
  o Arrow EZ-IO (Teleflex, Morrisville, NC)
  o FAST1 Intraosseous Infusion System (Pyng Medical, Richmond, BC, Canada)
  o NIO New Intraosseous Device (PerSys Medical, Houston, TX)
  o BIG Bone Injection Gun (PerSys Medical, Houston, TX)
- 10-mL syringe with saline flush, IV fluid of choice, and infusion setup (Luer-Lock catheter with a three-way stopcock)
- Pressure bag for IV
- Gauze sponges, adhesive tape
- Gloves and eye protection

Background

Intraosseous (IO) infusion is the infusion of fluids or medications into the bone marrow cavity of a large bone. IO infusion is an important vascular access route for both children and adults. It is used for emergency vascular access (fluids, medications, blood products) when other access methods have been attempted and failed or would be too time consuming such as in the presence of cardiac arrest, trauma, shock). Originally IO access was suggested only for children 6 yr or younger, but studies have demonstrated safety in older children and adults. Successful infusions in newborns have further suggested that access via the intraosseous route is faster than access via umbilical veins.

The bone medullary cavity does not collapse during circulatory failure or hypovolemia. IO access is an acceptable alternative in prehospital and emergency room settings. The infusion of medications and fluids has the same hemodynamic effect as medications and fluids infused by the intravenous route. Complications are infrequent (0.6%), and several sites are suitable for infusion. In children, the most commonly used site is the proximal tibia, just distal to the tibial tuberosity. Sites for IO line placement in adults include the proximal humerus, distal tibia, distal femur, or sternum. Sternal placement is contraindicated when using drill-type insertion devices.

Procedure*

The patient should be supine. If the proximal tibia is selected, the leg should be rotated slightly externally. The ideal insertion site on the tibia lies 1–2 cm distal to the tibial tuberosity on the anterior medial surface. On the femur it is 2–3 cm proximal to the lateral epicondyle in the midline.

A. Drill-Driver Type Devices (example using EZ-IO system)

1. Sterilize the skin using chlorhexidine or Betadine solution.
2. Select appropriately sized needle. Needles are color coded based on length of the needle, all with a 15-gauge bore.
   a. Children (3–39 kg): Pink/15-mm length.
   b. Adult: Blue/25-mm length.
   c. Adult (obese or proximal humerus access): Yellow/45-mm length.
3. Load the needle onto the driver device and ensure that it is securely seated. Remove the plastic cover from the needle.
4. Do not activate drill until in contact with bone. Insert the needle through the skin and soft tissue until it contacts bone. Ensure that at least one black band marking on the needle shaft is visible outside the skin when in contact with bone; if line is not visible, select a larger size needle and repeat process.
5. Exert firm pressure at 90 degrees to the bone cortex and squeeze trigger to activate drill. Maintain firm pressure as the needle advances. Release the trigger when you feel a sudden decrease in resistance; the needle hub need not be against the skin.
6. Remove the driver from the needle. Remove the inner stylet from the needle by holding the needle in place and unscrewing the top stylet hub and then pulling straight out.
7. Attach a piece of primed IV tubing to the hub of the needle and withdraw. Aspiration of blood and marrow contents confirms needle-tip placement in the marrow.
8. If the patient is conscious or responsive to pain, consider slowly infusing increments of 2% lidocaine through the syringe to decrease pain

19

*Adapted with permission from Stone CK and Humphries RL, eds. Chapter 7: Emergency Procedures. In CURRENT Diagnosis & Treatment: Emergency Medicine, 8e, New York, NY: McGraw Hill Education; 2017.

on injection. A standard dose is 0.5 mg/kg (up to 40 mg) in children and 40 mg in adults. Allow lidocaine to dwell for 60 sec in the marrow space prior to flushing.

9. Forcefully flush 10-mL saline (from a syringe) through the system to clear debris. This will cause significant pain in a conscious patient if lidocaine has not been infused first. Monitor for swelling in the soft tissue (a sign of infiltration). If soft tissue swelling occurs with flushing, or if unable to flush, discontinue usage and attempt insertion at a different site.

10. Secure needle hub to extremity using commercially available kit, or by using rolls of 4 × 4 in gauze rolled and taped around the device to buttress it against movement.

11. IO infusions must be maintained under pressure, as simple gravity will not overcome the resistance of the marrow cavity. IV bag should be placed in a pressure sleeve.

B. Manual IO Access

1. Sterilize the skin at insertion point.

2. Using sterile technique, locate the desired insertion site and infiltrate the skin with 1% lidocaine over a 2- to 3-cm area. Lidocaine should also be infiltrated along the anticipated course of insertion, down to and including the periosteum. For patients that are unconscious or obtunded, no local anesthetic is needed.

3. Using the bone marrow needle or IO infusion needle, penetrate the skin perpendicularly. Advance the needle toward the bone at a 6-degree angle (directed away from the growth plate, caudal at the tibia, and rostral at the femur).

4. Use firm pressure to penetrate the cortex, employing a rotating or twisting motion. Upon entry into the marrow space, a sudden "give" will be felt. *Caution*: Errant placement of the needle can cause injury to the growth plate with resultant growth deformity.

5. Remove the trocar from the needle and attach a 10-mL syringe. Aspiration of blood and marrow contents confirms needle-tip placement in the marrow.

6. Connect a fluid-filled syringe or intravenous tubing to the needle and infuse under pressure.

7. Apply gauze against the skin at the entry site, surrounding the needle. Occasionally, deep penetration of the needle through the bone cortex on the opposite side can occur, with delivery of infusion into surrounding tissue spaces. This can also occur if the needle becomes dislodged and withdrawn from its intramedullary position; tape the needle firmly in place. (Commercially available IO infusion needles may have a lip to which tape can be attached or a screw mechanism for securing the needle to the skin surface.)

Complications

1. Most common is extravasation.
2. Infections. Localized cellulitis, subcutaneous abscess, periostitis, and sepsis have all been reported. Osteomyelitis is rare (<0.6%). To prevent osteomyelitis, hypertonic and alkaline solutions and all medications should be diluted.
3. Clotting of bone marrow with loss of vascular access.
4. Iatrogenic bone fracture. Radiograph confirmation of the needle should be done to confirm position and rule out fracture (tibial fracture is most common).
5. Compartment syndrome. Due to prolonged infusion and extravasation. The leaking fluid collects in the spaces between the muscles of the leg.
6. Others: Blasts in the peripheral blood; fat embolism; extremity amputation; needle dislodgement.

19

Specialized Diagnostics

20

- Amniocentesis
- Ankle-Brachial Index
- Audiometry and Tympanometry
- Bone Marrow Aspiration and Biopsy
- Capsule Endoscopy
- Cardiac Monitor, Implantable
- Cardiac Monitor, External (Holter)
- Cardiac Stress Testing
- Chorionic Villus Sampling (CVS)
- Colposcopy
- Coronary Artery Calcium Scoring

- Cystoscopy
- Electroencephalogram (EEG)
- Electromyography (EMG) and Nerve Conduction Studies (NCV)
- Endoscopic Ultrasound
- Esophageal Manometry
- Fetal Heart Rate Monitoring
- Loop Electrosurgical Excision Procedure (LEEP)
- Polysomnography
- Urodynamics

A variety of diagnostic testing, both invasive and noninvasive, is performed in the inpatient and outpatient settings. This is a brief overview of some of the specialized diagnostic testing commonly used in daily patient care. Note that specific procedure details and preparations can vary by facility and by provider.

AMNIOCENTESIS

Description: A spinal needle is inserted transabdominally into the amniotic sac of a developing fetus under ultrasound guidance. Amniotic fluid is aspirated and sent to the laboratory for analysis. This procedure is typically performed in an ultrasound suite or on labor and delivery. Amniotic fluid can be analyzed for prenatal diagnosis of karyotypic abnormalities, genetic

Chapter update by Babak Abai, MD, FACS, Mark B. Chaskes, MD, MBA, Stephanie Chen, MD, Rebecca Chiffer, MD, Mitchell Conn, MD, Tricia Gomella, MD, Ritu Grewal, MD, Colin Huntley MD, Kathryn Landers, MD, Yair Lev, MD, Aaron Martin, MD, and, Alana Murphy, MD, FACS, Allyson Pickard, MD, Michael Sperling, MD, William Tester, MD, FACP, Stephanie Thomas, MD

disorders (for which testing is available), fetal blood type and hemoglobinopathies, fetal lung maturity, and monitoring the degree of isoimmunization by measurement of the content of bilirubin in the fluid, and for the diagnosis of chorioamnionitis. Testing for karyotypic abnormalities is usually done at 15- to 20-wk gestation. Amniocentesis also provides a useful tool later in pregnancy, is low risk, and can be used for diagnosis of intraamniotic inflammation and infection as a risk factor for preterm labor and adverse outcome.

Common Indications: Diagnosis of fetal genetic abnormalities; women at an increased risk of aneuploidy or genetic abnormalities (either by history or abnormal first- or second-trimester screening tests) and fetal structural abnormalities identified on ultrasound; and evaluation for intraamniotic infection when clinical findings are not sufficient to guide management. The American College of Obstetricians and Gynecologists' policy is that invasive diagnostic testing should be available to all women, regardless of age or risk.

General Preparation: Informed consent, counseling on the risks and limitations of the procedure; confirmation of gestational age and placental location and selection of a needle insertion site using ultrasound; antiseptic technique; local anesthetic is usually not necessary.

Potential Complications: Intraamniotic infection (<0.1%); fetal loss (<0.5%); risk of vertical transmission of maternal infection (HIV, hepatitis B and C).

Notes: Typically performed at 15-wk gestation or later. Early amniocentesis (before 15 wk) is generally not recommended because it is associated with a significantly higher rate of fetal loss, preterm premature rupture of membranes, and failed amniotic fluid cultures. Rh-negative patient should receive Rh immune globulin after this procedure.

References: 1. American College of Obstetricians and Gynecologists. ACOG Practice Bulletin No. 88, December 2007. Invasive prenatal testing for aneuploidy. Obstet Gynecol 2007;110(6):1459.

2. Shulman LP, Elias S. Amniocentesis and chorionic villus sampling, In Fetal Medicine [Special Issue]. West J Med 1993;159:260–268.

ANKLE-BRACHIAL INDEX

Description: The ankle-brachial index (ABI) is a simple, noninvasive, and reproducible bedside test to assess the patency of the distal arteries in the lower extremities (dorsal pedis [DP] and posterior tibial [PT] arteries). It compares the blood pressure in the ankles to the blood pressure in the arms. Since vascular pathology and atherosclerosis tend to affect the lower extremities predominantly, this comparison of lower extremity blood flow proves very useful. This test should be a part of the bedside exam in patients suspected of having peripheral arterial disease or decreased blood flow to the lower extremities. It is also helpful since the examination of pulses can be unreliable and is more subjective in patients with compromised blood flow or edema.

- $ABI = \dfrac{\text{Systolic BP lower extremity DP or PT}}{\text{Systolic BP Arm}}$

- Use the higher of DP or PT systolic occlusion pressure

Common Indications: Patients who are suspected of having a diagnosis of peripheral arterial disease (PAD); patients with nonpalpable pulses due to embolism, trauma, and atherosclerosis; and patients with questionable palpable pulses. Some symptoms of PDA include claudication, skin changes in the lower extremities, hair loss on legs, poorly healing wounds over pressure points, gangrene, numbness, weakness or heavy feelings in the legs, erectile dysfunction (males).

General Preparation: A bedside Doppler ultrasound and a blood pressure cuff are all that are needed for this test. The patient must be supine. The test is performed by placing the cuff on the arm. Then the cuff is inflated while the Doppler US signal is placed at the level of radial artery. Repeat on the other arm. The higher of the two brachial BPs at which the signal disappears is the systolic closing pressure of the brachial artery. The cuff is then placed above the ankle. While checking the dorsal pedal and subsequently posterior tibial signal, the cuff is inflated. The closing pressure is similarly recorded as above (Figure 20-1)

The ABI for a limb is the higher of the ratio of DP or PT systolic pressure over the higher brachial pressure. A ratio is obtained for each leg. The results then can be interpreted as in Table 20-1.

Potential Complications: This test is noninvasive and does not have any serious adverse effects for patients. Typically the blood pressure cuff is not

20

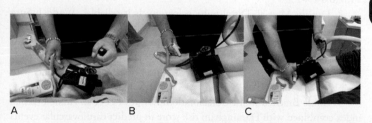

A   B   C

Figure 20-1. Technique to determine the ankle-brachial index (ABI) using a Doppler and blood pressure cuff. Some sources recommend the ABI be determined in the supine position. A. Measurement of brachial artery systolic pressure. B. Measurement of anterior tibial artery systolic pressure. C. Measurement of posterior tibial artery systolic pressure. (Courtesy of Babak Abai, MD, FACS)

Table 20-1. Interpretation of Ankle-Brachial Index (ABI)

ABI Value	Interpretation	Therapy
>1.3	Calcified blood vessels that are noncompressible	Formal pulse volume recordings (PVRs) along with toe pressures should be measured at the vascular laboratory of your hospital
0.9–1.29	Normal range	None
0.81–0.89	Mild disease	Medical therapy and risk factor modification.
0.4–0.80	Moderate disease	Referral to vascular specialist
<0.4	Severe disease	Urgent referral to vascular specialist

inflated above 250 mm Hg to prevent trauma to the area. If the artery does not close at 250 mm Hg, it is deemed nonocclusive.

Notes: Due to this limitation, whenever there is any doubt in regard to the digital palpation of the routine pulse exam, it is important to perform this bedside test. Abnormal results of ABI are an independent predictor of myocardial infarction and stroke due to atherosclerosis; therefore, a diagnosis of PAD (even if asymptomatic) portends a higher rate of morbidity and mortality. An abnormal test may require more formal studies such as arteriography.

References: 1. Johnston KW et al. Reproducibility of noninvasive vascular laboratory measurements in the peripheral circulation. J Vasc Surg 1987;6:147–151.

2. Lundin M et al. Distal pulse palpation: Is it reliable?. World J. Surg 1999;23:252–255.

3. American Diabetes Association. Peripheral arterial disease in people with diabetes. Diabetes Care 2003;26:3333–3341.

4. Criqui MH et al. Mortality over a period of 10 years in patients with peripheral arterial disease. N Engl J Med 1992;326:381–386.

5. Ankle Brachial Index Collaboration. Fowkes FG et al. Ankle brachial index combined with Framingham risk score to predict cardiovascular events and mortality: A meta-analysis. JAMA 2008;300:197–208.

AUDIOMETRY AND TYMPANOMETRY

Description: Pure-tone audiometry is performed to test a patient's hearing. During this test, sounds at various frequencies are presented to each ear independently, and the loudness or intensity required for the patient to perceive a sound 50% of the time is reported as the threshold. The typical frequencies tested range from 250 to 8000 hertz, which represent the most important frequencies for understanding speech. Audiometry tests hearing through air conduction as well as bone conduction. Air conduction is tested using headphones or inserting earphones to allow isolation of each individual ear during testing. Bone conduction is tested using a bone oscillator or vibrator placed on the mastoid tip just behind the ear. Thresholds for air and bone conduction are reported on an audiogram with frequency in hertz on the x-axis and intensity in decibels plotted downwards on the y-axis. Air conduction thresholds are conventionally represented using an "O" symbol for the right ear and an "X" symbol for the left ear. Bone conduction thresholds are represented using a "<" symbol for the right ear and a ">" symbol for the left ear. A patient with normal hearing should have air conduction thresholds ≤25 decibels and bone conduction thresholds ≤15 decibels. Elevated, or worsened, air conduction thresholds with normal bone conduction thresholds are indicative of a conductive hearing loss. Elevated air and bone conduction thresholds are consistent with a sensorineural or mixed hearing loss. The degree of hearing loss is measured using the pure tone average, which is the mean of the air conduction thresholds at three frequencies, usually 500, 1000, and 2000 hertz. A pure tone average ≤25 decibels is considered normal. Mild hearing loss is defined as a pure tone average of 25–40 decibels, moderate hearing loss as 40–55 decibels, moderately severe hearing loss as 55–70 decibels, severe hearing loss as 70–90 decibels, and profound hearing loss as ≥90 decibels.

At a certain intensity level, the signal presented to the test ear is conducted through the skull and perceived by the nontest ear. This phenomenon is called crossover. In order to prevent this bone conduction to the nontest ear from confounding the results of the study, a masking noise is presented to the nontest ear to prevent this ear from perceiving signals intended for the test ear. Audiograms traditionally report masked air and bone conduction thresholds in addition to unmasked thresholds.

In addition to pure tones, audiometry tests a patient's ability to hear and understand speech. Patients are presented with two-syllable spondee words, such as baseball or railroad, at varying intensities. The speech reception threshold is the lowest intensity in hertz at which a person can correctly repeat two-syllable spondee words 50% of the time. Once the speech reception threshold is determined, patients are presented monosyllabic words at an intensity level 35–40 decibels above their speech reception threshold. The percentage of words correctly repeated at this suprathreshold intensity level is reported as the word recognition score, or speech recognition score, for each ear (Figure 20-2).

Audiometry is usually accompanied by **tympanometry**, which measures pressure changes in the ear canal and middle ear as well as the compliance of the tympanic membrane. A tympanometry probe is placed in the external ear canal and emits a single tone while creating variations in air pressure. Some of the energy from the probe enters the middle ear, while the rest is reflected by the tympanic membrane. The amount of energy reflected back to the probe

20

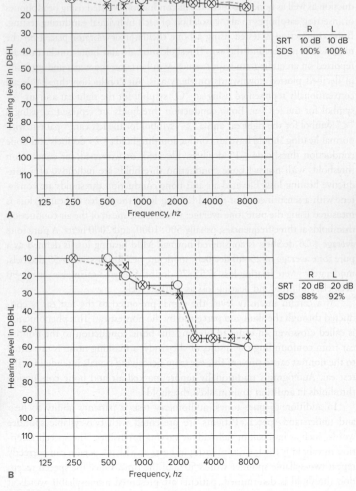

Figure 20-2. Audiogram. A. Normal bilateral hearing. B. Symmetric high-frequency hearing loss. Bone conduction thresholds (R = [and L =]) are measures of auditory function of the cochlea and proximal neural pathway, whereas air conduction thresholds (R = circle, L = X) measure function of the entire auditory system. SRT, speech reception threshold; SDS, speech discrimination score. (Reproduced with permission from Stone JH, Francis HW. Chapter 68. Sensorineural hearing loss (Immune-mediated inner ear disease). In Imboden JB, Hellmann DB, Stone JH [eds.]. *CURRENT Diagnosis & Treatment: Rheumatology*, 3e, New York, NY: McGraw-Hill; 2013.)

20

provides information about the tympanic membrane and middle ear. The various types of tympanograms are illustrated in Figure 20-3. A type A tympanogram is a normal tympanogram. Type A_s indicates stiffening of the tympanic membrane, which can be seen with tympanosclerosis or scarring. Type A_D indicates a flaccid tympanic membrane or ossicular chain discontinuity. A type B tympanogram appears flat and suggests decreased compliance of the tympanic membrane, which can be seen with stiffening middle ear pathology or middle ear effusions. A type B tympanogram can also indicate that there is a tympanic membrane perforation or patent tympanostomy tube. Type C tympanograms indicate negative pressure in the middle ear space, which is commonly seen with eustachian tube dysfunction.

Tympanometry also measures the volume of the external ear canal, which can be artificially increased if a perforation in the tympanic membrane allows inclusion of the middle ear volume in this calculation. Reported ear canal volumes greater than 2.5 cm³ in adults and 2.0 cm³ in children suggest a tympanic membrane perforation or patent tympanostomy tube.

Common Indications: Any patient complaining of decreased hearing in one or both ears should undergo audiometry. Patients with vertigo or tinnitus can also benefit from audiometry to assess hearing, as decreased hearing may

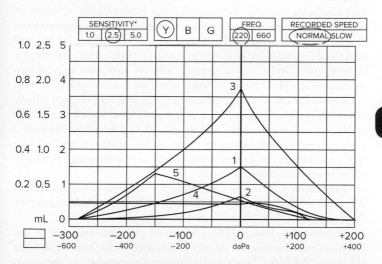

Figure 20-3. The historical tympanogram types. "1" is a type A tympanogram. "2" is a type A_s tympanogram. "3" is a type A_D tympanogram. "4" is a type B tympanogram. "5" is a type C tympanogram. See descriptions in the text above regarding the causes of the types of tympanograms. (Reproduced with permission from Silverman CA, Silman S. Audiologic testing. In Lalwani AK [ed.]. *CURRENT Diagnosis & Treatment Otolaryngology—Head and Neck Surgery*, 4e, New York, NY: McGraw-Hill; 2011.)

be associated with these symptoms. Patients with chronic ear infections should be monitored with audiometry. Infants who fail the initial newborn hearing screen or have known or suspected congenital abnormalities related to the ears should have additional audiometric testing. Patients with regular exposure to loud noises should be followed with audiometry. Audiograms can be useful for ototoxicity monitoring in patients taking ototoxic medications, including some antibiotics and chemotherapeutic agents, among others. Any patient with a sudden-onset hearing loss should obtain an audiogram to rule out a sudden sensorineural hearing loss, which can be an emergency and require radiologic imaging.

General Preparation: Generally, no preparation is needed for audiometry. A qualified provider may need to remove obstructive or impacted cerumen from the external ear canal prior to testing.

Potential Complications: There is very little risk associated with audiometry and tympanometry. Patients may have mild discomfort from the insert earphones or tympanometry probe, but this procedure is generally very well tolerated.

Notes: Children under the age of 5 are not able to participate reliably in conventional audiometric testing. Variations on pure tone audiometry have been developed for the pediatric population. In children less than 6 mo old, behavioral observation audiometry involves presenting sounds and observing the infant for signs of recognition, including eye turns, eye widening, or becoming more alert. The ears are not tested independently in behavioral observation audiometry, but a normal test suggests no worse than moderate hearing loss in at least one ear. From age 6 mo to 2.5 yr, children can be tested with visual reinforcement audiometry. Sound is introduced via a loudspeaker or headphones, and the child responds with eye movement or head turn towards the side of the presented sound where they are rewarded with visual reinforcement such as flashing lights or a toy. Sounds are presented initially at a clearly audible level and then at progressively lower intensities while the child's response is observed. Children ages 2.5 to 4 yr old can undergo a variant of conventional audiometry known as play audiometry, during which they are conditioned to perform a simple task, such as throwing a block into a box, in response to hearing a tone.

References: 1. Silverman CA, Silman S. Audiologic testing. In Lalwani AK (ed.). *CURRENT Diagnosis & Treatment Otolaryngology—Head and Neck Surgery,* 4e, New York, NY: McGraw-Hill; 2022.

2. Stone JH, Francis HW. Chapter 68. Sensorineural hearing loss (Immune-mediated inner ear disease). In Imboden JB, Hellmann DB, Stone JH (eds.). *CURRENT Diagnosis & Treatment: Rheumatology,* 3e, New York, NY: McGraw-Hill; 2013.

BONE MARROW ASPIRATION AND BIOPSY

Description: To obtain an adequate bone marrow specimen for determination of cellular morphology; marrow cellularity; presence of abnormal cells;

determination of iron stores; material for special studies, such as flow cytometry or infectious diseases.

Common Indications: Evaluation of unexplained anemia, thrombocytopenia, leukopenia; evaluation of unexplained leukocytosis, thrombocytosis; search for malignancy primary to the marrow (leukemia, myeloma) or metastatic to the marrow (small-cell lung cancer, breast cancer); diagnosis and/or staging of lymphoma, solid tumors, plasma cell disorders and leukemias; evaluation of suspected deposition or storage diseases (e.g., Gaucher disease, amyloidosis); evaluation of unexplained splenomegaly; evaluation of iron stores; evaluation of possible disseminated infection (tuberculosis, fungal disease); bone marrow donor harvesting (aspiration).

General Preparation: Kits are available that have all the materials necessary. A technician from the hematology lab or BMT facility must be present to ensure delivery and proper processing of specimens. Explain the procedure to the patient or the legally responsible surrogate in detail and obtain informed consent. Local anesthesia usually is all that is needed; if a patient is extremely anxious, premedication with an anxiolytic or sedative such as diazepam (Valium) or midazolam (Versed) or an analgesic is reasonable. Bone marrow can be obtained from numerous sites, such as the sternum, tibia, and anterior or posterior iliac crest. The posterior iliac crest is the safest and usually the site of choice. Position the patient on either the abdomen or on the side opposite the side from which the biopsy specimen is to be taken. Use sterile gloves, mask, and gown, and follow strict aseptic technique. Approximately 1 cc marrow is aspirated and quickly placed on slides prior to clotting of specimen. A thin smear of marrow is made by an assistant, and the slides are allowed to dry. A marrow biopsy needle is placed in a similar fashion, at a different angle than the marrow aspirate. A marrow core specimen is obtained, preferably 2 cm in length. The marrow core is removed, and touch prep can be made by rolling specimen onto glass slide and is then placed in formalin. After the procedure, observe for excess bleeding and apply local pressure for several minutes. Clean the area with alcohol and apply an adhesive bandage or gauze patch. Recommend (not required unless coagulopathic) that the patient assume a supine position and place a pressure pack between the bed or examination table and the biopsy site and apply pressure for 10–15 min. The site should then be inspected to ensure that there is no further bleeding. A patient who is stable at this point may resume normal activities.

Potential Complications: Local bleeding and hematoma, retroperitoneal hematoma, pain, bone fracture, infection, tumor seeding

Notes: Contraindications include infection, osteomyelitis near the puncture site; relative contraindications include severe coagulopathy and thrombocytopenia (may be corrected by platelet transfusion); previous radiation to the region.

Reference: Malempati S et al. Bone marrow aspiration and biopsy. N Engl J Med 2009;361:e28.

20

CAPSULE ENDOSCOPY

Description: Capsule endoscopy is a diagnostic procedure used to visualize the lumen of the small bowel not examined during upper endoscopy and colonoscopy. The patient swallows a disposable capsule containing a small camera, which captures images at several frames per second as the capsule passes through the bowel. The images are wirelessly transmitted to a recorder worn by the patient. Images can be obtained until the capsule's battery is exhausted or the capsule is excreted by the patient. The procedure takes approximately 9.5 hr to complete. Once the study is complete, a video is created using the uploaded images and reviewed by a gastroenterologist.

Common Indications: Evaluation of recurrent or continued GI bleeding after negative endoscopy and colonoscopy; evaluation of iron-deficiency anemia after negative endoscopy and colonoscopy; diagnosis of suspected Crohn disease or evaluation of known Crohn disease; suspected small bowel tumor; surveillance of polyposis syndromes; suspected or refractory malabsorptive syndrome (celiac disease).

General Preparation: Obtain focused history and physical concerning symptoms/signs of bowel obstruction. Patient should take a full or partial bowel prep the evening before the procedure. Patient should be NPO for at least 8–10 hr before swallowing the capsule. Sensing pads/belt with an attached external receiver need to be placed on the patient prior to swallowing the capsule.

Potential Complications: Incomplete examination (20.0%): Capsule battery runs out prior to the capsule reaching the ileocecal valve; thus, the small bowel is not completely visualized. Capsule retention (1.0 %): Passage of the capsule is impeded by a stricture or mass. The patient may require surgery to remove the capsule. Missed lesions.

Reference: Enns RA et al. Clinical practice guidelines for the use of video capsule endoscopy. Gastroenterology 2017;152(3):497–514.

CARDIAC MONITOR, IMPLANTABLE

Description: Implantable monitors known as implantable loop recorders (ILR) are becoming smarter, smaller, and easier to implant. When patients have events such as abrupt syncope or acute strokes, often an arrhythmogenic event is suspected. Ambulatory electrocardiogram (ECG) monitoring is useful for diagnosis and may alter the treatment of these events. As an example, if a patient had a stroke, and we diagnose atrial fibrillation, this will likely result in initiation of systemic anticoagulation. If a patient had true syncope, and we diagnose third-degree heart block, there is an indication for a pacemaker. Sometimes, an external monitor (requiring multiple leads and an external device, e.g., Holter monitor) for a few days/weeks is not enough if the suspected event is infrequent or the external device is inconvenient. The implantable devices continuously monitor heart rhythms and record them automatically or during an event with a handheld patient activator. These devices are the size of a hair clip or a flat AAA battery, have self-contained electrodes, and can provide continuous monitoring and detection of potential arrhythmias for up to 3 yr. Implanting these devices can easily be done in the cardiac electrophysiology lab or now more commonly in the cardiologist's office.

Common Indications: Suspected arrhythmias; infrequent symptomatic palpitations; acute idiopathic stroke (for detection of atrial arrhythmias); suspected arrhythmogenic syncope.

General Preparation: Can be done in an outpatient setting with local anesthesia for the subcutaneous insertion of the device. Insertion of the device is usually at the left side of the chest, around the fourth intercostal space (i.e., near the V2–V4 precordial lead positions where P waves can be easily detected). Wound closure can include sutures, adhesive strips, or surgical glue.

Potential Complications: Infrequently insertion site pain; rareley wound infection or minor bleeding.

Notes: If symptoms occur daily, an external Holter monitor may be adequate (see below). In the future, these devices will become even more prevalent as they are becoming smaller, more sophisticated, and easily evaluated with the patient's handheld device. Moreover, current technology still requires small incisions, but future technologies might involve other techniques such as a tattoo-like implantation, small patches, and others.

Reference: Steinberg et al. 2017 ISHNE-HRS expert consensus statement on ambulatory ECG and external cardiac monitoring/telemetry. Heart Rhythm 2017;14(7):e55–e96.

CARDIAC MONITOR, EXTERNAL (HOLTER)

20

Description: Ambulatory ECG monitoring is useful in the setting of frequently occurring cardiac events. The "Holter monitor" (in honor of Dr. Norman J. Holter) is a widely available tool that records the ECG continuously, typically over 24 hr to 7 days, and improves the sensitivity for detecting arrhythmic events over a standard ECG or exercise testing. Its monitoring duration makes the Holter ideal for daily or several-times-per-week arrhythmias, whether they are symptomatic or asymptomatic. The device is returned for analysis after use. In the in-patient telemetry setting, it can be used to detect arrhythmias during hospitalization for conditions such as MI or syncope. It can also document response to therapy, such as with antiarrhythmic medications. External cardiac monitoring devices are not ideally suited to detect infrequent events unlikely to occur during 1- to 7-day recordings. Implantable devices (see page 686) may be more useful.

Common Indications: Suspected arrhythmias when the routine ECG is not diagnostic; unexplained syncope, near syncope, or episodic dizziness;

unexplained recurrent palpitations; assessment of the adequacy of antiarrhythmic therapy.

General Preparation: Holter monitoring is the preferred ambulatory
ECG test for patients with daily or near-daily symptoms and in whom a
comprehensive or continuous assessment of all cardiac activity is required.
Holter-based technology uses small, lightweight, battery-operated recorders.
The typical configuration records two or three channels of ECG data from
electrodes placed on the patient's chest. More comprehensive 12-lead monitoring systems are also available.

Potential Complications: Rare skin irritation from surface electrodes.

Reference: Pevnick JM et al. Wearable technology for cardiology: An update
and framework for the future. Trends Cardiovasc Med 2018;28(2):144–150.

CARDIAC STRESS TESTING

Description: Numerous studies have validated the prognostic utility of
cardiac stress testing (also called ECG treadmill testing). Because ischemia
represents an imbalance between myocardial oxygen supply and demand,
exercise or pharmacologic stress increases myocardial oxygen demand and
reveals an inadequate oxygen supply (hypoperfusion) from diseased coronary arteries. Stress testing can thus induce detectable ischemia in patients
with no evidence of ischemia at rest. It is also used to determine cardiac
reserve in patients with valvular and myocardial disease. The most commonly used stress testing techniques are exercise electrocardiography (ECG
based using treadmill or stationary bicycle) and exercise or pharmacologic
stress combined with an imaging modality (stress echocardiography or stress
radionuclide myocardial perfusion imaging [MPI]/ SPECT or PET-CT). In
patients with normal resting ECGs, diagnostic ST depression of myocardial
ischemia has a high sensitivity and specificity for detecting coronary artery
disease in symptomatic patients if adequate stress is achieved (peak heart
rate at least 85% of the patient's maximum predicted rate, based on age
and sex). Exercise ECG testing is an excellent low-cost screening procedure
for patients with chest pain consistent with coronary artery disease, normal
resting ECGs, and the ability to exercise to maximal levels. Protocols such
as the "Bruce protocol" standardize the stress testing parameters (see Notes
below, page 689).

Common Indications: Evaluation of exertional chest pain; assess significance of known coronary artery disease; risk stratification of ischemic
heart disease; determine exercise capacity; evaluate other exercise symptoms; detect exercise-induced pulmonary hypertension; evaluate the severity
of valvular heart disease; determine maximum oxygen consumption; and
precipitate exercise-induced arrhythmias. Exercise stress testing is generally inappropriate for detection of ischemia in asymptomatic patients with
no history of revascularization. Absolute contraindications to stress testing
include within two days of an acute myocardial infarction; ongoing unstable

angina; uncontrolled cardiac arrhythmia with hemodynamic compromise; active endocarditis; symptomatic severe aortic stenosis; decompensated heart failure; acute pulmonary embolism, pulmonary infarction, or deep vein thrombosis; acute myocarditis or pericarditis; acute aortic dissection; physical disability that precludes safe and adequate testing and other relative contraindications.

General Preparation: If the patient can exercise (achieve at least five METs [mean exercise test] see below), exercise stress testing (bicycle or treadmill) is preferred, as it is more physiologic and gauges functional capacity. If the patient cannot exercise, use pharmacologic stress testing. Choice of agents for pharmacologic stress testing is based on several factors. Dobutamine (an inotrope) increases cardiac workload and is contraindicated in patients with severe baseline hypertension, ventricular arrhythmias, recent MI, or unstable angina. Vasodilators (adenosine, regadenoson, and dipyridamole) induce selective coronary vasodilation of less diseased vessels, causing hypoperfusion of areas at ischemic risk, and is contraindicated in patients with bronchospastic airway disease or hypotension. Adenosine can be used and is contraindicated in patients with sick sinus syndrome or high-degree AV block. See Figure 20-4 for an algorithm for determining appropriate stress test modality.

Potential Complications: One in 10,000 exercise stress tests result in sudden cardiac death or hospitalization. Major reasons to stop stress testing: ST-segment elevation (>1.0 mm) in leads without preexisting significant Q waves secondary to myocardial infarction; decrease in systolic blood pressure >10 mm Hg; moderate-to-severe angina; CNS symptoms (e.g., ataxia, dizziness, near syncope); signs of poor perfusion (cyanosis or pallor); sustained ventricular tachycardia (VT) or other arrhythmia; technical difficulties in monitoring the electrocardiogram or systolic blood pressure; the subject's request to stop; and others.

Notes: Exercise testing is done on a motorized treadmill or with a bicycle ergometer. A variety of exercise protocols are utilized, the most common being the **Bruce protocol**, which increases the treadmill speed and elevation every 3 min until limited by symptoms. At least two ECG leads should be monitored continuously. Exercise capacity is reported in terms of estimated **metabolic equivalents of task** (**METs**). The MET unit reflects the resting volume of oxygen consumption per minute (VO_2) for a 70-kg, 40-yr-old man, with 1 MET equivalent to 3.5 mL/min/kg of body weight.

In the standard Bruce protocol, the starting point (i.e., stage 1) is 1.7 mph at a 10% grade (equivalent to five METs). Stage 2 is 2.5 mph at a 12% grade (equivalent to seven METs). Stage 3 is 3.4 mph at a 14% grade (equivalent to nine METs). This standard Bruce protocol includes 3-min periods to allow achievement of a steady state before workload is increased.

References: 1. Kumar N, Law A, Choudhry NK (eds.). *Teaching Rounds: A Visual Aid to Teaching Internal Medicine Pearls on the Wards.* New York, NY: McGraw-Hill; 2016.

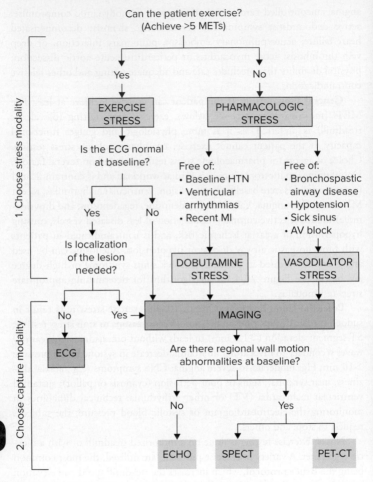

Figure 20-4. Cardiac stress testing. Protocol for determining appropriate stress test modality. (Reproduced with permission from Kumar N, Law A, Choudhry NK [eds.]. *Teaching Rounds: A Visual Aid to Teaching Internal Medicine Pearls on the Wards.* New York, NY: McGraw-Hill, 2016.)

2. McLaughlin M. Rehabilitation of the patient with coronary heart disease. In Fuster V, Harrington RA, Narula J, Eapen ZJ (eds.). *Hurst's The Heart*, 14e, New York, NY: McGraw-Hill; 2017.

CHORIONIC VILLUS SAMPLING (CVS)

Description: CVS is usually performed between 10- and 13-wk gestation. Chorionic villi are withdrawn from the placenta, either through a needle inserted through the abdomen or through a transcervical catheter, and the cells obtained are grown and analyzed for prenatal diagnosis of karyotypic abnormalities or genetic disorders for which testing is available. The benefit of CVS over amniocentesis is its availability earlier in pregnancy.

Common Indications: The American College of Obstetricians and Gynecologists' policy states that invasive diagnostic testing should be made available to all women, regardless of age or risk (ACOG Practice Bulletin No. 88). Some common indications include maternal age >35 yr or older at delivery date; previous pregnancy with a chromosome abnormality or genetic disorder; parental carrier of chromosome disorder; parents are carriers of autosomal recessive disease; congenital abnormality in first-trimester fetal ultrasound exam; aneuploidy screen with abnormal results (maternal serum with/without ultrasound markers of aneuploidy using cell-free DNA).

General Preparation: CVS is not recommended prior to 10-wk gestation due to the increased rate of limb anomalies reported. For both transabdominal and transvaginal CVS, an antiseptic preparation is used. Antibiotics are not standard. Minor spotting postprocedure is normal, and strenuous physical activity and intercourse are to be avoided for 1–2 days.

Potential Complications: Pregnancy loss rates after CVS are similar to those for amniocentesis but are highly operator dependent. There is a risk of vertical transmission of maternal infection, such as from human immunodeficiency virus (HIV), and hepatitis B and C; inconclusive genetic testing results; delayed rupture of membranes; also increased rate of transverse limb abnormalities can result with CVS before 9 wk of gestation.

Note: One disadvantage of CVS is that, unlike amniocentesis, it does not allow diagnosis of neural tube defects. Fetomaternal bleeding can cause alloimmunization and can cause a rise in maternal serum alpha-fetoprotein. RhD-negative women without alloimmunization should receive anti-D Rh immunoglobulin prophylaxis after the procedure.

References: 1. American College of Obstetricians and Gynecologists. ACOG Practice Bulletin No. 88, December 2007. Invasive prenatal testing for aneuploidy. Obstet Gynecol 2007;110(6):1459.

2. Mehta SH, Sokol RJ. Assessment of at-risk pregnancy. In DeCherney AH, Nathan L, Laufer N, Roman AS (eds.). *CURRENT Diagnosis & Treatment: Obstetrics & Gynecology*, 12e, New York, NY: McGraw-Hill; 2019.

COLPOSCOPY

Description: A colposcope, a binocular microscope, is used for direct visualization of the cervix, vagina, or vulva for abnormal cells to diagnose precancerous or cancerous disease (Figure 20-5). Colposcopy does not replace other methods of diagnosing abnormalities of the cervix; rather, it is an additional and important tool. The two most important groups of patients who can benefit by its use are (1) patients with an abnormal Pap smear and (2) DES-exposed daughters, who may have dysplasia of the vagina or cervix. The colposcope has reduced the need to perform blind cervical biopsies for which the rate of abnormalities is low. In addition, the need for a cone biopsy,

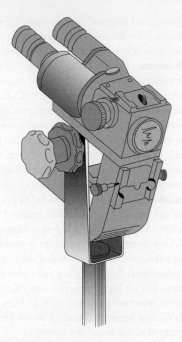

Figure 20-5. The colposcope is a binocular microscope used for direct visualization of the cervix. Magnification as high as 60× is available, but the most popular instrument in clinical use has 13.5× magnification, which effectively bridges the gap between what can be seen by the naked eye and by the microscope. Some colposcopes are equipped with a camera for single or serial photographic recording of pathologic conditions. (Reproduced with permission from Kawada C, Hochner-Celnikier D. Gynecologic history, examination, & diagnostic procedures. In DeCherney AH, Nathan L, Laufer N, Roman AS [eds.]. *CURRENT Diagnosis & Treatment: Obstetrics & Gynecology*, 12e, New York, NY: McGraw-Hill; 2019.)

20

a procedure with high morbidity, has been greatly reduced. Biopsies may be taken of any abnormal-appearing areas, and an endocervical curettage can be performed to sample the cervical canal. Colposcopy is usually performed in an office setting. Colposcopy can be performed during pregnancy; however, an endocervical curettage is contraindicated during pregnancy.

Common Indications: Abnormal cervical or vaginal Pap smear.

General Preparation: The cervix, vagina, and/or vulva is swabbed with acetic acid and/or Lugol solution to highlight abnormal cells prior to examination with a colposcope.

Potential Complications: Bleeding form biopsy site.

Reference: Kawada C, Hochner-Celnikier D. Gynecologic history, examination, & diagnostic procedures. In DeCherney AH, Nathan L,

Laufer N, Roman AS (eds.). *CURRENT Diagnosis & Treatment: Obstetrics & Gynecology*, 12e, New York, NY: McGraw-Hill; 2019.

CORONARY ARTERY CALCIUM SCORING

Description: This is a very rapid, low radiation, dedicated cardiac CT scan that is gated to the cardiac cycle. It quantifies the amount of calcium in the coronary arteries, which is a surrogate marker for plaque burden. This is not a CT angiography or stress test, and it is not utilized for chest pain assessment. It is a study that can help assess patients' risk for future cardiovascular events through assessment of cardiovascular vessel calcification. The main reason to perform this study is to determine if there is an indication for significant lifestyle modification and initiation of cardioprotective medications such as statin therapy and aspirin.

   Common Indications: Borderline or intermediate atherosclerotic cardiovascular disease (ASCVD) risk. As an example, if the patient has some risk factors and the provider and patient are debating whether to initiate statin therapy, the coronary calcium score can inform the decision. If the test result is 0, meaning there is no detectable calcium in the coronary arteries, this indeed supports not using statin therapy or aspirin. However, if a patient has a very high calcium score (above 400), there is a clear indication to initiate statin therapy and perhaps aspirin as well. Another indication is to assist the decision-making with patients with a relatively low ASCVD score and with a very strong family history of cardiovascular disease.

   General Preparation: No need for routine labs or any preparation; this study is low radiation exposure and does not require contrast administration.

   Potential Complications: Detection of other incidental findings that could lead to further unnecessary workup. Very low dose radiation that is clinically insignificant.

   Notes: The calcium score is measured by **Agtston units**, and can be automatically calculated by dedicated software. Only if the score is 0 is it truly a negative result. A calcium score above 100 suggests moderate coronary plaque burden, and a score above 400 suggests severe disease.

   Reference: Hecht H et al. Clinical indications for coronary artery calcium scoring in asymptomatic patients: Expert consensus statement from the Society of Cardiovascular Computed Tomography. J Cardiovasc Comput Tomogr 2017;11(2):157–168.

20

CYSTOSCOPY

Description: Cystoscopy is the visual inspection of the lower urinary tract with the use of a fiber-optic scope. A small camera is passed per the urethral meatus in a retrograde fashion to evaluate the urethra, bladder neck region, trigone, and bladder. In male patients, cystoscopy also allows for the evaluation of the prostatic urethra. The primary indication for cystoscopy is to diagnosis lower urinary tract pathology. Cystoscopy can be performed with either a flexible or rigid cystoscope. Cystoscopy can also be used to access the upper urinary tracts (ureters, kidneys) using an endoscopic approach through the injection of contrast into the ureters (retrograde pyelogram).

Common Indications: Direct visualization of the lower urinary tract through cystoscopy is primarily used to determine how urinary signs and symptoms are related to lower urinary tract anatomy and pathology. Cystoscopy is commonly used for the evaluation of both gross and microscopic hematuria. In conjunction with genitourinary tract imaging, cystoscopy can help determine the source of hematuria. Other common indications for cystoscopy include voiding symptoms, overactive bladder symptoms, bladder pain symptoms, incontinence, and dysuria.

General Preparation: Patients should receive preprocedure counseling that explains the indication for the procedure and how cystoscopy will aid in the diagnosis and possible treatment. Before performing a cystoscopy, it is important to check a urinalysis to determine if a patient has an active urinary tract infection. In most cases, cystoscopy should be deferred if a patient's lower urinary tract is acutely infected. Patients should also be counseled that they will be asked to undress from the waist down, they will be placed in a supine or lithotomy position, and their urethral meatus will be prepped with a cleansing solution. During the procedure, patients should be informed that they may feel a sense of bladder fullness or an urgency to void.

Potential Complications: Instrumentation of the lower urinary tract during cystoscopy can lead to a urinary tract infection. If a patient has an active infection, cystoscopy can exacerbate the UTI. Other potential complications include hematuria secondary to mechanical trauma of the lower urinary tract by the cystoscope and urethral or bladder injury. Such complications are rare.

Reference: Matulewicz RS, et al. Cystoscopy. JAMA 2017;317(11):1187.

ELECTROENCEPHALOGRAM (EEG)

Description: An electroencephalogram (EEG) assesses brain function by measuring the electrical activity of the brain. An array of electrodes (typically 21 electrodes) is placed on the scalp in standard positions to record the electrical fields generated by neurons. These fields represent summated excitatory and inhibitory postsynaptic potentials, which change from moment to moment and vary with level of arousal (wake/sleep cycles). An EEG recording can last from 20 to 30 min (routine EEG) to weeks or years (continuous inpatient or outpatient ambulatory EEG) depending on the indication and device. Activation techniques such as hyperventilation and photic stimulation with flashing lights may be performed during routine recordings to help elicit an abnormality. Simultaneous video recording can be performed so that physicians can review and characterize any abnormal movements or behaviors.

Common Indications: The most common use is in diagnosing seizures and epilepsy. Interictal epileptiform discharges, termed spikes or sharp waves, are produced by neuronal paroxysmal depolarization shifts and usually indicate a propensity for seizures. Seizures can be directly recorded with EEG, providing confirmation of the diagnosis. Recording these abnormalities aids in diagnosing the specific epilepsy syndrome, planning therapy, and assessing efficacy of treatment. In critically ill patients, EEG is essential for diagnosing status epilepticus and monitoring therapy. EEGs are also useful aids when diagnosing patients with altered consciousness, helping to differentiate between various causes of encephalopathy and coma, and can provide important prognostic information. EEG can sometimes help diagnose causes of dementia, mainly Creutzfeldt-Jakob disease. Also, EEG can detect focal brain abnormalities caused by stroke, tumors, and other causes, though imaging techniques such as MRI are superior for that purpose.

General Preparation: EEGs are performed in outpatient and inpatient settings. Patients may be instructed to restrict sleep to 3–4 hr the night prior to the test so they more readily fall asleep during the EEG. This increases the likelihood of detecting interictal epileptiform discharges (spikes, sharp waves). Patients should wash and dry their hair prior to the study to optimize recording quality.

Potential Complications: Complications are quite rare. It is possible to abrade the scalp when preparing an area for electrode placement. The electrode glue used in long-term recording infrequently causes transient hair loss where the electrodes are placed. Rarely, seizures can be provoked by hyperventilation or photic stimulation. Finally, although rare, electrical shocks may occur should the recording equipment be improperly grounded in the setting of equipment failure.

Notes: Fellowships in clinical neurophysiology and epilepsy provide training for advanced EEG interpretation. EEGs must be interpreted in the context of the clinical history and examination.

Reference: Marcuse LV, et al. *Rowan's Primer of EEG.* New York, NY: Elsevier Health Sciences; 2016.

ELECTROMYOGRAPHY (EMG) AND NERVE CONDUCTION STUDIES (NCV)

Description: Electromyography (EMG) and nerve conduction studies (NCS) are two procedures typically performed together that assess peripheral nervous system function. With EMG, a fine needle electrode is inserted into different muscles to evaluate the muscle action potentials evoked by motor

20

neurons. These potentials are assessed in terms of amplitude, morphology, and frequency during electrode insertion, muscle rest, and muscle contraction to identify abnormalities in the motor unit. During NCS, sensory and motor nerves are electrically stimulated. Responses to this stimulation are recorded in terms of amplitude and conduction velocity to identify an abnormality within the axon or its surrounding myelin sheath. NCS largely assesses large, myelinated nerve fibers rather than small, unmyelinated nerve fibers. These procedures supplement the clinical examination and they are interpreted only in the context of that examination.

Common Indications: EMG/NCS are used to assess neurological disorders involving muscle, nerve (including nerve root), or neuromuscular junction. It may be used to evaluate pain, sensory loss or tingling, weakness, or cramping. Commonly evaluated nerve disorders include polyneuropathies, carpal tunnel syndrome, radiculopathy, peroneal neuropathy (foot drop), and amyotrophic lateral sclerosis. Neuromuscular junction disorders include myasthenia gravis and Lambert-Eaton myasthenic syndrome. Myopathies include inflammatory myopathies, toxic myopathies, myotonic dystrophy, and hereditary myopathies such as muscular dystrophies.

General Preparation: The skin is cleaned and dried when starting the procedure. Surface electrodes are placed on the skin to stimulate underlying nerves. A sterile fine needle electrode is placed intramuscularly to record muscle action potentials. An oscilloscope displays the nerve and muscle potentials during the study, and an amplifier is used during EMG for auditory evaluation. Multiple needle insertions or electrical stimulations are typically required to comprehensively evaluate the relevant nerves and muscles.

Potential Complications: Needle insertion and electrical stimulation usually produce mild pain and discomfort, which may limit a patient's ability to fully cooperate with the study through inability to relax a muscle or resist movement. The discomfort is particularly limiting in children, who rarely undergo this procedure. Use of aseptic technique when inserting needles minimizes risk of infection, which is quite rare. Bleeding is very rarely provoked by needle examination of the muscles, and there is no convincing evidence that either antiplatelet or anticoagulant drugs pose a greater bleeding risk.

Notes: Fellowships in clinical neurophysiology and neuromuscular disorders provide training in advanced EMG/NCS testing and interpretation. Findings must be interpreted in light of the history and neurological examination, as asymptomatic, incidental abnormalities are quite common, particularly with advancing age.

Reference: Daube JR, Rubin DI. *Clinical Neurophysiology*, 4e, Oxford UK: Oxford University Press; 2018.

ENDOSCOPIC ULTRASOUND

Description: Endoscopic ultrasound (EUS) uses an ultrasound transducer attached to the tip of an endoscope to obtain ultrasound images from within the upper gastrointestinal tract. EUS allows physicians to visualize extraluminal organs and structures not visible during regular endoscopy, such as the layers of the gastrointestinal wall, the liver, pancreas, bile ducts, and adjacent lymph nodes. Endoscopic ultrasound with fine needle aspiration (EUS-FNA) uses real-time EUS guidance to advance a needle into these structures in order to aspirate fluid or obtain tissue samples.

Common Indications: Staging of esophageal, gastric, pancreatic, and rectal malignancies; diagnosis and characterization of submucosal gastrointestinal lesions; diagnosis of choledocholithiasis, gallbladder/biliary disease, and chronic pancreatitis; direct fine-needle aspiration (FNA) or core biopsy of pancreatic masses, cystic lesions of the pancreas, submucosal gastrointestinal lesions, and lymphadenopathy adjacent to the GI tract; aid in the drainage of abdominal abscesses, pancreatic pseudocysts, and pancreatic necrosis.

General Preparation: Patients should be NPO for at least 8 hr before the procedure. Preprocedure antibiotics are given if draining a cyst or fluid collection.

Potential Complications: Esophageal or duodenal perforation (0.03–0.06%) EUS with FNA; bleeding (0.5%); infection (<1%); pancreatitis (<2%).

Reference: Wani S, et al. Quality indicators for EUS. Gastrointest Endosc 2015;81(1):67–80.

ESOPHAGEAL MANOMETRY

Description: Esophageal manometry is a procedure used to evaluate the motility of the esophagus. The procedure involves placing a soft, flexible, pressure-sensing catheter through the nose into the patient's esophagus. The patient is then instructed to swallow with the catheter in place, and the muscular contractility of the esophagus is measured. The catheter is able to measure the relaxation of the upper and lower esophageal sphincters as well as the intersphincteric peristaltic contractions of the esophagus.

Common Indications: Evaluation of difficulty swallowing (dysphagia) after mechanical obstruction has been ruled out. Preoperative assessment of patients being considered for antireflux surgery.

General Preparation: Patient cannot eat solid food for 4 hr before testing. Patients must discontinue the following medications 24 hr prior to the procedure: promotility medications (metoclopramide), calcium channel blockers, nitrates, anticholinergic medications, tricyclic antidepressants, and benzodiazepines.

Potential Complications: Sore throat; epistaxis; lightheadedness or dizziness during the study; accidental insertion into the larynx may cause coughing or aspiration.

Reference: Kahrilas PJ, Hirano I. Diseases of the esophagus. In Jameson JL et al. (eds.). *Harrison's Principles of Internal Medicine*, 20e, New York, NY: McGraw-Hill; 2018.

20

FETAL HEART RATE MONITORING

Description: A variety of techniques are available to assess fetal distress during labor and delivery with emphasis on fetal heart rate changes. Traditional intermittent stethoscope/Doppler auscultation of fetal heart rates have long served as an indirect measure of fetal well-being. Contemporary electronic fetal heart rate monitoring (EFM) may be internal, with a spiral electrode attached to the fetal scalp, or external, with a monitor that uses Doppler technology attached to the maternal abdomen. These techniques have been shown to improve outcomes. For a low-risk patient, intermittent auscultation of the fetal heart may be acceptable; however, for most high-risk deliveries, continuous electronic EFM is recommended. The nomenclature and interpretation of EFM are based on the 2008 National Institute of Child Health and Human Development (NICHD) workshop report (J Obstet Gynecol Neonatal Nurs 2008;37(5):510–515) and are as follows (see also Figure 20-6):

- **Baseline fetal heart rate (FHR):** The rate maintained for at least 2 min apart from periodic variations, rounded to the nearest 5 beats/min (BPM) over a 10-min period. The normal FHR is 110 to 160 beats/min. Bradycardia mean FHR <110 BPM; tachycardia mean FHR >160 BPM.
- **Variability:** Indicates a functioning sympathetic–parasympathetic nervous system and is the most sensitive indicator of fetal well-being.
- **Accelerations:** Associated with fetal movement and are an indication of fetal well-being.
- **Early decelerations:** Result from physiologic head compression; these are benign and are not associated with fetal compromise.
- **Late decelerations:** Are a result of uterine placental insufficiency and indicate fetal hypoxia.
- **Variable decelerations:** Result from abrupt compression or stretch of the umbilical cord. Many of these decelerations are benign and not predictive of an acidotic fetus. However, severe variable decelerations (those lasting >60 sec) suggest a compromised fetus.

Common Indications: Assess fetal well-being during labor and delivery.

General Preparation: None specifically for the external monitor. The mother must have ruptured membranes with a sufficiently dilated cervix for the fetal scalp monitor. The fetal scalp electrode should NOT be applied in the following settings: when it is not possible to identify the fetal presenting part, malpresentation, placenta previa, excessive vaginal bleeding, genital infections (e.g., herpes, group B strep, gonorrhea), or bloodborne diseases (e.g., hepatitis B and C, HIV). No special prep is needed for the external monitoring device.

Potential Complications: For the fetal scalp monitor: maternal vaginal or cervical laceration; fetus scalp laceration or other body part trauma,

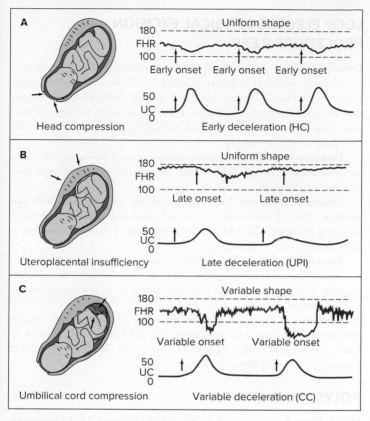

Figure 20-6. Examples of fetal heart rate monitoring. CC, cord compression; FHR, fetal heart rate (beats/min); HC, head compression; UC, uterine contraction (mm Hg); UPI, uteroplacental insufficiency. (Reproduced with permission from Gomella, TL [ed.]. *Gomella's Neonatology*, 8e, New York, NY: McGraw-Hill; 2020.)

20

neonatal infection, vertical transmission of infection from mother to infant (avoid scalp monitoring as noted in General Preparation above, page 698); provider self-injury related to placement. Conversion to C-section with a fetal scalp monitor in place may require antibiotics.

Notes: In the United States, fetal heart rate monitoring in labor has become the standard of care in most facilities.

Reference: Gomella, TL (ed). Intrapartum tests of fetal well-being: Prenatal, labor, delivery and transport management. In *Gomella's Neonatology*, 8e, New York, NY: McGraw-Hill; 2020.

LOOP ELECTROSURGICAL EXCISION PROCEDURE (LEEP)

Description: Loop electrosurgical excision procedure (LEEP) is one modality of therapy for vulvar and cervical lesions. LEEP uses a low-voltage, high-frequency alternating current that limits thermal damage but at the same time has good hemostatic properties. It has displaced sharp knife and laser cone biopsies for treatment of most cervical dysplasias. LEEP is usually performed in an office setting.

Common Indications: It is most commonly used for excision of vulvar condylomata and cervical dysplasias and for cone biopsies of the cervix (cervical intraepithelial neoplasia [CIN] 2 or 3).

General Preparation: The cervix is injected with lidocaine with epinephrine. The cervix is swabbed with acetic acid and/or Lugol solution to highlight abnormal cells, and the cervix is examined with a colposcope to determine the area of excision.

Potential Complications: Bleeding from the surgical bed.

Notes: The major advantages of LEEP are its usefulness in an office setting with lower equipment cost, minimal damage to the surrounding tissue, and low morbidity.

Reference: Kawada C, Hochner-Celnikier D. Gynecologic history, examination, & diagnostic procedures. In DeCherney AH, Nathan L, Laufer N, Roman AS (eds.). *CURRENT Diagnosis & Treatment: Obstetrics & Gynecology*, 12e, New York, NY: McGraw-Hill; 2019.

POLYSOMNOGRAPHY

Description: Polysomnography (PSG) is a diagnostic test, commonly referred to as a "sleep study," and is often performed when the clinical history suggests a sleep disorder. During PSG, the patient sleeps while connected to a variety of monitoring devices that record physiologic variables. It is typically performed in a sleep lab with the patient being monitored by a sleep technologist. In selected patients, it can be performed at home to diagnose obstructive sleep apnea. This is called home sleep apnea testing (HSAT).

Following a night of monitored sleep, the PSG is evaluated in 30-sec intervals, called "epochs." A number of sleep variables are measured and scored, including sleep-onset latency, sleep efficiency, time spent in each sleep stage, breathing irregularities including apneas and hypopneas, arousals, cardiac rhythm abnormalities, leg movements, body position, and oxygen saturation levels. The information gathered is evaluated and interpreted by the polysomnography technologist and the sleep lab physician.

The diagnosis of obstructive sleep apnea (OSA) is confirmed when the apnea-hypopnea index (AHI) is equal to or greater than 5 (mild OSA: $5 \geq$ AHI <15; moderate OSA: $15 \geq$ AHI <30; severe OSA: AHI ≥ 30). AHI is defined as the sum of apneas and hypopneas per hour of sleep. Apnea is defined as a near-complete cessation of airflow for at least 10 sec. A hypopnea is defined as decrease in airflow for at least 10 sec followed by an oxygen desaturation.

Common Indications: The most common indication to perform a sleep study is for suspected obstructive sleep apnea when the upper airway closes while sleeping leading to absent or reduced airflow. This leads to snoring, hypoxemia, and disrupted sleep. Other indications are suspected narcolepsy, which leads to excessive daytime sleepiness; parasomnias like sleepwalking or dream enactment behavior; and sleep-related movement disorders like periodic limb movement disorder and nocturnal seizures.

General Preparation: Consumption of alcohol and caffeine is generally avoided on the evening of the study, as both can severely disrupt sleep and in the case of alcohol make sleep apnea worse. Patients are advised to continue their usual medications. For patients who are very anxious and nervous about sleeping in a strange environment, a low-dose sedative may be prescribed by their physician. It may be helpful for them to take a brief tour of the laboratory before the study. Patients can be encouraged to bring their own pillow if they use a special pillow to sleep.

Potential Complications: Complications of PSG are rare. The most common complication is skin irritation caused by adhesive used to attach electrodes to the patient. Drawbacks include inconvenience, difficulty sleeping in the laboratory setting, strange surroundings, and discomfort related to the monitoring equipment or bed. As patients can and do experience medical emergencies while undergoing testing, laboratories must be prepared with ready access to resuscitation equipment and appropriately trained staff with an established protocol for access to emergency medical services.

Notes: Polysomnography is an expensive procedure, and the monitoring and the interpretation of these physiologic variables should be performed in an accredited facility with well-trained and certified staff and physicians. For patients diagnosed with OSA, continuous positive airway pressure (CPAP) is considered first-line therapy. PSG can be used to titrate CPAP. If patients are not adequately benefitting from CPAP or would like to explore therapeutic surgical options, **drug-induced sleep endoscopy (DISE)** can be performed. DISE refers to flexible laryngoscopy performed during a pharmacologically induced sleep state. This allows for dynamic physiological assessment of upper airway collapse during sleep.

References: 1. Kushida CA et al. Practice parameters for the indications for polysomnography and related procedures: An update for 2005. Sleep 2005;28(4):499–521.

2. Berry RB et al. for the American Academy of Sleep Medicine. The AASM Manual for the Scoring of Sleep and Associated Events: Rules, Terminology and Technical Specifications, Version 2.5, www.aasmnet.org, American Academy of Sleep Medicine, Darien, IL; 2018.

3. Kezirian EJ, et al. Drug-induced sleep endoscopy: The VOTE classification. Eur Arch Otorhinolaryngol 2011;268:1233–1236.

20

URODYNAMICS

Description: Urodynamics is a bladder function test that evaluates the storage and emptying phases of the lower urinary tract. During a urodynamic evaluation, small catheters are placed in the bladder and the rectum to obtain pressure measurements. Patch or needle electrodes are also placed in the pelvic region to obtain an electromyography tracing of the pelvic floor muscles and urethral sphincter. Urodynamics can be utilized to investigate the following lower urinary tract parameters: bladder sensation, bladder compliance, type of incontinence, presence of involuntary bladder contractions, bladder capacity, detrusor function, and presence of obstructed voiding. Fluoroscopy of the lower urinary tract can be added when there is suspicion for concomitant upper tract dysfunction or obstructed voiding.

Some specific elements of urodynamics include:

- Cystometry, leak point pressure measurement and pressure flow study.
- Electromyography.
- Pressure flow study.
- Uroflometry.
- Postvoid residual measurement.
- Video urodynamic tests

Common Indications: Patients should undergo urodynamic evaluation if they have persistent bothersome lower urinary tract symptoms that have failed to respond to therapies based on clinical symptomatology alone. Clinical problems that might benefit from urodynamic testing include: urine leakage or incontinence, sudden urges to urinate, frequent urination, pain with urination, recurrent UTI, urinary hesitancy or inability to fully empty the bladder. Urodynamics is also indicated in patients being considered for invasive treatment or therapies with significant side effects. Finally, urodynamics is a crucial step in evaluating patients with neurologic pathology that may affect lower urinary tract function. The decision to pursue urodynamic testing should be made by a urologist or urogynecologist.

General Preparation: Most patients are unfamiliar with urodynamic testing and do not have a clear understanding of what the evaluation involves. Patients should receive preprocedure counseling to review the indication for the evaluation and to inform them that they will sit in a special testing chair, be asked to undress from the waist down, have catheters placed in both their urethra and rectum, and have electrodes placed in their pelvic region. Due to the sensitive nature of urodynamic testing, it is important to conduct the test in a private setting and have an empathetic and knowledgeable medical professional conduct the evaluation. Before performing urodynamics, it is important to check a urinalysis to determine if a patient has an active urinary tract infection. Urodynamics should be deferred if a patient's lower urinary tract is acutely infected.

Potential Complications: Instrumentation of the lower urinary tract during urodynamics can lead to a urinary tract infection. If a patient has an active infection, urodynamics should be avoided since it can exacerbate the UTI. Other potential complications include hematuria secondary to catheterization.

Reference: Roseir PF et al. International Continence Society Good Urodynamic Practices and Terms 2016: Urodynamics, uroflowmetry, cystometry and pressureflow study. Neurourol Urodyn 2017;36.

Pain Management **21**

- Defining Pain and Educating the Patient
- Classification of Pain
  - Nociceptive Pain
  - Neuropathic Pain
- Effects of Pain on the Body
- Assessing Pain
  - Measuring Pain Intensity
- Essentials of Pain Management
  - Nonopioid Analgesics
- Opioid Analgesics
- Pain Management in the Opioid-Tolerant Inpatient
- Patient-Controlled Analgesia (PCA)
  - PCA Ordering Parameters
- Nonpharmacologic Approaches to Pain
- Pain Management with Substance Use Disorder (SUD)

DEFINING PAIN AND EDUCATING THE PATIENT

The International Association for the Study of Pain defines pain as an "unpleasant sensory and emotional experience associated with actual or potential tissue damage, or described in terms of such damage." Acute pain is the most common symptom that brings a patient to see a physician, and it is frequently the first sign of an ongoing pathologic process. Chronic pain, defined as pain lasting longer than 3 mo or a greater duration than expected, often has an unclear etiology that includes tissue injury and psychosocial factors. Whenever possible, inform the patient beforehand about the nature and the degree of pain to be expected during a hospital stay. Hospitalized patients, especially those with acute-on-chronic pain, should be made aware that his or her pain might not completely go away with treatment. Rather, the goal of pain management should be to achieve improved pain control to allow adequate function for recovery and performance of daily activities.

Chapter update by William Denk, MD, and Eugene R Viscusi, MD

CLASSIFICATION OF PAIN

Nociceptive Pain

Pain due to stimulation of pain receptors, i.e., nociceptors. Nociceptive pain can be further characterized as somatic or visceral pain. Somatic pain is sharp, constant, well-localized, and is caused by injury to skin, subcutaneous tissue, muscle, blood vessels, or bones. Examples include incisional pain, bone fractures, phlebitis, and osteoarthritis. Visceral pain originates from nociceptors within the internal organs (viscera), and is poorly localized, crampy, and intermittent in frequency. Some examples are intestinal colic, bladder spasm, gastroesophageal reflux, urolithiasis, and angina.

First-line treatment for nociceptive pain includes nonsteroidal anti-inflammatory drugs (NSAIDs) and acetaminophen. When these medications fail to relieve symptoms, opioids may be considered. While NSAIDs are best at treating inflammatory pain exacerbated by movement, e.g., osteoarthritic joint pain, opioids are useful for treating pain at rest.

Neuropathic Pain

Pain resulting from damage of the nervous system. Neuropathic pain is typically described as "shooting" or "burning," is poorly localized, and frequently occurs spontaneously. In addition, the pain can be accompanied by abnormal sensations (dysesthesias), including an exaggerated response to a painful stimulus (hyperalgesia) or the sensation of pain due to a nonpainful stimulus (allodynia). Sympathetic nerve stimulation may further exacerbate neuropathic pain. Examples include radiculopathy, postherpetic neuralgia, diabetic polyneuropathy, phantom limb pain, and nerve compression.

Neuropathic pain is best treated with anticonvulsants (e.g., gabapentin, pregabalin), antidepressants (e.g., duloxetine, amitriptyline, nortriptyline), or topical anesthetics (e.g., lidocaine, capsaicin). Opioids are not effective at treating neuropathic pain.

21

EFFECTS OF PAIN ON THE BODY

Table 21-1, page 707, shows adverse effects of pain as they relate to specific organ systems.

ASSESSING PAIN

Pain assessment involves consideration of physiologic, emotional, and psychological aspects. First, observe the patient and try to gauge his or her level of distress. Ask the patient about discomfort and how it impairs his or her functional status. Conduct a detailed interview to classify the pain and the underlying disease process. Here are some important questions to consider:

Table 21-1.   Adverse Effects of Pain as They Relate to Specific Organ Systems

Organ System	Adverse Effect
RESPIRATORY	
Increased skeletal muscle tension	Hypoxia, hypercapnia
Decreased total lung compliance	Ventilation–perfusion abnormality, atelectasis, pneumonitis
ENDOCRINE	
Increased adrenocorticotropic hormone	Protein catabolism, lipolysis, hyperglycemia
Decreased insulin	Decreased protein anabolism
Decreased testosterone	Decreased sex drive
Increased aldosterone, increased antidiuretic hormone	Salt and water retention, congestive heart failure, edema
Increased catecholamines	Vasoconstriction, hypertension
Increased angiotensin II	Increased myocardial contractility
CARDIOVASCULAR	
Increased myocardial work	Dysrhythmias, angina, ischemia
IMMUNOLOGIC	
Lymphopenia, depression of the reticuloendothelial system, leukocytosis, reduced killer T-cell cytotoxicity	Decreased immune function, increased susceptibility to infection
COAGULATION EFFECTS	
Increased platelet adhesiveness, diminished fibrinolysis, Activation of coagulation cascade	Increased incidence of thromboembolic phenomena
GASTROINTESTINAL	
Increased sphincter tone, Decreased smooth muscle tone	Ileus
GENITOURINARY	
Increased sphincter tone, Decreased smooth muscle tone	Urinary retention

21

- Where is the pain located?
- How severe is the pain? How does this compare to the pain level at baseline? Has the pain progressively worsened?
- How is the pain characterized?
- When did the pain start? Were there any previous episodes of the pain?
- Is the pain constant or intermittent?

- What relieves the pain and what worsens the pain?
- How is the pain managed at home? Is there any history of chronic opioid use?
- Are there any associated symptoms, e.g., nausea, vomiting, swelling, numbness?
- Does the pain radiate?
- Is the pain referred from an internal source?

An example of pain radiating to an extremity is leg pain following lumbar disk herniation. An example of referred pain is a ureteral calculus with pain referred to the ipsilateral testicle. A thorough physical exam may reveal more clues to identify the internal cause of acute pain. Despite this, many chronic pain syndromes have no known anatomic cause, and physical exam is less informative in these cases.

Measuring Pain Intensity

There are a number of scales and questionnaires available to assess a patient's pain level and disability. These tools are particularly useful for monitoring pain over time and assessing the efficacy of pain management interventions. The most common scales and questionnaires are shown below.

Numerical Rating Scale (NRS): An 11-point scale where 0 is the absence of pain and 10 is the worst pain imaginable. NRS is a quick verbal method to assess pain, and it is sensitive for detecting daily changes in pain. A disadvantage is that patients may report a number higher than 10 when asked to describe pain that has worsened from what he or she previously described as a "10 out of 10," which is difficult to interpret. Another disadvantage is that the NRS oversimplifies pain to a single number and does not give information about the patient's functional status. Pain scores are ultimately subjective, so the same score will mean different things to different patients. A good rule of thumb is that a 2-point reduction or 30% decrease in pain scores demonstrates a clinically significant improvement.[1]

Visual Analogue Scale (VAS) and Wong-Baker Faces Pain Rating Scale: See Figure 21-1. The VAS is a visual representation of the NRS, which allows it to be administered to nonverbal and mechanically ventilated patients. The Wong-Baker Scale depicts a series of faces ranging from a happy face (no pain) to a crying face (worst possible pain). Since this scale is intuitive and requires no verbal or written instructions, it can be administered to children, neurologically impaired patients, or those facing language barriers.

Short Form 12-Item Health Survey (SF-12): The SF-12 measures health-related quality of life, including the impact of pain on performing daily activities. This form assesses the impact of chronic conditions on mood, well-being, and functional status. Consider using this tool during follow-up appointments for chronic pain patients to monitor response to pain control interventions.

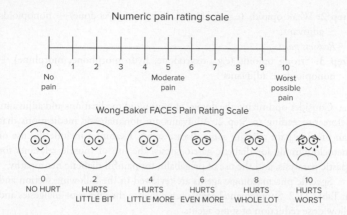

Figure 21-1. Scales used to determine pain intensity. The patient is asked to indicate where on the scale his or her pain would fall. (From Clinical Practice Guidelines Number 9: Management of Cancer Pain, Rockville, MD: U.S. Department of Health and Human Services, ICCPR publication 94-0592.)

McGill Pain Questionnaire (MPQ): The MPQ[2] is a checklist of words describing symptoms. It analyzes scores in various sensory and affective dimensions to identify the quality of pain. Consider using this tool in the detailed management of pain syndromes.

ESSENTIALS OF PAIN MANAGEMENT

The goal of pain management is to provide adequate relief with minimal side effects. When beginning therapy always start with the lowest dose of pain medicine that provides relief. If rapid pain control is necessary, utilize an intravenous analgesic rather than an oral one. However, it is important to be aware that even IV analgesics do not work instantly. In order to avoid unnecessary doses, one should wait until the medication's time to peak analgesic effect has been reached before considering whether to redose the medication. If pain remains uncontrolled despite appropriate dosing of one analgesic, then consider adding another agent from a different medication class. This technique is commonly known as *multimodal analgesia*. Multimodal analgesia starts with a foundation of around-the-clock nonopioid analgesics (typically acetaminophen and NSAIDs) before adding an opioid.

The World Health Organization Pain Ladder serves as a useful model to guide pain management. Although it was originally developed for cancer pain, the Pain Ladder can be used in any clinical setting. There are three steps in the Pain Ladder:

Step 1: Nonopioid (e.g., NSAIDs, acetaminophen) ± adjuvants
   Reassess pain

Step 2: Weak opioids (e.g., tramadol, low-dose oxycodone) + nonopioids ± adjuvants
Reassess pain
Step 3: Strong opioids (e.g., oxycodone, hydromorphone, morphine) + nonopioids ± adjuvants

Consider optimizing the dosage of nonopioid medications and adjuvants before proceeding to Step 2. Adjuvants are nonanalgesic medications that can provide pain relief in some disease states. Examples include the use of metoclopramide for diabetic gastroparesis, the use of muscle relaxants for spastic paralysis, and the use of pregabalin for painful diabetic neuropathy.

Specific pharmacologic agents are reviewed in the following section and in Table 21-2. Supplemental agents can enhance the effects of analgesics and allow dose reduction of some agents.

Nonopioid Analgesics

Acetaminophen: One of the most commonly used analgesics and a good choice for mild-to-moderate pain due to its favorable side effect profile. The mechanism of action of acetaminophen is not well-understood, but it may act on cyclooxygenase (COX) receptors within the CNS. Because it does not act on peripheral COX receptors, acetaminophen can be safely administered with NSAIDs. Acetaminophen is available in oral, rectal, or IV forms. The drug is generally safe in patients with renal impairment, but should be used with extreme caution in patients with hepatic impairment or cirrhosis. Healthy adults can generally tolerate up to 4 g/day without issue. **Side effects:** Nausea, vomiting, skin rash, hypersensitivity reactions, acute liver failure (with overdose).

NSAIDs: Bind to peripheral COX receptors, where they inhibit the production of prostaglandins, which are important mediators of pain and inflammation. Commonly used NSAID analgesics include ibuprofen, ketorolac, and naproxen. Aspirin is an NSAID that has a relatively higher affinity to COX receptors on platelets, where it acts to inhibit platelet aggregation. Because this is an unwanted side effect that can worsen risk of bleeding, aspirin is no longer widely used as an analgesic. NSAID dosage is usually limited by renal function since these medications decrease blood flow to the kidneys. For this reason, they should be avoided in patients with renal impairment, even if the patient is on dialysis. **Side effects:** Headache, dyspepsia, bleeding, dizziness, skin rash, gastroesophageal reflux, nausea, cardiovascular thrombosis (e.g., MI, stroke), GI ulcers or perforation, acute kidney injury. Celecoxib is an NSAID that binds preferentially to the COX-2 receptor subtype, meaning that it carries a lower risk of GI ulcers or platelet dysfunction. However, celecoxib is not widely used because it has a significantly higher risk of cardiovascular thrombosis compared to traditional NSAIDS.

Table 21-2. Commonly Used Analgesic Agents. Many of these agents have Black Box Warnings on their FDA label. Name and formulation include generic and some common brand names.

Name and Formulation	Dose Range/ Interval (Adults)	Dose Range/ Interval (Children)	Pharmacokinetics	Precautions	Comments
Acetaminophen (IV, PO)	650–1000 mg q4–6h; daily max 4000 mg	6–11 yr: 325 mg q4–6h; daily max 1625 mg >11 yr: as adult	Onset 5–10 min (IV), <1h (PO) Peak: ° h (IV) Duration: 4–6h	Use with caution in liver disease or history of alcohol abuse	No peripheral antiinflammatory effects, unlike NSAIDs
NONSTEROIDAL ANTIINFLAMMATORY DRUGS (NSAIDS)					
Ibuprofen (Advil, Motrin, Nuprin, Mediprin, Rufen; IV, PO)	IV: 400–800 q6h; daily max 3200 mg PO: 200–800 mg q6–8h; daily max 3200 mg	6 mo–12 yr: 4–10 mg/kg q6–8h; daily max 40 mg/kg >12 yr: 400 mg q6–8h, daily max 400 mg	Onset: 30–60 min Peak: 1–2h (PO) Duration: 6–8h	Avoid in history of NSAID hypersensitivity, severe kidney disease, GI bleeding, ulcers, or perforation	Causes platelet dysfunction and may increase bleeding time. Increases risk of HTN, MI, stroke. Should be administered with food.
Indomethacin (PO, rectal)	25–40 mg q8–12h; daily max 200 mg	>2 yr: 0.25–0.5 mg/kg PO q6–12h; daily max 4 mg/kg or 200 mg	Onset: 30 min Peak: 2h Duration: 4–6h	Refer to *Ibuprofen Precautions*	Increased risk of vascular, GI, and CNS sensory adverse effects

(Continued)

Table 21-2. Commonly Used Analgesic Agents. Many of these agents have Black Box Warnings on their FDA label. Name and formulation include generic and some common brand names. (*Continued*)

Name and Formulation	Dose Range/ Interval (Adults)	Dose Range/ Interval (Children)	Pharmacokinetics	Precautions	Comments
Ketorolac (Toradol; IV, IM, PO)	IV: 15–30 mg q6h; daily max 120 mg IM: 30 mg q6h; daily max 120 mg PO: 20 mg initial, then 10 mg q4–6h; daily max 40 mg **Treatment should be limited to 5 days max.**	IV, IM: 0.5 mg/kg q6–8h **Treatment should be limited to 3 days max.**	Onset: 30 min (IV, IM), 30–60 min (PO) Peak: <2h (IV, IM), 2–3h (PO) Duration: 4–6h	Refer to *Ibuprofen Precautions*	PO ketorolac intended only as continuation of IM or IV therapy
Naproxen (Aleve, Anaprox, Naprosyn; PO)	500 mg initial, then 250 mg q6–8h; daily max 1250 on day 1, then 1000 mg subsequently	<60 kg: 5 mg/kg q12h ≥60 kg: 250 q12h Daily max 600 mg	Onset: 30–60 min Duration: <12h	Refer to *Ibuprofen Precautions*	Naproxen sodium has faster onset (1–2h) than base formulation
Celecoxib (Celebrex; PO)	400 mg initial, then 200 mg q12h	≥10 to ≤ 25 kg: 50 mg q12h >25 kg: 100 mg q12h	Peak: 3h	Refer to *Ibuprofen Precautions*. Recent data show the incidence of MI and stroke is comparable to other NSAIDs	COX-2 -selective blocker. Does not inhibit platelet aggregation

MUSCLE RELAXANTS				
Metaxalone (Skelaxin, Metaxall; PO)	800 mg q6–8h	Not indicated	Peak: 3h	CNS depressant. May cause additive depression when used with other sedatives. May cause serotonin syndrome	Avoid in geriatric patients and with hepatic or renal impairment
Cyclobenzaprine HCl (Flexeril, Amrix, Fexmid; PO)	5–10 mg q8h; daily max 30 mg	Not indicated	Onset: <1h Peak: 4h Duration: 12–24h	Additive CNS depression with other agents. May cause serotonin syndrome	Avoid in geriatric patients and with hepatic or renal impairment. Do not use longer than 3 weeks
OPIOID ANALGESICS (Continued on next page)				
Hydromorphone (Dilaudid; IV, PO, rectal)	IV: 0.01–0.015 mg/kg q3–6h PO: 0.03–0.06 mg/kg q3–6h	IV: 0.2–1 mg q2–3h PO: 2–4 mg q4–6h	Onset: 5 min (IV), 15–30 min (PO) Peak: 10–20 min (IV), 30–60 min (PO) Duration: 3–4h (IV, PO)	May cause additive CNS depression with other sedatives; also respiratory depression, hypotension, constipation, other opioid adverse effects	Use a lower starting dose in elderly patients or those with renal or hepatic impairment

21

(Continued)

713

Table 21-2. Commonly Used Analgesic Agents. Many of these agents have Black Box Warnings on their FDA label. Name and formulation include generic and some common brand names. (*Continued*)

Name and Formulation	Dose Range/ Interval (Adults)	Dose Range/ Interval (Children)	Pharmacokinetics	Precautions	Comments
Morphine IR (Avinza, Kadian, MSIR; IV, PO)	IV: 2.5–5 mg q3–4h PO: 10–30 mg q3h Oral form given q4h to establish daily opioid requirement	Various dosing schedules exist based on weight, age, and morphine formulation	Onset: 5–10 min (IV), 30 min (PO) Duration: 3–5h (IV, PO)	Refer to *Hydromorphone Precautions*. May also cause hypersensitivity, severe bronchial asthma	Avoid in renal insufficiency (use alternate opioid). Consider antihistamine for morphine-induced pruritus. Avoid ER form (i.e., MS-Contin) in inpatient setting.
Oxycodone IR (OxyIR, Roxicodone; PO)	5–15 mg q4–6h	>6 mo, <50 kg: 0.1–0.2 mg/kg q4–6h	Onset: 10–15 min Peak: 0.5–1h Duration: 3–6h	Refer to *Hydromorphone Precautions*	Use a lower starting dose in elderly patients or those with renal or hepatic impairment. Avoid ER form (i.e., OxyContin) in inpatient setting
Tramadol (Ultram; PO)	50–100 mg q4–6h; daily max 400 mg	Not recommended under age 16	Onset: <1h Peak: 2–3h	Refer to *Hydromorphone Precautions*. May also cause seizures or serotonin syndrome	Seizure and serotonin syndrome risk is increased with SSRIs, SNRIs, TCAs, MAO inhibitors, neuroleptics, CYP450 inhibitors

21

ANTIEPILEPTICS

Gabapentin (Neurontin, Gralise; PO)	100–300 mg q8–24h	Not recommended	Peak: 2–4h	May cause CNS depression, neuropsychiatric effects, DRESS syndrome, physical dependence	Decrease dose and frequency in renal impairment
Pregabalin (Lyrica; PO)	25–150 mg q12–24h	Not recommended	Peak: 1.5h	May cause CNS depression, suicidal ideation, peripheral edema, visual disturbances, rhabdomyolysis	Decrease dose and frequency in renal impairment

DRESS: Drug rash with eosinophillia and systemic symptoms; ER: Extended release; IR: Intermediate release; MAO: Monoamine oxidase; MSIR: Brand name for morphine solution and tablets; SNRI: Serotonin-norepinephrine reuptake inhibitor; SSRI: Selective serotonin reuptake inhibitors; TCA: Tricyclic antidepressant.

21

Anticonvulsants: Gabapentin and pregabalin are structural analogues of GABA, the principal inhibitory neurotransmitter in the CNS. Despite this similarity, they do not bind to GABA receptors and instead inhibit excitatory neurons involved in pain pathways. Due to their favorable side effect profile, the gabapentinoids have largely replaced tricyclic antidepressants (TCAs) in the treatment of neuropathic pain. A main disadvantage of these medications is that they are only available in oral formulation. Both gabapentin and pregabalin are renally cleared, and require dose adjustment in renal impairment. **Side effects:** Dizziness, sedation, edema, weight gain, blurred vision, rhabdomyolysis. Because pregabalin has a significantly higher bioavailability than gabapentin, time to onset is generally faster.

Antidepressants: SNRIs (e.g., duloxetine) and the older TCAs (e.g., amitriptyline) work well as adjuvant therapy and are an appropriate consideration mostly for chronic pain associated with diabetic neuropathy, postherpetic neuralgia, and chemotherapy. **Side effects to TCAs:** Antimuscarinic effects (e.g., dry mouth, blurred vision, urinary retention), antihistaminic effects (e.g., sedation), and alpha-adrenergic blockade (e.g., hypotension). Also, see Table 22-7, pages 743–747.

Local Anesthetics: Bind to sodium channels, exerting an effect on the cellular level. Effect is usually localized to the area where the drug is injected. **Side effects:** Relatively few side effects. Allergic reactions usually due to PABA-like (Para-aminobenzoic acid) preservatives in the solution and not the agents themselves. Toxicity (usually due to overdose) includes tonic-clonic seizures, respiratory arrest, and subsequent cardiovascular collapse. Topical local anesthetics (lidocaine patch) have specific efficacy for neuropathic pain.

Opioid Analgesics

Opioids act on opioid receptors located throughout the body, including the spinal cord, brainstem, thalamus, and cortex, where they exert their analgesic effects. There are three major receptor subtypes: μ, κ, and δ. Of these, binding at the μ-opioid receptor produces the strongest analgesic effect, which is the target of the most commonly used opioids. This includes hydrocodone, oxycodone, hydromorphone, oxymorphone, morphine, codeine, and fentanyl. Opioids are quite effective at treating the slower onset, throbbing, "second pain" that occurs at rest after an initial nociceptive stimulus. However, opioids are less effective at treating visceral signaling and neuropathic pain or reducing sudden-onset, sharp "first pain." When taken on a long-term basis, opioids are not found to be superior to NSAIDs or acetaminophen in improving pain outcomes. In fact, they can induce a state of nociceptive sensitization to lower pain tolerance, a finding referred to as opioid-induced hyperalgesia.

Adverse effects of opioids include euphoria, nausea, constipation, urinary retention, delayed gastric emptying, miosis, pruritus, muscle rigidity, bradycardia, cough suppression (may be an intentional effect), and respiratory depression that may lead to apnea and death. The risk of respiratory depression is greatest for extended-release opioids, and for this reason their routine use is discouraged. Life-threatening respiratory depression can be reversed with emergency administration of naloxone, which blocks μ-opioid receptors and rapidly increases the respiratory rate. Long-term use of opioids is associated with hypogonadism, decreased cellular immunity, tolerance, and eventually hyperalgesia and dependence.

Most opioids have similar mechanism of action, but differ significantly in their pharmacokinetics. Morphine and meperidine are two opioids that are cleared by the kidneys, and these drugs should be avoided in renal failure to prevent overdose. Most other opioids are safely metabolized by the liver, even in cases of hepatic impairment. Codeine is a prodrug that has no effect until it is converted to morphine in the liver. Because this metabolism can be slowed in some individuals due to genetic differences, morphine levels may not rise quickly enough to produce significant analgesia. Tramadol is a unique opioid that produces weak analgesia by activating all three opioid receptor subtypes and may have a primary mode of action by blocking serotonin reuptake in the CNS. In addition to its other side effects, tramadol may cause serotonin syndrome or seizures.

All opioids have a broad and flat dose-response curve exhibiting a wide range of dose related efficacy across individuals. Hence, careful dose titration is critical when using opioids. Further, most patients reach a ceiling effect above which there is little benefit to dose escalation. The rule of opioid prescribing is that every dose should have a clear benefit in pain relief and functionality, or opioids should not be employed or escalated.

Pain Management in the Opioid-Tolerant Inpatient

Opioids are among the most commonly prescribed medications in the United States, with a significant amount of the population on chronic opioid therapy. Approximately 21–29% of patients misuse their prescribed opioids. Of these, 4–6% transition to heroin. Managing an acute episode of pain in an opioid-tolerant patient is a challenging task due to opioid tolerance and increased pain sensitivity. Many providers are rightfully cautious to administer high doses of opioids capable of causing respiratory depression in an opioid-naive patient, but such doses may be necessary in some opioid-tolerant individuals.

1. Start by obtaining a thorough history of past opioid use. This includes the duration, dosage, and frequency of prescription opioids used and any nonprescription or illicit use (e.g., heroin).
2. Ensure that the prescriptions are correct by verifying the information in the patient's chart and through your state's prescription drug monitoring program.

3. Choose one of the following:

    a. If you are confident in the patient's safety on his or her opioid regimen, you may choose to either continue the patient's home regimen or convert the regimen to an equianalgesic dose of a single, as needed, immediate release oral opioid (e.g., oxycodone IR q4h PRN). See Table 21-3 for opioid dose conversions. In either case, first optimize all nonopioid analgesics and adjuvants. If the patient was taking an acetaminophen–opioid combination medication (e.g., Vicodin, Percocet), these should be given separately in order to maximize the acetaminophen component.

    b. If you are not confident in the safety of the home regimen, the patient takes uncertain quantities of opioids (e.g., heroin use), or pain continues to be uncontrolled despite therapy, stop **all** opioids and start a standard IV opioid PCA (see PCA section, page 719).

Table 21-3. Equianalgesic Opioid Conversion Chart. Note: All opioid conversions are approximate at best, and there is great variability among patients. Hence, always start the new opioid at a substantially lower dose (approx. 50%) and titrate upward as needed. Extended-release or long-acting opioids should only be used with stable, chronic, long-term pain with stable opioid doses and never in the setting of acute pain or acute on chronic pain.

Agent	Equianalgesic Doses (mg)	
	Parenteral	Oral
Morphine	10	30
Morphine Controlled-Release (MS Contin)	—	30
Oxycodone Immediate (OxyIR) or Controlled-Release (OxyContin)	—	20
Fentanyl (Sublimaze)	0.1	—
Hydromorphone (Dilaudid)	1.5	7.5
Meperidine (Demerol)	75	300
Note: Routine or chronic use not recommended		
Oxymorphone Immediate (Opana) or Extended-Release (Opana ER)	—	10
Hydrocodone	—	30
Codeine	120	200
Note: Efficacy highly variable; based on differences in metabolism of the prodrug		

PATIENT-CONTROLLED ANALGESIA (PCA)

Most commonly used after surgery, a PCA allows the patient to self-administer small boluses of narcotics with an IV pump. PCAs have a lockout interval, typically 6 min, in order to prevent multiple concurrent doses that may lead to oversedation. Breakthrough pain may be managed with nurse-administered boluses as needed, which typically are double the dose of a patient bolus. Although they were once commonly used in PCAs, basal infusions are no longer recommended. Opioid basal infusions are linked to respiratory depression without improving analgesia. PCA opioid concentrations are standardized in order to prevent medication error, meaning that an adjustment in dose comes from adjusting the volume administered. A central requirement for PCA use is a patient's ability and cooperation. For example, a PCA would be inappropriate for an encephalopathic patient or one unable to use the upper extremities to push the button.

A PCA is useful in the opioid-tolerant patient because it allows the patient to safely titrate the opioid to his or her requirements. The amount of opioid dispensed by the PCA should be monitored daily to assess pain control requirements. Once PCA use declines and stabilizes, the patient can be placed back on the home regimen or an equivalent dose of immediate release oral opioid prior to discharge.

PCA Ordering Parameters

Table 21-4, below, shows examples of PCA orders.

NONPHARMACOLOGIC APPROACHES TO PAIN

Physical Therapy: Heat and cold can provide pain relief by alleviating muscle spasm. Heat decreases joint stiffness and increases blood flow; cold causes vasoconstriction and reduces tissue edema.

21

Table 21-4. Examples of PCA Orders Using Different Agents

Opioid in PCA	Concentration	Standard Patient Bolus	Lockout Interval	PRN Nursing Bolus	Hourly Max Dose
Morphine	1 mg/mL	1 mg	6 min	2 mg q2h PRN	10 mg
Hydromorphone	0.2 mg/mL	0.2 mg	6 min	0.4 mg q2h PRN	2 mg
Fentanyl	10 mcg/mL	10 mcg	6 min	20 mcg q2h PRN	100 mcg

Osteopathic or Chiropractic Treatment: Physical manipulation can relax soft tissues, increase range of motion, and alleviate pain. Biweekly or monthly treatments are recommended and are best for chronic pain. Acute treatment minimizes musculoskeletal pain.

Psychological Intervention: Cognitive therapy, behavioral therapy, or biofeedback relaxation techniques. Pain is often associated with depression, especially when it becomes chronic.

Acupuncture: Needles are inserted into discrete anatomically defined points or meridians and stimulated by mild electric current. This method is believed to release endogenous opioids.

PAIN MANAGEMENT WITH SUBSTANCE USE DISORDER (SUD)

With the prevalence of opioid abuse, anyone treating pain must have a basic understanding of the specific considerations in these patients. Patients with SUD are typically and profoundly opioid tolerant. Hence, opioids will likely not be very effective. Opioid escalation is discouraged, and reliance on non-opioid analgesics is critical. Avoidance of opioid withdrawal is important, as it can be the driver for early termination of care by the patient. Opioid withdrawal can be managed by modest amounts of an opioid, clonidine, and a benzodiazepine, as well as other agents.

Whenever possible, patients with SUD should be started on medication-assisted treatment (buprenorphine or methadone) in the hospital setting with outpatient follow-up. Patients with SUD have a high incidence of death in the 28 days following hospital discharge if left untreated. Buprenorphine is a viable analgesic for these individuals while preventing opioid withdrawal. With appropriate titration by a specialist, buprenorphine can minimize opioid craving and help maintain abstinence. Lastly, patients in recovery on stable buprenorphine doses should virtually NEVER have their buprenorphine held in the acute care setting, as it may lead to return to opioid abuse.

21

References

1. Malzack RR. The McGill Pain Questionnaire: Major properties and scoring methods. *Pain.* 1975;1:227–299.
2. Farrar JT, et al. Clinical importance of changes in chronic pain intensity measured on an 11-point numerical pain rating scale. *Pain.* 2001 Nov;94(2):149–158.

Further Reading

1. Kato K, et al. A study of transdermal fentanyl in cancer pain at Aichi-Cancer Center. *Yakugaku Zasshi.* 2004. 124(5): 287–291.

2. Treillet, E, et al. Practical management of opioid rotation and equianalgesia. *Journal of Pain Management*. 2018. 11: 2587–2601.

3. Gabrail NY, et al. Establishing the dosage equivalency of oxymorphone extended release and oxycodone controlled release in patients with cancer pain: A randomized controlled study. *Current Medical Research and Opinion*. 2004. 20: 911–918.

4. Rennick A, et al. Variability in opioid equivalence calculations. *Pain Medicine*. 2016. 17: 892–898.

5. Clinical Practice Guidelines Number 9: Management of Cancer Pain, Rockville, MD: U.S. Department of Health and Human Services, ACHPR publication 94-0592.

Palliative Care and Nonpain Symptom Management

22

INTRODUCTION

Palliative care is defined by the World Health Organization as an approach to end-of-life healthcare "that improves the quality of life of patients and their families facing the problems associated with life-threatening illness through

Original chapter by Miguel Paniagua, MD, FACP, FAAHPM and Tanya J. Uritsky, PHARMD, BCPS, Steven A Haist, MD, MS

the prevention and relief of suffering by means of early identification and impeccable assessment and treatment of pain and other problems, physical, psychosocial, and spiritual."[1] Palliative care is provided by a wide array of healthcare professionals in a wide spectrum of settings, from the patient's home to an acute care hospital. Hospice is an approach to providing palliative care in the patient's home or a home-like setting involving the patient's family in the care of the terminal patient. Hospice care is generally reserved for the last 6 months of life; however, it is often difficult to predict the date a patient will die, and often hospice care is instituted too late for the patient and the patient's family to receive the full benefits of hospice care. Hospice care is provided by physicians, nurses, social workers, clergy/chaplains/spiritual guides, and volunteers, all of whom are often specifically trained in end-of-life care. There are over 4,000 hospice agencies across the United States, and over 60% are nonprofit organizations. Two major differences between hospice care and palliative care are that the patient's life expectancy in hospice care is months and treatment involves relief of symptoms to reduce suffering, and there is no treatment directed at curing the underlying terminal disease. There is no expected life expectancy for patients receiving palliative care, and patients may continue to receive treatment for their underlying disease. This chapter focuses on overall palliative care management, including non-pain symptom management. Principles of pain management are discussed in Chapter 21, Pain Management, page 705.

Whether engaged in the co-management of symptoms of a patient with restorative or disease-oriented goals, or a patient who has prioritized symptom management over curative treatments, the methodological assessment of symptoms is essential. Using objective and validated instruments is beneficial. The Revised Edmonton Symptom Assessment Scale (ESAS) is a useful symptom assessment tool that allows for simple and rapid documentation of multiple patient-reported symptoms simultaneously (see Table 22-1[2], page 725).

GOAL-ORIENTED DECISION-MAKING[3]

Effective Communication Strategies

End-of-life goal setting is a critically important procedure in medicine that typically occurs as part of a family meeting. After discussing the patient's current condition, questions to help establish patient-centered goals include:

1. What are you hoping for now?
2. What is important to you?
3. What do you need to accomplish?
4. Who do you need to see in the time that is left?

Ensure that you leave time for responses and for questions. Then restate your understanding:

"What I hear you saying is that you desire…."

Table 22-1. Edmonton Symptom Assessment Scale (Revised Version)

No pain	0	1	2	3	4	5	6	7	8	9	10	Worst possible pain
No tiredness (tiredness = lack of energy)	0	1	2	3	4	5	6	7	8	9	10	Worst possible tiredness
No drowsiness (drowsiness = feeling sleepy)	0	1	2	3	4	5	6	7	8	9	10	Worst possible drowsiness
No nausea	0	1	2	3	4	5	6	7	8	9	10	Worst possible nausea
No lack of appetite	0	1	2	3	4	5	6	7	8	9	10	Worst possible lack of apppetite
No shortness of breath	0	1	2	3	4	5	6	7	8	9	10	Worst possible shortness of breath
No depression (depression = feeling sad)	0	1	2	3	4	5	6	7	8	9	10	Worst possible depression
No anxiety (anxiety = feeling nervous)	0	1	2	3	4	5	6	7	8	9	10	Worst possible anxiety
Best well-being (well-being = how you feel overall)	0	1	2	3	4	5	6	7	8	9	10	Worst possible well-being
No other problem (for example, constipation)	0	1	2	3	4	5	6	7	8	9	10	Worst possible _____

Note: Please circle the number that best describes how you feel NOW.

Source: From Watanabe SM, et al. A multicenter study comparing two numerical versions of the Edmonton Symptom Assessment System in palliative care patients. J Pain Symptom Manag 2011;41(2):456–466.

22

Recommend a care plan based on the goals stated, then review the patient's treatment, including planned interventions, diagnostic tests and/or procedures, symptom monitoring, and medications and, if practical and feasible, collaboratively decide how to meet the patient's goals. Depending on the clinical situation, the discussion should include:

1. Whether to forgo cardiopulmonary resuscitation, a "do not attempt resuscitation" (DNAR) or "allow natural death" (AND).
2. Further treatments such as transfusions, antibiotics, hydration, or nutrition.
3. If relevant, address avoidance or discontinuation of cardiac devices and hemodialysis.
4. Discuss role of future hospitalizations, ICU-level care, and other laboratory and radiology tests.
5. Discuss what disposition options best meet the patient and their family needs/goals.

DO NOT offer treatments as a checklist of options for them to consider ("Do you want antibiotics?"), but rather make recommendations about what should and should not be done as appropriate based on sound clinical judgment and the patient's goals. If uncertain, it is optimal to disclose the uncertainty in the discussions with the patient and the patient's family. Considerations when communicating with the patient and the patient's family should include the following:

1. Reinforce the notion that family is part of the team in advocating for the patient (if the patient cannot do so for themselves).
2. "Hope for the best, but prepare for the worst" in case plans to continue curative or restorative treatments are maintained.
3. NEVER abandon the patient and family. NEVER say "there is nothing more we can do" or "we can just do nothing." You can always attempt to maximize quality of life with aggressive pain and symptom management and support.
4. Reinforce that the team will not abandon the patient and family even if the decision is not what is being recommended.
5. Always close an encounter or meeting with two questions:
   a. Do you have any questions or concerns (and if so, be sure to fully address)?
   b. Is there anything you need before I leave?

Compassionate Withdrawal of Care[4]

Compassionate withdrawal of care should be based on the following:

1. The goal of withdrawing life-sustaining treatments is to remove treatments that are no longer desired or do not provide comfort to the patient.
2. Withholding life-sustaining treatments is morally and legally equivalent to withdrawing them.

3. Actions whose sole goal is to hasten death are morally and legally problematic.
4. Any treatment can be withheld or withdrawn.
5. Withdrawal of life-sustaining treatment is equivalent to a medical procedure.
6. Corollary to 1 and 2: When circumstances justify withholding one indicated life-sustaining treatment, strong consideration should be given to withdrawing all life-sustaining treatments.

Procedure for withdrawal of care should include the following:

1. Separate the patient from the commotion of the ICU by moving the patient to a separate area or an isolated room. In open units, curtains should be closed.
2. Turn off monitors and, if possible, remove them from the room. Remove electrocardiographic leads, pulse oximeter, and hemodynamic monitoring catheters.

There is no point to monitoring physiologic parameters when the data generated will not alter the care provided. Families attending the dying patient can become preoccupied with irrelevant numbers and waveforms instead of focusing their attention on the patient.
3. Remove all tubes, lines, and drains if this can be done without causing significant discomfort.
4. Liberalize visitation to the extent that it does not interfere with the delivery of care to other patients.
5. Do not obtain further laboratory or imaging studies.

The following will guide the provision of sedation and analgesia:

1. Before patients are removed from life support, they should be completely comfortable, as judged by the cessation of tachypnea, grimacing, agitated behavior, and autonomic hyperactivity.
2. Doses should not be increased in the absence of demonstrable signs of discomfort or for behavior that cannot plausibly be interpreted as distress.
3. Specific doses of medication are less important goals than titration to achieve the desired effect.
4. Continuous infusion is the route of choice for drug delivery when the goal is sedation. Increases in dosage should be preceded by a bolus so that steady-state levels can be rapidly achieved. For example, the order might read: "Titrate morphine drip to keep respiratory rate <30, heart rate <100, and eliminate grimacing and agitation."

The following will guide the withdrawal of mechanical ventilation:

1. Sedation and analgesia sufficient to prevent grimacing or response to painful stimuli should be provided before withdrawing mechanical ventilatory support.
2. When adequate sedation is achieved, reduce the inspired oxygen concentration to 0.21, remove positive end-expiratory pressure, and set the

22

ventilator at an intermittent mandatory ventilation (IMV) rate equal to the spontaneous respiratory rate or at a level of pressure support (PS) sufficient to fully meet ventilatory requirements.

3. Air hunger, as manifested by tachypnea or agitation, should be treated with a bolus of the chosen medication followed by an increase in the continuous infusion.

4. After the patient is comfortable, ventilatory support is weaned rapidly in either IMV or PS mode until the patient is comfortable with an IMV rate of zero or a PS of zero cm H_2O at which point the patient can be placed on a T-piece on humidified air.

5. The transition from full ventilatory support to T-piece or extubation should take no more than 15–30 min.

6. It may be appropriate to extubate the patient, particularly when the patient may be able to communicate or when prolonged survival off of life support is possible. Some families or providers may feel strongly about whether to remove the endotracheal tube. These wishes should be respected.

7. If the endotracheal tube is removed, specific plans should be formulated to anticipate secretion problems and agonal airway obstruction, and the family should be prepared for these possibilities.

8. The time course leading to death will vary according to the clinical situation, and cannot be predicted accurately in every case.

COMPLEMENTARY AND ALTERNATIVE MEDICINE (CAM)

As part of your initial history, you should always inquire about CAM. Natural and herbal agents can inhibit or induce certain cytochrome P450 enzymes, inhibiting or inducing the metabolism of prescribed medications, thus leading to toxicity from or reducing the efficacy of the prescribed medication(s). Additionally, patients who are seeking palliative care may have renal or hepatic insufficiency or failure related to their underlying disease. You must be aware of how natural and herbal agents are metabolized. For instance, patients receiving palliative care may take St. John's wort for depression, an anxiety disorder, or insomnia. St John's wort is an inducer of CYP3A4, CYP2C9, and CYP1A2. Any prescribed medications that are metabolized by these enzymes may become less effective because of the induction of the enzyme. Kava kava extract is a potent inhibiter of CYP1A2, 3A4, 2C19, and others and has the potential to increase the concentrations of any prescription medications metabolized by these enzymes.

Refer to your state, local, and hospital policies for guidance on the use of medical marijuana in your practice setting. As many institutions do not permit medical marijuana on site, clinicians may encounter having to discontinue therapy when the patient is admitted. FDA-approved formulations of cannabis include isolated tetrahydrocannabinol (THC) or cannabidiol (CBD) products, and will likely not provide the same symptomatic relief or completely replace medicinal cannabis therapies. There is a paucity of data on the evidence of cannabis for the management of many symptoms, with the strongest evidence supporting its benefit in the management of neuropathic pain, nausea and vomiting, spasticity, and intractable seizures/epilepsy. For considerations on medical marijuana adverse effects, refer to Anorexia-Cachexia (Table 22-2, Medications for the Stimulation of Appetite in Palliative Care) and Nausea and Vomiting (Table 22-14, Antiemetic Medications), pages 763–764.

ANOREXIA-CACHEXIA

Definition and Etiology

Anorexia is an appetite reduction that can be psychogenic or secondary to an underlying advanced illness, whereas cachexia is defined as >5% weight loss over 6 months in the absence of starvation or a BMI <20 and weight loss >2%; or appendicular skeletal muscle index consistent with sarcopenia and weight loss >2%. Cachexia may be refractory in the context of a progressive, advanced, incurable illness, or as a manifestation of advanced untreatable cancer. The prognosis with refractory cachexia is less than 3 months.

There may be many contributing etiologies beyond just a loss of appetite, such as nausea, glucose intolerance, early satiety, and changes in taste or smell. Anorexia is driven by a hyperinflammatory state with an influx of inflammatory mediators (TNF-alpha, IL-1, IL-6, IL-8, INF-alpha, others) and hormonal changes leading to an increase in oxidative stress and protein breakdown, a decrease in response to appetite hormones, and an increase in resting energy expenditure.

Assessment and Management

There are validated tools to assess anorexia/cachexia. The Functional Assessment of Anorexia questionnaire is an example of an assessment tool. There is no additional testing needed to confirm the diagnosis beyond meeting the criteria for weight loss and advanced illness. Uncontrolled symptoms or physical barriers to oral consumption should be treated to minimize external factors. Potential treatable factors contributing to anorexia/cachexia include the following:

- Uncontrolled symptoms (e.g., nausea/vomiting)
- Dental issues (e.g., thrush, dental caries)
- Social factors (e.g., access to food, social isolation, etc.)
- Dysphagia (e.g., obstructive tumor)
- Gastrointestinal etiologies (e.g., diarrhea, constipation)
- Electrolyte or metabolic changes (e.g., uremia, hypercalcemia, hyperthyroidism, hyponatremia, etc.)

22

Table 22-2. Medications for the Stimulation of Appetite in Palliative Care

Medication	Adverse Effects	Considerations
Medical cannabis	Tachycardia, dry mouth, cough, confusion, hyperactivity/psychosis, nausea, fatigue	Efficacy of inhaled cannabinoids in AIDS wasting syndrome
Dronabinol 2.5 mg (2.1 mg solution) PO BID	Euphoria, confusion, lethargy/drowsiness	FDA approved for AIDS cachexia; has limited benefit in weight gain beyond water weight and has limited evidence in cancer cachexia; utility includes improved enjoyment of food, increased protein intake, and improved appetite before meals
Megestrol acetate (Megace) 160–800 mg PO Daily	Thromboembolic events; nausea, diarrhea, impotence, peripheral edema, hypertension, hyperglycemia, breakthrough uterine bleeding, and skin photosensitivity; can precipitate adrenal insufficiency	1 in 4 patients will have an increase in appetite and 1 in 12 will have an increase in weight; no more effective than dexamethasone and no optimal dose has been determined
Mirtazapine 7.5–15 mg PO qhs	Sedation, daytime sleepiness, dry mouth, constipation	No well-designed studies in advanced cancer; in a small study, weight gain of >1 kg following 4 wk of therapy was found in only 4 of 17 (24%) cancer patients with only 24% of patients experiencing improvements in appetite and 6% in health-related quality of life
Dexamethasone 4 mg PO daily	Include hyperglycemia, hyperactivity/psychosis, and adrenal axis suppression	Dexamethasone has the most potent antiinflammatory activity, not associated with sodium or water retention; should be dosed in AM; equal efficacy in improving appetite and weight gain as megestrol acetate
Olanzapine 2.5–5 mg PO qhs	Anticholinergic effects include dry mouth, sedation, orthostatic BP changes; long-term use can cause metabolic changes	Weight gain and appetite stimulation when olanzapine 5 mg/day added to megestrol acetate therapy; doses of 2.5 to 20 mg attenuated the weight loss of advanced cancer patients when used as monotherapy

- Infection (e.g., *Candida* or viral infection in the mouth or esophagus; any febrile illness)
- Mental health disorders (e.g., anorexia nervosa, depression, anxiety)
- Medications (e.g., antibiotics, anticholinergics, chemotherapy, etc.)

Nonpharmacologic management should focus on patient and family education. Fluids and artificial nutrition have not demonstrated a mortality or quality of life benefit unless there is an isolated irreversible obstructive issue involving the proximal GI tract and possibly in select patients with HIV or ALS. Potential nonpharmacologic interventions include:

1. Education of the patient and family about the inflammatory etiology of anorexia/cachexia in advanced disease.
2. Comfort eating and not artificial nutrition.
3. Nutritional counseling in pre-cachexia to offer creative solutions to taste changes and suggestions for increasing tolerability with feedings.
4. Fluid administration should be goal-directed and carefully considered. Fluids can lead to fluid retention and may increase pain and discomfort as well as cause pulmonary edema.

Pharmacological interventions include a variety of appetite stimulants. Appetite stimulation may result in an increase in oral intake, and potentially an increase in fat storage and not in lean muscle, which is required for strength and longevity. Additionally, there is no mortality benefit to increasing appetite and resultant weight gain. The inflammatory process at the end of life is itself an appetite suppressant. The body is utilizing its energy to sustain life-preserving organ function, leaving minimal energy to digest food. The resultant decrease in appetite is a normal part of severe illness, and while the patient may not feel hungry, it is difficult for loved ones to no longer feed them.

If it is determined to use an appetite stimulant, it is important to consider other compelling indications to maximize the utility of the selected agent. Please see Table 22-2 for possible appetite stimulants and selection considerations.

ANXIETY (See DEPRESSION AND ANXIETY, page 741)

BOWEL OBSTRUCTION

Etiology

Malignant bowel obstruction (MBO) is a common complication in gastrointestinal cancers and can occur in other cancers, such as lymphomas. Ovarian and colon cancer are the most common cancers associated with MBO. MBO is a poor prognostic indicator suggesting a shortened life expectancy of weeks to months.

Assessment and Management

MBO can present with nausea, vomiting, and abdominal pain, which can be either constant and/or colicky in nature. MBO is diagnosed clinically and radiographically. Treatment options are based on the site of obstruction, functional status, patient values and goals of care, and prognosis. Options can include surgical intervention, placement of a venting gastrostomy tube, and medical management.

Surgical

Surgical goals are to relieve nausea and vomiting, allow oral intake, alleviate pain, and permit the patient to return to their preferred care setting. Improvement in quality of life is variable after surgery, but it may offer a survival advantage. Poor prognostic indicators for surgical success include ascites, carcinomatosis, palpable abdominal masses, multiple obstructions, prior obstructions, and very advanced disease. Less invasive endoscopic interventions such as stents may be an option for symptom relief. PEG tubes can alleviate intractable vomiting from upper GI obstructions.

Nutritional Support

Nutritional support via total parenteral nutrition may be beneficial to a subset of patients who may die from malnutrition or starvation before succumbing to the cancer. Even with interventional treatment, medication management of symptoms is essential. The goal of medication management is symptom relief and to avoid the need for decompression with a nasogastric tube or PEG tube placement and IV hydration. If an NG tube is placed for temporary relief, once the output is less than 100 cc/day, the tube can be clamped for 12 hr and then removed. Intravenous hydration should only be considered for patients who are dehydrated despite oral intake or when such measures are consistent with the patient's goals of care.

Medication

Medication management is outlined in Table 22-3. For all medications, consider alternative delivery routes for PO medications if the patient is not tolerating IV medications or if unable to clamp venting G-tube.

CONSTIPATION

Definition and Etiology

Constipation has many definitions. In palliative care, the diagnosis is different than in other chronic settings. There are many possible etiologies of constipation in this setting. The most common offender is an opioid, but there are many other causes. Addressing reversible factors and eliminating any offending medications is essential to management. Risk factors for constipation in palliative care include the following:

- Advanced disease
- Older age
- Decreased activity
- Low-fiber diet
- Depression
- Cognitive changes
- Physical impediments (e.g., rectal mass, hemorrhoids, abdominal pain)
- Polypharmacy: opioids, iron, calcium channel blockers, diuretics, anticholinergics, serotonin antagonists, chemotherapy (vinca alkaloids)
- Metabolic changes: hypercalcemia, hypothyroidism
- Neural changes: spinal cord compression, hypercalcemia of malignancy

Assessment and Management

The assessment of any problem begins with a thorough history, and the history of a patient with constipation should include inquiry regarding the following:

- Description of the stool (hard, small, infrequent)
- Bloating
- Abdominal pain
- Diarrhea in the form of stool leakage around impacted stool or a mass
- Nausea
- Vomiting
- Confusion
- Assessment for irritable bowel syndrome (abdominal pain on average 1 day a week for 3 months and two of the following: (1) associated with BM, (2) change in frequency of BM, and (3) change in the stool appearance)[3]
- Physical dysfunction impeding defecation
- Subjective symptoms of fullness or incomplete evacuation
- Objective changes in the frequency and consistency of stools

A physical examination should be performed to assess for the presence of constipation, including a rectal exam to palpate for hard stool, assess for masses, anal fissures, hemorrhoids, sphincter tone, push effort during attempted defecation, prostatic hypertrophy in males, and posterior vaginal masses in females. Rectal examination may demonstrate impaction, or the rectal vault may be empty. If a diagnosis of malignant bowel obstruction is suspected, radiographic imaging with abdominal radiographs or CT scan is indicated. Radiographs may also be indicated in the setting of possible toxic

22

Table 22-3. Medications for the Management of Malignant Bowel Obstruction

Medication Class	Agent	Adverse Effects	Considerations
Corticosteroids	Dexamethasone 6–16 mg IV or SC in the AM or in divided doses in AM and early afternoon	Hyperglycemia, hyperactivity/psychosis, adrenal axis suppression	For visceral and colicky pain, also for nausea. Decreased inflammation may help relieve partial obstruction
Opioids	Morphine, hydromorphone, oxycodone, etc.	Constipation, sedation, respiratory depression, pruritus, nausea/vomiting	For management of constant visceral pain
Antiemetics	Antidopaminergic (haloperidol, prochlorperazine) Serotonin antagonist (ondansetron) Olanzapine	For agent-specific considerations see Table 22-14	First line are the antidopaminergics; olanzapine may be preferred if tolerating PO for once-daily dosing and concomitant anticholinergic action to treat cramping
Antisecretory	Octreotide 100–200 mcg SQ/IV TID, or continuous infusion 10–20 mcg/hr; titrate q24h to symptom relief; avoid rapid IV push as this may increase nausea/vomiting	Nausea/vomiting, constipation, bradycardia, abdominal/back pain, injection site reactions, myalgias, alopecia	Decrease peristalsis and endocrine secretion leading to gastric acid production

(Continued)

Table 22-3. Medications for the Management of Malignant Bowel Obstruction (*Continued*)

Medication Class	Agent	Adverse Effects	Considerations
Anticholinergic	Scopolamine 1.5 mg patch q72h; hyoscyamine 0.125 PO/SL q4hPRN; atropine eye drops 0.5–1 mg drops SL/PO/buccal mucosa q4h PRN; glycopyrrolate 0.2–0.4 mg IV/SQ qh PRN	Sedation, urinary retention, constipation, confusion, blurry vision, risk of falls	Decrease cramping from smooth muscle contraction and bowel wall distention, and associated colicky pain; onset of scopolamine is up to 24 hr; atropine is used at end of life; glycopyrrolate is less likely to cause delirium compared to atropine
Antacid	H2-blockers (e.g., ranitidine, famotidine); proton pump inhibitors (e.g., pantoprazole, omeprazole, etc.)	Dizziness, headache	For reflux symptoms due to obstruction or steroid therapy; together with metoclopramide and dexamethasone may help relieve partial obstruction
Prokinetic	Metoclopramide: 5–10 mg IV/PO q6h	Increased cramping, sedation, extrapyramidal symptoms	Contraindicated in complete obstruction; concomitant use with H2 blocker and dexamethasone may help resolve a partial obstruction

22

megacolon, presumed severe impaction with liquid stool, and occasionally in the setting of fecal retention.

The Constipation Assessment Scale is a self-administered and subjective tool that can be used to assess changes in constipation over time. This scale has been validated with cancer patients treated with vinca alkaloids or morphine; thus, it will be helpful in assessing the effect of medications that induce constipation in this population (see Table 22-4[6]). The scale does not account for objective information about the volume of stool.

Management of Constipation

The goal of treatment should always account for what is considered normal bowel function for the patient. A goal of once daily is likely too ambitious for a patient who normally has a bowel movement three times weekly, in whom a goal of twice weekly may be more reasonable. Treatment option considerations are in Table 22-5.

Table 22-4. Constipation Assessment Scale

ITEM	No Problem	Some Problem	Severe Problem
1. Abdominal distension or bloating	0	1	2
2. Change in amount of gas passed rectally	0	1	2
3. Less frequent bowel movements	0	1	2
4. Oozing liquid stool	0	1	2
5. Rectal fullness or pressure	0	1	2
6. Rectal pain with bowel movement	0	1	2
7. Small volume of stool	0	1	2
8. Unable to pass stool	0	1	2

Note: Circle the appropriate number to indicate whether, during the past 3 days, you have had NO PROBLEM, SOME PROBLEM, or a SEVERE PROBLEM with each of the listed items above.
Total the number in each row and 0 = no problem with constipation within the last week and 16 = severe constipation in the last week
Source: From McMillan SC, Williams FA. Validity and reliability of the Constipation Assessment Scale. Cancer Nurs 1989;12(3):183–188.

DELIRIUM

Definition and Etiology

Delirium is one of the most common neuropsychological diagnoses in palliative care, in advanced cancer, and in older individuals. It may be an indicator

Table 22-5. Treatment of Constipation

Drug	Standard Dose	Onset	Clinical Considerations
Emollients (Softening)			
Docusate	50–500 mg in divided doses, Q day up to QID	1–3 days	Does not appear to provide benefit in palliative care patients
Osmotic Stimulants			
Magnesium citrate	150–300 mL once	3–6 hr	For rescue use only; caution in patients with renal impairment; associated with significant cramping
Magnesium hydroxide	1200–2400 mg QHS or in 2–3 in divided doses	30 min–6 hr	Avoid regular dosing in renal impairment; fast onset allows for frequent dosing without dose-stacking
Polyethylene glycol	17 gm in 8 oz of water, daily to twice daily	24–96 hr	Maximum effective dose is 68 grams; requires ability to tolerate 8 ounces of fluid; less GI discomfort than lactulose and sorbitol
Lactulose	30–60 mL in divided doses 2–4 times daily	24–48 hr	Maximum effective daily dose is 60 mL; associated with *explosive* bowel movements when used more frequently than recommended dosing
Sorbitol	30 mL every 2 hr ×3, then as needed	30 min–1 hr	Maximum effective daily dose is 150 mL; also found in chewing gum, sugar-free candies; associated with bloating and cramping
Contact Stimulants			
Bisacodyl	5–15 mg daily up to 3 times daily (up to 30 mg/day)	6–12 hr	May be associated with more cramping than senna; cramping may be alleviated by smaller, more frequent dosing
Senna	2 tabs daily up to max 12/ day in divided doses	6–12 hr	First line; can be used alone for initial prophylaxis or treatment

22

(Continued)

Table 22-5. Treatment of Constipation (*Continued*)

Drug	Standard Dose	Onset	Clinical Considerations
Rectal			
Suppositories/ Enemas	Use as directed	Minutes to hours	Avoid in patients with thrombocytopenia or neutropenia; avoid using magnesium-based enemas in renal insufficiency
Peripherally Acting Mu Opioid Receptor Antagonists			
Methylnaltrexone	Weight-based dose SQ every other day as needed	Within 4 hours	For use with opioid-induced constipation; contraindicated in bowel obstruction

of shortened survival and can lead to significant distress in patients, family members, and loved ones. Delirium may be hyperactive, which is characterized by increased level of arousal, restlessness, and agitation, possibly with hallucinations and psychosis; or hypoactive and characterized by psychomotor retardation, lethargy, and decreased level of arousal; or a mix of both states.

The American Psychiatric Association's *Diagnostic and Statistical Manual of Mental Disorders, Fifth Edition* (DSM-5) requires each of the following criteria for the diagnosis of delirium: (1) rapid onset disturbance in attention and awareness, developing over hours to days; (2) fluctuating throughout the day; (3) cognitive changes in memory, language, orientation, perception, and visual spatial ability; and (4) there is no other explanation for the changes, which are evidenced to be caused by the general medical condition, substance intoxication or withdrawal, or a medication side effect. Some common etiologies of delirium in this population include:

1. Infections (e.g., meningitis, encephalitis, UTI, pneumonia, intra-abdominal sources, sepsis)
2. Medication-related (e.g., anticholinergics, opioids, benzodiazepines, toxic drug levels)
3. Withdrawal from a CNS active substance (e.g., alcohol)
4. Brain etiology (e.g., primary CNS tumor or metastasis)
5. Cancer treatments
6. Metabolic (e.g., hypercalcemia, hypoglycemia, hyperglycemia, hyponatremia, hypernatremia, hyperammonemia, hypoxemia)
7. Altered sleep–wake cycles
8. Neurologic (e.g., cerebrovascular accident, increased intracranial pressure, see above)

Assessment and Management

The standard assessment and diagnostic tool is the Confusion Assessment Method (CAM), sometimes referred to by the mnemonic **FACT**, which provides a summary of the diagnostic criteria of delirium:

Confusion Assessment Method
1. **F**luctuating cognitive deficit(s) with acute onset
2. **A**ttention deficits and either:
3. **C**onsciousness level disturbance, **or**
4. **T**hought disorganization

Multiple instruments have been developed for screening for delirium:

1. CAM (above) is the gold standard.
2. Memorial Delirium Assessment Scale (MDAS) is able to distinguish patients with delirium from those with other cognitive or noncognitive psychiatric disorders.
3. The bedside confusion scale involves asking the patient to recite the 12 months in reverse order and also includes the assessment of the patient's consciousness state. The bedside confusion scale can be used longitudinally. Serial-sevens and spelling a word such as "farm" or "world" backward are other simple tests of attention.

The first line of therapy for all types of delirium is to implement nonpharmacologic strategies.

Nonpharmacologic interventions for management of delirium should include:

1. Minimizing sensory stimulation
2. Having familiar visitors and frequent reorientation
3. The acronym **ABCDE** is used in intensive care settings:
   Awakening
   Breathing
   Coordination
   Delirium monitoring
   Early exercise/mobility

22

Pharmacologic management is second-line therapy because there is mixed evidence on using antipsychotics to treat delirium, and there are known risks associated with the regular use of these agents, including a black box warning about increased risk of stroke and death in dementia-related psychosis. Pharmacologic agents should be considered when the patient experiences distress from the altered mental status or is a potential hazard to themselves or others. Benzodiazepines are contraindicated in the management of delirium unless being used for the treatment of terminal or agitated delirium. For consideration on antipsychotics for the management of delirium, please refer to Table 22-6. There is no benefit of atypical antipsychotic drugs over typical drugs and as such, they are considered second line in the pharmacologic treatment of delirium.

Table 22-6. Pharmacologic Management of Delirium

Medication	Dose	Adverse Effects	Considerations
Typical Antipsychotics			
Haloperidol	0.5–1 mg, higher doses may be needed for severe agitation	Extrapyramidal symptoms (EPS), QT prolongation	Dose titration can occur hourly if needed based on peak effect of medication; QT prolongation associated with higher doses and IV administration
Chlorpromazine	25–50 mg	Sedation, EPS, QT prolongation	Much more sedating than haloperidol due to antihistaminergic effects; low doses can also be used to treat hiccups
Atypical Antipsychotics			
Quetiapine	25 mg daily, titrate q3 days	Less EPS than other agents	Agent of choice for delirium in patients with Parkinson or Lewy body dementia
Risperidone	1–2 mg PO qhs, titrate up to 1 mg every 2–3 days; becomes selective dopamine antagonist at doses >6 mg daily	Least sedating at doses less than 6 mg/day	Available as tablets or solution
Olanzapine	2.5–5 mg PO daily, up to 20 mg daily at bedtime	Anticholinergic symptoms, sedation, orthostasis	Compelling indication for nausea and vomiting (second-line antiemetic in cancer patients); available as an orally disintegrating tablet (ODT) (Zydis)

(Continued)

22

Table 22-6. Pharmacologic Management of Delirium (*Continued*)

Medication	Dose	Adverse Effects	Considerations
Aripiprazole	2 mg PO daily every 4–6 hr as needed, up to 15 mg daily	Least likely to cause QT prolongation and orthostasis	Available as a solution and orally dissolving tablet (ODT)
Benzodiazepines			
Lorazepam	0.5–1 mg IV/SQ	Sedation, amnesia, confusion	Avoid unless in the setting of agitated or terminal delirium; higher doses may be needed in severe agitation
Midazolam	0.5–1 mg/hr, titrate as needed	Sedation, amnesia, confusion	Avoid unless in the setting of agitated or terminal delirium; should be used in consultation with a palliative care specialist

DEPRESSION AND ANXIETY

Prevalence and Presentation

Depression and anxiety symptoms are common comorbidities associated with life-limiting illness. In this setting, the prevalence of depression is greater than in the general population, as is the risk of suicide. The prevalence of depression in terminally ill cancer patients is 15–25% and varies widely across many studies. Depressive symptomatology in this population is even more common with about one-half of patients reporting such and anxiety is just as prevalent. While most of the patients with cancer do adjust normally, about 30% have an adjustment disorder with a depressive or anxious mood.[7] Despite these figures, only about one-half of the cancer patients who have major depressive disorder (MDD) are diagnosed with it.

A thorough history will assist in making the diagnosis of MDD. Cancer patients with depression are more likely to have pain, and cancer patients with pain are more likely to be diagnosed with MDD. Besides pain, hopelessness is a significant contributor to depression as well as to the severity of depression. Also, patients with low religiosity and limited social networks are prone to develop MDD in this setting.[8] Additionally, asking patients regarding their perceptions may point to those who have MDD; fear of a painful death, loss of independence, loss of body function, and change in appearance are but a few factors that increase stress in terminally ill cancer patients.[7] The use of certain medications and chemotherapeutic agents can cause depressive symptomology (opioids) or depression (corticosteroids, vin-blastine, vincristine, interferon, tamoxifen). In diagnosing depression in a terminally ill patient with cancer, one should rely more on the psychological symptoms (feeling helpless or hopelessness, low self-esteem, anhedonia) than somatic symptoms (anorexia, insomnia, weight loss), since somatic symptoms are often caused directly by the malignancy via tumor-related effects (e.g., production of certain cytokines induce anorexia leading to weight loss), or disease-directed treatments. It is important to realize that the diagnosis of MDD in the setting of pain should not be made until the pain is controlled.

Anxiety can be as debilitating as depression in the palliative care setting. Anxiety as a symptom and anxiety-related disorders as defined by DSM-5 are very common. The fear of death, also called death anxiety, loss of control, loss of independence, and pain can elicit anxiety. Death anxiety must be addressed; otherwise, many patients desire a hastened death.[9] Additionally, surgery, chemotherapy, and radiotherapy can all increase anxiety in patients with cancer. It should be noted that in one study of the 13.9% of individuals who were diagnosed with an anxiety disorder, 66% also met the criteria for depression.[8]

Since the treatment is different, it is important to differentiate MDD from anxiety symptomology versus a primary anxiety disorder. Furthermore, anxiety, depression, and pain all can independently affect the quality of life in terminally ill patients; treatment of anxiety and depression as well as pain improves the quality of life.[10]

Assessment and Management

Assessment for MDD or a primary anxiety disorder begins with a careful history and physical examination. There are questionnaires available to assist in the diagnosis of depression in palliative care.[11] One single question that has excellent sensitivity and specificity: "Have you felt down, depressed, or hopeless most of the time over the last 2 weeks?"[12]

Treatment should include psychotherapy in addition to pharmacotherapy. In palliative care, a number of considerations can help direct which therapeutic agent is the most appropriate. For instance, if the patient has MDD and is only expected to live for another 4–6 weeks, using a psychostimulant (e.g., morning dose of methylphenidate) would be a better choice than a more traditional antidepressant, such as an SSRI that may take 4 weeks to have a therapeutic effect. With patients who have anorexia and/or weight loss, choosing an antidepressant that has appetite stimulant properties, such as mirtazapine, would be a better choice than choosing an antidepressant that has no effect on appetite or is associated with weight loss or anorexia, such as bupropion. Refer to Table 22-7 for therapeutic agents to treat MDD and Table 22-8 for agents to treat anxiety disorders. Obviously, one should pay particular attention to the side-effect profile when choosing a therapeutic agent to treat depression or an anxiety

Table 22-7. Pharmacologic Management of Depression

Medication	Starting Dose (Usual Therapeutic Dose)	Adverse Effects	Comments/Considerations
Selective Serotonin Reuptake Inhibitor (SSRIs): First-line therapy for depression and anxiety disorders; increases serotonin levels for the treatment of depression and anxiety disorders; BLACK BOX WARNING: Closely monitor for worsening depression or emergence of suicidality, especially children and young adults; DO NOT use if MAOI administered within the last 14 days and concomitant use of SNRI, haloperidol, linezolid, and other serotonin antagonists may induce serotonin synd; side effects for the class include HA, nausea, diarrhea, sexual dysfunction, long-term weight gain, short-term weight gain or loss, insomnia or somnolence, tremor; if bipolar, may induce mania; SIADH ($\downarrow$ Na$^+$ worse in elderly), plt dysfunction, QT prolongation.			
Citalopram	10 mg/day (10–60 mg/day, 20 mg elderly)	QT prolongation more likely with citalopram and escitalopram	Relatively few drug interactions; $\downarrow$ dose hepatic or renal impair; can be used to treat interferon-α induced depression
Escitalopram	5–10 mg/day (10–20 mg/day, 10 mg elderly)	QT prolongation more likely with citalopram and escitalopram	Relatively few drug interactions; $\downarrow$ dose hepatic or renal impair
Fluoxetine	10–20 mg (20–60 mg; 80 mg doses given 40 mg BID)	Least likely to cause weight gain, may induce weight loss	Long half-life decreases risk of withdrawal symptoms; stimulating effect may be benefit in this setting; $\downarrow$ dose hepatic impair; can be used to treat interferon-α induced depression; only SSRI approved for use in children; inhib CYP2D6, CYP1A2, CYP2C19, CYP3A4, many drug–drug interactions
Paroxetine	5–10 mg (10–60 mg)	Weight gain, most sedating	Weight gain may be a benefit; concomitant use of paroxetine reduces risk of depression from interferon-2; can be used in panic disorder, social anxiety disorder, OCD
Sertraline	25–50 mg (50–200 mg/day)	Diarrhea more common than with other SSRIs	Relatively few drug interactions; use with caution with hepatic impair; can be used in panic disorder, social anxiety disorder, OCD, interferon-α induced depression

(Continued)

22

Table 22-7. Pharmacologic Management of Depression *(Continued)*

Medication	Starting Dose (Usual Therapeutic Dose)	Adverse Effects	Comments/Considerations
Serotonin–Norepinephrine Reuptake Inhibitors (SNRIs): In addition to SSRIs, first-line therapy for depression and anxiety disorders, generally preferred in patients with concomitant pain synd; serotonin and norepinephrine reuptake inhibition increases these neurotransmitters for the management of depression and anxiety disorders; BLACK BOX WARNING: Closely monitor for worsening depression or emergence of suicidality, especially in children and young adults; DO NOT use if MAOI administered within the last 14 days and concomitant use of SSRI, haloperidol, linezolid, and other serotonin antagonists may induce serotonin synd; side effects: nausea and vomiting, constipation, tachycardia, sexual dysfunction, diaphoresis.			
Duloxetine	20–40 mg/day in 2 divided doses (40–120 mg/day in 2 divided doses)	Urinary retention; hepatotoxicity with alcohol ↑ intake	May help with neuropathic pain; cannot be administered through G-tubes but can be opened and sprinkled on applesauce; may be preferred in comorbid pain syndromes; do NOT use if CrCl <30 mL/min; use with caution with hepatic impair
Venlafaxine	37.5 mg/day (75–375 mg/day in 2–3 divided doses)	If dose missed, can induce abrupt withdrawal syndrome; QT prolongation; ↑ BP at higher doses; N/V	May help with neuropathic pain, immediate release can be administered through G-tube
Tricyclic Antidepressants (TCAs): Third-line therapy, effective especially in severe depression but seldom used because of side-effect profile and in the elderly can be even more worrisome; blocks reuptake of norepinephrine and serotonin; BLACK BOX WARNING: Closely monitor for worsening depression or emergence of suicidality, especially in children and young adults; side effects: anticholinergic effects (dry mouth, constipation, urinary retention, blurred vision), ↑weight, orthostatic hypotension, sexual dysfunction, QT prolongation, and cardiac conduction delays; narrow therapeutic window (toxicity can occur just above therapeutic dosing), therapeutic drug monitoring is needed at antidepressant dosing.			
Amitriptyline	25–50 mg/day (100–300 mg/day once a day or 2 divided doses)	Most anticholinergic, most sedating of the TCAs, weight gain, urinary retention, photosensitivity; DO NOT use during recovery from MI, QP may be fatal	Give first dose at night; therapeutic level 150–250 ng/mL, toxic >500 ng/mL

22

Desipramine	25–50 mg once/day or divided doses (100–300 mg once/day or divided doses)	↑ risk serotonin synd; photosensitivity; DO NOT use during recovery from MI	Therapeutic level 100–250 ng/mL; least anticholinergic of TCAs, least sedating; causes blue-green urine
Doxepin	25–50 mg (150–300 mg daily 2–3 divided doses)	Contraindicated with glaucoma, urinary retention; DO NOT use during recovery from MI	Therapeutic level 150–250 ng/mL; treats pruritus as well
Imipramine	25–50 mg/day (100–300 mg/day once a day or 2 divided doses)	Weight gain, orthostat c hypotension; DO NOT use during recovery from MI	Therapeutic level 150–250 ng/mL; less sedation than amitriptyline
Nortriptyline	25 mg/day (50–200 mg, once a day or in 2 or 3 divided doses); elderly 10–25 mg qhs	↓ dose with hepatic dysfunction	Least anticholinergic of the TCAs; therapeutic level 50–150 ng/mL

Antipsychotics: Adjunct in treating depression with psychotic or anxiety symptoms (quetiapine has been used as a single agent); D_2 receptor antagonism, other receptors targeted depending on the drug and the degree varies from drug to drug; side effects: weight gain, DM type 2, extrapyramidal side effects (EPS) (akathisia, acute dystonia, parkinsonism [rigidity, tremor, bradykinesia, shuffling gait], and tardive dyskinesia), QT prolongation, ↑ prolactin. * = also in IV or IM formulation

Aripiprazole	5–10 mg once a day (5–20 mg once a day)	Orthostatic hypotension, EPS, HA, nausea, anxiety; loss of impulse control (compulsive eating, gambling, sexual activity)	Second-generation antipsychotic; minimal sedation; low risk DM; lowest risk for QT prolongation; may be more effective in the elderly
Olanzapine*	2.5–5 mg once a day (5–20 mg once a day)	↑↑ weight, ↑↑ DM, dose-related lowering of seizure threshold, ↑ chol, orthostasis, sedation	Second-generation antipsychotic; less likely to cause EPS; receptor binding profile advantageous in refractory nausea or if weight loss present
Quetiapine	25 mg BID (titrate up to 150–300 mg/day in 2 or 3 divided doses)	Orthostatic hypotension, sedation, ↑ weight, ↑ DM	Second-generation antipsychotic; less likely to cause EPS – **preferred antipsychotic in Parkinson disease and Lewy body dementia**

22

(Continued)

745

Table 22-7. Pharmacologic Management of Depression (Continued)

Medication	Starting Dose (Usual Therapeutic Dose)	Adverse Effects	Comments/Considerations
Risperidone*	0.25–0.5 mg once a day (if needed, titrate up 1–2 mg/day)	EPS, ↑↑ prolactin, ↑ weight, insomnia, ↓ BP with higher doses	Second-generation antipsychotic; fewer anticholinergic side effects (less sedation), doses >6 mg daily are more D2 selective and similar in mechanism of action as haloperidol
Ziprasidone*	20–40 mg BID (20–80 mg BID)	Sedation, fatigue, QT prolongation; rarely severe drug reaction with fever, rash, ↑ eosinophils	Second-generation antipsychotic; lowest risk DM and weight gain; less likely to cause EPS

Psychostimulants: Used in palliative care to treat certain depressive symptoms such as fatigue and vegetative symptoms; increased alertness may improve oral intake; rapid onset of action is an advantage over traditional antidepressants, especially in patients with weeks to live; do not use with ischemic heart disease or with delirium. Side effects include insomnia, anxiety/agitation, confusion, tremor, tachycardia, decrease in seizure threshold, nightmares, ↑BP, arrhythmias.

Dextroamphetamine (short-acting)	5 mg BID (60 mg divided dose BID)	Anorexia, weight loss, diarrhea, HA, insomnia, ↑ BP, ↑ HR, tremor, restlessness, psychosis	↑ dopamine, norepinephrine release; schedule II controlled substance, do not dose at night
Dextroamphetamine (long-acting)	5 mg/day or BID (60 mg qAM or divided dose BID)	Contraindicated: advanced CAD or poorly controlled ↑ BP or hyperthyroidism or glaucoma	
Methylphenidate (short-acting)	2.5–5 mg (5–10 mg at 8 AM and 12 noon; up to 60 mg/day)	Anorexia, weight loss, diarrhea, N, V, HA, insomnia, ↑ BP, ↑ HR, tremor, restlessness, irritability, psychosis	↑ dopamine, norepinephrine by blocking reuptake; schedule II controlled substance

22

Methylphenidate (intermediate acting)	10 mg BID (up to 60 mg in BID or TID divided doses)	Contraindicated: advanced CAD or poorly controlled ↑ B° or hyperthyroidism or glaucoma	↑ dopamine, norepinephrine, serotonin, and glutamate and ↓ GABA; primarily used to treat narcolepsy; schedule IV controlled substance
Modafinil	100–200 mg qAM (400 mg qAM) dose 100 mg in elderly	Rash including Stevens-Johnson synd, HA, nausea, diarrhea, agitation	

Miscellaneous antidepressants: Bupropion and mirtazapine, both second-line therapy; side-effect profile may make these drugs preferred over other antidepressants depending on the individual patient and their symptoms.

Bupropion HCL	75–100 mg BID (200–300/day in BID to TID dosing)	Decreases seizure threshold; HA, insomnia, tremor, agitation, anxiety, anorexia, nausea	Inhibition of dopamine and norepinephrine reuptake and increased presynaptic release of catecholamines; NOT associated with sexual dysfunction, NOT sedating; avoid if anxiety present; may induce or worsen anorexia. Urine drug screen false-positive methylenedioxyethylamphetamine (MDEA) (ecstasy) and amphetamine
Bupropion SR	150 mg/day (150 mg BID)		
Bupropion XL	150 mg/day (300–450 once a day)		
Mirtazapine (tetracyclic antidepressant)	15 mg qhs (15–45 mg PO qhs)	Antihistaminergic side effects, including sedation, daytime sleepiness, dry mouth, dizziness, blurred vision, constipation, weight gain	Enhances release of norepinephrine and serotonin; also 5-HT3 antagonist; may have antiemetic effect; few drug interactions; maybe preferred if insomnia or if weight loss is present; can be used to treat interferon-α induced depression; ↑ risk for serotonin synd; most sedation and weight gain associated with doses ≤15 mg.

Source: From Drugs for Depression. Med Lett 2020;62(1592):25–32

22

22

Table 22-8. Pharmacologic Management of Anxiety

Medication	Starting Dose (Usual Therapeutic Dose)	Adverse Effects	Comments/Considerations
Selective Serotonin Reuptake Inhibitor (SSRIs): First-line therapy for anxiety disorders and depression; increases serotonin levels for the treatment of anxiety disorders and depression; BLACK BOX WARNING: Closely monitor for worsening depression or emergence of suicidality, especially children and young adults; DO NOT use if MAOI administered within the last 14 days and concomitant use of SNRI, haloperidol, linezolid, and other serotonin antagonists may induce serotonin synd; side effects for the class include HA, nausea, diarrhea, sexual dysfunction, long-term weight gain, short-term weight gain or loss, insomni or somnolence, tremor; if bipolar, may induce mania; SIADH (↓ Na⁺ worse in elderly), plt dysfunction, QT prolongation.			
Escitalopram	5–10 mg/day (10 mg/day)	QT prolongation more likely with escitalopram and citalopram	FDA approved to treat generalized anxiety disorder (GAD); relatively few drug interactions; ↓ dose hepatic or renal impair
Fluoxetine	10–20 mg (20–60 mg)	Least likely to cause weight gain, may induce weight loss	FDA approved to treat panic disorder; long half-life decreases risk of withdrawal symptoms; stimulating effect may be benefit in this setting; ↓ dose hepatic impair; inhib CYP2D6, CYP1A2, CYP2C19, CYP3A4, many drug–drug interactions; only SSRI approved for use in children
Paroxetine	5–10 mg (10–60 mg)	Weight gain, most sedating	FDA approved to treat generalized anxiety disorder (GAD), panic disorder, and social anxiety disorder; weight gain may be a benefit
Sertraline	25–50 mg (25–200 mg/day)	N/V/D more common than with other SSRIs	FDA approved to treat panic disorder and social anxiety disorder; relatively few drug interactions; use with caution with hepatic impair

Serotonin–Norepinephrine Reuptake Inhibitors (SNRIs): First-line therapy for anxiety disorders and depression; serotonin and norepinephrine reuptake inhibition increases these neurotransmitters for the management of depression and anxiety disorders; BLACK BOX WARNING: Closely monitor for worsening depression or emergence of suicidality, especially children and young adults; DO NOT use if MAOI administered within the last 14 days and concomitant use of SSRI, haloperidol, linezolid, and other serotonin antagonists may induce serotonin synd; side effects: nausea and vomiting, constipation, tachycardia, sexual dysfunction, diaphoresis.

| Duloxetine | 20–40 mg/day in 2 divided doses (60–120 mg/day in 2 divided doses) | Urinary retention; hepatotoxicity with alcohol ↑ intake | Approved for use for generalized anxiety disorder (GAD); may help with neuropathic pain; cannot be administered through G-tubes but can be opened and sprinkled on applesauce; may be preferred in comorbid pain syndromes; do NOT use if CrCl <30 mL/min; use with caution with hepatic impair |
| Venlafaxine | 37.5 mg/day (75–225 mg/day) in 2–3 divided doses) | If dose missed, can induce abrupt withdrawal syndrome; QT prolongation; ↑ BP at higher doses | FDA approved to treat generalized anxiety disorder (GAD), panic disorder, and social anxiety disorder; may help with neuropathic pain |

Benzodiazepines: Can provide immediate relief from symptoms; binds to gamma-aminobutyric acid (GABA) receptor sites, potentiating the inhibitory effect; schedule IV controlled substance; concomitant use of other sedatives, opioids and alcohol can lead to respiratory depression; ensure appropriate monitoring and shared decision-making; reduces anxiety associated with dyspnea; may help with associated anticipatory nausea/vomiting associated with chemotherapy; side effects: affects cognitive and motor skills, falls, ↓ reaction time, avoid driving; withdrawal symptoms including seizures are possible; also sedation, amnesia, confusion.

| Lorazepam | 0.5–1 mg 3 times/day (1–1.5 mg 3–4 times/day) | Shorter half-life ↑ risk for withdrawal symptoms | Higher doses may be needed in severe agitation |
| Alprazolam | 0.25–0.5 mg 3 times/day (0.5–1 mg 3 times/day max of 4 mg/day) | Shorter half-life ↑ risk for withdrawal symptoms | Metabolized by CYP3A4, CYP3A4 inhibitors can increase toxicity and CYP3A4 inducers can decrease effectiveness |

22

(Continued)

Table 22-8. Pharmacologic Management of Anxiety (*Continued*)

Medication	Starting Dose (Usual Therapeutic Dose)	Adverse Effects	Comments/Considerations
Clonazepam	0.25 mg 2 times/day (0.5–2 mg 2 times/day)		Metabolized by CYP3A4, CYP3A4 inhibitors can increase toxicity and CYP3A4 inducers can decrease effectiveness; while the max dose per day is 4 mg, generally doses above 1 mg/day are no more effective than 1 mg/day for panic disorder
Diazepam	2.5–5 mg 1–2 times/day; elderly start with 2–2.5 mg 1–2 times/day (5–10 mg PO 2–4 times/day)	Use caution or avoid in liver dysfunction	Metabolized by CYP3A4, CYP3A4 inhibitors can increase toxicity and CYP3A4 inducers can decrease effectiveness; active metabolite with extended half-life up to 150 hr

Tricyclic Antidepressants (TCAs): Can be used to treat anxiety disorders not responsive to SSRI or SNRIs; BLACK BOX WARNING: Closely monitor for worsening depression or emergence of suicidality, especially in children and young adults; side effects: anticholinergic effects (dry mouth, constipation, urinary retention, blurred vision), ↑weight, orthostatic hypotension, sexual dysfunction, QT prolongation, and cardiac conduction delays; narrow therapeutic window (toxicity can occur just above therapeutic dosing), since doses to treat anxiety disorders are considerably lower than used to treat depression, very unlikely to cause toxicity.

Medication	Starting Dose (Usual Therapeutic Dose)	Adverse Effects	Comments/Considerations
Amitriptyline	25–50 mg/day (50–100 mg/ day once a day)	Most anticholinergic, most sedating of the TCAs, weight gain, urinary retention, photosensitivity; DO NOT use during recovery from MI; OD may be fatal	Give first dose at night
Doxepin	25–50 mg (75–150 mg once a day)	Contraindicated with glaucoma, urinary retention; DO NOT use during recovery from MI	Can be helpful in treatment of pruritus

22

Imipramine	25–50 mg/day (50–100 mg/day once a day)	Weight gain, orthostatic hypotension; DO NOT use during recovery from MI	Less sedation than amitriptyline
Miscellaneous*			
Buspirone	5–7.5 mg BID (15–60 mg per day, divided into 2–3 doses)	Dizziness, sedation, headache, nausea; ↑ risk for serotonin synd if used with an SSRI or SNRI	5-HT$_{1a}$ receptor partial agonist; usually used as an adjunct treatment; indicated for GAD; reduces acute anxiety associated with shortness of breath; metabolized by CYP3A4, CYP3A4 inhibitors can increase toxicity and CYP3A4 inducers can decrease effectiveness
Pregabalin	150–600 mg/day, divided into 2–3 doses	Dizziness, sedation, confusion, weight gain, edema; withdrawal symptoms with discontinuation (HA, diarrhea, nausea, insomnia)	Inhibits release of glutamate; NOT FDA approved in United States for use in anxiety disorders, however, widely used in Europe for such. Clinical trials in the United States have been positive; rapid onset of action; schedule V controlled substance
Mirtazapine (tetracyclic antidepressant)	15 mg qhs (15–45 mg PO qhs)	Antihistaminergic side effects, including sedation, daytime sleepiness, dry mouth, dizziness, blurred vision, constipation, weight gain	Tetracyclic antidepressant; enhances release of norepinephrine and serotonin, also 5-HT3 antagonist; may have antiemetic effect; few drug interactions; maybe help if insomnia or weight loss is present; ↑ risk for serotonin synd; may need dose adjustment in the elderly and in hepatic or renal dysfunction; most sedation and weight gain associated with doses ≤15 mg
Quetiapine	25 mg once a day (titrate up to 50–150 mg once a day)	Orthostatic hypotension, sedation, ↑ weight, ↑ DM, akathisia, QT prolongation, cataracts	Second-generation antipsychotic; antagonist at multiple neurotransmitter receptors including serotonin (5HT1A and 5HT2), dopamine (D1 and D2), histamine (H1), and adrenergic (α1 and α2); one of the second-generation antipsychotics to less likely cause EPS; reduce dose in hepatic dysfunction

*Diphenhydramine and hydroxyzine can be used as anxiolytics, commonly used in patients with substance use disorder so as to avoid using benzodiazepines.

Sources: From Drugs for anxiety disorders. Med Lett 2019;61(1578):121–128; Drugs for anxiety. In Drugs of Choice 2020, 21e. New Rochelle, NY: The Medical Letter.

disorder. Also, the agent chosen will vary if you are treating MDD versus MDD with a significant anxiety component versus a primary anxiety disorder. Selective serotonin reuptake inhibitors (SSRIs) and serotonin-norepinephrine reuptake inhibitors (SNRIs) are first-line agents to treat MDD and/or anxiety disorders. Improvement in symptoms may occur as soon as 2 weeks but it usually takes 4–8 weeks for a significant improvement.

In a meta-analysis of psychotherapy targeting depression and anxiety in palliative care, psychotherapy decreased symptoms of both depression and anxiety and improved quality of life.[12] Many types of psychotherapy have been shown to be effective in treating patients with terminal illnesses, including cognitive behavioral therapy (mindfulness-based stress reduction [MBSR] and acceptance and commitment therapy), and problem-solving therapy has shown to be successful in some palliative care settings. Psychotherapy and pharmacotherapy together have better outcomes than either modality as a single form of treatment.

DIARRHEA

Etiology

There are a wide variety of causes of diarrhea in the palliative care setting, including:

1. Chemotherapy
2. Disease-related (e.g., neuroendocrine tumors)
3. Radiation therapy to the pelvis
4. Medications (e.g., antibiotics, magnesium)
5. Fecal impaction
6. Dietary changes
7. Infection (e.g., *C. difficile*)

Assessment and Management

Refer to Table 22-9 for the assessment and supportive care for patients with diarrhea.

For any diarrhea, assess cause and treat accordingly. For specific medications refer to Table 22-10.

DYSPHAGIA

Definition and Etiology

Difficulty swallowing can be part of the end-of-life process. It can be distressing for caregivers and loved ones who desire to nurture their loved one with

Table 22-9. Assessment and Supportive Care Considerations for the Treatment of Diarrhea

Grade	Definition	Treatment
1	<4 stools/day over baseline; mild ostomy output increase over baseline	Oral hydration and electrolyte replacement; initiate antidiarrheal bland diet/**BRAT** (**B**ananas, **R**ice, **A**pplesauce, **T**oast)
2	4–6 stools/day over baseline; moderate ostomy output increase over baseline	IV fluids if not tolerating PO; initiate antidiarrheal bland/BRAT diet; oral hydration and electrolyte replacement; consider anticholinergic medications
3	>7 stools/day over baseline; severe ostomy output increase over baseline; limiting ADLs	As above with grade 1 and 2; consider octreotide
4	Life-threatening consequences	Admit to or transfer to the intensive care unit

Table 22-10. Pharmacologic Treatment of Diarrhea

Medication Class	Agents	Adverse Effects
Antidiarrheals	Loperamide 4 mg PO × 1, then 2 mg PO after each loose stool, up to 16 mg/day If not already on opioids: atropine/diphenoxylate 1–2 tabs PO q6h PRN, max 8/day; tincture of opium (10 mg/mL) 10–15 drops PO q4h PRN	Constipation, abdominal cramps, nausea
Anticholinergics	Hyoscyamine 0.125 mg PO/SL q4h PRN, max 1.5 mg/day; atropine 0.5–1 mg SQ/IV/SL q4–6h PRN	Sedation, urinary retention, constipation, confusion, blurry vision, risk of falls
Antisecretory	Octreotide 100–500 mcg SQ/IV daily, divided q8h or by continuous infusion; avoid rapid IV push, may cause nausea/vomiting	Nausea/vomiting, constipation, bradycardia, abdominal/back pain, injection site reactions, myalgia, alopecia
Bulk-forming fiber agents	Psyllium or cholestyramine	For administration through G-tubes as tolerated; may be difficult to administer, and dosing frequency may be a challenge to tolerate orally

22

food. Dysphagia in advanced illness indicates that life expectancy is short and should entail revisiting the goals of care. A speech-language pathologist can assess swallowing potential and assist in prognostication, as well as increase the likelihood of safe feeding and provide medication guidance.

Assessment and Management

Assessment of dysphagia should include the following:

1. Oral hygiene and secretion management, assess for xerostomia, thrush
2. Cranial nerve examination—V, VII, IX, X, XII
3. Direct patient observation of swallowing
4. Evaluation for silent aspiration
5. Video fluoroscopy, endoscopy, barium swallow study — if aligned with patient's goals and clinical status

Management is based on overall treatment goals, values, and prognosis. The goal is to facilitate safe and effective oral feeding for as long as possible. Food may be altered in consistency, and alternative routes can be considered. In the setting of dysphagia, the risk of aspiration and possible consequences must be explained to the patient and caregivers to allow for informed decision-making and decrease the risk of the family or patient causing aspiration by feeding, etc. The risk of aspiration is not eliminated by the placement of a feeding tube. Longevity in advanced dementia patients is not compromised when hand-feeding is used versus total enteral nutrition. With hand-feeding, there is the added benefit of an intimate human interaction and decreased risk of infection and complications.

DYSPNEA

Etiology and Principles of Treatment

There are a wide array of causes of dyspnea in terminally ill patients. Causes of dyspnea and principles of treatment in this population include the following:

Bronchospasm. Consider nebulized albuterol and ipratropium and/or an inhaled steroid such as beclomethasone. Systemic steroids can be useful in cases of superior vena cava obstruction or tumor mass effect in the lung.

Effusions. Thoracentesis may be effective, and if the effusion recurs, pleurodesis or indwelling chest tube drainage may be appropriate based on goals of care and an anticipated life expectancy of at least several weeks to months.

Airway obstruction, aspiration. Make sure that tracheostomy appliances are cleaned regularly. If aspiration of food is likely, purée solids and thicken liquids with cornstarch. Educate the family about how to position the patient during feeding. Suction the patient when appropriate.

Cough, congestion, and secretions. Cough may have many different causes, for instance, infection, structural lung disease (e.g., COPD or asthma), lung cancer and/or cancer treatments, medications (ACE inhibitors), throat or airway irritation or secretions. If the underlying cause can be treated, this is optimal. Symptomatic relief can be provided via cough suppression through the use of opioids and dextromethorphan. For productive cough, anticholinergics, expectorants, and nebulizers may provide relief of secretions. For details of medications used to treat cough, see Table 22-11.

If the cough reflex is still strong, loosen thick secretions with nebulized saline and guaifenesin. If the cough is weak, treat thin secretions with atropine, 1% ophthalmic solution, 1–4 drops SL every 4 hr or as needed; 1–3 patches of topical scopolamine (1.5 mg/patch) behind the ear(s) every 3 days; or glycopyrrolate, 0.2–0.4 mg SC or IV bolus every 3 hours as needed; use with caution due to the significant anticholinergic effects.

Upper airway secretions can be troublesome for both patients and families. Anticholinergics are most often used because they can be relied on to dry up secretions and congestion; different formulations can be chosen based on a patient's clinical scenario.

Anxiety. Anxiety is a common and often overlooked cause of dyspnea. Sitting upright, using a bedside fan, listening to calming music, and practicing relaxation techniques can be effective, as can skillful counseling and the presence of calming caregivers. When chronic anxiety is believed to be a trigger for dyspnea, clonazepam or antidepressants may be helpful. Keeping this in mind, dyspnea is a potent trigger for anxiety and may best be treated first with opioids and then a benzodiazepine. If the opioid dosage is limited by drowsiness, reduce the benzodiazepine dosage and then attempt to increase the opioid dosage. See also Depression and Anxiety, page 741.

22

Management

General measures include:

- Reduce the need for exertion and arrange for readily available assistance with transfers, ambulation, activities of daily living, feeding, or any other activities known to trigger dyspnea.
- Reposition the patient, usually to a more upright position or if recumbent, with the compromised lung inferior or below the good lung.
- Remember to provide skin care for the buttocks if the patient cannot stand or turn to make sitting more comfortable.

Table 22-11. Medications for the Management of Dyspnea, Secretions, and Cough

Medication	Mechanism of Action	Adverse Effects	Comments
Opioids			
Morphine Hydromorphone Fentanyl, others	Decreases the chemoreceptor response to hypercapnia, increases peripheral vasodilatation with a decrease in cardiac preload, or a decrease in anxiety and the subjective feeling of dyspnea	Constipation, sedation, respiratory depression, pruritus, nausea/vomiting	First-line pharmacologic agent in advanced disease; refer to Chapter 21, Pain Management for opioid selection considerations
Anxiolytics			
Benzodiazepines: Lorazepam PO/IV 0.5–1 mg Midazolam 0.5–1 mg IV/SQ/IN Alprazolam 0.5–1 mg Clonazepam 0.5–1 mg	Reduces acute anxiety associated with shortness of breath	Concomitant sedatives and opioids can lead to respiratory depression, ensure appropriate monitoring and shared decision-making	For breakthrough dyspnea or refractory dyspnea compounded by anxiety symptoms or when undue side effects limit titration of opioids; Lorazepam is anxiolytic of first choice because of short duration of action and in the setting of liver dysfunction because of renal excretion; Midazolam may be preferred in inpatient hospice or critical care settings
Miscellaneous: Buspirone 10–15 mg per day in divided doses	Reduces acute anxiety associated with shortness of breath	Dizziness, sedation, headache, nausea	Indicated for general anxiety disorder

Anticholinergic

Glycopyrrolate 0.2–0.4 mg IV Scopolamine 1.5 mg patch Atropine 1–2 drops	Decreases secretions in respiratory tract	Sedation, urinary retention, constipation, confusion, sedation, blurry vision, risk of falls	Glycopyrrolate can be given SQ if needed; atropine eye drops given SL/buccal mucosa at end of life; scopolamine is a transdermal patch, takes up to 24 hours for effect. If weak cough reflex, can help dry up thin secretions

Antidepressant

SSRI* (e.g., sertraline, citalopram, escitalopram)	Selective serotonin reuptake inhibition increases serotonin levels for management of chronic anxiety	Insomnia, diarrhea, N&V, dizziness, agitation, HA, sexual dysfunction	SSRIs are first-line agents for the management of chronic anxiety; missing a couple of doses can cause withdrawal syndrome
SNRI** (e.g., venlafaxine, duloxetine)	Serotonin and norepinephrine reuptake inhibition increases these neurotransmitters for the management of chronic anxiety	Nausea and vomiting, tachycardia, urinary retention (duloxetine), sexual dysfunction	Venlafaxine associated with abrupt withdrawal syndrome if dose is missed; duloxetine cannot be administered through G-tubes but can be opened and sprinkled on applesauce; may be preferred in comorbid pain syndromes
Other (e.g., mirtazapine)	Tetracyclic antidepressant; for management of chronic anxiety	Antihistaminergic side effects, including sedation, constipation; weight gain	Mirtazapine preferred when need sleep or appetite benefit; doses 15–45 mg for antidepressant effect

(Continued)

22

22

Table 22-11. Medications for the Management of Dyspnea, Secretions, and Cough (*Continued*)

Medication	Mechanism of Action	Adverse Effects	Comments
Nebulizers			
Albuterol Ipratropium 3% Hypertonic saline Corticosteroids	Dilate bronchioles, results in dry secretions, less viscous secretions, and decrease in inflammation	Albuterol may be associated with increased anxiety Ipratropium can cause bronchospasm and increased secretions	Sensation of air blowing over the nose/mouth contributes to effect of relieving dyspnea; dry powder inhalers take significant strength to use effectively, therefore nebulizers may be preferred for ease of administration; also can thin secretions in patients with a strong cough reflex
Systemic corticosteroids			
Dexamethasone Prednisone Methylprednisolone	Decrease inflammation	Includes hyperglycemia, hyperactivity/psychosis, adrenal axis suppression	Dexamethasone has most potent anti-inflammatory activity, not associated with sodium or water retention; dose in morning/early in day to avoid insomnia
Expectorant			
Guaifenesin	Increase volume and reduce viscosity of secretions from the airway	Generally well tolerated; headache, nausea, vomiting, upset stomach	If strong cough reflex, will help with expectoration of secretions
Cough suppressant			
Dextromethorphan	N-methyl-D-aspartate (NMDA) receptor antagonist, depresses the medullary cough center and decreases the sensitivity of cough receptors; interrupts cough impulse transmission	Generally well tolerated; dizziness, drowsiness	Indicated to suppress dry cough due to irritation of the airway; many formulations including extended release suspension with twice daily dosing; may be preferred for relief of cough at night

*SSRI – Selective serotonin reuptake inhibitor; for specific medications, see Table 22-8, page 748.

- Improve air circulation:
  - o Provide a draft by using fans or open windows.
  - o Adjust humidity with a humidifier or air conditioner.
  - o Avoid strong odors, fumes, and smoke.
  - o Increase flow of oxygen temporarily until symptoms improve.
- Address anxiety and provide reassurance:
  - o Discuss the need for companionship and spiritual support because isolation and spiritual concerns can exacerbate symptoms.
  - o Discuss the meaning of symptoms and other patient or family concerns.
  - o Anticipate and rehearse with the patient and family their responses when symptoms worsen.
  - o Identify situational components (such as things that trigger increased dyspnea).
  - o Teach relaxation interventions such as abdominal breathing or hypnosis.
  - o Consider rehabilitative strategies such as breathing training, relaxation, and adaptive strategies.
  - o Discuss any patient, family, or staff concerns about using opioids to relieve dyspnea.
  - o Consider noninvasive positive pressure devices, which can provide continuous or intermittent positive pressure breathing.

For use of specific medications refer to Table 22-11.

Noninvasive Positive Pressure Ventilation

Noninvasive positive pressure ventilation (NPPV) decreases the work of breathing and dyspnea in conditions such as COPD, heart failure, and ALS, allowing respiratory muscle rest during inspiration. This can be initiated in patients who desire full restorative care and who may end up intubated and ventilated. NPPV is used as an alternative to intubation or purely for palliation of dyspnea symptoms or to maintain wakefulness at the end of life. For patients requiring opioids at the end of life for dyspnea and who desire to be awake as much as possible, NPPV could be offered if congruent with goals; however, NPPV can be uncomfortable and could disrupt sleep and the ability to communicate.

22

FATIGUE
Definition and Etiology

Fatigue is the persistent sense of tiredness and lack of energy, most commonly described in cancer literature in relation to cancer and its treatments. Fatigue is not relieved by rest and is associated with decreased function and decreased quality of life. The etiology is generally multifactorial, consisting of physical, psychological, biochemical, and behavioral elements. Fatigue may be associated with decreased memory, cognition, concentration, and motivation, as well as hypersomnia or insomnia and emotional lability.

Possible causes of reversible fatigue in the palliative care setting include the following:

- Effect of a disease or its treatment (e.g., ESRD/hemodialysis, cancer/chemotherapy)
- Medications (e.g., opioids, benzodiazepines)
- Hypoxemia
- Severe anemia
- Infection
- Psychiatric comorbidities (e.g., depression)
- Organ dysfunction (e.g., renal or liver dysfunction)
- Electrolyte alterations (e.g., hyponatremia, hypercalcemia)
- Insomnia
- Pain
- Immobility

Assessment and Management

Assessment includes evaluating for reversible causes of the above symptoms and treatment when able to do so.

Other general treatment options include:

- Education of patient and family regarding realistic goal setting, expectations, and planning and pacing of activities.
- Light to moderate intensity exercise, aiming for 20–30 minutes of exercise three times weekly.
- Consider acupuncture; however, more research is needed.
- Medications have limited evidence for use with variable outcomes in treating fatigue.
  - o Increased alertness when on a low-dose psychostimulant minimizes the effect on appetite suppression and may actually improve overall oral intake.
  - o See Table 22-12 for medication considerations.

NAUSEA AND VOMITING

Etiology

Nausea and vomiting are a common symptom in palliative care. They frequently have multiple etiologies and often require more than one agent to treat effectively. In order to treat nausea and vomiting, an understanding of

Table 22-12. Medications with Stimulant Properties for the Treatment of Fatigue

Medication Class	Agents	Adverse Effects	Considerations
Psychostimulants	Methylphenidate 2.5–5 mg qAM up to 15–30 mg PO qAM and noon; Modafinil 50 mg PO qAM up to 400 mg PO qAM	Insomnia, headache, irritability, dry mouth, decreased appetite, tachycardia	Methylphenidate shown to be superior to placebo; Modafinil inconsistent evidence for treatment of fatigue in this setting
Corticosteroids	Dexamethasone up to 4 mg daily	Hyperglycemia, hyperactivity/psychosis, adrenal axis suppression	Limited evidence with risk of significant toxicity
Progesterone derivative	Megestrol acetate 160 mg PO TID	Thromboembolic events; nausea, diarrhea, impotence, peripheral edema, hypertension, hyperglycemia, breakthrough uterine bleeding, and skin photosensitivity; can precipitate adrenal insufficiency	Evidence for use in 2 double-blind crossover studies
Herbals/supplements	Ginseng 2000 mg	Well tolerated at therapeutic doses	Significant improvement versus placebo at 8 weeks

22

the receptors involved in the etiology is critical to select the most effective therapy. Table 22-13 lists the causes of nausea and vomiting, which can be remembered using the mnemonic VOMIT.

Management

Assessment includes evaluating for possible reversible causes and treating appropriately. Principles for the management of nausea include the following:

• Prevention of nausea is paramount; antiemetics should be scheduled in this setting.

- Antiemetic selection should be based on the suspected underlying etiology.
- Account for risks of adverse effects based on underlying mechanisms of action.
- Layer agents on one at a time until symptom relief is achieved.
- De-escalate therapy by subsequently removing one agent at a time.
- For antiemetic considerations please refer to Table 22-14.

Table 22-13. Possible Causes of Nausea and Vomiting and Related Receptor Involvement

---

Vestibular — cholinergic and histaminergic
Obstruction of the bowel (constipation) — cholinergic/muscarinic, histaminergic, possibly 5HT3
Dys**M**otility — cholinergic, histaminergic, 5HT3, 5HT4
Infection, **i**nflammation — cholinergic, histaminergic, 5HT3, neurokinin-1
Toxins stimulating the chemoreceptor trigger zone — dopamine 2, 5HT3

PRURITUS

Etiology

It is hypothesized that pruritus is the result of stimulation of peripheral and central "itch" neurons. The neurotransmitters involved in the development of pruritus include histamine, serotonin (5HT3), substance P, trypsin, opioid, and prostaglandin E2. Opioid-induced pruritus is likely mediated through the central mu-opioid receptor.

Possible etiologies include:

- Dermatologic (e.g., dry skin, atopic dermatitis, eczema, infestation [lice], seborrheic dermatitis)
- Metabolic (e.g., hyperbilirubinemia, uremia, hypothyroidism, hyperthyroidism)
- Hematologic (e.g., iron deficiency, polycythemia vera, lymphoma, leukemia, multiple myeloma)
- Medications (e.g., opioids, allopurinol, BCPs, cephalosporins, penicillins, diuretics, statins, phenytoin)
- Infections (e.g., *Candida*; many parasitic infections: *S. stercoralis, E. vermicularis, T. trichiura*, others)
- Allergy (e.g., contact dermatitis, urticarial reaction)
- Psychogenic (e.g., depression, psychosis, OCD)

Management

Treatment includes addressing the underlying etiology when possible. Symptomatic relief can be attempted with many different approaches, depending on the presumed etiology. Nonpharmacologic measures should be tried first, especially when there is a dry skin component to the symptomatology.

22

Table 22-14. Antiemetic Medications

Class	Mechanism of Action	Agents	Adverse Effects	Considerations
Antidopamine	Block dopamine 2 receptor	Prochlorperazine 5–10 mg, haloperidol 0.5–1 mg, metoclopramide 5–10 mg, chlorpromazine 25 mg IV/PO	Extrapyramidal symptoms, QT prolongation, sedation, anticholinergic effects (chlorpromazine)	Low dose, PO route associated with lower risk of QT prolongation; IV route associated with increased risk of QT prolongation; metoclopramide is a prokinetic and not an antiemetic at usual dosing
Serotonin antagonists	Block 5HT3 receptor	Ondansetron 4–8 mg PO/IV q8h	Constipation, headache, QT prolongation	Available as orally disintegrating tablet
Anticholinergic	Block muscarinic receptor	Scopolamine patch 1.5 mg q72h	Sedation, urinary retention, constipation, confusion, blurry vision, risk of falls	Takes up to 24 hr for effect
Antihistamine	Block histamine receptor	Diphenhydramine 25–50 mg IV/PO, promethazine 12.5–25 mg IV/PO	Sedation, urinary retention, constipation, confusion, blurry vision, risk of falls	Caution with concomitant opioids, increased risk of respiratory depression
Cannabinoids	Cannabinoid receptor 1/2	Dronabinol 2.5–5 mg, medicinal marijuana	Tachycardia, dry mouth, cough, confusion, hyperactivity/psychosis, nausea, fatigue	Dronabinol also available in solution formulation. For medicinal marijuana, refer to state/local/hospital laws or guidelines

(Continued)

22

Table 22-14. Antiemetic Medications *(Continued)*

Class	Mechanism of Action	Agents	Adverse Effects	Considerations
Corticosteroids	Anti-inflammatory	Dexamethasone 4 –16 mg daily in once-daily or divided doses	Include hyperglycemia, hyperactivity/psychosis, adrenal axis suppression	Indicated for increased cerebrospinal pressure, malignant bowel obstruction, superior vena cava syndrome, and refractory cases. May cause hiccups**
Benzodiazepine	GABA receptor	Lorazepam 0.5 mg IV/PO	Amnesia, sedation, confusion, risk of falls	Only for anticipatory nausea, caution with concomitant opioid, increased risk of respiratory depression
Mixed mechanism of action	Dopamine antagonism, anticholinergic, antihistaminergic, serotonin blockade	Olanzapine 2.5–5 mg PO	Anticholinergic effects including dry mouth, sedation, orthostatic BP; long-term use can cause metabolic changes	Effective in chemotherapy-induced N/V and palliative care; dose at bedtime; generally second-line therapy due to cost and adverse effect profile

**For treatment of medication-related hiccups, if not self-limiting; nonpharmacologic approaches are seldom successful. Chlorpromazine (low dose) 10–25 mg or baclofen 5–10 mg can be used for the treatment of refractory, persistent hiccups.

22

Nonpharmacologic options include moisturizers—preferably ointments for maximum hydration—and oatmeal topical preparations or baths. For medication treatment options for the management of pruritus, refer to Table 22-15.

Table 22-15. Pharmacologic Treatment of Pruritus

Medication Class	Mechanism of Action	Agents	Considerations
Antihistamines	Histamine (H1) receptor blockade	First generation: diphenhydramine 25–50 mg or hydroxyzine 25–50 mg; second generation: loratadine 10 mg or cetirizine 5–10 mg	First-generation agents more likely to yield greater sedation
Antidepressants	Histamine and serotonin blockade	Tricyclic antidepressants, doxepin 10–25 mg; mirtazapine 7.5–15 mg; paroxetine 10 mg	Anticholinergic effects likely contribute to symptom relief, best to dose at bedtime; monitor for anticholinergic effects; may result in daytime sleepiness and increased risk for confusion and falls
Corticosteroids	Anti-inflammatory	Hydrocortisone comes in varying strengths; low potency preferred unless severe or refractory cases	Topical in an ointment is preferred for local treatment to minimize systemic effects; reserve systemic corticosteroids for refractory cases
Serotonin antagonist	Serotonin blockade	Ondansetron 4–8 mg IV/PO q8h	Efficacy in opioid-induced and cholestasis-related pruritus
Opioid antagonists	Mu-receptor mediated pruritus	Low-dose IV naloxone infusion <2 mcg/kg/h; nalbuphine 2.5–5 mg IV	Dose low to avoid reversing analgesia or precipitating withdrawal
Anticonvulsants	Alter neurological response to pain pathway mediators (e.g., bradykinin)	Gabapentin 100 mg PO TID up to 1200 mg PO TID	Gabapentin only agent with evidence; associated with sedation, start low dose and titrate as tolerated
Bile salt sequestrants	Bind bile acid salts	Cholestyramine 4 gm/day, increase up to 24 gm/day in 6 divided doses	Indicated for cholestasis-related pruritus; 4 gm mixed with 2–6 ounces of noncarbonated drink

22

References

1. https://www.who.int/cancer/palliative/definition/en/, accessed January 20, 2020.
2. Watanabe SM, et al. A multicenter study comparing two numerical versions of the Edmonton Symptom Assessment System in palliative care patients. *J Pain Symptom Manag.* 2011;41:456.
3. Bernacki R, et al. Communication about serious illness care goals: A review and synthesis of best practices. *JAMA Intern Med.* 2014;174(12):1994–2003.
4. Rubenfeld GD. Principles and practice of withdrawing life-sustaining treatments. *Crit Care Clin.* 2004;20(3):435–452.
5. Lacy BE, et al. Rome criteria and a diagnostic approach to irritable bowel syndrome. *J Clin Med.* 2017;6(11):99.
6. McMillan SC, et al. Validity and reliability of the constipation assessment scale. *Cancer Nurs.* 1989;12(3):183–188.
7. Miller K, et al. Depression and anxiety. *Cancer J.* 2006;12:388–397.
8. Wilson KG, et al. Depression and anxiety disorders in palliative cancer care. *J Pain Symptom Manag.* 2007;33(2):118–129.
9. Grossman CH, et al. Death anxiety interventions in patients with advanced cancer: A systematic review. *Palliat Med.* 2018;32(1):172–184.
10. Smith EM, et al. Assessing the independent contribution to quality of life from anxiety and depression in patients with advanced cancer. *Palliat Med.* 2003;17:509–513.
11. Lloyd-Williams M, et al. Which depression screening tools should be used in palliative care. *Palliat Med.* 2003;17(1):40–43.
12. Fulton JJ, et al. Psychotherapy targeting depression and anxiety for use in palliative care: A meta-analysis. *J Palliat Care* 2018;21(7):1024–1037.

Imaging Studies **23**

- ➤ Radiology Workflow
- ➤ Reading Radiology Reports
- ➤ Common Radiographic Studies: Noncontrast
- ➤ Common Radiographic Studies: Contrast
- ➤ Intravenous Contrast Studies
- ➤ Computed Tomography (CT)
- ➤ Ultrasonography (US)

- ➤ Magnetic Resonance Imaging (MRI)
- ➤ Nuclear Scans
- ➤ Positron Emission Tomography (PET)
- ➤ Radiation and Medical Imaging
- ➤ Ordering Imaging Tests
- ➤ How to Read a Chest Radiograph

RADIOLOGY WORKFLOW

1. Provider orders an imaging study for the patient to support or disprove his or her working clinical diagnosis. The clinician should provide a brief description of the patient's symptoms and the indication for the study, considering any preparations the patient may need (such as bowel prep).
2. The study is performed by the radiology department according to standardized and specialized protocols. The images are uploaded into PACS (picture archiving and communication system) on a computer where they will be visible to anyone with access, as well as placed into a work queue for the radiologists to interpret and issue reports.
3. A radiologist then interprets the findings in the study with attention to the indication and dictates a report, which is uploaded into the PACS system. In general, if there are any critical or urgent findings the radiologist calls the ordering physician directly.

READING RADIOLOGY REPORTS

Radiology reports are written with a specific language with terms to accurately convey the findings in the imaging studies and to interpret their

---

Chapter update by Andrew A. Gomella, MD, and Oksana H. Baltarowich, MD

meaning in the clinical context. For instance, the term "hyperdensity" on a CT image appears bright on a monitor, reflecting the fact that it corresponds to increased atomic density in the region on the image. Below is a brief selection of some of these key terms:

Artifact: A visual finding in the image that does not reflect actual anatomy or anatomic abnormality, but rather an artificial process generated by the computer, for example, from reconstruction algorithms (streak artifact in CT imaging), issues with technique (such as heart appearing larger in AP vs. PA views), motion artifact from breathing in any technique, or shadowing from bowel gas obscuring structures on ultrasound.

Air–fluid level: A pattern in which fluid rests in a gravity dependent position with overlying air/gas ("fluid sinks, air rises").

Enhancement: When intravenous contrast administration causes an organ or region of tissues to be "brighter" or have more contrast with surrounding structures, implying increased blood flow to the area (Table 23-1).

COMMON RADIOGRAPHIC STUDIES: NONCONTRAST

Although you will see the term "chest x-ray" and "chest radiograph" used interchangeably, the proper terminology is "chest radiograph" because "x-rays" are the electromagnetic waves that are generated by an x-ray tube.

Chest Radiograph

(See also How to Read a Chest Radiograph, page 791)

Chest Radiograph (Routine): The standard radiograph of the chest is a PA (posteroanterior) and a lateral view. PA means the image receptor (film cassette, digital cassette, or flat panel x-ray detectors) is placed in front of the patient with the beam entering from the back (a frontal image). The patient is

23

Table 23-1. Terminology Used in the Different Imaging Modalities to Report Brighter and Darker Areas on an Image

Modality	Brighter	Darker
Radiography ("plain-film" or x-ray)	Opacity/radiodensity Increased density	Lucency/radiolucency Decreased density
CT	Hyperdense Increased attenuation	Hypodense Decreased attenuation
Ultrasound	Hyperechoic	Hypoechoic Anechoic
MRI	Hyperintense Increased signal	Hypointense Decreased signal

in an upright position, and takes a maximal inspiration with arms on the hips and shoulders rotated forward to move the scapulae out of the way. In this view the heart is closer to the image receptor and causes less magnification. (**Principle: The greater the distance between an anatomic structure and the x-ray detectors, the greater the degree of magnification.**) The PA (versus the AP, anteroposterior) view gives much more detail and is always preferred over the AP view. In the lateral view the left side of the chest is usually placed adjacent to the image receptor and the patient raises both arms over the head.

Used for evaluation of pulmonary, cardiac, and mediastinal diseases and traumatic injury as well as presurgical evaluation. Best position for finding a pneumoperitoneum under the diaphragm (handy rule: air rises, fluid sinks).

Expiratory Chest X-ray: Can improve visualization of a small pneumothorax. Evaluates for air trapping.

Lateral Decubitus Chest X-ray: Patient lies on right or left side; x-ray beam passes through the patient's body AP (anterior to posterior). Allows small amounts of pleural effusion to layer out on the downside between the ribs and the edge of the lung. Also allows air collected in a pneumothorax to rise to the upside, between the ribs and the lung.

Portable Chest X-ray (All Are AP): For imaging of critically ill patients who cannot stand or even sit up for a routine PA CXR. A portable x-ray machine is brought to the patient's bedside. The image receptor is placed *behind* the patient, and x-rays pass through the patient from anterior to posterior. This is also a frontal view of the chest. The AP projection is less optimal than obtaining the PA film. One of the reasons is that the heart is farther from the film and looks larger, which interferes with visualization of other structures.

Used for diagnosis of pneumothorax, pneumonia, and edema; verification of vascular line or tube placement. Not accurate in evaluation of heart or mediastinal size due to magnification and lung volumes are lower due to pressure from abdominal contents.

Rib Series: Delineation of rib abnormalities in several positions when plain frontal CXR or bone scan findings suggest fracture, metastatic lesions, or are inconclusive. Note: With rib fractures it is more important to assess complications, such as pneumothorax, pleural fluid/hemothorax, and lung contusion, than to find the rib fracture itself, which is more of a clinical diagnosis. (Note: Scanning over an area of focal pain with ultrasound may be very helpful in finding a rib fracture in some cases.)

23

Abdominal Radiograph

Abdominal Plain Film/Radiograph (Flat plate is considered an outdated term): Obtained supine, upright, occasionally prone. Image receptor is under the patient on the x-ray table. No prep. In adult, usually cannot include both domes of diaphragm and symphysis pubis on one image. Used for evaluation of the gas pattern, calcifications, foreign bodies, psoas shadows, renal and liver shadows, flank stripes, vertebral bodies, and pelvic bones.

KUB: Short for "kidneys, ureter, and bladder"; x-ray beam is centered lower on the abdomen to include these structures. For initial evaluation of the urinary tract (29–59% of kidney stones and 20% of gallstones are visualized on KUBs).

Abdominal Decubitus Radiograph: Obtained instead of upright abdominal film for imaging of debilitated patients. Patient's left side is down to show free air accumulating between the liver surface and parietal peritoneum.

Obstruction Series: Includes supine, upright, left lateral decubitus views of the abdomen, and chest PA and lateral views. Useful when the patient has acute abdominal pain or distention to look for bowel obstruction and free air (pneumoperitoneum). On the upright views, look for air–fluid levels of mechanical obstruction and adynamic ileus and for free air under the diaphragm, which suggests a perforated viscus or recent surgery; an upright CXR is often best for spotting pneumoperitoneum.

Cross-Table Lateral Abdominal Radiograph: Used when patient is too ill to move, lies supine, and x-ray beam is shot from side to side through the abdomen. Usually a very limited view because of poor beam penetration through the torso. Used for identification of free air between the anterior abdominal wall and bowel loops.

Other Noncontrast Radiographs

C-Spine Radiographs: Usually includes AP, lateral, and oblique views. Evaluation of trauma, neck pain, disc disease, neurologic evaluation of the upper extremities, and postoperative findings. All seven cervical vertebrae must be seen for this study to be acceptable. Add an "open mouth" view to identify odontoid fractures in trauma.

Thoracic, Lumbar, Sacral Vertebral Radiographs: Usually includes AP, lateral, and oblique views. Evaluation for fractures, disc disease, the effects of arthritic and metabolic disorders of the spine, and postoperative findings.

Skull Films: Have generally been replaced with other imaging modalities (CT and MRI). May be used to assess position of a VP (ventriculoperitoneal) shunt in head, metallic foreign body presence/location, or nasal fracture in a young patient.

Sinus Films (Paranasal Sinus Radiographs): Have largely been replaced with sinus CT scans.

Extremities: Studies performed on the bones and joints of the upper and lower extremities to evaluate for fractures, joint space irregularities, dislocations, foreign bodies. Two or more views are required depending on which bone or joint is being imaged, usually AP and lateral. Certain joints need to be imaged in flexion, extension, or other positions for ideal visualization. For example, a foot series usually includes a weight-bearing view taken from a lateral approach.

Mammography: An x-ray technique dedicated to breast imaging. Mammography studies are generally ordered and performed in two categories; screening and diagnostic. **Screening mammography** includes two views of each breast (craniocaudal [CC] and mediolateral oblique [MLO]). Patients are recalled for **diagnostic mammography** when there are abnormal findings on a screening mammogram or when a patient has signs or symptoms suspicious for breast cancer. Additional views of the breast may include spot views, compression views, and others, including using ultrasound.

- *Digital Mammography*: Has generally replaced film mammography for its improved resolution and improved accuracy when used on nonfatty, denser breasts, which is more common in premenopausal women. Images are taken in standard views and manipulated on a computer.
- *Digital Breast Tomosynthesis (DBT), also called 3-D Mammography:* A sequence of images of the breast is scanned in an arc and then reconstructed to give images corresponding to tissue depth, which improves visualization of lesions in overlapping tissues. When used in addition to digital mammography, it results in significantly decreased recall rates for routine cancer screening.

COMMON RADIOGRAPHIC STUDIES: CONTRAST

Oral and Rectal Contrast: Includes barium and iodine-based, water-soluble agents (e.g., Gastrografin, Gastroview, and selective use of IV contrast solution).

- **Barium** is an inert, tasteless, white powder mixed with water that coats the lining of intestines after it is swallowed or introduced per rectum. If a GI tract fistula or perforation is present or suspected, then barium can cause "barium peritonitis or mediastinitis" and should be avoided. Barium is not harmful to lungs or kidneys.
- **Gastrografin and Gastroview** are water-soluble contrast agents that contain iodine. They are safe to use in the case of perforation or fistula, but are very harmful to the lungs if aspirated.
- **A solution of IV contrast** is an excellent choice if there is suspicion of a perforation and the patient is at risk of aspiration. Usage requires considerations of allergy to IV contrast agents and cost.

23

    Fluoroscopy: General term to describe acquisition of single spot and rapid sequence x-ray images being performed during a diagnostic or interventional procedure. Used during GI/GU and angiography studies. Most fluoroscopy machines are shaped in a C configuration ("C-arm") allowing the C-arm to slide over the patient bed at different angles.

    Barium Swallow (Esophagogram): Evaluation of swallowing mechanism, esophageal lesions, and abnormal motility.

    Upper GI (UGI) Series: Includes esophagogram and imaging of stomach and duodenum. Visualization of ulcers, masses, hiatal hernia and to evaluate heme-positive stools, upper abdominal pain, and reflux.

Small Bowel Follow-Through (SBFT): Done after an UGI series. Delayed films show jejunum and ileum. Evaluation of diarrhea, abdominal cramps, malabsorption, and masses. Rarely ordered (CT or MR enterography, and capsule endoscopy are more informative).

Barium Enema (BE): Examination of colon and rectum. Used when standard (optical) colonoscopy is contraindicated or CT colonography is not feasible. Indications include diarrhea, crampy abdominal pain, heme-positive stools, change in bowel habits, unexplained weight loss, and rarely incomplete colonoscopy when CT colonography cannot be performed. Usually performed as a double-contrast study with barium and air introduced through a rectal tube for better visualization of the lining and intraluminal masses.

Iodine-Based, Water Soluble Enema: Similar to barium enema, but water-soluble contrast agent is used (clears colon more quickly than barium). Safer than barium to use in cases of bowel perforation, fistulae, and anastomotic leaks. Can be therapeutic in evaluation of obstipation and colonic volvulus.

Catheter Angiography: A rapid series of images is obtained after a bolus contrast injection through a percutaneous catheter, usually done in a fluoroscopy suite. For imaging of aorta, major arteries and branches with late "run-off" images, tumors, and venous drainage. Angiography is performed as a procedure by interventionalists in radiology, cardiology, vascular surgery, and neuroradiology. Some angiographic contrast studies are listed here. CT angiography is another technique.

- **Digital subtraction angiography (DSA):** A computational technique performed with all types of angiography. A precontrast image is subtracted from the contrast images to allow vasculature and other contrast containing structures to be better visualized.
- **Coronary angiography:** Definitive for diagnosis and assessment of severity of CAD. Stenoses including significant stenotic lesions (>70% occlusion) can be identified.
- **Cerebral angiography:** Evaluation of intracranial and extracranial vascular disease, atherosclerosis, aneurysms, and AV malformations. Not used for detection of cerebral structural lesions (use MRI or CT instead).
- **Pulmonary angiography:** Most accurate diagnostic procedure for pulmonary embolism, but due to its invasive nature, is only used if findings on CT-PA are not diagnostic. Visualization of vascular abnormalities, AV malformations, and bleeding from tumors.
- **Bronchial angiography:** Visualization of bleeding vessels from the systemic circulation in cases of massive hemoptysis in which embolization is planned.

Lymphangiography: Iodinated oil is injected to opacify lymphatics of the leg, pelvis, retroperitoneum, cisterna chyli, or thoracic duct; for example, to evaluate chylous pleural effusions. Test of the integrity of the lymphatic system, evaluation for metastatic tumors (e.g., testicular) and lymphoma.

Hysterosalpingography (HSG): Evaluation of uterine abnormalities (congenital anomalies, fibroids, adhesions) or tubal abnormalities (occlusion or adhesion), often as part of infertility evaluation. Contraindicated during menses and if there is undiagnosed vaginal bleeding, acute PID, or pregnancy is suspected. Patient is placed in pelvic exam position, a speculum is inserted, the cervix is cannulated, and contrast material is injected into the endometrial canal and fallopian tubes.

Cystogram: Fluoroscopy study during which the bladder is filled and emptied with a catheter in place. Used to evaluate bladder filling defects (tumors), outpouchings (diverticula), and bladder perforation (**CT cystogram** is more sensitive for perforation with trauma).

Voiding Cystourethrography (VCUG): Fluoroscopy study in which bladder is filled with contrast material through a catheter, then catheter is removed, and the patient voids. Used for diagnosis of vesicoureteral reflux, examination of urethral valves, and evaluation of recurrent UTIs.

Percutaneous Nephrostomy: A percutaneous catheter is placed through the renal parenchyma and into the collecting system for management of renal obstruction and to evaluate the level and cause of obstruction.

Retrograde Pyelography (RPG): Contrast material injected into the ureters during cystoscopy. Used for imaging upper urinary collecting system. Not used as a first-line study. Used if kidney or ureter cannot be visualized with other imaging techniques and in the presence of a renal mass, ureteral obstruction, or filling defects in the collecting system.

Retrograde Urethrography (RUG): Visualization of traumatic disruption of the urethra and urethral strictures.

Endoscopic Retrograde Cholangiopancreatography (ERCP): Contrast material is endoscopically injected into the ampulla of Vater to visualize the common bile and pancreatic ducts for obstruction, stones, and ductal pattern.

Percutaneous Transhepatic Cholangiography (PTHC): Visualization of biliary tree in patients unable to concentrate contrast medium (bilirubin >3 mg/dL). Needle inserted percutaneously into dilated biliary duct and contrast material is injected. If needed, a drain is left in place (percutaneous transhepatic biliary drain [PTBD]).

T-Tube Cholangiography: Contrast injection into T-tube placed in the common bile duct after gallbladder or bile duct surgery. Evaluation of bile duct for patency and drainage as well as residual stones.

Myelography: Evaluation of subarachnoid space for tumors, herniated discs, and other cause of nerve root injury. Lumbar puncture technique is used to inject contrast material into the subarachnoid space.

23

INTRAVENOUS CONTRAST STUDIES

Intravenous Contrast: Standard iodinated contrast media are nonionic agents, which have a generally safe profile. The main potential complications are contrast reactions and nephrotoxicity (in selected patients). Ionic agents are rarely used today, in part because of higher reaction rates. In general, for use of an IV contrast agent, the renal function should not be significantly impaired. GFR must be ≥ 30 mL/min/1.73 m². Creatinine should be $<1.8–2.0$ mg/dL and there should be no upward trend of the creatinine. (Confirm these acceptable ranges with your local radiology service.) Exceptions to this rule are patients with irreversible end-stage renal disease on dialysis. In rare instances, patients with significant renal disease may need contrast in a life-threatening condition where the risk outweighs the benefit. All patients, especially patients with underlying or suspected renal disease (including diabetes, hypertension, sickle cell, multiple myeloma, lupus, etc.) and with elevated creatinine, should be well hydrated to minimize nephrotoxicity (contrast-induced nephropathy). Other nephrotoxic drugs should be avoided if possible.

Contrast reactions to IV agents can occur. Allergic reactions to modern iodinated contrast agents are uncommon (0.6% aggregate and 0.04% severe). Patients who have had an allergic reaction to contrast medium have an approximately 5-fold increased risk of developing a future allergic reaction if exposed to the same class of medium. Reactions can be mild (nausea, vomiting, sneezing, diaphoresis, headache, vertigo), intermediate (urticaria, angioneurotic edema, wheezing/bronchospasm, fever, chills, palpitations, increased or decreased blood pressure), or severe (anaphylactoid, dyspnea, cardiovascular collapse, pulmonary edema, shock, asthma, laryngeal edema, respiratory arrest). Vagal reactions (hypotension and bradycardia) and periorbital edema are other adverse effects. A history of asthma is a risk factor, and if possible, the agent should be withheld until active wheezing is treated. Allergy to seafood or iodine (e.g., Betadine) is no longer considered an important risk factor. But patients who have severe or multiple allergies are at higher risk.

- **Premedication:** Institution dependent (check with your institution's radiology department for details). For example, premedication can be accomplished by one of two recommended methods. One is by administration of 32 mg methylprednisolone PO 12 hr before the scan and again 2 hr before the scan. The other method recommends three doses of PO prednisone 50 mg, 13 hr before, 7 hr before, and 1 hr before IV contrast injection, as well as oral antihistamines (diphenhydramine 50 mg 1 hr before). **Premedication may limit symptoms, but is not guaranteed to eliminate a breakthrough reaction (2.1%).**
- **Accelerated IV premedication** in urgent situations may be considered; however, this requires a minimum of 4–5 hr of preparation. Regimens less than 4–5 hr have not been shown to be effective. Unprepped patients with prior reactions should, in general, have a physician in attendance to treat a repeat reaction if necessary.
- A previous mild or moderate reaction to a contrast agent does not necessarily preclude use of IV contrast material. For patients with a known

history of allergic reaction to IV contrast, the likelihood of an adverse event should be balanced with the benefits of the examination. An alternative imaging technique should be considered. However, in a person with a known serious contrast reaction and a life-threatening situation (such as aortic dissection), IV contrast should not be withheld if the attending physician documents that the study is medically necessary. This is especially true after a previous anaphylactoid reaction, but in general, if contrast is given, physicians should be in attendance to treat a repeat reaction.

- There is no cross-reaction between gadolinium-based contrast used for MRI and iodinated contrast used for CT.

COMPUTED TOMOGRAPHY (CT)

How CT Works

Computed tomography (CT) utilizes x-rays and opposing detectors that spin around a patient who lies on a table that moves through the center of a large donut-shaped machine (hence a CT scan is called a multidetector CT, or **MDCT**). A computer processes the attenuation data from multiple different angles and produces cross-sectional images of the body. The computer acquires an entire volume of data that can be displayed in a variety of slice thicknesses, sagittal and coronal reconstructions, and 3-D reconstructions.

A CT can be performed with or without intravenous contrast and with or without oral contrast. IV contrast enhances vasculature and soft tissues. Check allergy history, GFR, and creatinine level to determine the suitability of IV contrast administration (see Intravenous Contrast section, page 773). Administration of a dilute oral contrast agent before abdominal or pelvic scans helps delineate the bowel. Any body part can be scanned depending on the indications, but CT is most helpful in evaluating the lung, mediastinum, retroperitoneum (pancreas, kidney, lymph nodes, aorta, adrenals), liver, spleen, brain, coronary arteries, and to a lesser extent pelvis, colon, and bone.

In CT, radiodensities are measured along a quantitative scale that transforms the attenuation coefficient measurements into **Hounsfield units (HU),** named for the developer of the CT scanner, Nobel Laureate Sir Godfrey N. Hounsfield. Water is assigned to 0 HU, air is −1000 HU, fat is −120 to −90 HU, soft tissue is +100 to +300 HU, and bone is +1000 HU. At the two extremes of the spectrum, air is depicted as black on the image and bone is white, with various shades of gray in between. Masses such as cysts, solid tumors, fat-containing tumors, and vascularized (contrast enhancing) and nonvascularized (nonenhancing) lesions can be differentiated. Iron, iodine, and calcium in organs can be identified. Metal and dense barium can cause artifacts and distortion of the image.

When viewing CT images it is imperative to properly **window** the image in order to visualize the structure you are viewing. The image contains far more

23

detail than the eye can see or that monitors can display (each pixel corresponds to a Hounsfield unit, and there are 2000 possible shades per pixel). Windowing enables us to view specific sections of this data depending on the intensity or brightness of the data point. For instance, a bone window will focus in on a higher range of Hounsfield units (e.g., 400–1800 HU) and stretch them such that they display the full range on a monitor and subtle variations in the bony structures become apparent. At this setting, all the detail below 400 HU will be lost, such that soft tissues and lung details are not displayed. Typically, routine CT images are viewed in the lung (air), soft tissue, and bone windows. Check with your specific PACS* viewing software to learn how to change the window.

Uses of CT

CT Abdomen and Pelvis: Scans begin above the dome of the diaphragm to include lung bases and end below the groin to include upper thighs. This includes imaging of intraabdominal/pelvic and retroperitoneal structures and disease processes and is accurate for tumors, fluid collections, extent of ascites, obstructions, calcifications, etc. The oral contrast agent that can be administered opacifies the entire small bowel in approximately 45 min before imaging and reaches the rectum in about 2 hr.

Abdominal CT: Scans begin above the dome of the diaphragm to include lung bases and end at the iliac crests. This includes imaging of the liver, biliary tree, spleen, pancreas, adrenal glands, kidneys, upper GI tract, abdominal aorta, and upper retroperitoneum.

Pelvic CT: Scans begin at the iliac crests and end below the groin to include upper thighs. This includes imaging of pelvic vessels, perirectal/perianal tissues (fistulas, abscesses), soft tissue masses, lymph nodes, bone tumors, and decubitus ulcers, and is used for staging of bladder, prostate, rectal, and gynecologic cancers.

Chest CT: For detection of lung parenchymal diseases, pulmonary nodules (<3 cm), pulmonary masses (>3 cm), and traumatic injury. Although calcifications suggest benign disease (e.g., granuloma), no definite density value can reliably separate malignant from benign lesions. Useful in differentiating hilar adenopathy from vascular structures seen on plain CXR, especially when contrast-enhanced images are obtained. Also useful for viewing mediastinal masses, vessels, trachea, and lymph nodes. High-resolution images with inspiration and expiration are useful for characterizing interstitial lung disease. Pulmonary embolism scans are obtained with contrast enhancement. CT is used in guiding biopsies and radiation planning.

CT for Lung Cancer Screening: The USPSTF has updated its lung cancer screening guidelines: annual screening for lung cancer with low dose computed

---

* PACS is an abbreviation for Picture Archiving and Communication System. This refers to a system used in medical imaging to store, retrieve, distribute, analyze, and digitally process medical images.

tomography (LDCT) in adults age 50 to 80 who have a 20 pack-year smoking history and currently smoke or have quit within the past 15 years.

Computed Tomographic Angiography (CTA): A CT scan taken with precisely timed injection of contrast by an automated injector ("power injector") during a preset vascular phase (pulmonary, arterial, venous). CTA can be performed for the chest, abdomen, pelvis, neck, and cerebral vessels. CT-PA (**CT pulmonary angiogram**), performed during the right heart phase, is the gold standard for detecting pulmonary embolism as it highlights clots in the pulmonary arteries. CTA of the aorta is performed in an early phase that highlights the aorta and its branches. CTA of the coronary arteries is optimized to highlight coronary arteries and is often performed with noncontrast calcium scoring CT to screen for risk of a coronary event. CTV (CT venography) is performed in a delayed phase for venous structures.

Head CT: For evaluation of head injuries, severe headaches, intracranial bleeding (ruptured or leaking aneurysms, subarachnoid, subdural, and epidural hematomas), brain tumors, hydrocephalus, and sinus and temporal bone abnormalities. Initial test of choice for trauma and stroke.

CT Urography: IV contrast study of the kidneys and ureters; limited usefulness for lesions inside of the bladder (better visualized with cystoscopy). Performed in noncontrast, nephrographic, and pyelographic phases (for calculi, renal masses, and collecting system abnormalities, respectively). Indications include flank pain, renal calculi, hematuria, recurrent UTI, trauma, obstruction, and malignancy. Note that a noncontrast CT may be ordered in the acute evaluation of renal colic and possible urolithiasis.

CT Cystogram: The bladder is filled retrograde with dilute IV contrast via a catheter to look for bladder perforation in trauma because it is more sensitive than a standard cystogram under fluoroscopy. Include a drainage film to evaluate for residual contrast outside of bladder with perforation.

CT Colonography: A screening technique where the colon is distended with gas (usually CO_2 instead of room air due to quicker absorption and less patient discomfort) and noncontrast CT images are reconstructed in 3-D to visualize polyps or masses. Rectal contrast and/or IV contrast may be used. Used as an alternative test when standard (optical) colonography is contraindicated.

Neck CT: Workup of soft tissue abnormalities such as neck masses and abscesses and other diseases of the throat and trachea. Usually performed with IV contrast.

Spinal CT: Used in trauma to assess for spinal fractures in the cervical, thoracic, or lumbosacral regions. MRI is preferred over CT for evaluation of soft tissues including spinal cord, disc space, and nerve roots; however, contraindications to MRI or artifact from metal may make CT the preferred test.

Dual-Energy (Spectral) CT: An emerging type of CT scan involving imaging of the patient with more than one x-ray energy (spectrum), which allows for better differentiation of tissue and its elemental composition when compared to conventional CT. This enables significantly improved "material separation" or delineation of IV contrast, uric acid (renal calculi, or in gout), arterial plaques and bone, and decreases streak artifact from metal implants.

23

With dual-energy CT, "virtual noncontrast" images can be reconstructed from a single contrast-enhanced scan by subtracting out the iodinated contrast and thereby generating noncontrast CT images without rescanning the patient, allowing for decreased overall radiation dose.

ULTRASONOGRAPHY (US)

How US Works

High-frequency sound waves are used to image internal organs. Ultrasonography uses sound waves (1–20 MHz) with frequencies higher than those audible to humans (20 Hz to 20 kHz). The sound waves are sent into the body from a transducer that both sends and receives returning echoes from the interfaces of tissues with dissimilar acoustic properties (the greater the difference in acoustic properties, the stronger the reflection at the interface). The amplitude, delay, and frequency of returning sound waves are measured. The transducer converts the returning sound waves into electrical signals that are digitally converted into images on a monitor.

With ultrasound, there is a constant trade-off between **resolution** and **depth** (beam penetration).

- The higher the frequency of the transducer, the higher the resolution of the image but the lower the penetration of the beam into the body.
- Lower frequency probes give lower resolution but better penetration into deeper structures (more depth).

Ultrasound Transducers (Probes)

There are different sizes, shapes, and frequencies of transducers with a variety of features designed to produce the best images for certain body parts. There are external (used on the body surface) and internal (endocavitary—vaginal, rectal, endovascular, esophageal) transducers. The more common ones are:

Curvilinear: Generally used for abdominal and obstetrical imaging, ideal for deeper structures.

Linear: Flat, rectangular surface (footprint). High frequency with increased detail of superficial structures, commonly used for abdominal wall masses, breast, thyroid, musculoskeletal studies, vascular studies in extremities (DVT, arteries, IV access).

Phased array: A small-faced transducer that can image in small spaces with the ability to change the focus of the ultrasound beam.

Ultrasound Modes

B-mode ("Brightness mode"): Also called 2D. Grayscale image. Most well-known type of ultrasound image, which displays the reflected ultrasound echoes of tissues in a two-dimensional cross-section image using grayscale.

M-mode ("Motion mode"): Uses ultrasound to track the motion of tissues over time, which is then displayed across the screen. The section corresponds to a specific line across the plane of the transducer's image, e.g., motion of the mitral leaflets during cardiac cycles.

Doppler Ultrasonography: Uses the Doppler effect to generate images of moving blood and tissues. By calculating the frequency shift of blood flow in an artery, its speed and direction can be calculated and displayed on an image. **Color Doppler** or **color flow Doppler** displays direction of flow towards or away from the probe by a color scale (note: although blue and red are often used, the colors are arbitrary and do not correspond to arterial and venous flow). **Power Doppler** displays amplitudes, but no direction of flow. There is also **pulsed Doppler or spectral Doppler**, by which Doppler information is sampled from a small sample volume rather than from a continuous line (**continuous wave Doppler**).

Duplex Ultrasonography: Combines color Doppler images with grayscale images that allow visualization of blood flow and anatomy simultaneously.

Ultrasound Advantages

- Noninvasive, safe, no ionizing radiation (safe to use in pregnancy and pediatrics)
- Multiplanar imaging in real time
  o Images are generally taken in two planes, along the sagittal and transverse planes of the body or along the longitudinal and transaxial planes of the organ being imaged, but any plane is obtainable by rotating the transducer and placing it anywhere on the body
- Relatively inexpensive imaging technology
- Widely available; point of care ultrasound becoming commonplace
- Portable, can be used at the bedside
- Good contrast of tissue layers in many organs

Ultrasound Disadvantages

- Relatively small field of view
- Operator dependent, inconsistent reproducibility
  o Depends on operator training, knowledge, skill, experience, and commitment to produce diagnostic images
- Dependence on acoustical properties
  o Air, metal, and bone strongly reflect sound and cause "acoustical shadows" that do not allow visualization of deeper structures
    ▪ Reflection by even a small pocket of air between the transducer and the skin is so strong, that a coupling agent (water, oil, or gel on the skin) is necessary to conduct the beam into the body.

23

o Depth is a challenge
  - Thick and deep structures attenuate the sound beam and compromise the images.
  - Better images are obtained from thin patients than from obese patients.

Uses of Ultrasound

Abdominal: Gallbladder (95% sensitivity in diagnosis of stones), cholecystitis (gallstones, dilated gallbladder, wall thickening >3 mm, presence of pericholecystic fluid, pain directly over gallbladder). Focal liver masses, diffuse liver disease (hepatic steatosis, infiltrative disorders), biliary tree obstruction, pancreas (pseudocyst, tumor, pancreatitis), kidneys (hydronephrosis, calculi, tumor, cyst, perirenal collections), abscesses, ascites, appendicitis in children and thin patients (difficult in adults due to body habitus and bowel gas).

Gynecologic Ultrasound

- Transabdominal pelvic US with a full bladder is no longer the preferred routine ultrasound method of evaluation of the female pelvis. Women are no longer instructed to come in with a full bladder. Full bladder US is only done in cases of a constricted or stenotic vaginal opening (virginal females, elderly postmenopausal women, inability to tolerate vaginal probe) or if patient refuses a transvaginal scan.
- Limited transabdominal scan with no particular bladder filling or emptying is often used as a survey scan before a transvaginal scan to judge the size of the uterus and to survey for large pelvic masses or fluid collections that may be out of the field of view of the transvaginal probe.
- Transvaginal pelvic US is the preferred method for evaluation of female pelvic organs. Diagnosis of abnormalities of the uterus, ovaries, fallopian tubes (e.g., tumors, cysts, fibroids), some vaginal masses, ectopic pregnancy, abscesses, ovarian torsion (with Doppler to assess blood flow).
- Sonohysterography (also called saline infusion sonography). The cervix is cannulated, and saline is instilled into the endometrial cavity under US guidance to delineate endometrial abnormalities such as polyps, submucosal fibroids, hyperplasia, cancer, adhesions. Also used to assess tubal patency.

Obstetrical Ultrasound

- ***First Trimester:*** Presence, size, location, and number of gestational sacs, presence of yolk sac and embryo(s), heartbeat, viability, evaluation of uterus, cervix, adnexa and cul de sac.
- ***Second and Third Trimester:*** Fetal number, cardiac activity, fetal anatomy survey, fetal biometry, determination of intrauterine growth, presentation, amniotic fluid volume, localization of placenta, evaluation of maternal cervix, uterus (fibroids), and adnexal masses.

Vascular: Assessment of blood flow speed with Doppler waveforms, abdominal aortic aneurysms, carotid artery plaques and stenosis (bruits), mesenteric ischemia (celiac and superior mesenteric arteries for stenosis), renal artery stenosis, peripheral arterial disease (stenoses, occlusions), pseudoaneurysms, follow-up of surgical interventions (bypasses, angioplasty, endarterectomy, stents, dialysis fistula and grafts), arterial and venous mapping. Presence of deep venous thrombosis (DVT) in leg veins and abdominal veins.

Contrast-Enhanced Ultrasound (CEUS): Microbubble-based IV contrast medium composed of specially formulated gas microbubbles injected intravenously into the blood stream and observed during an ultrasound exam. The microbubbles circulate in the blood vessels creating strong reflections and therefore delineate the vascular patterns, which are used in diagnostic criteria. After injection, the microbubbles remain in the vascular space for a short time and later dissolve and are exhaled. No special patient preparation. No lab tests required. Used in the evaluation of lesions of abdominal organs (in particular liver and kidney masses) as well as general delineation of vascular structures.

Thyroid and Parathyroid: Evaluation of thyroid nodules (cyst versus solid) and guidance for needle biopsy. US findings alone cannot be used to differentiate benign from malignant lesions, but certain features are more suspicious than others.

Bladder: Prevoid and postvoid residual volume is calculated for determination of bladder emptying, intraluminal abnormality, presence of ureteral jets with color Doppler, estimation of prostate size in males.

Scrotum: Evaluation for testicular and scrotal masses (e.g., tumor, cysts, hydrocele, varicocele), testicular torsion and epididymitis (with Doppler to assess blood flow).

Musculoskeletal: Pain evaluation, abnormalities of soft tissues (masses, fluid collections, swellings, foreign bodies), tendons, ligaments, muscles, joints (effusions, arthritis, synovitis, crystal deposits, intraarticular bodies), nerves (entrapment, injury, masses, neuropathy), anomalies, bone injury, guidance for diagnostic and therapeutic procedures.

Breast: Characterizations of breast masses (cyst versus solid, benign versus malignant features), breast mass in young patient <30 years old, dense breast tissue, asymmetrical breast tissue, lymph nodes, guidance for breast biopsy.

Solid Organ Transplants (Liver, Renal, Pancreas): Baseline scan following transplantation, abnormal bloodwork, evaluation of pain, fever, sepsis, white count, vascular patency, fluid collections, rejection, organ failure.

Point-of-Care Ultrasound

- *FAST* (**F**ocused **A**ssessment with **S**onography for **T**rauma): A type of point-of-care ultrasound that involves a rapid focused bedside exam used in trauma patients for detecting the presence or absence of free fluid in the perihepatic and perisplenic spaces, pericardium, and pelvis. Patients

23

with free fluid in these areas, as well as two of the following—penetrating injury, systolic blood pressures less than 90 mm Hg, or heart rate over 120 beats per minute—are likely to have a high mortality, trauma-induced coagulopathy, and require a massive transfusion.

- *Point-of-Care Ultrasound for Bedside Procedures:* See Chapter 19, page 503.

Transrectal: Prostate abnormalities (abnormal digital rectal exam), guidance for prostate needle biopsy for diagnosis of prostate cancer (trans rectal and trans perineal biopsy), determine prostate size, drainage of pelvic and prostatic abscesses. Evaluation of the rectal wall.

Intraoperative: Assist the surgeon in the operating room in identification, evaluation, resection of masses, and any possible complications. Probe is covered in a sterile sheath and can be used for open, laparoscopic and robotic procedures involving the abdomen.

Echocardiography: Performed from either a transthoracic (TTE) or transesophageal (TEE) approach, with TEE being superior, however requiring anesthesia. To assess for valvular vegetations (endocarditis), septal defects, wall motion, chamber size, pericardial effusion, valve motion, wall thickness. **Doppler mode:** Cross-valvular pressure gradients, blood flow patterns, and valve orifice area in work-up of cardiac valvular disease. **M-mode:** Valve mobility, opening, chamber size, pericardial effusions, septal thickness.

MAGNETIC RESONANCE IMAGING (MRI)

How MRI Works

Measurements of the magnetic movements of atomic nuclei are used to delineate tissues. When placed in a strong magnetic field, nuclei, such as hydrogen protons, resonate and emit radio signals when pulsed with radio waves. A defined sequence of magnetic field and radio pulses, or "pulse sequence," produces radiofrequency echoes that are measured and produce an MR image. There are many sources of tissue contrast on the resulting MR images, including differences in longitudinal (T1) and transverse (T2) relaxation times following excitation radiofrequency pulses.

Each tissue, normal or pathologic, has unique T1 and T2 for a given MRI field strength. T1 is usually longer than T2, but can never be shorter. At 1.5 Tesla (1.5 T), the most common field strength used, T1 and T2 for free water are both about 2–3 sec. T1 and T2 for everything else is shorter. An image is **T1-weighted** if it primarily depends on the differences in T1 measurements for visual contrast and **T2-weighted** if it depends primarily on T2 measurements. There are numerous other sources of tissue contrast, such as whether protons are in water or lipid, and magnetic field distortions caused by air, iron, other substances, or tissue movement.

The oldest pulse sequence is called spin echo (SE), but these are used less frequently due to their longer acquisition time. A faster version of SE has become more common, acquiring several echoes (rather than just one) after each excitation pulse. Gradient recalled echo is a faster sequence preferred when rapid imaging is needed to reduce motion artifact or capture rapidly changing physiologic events, such as enhancement following a bolus of a contrast agent. MR images can be obtained in any orientation.

MRI Contrast: **Gadolinium** is a paramagnetic agent that is included in a highly stable chelate to form contrast agents that are used to enhance vessels and characterize tissues based on differences in vascularity. It causes fewer anaphylactoid contrast reactions than iodinated contrast agents used in CT, and at clinically used doses has no nephrotoxicity. Gadolinium use in patients with GFR <30 mL/min/1.73 m² must be discussed with the radiologist, because nephrogenic systemic fibrosis (NSF) is a possible severe complication if relatively unstable gadolinium chelates or higher-than-recommended doses are used. Fortunately, there are several clinically available gadolinium contrast agents for which NSF has not been reported, even in patients with severe renal dysfunction. Another concern with gado-linium contrast is that trace amounts can remain in the body long-term, most notably in the brain parenchyma. There are no known adverse effects related to the retention of gadolinium; however, minimizing repeated gadolinium scans and weighing benefits versus risk of each scan is recommended.

Closed MRI, Open MRI, Wide-Bore MRI: Most older **closed MRI** units had a 60-cm opening. Some patients could not fit into the "tunnels" or experienced claustrophobia. *Open MRI* was devised to accommodate such patients by having three to four sides open. However, these systems have lower magnet strength and significantly reduced image quality, and many useful MRI techniques are not available on these systems. **Wide-bore MRI** was designed to solve the problem, and is the most common configuration for new MRI systems. It has a larger bore (70 cm), but still delivers high magnet strength for high image quality and shorter duration for image acqui-sition than open MRI, which makes it much more acceptable to patients.

Basic MR Images

23

- **T1-Weighted Images**: Provide good anatomic planes because of the wide variance in T1 values among normal tissues, particularly fat versus most other tissues. A separate pulse can be used to suppress the signal of fat, which is particularly helpful for showing enhancement following admin-istration of gadolinium contrast agent.
  - o Brightest (high signal intensity): Fat, blood, protein, and melanin.
  - o Dark or black (low signal intensity): Pathologic tissues, tumor or inflam-mation, fluid collections. Also respiratory tract, GI tract, bone and cal-cified tissues, blood vessels, heart chambers, and pericardial effusions

- **T2-Weighted Images**: Pathologic lesions often have long T2 values. Fluid also has high signal on these images.
  o Bright: Fat and fluid. Certain lesions such as cysts and liver hemangiomas.

Advantages of MRI

- No ionizing radiation, considered safe in children and pregnancy (although should be performed without IV contrast in pregnancy)
- Display of vascular anatomy without contrast
- Visualization of linear structures: spine and spinal cord, aorta, vena cava
- Visualization of posterior fossa and other difficult-to-see CT areas
- High-contrast soft tissue images

Disadvantages of MRI

- Claustrophobia because of confining magnet; **open MRI** systems may help, but some may have more motion artifact, limiting imaging for chest and abdomen; this is less of an issue for extremity imaging.
- Longer scanning time, resulting in motion artifacts
  o MRI is sensitive to motion artifact; anxious or agitated patients may have to be sedated for acquisition of optimal images.
  o Intramuscular glucagon can be used to suppress intestinal peristalsis on abdominal studies.
- Inability to image critically ill patients who need life support equipment that is not safe in or near the magnet, e.g., oxygen tank.
- MRI-noncompatible clinical settings: Metallic eye foreign bodies, some implants and devices (e.g., most pacemakers, CNS vascular clips, and cochlear implants) are contraindications because they may heat up, malfunction, or move. If metallic eye foreign bodies are likely, obtain screening x-rays of the orbits before MRI. The strong magnetic field can interact with electrical currents and cause programmable devices such as pacemakers, insulin pumps, cochlear implants, and neuro-stimulators to malfunction. Dental fillings, dental prostheses, artificial cardiac valves, IVC filters, IUDs, and large metallic devices in place for a while (hip prostheses, spinal hardware) are safe; however, they may cause artifacts.
- Recent concerns about gadolinium contrast agent deposition in the brain.

Uses of MRI

MRI provides better soft tissue contrast than CT. MRI also is generally better than CT for imaging of the brain, spinal cord, musculoskeletal soft tissues, and liver.

Abdomen: Evaluation of liver lesions, the biliary system **(MRCP – magnetic resonance cholangiopancreatography)** for strictures, dilatation, choledocholithiasis. Hepatobiliary contrast material that is excreted through the biliary system (and not the kidneys like other gadolinium-based agents) may be useful for biliary leaks (e.g., after cholecystectomy). Evaluation of liver fat and iron content. Quantification of liver fibrosis using MR elastography. Adrenal lesions (differentiation of benign adenoma from malignancy/metastasis), tumor staging (renal, GI, pelvic), evaluation of abdominal masses, examination of almost all intraabdominal and retroperitoneal structures. Appendicitis in children and pregnancy. Small bowel evaluation using MR enterography (the only scan for which oral contrast material is given).

Pelvis: Evaluation of all pelvic organs in male and female patients, evaluation of endometrial and ovarian masses, differentiation of myoma and adenomyosis, staging of cervical cancer, diagnosis of congenital uterine anomalies (e.g., bicornuate, septate uterus). Dedicated MRI of the prostate (due to improved signal to noise techniques, endorectal coils rarely used). Dedicated rectal MRI for evaluation of local extension of rectal tumors.

Chest: Evaluation of mediastinal masses. Dedicated cardiac MRI for evaluation of myocardial ischemia, myocarditis and infiltrative diseases such as sarcoidosis and amyloidosis. Chest MR angiography can be performed without contrast material using a time of flight technique to evaluate aortic dissection in patients allergic to iodinated contrast or young patients who need long-term follow-up for aortic dissection (such as Marfan syndrome) to reduce their exposure to ionizing radiation.

Head: Analysis of all intracranial lesions, identification of demyelinating diseases; some conditions, including acute trauma, are better evaluated with CT (see previous section). Magnetic resonance spectroscopy **(MRS)** provides a biochemical "fingerprint" of tissues in the brain and is performed in conjunction with MRI equipped with MRS capability. It is not routinely indicated; however, MRS can help differentiate primary brain tumors from other non-neoplastic conditions.

Musculoskeletal System: Detection of bone tumors and bone and soft tissue infection, osteomyelitis, evaluation of joint spaces (unless a prosthesis is in place), marrow disorders, aseptic necrosis, meniscal tears, tendon and ligament injuries.

Spine: Diagnosis of diseases of the spinal column (e.g., herniated disc, tumors).

NUCLEAR SCANS

How Nuclear Scans Work

Radioactive isotopes, called radiotracers, are designed to reach specific tissues or organs in the body. The radioactive material is usually injected into the bloodstream, but others are inhaled as a gas or swallowed. After appropriate uptake by the targeted tissue or organ, the emitted radiation energy, usually in the form of gamma rays, is detected by a special camera or device (usually gamma camera), and is processed by a computer to create images. This provides molecular and functional information, which aids in the diagnosis of certain conditions. Nuclear scan images can be fused with anatomic images, such as CT scans or MRIs, called fusion imaging, to more precisely localize the abnormal activity identified by the nuclear scan. Nuclear imaging utilizes gamma and positron. Gamma emitters, such as technetium-99m (99mTc) or iodine-123 (^{123}I), can be located using gamma cameras (planar imaging) or SPECT (single photon emission computed tomography). Improved resolution is seen via PET (positron emission tomography) using positron emitters, such as gallium-68 (68Ga) and fluorine-18 (^{18}F) (see PET Scans, page 788).

Uses of Nuclear Scans

The following are the more commonly used nuclear scans and their purposes. Most are contraindicated in pregnancy; check with your nuclear medicine department.

Hepatobiliary Scan (HIDA-Scan, BIDA-Scan): Differential diagnosis of biliary obstruction, acute cholecystitis, biliary atresia. Not good for stones unless cystic duct is completely occluded and acute cholecystitis is present.

Bone Scan: Metastatic work-ups (cancers most likely to go to bone: prostate, breast, lung); evaluation of delayed union of fractures, osteomyelitis, avascular necrosis of femoral head; evaluation for hip prosthesis; differentiation of pathologic and traumatic fractures.

Lung Scan ($\dot{V}$/$\dot{Q}$ Scan): Evaluation for pulmonary embolism (PE). Should be interpreted with a recent CXR. Performed with the injection of technetium-99m macroaggregated albumin ($\dot{Q}$ or the perfusion portion), and the inhalation of radioactive gas ($\dot{V}$ or the ventilation portion). Normal scan with low clinical suspicion excludes PE; indeterminate scan necessitates further study with chest CT-PA (CT pulmonary angiography); clear perfusion deficit coupled with a normal ventilation (mismatch) is highly suggestive of PE. Also shows evidence of pulmonary disease, COPD, and emphysema.

Cardiac Scans: Diagnosis of CAD, stress testing, measurement of ejection fractions and cardiac output.

- **Technetium-99m (^{99m}Tc)-Sestamibi:** Uses ^{99m}Tc-labeled RBCs. Used for stress myocardial perfusion imaging (SMPI) to detect stress-induced ischemia.
- **MUGA Scan (Multigated Acquisition Scan):** Portrays contractility of the left ventricle, i.e., ventricular wall motion. It is synchronized with an EKG to produce a "moving picture" of cardiac function and calculate the LV ejection fraction.

- **Thallium-201 (^{201}Tl):** Measurement of myocardial perfusion by uptake of ^{201}Tl by normal myocardium. Normal myocardium appears hot, and ischemic or infarcted areas cold. Useful for myocardial viability.
- **Technetium-99m (^{99m}Tc) Pyrophosphate:** For diagnosis of myocardial amyloid.
    Bleeding Scan: Detection of source of GI tract bleeding.
- **Technetium-99m (^{99m}Tc) Sulfur Colloid Scan:** Detection of bleeding of 0.1 mL/min, if patient is actively bleeding.
- **Technetium-99m (^{99m}Tc)-Labeled Red Cell Scan:** Same as sulfur colloid scan, but may be superior for localizing intermittent bleeding.
    DEXA Scan (Dual Energy X-Ray Absorptiometry, Bone Densitometry): Quantification of osteoporosis by measurement of bone mineral density (BMD). Used for assessment of hip or spine fracture risk and effect of drugs such as bisphosphonates and rank ligand inhibitors in osteoporosis. Central DEXA measures BMD in the spine or hip. Peripheral DEXA scans are for assessment of osteoporosis in wrists.
    Gastric Emptying Scintigraphy: Measurement of gastric transit of a radioactive isotope containing meal. Diagnostic of gastroparesis when gastric retention of meal is greater than 10% at 4 hr after meal and/or greater than 60% at 2 hr. In a healthy adult retention is 90% at 1 hr, 60% at 2 hr, 10% at 4 hr.
    Renal Scans: Agents are generally classified as functional tracers or morphologic tracers.
- **Technetium-99m (^{99m}Tc) Mercaptoacetyltriglycine (MAG3):** Renal function; imaging of the parenchyma within minutes of injection and with low radiation dose. Has nearly replaced other renal agents.
- **Technetium-99m (^{99m}Tc) DTPA (diethylenetriamine pentaacetic acid):** Renal function; renal blood flow studies, estimation of GFR, evaluation of collecting system
    Single-Photon Emission CT (SPECT): Multiple nuclear images are sequentially displayed as in CT; can be applied to many nuclear scans. SPECT/CT adds anatomic detail.
    Thyroid Scan: Most often technetium-99m pertechnetate. Evaluation of nodules (solitary cold nodules require a tissue diagnosis because 25% are cancerous). Scan patterns in correlation with lab tests may help diagnose hyperfunctioning adenoma, Plummer and Graves diseases, multinodular goiter; localization of ectopic thyroid tissues (especially after thyroidectomy for residual/recurrent cancer); identification of superior mediastinal thyroid masses.
    Adrenal Scan: Localization of pheochromocytoma when MRI or CT findings are equivocal. Performed with labeled **MIBG (metaiodobenzylguanidine)**, norepinephrine analog, labeled to iodine-123 or iodine-131.

23

Indium-111 (^{111}In) Octreotide (OctreoScan): Imaging of tumors with somatostatin receptors (pheochromocytoma, gastrinomas, insulinomas, small-cell lung cancer).

Brain Scan: Metastatic work-up, determination of blood flow (in brain death or atherosclerotic disease), evaluation of Parkinsonian syndromes.

Gallium Scan: Location of abscesses (5–10 days old) and chronic inflammatory lesions, such as sarcoidosis. Also useful for diagnosis of chronic osteomyelitis.

Liver–Spleen Scan: Used to identify accessory spleen.

POSITRON EMISSION TOMOGRAPHY (PET)

How PET Works

PET involves injection of a positron-emitting tracer that is attached to a metabolically active molecule and accumulates in areas of increased metabolic activity. Tomographic images localize the tracer within the body. PET is performed with CT and more recently with MRI, and the functional information obtained with PET scan is correlated with the precise anatomic detail obtained from CT or MRI as the images are fused. The most commonly used PET tracer is 18-fluoro-deoxyglucose (18-FDG). Fluorine-18 decays by positron emission. The positron emitters used in PET generally have a short half-life. The half-life of ^{18}F is 110 min. This short half-life results in a low dose to the patient but it also means that it must be delivered daily by a vendor.

Clinical applications of PET:

- **Cancer:** Because malignant tissue has a higher metabolic rate than benign tissue, PET tracers of glucose metabolism are selectively concentrated in living tumor. PET depicts small foci of cancer that may be missed with conventional CT or MRI. PET can also be used to differentiate live tumors from treated dead tissue and fibrosis. Any metabolically active tissue will "light up," however. Areas of inflammation can cause false-positive results. The tumors most commonly imaged with PET include colorectal cancer, lung cancer, brain cancer, breast cancer, lymphoma, and melanoma. PET can be used in both diagnosis and staging of these cancers. Due to the relatively slow metabolism of prostate cancer cells, routine 18-FDG PET is not usually used with specific PET imaging agents used in this cancer. Recently, the concept of **theranostics** has expanded PET scanning by combining one radioactive PET diagnostic agent with a second radioactive drug to deliver a lethal radioactive dose to the cancer cells.

- **Neurologic Imaging:** Localization of specific functions and definition of functional neuroanatomy, such as localization of epileptogenic foci in patients with a seizure and diagnosis of various brain disorders, including dementia, depression, and schizophrenia.

- **Cardiac Imaging:** Definition of myocardial viability; findings complementary to anatomic information obtained with cardiac angiography; may be used in treatment planning.

RADIATION AND MEDICAL IMAGING

Measuring Radiation Dosage

"Radiation dose" refers to the absorption of electromagnetic energy (x-rays and gamma rays) by the body. The amount of energy absorbed per unit mass of tissue is measured in grays (1 Gy = 1 joule/kg). Another radiation measure is "effective dose," in units of sieverts (Sv). This measure is intended to allow comparison of different radiation doses to different organs or tissues (for example, internal vs external radiation exposure, or exposure of different organs). Effective dose is sometimes used as an approximate indicator of radiation risk, although there are large uncertainties in radiation risk assessment at low dose and low dose rate.

Naturally Occurring "Background" Radiation Exposure

The average person in the United States receives an effective dose of about 3 mSv per year from naturally occurring radiation such as cosmic rays and terrestrial materials. This "natural background" level varies geographically—people living at high altitudes, such as Colorado, receive about 1.5 mSv more of radiation per year than those living at sea level. The largest overall worldwide source of background radiation comes from radon gas in homes (about 2 mSv per year); however, this also varies from region to region.

Radiation Exposure from Medical Imaging

In the last 25 yr, radiation from medical imaging has become a large contributor to the radiation exposure of the U.S. population, equaling the natural background (3 mSv) when averaged across the entire U.S. population. Radiation exposure from CT scans, nuclear medicine studies, and fluoroscopy accounts for nearly 90% of the radiation exposure from medical imaging. The increased utilization of medical radiation has raised concerns about the potential for future cancers in the population. As a result, the medical imaging community has responded with more radiation dose awareness and more dose-efficient imaging technology. Particular attention is paid to the radiation exposures in the pediatric population, as well as prenatal exposure (Table 23-2).

23

Table 23-2. Radiologic Procedure, Adult Effective Radiation Dose, and Approximate Risk of Fatal Cancer from the Examination

Procedure	Adult Effective Dose	Lifetime Risk Fatal Cancer
Chest x-ray	0.1 mSv	Negligible
Chest CT	7 mSv	Low
Lung cancer screening CT	1.5 mSv	Negligible
Abdominal and pelvic CT	10 mSv	Low
Abdominal and pelvic CT with and without contrast	20 mSv	Low
Upper GI	6 mSv	Low
Mammography screening	0.4 mSv	Negligible
Bone (extremity) x-ray	0.001 mSv	Negligible
Coronary artery CTA	12 mSv	Low
Cardiac CT (calcium scoring)	3 mSv	Negligible
Dental x-ray	0.005 mSv	Negligible
Bone densitometry (DEXA)	0.001 mSv	Negligible
PET/CT	25 mSv	Low
Nuclear bone scan	6 mSv	Low

It is very important to realize, however, that there is no conclusive evidence to indicate that effective doses below about 100 mSv cause cancer. Evidence of radiation-induced carcinogenesis comes only from high-dose incidents (>200 mSv) such as nuclear bombs and disasters. There is no proof that medical imaging doses cause cancer. However, out of an abundance of caution, radiologists practice by the ALARA principle, keeping radiation doses "As Low As Reasonably Achievable," because we do know that high doses are carcinogenic and carry other health risks.

23

ORDERING IMAGING TESTS

Based on concerns for radiation exposure, clinicians should order only necessary and appropriate diagnostic imaging tests for their patients. The American College of Radiology (ACR) has compiled evidence-based guidelines to assist clinicians in making the most appropriate decisions regarding diagnostic imaging for specific clinical conditions. The ACR Appropriateness Criteria (https://www.acr.org/Clinical-Resources/ACR-Appropriateness-Criteria) is constantly updated and ranks the appropriateness of the various radiologic studies for each clinical scenario. This is a very useful tool for providers ordering imaging tests to make sure that they are ordering the best test to yield the most information in establishing a diagnosis for their patient. A medically justified diagnostic test should never be avoided based on radiation dose concerns, if the risk outweighs the benefit. The immediate benefit to the patient of receiving the diagnostic information far outweighs the small theoretical increased cancer risk later (10–20 yr) in their lifetime.

HOW TO READ A CHEST RADIOGRAPH

A chest radiograph (CXR) is a basic part of the evaluation of an ill patient. Understanding the basic principles of CXR interpretation is considered a key learning step for all physicians. The key structures are shown in Figures 23-1 (PA chest radiograph) and 23-2 (lateral chest radiograph), page 792.

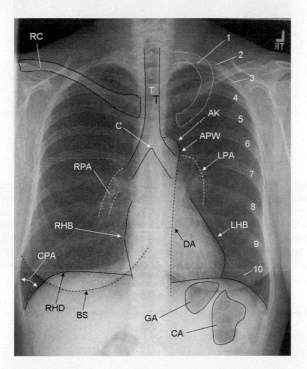

Figure 23-1.   Structures seen on a posteroanterior (PA) chest x-ray. 1 = first rib; 2–10 = posterior aspect of ribs 2–10; AK = aortic knob; APW = aortopulmonary window; BS = breast shadow (labeled only on right); C = carina; CA = colonic air; CPA = costophrenic angle; DA = descending aorta; GA = gastric air; LHB = left heart border (*Note:* Most of the left heart border represents the left ventricle; the superior aspect of the left heart border represents the left atrial appendage.); LPA = left pulmonary artery; RC = right clavicle (left clavicle not labeled); RHB = right heart border (*Note:* The right heart border represents the right atrium.); RHD = right hemidiaphragm (left hemidiaphragm not labeled); RPA = right pulmonary artery; T = tracheal air column.

23

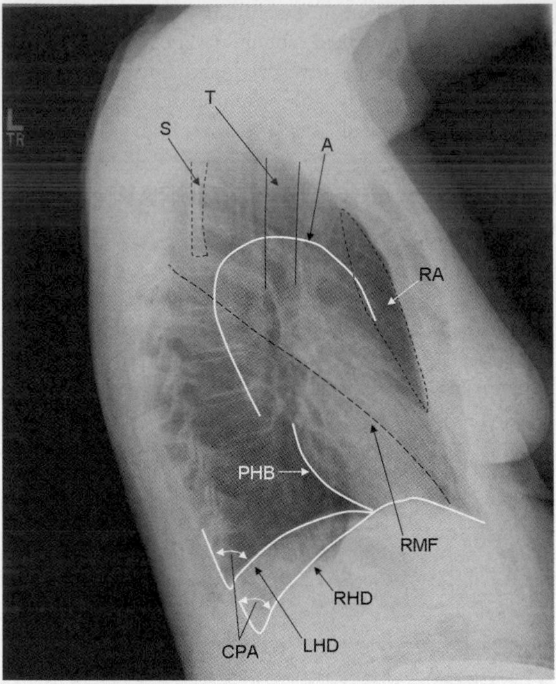

Figure 23-2. Structures seen on a lateral chest x-ray. A = aorta; CPA = posterior costophrenic angle; LHD = left hemidiaphragm; PHB = posterior heart border (*Note:* The posterior heart border represents the left atrium superiorly and left ventricle inferiorly; the anterior heart border is not clearly defined on this film but represents the right ventricle.); RA = retrosternal airspace; RHD = right hemidiaphragm; RMF = right major fissure (left major fissure and minor fissures not well visualized on these films but can occasionally be seen); S = scapula; T = tracheal air column.

Determine the Adequacy of a Chest X-ray

The first step in looking at a chest radiograph is to assess the quality of the image. You can remember this by the mnemonic **RIPPA**.

- **Rotation:** Clavicles should be equidistant from the midline spinous processes.
- **Inspiration:** Lungs should be inflated so that the diaphragm is at least at the level of posterior ribs 9-10.
- **Penetration:** Disc spaces are seen, but bony details of spine cannot be seen. Lung markings are visible.
- **Position:** Air–fluid level in the stomach confirms an erect/upright position.

- **Angulation:** Clavicles normally project over the apices. If they project over the supraclavicular soft tissues, then the patient is leaning back with respect to the detectors (view is called lordotic). If the clavicles project over the mid-lungs, the patient is kyphotic with respect to the detectors. Both lordotic and kyphotic views yield limited information.

PA Chest Radiograph

The image receptor is placed in front of the patient, and the x-ray beam passes from back to front (posterior to anterior). In this view, the heart is closer to the image receptor, and is therefore less magnified. The PA (versus the anterior posterior, or AP) view gives much more detail and is always preferred over the AP view. When you look at a PA radiograph, it is as if you are looking at the patient from the front, therefore the patient's right side is on your left, and vice-versa.

Lungs and Airways: The trachea should be straight, midline in location, and the carina and right and left main stem bronchi should be visible. Tracheal deviation suggests mass effect (pushed to one side by tumor, goiter, or air trapped in a tension pneumothorax, for example) or unilateral loss of lung volume (trachea deviated towards side of atelectasis).

Lung radiolucency should be symmetrical at the same level as one's eyes scan the lungs side to side, moving down the image from apices to bases. The entirety of the lungs should be clear with normal lung markings all the way to the edges bordered by the bony thorax. Asymmetrical increased density of lung may be seen with consolidation, a mass, or fluid. There are four main causes of a totally opacified (white) hemithorax: large pleural effusion, total lobar pneumonia, complete atelectasis of the lung, or pneumonectomy. Asymmetrical hyperlucency in the lungs may be seen in emphysema, pneumothorax, mastectomy, etc.

Heart and Mediastinum: The heart should be less than one-half the width of the widest internal diameter of the thoracic cavity on a PA film. Greater than one-half the width is consistent with cardiomegaly. If the heart shadow is markedly enlarged ("water bottle heart" or "giant Hershey Kiss heart"), consider pericardial effusion or multi-chamber cardiomyopathy. The right heart border represents the right atrium. The left heart border represents the left ventricle.

The ascending aorta makes a smooth arc that should not extend lateral to the right heart border. The aortic knob should be visible and distinct along the left superior mediastinal border. Widening of the mediastinum is seen with traumatic disruption of the thoracic aorta. Mediastinal masses can be associated with lymphomas (such as Hodgkin disease) and other tumors (thymomas, teratomas). In infants, do not mistake the normally prominent cardiothymic shadow for abnormal widening. Note any displacement of the right or left paraspinal lines, which represent the interface between the lung and posterior mediastinum (left paraspinal line is more commonly seen than the right).

23

Hilum: Inspect the hilar areas, where the roots of the lungs are found, containing the pulmonary arteries, veins, bronchi, and lymph nodes. The left hilum is usually higher than the right. Vessels have clear borders, taper, and divide until they become invisible. Look for vessel enlargement, increased density in the hilum, lobulated, rounded, or irregular borders of hilar structures (lymphadenopathy, masses), obliterated vessel borders, or calcifications.

Diaphragm: Both hemidiaphragms should be visible (obliteration or effacement suggests pathology in or around the lower lobes). Both hemidiaphragms should have rounded, dome-shaped configurations. The right hemidiaphragm is higher than the left in 90% of cases. A unilateral high diaphragm suggests paralysis (from nerve damage, trauma), eventration, hepatomegaly, lung mass, subpulmonic fluid accumulation, or loss of lung volume on that side because of atelectasis. A low, flat, or even inverted diaphragm is seen in COPD from hyperinflated lungs. Lateral costophrenic sulci/angles should be clear, sharp, and pointed downward. Blunting suggests fluid or scarring. It takes about 150 mL of pleural fluid to cause blunting of the lateral costophrenic sulcus. Check below the diaphragm for the gas pattern and free air.

Skeletal Structures: Examine the bones for symmetry and intact cortical outlines. Check clavicles, shoulder joints, scapulae, proximal humeri, and ribs. Look down the vertebral column to look for vertebral height loss, midline position of spinous processes, and intact bilateral pedicles. The sternum is superimposed over the spine and is usually not recognizable. Check for osteolytic or osteoblastic lesions, fractures, and arthritic changes.

Soft Tissues: Neck, supraclavicular, axillary soft tissues, breast shadows, upper abdomen. Check for symmetry, enlargement, loss of tissue planes, subcutaneous air, and calcifications.

Anything Else: Note the presence of any lines or tubes (endotracheal tubes, central venous lines, dialysis catheters, pulmonary artery catheters, enteric tubes, etc.). Look for surgical clips, sutures, stents, other metallic objects. Check the four corners of the image for markers placed by the technologist, which could provide clues about the patient's condition and positioning.

23

Lateral Chest Radiograph

For the lateral view of the chest, the image receptor is usually placed on the left side of the patient (called the left lateral chest radiograph) and the x-ray beam passes from right to left through the patient. In this view, the heart is closer to the image receptor, and is therefore less magnified. The patient's arms should be raised above the head as high as possible, so as not to obscure structures. The lateral radiograph may be viewed with the spine to the right or left of the image on the monitor, but whichever way you choose, you should always look at the images the same way each time to facilitate development of your eye-brain coordination.

Heart: The heart has an oval shape and occupies less than half of the thoracic diameter. The right ventricle is located directly behind the sternum. The inferior border of the heart represents the left ventricle. The posterior upper border is the left atrium. As the left atrium enlarges, it expands toward the spine. It is useful to remember that both the right middle lobe and the lingula project over the heart shadow.

Lungs: It is important to see a retrosternal clear space, because anterior mediastinal masses obliterate this space, most commonly due to lymphoma. Similarly, there should be a retrocardiac clear space, which could be obliterated by cardiomegaly, hiatal hernias, masses, or fluid. Localize lesions by thinking three-dimensionally with the frontal image.

Hila: Centered around the end of the trachea, the hilar structures have slightly increased density. The small, round air-filled structure in the center of this area is the left mainstem bronchus seen end on, with the left pulmonary artery curving over it. Lymphadenopathy would make the hilar region denser and more lobulated.

Hemidiaphragms: Both hemidiaphragms should be visible with rounded, dome-shaped contours (obliteration or effacement suggests pathology in the lower lobes or surrounding fluid). Posterior costophrenic sulci/angles/gutters, which are the deepest parts of the thoracic cavity, should be clear and sharp. Blunting suggests fluid (meniscus sign) or scarring. It takes over 50 mL of pleural fluid to cause blunting of a posterior sulcus, so it is the first to fill with pleural fluid (recall that it takes about 150 mL of pleural fluid to cause blunting of a lateral sulcus on the frontal radiograph). The right hemidiaphragm is identified by ending at the right ribs, which appear larger than the left ribs on a left lateral radiograph (patient's left side closest to the detector), because the right ribs are farther from the film/detector (magnified). Similarly the left hemidiaphragm ends at the smaller appearing left ribs, but it also has underlying stomach and splenic flexure gas.

Skeletal Structures: Examine the vertebrae for height, bone density, and cortical outlines. Check disc spaces. The apparent bone density of the spine from superior to inferior should give the impression that the spine gets darker, because the x-ray beam travels easily through the air-filled lower lobes and bone, whereas superiorly there is more density from bones of the shoulder girdles and soft tissues of the chest wall and axilla. Shadows from the ribs overlay the image and may cause extra shadows. Edge effects from the soft tissues of the raised arms may be in variable positions. Two parallel lines in the upper portion of the image are from the thin blades of the scapulae.

Other Structures: The aorta arises from the center of the heart and the arch is usually visible, but the descending aorta becomes invisible, unless there is density from calcified plaques. The esophagus is located anterior to the spine, but is normally not identifiable.

23

Common Chest X-ray Abnormalities

Opacities: Increased density in an area of lung.

- Consolidation: Airspace disease. Alveoli fill with fluid (edema), exudate or pus (pneumonia), blood (hemorrhage), gastric contents (aspiration), cells (bronchoalveolar carcinoma), abnormal protein (alveolar proteinosis), etc.
- Interstitial changes: Fluid, fibrosis, nodularity of the interstitium (supporting tissues) of the lung causes reticular, nodular, or reticulonodular densities on the radiograph.
- Atelectasis: Collapsed parts of lung that cause opacities and compensatory shifts of fissures, mediastinum, hemidiaphragms, and trachea.

Congestive Heart Failure (CHF)

- Initially the vessels in the lower lung should be larger than those in the upper lung. A reversal of this difference (called cephalization, equalization, redistribution) suggests pulmonary venous hypertension and heart failure.
- Then interstitial pulmonary edema manifests with increased lung markings and indistinct vessel borders. Fluid surrounds bronchi (peribronchial cuffing). A well-known sign of interstitial pulmonary edema is **Kerley B lines,** which are small linear densities seen at the lung bases perpendicular to the pleura that represent build-up of interstitial fluid in the interlobular septa. Pleural effusions begin to accumulate.
- As CHF progresses, alveolar edema causes fluffy air space opacities radiating out from the hila (perihilar haziness) and a "butterfly" appearance on the radiograph.

Pneumonia: Usually manifests as airspace (alveolar) disease, which can be patchy, segmental, or lobar in distribution. It has been described as fluffy, hazy, cloud-like opacities or consolidations that are confluent with indistinct margins. Air bronchograms can be seen (see Signs below, page 798). There is little or no mass effect on the heart and mediastinum. Aspiration pneumonia usually occurs in the dependent portions of the lungs (lower lobes and more so on the right compared to the left due to the more vertical orientation of the right main stem bronchus or posterior parts of the upper lobes)

Atelectasis: Is the incomplete expansion of a lung, lobe, or segment of the lung that becomes airless, resulting in volume loss. Atelectasis can range from areas of subsegmental atelectasis, manifested as linear opacities on the chest film, to complete collapse of a lung that appears dense. The adjacent thoracic structures shift in response to the volume loss, for example, shifting of the trachea, heart, and/or mediastinum toward the collapsed side, elevation of the ipsilateral hemidiaphragm, and compensatory hyperinflation of the contralateral lung or remaining lung segments on the same side. Collapse of an entire lobe (right upper/middle/lower lobe or left upper/lower lobe) has a specific appearance on chest radiographs, based on location. Collapse of an entire lung causes the most dramatic shifts in the thorax. In cases of atelectasis one must consider the underlying causes, which include obstructing malignancy, mucus plugs, or foreign bodies.

Pulmonary Nodules: By definition, a round or oval, well-defined density, completely surrounded by lung parenchyma, measuring ≤ 3 cm. May be benign (granuloma, hamartoma, infection, AVM) or malignant (carcinoma, metastasis). Ground-glass (nonsolid) nodules are nonspecific and may be infectious/inflammatory in etiology; however, partially solid nodules with ground-glass components are more likely to be malignant.

Masses: By definition, a lesion >3 cm is usually malignant. Masses may be rounded or irregular/spiculated in shape.

Cavitary Lesions: Caused by abscess, TB, cancer (especially squamous cell carcinoma), coccidioidomycosis, granulomatosis with polyangiitis (formerly known as Wegener granulomatosis).

Pleural Effusion: As fluid accumulates between the visceral and parietal pleura, it fills the most dependent part—the posterior costophrenic sulcus (>50 mL fluid needed to be visible), then fills the lateral costophrenic angle (>150 mL fluid needed to be seen), and proceeds to accumulate around the lung as it progresses superiorly (maximum 3 L). Presence and amount of fluid can be confirmed on the decubitus view. Free-flowing fluid will shift to the dependent position. Loculated fluid will be trapped in place, for example, by adhesions. A very large effusion (about 2–3 L) will opacify the entire hemithorax. Large amounts of fluid will collapse the underlying lung (compressive atelectasis) and cause mass effect with displacement of the trachea, heart, and mediastinum to the contralateral side. When air and fluid are present in the pleural space, there will be a visible air-fluid level, called a **hydropneumothorax.**

Pneumothorax: Occurs when air leaks out of the lung and enters the pleural space; however, the negative pressure in the pleural space is preserved. Air surrounds the partly collapsed lung and the visceral pleura becomes visible as a thin white line, because it is outlined by the air inside and outside the lung. The thin white line of the visceral pleura can be easily overlooked with grave consequences. Lung markings should not be visible lateral to the visceral pleura. When the trachea, heart, and /or mediastinum shift toward the side opposite of a pneumothorax, one must suspect a **tension pneumothorax**. In this case, air leaks into the pleural space through a check-valve mechanism, the normal negative pressure is lost, and pressure builds up that leads to compression, decreased venous return, and cardiovascular collapse, if not relieved.

Pneumomediastinum: Air abnormally tracking into the mediastinum, possibly from rupture of a mediastinal structure such as the esophagus.

Subcutaneous Emphysema: Air abnormally tracking into the subcutaneous soft tissues.

23

Common CXR Radiographic Signs

Silhouette Sign: One of the most important and useful radiographic signs. Normally, when two structures of different density are adjacent to each other, then their borders (or their silhouettes) are visible. **The silhouette sign occurs when two structures of similar density are adjacent to each other, causing their borders or silhouettes to be obscured.** For example, if two structures of water density are adjacent to each other, then their interface is obliterated and they cannot be identified as separate structures. If a lung filled with pneumonia, or a pleural space full of fluid, touches the diaphragm (equal in density to pneumonia and fluid), then their densities blend and their borders disappear.

Air Bronchogram Sign: A sign seen with airspace disease and consolidation. Small air-filled tubular structures within an opacified area, e.g., pneumonia, represent small air-containing bronchi that are usually too small to see, which become visible because of consolidation within the alveoli surrounding them.

Meniscus Sign: This occurs when the pleural space is intact and the negative pleural pressure is preserved. Fluid in the pleural space accumulates between the visceral and parietal pleura. First the posterior, then the lateral costophrenic sulci fill with fluid (increased density) that takes the shape of a meniscus. As fluid increases, it continues to track up around the lungs.

Spine Sign: Normally, the vertebral bodies appear darker as one looks down the spine. If the spine looks lighter or whiter as your eyes track more inferiorly, then this is called the **spine sign**, in which case an abnormality such as pneumonia, fluid, or mass is present in the area of the lower lung segments, causing increased radiodensity in line with the spine.

Common Lines and Tubes Seen on CXR

ET (endotracheal tube): The tube should be seen overlying the air-filled trachea, with the tip positioned 3–7 cm above the carina.

Central Venous Catheters (PICC, Internal jugular, subclavian, port): Tip of line should be at the level of the cavoatrial junction.

Swan-Ganz (pulmonary artery catheter): Tip should be in the proximal right or left main pulmonary artery (see Chapter 28, page 902).

Nasogastric Tube (NG): The tube should course below the diaphragm, curving slightly to the left of midline (as it crosses the GE junction), with the side hole overlying the stomach bubble, the tip ideally at least 10 cm past the GE junction. Commonly used for suction.

Dobhoff Tube: The weighted feeding tube should course below the diaphragm, curving slightly to the left of midline (as it crosses the GE junction), with the weighted tip located beyond the pylorus in the second or third portion of the duodenum to avoid reflux and aspiration since it is used for feeding.

23

Common Complications Related to Tubes and Lines: Include malposition, pneumothorax, hemothorax, atelectasis, perforation, vascular injury, thrombosis/occlusion, fragmentation/embolization, and infection.

Further Reading

American College of Radiology. ACR Appropriateness Criteria. Available at https://acsearch.acr.org/list. Accessed January 15, 2020.

National Council on Radiation Protection and Measurements (NCRP) Report #160, 2009.

http://www.radiologyinfo.org. Accessed September 20, 2021.

Introduction to the Operating Room

24

OR BASICS FOR STUDENTS

Prepare before you enter the operating room (sometimes referred as the "theatre" in the British Commonwealth countries) by knowing the patient thoroughly and having a basic understanding of what is planned. Review the medical history and read up on the basic anatomy and the procedure to be performed. Students are often quizzed on anatomy demonstrated in the OR during the operation. Avoid stereotyping the nurses as "cranky," the surgeons as "egotistical," and the medical students as "clueless" by learning the OR routine. Be alert, attentive, and, above all, patient. It is important to introduce yourself to the members of the operating room team when you are new to the operating room. Tell the scrub nurse and circulating nurse if you have never scrubbed into a procedure, and they will help you follow correct procedures.

STERILE TECHNIQUE

The members of the OR team include the surgeons, anesthesia staff, and the nursing staff. Members of the surgical team are the surgeon, surgical

---

Chapter update by Caitlyn Costanzo, MD, and Gerald Isenberg, MD, FACS assistants, students, and scrub nurse or technician responsible for the instruments, gowning the surgical team, and maintaining a sterile field. The circulating nurse acts as a go-between between the sterile and nonsterile areas.

Sterile areas include the front of the gown to the waist, gloved hands and arms to the shoulder, draped part of the patient down to the tabletop, covered part of the Mayo stand (the small table where the most commonly used instruments are kept), and the top of the back table where additional instruments are kept. The sides of the back table are not considered sterile, and anything that falls below the level of the patient table is considered contaminated.

ENTERING THE OR

In the OR, everything is geared toward maintaining a sterile field. Use of sterile technique begins in the locker room. Change into scrub clothing. Remove your T-shirt, tuck the scrub shirt into the pants, and tuck the ties of the scrub pants inside the pants. In some hospitals scrub clothes are allowed on the wards, provided they are covered by a coat or other form of gown; check your hospital's requirements, as there may be restrictions. If you wear scrub clothing out of the OR, be sure that it is not bloodstained.

Pass into the surgical anteroom to get your mask, cap, and shoe covers. The mask should cover your entire nose and mouth. Full hoods are necessary for men with beards. The cap must cover all of your hair. The cap may be a bouffant hat or skull cap. If you choose to wear a decorative fabric cap from home, most operating rooms require that it must be covered by a bouffant hat when in the sterile corridors and operating room. Because of universal precautions, protective eyewear is required while you are at the operative field. If you wear regular glasses, use a mask with adhesive at the bridge of the nose to prevent fogging. Tape the glasses to your forehead if you think they may be loose enough to fall onto the table during the operation. Do not wear nail polish, and remove any loose jewelry, watches, and rings before scrubbing. Make sure that shoelaces are tucked inside the shoe covers.

At most hospitals you do not have to wear the mask in the hallway of the OR suite, but you do have to wear everything else. The mask must be worn in the OR itself, near the scrub sinks, and in the sub sterile room between ORs. Be aware if there are any unusual infectious disease precautions beyond the basic standard precautions (page 391) that are used for all patients.

Find the OR where your patient's procedure is taking place, and assist in transport, if necessary. Introduce yourself to the intern or resident and nurse, and try to get an idea of when to begin scrubbing (usually when the first surgeon starts to scrub). If you have a pager or cell phone, follow local operating room protocols, and remove the pager or cell phone if you are going to scrub into the case. If the electronic device is allowed, keep it in the room, identifying it with your name and informing the circulating nurse about its presence.

SURGICAL HAND SCRUB

The purpose of the surgical scrub is to decrease the bacterial flora of the skin by mechanical cleansing of the arms and hands before the operation. Key points to remember: (1) If contamination occurs during the scrub, start over, and (2) in emergency situations exceptions are made to the time allowed for scrubbing (as in obstetrics, when the baby is brought out from the delivery room and the student is still scrubbing!). Properly position your cap and mask before starting the scrub.

Scrubbing technique depends somewhat on local policies. Some ORs require a timed scrub in which you determine the duration of scrubbing by watching the clock. Other ORs use an "anatomic" scrub in which the duration of scrubbing is determined by counting strokes. Some ORs use brush-free or waterless scrubs.

Brush Hand Scrub

There are a variety of antiseptics that come prepackaged with surgical brushes. These include, but are not limited to, chlorhexidine, povidone-iodine (Betadine), and parachlorometaxylenol (PCMX).

Timed Scrub

- Perform a general prewash with surgical soap and water up to 2 in (5 cm) above the elbows.
- Open the brush. Use the nail cleaner to clean under all fingernails. Wet the brush.
- Scrub both arms during the first 5 min. Start at the fingertips and end 2 in (5 cm) above the elbows; pay close attention to the fingernails and interdigital spaces.
- Discard the brush and rinse from fingertips to elbows with running water. Always allow water to drip off the elbows by keeping the hands above the elbows.
- Move into the OR to dry your hands and arms (back into the room to push the door open).
- Scrubbing times:
  o Ten minutes at the start of the day or with no previous scrub within the last 12 hr and on all orthopedic cases.
  o Five minutes with a previous scrub or between cases if you have not been out of the OR working with other patients.

Anatomic Scrub

- Perform a general prewash with surgical soap and water, up to 2 in (5 cm) above the elbows.
- Open the brush. Use the nail cleaner to clean under all fingernails. Wet the brush.

24

- Scrub each surface vigorously 10 times. Start with each finger (each of which has four surfaces), proceeding to the hand, the forearm, and the arm above the elbow. After finishing one extremity, scrub the other from fingers to above the elbow. Be sure to include all parts of your hand, especially the interdigital spaces.
- Rinse both arms and rescrub each extremity, this time not going above the elbow. The method is the same as that for step 3: 10 times on each surface from fingers to elbow.
- Discard the brush and rinse from fingertips to elbows with running water. Always allow water to drip off the elbows by keeping the hands above the elbows.
- Move into the OR to dry your hands and arms (back into the room to push the door open).

Brushless Hand Scrub

Chlorhexidine (Hibiclens) 6-Min Hand Scrub (Timed)

- Wet your hands and forearms to the elbows with water.
- Dispense about 5 mL of chlorhexidine into your cupped hands and spread it over both hands and arms to the elbows.
- Use your hands to scrub vigorously for 3 min without adding water. Pay particular attention to fingernails, cuticles, and interdigital spaces.
- Rinse thoroughly with running water.
- Dispense another 5 mL of chlorhexidine into your cupped hands.
- Repeat the steps.

Waterless Surgical Scrub (Handrub)

- Most waterless surgical handrubs are alcohol based (usually >60% ethyl alcohol with chlorhexidine). The CDC recommends that surgical staff prewash with nonantimicrobial soap and dry hands and arms completely before using an alcohol-based product, such as Avagard or Triseptin.
- Make sure your hands are visibly clear of any soiling (the same is true for subsequent scrubs), and clean the nails with the provided cleaner.
- **Apply the product to clean, dry hands.** Dispense one pump (2 mL) into the palm of one hand. Dip the fingertips of the other hand into the hand prep and work under the fingernails. Spread the remaining hand prep over the hand and up to just above the elbow.
- Dispense one pump (2 mL) and repeat the procedure with the other hand.
- Dispense the final pump (2 mL) of hand prep into either hand and reapply it to all aspects of both hands up to the wrists. Allow the prep to air dry; do not use towels. Air dry completely before gowning and gloving.

GOWNING AND GLOVING

1. If you have just completed the hand scrub, back into the room to push the door open; keep your hands above your elbows.

2. Ask the scrub nurse for a towel if you have completed a brush hand scrub. If you used a waterless hand scrub, the hands should air dry, and a towel is not needed. Do not be impatient; the scrub nurse is often very busy. Stick out one hand, palm up and well away from the body. The nurse drapes the towel over your hand.

3. Bend at the waist to maintain sterility of the towel. It should never touch your clothing.

4. With one half of the towel, dry one arm, beginning at the fingers; change hands and dry the other arm with the other half of the towel. Never go back to the forearm or hands after drying your elbows.

5. Drop the towel in the hamper as directed by the nursing staff. Again, remember to keep your hands above your elbows.

6. Ask for a gown and hold your arms out straight. The scrub nurse places the gown on you, and the circulator ties the back.

7. The nurse holds out a right glove with the palm toward you (usual custom to start with the right hand glove). Push your hand through the glove. Gloves come in several sizes—small (5½ 6½), medium (/–7½), and large (8–8½)—and materials: standard latex gloves, hypoaller-genic, reinforced (orthopedic), and latex free. Ask the resident or scrub nurse for guidance on the type of glove to request. It is good form to ask the circulating nurse to open your gloves before you actually begin to scrub. Talcum powder was once used for making the donning of gloves easier. However, in 2016 it was banned when it was linked to the development of postoperative scars and inflammation. It is no longer required to wipe off gloves before starting a case to remove powder.

8. Repeat the procedure with the left glove. It is easier if you use two fingers of your gloved right hand to help hold the left glove open.

9. Visually inspect the gloves for holes. Double gloving is becoming com-monplace because of increased awareness of universal precautions and may be mandatory depending on the procedure being performed.

10. Give the scrub nurse the long string of your front gown-tie. Hold the other string yourself and turn around in place. Tie the strings.

11. The nurse may offer you a damp sponge to clean the powder off the gloves (powder is implicated in some postoperative complications, e.g., adhesions); however, most gloves are powder free.

12. Wait patiently; stay out of the way, and keep your hands above your waist. Hold them together to prevent yourself from accidentally drop-ping them or touching your mask. This is one of the most difficult things to remember. Be attentive. The only sterile area is the front of your body from chest to waist and hands to shoulders. Your back is not sterile, nor is your body below the waist. Do not cross your arms.

24

PREPARING THE PATIENT

The patient prep technique begins prior to surgical hand scrub. Once the patient is asleep, the patient is positioned for the operation. The entire surgical team must ensure that joints and limbs maintain proper anatomical alignment and all pressure points are appropriately padded. In the setting of a longer case, forced air warmers are applied to prevent hypothermia during the operation. Sequential compression devices are applied to the lower extremities to help prevent blood clots from forming in the lower legs. The hair on the area of the body that is to be operated on is removed with an electric clipper. Excess free hair is removed from the body using long strips of tape. Next, the prep involves mechanically cleansing the patient's skin in the region of the surgical site to reduce bacterial flora. Ask the resident to guide you through the procedure; it is always better to prep a wider area than you think necessary. For example, for midline laparotomy, prep the patient from nipples to pubis and from the flank at table level on one side to the flank at table level on the other side.

Materials

Small prep table containing gloves, towels, povidone–iodine or other scrub soap (optional), povidone–iodine or other paint solution, 4 × 4 gauze squares or sponges, ring forceps (optional), chlorhexidine prep stick

Technique

1. Prep the patient before putting on the sterile gown. Using sterile technique, put on a pair of gloves, and scrub the area designated with the soap solution. At many centers, wound scrubbing is no longer routine and is used only in specific conditions, such as contaminated wounds.
2. Cover the area with a towel, and then gently pat the area dry if the wound was scrubbed. Gently peel off the towel from one side, being careful not to allow the towel to fall back on the prepped area.
3. Use either a chlorhexidine prep stick OR 4 × 4s soaked in povidone–iodine or other solution to paint the exposed area, using the proposed incision site as the center. Move circumferentially away from the incision site. Never bring the 4 × 4s/prep stick back to the center after they have painted peripheral areas. Paint in a series of concentric circles.
4. After the prep, remove the gloves using sterile technique and put on your gown.
5. It is mandatory to wait at least 3 min for chlorhexidine-based prep to dry and at least 10 min for povidone–iodine-based prep to dry PRIOR to draping the patient.

PATIENT POSITIONING

Patient positioning in the operating room is dependent on many factors such as the type and length of the procedure, proper anesthesia access to the patient, and access to any devices required. All members of the surgical team are responsible for ensuring patient safety by establishing and maintaining the correct patient positioning. The goals of patient positioning include making sure the patient's airway and circulation are maintained throughout the operation, allowing easy access to the surgical site, preventing soft tissue or nerve damage with proper padding, and making the patient as comfortable as possible. Some common patient positions are demonstrated in Figure 24-1.

A. **Supine.** Most common position for a variety of procedures.
B. **Trendelenburg.** Named for Dr. Friedrich Trendelenburg, a surgeon in the late 1800s. The patient is supine but the head is tilted 15–30 degrees downward. Used for lower abdominal, colorectal, gynecology, and genitourinary procedures and central venous catheter placement as it tends to engorge veins. Traditionally used to help support low blood pressure, although this practice has become controversial, as adverse effects may include increased intracranial pressure, decreased lung expansion/lung volumes, and an opposite effect on BP with baroreceptors causing paradoxical vasodilation.
C. **Reverse Trendelenburg.** The patient is supine with the table tilted with the feet downward and the head up to 30 degrees higher. Used for some head and neck procedures and ocular surgery.
D. **Sims position.** This is a variation of the left lateral position and provides access to the anus.
E. **Prone position.** Common surgical procedures include spine and neck surgeries, neurosurgery, colorectal surgeries, lower extremity tendon repairs, and others.
F. **Fowler position** (sitting position). Used frequently for shoulder and neurosurgical procedures.
G. **Lateral position.** Used for some back, kidney, colorectal, and hip surgeries. A modification is the kidney position where a lift is placed on the posterior abdominal wall to exaggerate retroperitoneal exposure.
H. **Lithotomy position.** Used for urology, gynecology, colorectal, and perineal procedures. The patient's legs can be placed in either a boot-style leg holder or in stirrups.
I. **Jackknife (Kraske) position.** Similar to a knee–chest or kneeling positions and is often used for colorectal surgery.

DRAPING THE PATIENT

Draping the patient is usually done by the surgeon and assistants. Watch how they do it and consider helping in a future procedure with the permission of the resident or attending. It is more difficult to keep sterile than it looks.

24

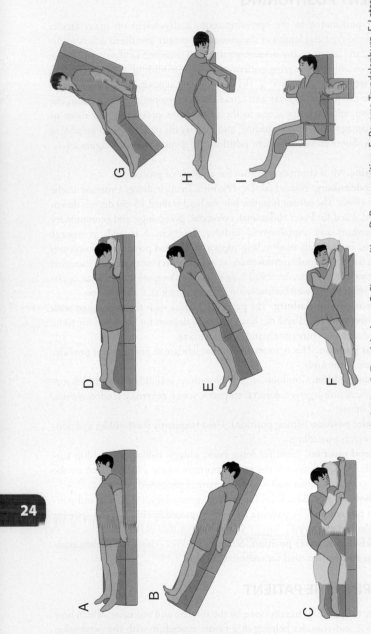

Figure 24-1. Some common surgical positions. A. Supine. B. Trendelenburg. C. Sims position. D. Prone position. E. Reverse Trendelenburg. F. Lateral position. G. Fowler position (sitting position). H. Jackknife (Kraske) position. I. Lithotomy position.

THE UNIVERSAL PROTOCOL AND THE "TIME-OUT"

The Joint Commission** has provided guidance known as the "Universal Protocol" that has been adopted by most healthcare organizations with the goal of "Preventing Wrong Site, Wrong Procedure, and Wrong Person Surgery." Most ORs have instituted this protocol, which comprises three steps.

1. **A preprocedure verification process.** This is to address missing information or discrepancies before starting the procedure.
2. **Marking the surgical site.** If possible, involve the patient in the site marking process. The site does not need to be marked for bilateral structures such as tonsils or ovaries. The mark is sufficiently permanent to be visible after skin preparation and draping.
3. **Performing a "time-out."** This is done in the operating room or procedure area before starting the invasive procedure or making the incision until all questions or concerns by any member of the OR team are resolved. The time-out involves the immediate members of the procedure team: the individual performing the procedure, anesthesia providers, circulating nurse, operating room technician, and other active participants who will be participating in the procedure from the beginning. During the "time-out" all attention is directed at reading the identified procedure on the surgical permit aloud and clearly identifying the patient, operation, and site of procedure to reduce medical errors. The attending surgeon is given the opportunity to confirm that he or she has reviewed all pertinent imaging and to voice any concerns he or she may have and to give an idea of the duration of the case and the postoperative destination. Likewise, the anesthesiologist has the opportunity to voice any of his or her concerns and to confirm appropriate perioperative antibiotics were given and if blood products are available if they may be needed. The scrub nurses will note any specific aspects of the surgical setup. An important component of the time-out is the declaration that anyone in the room is encouraged to speak up if he or she sees anything that could harm the patient or the operating room staff—and that includes YOU, the student! Note that in 2020 many organizations have added "COVID-19 Status: Positive/Negative/Unknown" to the surgical time-out process.

24

FINDING YOUR PLACE

As a student, stand where the senior surgeon or senior resident indicates. The first thing to remember is that once you are scrubbed, you must not

---

**The Joint Commission is a nonprofit organization that provides accreditation for healthcare facilities. Most U.S. state governments recognize Joint Commission accreditation as a condition of licensure for participation in Medicaid and Medicare programs (https://www.jointcommission.org/).

touch anything that is not sterile. Put your hands on the sterile field and do not move about unnecessarily. If you need to move around someone else, pass back to back. When passing by a sterile field, try to face it. When passing a nonsterile field, pass it with your back toward it. If you are observing an operation and are not scrubbed in, do not go between two sterile fields, and stay about 1 ft (30 cm) away from all sterile fields to avoid contamination (and condemnation!). When not scrubbed in, it is helpful to keep your hands behind your back, being careful not to back into the instrument table.

When scrubbed, do not drop your hands below your waist or table level. Do not grab at anything that falls off the side of the table—it is considered contaminated. If something falls, inform the circulating nurse. Do not reach for anything on the scrub nurse's small instrument stand (the Mayo stand); ask for the instrument to be given to you.

If someone tells you that you have contaminated a glove, light handle, or anything else, do not move and do not complain or disagree. Remember that the focus of the OR is maintaining a sterile field, so if anyone says, "You're contaminated," accept the statement and change gloves, gown, or whatever is needed. If a glove alone is contaminated, hold the hand out away from the sterile field, fingers extended and palms up, and a circulating nurse will pull the glove off. The same is true if a needle sticks you or if a glove tears. Tell the surgeon and scrub nurse and change gloves. For a skin break event such as a needlestick, follow local infectious disease policies.

If you have to change your gown, step away from the table. The circulator will remove first the gown and then the gloves. This procedure prevents the contaminated inside of the gown from passing over the hands. Regown and reglove without scrubbing again.

Always be aware of "sharps" on the field. When passing a potentially injurious instrument, alert the other members of the team that you are passing a sharp (e.g., "needle back," "knife back"). Learn the names and functions of the common instruments (see page 814). A knowledgeable student is more likely to actively participate in the operation.

At the end of the operation (once the dressing is on the wound), remove the gown and gloves but not the mask, cap, or shoe covers. To protect yourself, remove the gown first, and remove your own gloves last. This system keeps your hands clean of blood or fluids that got onto your gown during the procedure.

In accordance with the OSHA Bloodborne Pathogens Standard, **wash your hands with soap and water after the surgical procedure.** Assist in the transfer of the patient to the recovery room. Assist the resident with the postop orders and constructing a brief operative note immediately after the procedure before the formal operative note is dictated. (See Chapter 7, page 136, on how to write postop notes and orders.) Because of regulations that affect attending physicians at teaching hospitals, the attending may be required to write the note personally. At the very least, the attending of record annotates an "attestation" that the surgeon was "personally present during the critical portions of the procedure."

COMMON SURGICAL INCISIONS

Many procedures are performed today using laparoscopic or robotically assisted laparoscopic procedures. These require a variable number of small incisions in the abdomen or chest wall to place small trocars or "ports" that are used to pass instruments into the body cavity. These trocars are designed with a valve seal to maintain the carbon dioxide pneumoperitoneum necessary for abdominal distension and visualization by increasing the internal space available for manipulating surgical instruments. Size of the trocars varies from 3 mm up to 30 mm with 5, 10, and 12 mm the most common sizes. For many abdominal procedures, the umbilicus is a central site for laparoscopic camera port placement.

Many abdominal procedures are performed using traditional surgical incisions. The specific incision depends on many factors including the disease location, patient characteristics, and surgeon's preference. Many describe the location, while others are eponymous. Wherever possible the incisions should try to follow Langer lines,** and ideally muscles should be split and not cut. Familiarity with these incisions and common indications for their application is useful not only in the operating room but also when describing healed incisions as part of a physical examination (see Figure 24-2, page 812). Skin suturing techniques, surgical knot tying, and types of suture materials are reviewed in Chapter 25, Suturing Techniques and Wound Care, page 815.

1. **Battle incision.** A lower-right paramedian incision but placed more laterally than the standard paramedian incision; used for appendicitis.
2. **Kocher/subcostal incision.** Under the right rib cage, commonly used to access the gallbladder and biliary system. If extended to the opposite left subcostal incision, referred to as the chevron or rooftop incision.
3. **Lanz incision.** Transverse incision at McBurney's point (two-thirds from the umbilicus to the anterior superior iliac spine) used commonly for appendectomy.
4. **McBurney/gridiron incision.** Oblique muscle-splitting incision located one-third of the way from the iliac spine to the umbilicus used for appendectomy.
5. **Midline incision.** Allows the majority of the abdominal viscera and major vessels to be accessed. Can extend anywhere from the xiphoid process to the pubic symphysis.

24

**Langer lines are also called relaxed skin tension lines. Incisions made parallel to these lines of maximal tension will gap to a lesser extent.

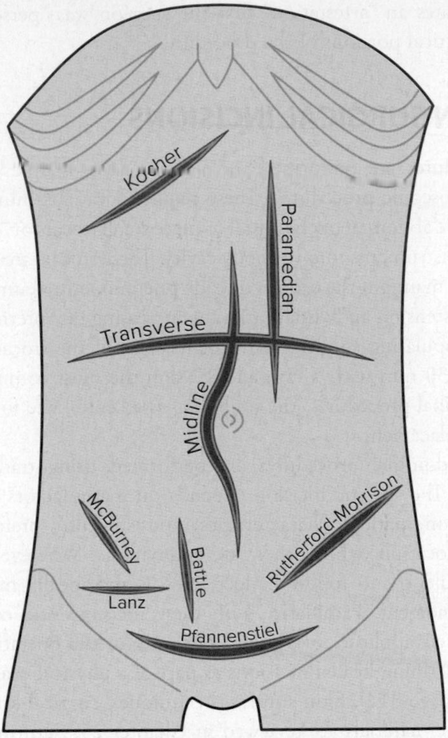

Figure 24-2.   Common abdominal surgical incisions (see text for descriptions).

6. **Paramedian incision.** Infrequently used to access kidneys, spleen, and adrenal glands.

7. **Pfannenstiel incision.** Lower abdominal transverse incision made below the umbilicus and 2–5 cm above the pubic symphysis. Used for pelvic surgery in females and males and for caesarean section; good cosmetic results.

8. **Rutherford-Morrison incision.** Can be performed in the right or left lower quadrant and often used for renal transplantation and colon procedures.

9. **Transverse incision.** Rarely used in adults to access the abdominal organs; more commonly used in the pediatric population.

UNIVERSAL PRECAUTIONS

All operating room personnel are at risk of infection with bloodborne infectious agents (e.g., HIV, hepatitis). To reduce the incidence of such transmission, the CDC has developed a set of guidelines called universal precautions. The underlying principle is that because patients cannot be routinely tested for HIV and are rarely tested preoperatively for transmissible diseases such as hepatitis, the safest policy is to treat all patients as though they have an infection. This approach ensures evenhanded treatment of all patients and the safest work environment for those exposed to the blood of others. (See also page 504).

Minimizing the risks to all who are in the OR requires constant vigilance. Movements must be coordinated among surgeon, assistant, and technician. Never use your fingers to pick up needles; pick them up only with another instrument. DO NOT use your fingers and hands as retractors. Two people should never be holding the same sharp instrument. Placing a sharp instrument down or handing it to another member of the team is always preceded by a verbal warning that notifies the recipient that a sharp object is about to be passed. Protective eyewear must be worn by all members of the operating team.

Double gloving is considered the best approach for universal precautions. This technique reduces the incidence of blood–skin contact, especially in light of the extraordinarily high incidence of unrecognized glove perforations. Until puncture-resistant gloves are developed, double gloving is the considered standard in most settings.

LATEX ALLERGY

People with medical conditions or occupations heavily exposed to products containing natural rubber latex may become sensitized to it and develop allergic reactions (~7% of healthcare workers). Some conditions, such as spina bifida, paraplegia, cerebral palsy, or allergy to bananas, chestnuts, avocados and others, predispose patients to an 18–40% incidence of allergy. Reactions vary from mild rash and itching to anaphylaxis and death. Latex products are found in a wide array of medical products, from gloves and drapes, to IV tubing and syringes. Some patients have documented latex allergy. Hospitals have latex allergy protocols in place and maintain an inventory of latex-free products that should be used in these cases. (See also page 514).

ASA PHYSICAL STATUS CLASSIFICATION SYSTEM

24

The American Society of Anesthesiologists (ASA) has developed the ASA Physical Status Scale. The system is used to assess and communicate a patient's preanesthesia medical comorbidities. The classification system alone does not predict the perioperative risks, but used with other factors (e.g., type of surgery, frailty, level of deconditioning), it can be helpful in predicting perioperative risks.

ASA I: Normal healthy patient; nonsmoker, no or minimal alcohol use

ASA II: Mild systemic disease; examples include current smoker, social alcohol consumption, pregnancy, obesity (BMI 30–40), well-controlled DM/HTN, mild pulmonary disease

ASA III: Severe systemic disease; has substantial functional limitations; examples include poorly controlled DM or HTN, COPD, morbid obesity (BMI ≥40), active hepatitis, alcohol dependence or abuse, pacemaker, reduced ejection fraction, on dialysis, premature infant, and history of greater than 3 mo since MI, CVA, TIA, or CAD/stents

ASA IV: Severe systemic disease that is a threat to life; examples include recent (<3 mo) since MI, CVA, TIA, or CAD/stents, ongoing cardiac ischemia, severe valvular heart disease, reduced ejection fraction, sepsis, DIC

ASA V: Moribund patient not expected to survive without the operation: ruptured abdominal/thoracic aneurysm, massive trauma, intracranial bleed with mass effect, ischemic bowel with significant cardiac disease

ASA VI: Brain-dead patient whose organs are being taken for donation purposes (https://www.asahq.org/standards-and-guidelines/asa-physical-status-classification-system, accessed May 19, 2020)

BASIC SURGICAL INSTRUMENTS

There are thousands of useful surgical instruments that can be found in an operating room. Among all of these tools, there are common items that are used in most cases regardless of the specialty. While a student in the operating room for the first time is not expected to be able to identify the name and use of surgical instruments, general familiarity will enhance your operating room experience and enhance your understanding of the procedure. Surgical instruments are often generally classified as cutting or incising, grasping, holding or clamping, suturing or stapling, retracting, suctioning, dilating, or measuring, to name a few broad categories. Common scalpels can be found in Chapter 19, Bedside Procedures starting on page 518. Suture and wound closure is discussed in Chapter 25 Suturing Techniques and Wound Care, page 815. Basic description and function of common surgical instruments can be found online at www.medicalstudentbook.com.

Suturing Techniques and Wound Care

- ➤ Wound Healing
- ➤ General Principles of Wound Closure
- ➤ Suture Materials
- ➤ Suturing Procedure
- ➤ Suturing Patterns
- ➤ Surgical Knots

- ➤ Suture Removal
- ➤ Skin Wound Stapling
- ➤ Tissue Adhesives
- ➤ Wound Closure Adhesive Tapes
- ➤ Wound Care
- ➤ Tetanus Prophylaxis
- ➤ Vacuum-Assisted Wound Closure

WOUND HEALING

The process of wound healing is generally divided into four stages: inflammation, fibroblast proliferation, contraction, and remodeling. There are three types of wound healing:

- **First intention**. The wound is closed by routine primary suturing, stapling, or gluing. Epithelialization occurs in 24–48 hr in an uninfected wound.
- **Secondary intention**. The wound is not closed by suturing, stapling, or gluing but closes by spontaneous contraction and epithelialization at a rate of 1 mm/day (granulation). Most often used for wounds that are infected and packed open.
- **Third intention**. (also called delayed primary closure). The wound is left open for a time and then sutured at a later date. Often used with grossly contaminated wounds.

GENERAL PRINCIPLES OF WOUND CLOSURE

The decision on how to close a wound is based on many factors. They include the nature of the wound (traumatic vs. intentional wounds such as in the operating room, crush, or puncture wounds), location (e.g., scalp,

Chapter update by Patrick Greaney, MD, FACS, and Leonard Gomella, MD, FACS

face, trunk, and joint), degree of contamination, patient factors (allergies, diabetes, and patient age), and physician preference. Primary closure of wounds is usually the preferred approach unless there is significant contamination, obvious infection (pus, severe inflammation, or redness), or delayed presentation of traumatic wounds (beyond 12 hr on the body or 24 hr on the face). Traumatic wounds with concerning characteristics can often be managed with oral antibiotics and packed with saline-soaked gauze packing using a wet-dry closure method that debrides the wound over several days with closure by either secondary (granulation) or third intention (delayed primary closure). Puncture wounds that cannot be irrigated and any wound associated with an abscess cavity should not be closed. Consideration is also given not to close certain animal or human bites due to the risk of infection. Bites that are closed should also be given antibiotics and re-evaluated for signs of infection.

Bleeding from the wound itself (not associated with major vascular injury) should be controlled with direct pressure or using 1% epinephrine with lidocaine topically or by infiltration. Caution is recommended in the use of epinephrine in digits, tip of the nose, ears, and the penis. Wounds can be closed by suture, staples, tissue adhesives, and wound closure adhesive strips.

SUTURE MATERIALS

(See Tables 25-1 and 25-2, Page 817)

Suture materials can be broadly defined as absorbable and nonabsorbable. **Absorbable sutures** can be thought of as temporary and include plain catgut, chromic catgut, and synthetic materials such as polyglactin 910 (Vicryl), polyglycolic acid (Dexon), and poliglecaprone (Monocryl). Left inside the body, these materials are resorbed after a variable period of time. Polydioxanone (PDS) is a longer-lasting absorbable suture. **Nonabsorbable sutures** can be thought of as "permanent" unless they are removed; these materials include silk, stainless steel wire, polypropylene (Prolene), and nylon.

The size of a suture is defined by the number of zeros. The more zeros in the number, the smaller the suture diameter. For example, a 5-0 suture (00000) is much smaller than a 2-0 (00) suture. Most sutures come prepackaged and mounted on needles ("swaged on"). **Cutting needles** are used for tough tissues such as skin, and **tapered needles** are used for more delicate tissues such as intestine. The most common needle for skin closure is the ⅜-circle cutting needle.

Additionally, some sutures are designed as "barbed" sutures, distributing tension along the entire length of the suture and without the need to tie knots to secure the wound. Examples include V-Loc and Stratafix sutures.

Table 25-1. Common Absorbable Suture Materials

Suture (Brand Names)	Description	Tensile Strength[a]	Absorbed	Common Uses
Fast catgut	Twisted/fast absorption	3–5 d	30 d	Facial lacerations in children
Plain catgut	Twisted/ rapidly absorbable	7–10 d	70 d	Vessel ligation, subcutaneous tissues
Chromic catgut	Twisted/ absorbable	10–14 d	90 d	Mucosa
Polyglycolic acid (Dexon)	Braided/ absorbable	14–21 d	60–90 d	GI, subcutaneous tissues
Polyglactin 910 (Vicryl Rapide)	Braided/ absorbable	5 d	42 d	Skin repair needing rapid absorption
Polyglactin 910 (Vicryl)	Braided/ absorbable	21 d	56–70 d	Bowel, deep tissue
Poliglecaprone 25 (Monocryl)	Monofilament/ absorbable	7–14 d	91–119 d	Skin, bowel
Polydioxanone (PDS)	Monofilament/ absorbable	28 d	6 mo	Fascia, GI
Polyglyconate (Maxon)	Braided/ absorbable	28 d	6 mo	GI, muscle, fascia
Panacryl	Braided/ absorbable	>6 mo	>24 mo	Fascia, tendons

[a]When suture loses approximately 50% strength.

Table 25-2. Common Nonabsorbable Suture Materials

Suture (Brand Names)	Description	Common Uses
Polytetrafluoroethylene (PTFE) (Gore-Tex)	Monofilament	Vascular grafts, hernia, valve repair
Nylon (Dermalon, Ethilon)	Monofilament	Skin, drains
Nylon (Nurolon)	Braided	Tendon repair
Polyester (Ethibond, Tycron)	Braided	Cardiac, tendon
Polypropylene (Prolene)	Monofilament	Vessel, fascia, skin
Silk	Braided	GI, vessel ligation, drains
Stainless steel	Monofilament	Fascia, sternum

25

SUTURING PROCEDURE

The following guidelines cover suture repair of lacerations in the emergency setting with similar principles holding true for closure of wounds in the operating room and for minor bedside procedures. The choice of suture material is based on many factors, including location, extent of the laceration, strength of the tissues, and preference of the physician. Some common suture choices:

- **Face**: 5-0 or 6-0 nylon or polypropylene when appearance is important
- **Scalp**: 3-0 nylon or polypropylene
- **Trunk and extremities**: 4-0 or 5-0 nylon or polypropylene

Use 3-0 and 4-0 absorbable sutures such as Dexon or Vicryl to approximate deep tissues. Close skin with interrupted sutures placed with good approximation and minimal tension or with a running subcuticular suture. Use tissue adhesives or stapling techniques selectively (see page 828 and 823). Suturing wounds is preferred where precise approximation is needed, such as lacerations involving the vermillion border of the lip. Sutures or staples should always be used in settings where the wound may be under tension, such as the hands, feet, or over joints. Suture patterns are discussed in the next section. Suture marks ("tracks") are the result of excessive tension on the tissue or leaving the sutures in too long. In most cases the length of time (see above) and the technique used are more important in determining the final result than is the type of suture used.

1. Prepare all necessary items, use sterile gloves, and drape the wound if possible.
2. Local anesthesia may be necessary before any of these steps. Remove all foreign materials and devitalized tissues by sharp excision (debridement). If all the debris is not removed, traumatic "tattooing" of the skin can result. If hair will interfere with the closure, shaving the site is discouraged as this increases the chance of infection. In these cases use a scissor to clip the hair. Alternatively, sterile lubricant can be applied and the hair combed away from the closure.
3. Obtain a surgical consultation before suturing infected or contaminated wounds, lacerations more than 6–12 hr old (24 hr on the face), missile wounds, and human or animal bites.
4. **A. Local anesthesia consideration in adults.** Anesthetize the wound by infiltrating it with an agent such as 0.5% or 1% lidocaine (Xylocaine). The maximum safe dose is 4.5 mg/kg (about 28 mL of a 1% solution in an adult). Lidocaine and other local anesthetic agents are available with epinephrine (1:100,000 or 1:200,000) added to produce local vasoconstriction that prolongs the anesthetic effect and helps decrease systemic side effects and bleeding. Use epinephrine with caution, particularly in treatment of patients with a history of hypertension, and do not use epinephrine on the fingers, toes,

Table 25-3. Local Anesthetic Comparison Chart for Commonly Used Injectable Agents

Agent	Proprietary Names	Onset	Duration	Maximum Dose mg/kg	Maximum Dose Volume in 70-kg Adult[a]
Bupivacaine	Marcaine, Sensorcaine	7–30 min	5–7 hr	3	70 mL of 0.25% solution
Lidocaine	Xylocaine, Anestacon	5–30 min	2 hr	4	28 mL of 1% solution
Lidocaine with epinephrine (1:200,000 or 1:100,000)	Xylocaine with epinephrine	5–30 min	2–3 hr	7	50 mL of 1% solution
Mepivacaine	Carbocaine	5–30 min	2–3 hr	7	50 mL of 1% solution
Procaine	Novocain	Rapid	30 min–1 hr	10–15	70–105 mL of 1% solution

[a]To calculate the maximum dose if the patient is not a 70-kg adult, use the fact that a 1% solution has 10 mg of drug per milliliter.

or penis (concern for vasoconstriction). One milliliter of 1:10 $NaHCO_3$ can be mixed with 9 mL of lidocaine to help minimize the discomfort of the injection, which is due to the relatively acidic nature of lidocaine. Commonly used local anesthetics are compared in Table 25-3, above. (Note that commercially available lidocaine cannot be buffered to a less acidic and less painful form as this increase in pH decreases the shelf life and degrades the product. Bupivacaine should not be buffered in this fashion.)

   B. Local anesthesia consideration in children. With smaller, uncomplicated lacerations in children, topical forms of anesthetic (gel or liquid) **lidocaine-epinephrine-tetracaine**, commonly referred to as **LET**, can be applied 20–30 minutes before the wound is sutured. Use up to 3 mL of either formulation. LET should not be used on mucosal surfaces or on the penis, digits, nose, or ears.

5. When using injectable local anesthetics, always aspirate before injecting to prevent intravascular injection of the drug. Anesthetize with a 26- to 30-gauge needle. Symptoms of toxicity from local anesthetics include twitching, restlessness, drowsiness, light-headedness, and seizures.

6. Clean the wound with plain saline solution or sterile water. A useful technique involves irrigation with at least 200 mL of saline through a 35-mL

25

syringe and a 19-gauge needle. If there is a grossly contaminated wound, bite wound, or for wounds that are several hours old, a dilute povidone/iodine solution diluted 1:10 with normal saline can be used for irrigation. In general, avoid other antiseptic solutions and povidone/iodine surgical scrub solution as these can result in impaired wound healing due to tissue toxicity.

7. Close the wound using one of the suturing patterns discussed in the next section. To decrease trauma, use a fine-toothed forceps (formally called Adson or Brown-Adson) with gentle pressure to handle the skin edges. Toothed forceps are *less damaging* to the skin than other forceps with flat surfaces that can crush the tissue, causing more damage.

8. Cover the wound and keep it dry for at least 24–48 hr. Dry gauze or Steri-Strips are sufficient. Antibiotic ointment can also prevent the dressing from sticking to the wound. On the face, simply cover the wound with antibiotic ointment, especially around the eyes and mouth. After that time, *epithelialization is complete* in healthy patients with uninfected wounds. The patient may shower and wet the wound without increasing the risk of infection but should not soak the wound in a bath.

9. Address tetanus and antibacterial prophylaxis, particularly for contaminated wounds (Table 25-4, page 832).

SUTURING PATTERNS

Opinions vary greatly on the ideal technique for skin closure. The following are the common techniques of skin approximation. Critical to any suturing technique is making certain that the edges of the wound closely approximate without overlapping or inversion and that there is no tension. Remember "approximation without strangulation" or eversion of the skin edges gives the best results (Figure 25-1). Figures 25-2 through 25-6 illustrate the commonly used suturing patterns. These include simple interrupted suture (Figure 25-2), running (locked or unlocked) suture (Figure 25-3), vertical mattress suture (Figure 25-4), horizontal mattress suture (Figure 25-5), and subcuticular suture (Figure 25-6).

SURGICAL KNOTS

There are three basic knot-tying techniques: one-handed and two-handed ties and the instrument tie. The most advanced knot-tying technique is a one-handed tie, not recommended for medical students or junior residents. Although one-handed ties can be more useful in certain situations (e.g., deep cavities or need for speed), the two-handed tie is easier to learn. Instrument ties are more useful for closing skin and for emergency department laceration repair. Figure 25-7, page 825, shows the technique for tying a two-handed square knot, the standard surgical knot that should be learned first.

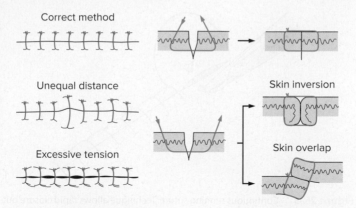

Figure 25-1. Proper method for simple interrupted suturing of a skin wound compared with incorrect techniques that result in poor or excessive scars from skin overlap, skin inversion, or necrosis of the skin edges due to excessive tension.

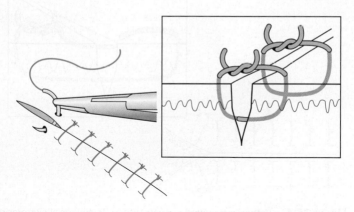

Figure 25-2. Simple interrupted sutures. "Bites" are taken through the thickness of the skin, and the width of each stitch should equal the distance between sutures to avoid inverting the skin edges.

25

Figure 25-8, pages 827 and 828, shows the technique for a one-handed tie. Figure 25-9, page 829, shows the technique for an instrument tie.

SUTURE REMOVAL

The longer a permanent suture is left in place in the skin, the more scarring it produces. Using a topical antibiotic ointment (e.g., Polysporin) on the wound is helpful in decreasing suture tract epithelialization. Epithelialization

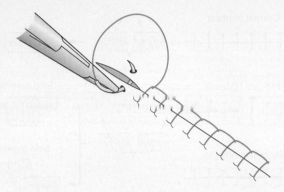

Figure 25-3. Continuous running suture. Technique allows rapid closure but depends on only two knots for security and may not allow precise approximation of the skin edges. "Locking" each stitch, as shown, may increase scarring.

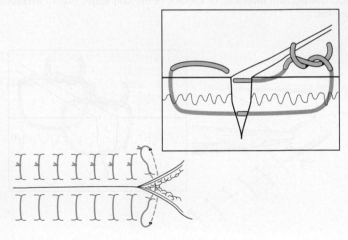

Figure 25-4. Vertical interrupted mattress sutures. Technique allows precise approximation of skin edges with little tension but can result in more scarring than simple stitches. Needle is placed in the skin in a "far, far, near, near" sequence.

25

results from crusting around the suture that increases suture marks and subsequent scarring. Sutures can be safely removed when a wound has developed sufficient tensile strength. Situations vary greatly, but general guidelines for removing sutures from different areas of the body are as follows: face and neck, 3–5 d; scalp and body, 5–7 d; and extremities, 7–12 d. Any suture material or skin clips can be removed earlier if they have been reinforced with a deep absorbable suture or with application of Steri-Strips after the suture is removed. Steri-Strips stay in place more securely if tincture of benzoin (spray or solution)

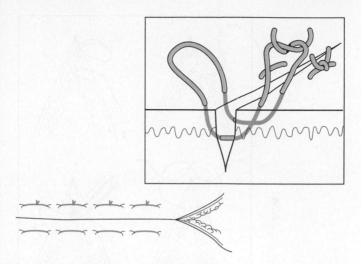

Figure 25-5.   Horizontal interrupted mattress sutures. This everting stitch is more frequently used in fascia than in skin. It is often used in calloused skin, such as the palms and soles.

is applied to the skin and allowed to dry before the Steri-Strips are applied. The length of time absorbable sutures remain in tissues is shown in Table 25-1.

1. Gently clear away any dried blood with saline solution and gauze. Verify that the wound is sufficiently healed to allow suture removal and there is no evidence of infection. Use a forceps to gently elevate the knot off the skin. This step can be uncomfortable for the patient.
2. Cut the suture as close to the skin as possible so that a minimal amount of "dirty suture" is dragged through the wound. When removing continuous sutures, cut and pull out each section individually. **Never** pull a knot through the skin. Often the suture material is pulled tight to the skin, and it is difficult to remove the stitch with thick scissors. A no. 11 scalpel (see page 518) with the blade pointed up is helpful in this situation.

SKIN WOUND STAPLING

25

Wound closure can be accomplished by several techniques based on the characteristics of the wound. Suturing and tissue adhesives are described elsewhere in this chapter. A common technique used in the operating room for clean linear incisions is through the use of a mechanical stapler. Use of skin staples is commonplace in the OR because of the rapidity of closure and the nonreactive nature of the steel staples. The stapling technique may also be appropriate for linear lacerations through the dermis in

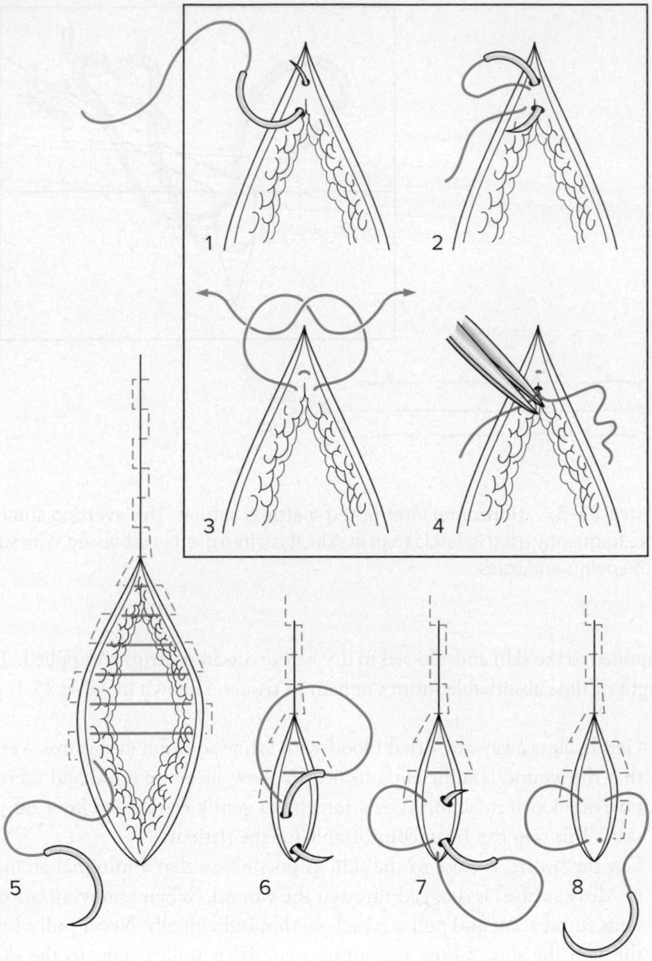

Figure 25-6. Subcuticular closure is usually performed with continuous, horizontally applied intradermal sutures. These sutures are ideal for linear cosmetic closure because they eliminate possible cross-hatching deformities. If nonabsorbable suture material (e.g., 5-0 or 6-0 Prolene) is used, the knot is placed on the skin and pulled taut. If absorbable (5-0 or 6-0 Dexon or Vicryl) is used, the knot is usually buried as shown. The knot is tied in step 8, the needle passed through the skin, and the suture material cut flush.

the outpatient setting and may provide superior outcomes for scalp lacerations when compared to routine suturing. Staples are not recommended in the following settings: where cosmetics are important (do not use on neck or face) or wounds on the hands or feet. Accidental needle sticks are avoided by the use of the stapler.

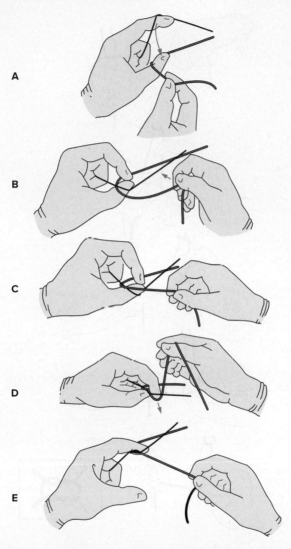

Figure 25-7. Technique for tying a two-handed square knot. Suture ends are uncrossed as step A begins. Two-handed square knot. Hands must be crossed at the end of the first loop tie (step F) to give a flat knot; hands are not crossed at the end of the second loop tie (step J). (Continued)

25

1. For emergency situations, follow the basic wound anesthesia and cleaning steps for suturing noted on page 818.
2. Using a fine-toothed forceps (Adson or Brown-Adson), evert the skin edges. In the operating room setting, an assistant can evert the skin edges.

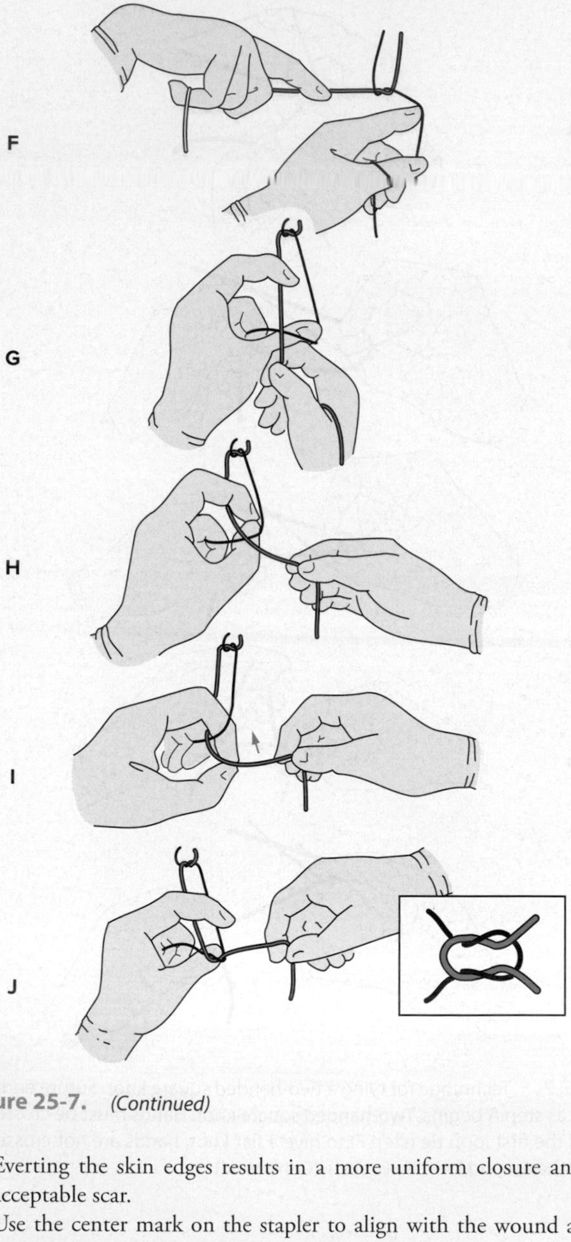

F

G

H

I

J

Figure 25-7. *(Continued)*

Everting the skin edges results in a more uniform closure and a more acceptable scar.

3. Use the center mark on the stapler to align with the wound and apply enough contact pressure without causing the skin to indent.

4. Fire the stapler by squeezing the handle. When properly placed, the staple should not be flush against the skin with a small space between the wound and staple. As a rule of thumb, staples should be placed no less than 0.5 cm apart.

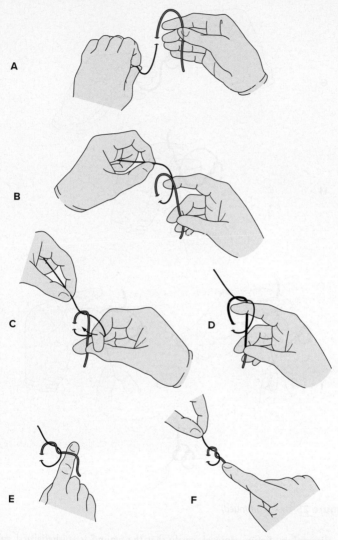

Figure 25-8. (A) One-handed tie. The right hand sets up the loop and manipulates the working strand. (B) One-handed tie technique continued.

5. Wound care is similar to standard suturing, including the duration of the removal.

6. Staples are typically removed 3–5 d after surgery (abdominal incisions). Reinforce the incision with Steri-Strips and benzoin. When removing skin staples, make sure that the staple is completely reformed (see Figure 25-10) before pulling it out of the skin to decrease patient

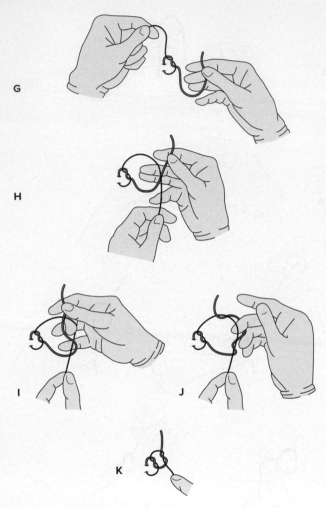

G

H

I

J

K

Figure 25-8. *(Continued)*

25

discomfort. Before removal, verify that the wound is epithelialized and that there is no sign of infection or wound leakage. If the wound gaps or if a discharge appears as the staples are removed, stop the removal procedure and ask a senior physician to evaluate the wound. Figure 25-10 demonstrates the technique for skin staple removal.

TISSUE ADHESIVES

2-Octyl cyanoacrylate (Dermabond/SurgiSeal) and *n*-2-butyl-cyanoacrylate (Indermil/Histoacryl/GluStitch/GluSeal/PeriAcryl/LiquiBand) are topical

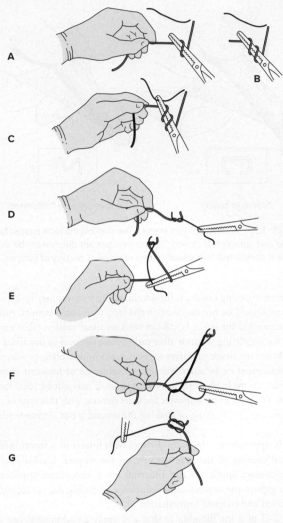

Figure 25-9. The instrument tie. Begin with either a single or double (illustrated) looping of the lower end of the suture around the needle holder. The first loop is laid flat without crossing the hands. Hands must be crossed after the second loop tie (step G) to produce a flat square knot.

25

skin adhesives similar to cyanoacrylate glue that hold wound edges together. These substances are useful in closure of topical skin incisions and lacerations in areas of low skin tension that are simple, thoroughly cleansed, and have easily approximated skin edges. Adhesives can be used in conjunction with, but not in place of, deep dermal stitches. They are particularly useful

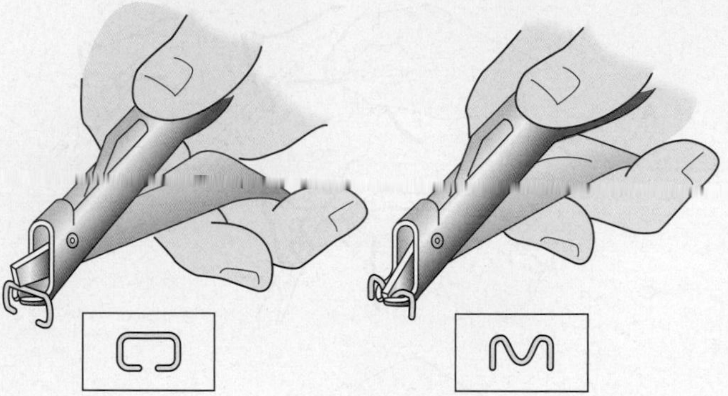

Staple in place   Removed staple "reformed"

Figure 25-10. Removal of skin staples. The staple remover is passed beneath the staple and completely closed. To decrease patient discomfort, be sure that the staple is completely "reformed" before removal. (Courtesy of Ethicon, Inc.)

in treatment of young children, for whom suture removal may be a problem. The wound should be nonmucosal on the face, torso, or extremity. Adhesives are recommended for wounds <8 cm with minimal tension (skin gap <0.5 cm) and for stabilizing wounds after early suture removal to minimize suture marks. Do not use tissue adhesives for puncture wounds, bites, or wounds that need debridement or in anatomic regions subjected to frequent movement (e.g., joints). Actively bleeding or oozing wounds may not be ideal for tissue adhesives. The patient may shower for brief periods with this type of closure and pat the site dry. Bathing or soaking the wound is not recommended.

1. Gently approximate the wound edges with fingers or a forcep and place a small coating of the glue directly on the wound. Dermabond has a direct-contact applicator tip; Indermil has a noncontact applicator tip. Small gaps in the wound can be ameliorated during the curing process if identified and coapted immediately.
2. Wait 2–3 min for the glue to dry, and apply an additional one or two coats if needed. The glue sheds in 5–10 d.
3. Once the glue is in place and stable, it is not necessary to use topical medication or ointment. If the adhesive remains tacky, too much glue has been applied.

WOUND CLOSURE ADHESIVE TAPES

Wound closure tapes such as Steri-Strips can be used in clean linear lacerations that are not subject to tension. They may be useful in the elderly and are useful to reinforce incisions after suture or staple removal.

WOUND CARE

Fresh properly closed incisions and lacerations epithelize superficially within 48 hr. Wounds may become primarily or secondarily infected and necrotic due to a variety of factors, such as wound dehiscence, pressure ulcers, diabetes, venous or arterial insufficiency, or other conditions that compromised healing. In these cases, wound management requires a multidisciplinary team approach relying on skilled nursing care and engagement of the patient and his/her family or caretaker. Some nurses have WOCN (**W**ound, **O**stomy, and **C**ontinence **N**ursing) advanced training to assist in wound management.

Chronic wounds tend to heal best in a "moist" environment with the exception of the wound that is ischemic and necrotic. The latter must be kept dry to minimize the development of gangrene. Examples of some wound care dressing products with some common brand names are shown here.

- **Wet to Dry Dressing Changes.** A wet or moistened gauze with normal saline or packing dressing is put on the wound and allowed to dry. The drainage and necrotic tissue is mechanically debrided when taking off the old dressing. If the dressing is adherent it can be moistened. The wound usually heals by granulation.
- **Hydrocolloids (e.g., DuoDERM, Exuderm).** Helps with wounds with minimal drainage that have necrosis and sloughing tissue.
- **Transparent films (e.g., 3M Tegaderm, ClearSite, OPSITE).** Most useful on delicate/fragile skin as a cover dressing for hydrocolloids and foams. Also secures IV and central line sites. Protects site but allows oxygen exchange. Not for infected wounds.
- **Foams (e.g., Polyderm, Lyofoam).** Foam covered by a hydrophilic polyurethane or gel that maintains a moist wound environment and is highly absorbent. Suitable for light to heavy draining wounds but not for wounds with a dry eschar.
- **Alginates (e.g., AQUACEL, KALGINATE).** Absorbs exudate and facilitates autolytic debridement.
- **Hydrogels (e.g., DermaGauze, Flexigel).** For dry or low exudate wounds. For low drainage wounds, may require a secondary dressing to secure. For all wound types including necrotic and dry wounds.

25

TETANUS PROPHYLAXIS

(See Table 25-4 below)

A tetanus toxoid–containing vaccine is indicated for wound management when >5 years have passed since the last tetanus toxoid–containing vaccine dose. If a tetanus toxoid–containing vaccine is indicated for persons aged

Table 25-4. Tetanus Prophylaxis

History of Absorbed Tetanus Toxoid Immunization	Clean, Minor Wounds		All Other Wounds[a]	
	Td[b]	TIG[c]	Td[b]	TIG[c]
Unknown or <3 doses	Yes	No	Yes	Yes
3 doses[d]	No[e]	No	No[f]	No

[a]Such as, but not limited to, wounds contaminated with dirt, feces, soil, saliva, etc.; puncture wounds; avulsions; and wounds resulting from missiles, crushing, burns, and frostbite.
[b]Td = tetanus–diphtheria toxoid (adult type), 0.5 mL IM.
  • For children <7 y of age, DPT (DT, if pertussis vaccine is contraindicated) is preferred to tetanus toxoid alone.
  • For persons >7 y of age, Td is preferred to tetanus toxoid alone.
  • DT = diphtheria–tetanus toxoid (pediatric), used for those who cannot receive pertussis.
[c]TIG = tetanus immune globulin, 250 U IM.
[d]If only three doses of fluid toxoid have been received, then a fourth dose of toxoid, preferably an absorbed toxoid, should be given.
[e]Yes, if >10 y since last dose.
[f]Yes, if >5 y since last dose.

≥11 years, Tdap is preferred for persons who have not previously received Tdap or whose Tdap history is unknown. If a tetanus toxoid–containing vaccine is indicated for a pregnant woman, Tdap should be used. For nonpregnant persons with documentation of previous Tdap vaccination, either Td or Tdap may be used if a tetanus toxoid–containing vaccine is indicated. Complete information on tetanus prophylaxis and the use of tetanus immunoglobulin when indicated for wound management is available at https://www.cdc.gov/mmwr/volumes/67/rr/rr6702a1.htm, accessed September 20, 2021.

VACUUM-ASSISTED WOUND CLOSURE

Vacuum-assisted closure (negative pressure wound therapy), commonly referred to as a "wound vac" or "vac," is used for healing both acute and chronic wounds. Continuous negative pressure is distributed over the wound surface. The system consists of a soft sponge cut to fit and occupy the volume of the wound, a plastic tube imbedded in the center of the sponge and extending out of the wound to a controlled suction pump, and a gas- and fluid-impermeable plastic outer film that adheres to the back of the sponge and the surrounding normal skin. Vacuum-assisted closure allows "active" removal of extracellular debris (exudate). Soft-tissue defects heal faster when subatmospheric pressure is applied. Used for wounds resulting from pressure, trauma, infection, IV extravasation, A-V insufficiency, and skin grafting. Newer "incisional VAC" devices are also available and are designed to be placed over closed incisions that continue to drain following stapled or sutured closures.

Respiratory Care 26

- ➤ Respiratory Therapy
- ➤ Pulmonary Function Tests (PFTs)
- ➤ Differential Diagnosis of PFTs
- ➤ Oxygen Supplementation
- ➤ Pulse Oximetry
- ➤ Postoperative Pulmonary Care
- ➤ Bronchopulmonary Hygiene
- ➤ Aerosol (Nebulizer) Therapy

- ➤ Topical Medications
- ➤ Inhalers
- ➤ Chest Physiotherapy
  - ▷ Incentive Spirometry
  - ▷ Flutter Devices (Acapella©, Aerobika©, Cornet©)
  - ▷ High Frequency Chest Wall Oscillation Device

RESPIRATORY THERAPY

Respiratory therapy is a vital component of healthcare. For any patient, initial medical care begins with assessment of the ABCs: **A**irway, **B**reathing, and **C**irculation. Respiratory therapy includes key components of airway and breathing management and support. The objective is the care of all types of patients with cardiopulmonary diseases. Functions of the respiratory therapist include emergency care, airway management, ventilatory support, oxygen therapy, aerosol therapies, chest physiotherapy (CPT), physiologic monitoring, and pulmonary diagnostics. Special precautions relating to disease transmission due to aerosol generating respiratory procedures are reviewed in Chapter 19 on page 508.

PULMONARY FUNCTION TESTS (PFTs)

Pulmonary function tests (PFTs) are essential in the diagnosis of a variety of pulmonary disorders. Common PFTs include spirometry, lung volume determinations, and diffusing capacity. Other components include maximal voluntary ventilation (MVV), maximal inspiratory effort (MIP), and maximal expiratory effort (MEP). Important spirometric measurements include forced vital capacity (FVC), forced expired volume in 1 s (FEV_1), and FEV_1/FVC. Spirometry results indicate the presence of obstructive airway diseases

---

Chapter update by Jessica Most, MD

such as asthma or chronic obstructive pulmonary disease (COPD) when the FEV_1/FVC ratio is <0.70 or <LLN (lower limit of normal). A fixed ratio of <0.70 should be used in adults 65 years or older who are at risk for COPD. The LLN should be used for younger patients or never smokers. Both methods can lead to over- and underdiagnosis. If the FVC is <LLN and the FEV_1/FVC ratio is normal, this suggests restrictive lung diseases such as interstitial lung disease or neuromuscular disease. Restrictive lung disease must be confirmed by lung volume testing.

Obtain spirometry before and after administration of bronchodilators unless contraindicated to evaluate for reversible obstruction. A bronchodilator response is considered significant if the FEV_1 or the FVC improves by 12% and at least 200 mL.

Order lung volumes, determined by helium dilution or body plethysmography, to definitively diagnose restrictive lung disease. Restriction is present when TLC <80% of predicted normal. Hyperinflation is present if TLC >120%, and air trapping is present if residual volume (RV)/TLC is >50%. A reduction in diffusing capacity is used in the diagnosis of interstitial lung disease and pulmonary vascular disease. Spirometry and diffusing capacity should be measured in all patients being considered for lung resection surgery.

Normal PFT values vary with age, sex, race, and body size. Normal values for a given patient are established from studies of healthy populations and are provided along with the results. The most commonly used data set is from the Third National Health and Nutrition Examination Survey (NHANES III) or the Global Lung Function Initiative (GLI). Typical volumes and capacities are illustrated in Figure 26-1, page 835, with normal values in Table 26-1.

- **Tidal Volume (TV):** Volume of air moved during a normal breath on quiet respiration
- **Functional Residual Capacity (FRC):** Volume of air in the lungs after a normal tidal expiration (FRC = residual volume + expiratory reserve volume)
- **Total Lung Capacity (TLC):** Volume of air in the lungs after maximal inspiration
- **Forced Expired Volume in 1 Second (FEV_1):** Measured after maximum inspiration, the volume of air that can be expelled in 1 s
- **Forced Vital Capacity (FVC):** Maximum volume of air that can be forcibly expired after full inspiration
- **Vital Capacity (VC):** Maximum volume of air that can be exhaled from the lungs after a maximal inspiration
- **Residual Volume (RV):** The volume of air remaining in the lungs at the end of a maximal exhalation

DIFFERENTIAL DIAGNOSIS OF PFTs

Table 26-1 shows the differential diagnosis of various PFT patterns. When interpreting PFTs, remember that some patients may have combined

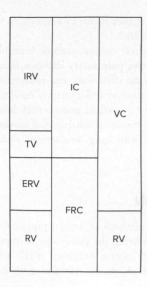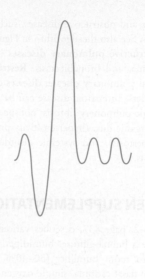

VC = vital capacity
RV = residual volume
FRC = functional residual capacity
TV = tidal volume

ERV = expiratory reserve volume
IRV = inspiratory reserve volume
IC = inspiratory capacity

Figure 26-1. Lung volumes used in the interpretation of pulmonary function testing.

Table 26-1. Differential Diagnosis of Pulmonary Function Tests

Test	Restrictive Disease	Obstructive Disease	
FVC	↓	N or ↓	
TLC	↓	↑	
FEV₁/FVC	N or ↑	↓	
FEV₁	↓	↓	
OBSTRUCTIVE AIRWAYS DISEASE (COPD)			
Test	Normal	Mild	Moderate	Severe
FEV₁ (% of VC)	>75	60–75	40–60	<40
RV (% of predicted)	80–120	120–150	150–175	>200
RESTRICTIVE LUNG DISEASE			
Test	Normal	Mild	Moderate	Severe
FVC (% of predicted)	>80	60–80	50–60	<50
FEV₁ (% of VC)	>75	>75	>75	>75
RV (% of predicted)	80–120	80–120	70–80	<70

N = normal; ↑ = increased; ↓ = decreased; FVC = forced vital capacity; TLC = total lung capacity; RV = residual volume; FEV₁ = forced expiratory volume in 1 s; VC = vital capacity

26

restrictive and obstructive diseases, such as coexistence of emphysema and asbestosis. See also the algorithm in Figure 26-2.

Obstructive pulmonary diseases include asthma, chronic bronchitis, emphysema, and bronchiectasis. **Restrictive pulmonary diseases** include interstitial pulmonary disease, diseases of the chest wall, and neuromuscular disorders. Interstitial disease can be caused by inflammatory conditions (idiopathic pulmonary fibrosis, nonspecific interstitial pneumonia), inhalation of organic dust (hypersensitivity pneumonitis), inhalation of inorganic dust (asbestosis), and systemic disorders with lung involvement such as sarcoidosis.

OXYGEN SUPPLEMENTATION

Table 26-2, page 837, describes various methods of oxygen supplementation. Use a bubble-diffuser humidifier to bring the percentage of inspired gas up to room humidity (30–40% of relative humidity [RH]) when using the nasal cannula, simple oxygen mask, partial rebreathing mask, or

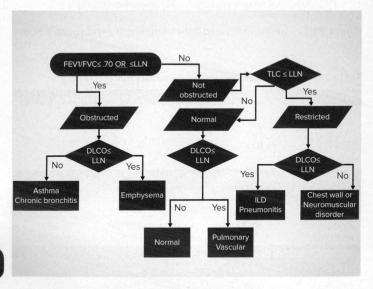

Figure 26-2. Assessment of lung functions associated with various pulmonary disorders. Based on guidelines from the American Thoracic Society (https://www.thoracic.org/statements, accessed December 24, 2019). LLN: lower limit of normal, TLC: total lung capacity, DLCO: diffusing capacity for carbon monoxide, FEV$_1$: forced expired volume in 1 s, ILD: interstitial lung disease, VC: vital capacity.

Table 26-2. Various Methods of Oxygen and Humidity Supplementation (Illustrative Oxygen Delivery Devices Are Shown in Figure 26-3)

Type of O_2 Delivery	Flow Rates	FiO_2	How to Titrate	Notes
Low-flow nasal cannula	1–6 L/min	Each L/min adds ~4% FiO_2 above room air[a] 1 L/min = 24% 2 L/min = 28% 3 L/min = 32% 4 L/min = 36% 5 L/min = 40% 6 L/min = 44%	Titrate flow rate only	Best for patients with normal respiratory rates and tidal volumes
Simple face mask	~6–12 L/min	35–60%[a]	Titrate flow rate only	Minimum of 6 L/min flow is required to prevent re-breathing CO_2
Venturi mask	Fixed flow based on adapter chosen	Adapters are usually available in 24%, 28%, 31%, 35%, 40%	Titrate FiO_2 only	Adapter entrains a set amount of ambient air to deliver a fixed FiO_2
Non-rebreather mask	10–15 L/min	100%	Nontitratable	Short-term bridge therapy only
High-flow nasal cannula	Up to 60 L/min	30–100%	Titrate flow rate and FiO_2	Administers PEEP with high flow rate

[a]FiO_2 varies with fluctuations in the patient's minute ventilation with use of a nasal cannula. This is not true with use of a Venturi mask because it is a "high-flow oxygen enrichment system" that supplies three times the patient's minute ventilation, thus providing an exact FiO_2.
COPD = chronic obstructive pulmonary disease; FiO_2 = fraction of inspired oxygen.
Source: Navin Kumar, Anica Law. Teaching Rounds: A Visual Aid to Teaching Internal Medicine Pearls on the Wards, McGraw-Hill Education, www.accessmedicine.com (Reproduced with permission)

26

non-rebreathing mask. This helps to prevent nasal dryness. High-flow oxygen therapy can deliver high-flow air/oxygen blend with humidification. This has reduced the need for noninvasive ventilation and intubation in patients with type I respiratory failure. (Type I respiratory failure involves low oxygen, and normal or low carbon dioxide levels. Type II respiratory failure involves low oxygen, with high carbon dioxide.) Some commonly used devices for delivering oxygen supplementation are shown in Figure 26-3.

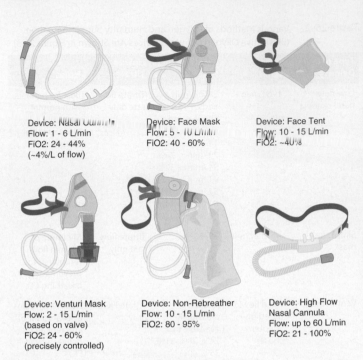

Device: Nasal Cannula
Flow: 1 - 6 L/min
FiO2: 24 - 44%
(~4%/L of flow)

Device: Face Mask
Flow: 5 - 10 L/min
FiO2: 40 - 60%

Device: Face Tent
Flow: 10 - 15 L/min
FiO2: ~40%

Device: Venturi Mask
Flow: 2 - 15 L/min
(based on valve)
FiO2: 24 - 60%
(precisely controlled)

Device: Non-Rebreather
Flow: 10 - 15 L/min
FiO2: 80 - 95%

Device: High Flow
Nasal Cannula
Flow: up to 60 L/min
FiO2: 21 - 100%

Figure 26-3. Commonly used delivery devices for oxygen supplementation. (Reprinted with permission from Rishi Kumar, MD (https://rk.md).)

PULSE OXIMETRY

Considered an additional vital sign by some providers, pulse oximetry ("pulse ox") is a measure of peripheral arterial oxygen saturation or SpO_2. It allows relatively rapid noninvasive continuous monitoring of oxygenation. It relies on spectrophotometry to determine the proportion of oxyhemoglobin (hemoglobin saturated with oxygen) in the peripheral arterial blood. Before the widespread use of pulse ox, direct arterial puncture was the only method available to assess oxygenation. The device consists of an emitter and detector and is usually placed on the fingers, toes, or ear lobes with other sites such as the forehead sometimes used. Complications of the use of pulse ox are extremely rare. Pulse ox techniques can also be used in neonates to detect congenital heart disease. It is indicated when there is concern about hypoxemia.

There are some limitations to the use of pulse ox in clinical care. There is a delay in the processing of the value due to multiple determinations and signal averaging over several seconds. This may cause a delay of up to 1 min that can be important in situations such as emergency resuscitation. Since $PaCO_2$ is not measured, the pulse ox cannot measure the adequacy of ventilation and it cannot detect hyperoxemia. The pulse ox does not directly measure arterial oxygen tension or PaO_2, and significant changes in oxygen saturation (SpO_2) in children and in adults on supplemental oxygen may not be apparent until extreme hypoxia is present.

There is no uniform consensus as to the "normal" values of pulse ox as the findings can vary by patient characteristics (such as COPD), temperature, pH, and other variables. **A common definition of normal at sea level on room air at rest is a SpO_2 >95%. With exertion or exercise the value should not decrease by more than 5%.** Errors in pulse ox can be caused by carboxyhemoglobin in carbon monoxide (CO) poisoning, methemoglobinemia, sickle cell disease, applying nail polish on the fingers, artifacts (poor probe positioning), and other conditions.

POSTOPERATIVE PULMONARY CARE

After a surgical procedure with general anesthesia, the patient needs close observation and good respiratory support. This care includes good suctioning and lateral turning of the head to prevent aspiration. The airway must be patent, and ensure adequate oxygenation and ventilation. For high-risk patients, including those with obstructive sleep apnea, maintain intubation until it has been clearly determined that the patient can maintain spontaneous ventilation and wakefulness. Determine the capability for maintaining spontaneous ventilation by using the following parameters. (Issues related to extubation are also reviewed in Chapter 28.)

- Ability to follow commands
- Vital capacity >15 mL/kg
- Inspiratory force >20 cm water
- Expiratory force >25 cm water
- Blood gases with normal $PaCO_2$ (<44 mm Hg) and pH (>7.35) during spontaneous breathing
- Adequate PaO_2

Administer a judicious regimen of analgesics to control pain but not inhibit the respiratory center. Avoid dressings that restrict chest wall and abdominal excursion. The implementation of the **I COUGH program** has reduced postoperative pulmonary complications including pneumonia and respiratory failure (AMA Surg. 2013 Aug; 148(8):740–5). I COUGH includes: **I**ncentive spirometry, **c**oughing and deep breathing, **o**ral care (brushing teeth twice daily), **u**nderstanding (patient and family education), **g**etting out of bed three times daily, and **h**ead of bed elevation.

26

BRONCHOPULMONARY HYGIENE

Bronchopulmonary hygiene techniques are used by the respiratory care and nursing services of most hospitals to maintain clear airways and removal of secretions from the tracheobronchial tree. This is often referred to as "pulmonary toilet." This therapy is important for routine postoperative surgical patients, medical patients with obstructive pulmonary diseases, patients with neuromuscular weakness, and any patient with excessive respiratory secretions. The techniques used include nebulizer therapy, inhalers, CPT, incentive spirometry, flutter devices, and the use of high frequency chest wall oscillation. These techniques are reviewed beginning in the next section.

AEROSOL (NEBULIZER) THERAPY

Aerosolized medications such as bronchodilators and mucolytic agents can be delivered via nebulizer to spontaneously breathing, awake patients or intubated patients. The function of a nebulizer is to convert medications into a mist that is more easily inhaled and delivered to the distal airways. Nebulizer therapy is less dependent on the patient's coordination and cooperation. However, it is more time-consuming, less efficient, and more costly than delivery through a smaller hand-held metered-dose inhaler (MDI) or dry powder inhaler. **(NOTE: Nebulizer therapy is considered an aerosol generating procedure requiring additional precautions. See Chapter 19, page 508.)**

Indications
- Management of COPD, acute asthma, cystic fibrosis, and bronchiectasis
- Inducing sputum for diagnostic tests

Goals
- Relief of bronchospasm
- Decreasing the viscosity to enable clearing of secretions

To Order: Specify the following:
- Frequency
- Heated or cool mist
- Medications: In sterile water or normal saline
- FiO_2
- *Example:* Albuterol 2.5 mg in 3 mL of sterile saline, FiO_2 0.28

TOPICAL MEDICATIONS

The following agents can be added to aerosol therapy to prevent or manage pulmonary complications caused by bronchospasm, mucosal congestion, and inspissated secretions. Even though these are primarily topical agents, systemic absorption can occur. Medications noted here are typically delivered via a nebulizer. A more comprehensive listing of inhaled agents suitable for hand-held devices or nebulizer can be found in Table 26-3.

Albuterol (Ventolin, Proventil): A short-acting selective bronchodilator with principally beta-2 activity; can cause tachycardia. It can also be used to treat acute hyperkalemia. Albuterol can cause a lactic acidosis. Onset 15 min after administration. Peak effect at 0.5–1 hr, duration 3–5 hr. *Usual Adult Dosage:* 2.5 mg in 3 mL NS q4h.

Levalbuterol (Xopenex): L-isomer of short-acting albuterol; more expensive but this form causes less tachycardia. If used more often than every 6 hr, it loses the selective effect that decreases tachycardia. Onset 15 min after administration. Peak effect at 0.5–1 hr, duration 3–5 hr. *Usual Adult Dosage:* 0.63–1.25 mg in 3 mL NS q6h.

Racemic Epinephrine: Contains both D- and L-forms of epinephrine. Alpha-adrenergic effects cause mucosal vasoconstriction to reduce mucosal engorgement, and bronchodilation lessens the risk of hypoxemia. Most useful for laryngotracheobronchitis, immediately after extubation in children, and in the treatment of acute laryngeal edema. *Usual Adult Dosage:* 0.125–0.5 mL (3–10 mg) in 2.5 mL NS.

Ipratropium Bromide (Atrovent): A parasympatholytic agent that causes bronchodilation and decreases secretions with "drying" of the respiratory mucosa. Minimally absorbed and rarely causes tachycardia. Onset 45 min after administration. Duration 4–6 hr. *Usual Adult Dosage:* 0.5 mg in 3 mL NS every 6 hr.

Hypertonic Saline: Concentrated sodium chloride comes in either 3% or 7% concentrations and is used to thin secretions. It can cause coughing as well as bronchospasm and is often used with albuterol. It is used for patients with mucus plugging or to induce sputum production. *Usual Adult Dosage:* 4 mL of 3% or 7% sodium chloride nebulized every 8–12 hr.

INHALERS (See Table 26-2, page 837)

All bronchodilating agents and inhaled corticosteroids can be effectively delivered by **metered-dose inhaler (MDI)** or **dry powdered inhaler (DPI)** as long as the patient can cooperate and proper technique is used. For these devices to be successful, inpatients must be well trained or have the assistance of a nurse or respiratory therapist. Albuterol and ipratropium bromide (Atrovent) can be delivered two puffs q4h. A combination bronchodilator (Combivent) containing the equivalent of one puff of each provides synergistic bronchodilation. The use of a holding chamber (spacer) can improve drug deposition when using MDIs, especially in patients with poor inhaler technique. Some inhalers are taken daily and are "controllers" or maintenance medications.

26

26

Table 26-3. Some Inhaled Drugs for Treatment of Asthma. Inhaled short-acting beta-2 agonists (SABAs) such as albuterol are the drugs of choice for acute asthma symptoms. With persistent symptoms, maintenance treatment with an inhaled corticosteroid (ICS) is recommended. For patients who remain symptomatic, adding of an inhaled long-acting beta-2 agonist (LABA) is recommended. (Based on data from: Drugs for Asthma. Med Lett Drugs Ther 2017;59:139; updated April 25, 2019.)

Drug	Common Formulations	Delivery Device	Usual Adult Dose
Short-Acting Beta -2 Agonists (SABAs)			
Albuterol—*ProAir HFA*	90 mcg/inh	HFA MDI (200 inh/unit)	1–2 inh q4-6h PRN
• *Proventil HFA*			
• *Ventolin HFA*			
• *ProAir Respiclick*	90 mcg/inh	DPI (200 inh/unit)	1–2 inh q4-6h PRN
• generic—single-dose vials	0.63, 1.25, 2.5 mg/3 mL soln	Nebulizer	1.25–5 mg q4-6h PRN
Levalbuterol—*Xopenex HFA*	45 mcg/inh	HFA MDI (200 inh/unit)	2 inh q4-6h PRN
• *Xopenex*			
• generic	0.31, 0.63, 1.25 mg/3 mL soln	Nebulizer	0.63–1.25 mg q6-8h PRN
Inhaled Short-Acting Muscarinic Antagonist (SAMA)			
Ipratropium—(Not FDA-approved to treat asthma)	17 mcg/inh	HFA MDI (200 inh/unit) Nebulizer	2 inh (34 mcg) qid PRN
• *Atrovent HFA*	200 mcg/mL		500 mcg qid PRN
• generic—single-dose vials			
Inhaled Corticosteroids (ICSs)			
Beclomethasone dipropionate—*QVAR Redihaler*	40, 80 mcg/inh	HFA MDI (120 inh/unit) Breath-activated MDI that does not require hand/breath coordination or priming and should not be used with a spacer	40–320 mcg bid Low: 80–160 mcg/d Medium: >160–320 mcg/d High: >320 mcg/d

(Continued)

Budesonide— • *Pulmicort Flexhaler*	90, 180 mcg/inh	DPI (60, 120 inh/unit)	180–720 mcg bid Low: 180–360 mcg/d Medium: >360–720 mcg/d High: >720 mcg/d
• *Pulmicort Respules generic*	0.25, 0.5, 1 mg/2 mL single-dose ampules	Nebulizer	—
Ciclesonide—*Alvesco*	80, 160 mcg/inh	HFA MDI (60 inh/unit)	80–320 mcg bid Low: 80–160 mcg/d Medium: >160–320 mcg/d High: >320 mcg/d
Flunisolide—*Aerospan HFA*	80 mcg/inh	HFA MDI (120 inh/unit)	160–320 mcg bid Low: 320 mcg/d Medium: >320–640 mcg/d High: insufficient data
Fluticasone furoate—*Arnuity Ellipta*	100, 200 mcg/inh	DPI (30 inh/unit)	100–200 mcg once/d Low: Not available Medium: 100 mcg/d High: 200 mcg/d
Fluticasone propionate— • *Flovent Diskus*	50, 100, 250 mcg/blister	DPI (60 inh/unit)	100–1000 mcg bid Low: 100–250 mcg/d Medium: >250–500 mcg/d High: >500 mcg/d

(Continued)

26

843

Table 26-3. Some Inhaled Drugs for Treatment of Asthma. Inhaled short-acting beta-2 agonists (SABAs) such as albuterol are the drugs of choice for acute asthma symptoms. With persistent symptoms, maintenance treatment with an inhaled corticosteroid (ICS) is recommended. For patients who remain symptomatic, adding of an inhaled long-acting beta-2 agonist (LABA) is recommended. (Based on data from: Drugs for Asthma. Med Lett Drugs Ther 2017;59:139; updated April 25, 2019.) (Continued)

Drug	Common Formulations	Delivery Device	Usual Adult Dose
• *Flovent HFA*	44, 110, 220 mcg/inh	HFA MDI (120 inh/unit)	88–880 mcg bid Low: 88–220 mcg/d Medium: >220–440 mcg/d High: >440 mcg/d
• *ArmonAir Respiclick*	55, 113, 232 mcg/inh	DPI (60 inh/unit)	55–232 mcg bid Low: 110 mcg/d Medium: 226–464 mcg/d High: >464 mcg/d
Mometasone furoate— • *Asmanex HFA*	100, 200 mcg/inh	HFA MDI (120 inh/unit)	200–400 mcg bid Low: 100–200 mcg/d Medium: >200–400 mcg/d High: >400 mcg/d
• *Asmanex Twisthaler*	110, 220 mcg/inh	DPI (30, 60, 120 inh/unit)	220–880 mcg once/d in evening or 220 mcg bid Low: 110–220 mcg/d Medium: >220–440 mcg/d High: >440 mcg/d
Long-Acting Beta-2 Agonist (LABA)			
Formoterol—*Perforomist*	20 mcg/2 mL	Nebulizer	20 mcg bid
Salmeterol—*Serevent Diskus*	50 mcg/blister	DPI (28, 60 inh/unit)	1 inh bid
Aformoterol—*Brovana*	15 mcg/2 mL	Nebulizer	15 mcg bid

Inhaled Corticosteroids/Long-Acting Beta-2 Agonist (LABA) Combinations

Budesonide/formoterol—*Symbicort*	80, 160 mcg/4.5 mcg/ inh	HFA MDI (60, 120 inh/unit)	2 inh bid
Fluticasone furoate/vilanterol—*Breo Ellipta*	100, 200 mcg/25 mcg/ʳnh	DPI (30 inh/unit)	1 inh once/d
Fluticasone propionate/salmeterol—			
• *Advair Diskus* (GSK) *Wixela Inhub*	100, 250, 500 mcg/ 50 mcg/ blister	DPI (60 inh/unit)	1 inh bid
• *Advair HFA*	45, 115, 230 mcg/21 mcg/inh	HFA MDI (60, 120 inh/unit)	2 inh bid
• *AirDuo Respiclick* generic	55, 113, 232 mcg/14 mcg/inh	DPI (60 inh/unit)	1 inh bid
Mometasone/formoterol— *Dulera*	100, 200 mcg/5 mcg/ inh	HFA MDI (60, 120 inh/unit)	2 inh bid

Long-Acting Muscarinic Antagonist (LAMA)

Tiotropium—*Spiriva Respimat*	1.25 mcg/inh 2.5 mcg/inh	ISI (60 inh/unit) is also available as a DPI, which is FDA-approved only for use in patients with COPD	2 inh once/d
Aclidinium—*Tudorza*	400 mcg/inh	DPI	1 inh bid
Umeclidinium—*Incruse*	62.5 mcg/inh	DPI	1 inh bid
Revefenacin—*Yupelri*	175 mcg/3 mL	Nebulizer	175 mcg daily

(Continued)

26

Table 26-3. Some Inhaled Drugs for Treatment of Asthma. Inhaled short-acting beta-2 agonists (SABAs) such as albuterol are the drugs of choice for acute asthma symptoms. With persistent symptoms, maintenance treatment with an inhaled corticosteroid (ICS) is recommended. For patients who remain symptomatic, adding of an inhaled long-acting beta-2 agonist (LABA) is recommended. (Based on data from: Drugs for Asthma. Med Lett Drugs Ther 2017;59:139; updated April 25, 2019.) (Continued)

Drug	Common Formulations	Delivery Device	Usual Adult Dose
LABA/LAMA			
Glycopyrrolate/formoterol fumarate—*Bevespi*	9 mcg/ 4.8 mcg/inh	MDI	2 inh bid
Tiotropium/olodaterol—*Stiolto*	2.5 mcg/2.5 mcg/inh	ISI	2 inh daily
Umeclidinium/vilanterol—*noro*	62.5 mcg/25 mcg/inh	DPI	1 inh daily
Triple therapy: LAMA/LABA/ICS			
Budesonide/glycopyrrolate/formoterol fumarate—*Breztri*	160 mcg/9 mcg/4.8 mcg	MDI	2 inh bid
Fluticasone/umeclidinium/vilanterol—*Trelegy*	100 mcg/62.5 mcg/25 mcg/inh 200 mcg/62.5 mcg/25 mcg/inh	DPI	1 inh daily
Nonselective Alpha and Beta Agonist			
Racemic epinephrine (generic)	(3–10 mg) in 2.5 mL NS	Inh nebulizer	0.125–0.5 mL
Epinephrine—Primatene Mist (OTC)	0.125 mg/inh	HFA inhaler	1–2 inh every 4 hr; Max 8 inh/24 hr

DPI = dry powder inhaler; HFA = hydrofluoroalkane; ICS = inhaled corticosteroid; inh = inhalation; ISI = inhalation spray inhaler; LABA = long-acting beta-2 agonist; LAMA = long-acting beta-2 agonist; MDI = metered-dose inhaler; SABA = short-acting beta-2 agonist; soln = solution; OTC = over the counter

These should be continued when admitted to the hospital. Some medications are taken on an as needed basis and are considered "rescue" medications. See Table 26-3 for a listing of some of the common inhaled drugs for the treatment of conditions such as asthma or used for bronchopulmonary hygiene.

CHEST PHYSIOTHERAPY

CPT can include both manual techniques: percussion and postural drainage (P&PD) along with cough and deep breathing exercises (TC&DB) and use of devices. CPT is used to mobilize or loosen secretions in the lungs and respiratory tract and is especially helpful for patients with large amounts of secretions or ineffective cough. Manual CPT positions the patient so that the involved lobes of the lung are in a dependent drainage position. A cupped hand or vibrator is used to percuss the chest wall. Nasotracheal (NT) suctioning is quite uncomfortable for patients but is still useful in the appropriate clinical setting in the absence of severe coagulopathy especially in those with a weak cough reflex. Other types of CPT include the use of high-frequency chest wall oscillation (HFCWO) devices, flutter devices, and positive expiratory pressure (PEP) devices. PEP and flutter devices may be superior to standard CPT. HFCWO and incentive spirometry are as effective as standard chest PT. (NOTE: CPT is considered an aerosol generating infection control procedure requiring additional infection control precautions. See Chapter 19, page 508.)

Indications
• Management of pneumonia, mucus plugging, atelectasis, and diseases resulting in weak or ineffective coughing

To Order
1. **P&PD:** Specify the following:
   o Frequency
   o Segments or lobes involved (e.g., right upper lung [RUL])
   o Duration
   o Drainage only
2. **TC&DB:** Order on a timed schedule or as needed
   o *Example:* P&PD four times daily of RUL and RML, 5 min/lobe or TC&DB q4h

Incentive Spirometry

Encourages the patient to make a maximal and sustained inspiratory effort to help reinflate the lungs or prevent atelectasis.

Indications
- Treatment of patients at risk of postoperative pulmonary complications
- Management and prevention of atelectasis, especially in the postoperative setting

Goals: Set for the patient depending on the device used:
- Moving "Ping Pong" balls while inhaling using the respiratory therapy device

To Order: Specify the following:
- Frequency (e.g., 10 min q1-2h while patient is awake or 10 repetitions q1h while patient is awake)
- Device (if you have a preference)
- *Example:* Incentive spirometry 10 repetitions every hour while awake

Flutter Devices (Acapella©, Aerobika©, Cornet©)

While patient exhales into the device, positive expiratory pressure and cyclic oscillations are generated through the airways. This leads to mucus loosening and movement into the central airways.

Indications
- Mucus plugging
- Bronchiectasis

To Order
- Frequency (every 4–6 hr while awake). Three sets of 15 exhalations performed over 10–15 min. Each set should be followed by "huff" cough (deep coughing).
- Device (depends on availability)
- *Example*: Acapella 3 sets of 15 exhalations Q6 hours while awake

High-Frequency Chest Wall Oscillation Device

This device is made up of an air-pulse generator and an inflatable vest. The vest inflates and deflates rapidly to help loosen secretions. It is often used in the treatment of cystic fibrosis.

Indications
- Mucus plugging
- Bronchiectasis

To Order
- Frequency: two to four times per day

26

- Duration: 10–30 min with breaks for "huff" coughing, frequently used with nebulized medication
- Specifications: indicate pressure and frequency of oscillations
- *Example:* HFCWO @ 50 cm H20 and 525 HZ or as tolerated by patient every 8 hr for 20 min while receiving albuterol via nebulizer

Basic ECG Interpretation

27

BASIC PRINCIPLES

The formal procedure for obtaining an electrocardiogram (ECG) is given in Chapter 19, page 563. Every ECG should be approached in a systematic, stepwise manner. Many automated ECG machines can give a preliminary interpretation of a tracing; however, all automated interpretations require analysis and sign-off by a physician. When reading an ECG determine each of the following:

- **Standardization.** With the ECG machine set on 1 mV, a 10-mm standardization mark (0.1 mV/mm) is evident (Figure 27-1).
- **Axis.** If the QRS is upright (more positive than negative) in leads I and aVF, the axis is normal. The normal axis is −30 degrees to +105 degrees.
- **Intervals.** Determine the PR, QRS, and QT intervals (Figure 27-2). Intervals are measured in the limb leads. The PR should be 0.12–0.20 s, and the QRS, <0.10 s (0.10–<0.12) incomplete bundle branch block (BBB), ≥0.12 s complete BBB. The QT interval increases with decreasing heart rate, usually <0.44 s. The QT interval usually does not exceed one half of the RR interval (the distance between two R waves).

Chapter update by Allison L. Bailey, MD, FACC, FAACVPR and Steven A Haist, MD, MS

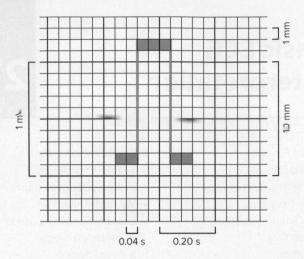

Figure 27-1. Examples of 10-mm standardization mark and time marks and standard ECG paper running at 25 mm/s.

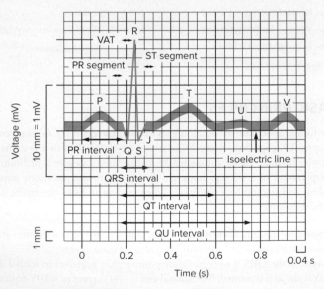

Figure 27-2. Diagram of the ECG complexes, intervals, and segments. The U wave is normally not well seen. VAT = ventricular activation time

27

- **Rate.** Count the number of QRS cycles on a 6-s strip and multiply that number by 10 to roughly estimate the rate. If the rhythm is regular, you can be more exact in determining the rate by dividing 300 by the number of 0.20-s intervals (usually depicted by darker shading) between two QRS complexes and then extrapolating for any fraction of a 0.20-s segment.

- **Rhythm.** Determine whether each QRS is preceded by a P wave, look for variation in the PR interval and RR interval (the duration between two QRS cycles), and look for ectopic beats.
- **Hypertrophy.** One way to detect LVH is to calculate the sum of the S wave in V_1 or V_2 plus the R wave in V_5 or V_6. A sum ≥ 35 mm indicates LVH. Additional criteria for LVH are R >11 mm in aVL or R in I + S in III >25 mm.
- **Infarction or Ischemia.** Check for ST-segment elevation or depression, Q waves, inverted T waves, and poor R wave progression in the precordial leads (see page 868, Myocardial Infarction).

Equipment

Bipolar Leads
- Lead I: Right arm (–) to left arm (+)
- Lead II: Right arm (–) to left leg (+)
- Lead III: Left arm (–) to left leg (+)

Augmented Unipolar Limb Leads
- aVR: Right arm and the average potential between L arm and L leg
- aVL: Left arm and the average potential between R arm and L leg
- aVF: Left leg and the average potential between L arm and R arm

Precordial Leads: V_1 to V_6 across the chest (see Figure 19-16, page 564).

ECG Paper: With the ECG machine set at 25 mm/s, each small box represents 0.04 s, and each large box 0.2 s (see Figure 27-1). ECG machines automatically print a standardization mark. Normal standard is considered 10 mm per 1 mV.

Normal ECG Complex

Note: A small amplitude in the Q, R, or S wave is represented by a lowercase letter. A large amplitude is represented by an uppercase letter. The pattern shown in Figure 27-2 can also be noted qRs.

- **P Wave.** Caused by depolarization of the atria. With normal sinus rhythm, the P wave is upright in leads I, II, aVF, V_4, V_5, and V_6 and inverted in aVR.
- **QRS Complex.** Represents ventricular depolarization.
- **Q Wave.** The first negative deflection of the QRS complex (not always present and, if present, may be pathologic). To be significant, the Q wave should be $>25\%$ of the QRS complex.
- **R Wave.** The first positive deflection; sometimes occurs after the Q wave.
- **S Wave.** The negative deflection following the R wave.
- **T Wave.** Caused by repolarization of the ventricles and follows the QRS complex, normally upright in leads I, II, V_3, V_4, V_5, and V_6 and inverted in aVR.

27

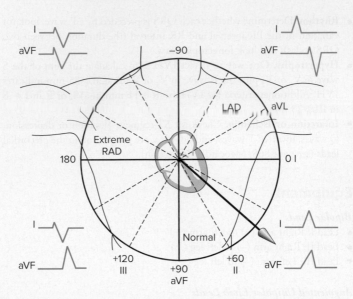

Figure 27-3. Graphic representation of axis deviation. ECG representations of each type of axis are shown in each quadrant. Large arrow indicates normal axis.

AXIS DEVIATION

Axis represents the sum of the vectors of the electrical depolarization of the ventricles and gives an idea of the electrical orientation of the heart in relation to the body. In a healthy person, the axis is downward and to the left (Figure 27-3). The QRS axis is midway between two leads that have QRS complexes of equal amplitude, or the axis is 90 degrees to the lead in which the QRS is isoelectric (i.e., R wave amplitude equals S wave amplitude).

- **Normal Axis.** QRS positive in I and aVF (0–90 degrees). Normal axis is −30 to 105 degrees.
- **Left Axis Deviation (LAD).** QRS positive in I and negative in aVF, −30 to −90 degrees
- **Right Axis Deviation (RAD).** QRS negative in I and positive in aVF, +105 to +180 degrees
- **Extreme RAD.** QRS negative in I and negative in aVF, +180 to +270 or −90 to −180 degrees

Clinical Correlations

- **RAD.** Seen with RVH, RBBB, COPD, and acute PE (a sudden change in axis toward the right) and occasionally in healthy persons
- **LAD.** Seen with LVH, LAHB (−45 to −90 degrees), LBBB, and obesity and in some healthy persons

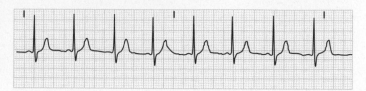

Figure 27-4.   Sample strip for rapid rate determination. In method 1, estimate the rate by counting the number of beats (eight) in two 3-s intervals. The rate is 8 × 10, or 80 beats/min (method 1). In method 2, each beat is separated from the next by four 0.20-s intervals, so divide 300 by 4, and the rate is 75 beats/min. Because the beats are separated by exactly four beats, extrapolation is not necessary.

HEART RATE

Bradycardia: Heart rate <60 beats/min
Tachycardia: Heart rate >100 beats/min
Rate Determination: Figure 27-4, above

- **Method 1.** Note the 3-s marks along the top or bottom of the ECG paper (15 large squares). The approximate rate equals the number of cycles (i.e., QRSs) in a 6-s strip × 10.
- **Method 2** (for regular rhythms). Count the number of large squares (0.2-s boxes) between two successive cycles. The rate equals 300 divided by the number of squares between two QRS complexes. Extrapolate if the QRS complex does not fall exactly on the 0.2-s marks (e.g., if each QRS complex is separated by 2.4 0.20-s segments, the rate is 120 beats/min. The rate between two 0.20-s segments is 150 beats/min, and between three 0.20-s segments is 100 beats/min). Each of the five smaller 0.04-s marks between the second and third 0.20 mark would be 10 beats/min (150 − 100 = 50 ÷ 5). Because the rate is three of the 0.04-s marks from the second 0.20-s segment (or two of the 0.04-s marks from the third 0.20-s segment, depending on which way you count), the rate is 150 − 30 (or 100 + 20), or 120 beats/min.

Remember that the number of beats per minute for each 0.04-s mark varies depending on which two 0.20 marks they are associated with (e.g., between the fifth and sixth 0.20-s mark each 0.04 mark is 2 beats/min).

RHYTHM

Sinus Rhythms

27

Normal: Each QRS preceded by a P wave (which is positive in II and negative in aVR) with a regular PR and RR interval and a rate between 60 and 100 beats/min (Figure 27-5, below)

Sinus Tachycardia: Normal sinus rhythm with a heart rate >100 beats/min (Figure 27-6, below)

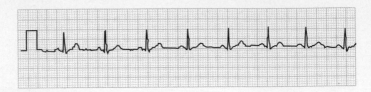

Figure 27-5. Normal sinus rhythm.

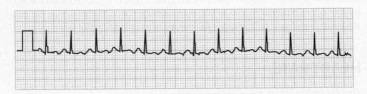

Figure 27-6. Sinus tachycardia. The rate is 120–130 beats/min.

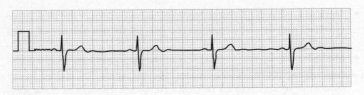

Figure 27-7. Sinus bradycardia. Rate is approximately 38–40 beats/min.

Clinical Correlations. Anxiety, exertion, pain, fever, hypoxia, hypotension, increased sympathetic tone (secondary to drugs with adrenergic effects [e.g., epinephrine]), anticholinergic effects (e.g., atropine), PE, COPD, AMI, CHF, hyperthyroidism, and others; inappropriate sinus tachycardia is a HR >100 for 24 hr with symptoms and not due to any of the above causes or as a physiologic response.

Treatment

- Treat the underlying problem; the tachycardia is a physiologic response to the underlying problem.
- Inappropriate sinus tachycardia: beta-blockers often ineffective; ivabradine effective but off-label use.

Sinus Bradycardia: Normal sinus rhythm with heart rate <60 beats/min (Figure 27-7)

Clinical Correlations. Well-trained athlete, normal variant, secondary to medications (e.g., amiodarone, beta-blockers, cimetidine, clonidine, digitalis, ivabradine, lithium, nondihydropyridine calcium channel blockers [verapamil, diltiazem], opioids, paclitaxel, thalidomide), acute myocardial infarction (inferior wall MI), hypothyroidism, hypothermia, sleep apnea, sick sinus syndrome (tachy–brady syndrome), disease and others.

Treatment

- If asymptomatic (good urine output, adequate BP, and normal sensorium), no treatment.
- If hypotension, support blood pressure, atropine, temporary pacing or permanent pacing if on critical medication causing the symptomatic sinus bradycardia (see Chapter 29, page 984).

Sinus Arrhythmia: Normal sinus rhythm with irregular heart rate. Inspiration causes a slight increase in rate; expiration decreases rate. Normal variation between inspiration and expiration is 10% or less.

Atrial Arrhythmias

Premature Atrial Contractions (PACs): Ectopic atrial focus firing prematurely followed by a normal QRS (Figure 27-8). The compensatory pause following the PAC is partial; the RR interval between beats 4 and 6 is less than between beats 1 and 3 and beats 6 and 8.

Clinical Correlations. Usually no clinical significance; caused by stress, caffeine, and myocardial disease.

Treatment

- Seldom needs treatment; if the patient is symptomatic, a beta-blocker can be used

Supraventricular Tachycardia (SVT): A run of three or more consecutive PACs. The rate is usually 140–250 beats/min. The P wave may not be visible, but the RR interval is very regular (Figure 27-9). SVT

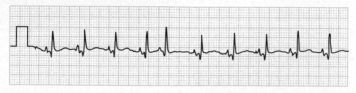

Figure 27-8.   Premature atrial contraction (PAC). Fifth beat is PAC.

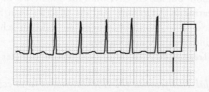

Figure 27-9.   Paroxysmal atrial tachycardia.

27

can be classified as **AV nodal reentrant tachycardia (AVNRT), AV reentrant tachycardia (AVRT)**, use of accessory pathway, narrow QRS complex vs wide QRS complex (delta wave present with anterograde conduction), and **atrial tachycardia** (secondary to increased automaticity of a group of atrial cells).

Clinical Correlations. Some healthy persons; heart disease. Symptoms: palpitations, light-headedness, syncope, dyspnea, chest pounding, and anxiety.

Treatment AVNRT

- **Cardioversion with Synchronized DC Shock.** In hemodynamically unstable conditions felt due to elevated heart rate (see Chapter 29, pages 976 and 990).
- **Increase Vagal Tone.** Valsalva maneuver, carotid massage, or cold water facial immersion.
- **Medical Treatment.** Can use adenosine, verapamil, IV beta-blockers (metoprolol, esmolol). Use verapamil and beta-blockers cautiously together because asystole can occur.

Treatment AVRT w Narrow QRS Complex

- **Cardioversion with Synchronized DC Shock.** In hemodynamically unstable conditions felt due to elevated heart rate (see Chapter 29, pages 976 and 990).
- **Increase Vagal Tone (first line).** Valsalva maneuver, carotid massage, or cold water facial immersion
- **Medical Treatment (second line).** Adenosine, verapamil, or diltiazem; IV beta-blockers or, IV procainamide can be used.
- **Long-Term Treatment.** Catheter ablation preferred

Treatment AVRT w Wide QRS Complex

- **Cardioversion with Synchronized DC Shock.** In hemodynamically unstable conditions felt due to elevated heart rate (see Chapter 29, pages 976 and 990).
- **Medical Treatment.** IV Ibutilide or IV procainamide. *Avoid use of medications that slow nodal conduction (adenosine, beta-blockers, verapamil)*
- **Long-Term Treatment.** Catheter ablation preferred

Treatment of Atrial Tachycardia

- **Address precipitating factors such as hypokalemia**
- **Increase Vagal Tone.** Valsalva maneuver, carotid massage, or cold water facial immersion, but less effective than for other types of SVT
- **Medical Treatment.** Adenosine but less effective than for other SVTs; IV beta-blockers or nondihydropyridine calcium channel blockers (verapamil, diltiazem); IV amiodarone
- **Long-Term Treatment.** Medications or consider catheter ablation

27

Multifocal Atrial Tachycardia (MAT): Originates from ectopic atrial foci; characterized by varying P wave morphology and PR interval and irregular rhythm (Figure 27-10).

Clinical Correlations. COPD, advanced age, CHF, diabetes, and theophylline use. Antiarrhythmics are often ineffective. Manage the underlying disease.

Treatment

- Treat underlying disease
- Must replace Mg^{++} and K^+ if low
- If rate control needed, beta-blockers (use with caution with COPD and CHF) or verapamil (use with caution with CHF)

Atrial Fibrillation: Irregularly irregular rhythm with no discernible P waves. Ventricular rate varies from 100–180 beats/min (Figure 27-11). The ventricular response may be <100 beats/min if the patient is taking digoxin, verapamil, or a beta-blocker or has AV nodal disease.

Clinical Correlations. Some healthy persons; CAD, hypertensive heart disease, valvular heart disease, cardiomyopathies, myocarditis, pericarditis, pre-excitation syndromes (WPW), cardiothoracic surgery, thyrotoxicosis, alcohol abuse, PE, and postoperative state.

Treatment

- **Cardioversion with Synchronized DC Shock.** In hemodynamically unstable conditions felt due to elevated heart rate (see Chapter 29, pages 976 and 990).
- **If unknown onset, recurrent, paroxysmal, or onset greater than 24–48 hr, or presence of left atrial thrombus, rheumatic/valvular dx, severe left ventricular dysfunction, CHF, DM, or prior thromboembolism, the patient should be anticoagulated before cardioversion unless hemodynamically unstable.**

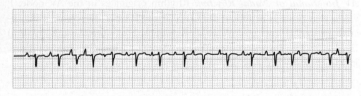

Figure 27-10. Multifocal atrial tachycardia.

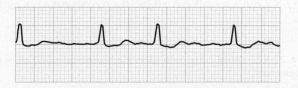

27

Figure 27-11. Atrial fibrillation (slow atrial fibrillation).

- **Pharmacologic Therapy (rate control).** IV verapamil or diltiazem (if ejection fraction normal and not hypotensive), beta-blockers (propranolol, metoprolol, esmolol), amiodarone, digoxin
- **Pharmacologic Therapy (rhythm control).** Amiodarone, sotalol, and dofetilide can be used to maintain or convert to sinus rhythm (see individual agents in Chapter 29, Common Medical Emergencies); catheter ablation effective in restoring sinus rhythm in select candidates

Atrial Flutter: Sawtooth flutter waves with an atrial rate of 250–350 beats/ min; rate may be regular or irregular depending on whether the atrial impulses are conducted through the AV node at a regular interval or at a variable interval (Figure 27-12).

Example. One ventricular contraction (QRS) for every two flutter waves = 2:1 conduction. A flutter wave may be buried within each QRS complex so if you see two flutter waves before each QRS complex, there is 3:1 flutter; one flutter wave before each QRS complex is 2:1 flutter (the second flutter is hidden in the QRS complex or the T wave).

Clinical Correlations. CAD, hypertensive heart dx, congenital heart dx, valvular heart dx, pericarditis, sick sinus syndrome, cardiothoracic surgery, thyrotoxicosis, alcohol abuse, PE, pulmonary disease.

Treatment
- **Rate Control:** Beta-blockers, calcium channel blockers (verapamil or diltiazem)
- **Conversion to NSR:** Ablation is preferred or ibutilide

Nodal Rhythm

AV Junctional or Nodal Rhythm: Rhythm originates in the AV node. P waves that precede or follow the QRS. If the P wave is present, it is negative in lead II and positive in aVR (opposite of normal sinus rhythm) (Figure 27-13). Three or more premature junctional beats in a row constitute junctional tachycardia, which has the same clinical significance as PAT.

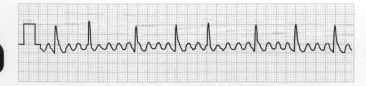

Figure 27-12. Atrial flutter with varying atrioventricular (AV) block (3:1 to 5:1 conduction).

Ventricular Arrhythmias

Premature Ventricular Contractions (PVCs): A premature beat arising in the ventricle. P waves may be present but there is no relation to the QRS of the PVC. The QRS is usually ≥0.12 s with a LBBB pattern. A compensatory pause follows a PVC that is usually longer than after a PAC (Figure 27-14). In the example below, the RR interval between beats 2 and 4 is equal to that between beats 4 and 6. Thus the pause following the PVC (the third beat) is fully compensatory. The following patterns are recognized:

- **Bigeminy.** One normal sinus beat followed by one PVC in an alternating manner (Figure 27-15).
- **Trigeminy.** Sequence of two normal beats followed by one PVC.
- **Unifocal PVCs.** Arise from one site in the ventricle. Each PVC has the same configuration in a single lead (see Figure 27-14).
- **Multifocal PVCs.** Arise from different sites and therefore have various shapes (Figure 27-16, below).

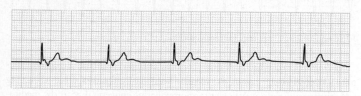

Figure 27-13. Junctional rhythm with retrograde P waves (inverted) following QRS complex.

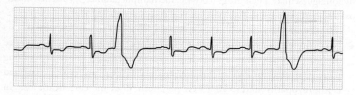

Figure 27-14. Premature ventricular contractions (PVCs). Third and seventh beats are PVCs.

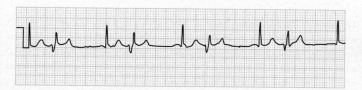

27

Figure 27-15. Ventricular bigeminy.

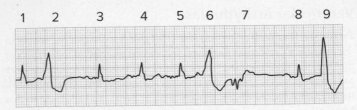

Figure 27-16. Multifocal PVCs. Second, sixth, and ninth beats are PVCs. Second and sixth PVCs have the same morphology.

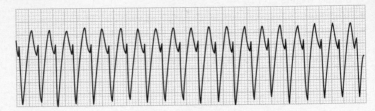

Figure 27-17. Ventricular tachycardia.

Clinical Correlations. Healthy persons, excessive caffeine ingestion, anemia, anxiety, ischemic heart dx, valvular heart dx, cardiomyopathies including arrhythmogenic right ventricular cardiomyopathy, congenital heart dx, medications (epinephrine, isoproterenol, digitalis, and amphetamines and theophylline toxicity), metabolic abnormalities (hypoxia, hypokalemia, acidosis, alkalosis, hypomagnesemia); illicit drugs (cocaine, methamphetamine, 3,4-Methyl enedioxy methamphetamine [MDMA, also called ecstasy and Molly]).

Treatment

- No treatment if **asymptomatic.** PVCs are generally benign in the absence of heart disease, and studies have shown increased mortality among patients treated for PVCs. However, frequent PVCs can result in a dilated cardiomyopathy and >10 PVCs per hour does increase death risk in patients with heart disease.
- If **symptomatic,** beta-blockers. Radiofrequency ablation for **right ventricular outflow tract (RVOT) tachycardia** in structurally normal hearts.

Ventricular Tachycardia: Three or more PVCs in a row (Figure 27-17). A wide QRS usually with a LBBB pattern (vs narrow complex seen with supraventricular tachycardia). May occur as short paroxysm or sustained run (>30 s) with rate of 120–250 beats/min. Can be life-threatening (hypotension and degeneration into ventricular fibrillation).

Clinical Correlations. See PVCs. Patients with a ventricular scar or aneurysm are more susceptible to arrhythmias, especially in the presence of other cardiac disease.

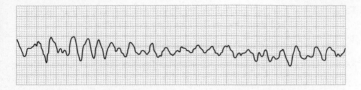

Figure 27-18.   Ventricular fibrillation.

Treatment. Management of nonsustained VT is controversial. If symptomatic, beta-blockers, then nondihydropyridine calcium channel blockers, and then amiodarone. If EF is decreased (<35%) implantable cardioverter defibrillator is recommended.

For sustained VT, to terminate rhythm and prevent recurrence beta-blockers, verapamil, amiodarone, sotalol, lidocaine. If EF is decreased (<35%) implantable cardioverter defibrillator is recommended.

See Chapter 29, pages 981 and 988.

Ventricular Fibrillation: Erratic electrical activity from the ventricles, which fibrillate or twitch asynchronously; no cardiac output (Figure 27-18).

Clinical Correlations. One of two patterns seen with cardiac arrest (the other is asystole/flat line).

Treatment. See Chapter 29, page 981.

Atrioventricular Block

Clinical correlations for atrioventricular block (first-, second-, third-degree, and high-degree AV block): (See Table 27-1)

First-degree: (see Figure 27-19): PR interval is ≥0.20 s

This is usually a benign finding.

Treatment. No treatment is needed; treat any underlying cause such as hypothyroidism

Second-degree: Periodic atrial impulses not conducted resulting in a P wave without an accompanying QRS complex

Mobitz type I **(Wenckebach)** (see Figure 27-20): PR interval progressively increases and then there is a dropped QRS (P wave without a QRS complex); usually this cycle will repeat with the next PR interval being similar to the first one in the previous cycle. A 3:2 conduction would be a cycle of three P waves with the first two PR intervals increasing from the first to the second PR interval, and then the third P wave is not conducted and then the pattern repeats.

Treatment. No treatment is needed; treat any underlying cause such as hypothyroidism

Mobitz type II. This is **NOT** considered a benign finding. PR interval between conducted P waves is constant and then a dropped QRS complex (P wave w/o a QRS complex) occurs. As with Mobitz type I, there is usually

27

Table 27-1. Clinical Correlations for Atrioventricular Block (first-, second-, and third-degree, and high-degree AV block)

Autonomic: increased vagal tone and carotid hypersensitivity

Cardiac surgery and procedures especially aortic value replacement and catheter ablation therapy

Congenital heart disease: left atrial isomerism, atrial septal defects (ASDs), transposition of the great arteries, endocardial cushion defects

Coronary artery disease: transient 3rd degree seen with inferior wall MI, while less common also seen with anterior wall MI, which often requires a permanent pacemaker and has a worse prognosis

Degenerative: usually seen in the elderly, also associated with chronic HTN and DM

Electrolyte abnormalities: hyperkalemia and hypermagnesemia (rare, usually iatrogenic)

Endocrine: hypothyroidism

Infectious: Lyme disease, Chagas disease, COVID-19, TB, bacterial abscess associated with infective endocarditis, viral myocarditis, acute rheumatic fever

Inflammatory: Rheumatoid arthritis (usually severe – erosive nodular disease), systemic lupus erythematosus (SLE), mixed connective tissue disease (MCTD), scleroderma

Infiltrative: amyloidosis, hemochromatosis, sarcoidosis

Medication induced: beta-blockers, dihydropyridine calcium channel blockers (verapamil and diltiazem), digoxin (especially with serum levels above therapeutic), class 1A antiarrhythmic drugs (disopyramide, procainamide, quinidine), class 3 antiarrhythmic drugs (amiodarone, dofetilide, ibutilide, sotalol), lithium

Neoplastic: lymphoma, carcinoma metastatic to the heart, multiple chemotherapeutic agents, radiation treatment

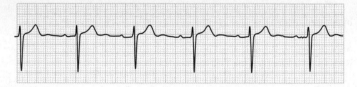

Figure 27-19. First-degree AV block. PR interval is 0.26 s.

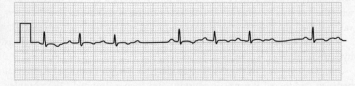

Figure 27-20. Second-degree AV block, Mobitz type I (Wenckebach) with 4:3 conduction.

a repetitive cycle. A 3:2 conduction would be a cycle of three P waves with the first two PR intervals being the same and then a third P wave without a QRS complex and then the pattern repeats. Mobitz type II is more malignant than type I and there is a significant risk of developing complete heart block.

Treatment. Frequently requires permanent pacing unless underlying reversible cause. **Symptomatic and hemodynamically unstable**: Atropine and then pacing (transcutaneous or transvenous); if hypotensive, add a pressor (dopamine) and treat any underlying cause. **Symptomatic and hemodynamically stable**: Monitor with pacing device available for immediate use and treat any underlying cause. **Asymptomatic**: Treat any underlying cause.

2:1 conduction of second-degree AV block. Cannot be easily differentiated as Mobitz type I or Mobitz type II based on a 12 lead ECG. A prolonged PR interval increases the likelihood of Mobitz type 1; however, this is not definitive.

High-degree AV block: Conduction is less than 2:1, meaning two or more P waves without conducted QRS complexes. Should be treated as complete heart block. Usually symptomatic.

Third-degree (complete heart block): (see Figure 27-21): The P waves are not conducted and there is no relationship between the P waves and the QRS complexes. The ventricular rate is usually 20–40 BPM and is the result of ventricular escape (the intrinsic ventricular rate) and the QRS complex will be wide and resemble PVCs. The ventricular rate can be faster if the rhythm originates from an ectopic focus in the AV node resulting in a junctional escape rhythm with a rate of 40–60 BPM as in the figure below. Usually symptomatic.

Treatment, symptomatic and hemodynamically unstable: Atropine and then pacing (transcutaneous or transvenous); if hypotensive, add a pressor (dopamine), and treat any underlying cause.

Treatment, symptomatic and hemodynamically stable: Monitor with pacing device available for immediate use; permanent pacemaker is often required unless reversible underlying cause.

Bundle Branch Block (BBB): Complete BBB is present when the QRS complex is >0.12 s (or three small boxes on the ECG) and incomplete BBB is when the QRS interval is 0.10 − >0.12. Look at leads I, V_1, and V_6. Degenerative changes and ischemic heart disease are the most common causes.

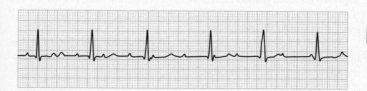

27

Figure 27-21.   Third-degree AV block (complete heart block). Atrial rate is 100 beats/min; ventricular rate is 57 beats/min.

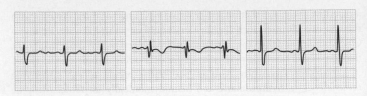

Figure 27-22. Leads I, V$_1$, and V$_6$ show right bundle branch block (RBBB) pattern.

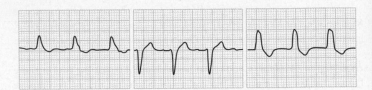

Figure 27-23. Leads I, V$_1$, and V$_6$ show left bundle branch block (LBBB) pattern.

Right Bundle Branch Block (RBBB): The RSR pattern seen in V$_1$, V$_2$, or both. Also a wide S in leads I and V$_6$ (Figure 27-22).

Clinical Correlations. Healthy persons; diseases affecting the right side of the heart (pulmonary hypertension, atrial septal defect (ASD) ischemia); sudden onset associated with PE and acute exacerbation of COPD.

Left Bundle Branch Block (LBBB): RR' in leads I, V$_6$, or both. QRS complex may be more slurred than double-peaked as in RBBB. A wide S wave is seen in V$_1$ (Figure 27-23).

Clinical Correlations. Heart disease (hypertensive, valvular, and ischemic), severe aortic stenosis. If new LBBB, consider MI until proven otherwise.

CARDIAC HYPERTROPHY

Atrial Hypertrophy

P wave >2.5 mm in height and >0.12 s wide (three small boxes on the ECG) ***Right Atrial Enlargement (RAE):*** Tall (>2.5 mm), slender, peaked P waves (P pulmonale pattern) in leads II, III, aVF (Figure 27-24). Tall (>1.5 mm) P may be present in V$_1$ and V$_2$.

Clinical Correlations. COPD with cor pulmonale, pulmonary arterial hypertension (primary, PE, others), tricuspid regurgitation, tricuspid stenosis, ASD, dilated cardiomyopathy.

Left Atrial Enlargement (LAE): Notched P wave (P mitrale pattern) in leads I and II. Wide (≥0.11 s), slurred biphasic P in V$_1$ with wider terminal than initial component (negative deflection) (Figure 27-25).

27

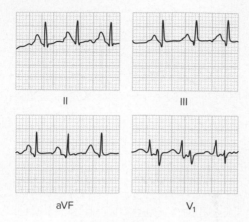

Figure 27-24.   Right atrial enlargement, leads II, III, aVF, and V₁. Note tall P waves in II, III, and aVF and tall, slender P waves in V₁.

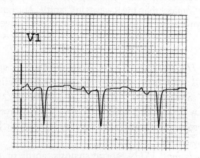

Figure 27-25.   Left atrial enlargement.

Clinical Correlations. Aortic and mitral stenosis, mitral regurgitation, ventricular septal defect (VSD), patent ductus arteriosus (PDA), arteriovenous fistula, HTN, and left ventricular systolic or diastolic heart failure.

Ventricular Hypertrophy

Right Ventricular Hypertrophy (RVH): Tall R wave in V_1 (R wave > S wave in V_1), persistent S waves in V_5 and V_6, progressively smaller R wave from V_1 to V_6, slightly widened QRS intervals (Figure 27-26), and strain pattern with ST segment depression and T wave inversion in V_1 to V_3. Pattern of small R waves with relatively large S waves in V_1 to V_6 may be present. Right axis deviation (>105 degrees) invariably present.

Clinical Correlations. Severe COPD, chronic recurrent PE, pulmonary arterial hypertension, tricuspid regurgitation, congenital heart disease (e.g., tetralogy of Fallot, VSD, ASD), biventricular hypertrophy (LVH and RVH, however LVH findings often predominating).

27

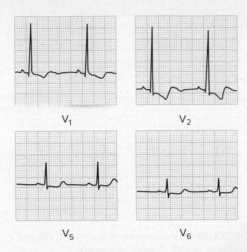

V_1 V_2

V_5 V_6

Figure 27-26. Right ventricular hypertrophy, leads V_1, V_2, V_5, and V_6. Note the tall R waves in V_1 and V_2, greater than the R waves in V_5 and V_6. Also note strain pattern in V_1 and V_2 with down-sloping ST segment depression and T wave inversion.

Left Ventricular Hypertrophy (LVH): Voltage criteria (>age 35 y): S wave in V_1 or V_2 plus R wave in V_5 or V_6 >35 mm, or R wave in aVL >11 mm or R wave in I + S wave in III >25 mm, or R wave in V_5 or V_6 >26 mm. QRS complex may be >0.10 s wide in V_5 or V_6. ST depression and T wave inversion in anterolateral leads (I, aVL, V_5 or V_6) suggest LVH with strain (Figure 27-27, page 869).

Clinical Correlations. HTN, aortic stenosis, aortic or mitral regurgitation, hypertrophic cardiomyopathy, dilated cardiomyopathy, some forms of congenital heart disease, and athlete heart.

MYOCARDIAL INFARCTION

(See also Chapter 29, page 992.)

Myocardial Ischemia: Inadequate myocardial oxygen supply (coronary artery blockage or spasm, severe anemia, hypoxia, many more). The ECG can show ST segment depression (ischemia) (Figure 27-28, page 869), ST elevation (injury) (Figure 27-29, page 869), or inverted (flipped) T waves (Figure 27-30, below). ST elevation or myocardial injury correlates with the territory involved while ischemia is a more diffuse finding and does not correlate with arterial territory (e.g., inferior injury seen in leads II, III, and F; anterior injury seen in leads V_1 to V_6; lateral injury seen in leads I, aVL; anterolateral injury seen in leads I, aVL, V_5, and V_6; anteroseptal injury seen in leads V_1, V_2, V_3, and V_4).

Acute Coronary Syndrome (ACS) and Acute Myocardial Infarction (AMI): Acute coronary syndrome (ACS) is due to myocardial ischemia and is

27

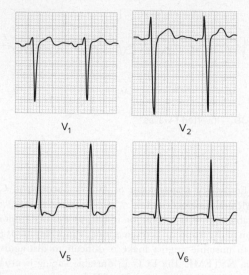

Figure 27-27. Left ventricular hypertrophy, leads V_1, V_2, V_5, and V_6. S wave in V_2 + R wave in V_5 is 55 mm. Note ST changes and T wave inversion in V_5 and V_6, suggesting strain. RAE is also seen in lead V_1.

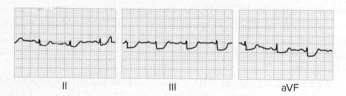

Figure 27-28. ST segment depression in leads II, III, and aVF in a patient with ischemic ECG changes.

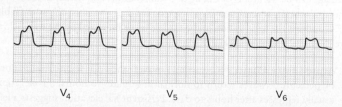

Figure 27-29. ST elevation in leads V_4, V_5, and V_6 in a patient with acute anterolateral myocardial injury.

27

usually described as pressure-like substernal pain (angina) at rest or with minimal exertion. The pain typically radiates to either arm, the neck, or the jaw. ACS can be due to **unstable angina, non-ST segment elevation myocardial infarction (NSTEMI) or the more classic ST segment elevation MI**

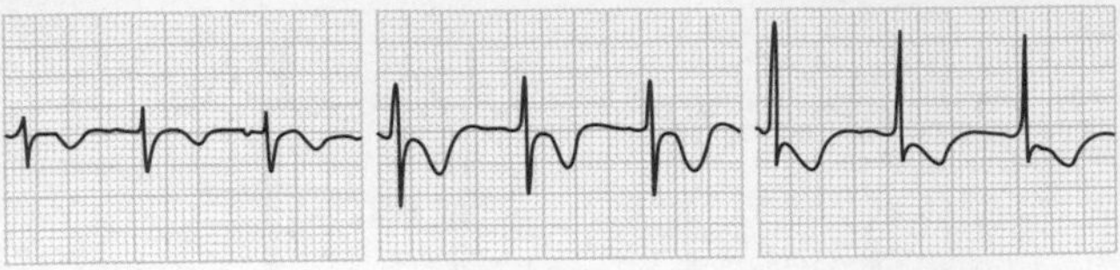

Figure 27-30. Inverted T waves.

(STEMI). Emergency management of ACS is discussed in Chapter 29, Common Medical Emergencies.

In unstable angina, it is common to have an elevated troponin though the elevation of the troponin is often minor. Minor elevations in troponin secondary to unstable angina make it difficult to distinguish unstable angina from NSTEMI. The ECG in unstable angina is usually normal whereas with NSTEMI there is often ST depression in more than one lead. Myocardial necrosis is absent in unstable angina, whereas there is myocardial necrosis with NSTEMI and with STEMI. The accompanying elevation in troponin in NSTEMI is usually greater than with unstable angina. In NSTEMI, the classic acute ST segment elevation in multiple leads on the ECG typically seen in STEMI is absent. Angina at rest associated with myocardial necrosis is identified by a markedly elevated troponin with ST segment elevation, hallmarks of the classic STEMI.

Myocardial infarction (MI) is necrosis of the myocardium caused by severe ischemia resulting in a NSTEMI or STEMI. This is usually a consequence of an acute coronary artery thrombus related to a disrupted coronary atherosclerotic plaque or coronary artery spasm. Sometimes the myocardial damage can be the result of a drug or toxin (cocaine, amphetamines, chemotherapy, others), severe anemia, or hypoxia from any number of causes. Table 27-2 outlines the localization of the cardiac tissue impacted by the MI. Below are the ECG findings associated with an evolving STEMI.

- **Acute Injury Phase.** Hyperacute T waves, then ST segment elevation. Hyperacute T waves return to normal in minutes to hours. ST elevation usually regresses after hours to days. Persistent ST elevation suggests a left ventricular aneurysm.
- **Evolving Phase.** Hours to days after MI. Deep T wave inversion occurs and then replaces ST segment elevation, and T waves may return to normal.
- **Q Waves.** Q wave is the initial negative deflection of the QRS complex. Q waves can be seen on a normal ECG but a significant/pathologic Q wave is 0.04 s in duration and >25% the height of the R wave (Figure 27-31).

Table 27-2.   Localization of Transmural Myocardial Infarction on ECG

Location of MI	Presence of Q Wave or ST Segment Elevation	Reciprocal ST Depression
Anterior	V_1 to V_6 (or poor R wave progression in leads V_1 to V_6)[a]	II, III, aVF
Lateral	I, aVL, V_5, V_6	V_1, V_3
Inferior	II, III, aVF	I, aVL, possibly anterior leads
Posterior	Abnormally tall R and T waves in V_1 to V_3	V_1 to V_3
Subendocardial	No abnormal Q wave. ST segment depression in the anterior, lateral, or inferior leads	

[a]Normally in V_1 to V_6, the R wave amplitude gradually increases and the S wave decreases with a "biphasic" QRS (R = S) in V_3 or V_4. With an anterior MI, there will be a loss of R wave voltage (instead of Q waves) and the biphasic QRS will appear more laterally in V_4 to V_6, hence the term *poor R wave progression*.

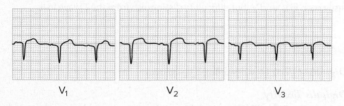

V_1 V_2 V_3

Figure 27-31.   Q waves in leads V_1, V_2, and V_3 in a patient with acute anteroseptal MI. Note ST elevation to determine acute nature of infarction or the presence of a ventricular aneurysm.

Abnormal Q waves develop within hours to days after a MI and may regress to normal after years.

ELECTROLYTE AND DRUG EFFECTS

Electrolyte Effects

Hyperkalemia: Narrow, symmetrical, diffuse, peaked T waves. In severe hyperkalemia, PR prolongation occurs, the P wave flattens and is lost, and the QRS widens and can progress to ventricular fibrillation (Figure 27-32).

Hypokalemia: ST segment depression with the appearance of U waves (positive deflection after the T wave) (Figure 27-33)

Hypercalcemia: Short QT interval

Hypocalcemia: Prolonged QT interval

27

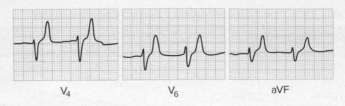

V_4 V_6 aVF

Figure 27-32. Diffuse tall T waves in leads V_4, V_6, and aVF with widened QRS and junctional rhythm (loss of P waves) secondary to hyperkalemia.

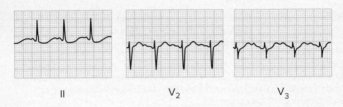

II V_2 V_3

Figure 27-33. Leads II, V_2, and V_3 in a patient with hypokalemia. A U wave is easily seen in V_2 and V_3 but difficult to distinguish from the T wave in II.

Drug Effects

Digitalis Effect: Down-sloping ST segment

Digitalis Toxicity:
- **Arrhythmias.** PVCs, bigeminy, trigeminy, ventricular tachycardia, ventricular fibrillation, PAT, nodal rhythms, accelerated junctional tachycardia, and sinus bradycardia
- **Conduction Abnormalities.** First-degree, second-degree, and third-degree atrioventricular block

Quinidine and Procainamide: With toxic levels, prolonged QT, flattened T wave, and QRS widening, ventricular tachycardia, ventricular fibrillation

MISCELLANEOUS ECG CHANGES

Pericarditis: Diffuse ST elevation concave upward, diffuse PR depression, diffuse T wave inversion, or a combination of these findings (Figure 27-34, page 873)

   Clinical Correlations. Idiopathic conditions; viral, bacterial, and fungal infections, such as TB; after AMI, postpericardiotomy syndrome, Dressler syndrome; collagen–vascular diseases (SLE); uremia; cancer

27

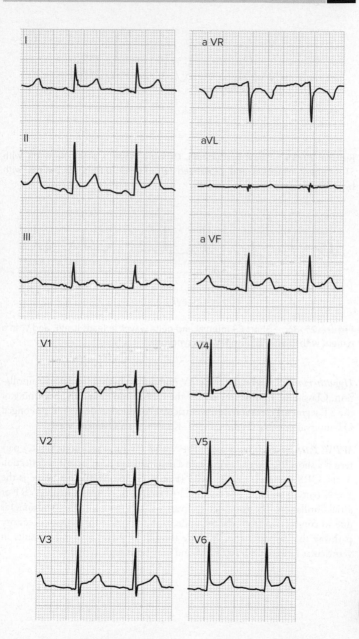

Figure 27-34. Acute pericarditis.

27

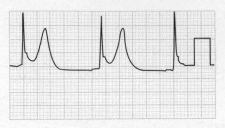

Figure 27-35. Sinus bradycardia, Osborne wave. J point elevation with ST segment elevation and prolonged QT interval (0.56 s) in patient with hypothermia.

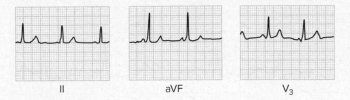

| II | aVF | V$_3$ |

Figure 27-36. Short PR interval and delta waves in leads II, aVF, and V$_3$ in a patient with Wolff–Parkinson–White syndrome.

Hypothermia: Sinus bradycardia, AV junctional rhythm, ventricular fibrillation. Classically, **J point** (the end of the QRS complex and the beginning of the ST segment) elevation, intraventricular conduction delay, and prolonged QT interval possible (Figure 27-35). Known as an **Osborne wave**.

WPW Pattern and Syndrome: The WPW (Wolff–Parkinson–White) pattern is a short PR interval along with a delta wave (a delay in initial deflection of the QRS complex) on the ECG (Figure 27-36). WPW syndrome is the WPW pattern on ECG *and* documented tachyarrhythmias, usually AVRT or atrial fibrillation. The associated tachyarrhythmia (preexcitation syndrome) is due to conduction from the SA node to the ventricle through an accessory pathway that bypasses the AV node (bundle of Kent) and often results in ventricular rates of 180-200 BPM and may be as high as 300 BPM.

27

Critical Care

Chapter update by J. Patton Robinette, MD, Luis C. Suarez-Rodriguez, MD, and John A. Morris, MD. Technical Contributor: Vanessa Gleason, PharmD. Original chapter and artwork by John A. Morris, MD.

ROUTINE CARE OF THE CRITICALLY ILL PATIENT

Patients admitted to the intensive care unit (ICU) often have multisystem disease, traumatic injuries, or are under intensive treatment regimens to manage end-organ dysfunction. The interactions between dysfunctional organ systems are complicated and can be overwhelming to students and new house officers. This chapter describes an organ-system approach to evaluate and treat critically ill patients and resultant complications.

The first part of this critical care chapter will address routine documentation and management of patients in the ICU. The second part of the chapter focuses on the physiologic approach to organ function and dysfunction in the ICU. The last section addresses complications and guidelines for treatment.

The field of critical care medicine is rapidly advancing and practice guidelines and protocols are being introduced to standardize care, reduce variation, and improve outcomes. Where available, national practice guidelines will be presented to frame the student's understanding of treatment options for the following domains:

- Sedation and analgesia
- Delirium and substance withdrawal
- Nutrition
- Intensive insulin therapy
- Deep venous thrombosis (DVT) and stress ulcer prophylaxis
- Weaning from mechanical ventilation
- Management of sepsis including:
  o Goal-directed therapy oxygen delivery; fluid resuscitation; transfusion; vasopressors; antibiotics
  o Adrenal insufficiency and use of steroids
  o Adult respiratory distress syndrome (ARDS)

We have divided the routine care of patients in the ICU into four parts:

- ICU Progress Note
- Routine ICU Monitoring
- The Risk of Transport
- End-of-Life Issues

ICU Progress Note

Understanding the complex care delivered in an ICU starts with a structured approach of the ICU progress note. The ICU progress note is a concise summary of the events of the past 24 hr, medications, physical exam, laboratory data, and the assessment and treatment plan. Although the information can be found elsewhere in the chart, the physician's interpretation of the data communicates the medical decision-making process. The structured ICU progress note includes the following:

1. Problem list and injury summary
   a. Active problems and major inactive problems
   b. Allergies
   c. Past medical or surgical history relevant to the present illness
   d. Notation of hospital day, posttrauma day, postoperative day, postadmission day, etc.
2. Events and procedures over the past 24 hr
3. Active medications
4. System-specific physical exam and pertinent flow sheet data
   a. **Central nervous system (CNS):** CNS functioning or other neurologic assessment and sedation level (e.g., Richmond Agitation–Sedation Scale [RASS], Confusion Assessment Method [CAM-ICU])
   b. **Cardiovascular system (CV):** cardiovascular function, including indicators of systemic perfusion, blood pressure, heart rate, and pulmonary artery (PA) catheter data if present
   c. **Pulmonary function:** including ventilator settings and ABG value
   d. **GI/Nutrition:** gastrointestinal function and nutrition
   e. **Fluids, electrolytes, and renal function**
   f. **Hematologic function:** including CBC, coagulation values
   g. **Infectious disease:** recent culture data, antibiotic regimen and duration
   h. **Prophylaxis:** DVT, ethanol withdrawal, stress gastritis management
   i. **Tubes, lines, and drains:** A summary of patient's current catheters including central lines, arterial lines, Foley catheter, surgical drains, endotracheal tube (ETT), chest tube, and their respective dates of insertion.
5. **Other relevant laboratory and radiographic data**
6. **Assessment and plan:** To include the specific plan for the day, the expected date of discharge, disposition, and if appropriate, probability of death.

Routine Monitoring in the Intensive Care Unit

The hallmark of critical care is the continuous monitoring and assessment of physiologic parameters. Basic physiologic monitoring includes:

1. **Continuous ECG:** Computerized arrhythmia detection systems facilitate rapid detection of rhythm abnormalities and increase the likelihood of successful resuscitation.
2. **Blood Pressure:** Intermittent (sphygmomanometer) or continuous (intravascular) assessment of BP (systolic, diastolic, mean arterial, and central venous pressures). Continuous monitoring required to assess the titration of vasoactive drugs or aggressive volume resuscitation.

28

3. **Pulse Oximetry:** Continuous, quantitative arterial O_2, saturation (SaO_2); ensures adequate oxygenation of systemic arterial blood for tissue delivery.

4. **Temperature:** Critically ill patients are at high risk of thermoregulatory disorders due to fluid resuscitation, burns, and sepsis. Accurate measurements of core temperature can be obtained by continuous temperature readings, either in the esophagus or the central venous compartment (utilizing the pulmonary artery catheter). Definitions of hypothermia are mild 35°C; moderate 32°C; and severe 28°C.

5. **Capnography:** Continuous measurement of expired CO_2. Changes imply alteration in clinical status (hypoventilation, overfeeding, fever, sepsis, loss of cardiac output [CO]).

Considerations When Transporting Critically Ill Patients

Because intensive monitoring is the hallmark of ICU care, the ICU is considered a "stable" environment. The only other stable environment outside the ICU is the operating room. Transporting patients to unstable environments such as radiology is often required for diagnostic or therapeutic services. However, you should assume whatever can go wrong will go wrong; this is especially true during the transportation of critically ill patients. Adherence to common sense guidelines helps to minimize the risk of adverse events during transport. **Perform the following "risk assessment":**

1. Does the benefit of transport and additional information that will be obtained outweigh the risk?
2. Assess the airway. If the airway is tenuous, consider intubating the patient.
3. Pay attention to IV catheters, pumps, drains, and connections that could be easily dislodged during the transport process.
4. Bring enough fluids, oxygen, sedation, and equipment.
5. Anticipate a crisis and ensure adequate support staff and nursing assistance to accompany the patient.
6. Expect the unexpected.

End-of-Life Considerations

It is estimated that at least 20% of patients admitted to ICU die during the hospital admission.[1] Thus, caring for the terminally ill and their family is an unfortunate but unavoidable part of managing the critically ill. Providers must understand the importance of establishing goals of therapy and the administration of comfort care.

Establishing **goals of care** is the most important, least appreciated, and common poorly performed aspect of ICU patient management. The ICU progress note should regularly include an assessment of the clinician's expectations for productive lifestyle, independent living, activities of daily living, survival, and resource utilization. These expectations should be clearly communicated to the family on a regular basis. The family conversations should include an understanding of the patient's wishes regarding return to an independent lifestyle.

Unfortunately, many families have not had this discussion prior to a catastrophic event. Family members legitimately may fail to agree on the patient's wishes, and the ICU patient is rarely able to contribute to the conversation. If this is the case, it is essential to determine if the patient has previously established their wishes through an advanced care plan (advanced care directive). If the patient has such a plan, it should be copied into the electronic medical record. Once documented, the clinical team is responsible for implementing that plan.

If no advance care plan exists, there may be person(s) with decision-making authority over the patient's medical care. This is officially known as a *surrogate decision maker*. If the patient has not directed a surrogate decision maker, the family should be consulted to establish one. The surrogate should base decisions upon their understanding of the patient's desires, not the surrogate's personal desires. These decisions are always difficult and made in a highly stressful environment. It is the responsibility of the critical care physician to assist (in what may be time-consuming conversations), making difficult decisions regarding additional resuscitation, intubation, or withdrawal of life support.

In all cases, the clinician must be objective and focus on the knowns and unknowns to provide the decision maker with balanced information and the emotional support needed to make appropriate decisions. There are several principles central to providing adequate comfort care for the terminally ill.

Chapter 22, Palliative Care and Nonpain Symptom Management, page 723, provides an overview of this area. The article "Comfort Care for Patients Dying in the Hospital," from NEJM in 2015 presents a succinct list of major conventions when caring for these patients.[2]

1. The clinician should assure the patient and family that comfort is a high priority and that troubling symptoms will be expertly treated.
2. The clinician should involve an interdisciplinary team that offers comprehensive, coordinated care for both the patient and the family, and promote good communication among the members of the clinical team.
3. Inquire about the patient's spiritual and religious needs and offer chaplaincy services when appropriate.
4. Discontinue diagnostic or treatment efforts that are likely to have negligible benefit or that may cause harm.
5. Discontinue unnecessary treatment with medications not intended for comfort.
6. Administer prophylactic analgesia or sedation before distressing procedures are performed.
7. Inform the patient and family about any proposed major changes in the management of the patient.

28

MANAGEMENT CONSIDERATIONS IN THE INTENSIVE CARE UNIT: CENTRAL NERVOUS SYSTEM (CNS)

Severe acute illness often results in altered mental status (AMS). AMS manifests a spectrum of disability from mild delirium to complex, life-threatening coma. Critically ill patients are often intubated, and medications must be administered for analgesia and sedation. Inadequate analgesia and sedation have adverse effects such as increased catabolism, tachycardia, higher myocardial O_2 consumption, immunosuppression, hypercoagulability, and severe anxiety. Consequently, great care must be taken in finding the proper balance of medications used for sedation and analgesia.

The first step in evaluating acute agitation is to rule out life-threatening pathology. Closely assess vital signs, oxygenation and ventilation status (check for ETT occlusion), serum glucose, and electrolytes. After life-threatening pathology has been excluded, consider the administration of sedation and analgesia, according to unit protocols.

Analgesia and Sedation

Critically ill patients have a wide scope of pain-producing diagnoses, exacerbated by surgery, mechanical ventilation, and bedside procedures. It is estimated over 50% of ICU patients have failure of pain management. Guidelines for the management of pain, sedation, and delirium have been created by the Society of Critical Care Medicine.[3] These guidelines support monitoring pain employing the following commonly used tools:

- Self-report
- The behavioral pain scale (Table 28-1)
- The critical care pain observation tool (Table 28-2)

In patients who can self-report pain, a numeric scale from 1–10 is considered as the gold standard.

If the patient is unable to report pain, a behavioral pain score of greater than 5 or a critical care pain observation tool score of greater than 3 defines pain requiring therapy. The Society of Critical Care Medicine guidelines recommend:

- Preemptive analgesia and nonpharmacologic interventions prior to bedside procedures.
- Intravenous opioids are still first-line drugs to treat nonneuropathic pain in critically ill patients.
- Opioids should be supplemented by nonopioid medication to decrease opioid usage.

28

Table 28-1. The Behavioral Pain Scale

Item	Description	Score
Facial expression	Relaxed	1
	Partially tightened (e.g., brow lowering)	2
	Fully tightened (e.g., eyelid closing)	3
	Grimacing	4
Upper limbs	No movement	1
	Partially bent	2
	Fully bent with finger flexion	3
	Permanently retracted	4
Compliance with ventilation	Tolerating movement	1
	Coughing but tolerating ventilation for most of the time	2
	Fighting ventilator	3
	Unable to control ventilation	4

Note: A score of greater than 5 defines pain requiring therapy.
Source: Reproduced with permission from Wolters Kluwer Health. Payen J, et al. Assessing pain in critically ill sedated patients by using a behavioral pain scale. Crit Care Med 2001;29 (12);2258–2263.

- Gabapentin or carbamazepine are recommended as first line for neuropathic pain.
- Monitoring depth of sedation utilizing the RASS (Table 28-3) or the Sedation-Agitation Scale (SAS).
- Light sedation is preferred over deep sedation.
- Sedation strategies utilizing propofol or dexmedetomidine are suggested over any benzodiazepine strategy.

Analgesia

General principles of pain management are reviewed in Chapter 21. Despite the challenges associated with the current outpatient opioid crisis, opioid narcotic agents remain the preferred agents of choice for acute pain control in the ICU. Opioids can be administered through numerous routes: orally, continuous infusions, intermittent boluses, or as part of patient-controlled analgesia (PCA) regimen. Respiratory depression is exacerbated when opioids are combined with benzodiazepines. When combined with epidural anesthesia, the dosage of IV narcotics dramatically decreases. Doses reflect use in adults.

28

Table 28-2. The Critical Care Pain Observation Tool

Indicator	Description	Score	
Facial expression	No muscular tension observed	Relaxed, neutral	0
	Presence of frowning, brow lowering, orbit tightening, and levator contraction	Tense	1
	All of the above facial movements plus eyelid tightly closed	Grimacing	2
Body movements	Does not move at all (does not necessarily mean absence of pain)	Absence of movements	0
	Slow, cautious movements, touching or rubbing the pain site, seeking attention through movements	Protection	1
	Pulling tube, attempting to sit up, moving limbs/thrashing, not following commands, striking at staff, trying to climb out of bed	Restlessness	2
Muscle tension	No resistance to passive movements	Relaxed	0
Evaluation by passive flexion and extension of upper extremities	Resistance to passive movements	Tense, rigid	1
	Strong resistance to passive movements, inability to complete them	Very tense or rigid	2
Compliance with the ventilator (intubated patients)	Alarms not activated, easy ventilation	Tolerating ventilator or movement	0
	Alarms stop spontaneously	Coughing but tolerating	1
OR	Asynchrony: blocking ventilation, alarms frequently activated	Fighting ventilator	2
Vocalization (extubated patients)	Talking in normal tone or no sound	Talking in normal tone or no sound	0
	Sighing, moaning	Sighing, moaning	1
	Crying out, sobbing	Crying out, sobbing	2
Total, range			0–8

Note: A score of greater than 3 defines pain requiring therapy.

Source: Critical-Care Pain Observation Tool. Adapted with permission from the American Association of Critical-Care Nurses. Gelinas C, et al. Validation of the Critical-Care Pain Observation Tool in adult patients. Am J Crit Care 2006;15(4):420–427.

Table 28-3. The Richmond Agitation–Sedation Scale

Score	Term	Description
+4	Combative	Overtly combative or violent; immediate danger to staff
+3	Very agitated	Pulls on or removes tube(s) or catheter(s) or has aggressive behavior toward staff
+2	Agitated	Frequent nonpurposeful movement or patient-ventilator dyssynchrony
+1	Restless	Anxious or apprehensive but movements not aggressive or vigorous
0	Alert and calm	
−1	Drowsy	Not fully alert, but has sustained (more than 10 seconds) awakening, with eye contact to voice
−2	Light sedation	Briefly (less than 10 seconds) awakens with eye contact to voice
−3	Moderate sedation	Any movement (but no eye contact) to voice
−4	Deep sedation	No response to voice, but any movement to physical stimulation
−5	Unarousable	No response to voice or physical stimulation

Procedure
1. Observe patient. Is patient alert and calm (score 0)?
   Does patient have behavior that is consistent with restlessness or agitation (score +1 to +4 using the criteria listed above, under DESCRIPTION)?
2. If patient is not alert, in a loud speaking voice state patient's name and direct patient to open eyes and look at speaker. Repeat once if necessary. Can prompt patient to continue looking at speaker.
   Patient has eye opening and eye contact, which is sustained for more than 10 seconds (score −1).
   Patient has eye opening and eye contact, but this is not sustained for 10 seconds (score −2).
   Patient has any movement in response to voice, excluding eye contact (score −3).
3. If patient does not respond to voice, physically stimulate patient by shaking shoulder and then rubbing sternum if there is no response to shaking shoulder.
   Patient has any movement to physical stimulation (score −4)
   Patient has no response to voice or physical stimulation (score −5).

Source: Reproduced with permission from Sessler CN, et al. The Richmond Agitation-Sedation Scale: Validity and reliability in adult intensive care unit patients. Am J Respir Crit Care Med 2002;166(10):1338–1344.

28

- **Hydromorphone:** Mu-opioid receptor agonist can cause respiratory depression, sedation, and cough suppression. Its onset is between 15 and 30 min when administered orally and 5 min in IV formulation. It is metabolized in the liver and excreted in the urine.
  o Indicated for moderate to severe pain.

o Available as oral, subcutaneous, IM, and IV formulations.
o Dose – IV 0.2 mg to 1–2 mg.
o Maintenance infusion – 0.5–3 mg/hr.
- **Morphine:** IV opioid narcotic; commonly used (low cost, ease of use).
  o Indicated in moderate to severe pain, used in myocardial ischemia, palliative end-of-life situations. Causes respiratory depression.
  o Loading dose – 1–5 mg IV
  o Maintenance/infusion – 1–10 mg/hr, may titrate further to desired effect.
- **Fentanyl:** A synthetic opioid; more potent and shorter acting than morphine; less histamine release than morphine (less potential for drug-induced hypotension).
  o Indicated for moderate to severe pain. Used commonly as drip in mechanically ventilated patients.
  o Loading dose – 1–3 mcg/kg
  o Maintenance dose – 0.01–0.03 mcg/kg/hr
- **Oxycodone:** An oral semisynthetic, morphine-like opioid alkaloid with analgesic activity. Onset 10–15 min and a duration of 3–6 hr.
  o Indicated for moderate to severe pain; may be used to decrease parenteral analgesia requirement such as while transitioning to an oral regime.
  o Dose 10–30 mg orally/per oro/nasogastric tube every 4–6 hr.

Sedation

If a patient requires long-term sedation and analgesia, interruption of sedation decreases mechanical ventilation days and ICU length of stay. Neuromuscular paralysis is rarely indicated but may be necessary for patients with severe respiratory failure who cannot properly oxygenate or ventilate. It eliminates the muscular elastic recoil of the chest wall and ventilator dyssynchrony, thus improving pulmonary compliance.

   Benzodiazepines are potent inducers of sedation, amnesia, muscle relaxation, and anxiolysis. These properties make this class of drug ideal for short- to intermediate-term use in the ICU setting. However, these agents can place ICU patients at risk of life-threatening respiratory depression. "Sedation scales" have been developed to allow the proper titration of sedative agents such as benzodiazepines to optimize patient safety and comfort. One such objective sedation scale is the 10-point **RASS**. At one extreme, a RASS score of +4 is indicative of a severely combative or violent patient with the other extreme of a score of –5 representing a patient who is unarousable (see Table 28-3).

   Caution is needed to choose a sedative drug that will not accumulate in the patient's system if end-organ dysfunction is present. Choice of sedative agent and initial doses may vary according to the route of administration.

28

Listed here are some commonly employed agents and dose ranges for sedation in the ICU or periprocedural sedation and analgesia. The goal is to reach a light level of sedation or comfortable awareness (RASS 0 to −2) depending on the patient's current clinical setting. The reliability and validity of the RASS for titration of sedation has been validated in numerous studies.

Benzodiazepines Commonly Used for Sedation

Titration of benzodiazepines helps to achieve a sedation level according to the RASS. A RASS +2 to +4 indicates inadequate level of sedation, and the patient should be evaluated further for causes of delirium or pain. A score of −3 or less suggests the level of sedation is too high, and the regimen should be reduced with a target RASS between 0 and −2.

- **Lorazepam:** Good intermediate-duration benzodiazepine; metabolized by the liver with inactive metabolite excreted in the urine; very potent but has a long time to peak effect (ideal agent for longer-term sedation).
  o Loading dose – 0.5–2 mg
  o Maintenance/infusion – start at 1 mg/hr and titrate
- **Diazepam:** Intermediate – to long-acting benzodiazepine. Used frequently to treat alcohol withdrawal symptoms.
  o Loading dose – 5 mg
  o Maintenance/infusion – 5 mg/hr and titrate
- **Flumazenil:** If severe benzodiazepine oversedation occurs, stop the medication, prepare to institute cardiopulmonary support, and use flumazenil (antidote for benzodiazepine overdose) to reverse the overly sedated state. Contraindications include hypersensitivity to the benzodiazepines class of drugs, if benzodiazepines are used to control a life-threatening condition (e.g., reduce intracranial pressure or status epilepticus) or with cyclic antidepressant overdose. Flumazenil may cause seizures.
  o Loading dose – 0.2 mg IV over 15–30 s
  o Dose interval – no drip, repeat 0.2 mg IV every 1 min, maximum of 1 mg. Up to 3 mg if benzodiazepine overdose.

Other Drugs for Sedation and Analgesia

- **Propofol:** It is a nonbenzodiazepine, lipid-based sedative–hypnotic; minimal analgesic properties; potentiates GABA receptors, alkylphenol extremely short onset and half-life make accumulation unlikely (ultrashort-term drug); expensive; longer-term use has adverse financial and infectious consequences. One approach is to initiate at 10 mcg/kg/min and adjust by increments of 10–20 mcg/kg/min q5–15 min to achieve desired level of sedation (reconsider dosing >50 mcg/kg/min). To discontinue, decrease infusion 25% q10–15 min, then halt the infusion when the patient is conscious.

- o Loading dose: 1.5–3 mg/kg
- o Maintenance/infusion: 10–50 mcg/kg/min
- **Ketamine:** Produces dissociative anesthesia, blocks NMDA receptors; excellent for invasive procedures such as chest tube placement.
  - o Loading dose: 1–4.5 mg/kg
  - o Maintenance/infusion: 0.1–0.5 mg/min
- **Dexmedetomidine:** Selective alpha$_2$-adrenergic agonist with sedative properties.
  - o Loading dose: for IV sedation, loading doses are usually not administered but may use 1 mcg/kg in 10 min
  - o Maintenance/infusion: 0.2–1.4 mcg/kg/hr

Delirium

Delirium is a disturbance in attention and awareness that fluctuates and develops over a short period of time. Its prevalence can range up to 85% in the ICU. Delirium is associated with prolonged hospitalization, increased mortality, increased cost, increased functional and cognitive decline, and an increased risk of institutionalization posthospitalization.[4,5] Delirium, according to the DSM-V, is defined by the following criteria[6]:

1. Disturbance in attention and awareness
2. Disturbance in cognition: e.g., memory, disorientation, language, perception
3. Develops over a short period of time and tends to fluctuate during the day
4. Disturbances are NOT better explained by a preexisting, established, or evolving neurocognitive disorder and do NOT occur in the context of a severely reduced level of arousal such as coma.
5. There is evidence from the history and physical exam and/or labs that the disturbance is caused by a medical condition, substance intoxication or withdrawal, or medication/toxin side effect.

Associated symptoms of delirium in the ICU include hallucinations and delusions, abnormal activity such as agitation or lethargy, emotional disturbances, and sleep disturbances.

The Society of Critical Care Medicine (SCCM) guidelines recommend that all patients in the ICU be screened for delirium at least once per 8–12 hr shift using the Confusion Assessment Method for the ICU (CAM-ICU) (see Figure 28-1).

Prevention strategies focusing on optimizing the ICU environment include the following[7]:

28

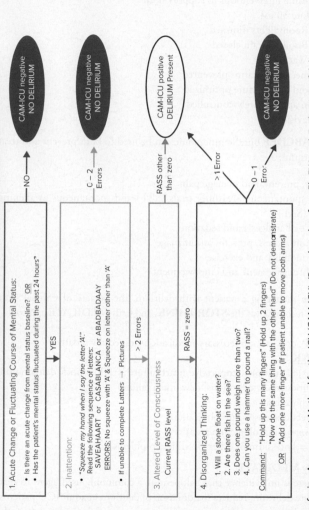

Confusion Assessment Method for the ICU (CAM-ICU) Flowsheet

1. Acute Change or Fluctuating Course of Mental Status:
- Is there an acute change from mental status baseline? OR
- Has the patient's mental status fluctuated during the past 24 hours?

→ NO → CAM-ICU negative NO DELIRIUM

→ YES

2. Inattention:
- "Squeeze my hand when I say the letter 'A.'"
  Read the following sequence of letters:
  SAVEAHAART or CASABLANCA or ABADBADAAY
  ERRORS: No squeeze with 'A' & Squeeze on letter other than 'A'
- If unable to complete Letters → Pictures

→ C – 2 Errors → CAM-ICU negative NO DELIRIUM

→ > 2 Errors

3. Altered Level of Consciousness
Current RASS level

→ RASS = zero → CAM-ICU negative NO DELIRIUM

→ RASS other than zero → CAM-ICU positive DELIRIUM Present

4. Disorganized Thinking:
1. Will a stone float on water?
2. Are there fish in the sea?
3. Does one pound weigh more than two?
4. Can you use a hammer to pound a nail?
Command: "Hold up this many fingers" (Hold up 2 fingers)
  "Now do the same thing with the other hand" (Do not demonstrate)
  OR "Add one more finger" (If patient unable to move both arms)

→ > 1 Error → CAM-ICU positive DELIRIUM Present

→ 0 – 1 Error → CAM-ICU negative NO DELIRIUM

Figure 28-1. Confusion Assessment Method for the ICU (CAM-ICU). (Based on data from Ely EW, et al. Evaluation of delirium in critically ill patients: Validation of the Confusion Assessment Method for the Intensive Care Unit (CAM-ICU). Crit Care Med 2001;29(7):1370–1379 and Adapted from Dr. Wes Ely [from icudelirium.org. Accessed March 20, 2020]).

- Day-time interventions to support wakefulness
  - Blinds raised
  - Less than 50% of the day napping
  - Avoid caffeine after 3 PM
- Night-time interventions to support sleep
  - Before 10 PM
    - Room lights dimmed
    - Room curtain closed
    - Warm bath
  - Unnecessary alarms prevented
  - Room temperature optimized
  - Pain appropriately controlled
  - Television off

The **ABCDEF** bundle mnemonic can be used to both prevent and treat ICU delirium[8]:

A. Assess, prevent, and manage pain
B. Both spontaneous breathing trials (SBT) and spontaneous awakening trials (SAT)
C. Choice of analgesia and sedation
D. Delirium: assess, prevent, and manage
E. Early mobility and exercise
F. Family engagement and empowerment

When managing a patient with delirium, the Society of Critical Care Medicine recommends the **STOP, THINK,** and lastly **MEDICATE** approach.

1. **STOP**, or wean, unnecessary medications, especially sedatives
2. **THINK**
   - **T**oxic situations (congestive heart failure [CHF], shock dehydration; deliriogenic medications, new organ failure)
   - **H**ypoxemia
   - **I**nfection/sepsis, immobilization
   - **N**onpharmacologic interventions
   - **K** = Potassium or other electrolyte problems

3. Lastly **MEDICATE**
   - There is no evidence that haloperidol, a commonly used agent to treat acute delirium, reduces the duration of delirium in adult ICU patients.
   - Atypical antipsychotics (e.g., quetiapine, olanzapine) may reduce the duration of delirium in adult ICU patients.
   - Sedation with dexmedetomidine or propofol improves clinical outcomes and has a lower prevalence of delirium compared to benzodiazepines.

MANAGEMENT CONSIDERATIONS IN THE INTENSIVE CARE UNIT: CARDIOVASCULAR SYSTEM

Cardiovascular instability is one of the most common problems encountered in the ICU. The first step in evaluating the cardiovascular system is a thorough physical exam.

Inspection

- Jugular venous distention (JVD) or neck vein visualization with the patient sitting at a 45-degree angle implies central venous pressure of >12–15 mm Hg. JVD in the presence of hypotension suggests life-threatening pathology including: tension pneumothorax, pericardial tamponade, or severe systolic cardiac dysfunction.
- Precordial contusion associated with blunt trauma from the steering wheel implies the possibility of underlying myocardial contusion. Treatment includes: continuous ECG monitoring (duration is subject to debate), monitor for and correction of arrhythmias, commonly sinus tachycardia, and right bundle branch block. If arrhythmias occur, obtain an echocardiogram to rule out anatomic injury or pericardial contusion or pericardial effusion.
- Extremity perfusion (pulse, color, temperature, and capillary refill) provides a window into the combined function of the cardiovascular and respiratory system. Pay special attention to distal sites, looking for: long bone fractures, joint dislocations, and indwelling arterial catheters that may affect perfusion.

Auscultation and Heart Murmurs

The presence of a premorbid cardiac murmur and, more important, the interval development of a new cardiac murmur is important in the care of a critically ill patient. Characterize all new murmurs by intensity, location, and variation with position and respiration as well as whether they are systolic or diastolic. In general, diastolic murmurs are always pathologic (see Chapter 6, History and Physical Examination, for more information on heart murmurs).

Blood Pressure

Over the short term, BP is considered adequate if renal perfusion is maintained. This is usually accomplished with a mean arterial pressure (MAP) >70 mm Hg in young and previously healthy persons. Premorbid medical problems and aging, however, may mandate a higher MAP. If the cuff is too small for the arm (i.e., the patient is obese), the measured systolic BP will be falsely elevated.

28

- **Systolic Hypertension:** It is defined as a systolic blood pressure greater than 130 mm Hg within normal diastolic blood pressure in the acute setting. This can be due to:
  - o Increased cardiac output
  - o Thyrotoxicosis
  - o Generalized response to stress
  - o Anemia
  - o Pain, anxiety, or both
- **Diastolic Hypertension:** It is defined as a diastolic BP >80 mm Hg and may be associated with:
  - o Intrinsic renal disease
  - o Endocrine disorders
  - o Renovascular hypertension
  - o Neurologic disorders
- **Treatment of Hypertension in the ICU:** Hypertension is of particular concern after acute coronary syndromes, subarachnoid hemorrhage, and vascular anastomosis (especially carotid artery surgery). *Malignant hypertension (BP >180/120 mm Hg) usually necessitates immediate treatment.*
  - o Commonly used agents in the treatment of hypertension include nitroprusside, nicardipine, metoprolol, labetalol, esmolol, hydralazine, and nitroglycerin. Use a rapid-acting and easily reversible beta-blocker (e.g., esmolol) to manage hypertension associated with ruptured aortic aneurysm or blunt traumatic aortic injury. Emergency management of malignant hypertension is discussed in Chapter 29.
- **Mean Arterial Pressure (MAP):** Mean arterial blood pressure is a better gauge of organ perfusion than systolic blood pressure. It is often calculated continuously in the ICU using an arterial line.
  - o MAP = DBP + [(SBP–DBP)/3] where SBP is systolic BP and DBP is diastolic BP.
- **Pulse Pressure:** Pulse pressure is the systolic BP minus diastolic BP (SBP – DBP). Normally the pulse pressure in adults is between 40 and 60 and increases slightly with age due to decreased vessel compliance.
  - o *Wide pulse pressure:* (>40–60 mm Hg) associated with:
    - ▪ Thyrotoxicosis
    - ▪ Arteriovenous fistula
    - ▪ Aortic insufficiency
  - o *Narrow pulse pressure:* (<25 mm Hg) associated with:
    - ▪ Significant tachycardia
    - ▪ Early hypovolemic shock
    - ▪ Pericarditis
    - ▪ Pericardial effusion or tamponade
    - ▪ Ascites
    - ▪ Aortic stenosis
- **Paradoxical Pulse:** Systolic BP changes during the respiratory cycle as a function of changes in intrathoracic pressure. Normally, systolic BP falls 6–10 mm Hg with inspiration.

28

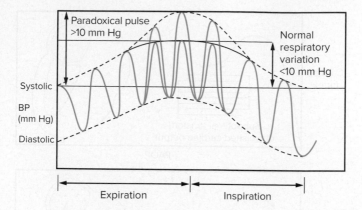

Figure 28-2.   Graphic representation of the paradoxical pulse.

  o If this variation occurs over a wider range (>10 mm Hg), the patient
    is said to have a paradoxical pulse (see Figure 28-2). Associated condi-
    tions include:
    ■ Pericardial tamponade
    ■ Asthma and chronic obstructive pulmonary disease (COPD)
    ■ Ruptured diaphragm
    ■ Pneumothorax

CARDIOVASCULAR PHYSIOLOGY

General Principles

• **Cardiac Output (CO):** Volume of blood pumped by the heart each minute; approximately 3.5–5.5 L/min (adult). CO is standardized to patient
  size by calculation of the cardiac index (CI).
• **Cardiac Index (CI)** = CO/BSA; normal CI ≈ 2.8–3.2 L/min/m². CI
  <2.5 L/min/m² may require pharmacologic intervention if O_2 delivery is inadequate. CO is the product of heart rate and stroke volume.
  Stroke volume is a function of preload, afterload, and contractility.
• **Preload:** Initial length of myocardial muscle fibers is proportional to
  left ventricular end-diastolic volume (LVEDV), which is governed
  by the volume of blood remaining in the left ventricle after systole. As
  LVEDV increases, the stretch on myocardial muscle fibers increases
  (Figure 28-3, top).
  o As LVEDV increases (i.e., stretch), the energy of contraction
    increases proportionally until an optimal tension develops (Starling
    law; Figure 28-3, middle). However, when the myocardial muscle
    fiber is overstretched, contractile strength decreases (Figure 28-3,
    bottom).

28

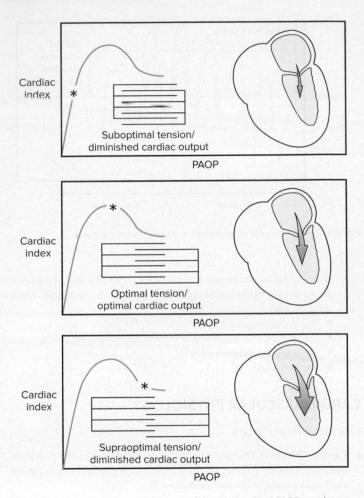

Figure 28-3. Graphic representation of the "Starling law." PAOP = pulmonary artery occlusion pressure, also known as pulmonary capillary wedge pressure (PCWP).

- **Afterload:** Resistance to ventricular ejection; measured clinically with aortic BP and calculation of systemic vascular resistance (SVR).
- **Contractility:** Ability of heart to alter its contractile force and velocity independent of fiber length (i.e., the intrinsic strength of the individual muscle fiber cells). Contractility may be increased by stimulation of beta-receptors in the heart (see following section).

28

Sympathetic Nervous System Influence on the Cardiovascular System

Cardiac output and its determinants (preload, afterload, and contractility) are influenced by the sympathetic nervous system (SNS). The SNS releases catecholamines (predominantly epinephrine and norepinephrine), which bind to end-organ receptors exerting a physiologic response. Adrenergic receptors are divided into two major classes: alpha (α) and beta (β). End-organ function after receptor activation is summarized in Table 28-4.

Understanding the adrenergic receptors is important because many of the cardiovascular drugs used in the ICU act through their sympathomimetic properties. Such drugs have a specific receptor affinity (i.e., α vs. β) and consequently differ in end-organ effects. For example, drugs that act on the $\alpha1$ receptors are called **vasopressors**, because they cause nonspecific systemic vasoconstriction.

Conversely, drugs that act on $\beta1$ receptors are called **inotropes** because they increase myocardial contractility and heart rate. Because each drug exerts receptor-specific effects, use of these agents provides differential activation of receptors and ultimately end-organ effects. Through tailoring pharmacologic support, physicians provide the necessary cardiovascular assistance to critically ill patients. Commonly used sympathomimetics and their relative receptor affinities are listed in Table 28-5, page 894.

Central Venous Pressure (CVP)

The central venous pressure (CVP) is determined through the use of a central venous catheter that can be used as a measuring device and to administer IV fluids and medications. The central venous catheter is one of two major devices used for invasive cardiovascular instrumentation in the ICU. The other, the pulmonary artery catheter (also called PA catheter), is discussed on page 895. For CVP monitoring, a 7 Fr or 9 Fr catheter is inserted into the central venous

Table 28-4. Adrenergic Receptors and Their Actions on the Cardiovascular System

Receptor	Location	Action
Alpha $(\alpha)_1$	Peripheral arterioles	Vasoconstriction (increased SVR)
Beta $(\beta)_1$	Myocardium	Increased contractility
	SA node	Increased heart rate
Beta $(\beta)_2$	Peripheral arterioles	Vasodilatation (decreased SVR)
	Bronchiolar smooth muscle	Bronchodilatation

SVR = systemic vascular resistance; SA = sinoatrial.

28

Table 28-5. Relative Actions of Sympathomimetic Drugs on Adrenergic Receptors

| Drug | Effect On | | | |
	α	β_1	β_2	D
Phenylephrine	++++	0	0	
Norepinephrine	++++	++	0	
Epinephrine	++++	++++	++	
Dobutamine	+	++++	++	
Isoproterenol	0	++++	+++	
Dopamine* (mcg/kg/min)	10–20	5–10		1–5

Key: + = Relative effect; 0 = no clinically significant effect; D = dopaminergic receptors.
* = predominate receptor activation is dose dependent.

Table 28-6. Interpretation of CVP Measurements

Reading (mm Hg)	General description	Clinical implications
<3	Low	Intravenous fluids may be administered
3–10	Midrange	Probable clinical euvolemia
>10	High	Suspect fluid overload, CHF, CP, COPD, tension PTX

CVP = central venous pressure; CHF = congestive heart failure; CP = cor pulmonale;
COPD = chronic obstructive pulmonary disease; PTX = pneumothorax.

circulation through the internal jugular or subclavian vein (see also Bedside Procedures, Chapter 19). A pressure transducer and monitor connected to the catheter provide the measured pressures. A chest x-ray (CXR) is required to confirm the proper position of the catheter in the superior vena cava. The zero point for the transducer is the level of the right atrium in a supine patient; 5 cm caudal to the sternal notch in the midaxillary line.

The transduced CVP reflects right atrial pressure, and by association, right ventricular filling pressure or preload. Although CVP is a relatively inaccurate indicator of preload, trends in relation to volume status and hemodynamics may be clinically useful. The general implications of CVP readings are listed in Table 28-6.

CVP Limitations

- CVP does not *entirely* reflect total blood volume or left ventricular function. CVP is altered by:
  o Changes in PA resistance
  o Changes in compliance of the right ventricle
  o Intrathoracic pressure (e.g., mechanical ventilation)

28

- Conditions that radically change intrathoracic pressure:
  - o Positive pressure ventilation, especially when high positive end-expiratory pressure (PEEP) is used
  - o Pneumothorax, hemothorax, hydrothorax, and tension pneumothorax
  - o Presence of intrathoracic tumors
- Sepsis or hypovolemia may be associated with spuriously normal CVP
- Left ventricular failure can occur in the presence of normal CVP
- Patients with COPD may need an elevated CVP to optimize CO

Technical Tips Regarding CVP Measurements

- CVP readings are inaccurate if they do not fluctuate with respiration.
- If appropriate, remove the patient from the ventilator when taking a CVP reading.
- To ensure comparable readings, have the patient positioned in the same manner for each measurement.
- Flatten the bed and use the same zero point for the transducer.

Pulmonary Artery Catheters (Swan–Ganz Catheter)

Pulmonary artery catheters (also called PA catheter, Swan–Ganz catheter, right-heart catheter, and balloon flotation catheter) are used for direct measurement of central cardiovascular pressures, used to calculate cardiac performance in critical care. The catheter is placed in a central vein (usually the subclavian or internal jugular with alternative sites being the femoral, antecubital, or brachial veins) and then passed into the right atrium, across the tricuspid valve, into the right ventricle, and through the pulmonic valve. The distal end is floated into the PA (pulmonary artery) where the balloon is normally left in the deflated state unless specific measurements are being made. The PA catheter is used to measure **PA pressure (PAP), PA occlusion pressure (PAOP, also known as pulmonary capillary wedge pressure [PCWP]), and CVP.**

Intravascular volume status, vascular resistance (both pulmonary and systemic), and the pumping ability of the heart (CO) are calculated, **mixed venous oxygen saturation** ($S\overline{v}o_2$) is continuously monitored, and **right ventricular ejection fraction (REF)** and **right ventricular end-diastolic volume index (RVEDVI)** are measured episodically. Table 28-7 indicates some of the normal PA catheter parameters. Figure 28-4 shows the relative positioning of PA catheter.

28

- **Key point:** The data obtained with a PA catheter are only as good as the initial setup and the *actual* measurements obtained (i.e., pressures). If patient data (height, weight, etc.) are incorrectly entered into the system, the subsequent calculations will be incorrect.

Table 28-7. Normal Parameters for a Properly Placed PA Catheter

Parameter	Range
Right atrial pressure	1–7 mm Hg
Right ventricular pressure	
Systolic	15–25 mm Hg
Diastolic	0–8 mm Hg
PAP	
Systolic	15–25 mm Hg
Diastolic	8–15 mm Hg
Mean	10–20 mm Hg
PAOP ("wedge pressure")	6–12 mm Hg
Cardiac output	3.5–5.5 L/min
Cardiac index	2.8–3.2 L/min/m²
Mixed venous O_2 saturation	65–85%

PAP = pulmonary artery pressure; PAOP = pulmonary artery occlusion pressure.

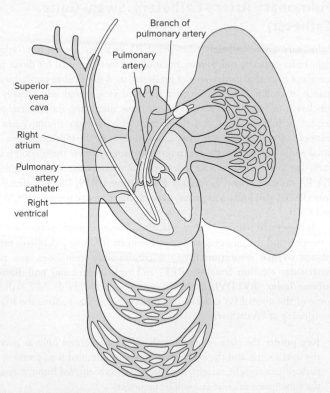

Figure 28-4. Relative positioning of a PA catheter.

Indications for PA Catheter Use: The PA catheter was first introduced in 1970. There has been ongoing debate concerning the utility of PA catheters[9] with an overall decline in its use. Prospective randomized trials report that in most circumstances, the routine use of balloon flotation catheters is not indicated. Balloon flotation catheters are diagnostic and not therapeutic tools with their overuse in critical care units resulting in many complications, including mortality.[10] However, many clinicians find these catheters an essential tool in the following settings:

- Acute heart failure
- Shock
- Suspected "pseudosepsis" (high CO, low SVR, elevated right atrial and pulmonary capillary wedge pressures)
- Complex circulatory and fluid conditions (massive resuscitation)
- Complicated MI
- Intraoperative management in high-risk cardiac patients (e.g., aneurysm repair, elderly patient undergoing a major operation)
- Select cases of cardiac/pulmonary transplantation workup

Contraindications to PA Catheter Use: While there are no absolute contraindications, patients with left bundle branch block may experience complete heart block (requiring temporary pacemaker) and presence of a ventricular assist device or active infection at the insertion site. Frequent manipulation may increase infection risk, as with any IV catheter. Complications tend to increase with the length of time the catheter is in place. The risks of bacteremia and spontaneous bacterial endocarditis (SBE) are high in severely ill patients undergoing long-term instrumentation. In the setting of unexplained fever, always remove and culture the PA catheter and sheath.

PA Catheter Description: The PA catheter generally consists of three or four lumens and a thermistor at the tip, so called thermodilution catheters. Thin black markings are typically in 10-cm increments with a thicker black band at 50 cm. The caliber is 5–8 Fr and the catheter is radiopaque. Length range is 100–110 cm in length. Pediatric catheters are available in 5 Fr and 75 cm length with only two infusion lumens (Figure 28-5). Catheter lumens are as follows:

- **Balloon port (red):** Usually a square port to inflate the balloon at the tip of the catheter; inflation of the balloon requires 1.0–1.5 mL of air.
- **Proximal port (blue):** Approximately 30 cm proximal to the tip; in proper position lies in the superior vena cava; may be used for fluid administration when not used for determination of CVP and CO.
- **Additional proximal port (white/clear):** In models with an additional infusion lumen in the right ventricle for infusion or pacing.

28

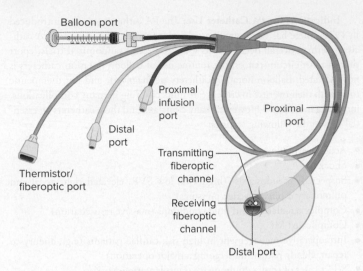

Figure 28-5. Typical pulmonary artery catheter ("Swan-Ganz catheter").

- **Distal port (yellow):** Lies in PA at the tip of the catheter just beyond the balloon; this port is attached to a pressure transducer for continuous PAP tracings and intermittent PAOP measurement. Can also be used to draw mixed venous blood gas. It can be used in the calculation of derived parameters such as oxygen consumption, oxygen utilization coefficient, and intrapulmonary shunt fraction.
- **Thermistor:** Temperature sensor that provides continuous core temperature measurements as well as measurements used in thermodilution CO techniques.

Additional Functions and Measurement Capabilities of PA Catheters

- **Pacing PA catheters:** Extra ports (approximately 19 cm from the tip) through which pacing wires can be passed into the right ventricle; other models contain electrodes along the surface of the catheter; capable of pacing both right atrium and right ventricle.
- **Oximetric PA catheter:** Standard PA catheter ports with fiberoptic components; emit light impulses to and from distal end of catheter; light impulses are then reflected by hemoglobin and measured; used for continuous O_2 saturation monitoring.
- **Right ventricular ejection fraction catheter:** Used to measure REF, which is then used to calculate RVEDVI (best indicator of preload).

28

Pulmonary Artery Catheterization Procedure

1. **Materials:** There are many versions of the flow-directed, balloon-tipped PA catheter; a generic representation is in Figure 28-6. A PA catheter introducer insertion kit usually contains an introducer sheath (cordis catheter), flexible J-tip guidewire, vessel dilator, catheter contamination shield, and other items needed to insert the catheter (Figure 28-7). The monitoring system (transducers, tubing, and stopcocks) and pressurized flush system are usually set up by the nursing staff and should be operational before catheter insertion.

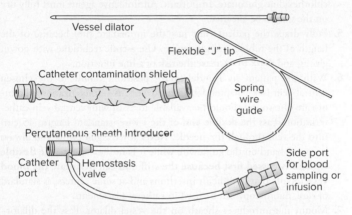

Figure 28-6. Some additional items used for PA catheter placement.

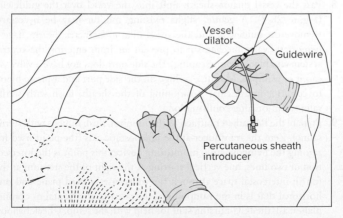

Figure 28-7. The introducer sheath and the vessel dilator are passed into the vessel.

2. Obtain informed consent from the patient or the patient's medical decision maker. Make sure that emergency resuscitation medications are on hand in the event of refractory arrhythmia.

3. Choose a site. In a patient who may receive thrombolytic therapy or who has a coagulopathy, femoral and internal jugular veins may be preferred because of their compressibility if a complication occurs. The easiest sites for floating the PA catheter are the right internal jugular and the left subclavian veins. Rationale: The PA catheter is packaged in a coiled position; these sites tend to the natural curve of the catheter as it assists in placement.

4. Widely prep the insertion site with a topical antiinfective agent such as chlorhexidine gluconate. Important: Antiinfective agents must fully dry on the skin to be effective.

5. Fully drape the patient (not just the immediate site) because of the length of the tubing and guidewire. Use aseptic technique with gown, gloves, and mask to decrease the risk of a line infection.

6. With the patient in Trendelenburg position, cannulate the chosen central vein (see Chapter 19, Central Venous Catheterization). Point-of-care ultrasound should be available to assist with central vein catheterization. Pass the flexible end of the J-wire (standard length, 45 cm) into the vein through the needle. **Never** force a guidewire, and always keep one hand on the guidewire while it is in the patient. **The flexible tip end is passed first because the stiff end can perforate the blood vessel.** Note that in difficult insertions and at some centers, as standard of care, fluoroscopy can be used in catheter placement.

7. Mount the introducer sheath on the vessel dilator. Pass the dilator–sheath unit over the wire. Make a full-thickness skin nick at the wire entry site with a no. 11 blade scalpel.

8. Pass the vessel dilator–sheath unit into the vessel over the guidewire (Figure 28-7). A gentle, slight twisting motion may be necessary. Remove the guidewire and the vessel dilator. Catheter sheaths have a hemostatic valve mechanism to prevent air from entering the central system and blood from escaping. The side port does not have a valve, so cap it or clamp it. Mount a syringe on the side port and aspirate blood to confirm intravascular positioning of the sheath; flush with sterile saline solution after confirmation.

9. Prepare the PA catheter (attach to the monitor, flush lumens with sterile saline). Zero the transducer at the phlebostatic axis (the point used for zeroing the hemodynamic monitoring device; this point is the intersection of two lines, one vertical starting at the right of the sternum at the fourth intercostal space through the transverse or axial plane and one horizonal that is in the midpoint of the chest in the frontal or coronal plane); ask the ICU nursing staff for help with the setup. Check balloon function and gently wave the catheter to ensure that an appropriate

28

waveform is present on the monitor. Note: Never fill the balloon with fluid; use only air. The volume is typically 1.5 mL. After placing the catheter through the contamination shield, check balloon function by insufflating with 1.5 mL of air.

10. Insert the prepared catheter (flushed, transduced, contamination shield in place) into the sheath (Figure 28-8). Once you have advanced approximately 15–20 cm and a CVP tracing is visible on the monitor, gently inflate the balloon with 1.0–1.5 mL of air using the volume-limiting syringe provided with the set. There should be no resistance to balloon inflation.

11. Once the balloon is inflated, advance the catheter to the level of the right atrium under the guidance of the pressure waveform and the ECG. Monitor the waveform and ECG at all times while advancing the balloon catheter. Figure 28-9 shows the normal pressures encountered as the catheter is advanced. Important: **Never** advance the catheter with the balloon deflated. Conversely, always withdraw the PA catheter with the balloon deflated.

12. Positioning of the PA catheter in the right atrium is probably best determined by watching for the characteristic waveform on the monitor (Figure 28-10). The right atrium is generally approximately 30 cm from the right internal jugular or subclavian vein insertion site and approximately 35–40 cm from the left subclavian vein insertion site.

13. An abrupt change in the pressure tracing occurs as the catheter enters the right ventricle (Figure 28-10). There is generally minimal ectopy on

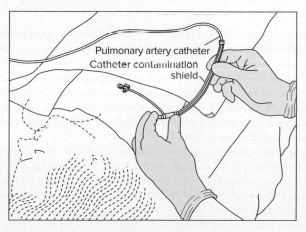

Figure 28-8. The fluid-filled pulmonary artery catheter is passed into the introducer sheath.

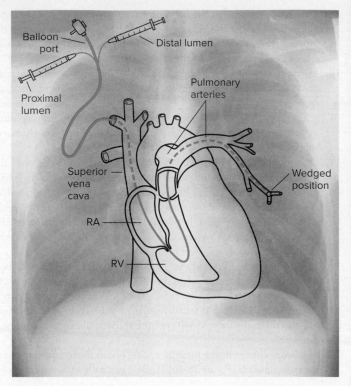

Figure 28-9. Relative positioning of the pulmonary artery catheter.

entry into the right ventricle; however, as the catheter advances into the right ventricular outflow tract, premature ventricular contractions may occur.

14. Steadily advance the catheter until ectopy disappears and the PA tracing (heralded by a rise in diastolic pressure) is obtained. If this does not occur by the time 60 cm is reached, deflate the balloon, withdraw the catheter to 20 cm, and make another attempt with the balloon inflated after slightly rotating the catheter.

15. Once the catheter is in the PA, obtain the PAOP (wedge pressure) after advancing the catheter another 10–15 cm. The final position of the catheter should be such that PAOP is obtained with no less than full balloon inflation and the PAP tracing is present with the balloon deflated. In the ideal position, transition from PAP to PAOP (and vice versa) occurs within three or fewer heartbeats. In an adult, the typical length to the PA position is 45–60 cm. Table 28-7 (page 896) shows normal PA catheter measurements important for patient evaluation and treatment.

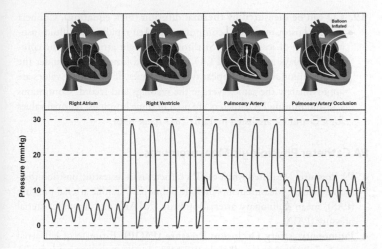

Figure 28-10. Characteristic pressure waveforms seen as the pulmonary artery catheter is advanced. RA = right atrium; RV = right ventricle; PA = pulmonary artery. The "wedge pressure" is the pulmonary artery occlusion pressure (PAOP) when the balloon is inflated. (Panel A: Internal Medicine on Call, 2e, Haist SA, et al. [eds.]. Appleton & Lange, Stamford, CT, 1996. Panel B: In: Brunicardi F, Andersen DK, Billiar TR, et al. [eds.]. Schwartz's Principles of Surgery, 11e. New York, NY: McGraw-Hill.)

16. Once the position is acceptable, lock the contamination shield onto the sheath. The catheter can be readjusted after the sterile field is taken down. Suture the sheath to the skin, secure the catheter in place, and dress the surgical site according to unit protocol. Connect catheters to the ports on the sheath. The inflow port on the sheath can be used for IV fluid and medication administration. The balloon should be kept deflated unless a PAOP is being measured.

17. Obtain a CXR to document the catheter position and to rule out pneumothorax or other complications. A properly positioned catheter should lie just beyond the vertebral bodies in the nonwedged position.

18. **Common problems:** Catheter placement is more difficult if severe PA hypertension is present. If there is significant cardiac enlargement, particularly dilatation of the right-heart structures, the catheter may coil in its path to the right ventricular outflow tract; fluoroscopy may be needed for correct positioning. Furthermore, under these conditions, the PA catheter may have difficulty holding its proper position. Because the balloon-tipped catheter depends on flow to carry it through the right-heart chambers, placement in the PA may be difficult if the patient has low CO.

28

19. **CO can be measured by thermal dilution (Fick equation).** Connect the thermistor to the CO computer and then rapidly inject fluid (usually 10 mL of ice-cooled NS) through the right atrial port. The computer displays a curve, and CO is calculated from the area under the thermal dilution curve. Repeat two more times. If all of these values are approximately the same, average the readings and record. Continuous CO-monitoring PA catheters are used in some hospitals. Normal values for CO and CI are listed in Table 28-7 (page 896).

PA Catheter Physiologic Measurements

- **PA Pressure:** Measured when the PA catheter is in its resting position (balloon deflated). Measurements include pulmonary systolic arterial pressure (PAS), mean pulmonary arterial pressure (MPAP), and diastolic arterial pressure (PAD).

- **Pulmonary Artery Occlusion Pressure (PAOP):** Estimate of left atrial pressure (LAP). Measured while the inflated balloon at the tip of the PA catheter occludes a branch of the PA. Important: To avoid pulmonary infarction, fully deflate the balloon when it is not in use. In the absence of mitral valvular disease, PAOP correlates closely with LAP and with the left ventricular end-diastolic pressure (LVEDP). This correlation exists because of the unobstructed continuity between the PA and the left side of the heart.

- **Left Ventricular End-Diastolic Pressure (LVEDP):** A measure of preload used to optimize fluid resuscitation and CO. For optimal stroke volume on the Starling curve, the preload must be adequate to stretch the wall of the left ventricle. Hypovolemia results in too little tension on the muscle fibers and therefore decreased stroke volume and CO. Too much preload stretches beyond the point of maximum tension and decreases CO. Clinically, LVEDP and PAOP are used to keep preload in an optimum range. The normal PAOP varies between 6 and 12 mm Hg but may be higher for different disease states and for preexisting cardiac disease leading to decreased chamber compliance.

- **Right Ventricular Ejection Fraction (REF)/Right Ventricular End-Diastolic Volume Index (RVEDVI):** RVEDVI, the optimal assessment of preload, is most helpful in patients with high intrathoracic pressure. A rapid-response thermistor and CO computer are used to calculate REF. Once REF and CO are known, RVEDVI can be calculated. RVEDVI is a more accurate assessment of volume status than PAOP. The normal range for EDVI is 80–120 mL/m^2.

- **Continuous Cardiac Output Measurement:** The specially designed PA catheter emits small pulses of energy that heat the surrounding blood for continuous CO measurement. CO is then calculated based on the magnitude and rate of temperature change. This continuous measurement, along with calculated derivatives, is intermittently updated and displayed on the device.

28

- **Continuous $S\bar{v}o_2$ Monitoring:** This is the most sensitive indicator of end-organ perfusion. Oximetric PA catheters are used for direct measurement of mixed venous Hgb saturation ($S\bar{v}o_2$). A microprocessor then displays a continuous graph of $S\bar{v}o_2$ measurements. Calibration is periodically confirmed with ABG measured from heparinized blood drawn from the distal port of the oximetric catheter.

- **Continuous SpO_2 Monitoring:** While pulse oximetry is not a standard part of the pulmonary artery catheter, the same fiberoptic technology used to measure $S\bar{v}o_2$ is used to measure SaO_2 (systemic arterial oxygen saturation). A SpO_2 <90% implies inadequate oxygenation and under most circumstances necessitates immediate intervention. *One exception* would be a patient with severe COPD whose usual O_2 saturation is in the upper 80% range. Conversely, SpO_2 >90% does not necessarily imply adequate O_2 delivery (see following section). Pulse oximetry is not useful in the setting of smoke inhalation and carbon monoxide poisoning because of the higher affinity of the hemoglobin molecule for carbon monoxide.

Differential Diagnosis of PA Catheter Abnormalities

Table 28-7 (page 896) indicates normal PA pressures and cardiovascular measurements. Perturbations of these values indicate a disease process and the differential diagnoses are shown in Table 28-8, page 906.

Clinical Applications of the PA Catheter

- **Cardiac output** provides an estimation of volume status and myocardial performance. It is a function of heart rate and stroke volume. Stroke volume depends on preload, afterload, and contractility.

- **Heart rate:** Heart rate is increased to maintain or increase CO in the face of inadequate tissue perfusion. Hence, tachycardia is an additional indicator of O_2 debt (i.e., delivery–demand deficit). Tachycardia >120 beats/min increases myocardial O_2 demand significantly and should be promptly treated; treatment often includes treating the underlying cause of the tachycardia (e.g., bladder outlet obstruction).

  The PA catheter is used to establish adequate myocardial filling pressures such that heart rate may be clinically manipulated to maximize CO. In a patient with adequate filling pressures, slow heart rate (<80 beats/min), and low CO, drugs that accelerate heart rate (chronotropes) can be used to increase CO. Alternatively, tachycardia >120 beats/min with an adequate PAOP can be pharmacologically slowed to decrease strain on the heart.

- **Preload:** Is indicated by PAOP or end-diastolic volume index (EDVI), a reflection of LVEDV. In simple terms, preload is the amount of blood in the heart before contraction. Consequently, preload represents the stretch placed on an individual myocardial cell. When PAOP is optimized, myocardial performance is optimized according to the Starling curve.

28

Table 28-8. Differential Diagnosis by Category Based on Perturbations in Hemodynamic Parameters[a]

Diagnosis	Systemic Blood Pressure	CVP	CO	PAOP/ LVEDP	PAP	PVR	SVR
Cardiogenic shock	↓	↑	↓	↑	↑	↑	↑
Cardiogenic tamponade	↓	↑	↓	↑	↑	–	↓
Pulmonary embolism (Typically massive/ saddle)	↓	↑	↓	– or ↓	↑	↑	↑
Hypovolemic shock	↓	↓	↓	↓	↓	↑	↑
Neurogenic shock	↓	↓	↓	↓	↓	↓	↓
Septic shock	↓	↓	↑	↓	↓	↓	↓

[a]These are the trends usually seen with the conditions noted. Clinical variables (medications, secondary conditions, etc.) may vary these trends somewhat.
Highlighted areas denote major differences between subgroups.
CVP = central venous pressure; CO = cardiac output; PAOP = pulmonary artery occlusion pressure; LVEDP = left ventricular end-diastolic pressure; PAP = pulmonary artery pressure; PVR = peripheral vascular resistance; SVR = systemic vascular resistance.
↑ = usually increased; ↓ = usually decreased; – = usually unchanged.

- o **Clinical implications.** Low PAOP or EDVI means suboptimal myocardial muscle stretch. CO can be increased first by administration of fluids. The result is an increase in LVEDV, an increase in myocardial muscle tension, and improved myocardial performance, thus shifting the Starling curve to the right. Consequently, a markedly elevated PAOP may be needed to optimize myocardial performance in a failing heart. It is common for patients who have just undergone heart valve replacement to need a PAOP of 20–25 mm Hg to optimize CO (because of decreased compliance of the postoperative heart muscle). Patients with a recent MI may similarly need a PAOP of 16–18 mm Hg to optimize output.
- **Afterload:** Resistance to ventricular ejection; measured clinically by calculating the SVR. Normal SVR = 900–1200 dynes/s/cm³.
  - o **Indications for afterload reduction.** Includes significant mitral regurgitation and increased PAOP with elevated SVR/decreased CI. Tereatment includes vasodilators (e.g., nitroprusside, nitrates, angiotensin-converting enzyme [ACE] inhibitors, hydralazine).

- **Contractility:** The ability of the heart to alter its contractile force and velocity independent of fiber length. This aspect is difficult to measure directly but can be estimated with surrogate markers. Correctable metabolic causes of depressed contractility include:

  o Hypoxia
  o Acidosis (pH <7.2)
  o Hypophosphatemia
  o Adrenal insufficiency
  o Hypothermia

  Improve contractility with inotropic agents such as dobutamine (inotropic agent; primary activity results from stimulation of the beta-receptors of the heart with mild chronotropic, hypertensive, arrhythmogenic, and vasodilative effects) or milrinone (positive inotrope and vasodilator, with little chronotropic activity).

- **Continuous $S\bar{v}o_2$ Monitoring**
  o Follows trends in O_2 supply–demand balance.
  o Because it is the best indicator of decreased peripheral O_2 delivery, a decrease in $S\bar{v}o_2$ is the earliest sign of organ dysfunction.
  o The effect of interventions (e.g., transfusions, fluid administration, inotropic agents) is best assessed using $S\bar{v}o_2$. $S\bar{v}o_2$ values between 65% and 75% represent adequate tissue O_2 delivery and extraction.
  o If $S\bar{v}o_2$ drops to <60%, immediately assess O_2 delivery, as organ perfusion is in jeopardy. See Figure 28-11.
- If $S\bar{v}o_2$ is <60% and SaO_2 is greater than 90%, hypoperfusion is a failure of cardiovascular performance.

  In summary, a decline of $S\bar{v}o_2$ prompts an emergent review of oxygen delivery (i.e., CO, [Hgb], SaO_2) and consumption ($SaO_2 - S\bar{v}o_2$). Potential treatments include:
  o Correction of hypoxia
  o Optimization of myocardial performance for decreased CO = SVR (MAP – CVP) × 80/ CO (L/min)
  o RBC transfusion for symptomatic anemia
  o Identification and management of conditions leading to increased metabolic demands (e.g., unrecognized seizures, shivering, and large tissue defects) because these conditions markedly increase in O_2 demand (Figure 28-11).

PULMONARY PHYSIOLOGY

28

The key to understanding pulmonary physiology and mechanical ventilation in the ICU is to differentiate oxygenation and ventilation (Figure 28-12).

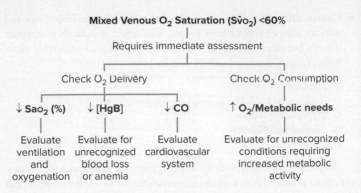

Figure 28-11. Algorithm for the assessment of decreased $S\bar{v}o_2$.

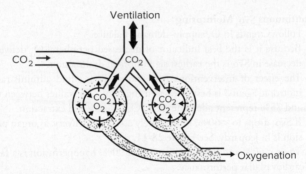

Figure 28-12. Ventilation and oxygenation in a typical alveoli.

Ventilation

Ventilation is the mechanical movement of air into and out of the respiratory system.

The result is the exchange of CO_2. Several parameters, such as volumes and capacities, are important in assessing the adequacy of ventilation. Spirometry gives both dynamic information (i.e., ability to move air into and out of the lungs) and static volume measurements. The lung volume subdivisions and capacities are shown on a spirometric graph in Figure 28-13.

Lung Volumes: Total lung capacity (TLC), or the maximum amount of gas in the lung at full inspiration, comprises four basic lung volumes:

1. **Tidal volume (TV):** The volume of inspired gas during a normal breath; approximately 6–8 mL/kg in resting, healthy adults.
2. **Inspiratory reserve volume (IRV):** The volume of gas that can be maximally inspired beyond a normal tidal volume inspiration.

28

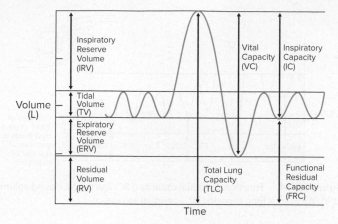

Figure 28-13. Spirometric graph with volumes and capacities of the lung.

3. **Expiratory reserve volume (ERV):** The volume of gas that can be maximally expired beyond a normal tidal volume expiration.

4. **Residual volume (RV):** The volume of gas that remains in the lung after a maximal expiratory effort (Figure 28-13).

Lung Capacity: The sum of two or more of these lung volumes makes up four divisions called lung capacities (Figure 28-13).

1. **Vital capacity (VC):** The volume of gas expired after a maximal inspiration followed by maximal expiration (VC = ERV + TV + IRV).

2. **Inspiratory capacity (IC):** The volume of gas expired from maximal inspiration to the end of normal resting TV (IC = TV + IRV).

3. **Functional residual capacity (FRC):** The amount of gas remaining in the lung after a normal tidal volume expiration (FRC = ERV + RV); acts as a buffer against extreme changes in alveolar PO_2 and consequent dramatic changes in arterial PO_2 with each breath.

Clinical Implications of Ventilation Abnormalities

These volumes and capacities are important factors in assessing ventilation because they can change under different conditions (e.g., atelectasis, obstruction, consolidation, and small airway collapse). For example, as *expiratory reserve volume (ERV)* decreases with small airway collapse, *functional residual capacity (FRC)* decreases (Figure 28-14). These alterations in lung volume affect respiratory reserve as well as oxygenation and ventilation.

Critical Closing Volume (CCV): Critical closing volume (CCV) is the minimum volume and pressure of gas necessary to prevent small airways from collapsing during expiration. When collapse occurs, blood is shunted around

28

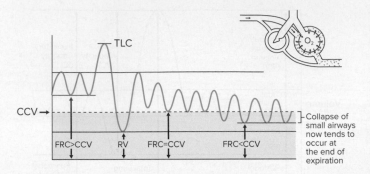

Figure 28-14. Functional residual capacity (FRC) and critical closing volume (CCV). TLC = total lung capacity; RV = residual volume.

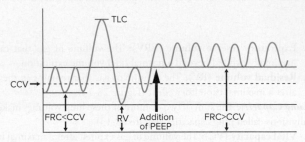

Figure 28-15. The effect of positive end-expiratory pressure (PEEP) is to increase functional residual capacity (FRC). CCV = critical closing volume; TLC = total lung capacity; RV = residual volume.

nonventilated alveoli. This phenomenon decreases the surface area available for gas exchange. CCV can vary as compliance changes. If CCV > FRC (air in the lung after tidal expiration), collapse tends to occur in a higher proportion of airways (Figure 28-14).

One method of overcoming CCV is to increase the amount of PEEP in the lung (see later, Ventilator Management, page 924). The effect of PEEP is to increase FRC by minimizing small airway collapse at the end of expiration. This maneuver improves alveolar ventilation, decreases shunting, and ultimately improves oxygenation (Figure 28-15).

Lung Compliance: Compliance is the *change* in lung volume (V) as a function of *change* in pressure (P) (Figure 28-16):

$$\text{Lung compliance} = \text{delta V/delta P}$$

This value can be measured at the bedside and reflects FRC and CCV.

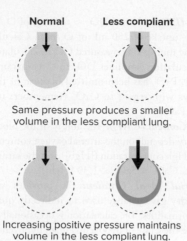

Normal   **Less compliant**

Same pressure produces a smaller
volume in the less compliant lung.

Increasing positive pressure maintains
volume in the less compliant lung.

Figure 28-16. The concept of pulmonary compliance.

Dynamic Compliance: Measure tidal volume (TV) and divide it by peak inspiratory pressure (PIP):

$$\text{Dynamic compliance} = \text{tidal volume/PIP minus PEEP}$$
$$\text{Normal: } 80\text{–}100 \text{ mL/cm water}$$

Static Compliance: Like dynamic compliance, except that *static* PIP is substituted for PIP. Measure static peak pressure (also called plateau pressure) by occluding the exhalation port at the beginning of exhalation (no flow = static pressure). Comparing *dynamic* with *static* compliance may indicate the type of processes causing changes in the elasticity of the lung. Dynamic compliance is affected by both elasticity and airway resistance. Static compliance reflects elasticity and is not affected by airway resistance because there *is no flow* (Figure 28-16).

1. Reduction in dynamic compliance *without* a change in static compliance indicates an airway resistance problem (obstruction, bronchospasm, or collapse of the small airways)
2. Reduction in *both* static and dynamic compliance indicates a decrease in lung elasticity (pulmonary edema, atelectasis, or excessive PEEP)

Oxygenation

Oxygenation is the process of transporting oxygen from the alveolus across the capillary membrane into the pulmonary circulation and subsequently distributing that oxygen to the body's tissues. O_2 delivery is a function of arterial O_2 content and CO.

28

Oxygen Delivery (DO₂): Normal $DO_2 \approx 600$ mL of O_2/min with an average normal O_2 uptake of 250 mL of O_2/min. Calculate DO_2 with PA catheter data by multiplying measured CO by calculated (CaO_2).

   Note: This calculation simplifies DO_2 to three parameters: CO, SaO_2, and [Hgb]. PaO_2 has been omitted because of the *extremely small role* it plays with regard to CaO_2 (remember: its contribution is $0.0031 \times PaO_2$).

Arterial Oxygen Content (CaO₂): The ability of the blood to carry oxygen to the periphery depends on the arterial oxygen content. CaO_2 is directly influenced by Hgb concentration ([Hgb]) and the saturation of Hgb with O_2 (SaO_2) (i.e., $CaO_2 = SaO_2 \times 1.39$ [Hgb]).

Alveolar-to-Arterial (A–a) Gradient: It provides an assessment of alveolar–capillary gas exchange used to indirectly quantify ventilation–perfusion abnormalities. The calculation is occasionally useful as a tool to help determine the cause of hypoxemia (e.g., hypoventilation).

Shunt Fraction: Normal <5%. Reflects the portion of CO that traverses the heart from right to left without increasing CaO_2 ($\approx 5\%$ of pulmonary capillary blood leaves the lung without being oxygenated). In an ideal state, the volume of lung ventilation equals the volume of pulmonary capillary blood flow (Figure 28-17).

   Alterations in these ventilation–perfusion relationships have two causes:

- Relative obstruction of alveolar ventilation (Figure 28-18).
- Relative obstruction of pulmonary blood flow (Figure 28-19).

1. **Perfusion greater than ventilation:** A common scenario is *pulmonary consolidation* due to infection or secretions (Figure 28-18). An alveolus receives no ventilation because of bronchiolar obstruction, yet normal

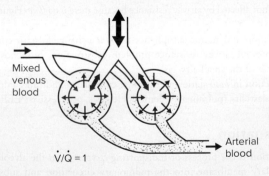

Figure 28-17. The ideal state where the volume of lung ventilation equals the volume of pulmonary capillary blood flow, resulting in a ventilation to perfusion ratio (V/Q) = 1.

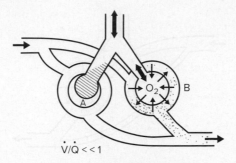

Figure 28-18. Perfusion greater than ventilation. Alveolus (A) receives no ventilation because of bronchiolar obstruction (B).

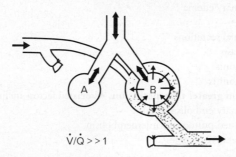

Figure 28-19. Ventilation greater than perfusion. Uniform ventilation continues to alveoli A and B but no blood flow passes alveolus A.

pulmonary capillary perfusion continues (i.e., complete pulmonary A–V shunt exists with respect to that alveolus).

2. **Ventilation greater than perfusion:** Impairment of pulmonary blood flow to the alveolar level occurs after lung surgery and after pulmonary embolism (Figure 28-19). Uniform ventilation continues to the alveoli, but no blood flow is associated with some of the alveoli. This situation increases the ventilated physiologic dead space *and* increases the shunt fraction.

3. **Compensation mechanism:** Local vasoconstriction results in diversion of blood flow to better ventilated alveoli. This mechanism is called hypoxic pulmonary vasoconstriction (Figure 28-20).

Principle: Recognize that at any given time, combinations of these situations exist *simultaneously* within the lung (remember that the normal shunt fraction is ≈ 5%). Therefore, alterations in either ventilation or perfusion can increase shunt fraction and seriously decrease oxygenation.

28

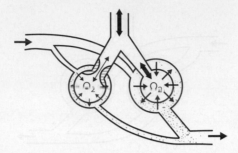

Figure 28-20. Compensation for ventilation perfusion mismatch.

1. **Perfusion greater than ventilation.** Associated factors include:
   o Pulmonary edema
   o ARDS
   o Bronchial secretions
   o Atelectasis
   o Pneumonia
   o Pneumonitis
2. **Ventilation greater than perfusion.** Associated factors include:
   o Pulmonary embolism (PE)
   o Continued pulmonary microembolism
   o Postoperative changes

Calculation of A–a Gradient and Shunt Fraction: The equations for determining A–a gradient and shunt fraction are in comprehensive textbooks
   on critical care.

GUIDELINES FOR AIRWAY MANAGEMENT IN THE ICU SETTING

Indications for Endotracheal Intubation

The decision to intubate is often a stress-provoking process but potentially
a life-saving measure that needs to be mastered by any physician caring for
critically ill patients. The primary objective of mechanical ventilation is to
decrease the work of breathing and reverse life-threatening hypoxia and
hypercapnia. The basic principles of endotracheal intubation and airway
management are presented in Chapter 19, Bedside Procedures, starting on
page 565. Common indications for endotracheal intubation and mechanical
ventilation in the ICU setting include:

- **Inability to adequately ventilate** (e.g., airway obstruction, severe chest
  trauma, excessive sedation, neuromuscular disease, and paralyzed or
  fatigued respiratory muscles)

28

- **Inability to adequately oxygenate** (e.g., pneumonia, PE, pulmonary edema, and ARDS)
- **Excessive work of breathing** (e.g., severe bronchospasm, airway obstruction)
- **Airway protection** (e.g., unconsciousness, altered mental status, massive resuscitation, and facial or head trauma)

A timely decision to intubate a decompensating patient can turn an otherwise chaotic intubation into a controlled, elective procedure. Diagnostic factors that help predict impending respiratory failure are listed in Table 28-9.

Noninvasive Ventilation (NIV)

Occasionally in patients with impending respiratory failure, endotracheal intubation with mechanical ventilation can be delayed or avoided using noninvasive ventilation (NIV) techniques. NIV positive pressure ventilation can be delivered by oronasal masks, or nasal prongs. NIV contraindications include cardiopulmonary arrest, impaired consciousness, inability to cooperate in clearing secretions or protecting the airway, facial trauma or deformity, and others. NIV is usually delivered using identical modes as invasive mechanical ventilation such as pressure support (PS) ventilation or assist control (see page 920). **Continuous positive airway pressure (CPAP)** is commonly used in patients with respiratory failure secondary to cardiogenic pulmonary edema. Another common mode for NIV is **bilevel positive airway pressure or BiPAP** that delivers both inspiratory positive airway pressure

Table 28-9. Indicators of Impending Respiratory Failure Necessitating Intubation and Mechanical Ventilation

Condition	Normal Range (Adults)
Respiratory impairment	
Tachypnea > 30 breaths/min	10–20 breaths/min
Dyspnea	
Use of accessory muscle to breath	
Neurologic impairment	
Loss of gag reflex	
Altered mental status (i.e., patient is unable to protect airway against aspiration)	
Gas exchange impairment	
$PaCO_2$ >60 mm Hg	35–45 mm Hg
PaO_2 <70 mm Hg (on 50% mask)	80–100 mm Hg (on room air)
SaO_2 <90%	

28

(IPAP) and expiratory positive airway pressure (EPAP) (Figure 28-21). In addition to alleviating the need for intubation and mechanical ventilation in some patients, NIV may be used to prevent recurrent respiratory failure following extubation.

Securing the Airway

An essential treatment component of respiratory failure is securing and maintaining a patent airway. The first step is a rapid assessment of the airway that includes history and physical exam. Most potential difficult airways can be recognized with a bedside evaluation. Indications of the difficult airway include limited mouth opening (<3 cm), mandibular protrusion, narrow dental arch, decreased thyromental distance, decreased submandibular compliance (inability to protrude the lower incisors past the upper incisor, decreased sternomental distance, limited neck extension [cervical spine limitations], dentures/poor dentition, and presence of a beard and obesity). A common system for evaluation of an airway is known as the Mallampati airway classification of oral opening (Figure 19-32, page 585). This test is used in the assessment of sleep apnea as well predicting the ease of endotracheal intubation. Class 1 suggests an easy intubation, whereas with increasing inability to visualize key laryngeal structures such as the soft palate, uvula, and anterior and posterior tonsillar pillars, Class IV suggests the most difficult airway management intubation.

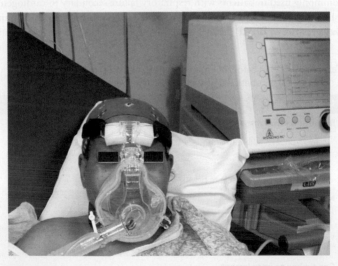

28

Figure 28-21. Example of a patient being treated with bilevel positive airway pressure or BiPAP noninvasive ventilation (NIV) technique by face mask. (Reproduced with permission from Knoop KJ, Stack LB, Storrow AB, Thurman RJ (eds.). The Atlas of Emergency Medicine, 4e. New York, NY: McGraw-Hill Medical.)

Temporary airway control is achieved using bag mask ventilation accompanied by the chin lift and jaw thrust maneuver (see Figure 19-25, page 575). Use caution in patients with possible cervical spine injury unless the neck has a stabilizing device. Difficulties using bag mask ventilation are associated with obesity, presence of a beard, lack of teeth, and history of sleep apnea or neck radiation. Use of a nasopharyngeal or oropharyngeal airway can keep the patient's tongue from obstructing the oropharynx. Alternatively, supraglottic airway (SGA) or laryngeal mask airway (LMA) can be used in the face of excessive gas leak or resistance to face mask ventilation and can be considered a "bridge procedure" to allow formal endotracheal intubation in a more controlled setting such as the critical care unit or operating room. (See Chapter 19, Bedside Procedures, for details.) Signs of inadequate temporary ventilation include absent chest movement, absent breath sounds, stridor, cyanosis, or decreasing oxygen saturation (SpO_2).

Definitive airway management includes oral or nasal endotracheal intubation. (Endotracheal intubation is also discussed in Chapter 19, Bedside Procedures, page 565.) A portable "**difficult airway kit**" containing specialized equipment must be immediately available (e.g., videolaryngoscope with monitoring, specialized blades, oropharyngeal airways, cricothyrotomy kit, etc.). Failure to intubate electively in the operating room, an ideal setting, occurs in 1–20 patients per 100,000 cases. Basic preparation for an awake ICU intubation is more challenging and involves the following:

1. Inform the patient (or responsible person) of the special risks and procedures pertaining to management of the difficult airway.
2. Confirm that there is at least one additional individual immediately available to serve as an assistant in difficult airway management.
3. Administer face mask preoxygenation before initiating management of the difficult airway. Anticipate that a hypoxic adult may be uncooperative, impeding preoxygenation.
4. Once the ETT has been placed, immediately confirm placement.
   o **Confirmation of endotracheal tube placement:** Use a colorimetric or capnographic end-tidal CO_2 detector (Figure 19-23, page 573) and auscultation of bilateral breath sounds (Figure 19-31, page 584). Consider obtaining a CXR to confirm the location of the distal tip of the ETT, which should reside 2–4 cm above the carina.
5. **Complications of endotracheal intubation:** Esophageal intubation; pneumothorax; pneumomediastinum; recurrent laryngeal nerve injury; hemorrhage; tracheal stenosis (can be avoided by keeping cuff pressures < 25 mm Hg); and ET tube dislodgement/self-extubation. A more extensive list of complications and potential management strategies can be found in Table 19-7, page 591.

28

Management of the intubated patient

1. Long-term endotracheal intubation (>7 days) can be associated with ventilator-associated pneumonia (VAP), sinusitis, vocal cord paralysis, tracheomalacia, and laryngotracheal stenosis. Intubated ventilator-dependent patients beyond 7 days should be considered for formal tracheostomy placement.

2. For patients on long-term ventilatory support, monitor ETT cuff pressures based on local protocols, but this should be done at least daily. The location of the ETT tube should be rotated from side to side daily to avoid pressure ulceration in one area of the lip or mouth. Once widespread, the daily practice of verifying ETT tube by chest radiograph has been largely abandoned and is only recommended if there is a concern for tube migration. The level of the ETT tube at the lip should be marked and used as a check for positioning.

3. Suctioning and oral hygiene care are important practices in patients on ICU ventilator support to limit ETT and ventilator-associated complications.

   a. Oral hygiene through decontamination with agents such as chlorhexidine is part of many nursing ICU protocols with some controversy concerning utility.

   b. Oral pharyngeal and ETT suctioning are critical since intubated patients cannot clear their own secretions. VAP is one of the most common healthcare-associated infections. To prevent this complication, aspiration of subglottic secretions using devices such as Hi-Lo Evac endotracheal tube (Evac ETT) is a recommended intervention in some units. The ETT has a dorsal lumen above the cuff, which is connected to suction to remove the secretions that pool above the cuff in the subglottic space. This type of ETT is often used in patients who are in the ICU setting on more long-term ventilation with the goal to reduce VAP. Their use, however, is not routine with studies conflicting on the utility of these special ETTs.

4. Enteric nutrition using the GI tract is the preferred mode of nutritional support. Nasogastric feeding tubes are commonly employed in ventilated patients. The practice of checking gastric residual volumes has been generally abandoned.

5. The use of sedation and analgesia and evaluation of pharmacologic intervention on the intubated and ventilated patient begins on page 880.

28 ## Surgical Options for Airway Management

- **Cricothyroidotomy (needle and surgical)** is an emergency surgical procedure used when nonsurgical attempts to secure the airway have failed. The procedures are discussed in Chapter 19, Bedside Procedures, pages 559–560. It is recommended to convert cricothyroidotomy to a tracheostomy within 72 hr to minimize long-term subglottic tracheal stenosis and tracheomalacia.

- **Tracheostomy** is used when long-term intubation is anticipated (greater than 5–7 days) and for patients with severe maxillofacial injuries. While tracheostomy is advocated by some as a bedside procedure, it is most commonly performed in the operating room on an elective basis. Cricothyroidotomy tends to be an emergent bedside procedure. Tracheostomy is most commonly performed in the operating room and percutaneous approaches have been reported. The incision is through the skin and into the trachea and not the cricothyroid membrane. The benefits of tracheostomy are suitability for long-term management, improved patient comfort, improved oral hygiene, secretion management, and a reduction in sedation requirements over endotracheal intubation.

PRINCIPLES OF MECHANICAL VENTILATION

On page 907 in reviewing pulmonary physiology, the anatomy of natural breathing was discussed. For a machine to re-create that anatomy, we need to introduce three new concepts and their underlying components. These concepts are: triggers (factors initiating a breath), target tidal volumes (pressure or flow rates are predefined), and cycles (factors terminating a breath).

1. **Triggers: factors initiating a breath**
   o **Time** – Defined by respiratory rate, where a breath is delivered at a predetermined number of times per minute.
   o **Pressure** – The patient attempts to breathe spontaneously, which is sensed by the ventilator as a fallen pressure and a complete breath is delivered by the ventilator.
   o **Flow** – The patient attempts to breathe spontaneously, flow is sensed by the ventilator, and the prescribed breath is delivered.
   o **Neural sensing** – This requires an esophageal sensor to determine an electromyographic signal from the diaphragm to initiate a prescribed breath.
2. **Target tidal volumes: based on either pressure or flow**
   o **Pressure** – The ventilator generates a breath until the predetermined pressure target is achieved. However, the tidal volume delivered is dependent on lung compliance and resistance. If these are deteriorating the patient may not be adequately oxygenated.
   o **Flow** – Ventilator delivers a breath based on inspiratory flow, independent of lung compliance or resistance and predetermined by the clinician.

28

3. **Cycle: factors that can terminate a breath**
   o **Volume** – Once the prescribed inspiratory volume is reached, the breath is terminated.
   o **Flow** – Flow decreases as the lungs fill up with gas. When the flow falls to about 30% of the initial flow, the ventilator terminates the breath.
   o **Neural sensing** – Termination of the electromyographic signal concludes the breath.

Mechanical Ventilation Modes

Combining the anatomy of a breath with factors that initiate and terminate a breath provides the physician with a menu of ventilator modes tailored to the patient's disease states. These modes include the following and are graphically represented in Figure 28-22, page 921.

1. **Assist-Control Ventilation (AC)**
   a. Volume Assist Control (VAC)
   b. Pressure Assist-Control Ventilation (PAC)
2. **Controlled Mechanical Ventilation (CMV)**
   a. Volume Control (VC)
   b. Pressure Control (PC)
3. **Synchronous Intermittent Mandatory Ventilation (SIMV)**
   a. Volume-Synchronized Intermittent Mandatory Ventilation (V-SIMV)
   b. Pressure-Synchronized Intermittent Mandatory Ventilation (P-SIMV)
4. **Pressure Support Ventilation (PSV)**
5. **Pressure-Regulated Volume Control (PRVC)**
6. **Airway Pressure Release Ventilation (APRV)**
7. **High-Frequency Oscillatory Ventilation (HFOV)**
8. **Neurally Adjusted Ventilatory Assist (NAVA)**
9. **Volume Diffusive Respirator (VDR)**

Detailed Description of Ventilator Modes

1. **Assist-Control Ventilation (AC):** The ventilator delivers a full tidal volume with each inspiratory effort. The respiratory rate can be determined by the patient, although a set rate ensures adequate minute ventilation.
   o **Advantages:** The patient can easily increase minute ventilation even with poor inspiratory effort. The result is a marked decrease in the work of breathing.

28

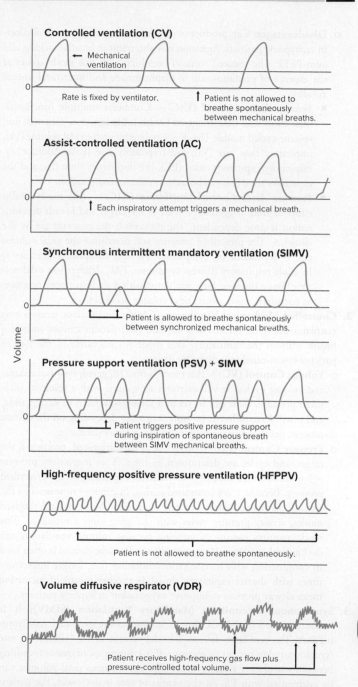

Figure 28-22. Graphic representation of different ventilator modes.

28

o **Disadvantages:** Can produce overventilation and respiratory alkalosis in tachypneic patients. Agitation can also result in breath-stacking and auto-PEEP. The reduced work of breathing with this mode comes at the expense of predisposition to diaphragmatic and intercostal muscle atrophy.

  ■ *Volume Assist Control (VAC)* – Combines multiple functionalities: effort and time-triggered breath initiation, flow-targeted, and volume-cycled modes. The clinician determines the tidal volume (Vt), inspiratory flow rate (Vi), and respiratory rate (RR). Additionally, inspiratory/expiratory ratios (I:E), the inspiratory time (It), and the expiratory time (Et) can be used to enhance oxygenation.

  ■ *Pressure Assist-Control Ventilation (PAC)* – This mode is also effort or time triggered; pressure is the target and breath determination is time dependent. The pressure is the constant set by the clinician. The prescribed pressure will determine the tidal volume and is dependent on compliance. As lung compliance declines as in adult respiratory distress syndrome, PAC delivers less tidal volume. For a diseased lung ventilated with a set inspiratory pressure, as compliance gets worse, tidal volume decreases.

2. **Controlled Mechanical Ventilation (CMV):** The patient receives *only* ventilator-delivered breaths at a set rate (i.e., patient cannot initiate a breath without the ventilator). This mode is used rarely in the care of patients intentionally paralyzed by drugs.

  o **Volume Control (VC)** – This mode is time triggered; flow is the target and volume cycled. It will deliver a set volume with a resultant measured pressure. Flow can be set at a square waveform or decelerating, and it will have different pressure outcomes depending on the disease process, decelerating typically resulting in lower pressures.

  o **Pressure Control (PC)** – This mode is time triggered, pressure is the target, and cycles are determined by time. A set inspiratory pressure will result in a tidal volume that is variable depending on the prescribed pressure. Because it is a controlled setting, inspiratory time is set by the settings on the ventilator and not the patient. With volume-targeted modes, airway pressure varies with changing lung compliance. This mode requires careful monitoring because minute ventilation can decline with worsening lung compliance. Pressure control is often used in conjunction with inverse-ratio ventilation (i.e., longer inspiratory times with shorter expiratory times) as another means of increasing mean airway pressure to improve oxygenation in hypoxic patients.

3. **Synchronous Intermittent Mandatory Ventilation (SIMV):** It is commonly used in the ICU for patients requiring extended ventilatory support. The ventilator delivers set tidal volume at a minimum set rate (synchronized to patient inspiratory effort) during spontaneous breathing between mandatory tidal volumes. The spontaneous tidal volumes can be augmented with PS. As the ventilator rate is decreased, the patient

assumes more and more work of breathing. This mode can either provide full support (with a high mandatory rate) or be used as a weaning mode by decreasing the rate over time.

o **Volume-Synchronized Intermittent Mandatory Ventilation (V-SIMV)** – It is a combination of VC + VA + PS and spontaneous breathing. Since VC is time triggered, flow or pressure targeted, and volume cycled and VA is effort triggered, flow targeted, and flow cycled so V-SIMV can be triggered, targeted, and cycled differently in each breath. Also, during spontaneous breathing it can provide PS set by the clinician to overcome the external resistance that is associated with the ETT and ventilator tubing. Depending on the timing of the effort trigger, it will deliver a spontaneous breath (if triggering occurs too fast) or a volume-assisted breath (if effort trigger occurs close to the prescribed RR).

o **Pressure-Synchronized Intermittent Mandatory Ventilation (P-SIMV)** – It is a combination of PC + PA + PS and spontaneous breathing. Since PC is time triggered, pressure targeted, and time and flow cycled and PA is effort triggered, pressure targeted, and flow cycled so this mode can be triggered, targeted, and cycled differently in each breath.

4. **Pressure Support Ventilation (PSV):** Flow cycled; patient determines tidal volume and cycle length. A preset level of positive pressure boost is turned on during inspiration and is off during expiration. The higher the PS, the less work the patient expends to take a breath. Because the patient can control the duration of lung inflation and tidal volume, PSV tends to be comfortable for most patients. PSV is useful for weaning because the PS can be turned down slowly, with changes as small as 1-cm water. Patient assumes additional work of breathing in small increments. PS is effort triggered; pressure is the target and flow cycled. Because it is only triggered by effort, it cannot be applied to patients without respiratory drive (e.g., deeply sedated or paralyzed patients). Clinician sets a PS level that will provide positive pressure ventilation and overcome the ventilator tubing and provide a tidal volume. Also, there is **volume support ventilation** in which the ventilator adjusts PS to achieve tidal volume prescribed in each effort triggered breath. Both inspiratory time and RR are determined by the patient. See Figure 28-22.

5. **Pressure-Regulated Volume Control (PRVC):** Used in the setting of increased airway pressures (e.g., acute lung injury, ARDS). A microprocessor in the ventilator minimizes the pressure needed to deliver the specified tidal volume by using decelerating flow during inspiration. PRVC can be thought of as dynamic pressure-controlled ventilation without the variation in tidal volumes associated with changing lung compliance. PRVC is both effort and time triggered with pressure target that will control volume and automatically adjust the pressure needed to achieve the tidal volume.

28

6. **Airway Pressure Release Ventilation (APRV):** In this mode pressure control, PS, and spontaneous breathing are combined. It is effort and time triggered, pressure is the target, and it is flow and time cycled. Characterized by very long inspiratory times, it is an inverse I:E ratio ventilation. The clinician sets both the high and low pressures and the times spent on each. Usually these settings are termed Pressure high (P high), Pressure low (P low), Time high (T high), and Time low (T low). PS can be added for the effort triggered breaths. P high usually is set at the plateau pressure limit and P low at zero. It is an alternative mode of ventilation that may assist to recruit lung during hypoxia caused by de-recruitment. Its use for specific diseases, such as ARDS, at this moment is controversial.

7. **High-Frequency Oscillatory Ventilation (HFOV):** Another alternative mode of ventilation where a mean airway pressure is set, and an oscillatory pump delivers small tidal volumes at very high rates. It may be protective since pressure is maintained and driving pressure is minimized due to the very low tidal volumes. Reducing frequency reduces PCO_2 since it will result in higher oscillatory volumes. In ARDS, two studies (OSCAR trial and HFOV in early ARDS) have determined that either it does not make a difference or actually increased mortality in ARDS. There has been some benefit for patients during de-recruitment with copious secretions and to minimize the large volume losses in bronchopleural fistulas.

8. **Neurally Adjusted Ventilatory Assist (NAVA):** Here the electrical activity of the diaphragm is measured by electrodes attached to a probe inserted as a nasogastric tube. It is a mode of ventilation that is electrically triggered, pressure targeted, and electrically cycled. NAVA requires a normal diaphragmatic anatomy and normal ventilatory drive and neural reflexes.

9. **Volume Diffusive Respirator (VDR):** This is a high-frequency time-cycled pressure ventilator that can provide ventilation, oxygenation, and promote the removal of secretions. It provides ventilation at lower airway pressures than those required for conventional ventilation in the pressure control mode.

Ventilator Management

Ventilator Orders

The following is a sample of typical initial ventilator settings for an adult:

- Mode (e.g., AC, SIMV)
- FiO_2 30–100%
- Rate 10–18 breaths/min
- Tidal volume 4–6 mL/kg

- PS (5–20 cm water)
- PEEP (5 cm water or higher, if needed)

Ventilator Setting Changes

Five basic respiratory parameters (FiO_2, minute ventilation, PS, PEEP, and I/E ratio) can be changed to improve ventilation, oxygenation, and compliance.

1. **FiO_2:** Choose an initial FiO_2 that ensures adequate arterial O_2 saturation (SaO_2 >90%). Increasing the level of PEEP is often a helpful means of decreasing the FiO_2 requirement while maintaining adequate oxygenation. Once adequate oxygenation is established, decrease the FiO_2 to avoid O_2 toxicity (avoid FiO_2 >60%).
   - **Oxygen toxicity:** Damage to lungs occurs if the interalveolar O_2 concentration is >60% (injury occurs after a few hours if $FiO_2 = 1.0$). The mechanism probably involves generation of reactive O_2 species that oxidize the cell membranes. O_2 toxicity has not been documented if FiO_2 is maintained <60%.
2. **Minute ventilation:** Adjust to maintain PCO_2 within a normal range (35–45 mm Hg). Because minute ventilation is the product of rate and tidal volume, make this adjustment by varying either of these values. Once a tidal volume is chosen, set the respiratory rate ($\approx$8–16 breaths/min) for adequate minute ventilation. For a spontaneously breathing patient, PS can be increased to achieve a target minute ventilation.
3. **Pressure support:** After the patient's respiratory pattern is established on SIMV, add PS at an initial level of 5–10 cm water. Increase PS to the level at which the patient can achieve reasonable tidal volume and breathe at a comfortable rate (<30 breaths/min). Depending on the overall stability and mental status of the patient, turn down the number of SIMV backup breaths so that the patient assumes more control of ventilation. PS *rarely* exceeds 20 cm water.
4. **PEEP:** With the addition of PEEP, the ventilator maintains positive airway pressure at the end of expiration even though net airflow is zero. PEEP increases alveolar ventilation by preventing small-airway collapse, thereby improving lung compliance and FRC. Increasing levels of PEEP are typically used in the care of hypoxemic patients who need FiO_2 > 50%. With PEEP, FiO_2 can be reduced and O_2 toxicity limited. PEEP $\approx$ 5 cm water is considered physiologic. If oxygenation remains marginal, PEEP is added in 2- to 3-cm increments until oxygenation is improved. In acute lung injury, the PEEP at which lung compliance is optimized can be determined by observation of pressure-volume loops.
   - **High-dose PEEP:** The elevated intrathoracic pressure associated with high PEEP can compromise venous return and thus decrease stroke volume and CO, particularly in hypovolemic patients. The result is

28

decreased oxygen delivery. Because ICP can become elevated, titrate PEEP upward with caution in patients with intracranial hypertension.

5. **Inspiratory to expiratory (I/E) ratio:** The normal I/E ratio is 1/2 or 1/3. Inverse-ratio ventilation (e.g., 2/1) results in progressive recruitment of alveoli and elevation of mean airway pressure, which improves oxygenation. This beneficial effect on oxygenation is lost if "breath stacking" or auto-PEEP occurs. *Note:* This technique may be inappropriate in the care of patients with obstructive lung disease, in which longer expiratory times are required. Inverse-ratio ventilation is poorly tolerated by awake patients and typically requires heavy sedation. Shorter expiratory times can result in hypercapnia; this "permissive hypercapnia" is sometimes acceptable to improve oxygenation. Balance FiO_2 and peak pressure to keep peak pressure <35 cm water. If unable to do so, move to PS ventilation.

Ventilator Dyssynchrony

Dyssynchrony is present when the patient is not synchronized with the ventilator in one or more of its three phases: trigger, flow delivery, or cycling. It occurs due to inappropriate ventilator settings, a patient with high ventilatory demand, or other factors such as mechanical tubing problems, condensation, or airway trauma. Types of dyssynchrony include:

1. **Trigger phase**
   o **Ineffective trigger**—The most common form of ventilator dyssynchrony in which the patient effort does not trigger a breath. Causes are hyperinflated lungs, low respiratory drive, high-pressure support, or the trigger sensing settings are set too high.
   o **Extra-triggering**—A breath may be automatically triggered if the triggering thresholds are too low, from circuit leaks or even a strong cardiac impulse or condensation in the ventilator tubing. Double triggering is two consecutive breaths without full expiration. It may happen if patient inspiratory period is longer than the set inspiratory time. Extra-triggering may be suppressed by increasing minute ventilation or prolonging inspiratory pause. Entrainment or reverse triggering will happen after a ventilator breath and by vagal pathways or if a spontaneous breath is immediately generated.
2. **Flow delivery phase**
   o **Flow dyssynchrony**—When the delivered flow is insufficient to meet the patient's demands. Usually seen in VA ventilation. Identified by examining the pressure-time wave form, there is a concave appearance of the wave. Increasing flow may resolve this as will switching to pressure ventilation.

o **Excessive flow asynchrony**—When too much flow is being delivered or expiratory muscles are activated or from discomfort. Reducing flow or pressure depending on the mode will help against this dyssynchrony.

3. **Cycling phase**
   o **Premature cycling**—When the patient's inspiratory time is longer than the machine is providing and prolongs the expiratory phase of the flow curve. May lead to double triggering of the breath.
   o **Delayed cycling**—When the ventilator inspiratory time is longer than the patient's. As the breath is still in its inspiratory phase, a rise in pressure can be noted since patient tries to exhale against the ventilator. It can be seen when flow suddenly cycles off instead of gradually tapering.

General Principles of Ventilator Management

1. Keep patients' semirecumbent position (30–45 degrees) to minimize aspiration.
2. Sedation and analgesia should be used based on standard protocols to reduce anxiety and pain while on mechanical ventilation. Avoid excess use of sedatives and analgesics. This may interfere with neurologic assessments and prolong the duration of mechanical ventilation. (Sedation and analgesia in the ICU setting are discussed on page 880).
3. Administer stress ulcer prophylaxis and consider DVT prophylaxis unless contraindicated (see page 940).
4. Enteral feeding is the preferred mode of nutritional support (Chapter 18, Enteral and Parenteral Feeding).

Ventilator Weaning

Before weaning the patient from the ventilator, assess pulmonary mechanics and oxygenation (Table 28-10, page 928).

Pulmonary Mechanics: These provide information about the patient's ability to perform the work of respiration. Routine pulmonary mechanics consist of:

- Vital capacity
- Tidal volume
- Spontaneous respiratory rate
- Lung compliance

(Note: Routine noncritical care pulmonary function [spirometry] testing is discussed in Chapter 26, Respiratory Care.)

Inspiratory Force: The maximum negative pressure that can be exerted against a completely closed airway (a function of respiratory muscle strength). An inspiratory force between 0 and –25 cm water suggests that the patient

28

Table 28-10. Criteria for Extubation from Mechanical Ventilation

Parameter	Value
Pulmonary mechanics	
Vital capacity	>10–15 mL/kg
Resting minute ventilation (tidal volume × rate)	>10 L/min
Spontaneous respiratory rate	<33 breaths/min
Lung compliance	>100 mL/cm water
Negative inspiratory force (NIF)	>−25 cm water
Oxygenation	
A–a gradient	<300–500 mm Hg
Shunt fraction	<15%
PO_2 (on 40% FIO_2)	>70 mm Hg
PCO_2	<45 mm Hg

may be incapable of generating adequate inspiratory effort for successful extubation.

Weaning Modes: Ventilators are designed to facilitate weaning. Although there is no mode that will expedite weaning, once the preceding criteria have been met, select a ventilator mode appropriate to the clinical situation. SIMV and PSV are considered weaning modes because the patient assumes more of the workload of breathing as mechanical support is reduced.

Order of Weaning: Take the following steps to wean the patient from the ventilator:

1. Reduce FiO_2 to 40% while monitoring SpO_2.
2. Sequentially reduce the IMV rate to a level of 4–8 breaths/min. Add PS to maintain adequate minute ventilation. Closely monitor minute ventilation (on ventilator display).
3. Sequentially reduce PEEP in increments of 2–3 cm water while maintaining SpO_2 >90% until a level of 5 cm water is achieved.
4. Sequentially reduce PS by increments of 2–3 cm water while maintaining minute ventilation (goal: 5–10 cm water); monitor respiratory rate, work of breathing, and minute ventilation.

Checklist for Extubation

28

- Correction of primary problem that prompted intubation and mechanical ventilation (e.g., successfully treated pneumonia, returned hemodynamic stability)

- Level of consciousness stable or improved
- Stable vital signs
- Pulmonary mechanics and oxygenation meet acceptable criteria (see Table 28-10)

Extubation Trials: Once weaning has been achieved, attempt trials with minimal mechanical support while the patient is still intubated. CPAP trials (with 5-cm water positive pressure) is the most commonly used method. A CPAP trial with an FiO_2 of 40% should result in a PaO_2 of >70 mm Hg, and a respiratory rate <25 breaths/min. One of the best predictors of successful extubation is the ratio of respiratory rate to tidal volume (f/Vt, or Tobin index). Extubation is frequently unsuccessful in patients with a rapid–shallow breathing pattern. A ratio >100 has been shown in some studies to be predictive of extubation failure. Extubation trials may vary in duration from 30 min to several hours and are used primarily as the last test before extubation.

Extubation: A patient who can maintain a PO_2 >70 mm Hg, a PCO_2 <45 mm Hg, and a respiratory rate <25 breaths/min for 1–2 hr on a CPAP on a trial with minimal ventilator support is ready for extubation. Criteria are summarized in Table 28-10. Next:

1. Disconnect the ET tube from the ventilator or T-piece.
2. Suction the ET tube and oropharynx.
3. Have the patient take a deep breath.
4. As the patient expires forcefully, deflate the cuff and remove the tube.
5. Suction any secretions and administer O_2 through a nasal cannula at 2–4 L/min.
6. Check postextubation ABG if adequate ventilation and oxygenation are in doubt.

NUTRITION AND THE ICU PATIENT

The nutritional support of critically ill patients is crucial to their survival. Restoring an anabolic state hastens recovery and avoids complications. General approaches for nutritional support are covered in Chapters 17 and 18. Remember the following two rules:

1. **The "2-day" rule applies to most patients.** If you believe the critically ill patient will not be able to take nutrition for 2 days because of conditions such as postoperative ileus and intubation, you should arrange for nutritional support consultation. In the first few days of the ICU episode, it is not necessary to immediately replace 100% of the estimated caloric needs.

28

2. **"If the gut works, use it."** Use enteral nutrition (oral, NG tube, jejunostomy tube) in all patients with a functioning intestinal tract (see Chapter 18, Enteral and Parenteral Nutrition). Some studies suggest this approach of using enteral nutrition may reduce overall infections and rates of pneumonia; however, the same may not be said for the early use of parenteral nutrition. Caution as to the use of enteral feeding in critically ill patients who are hemodynamically unstable and volume depleted is needed as some of these patients are predisposed to bowel ischemia.

COMPLICATIONS AND SPECIAL CONDITIONS IN CRITICAL CARE

By definition, patients with critical illness are subject to an increased rate of complications of various organ systems. Vigilance, anticipation, and early treatment lead to improved outcomes. Common complications and conditions encountered in the ICU include:

- Abdominal compartment syndrome
- Acalculous cholecystitis
- Acute renal failure
- Acute adrenal insufficiency
- Acute respiratory distress syndrome (ARDS)
- COVID-19 ICE management
- DVT and PE
- Gastrointestinal bleeding
- Infectious complications
- Shock

Abdominal Compartment Syndrome

This is a consequence of an increase in intraabdominal pressure or hypertension resulting in symptomatic organ dysfunction. Caused by resuscitation-related bowel edema and fluid sequestration, or retroperitoneal hemorrhage causing mass effect, increased intraabdominal pressure directly decreases visceral perfusion and results in organ dysfunction and respiratory compromise.

- *Diagnosis:* Consider the diagnosis in the setting of worsening lung compliance, abdominal distention, and oliguria. Hypotension is a late finding. Measurement of bladder pressure with a pressure balloon confirms the diagnosis. Although the clinical scenarios can be highly variable, organ dysfunction may be present with pressures as low as 10 mm Hg.

Consider abdominal decompression when abdominal pressure exceeds 20–25 mm Hg.

- *Treatment:* Early decompressive laparotomy. Close the abdominal fascia when edema and organ dysfunction resolve.

Acalculous Cholecystitis

Cholecystitis in the absence of gallstones is common among ICU patients. Related to diminished blood flow to the gallbladder during critical illness and to bacterial overgrowth secondary to bile stasis.

- *Diagnosis:* Signs are like those in noncritical patients with cholecystitis and include right upper quadrant pain, fever, and leukocytosis. Perform right upper quadrant ultrasonography. Add a hepatobiliary iminodiacetic acid (HIDA) scan if the sonographic findings are not diagnostic (lack of visualization of the gallbladder is highly suggestive of acalculous cholecystitis).
- *Treatment:* Treatment is open surgical removal of the gallbladder (cholecystectomy). Percutaneous cholecystostomy is an alternative in the care of critically ill patients who may not tolerate operative intervention. Interval cholecystectomy is performed when the patient's condition improves.

Acute Adrenal Insufficiency

Adrenal crisis may be precipitated in patients with primary adrenal insufficiency in the setting of severe infection or surgical stress. It may also arise because of bilateral adrenal infarction or hemorrhage. Clinical manifestations include sudden cardiovascular collapse, hyponatremia, hyperkalemia, fever, abdominal pain, and nonspecific findings such as malaise, anorexia, nausea, and decreased mental status. Initial treatment is directed at correcting hypotension and electrolyte abnormalities, as well as cortisol replacement.

- Initiate resuscitation with normal saline solution; large volumes may be required. Administer IV dexamethasone (4 mg) or hydrocortisone (100 mg) empirically if adrenal insufficiency is suspected.
- Dexamethasone may be preferable initially because it is longer acting than hydrocortisone and does not interfere with ACTH stimulation tests. Do not delay empiric treatment awaiting the results of an ACTH simulation test.
- Determine the factor that precipitated the adrenal crisis (e.g., infection) and correct it promptly.
- Once the crisis resolves, administer oral glucocorticoids and taper them over several days. Consider adding mineralocorticoid (e.g., fludrocortisone) replacement.

28

Acute Renal Failure (ARF)

This is the sudden development of renal insufficiency resulting in retention of nitrogenous wastes (blood urea nitrogen [BUN], creatinine), variable effects on fluid balance, oliguria and anuria, and progressive azotemia. Acute renal failure (ARF) is usually divided into prerenal, intrarenal, and postrenal causes (see Chapter 12). Once ARF is recognized, the primary objective is to *correct the underlying cause.* The most common causes of renal failure in the ICU are acute tubular necrosis (ATN) and prerenal disease. Among the many causes of ATN are nephrotoxic medications, ischemia, and hypotension. Prerenal causes include intravascular volume depletion and CHF. **Contrast nephropathy** is an iatrogenic cause of ARF. If use of contrast agents is unavoidable in high-risk patients (e.g., diabetic patients with chronic renal insufficiency), avoiding volume depletion and the use of nonsteroidal anti-inflammatory drugs (NSAIDs) has been the only consistently proven intervention that provides protection against contrast nephropathy.

Indications for hemodialysis include:

- Refractory fluid overload
- Severe metabolic acidosis
- Hyperkalemia
- Severe uremia
- Toxic accumulation of drugs

Acute Kidney Injury (AKI): It is defined by the Kidney Disease – Improving Global Outcomes (KDIGO) board as an increase in serum creatinine by 0.3 mg/dL or more within 48 hr, increase in serum creatinine to 1.5 times baseline that is presumed to have occurred within the previous 7 days, or urine volume of less than 0.5 mL/kg/hr for 6 hr. Increases in creatinine as low as 0.3 mg/dL have been demonstrated to correlate with worse outcomes and mortality. Sepsis is the most common condition associated with renal failure in the ICU. Oliguria is not always present in acute kidney injury (AKI). Normal urine output may be present in the setting of renal dysfunction. (KDIGO guidelines are available at https://kdigo.org/guidelines/; Accessed January 10, 2020.)

The Acute Dialysis Quality Initiative, a group that studied AKI, developed the **RIFLE criteria** to describe kidney dysfunction in increasing severity classes.[11] The acronym stands for:

- RISK is defined as increase in serum creatinine of 1.5× baseline, glomerular filtration rate (GFR) decrease of >25%, or urine output <0.5 mL/kg/hr.
- INJURY is defined as serum creatinine increase of two times baseline, GFR decrease of >50%, or urine output <0.5 mL/kg/hr for 12 hr.

- <u>FAILURE</u> is defined as serum creatinine 3× baseline, GFR decrease of >75%, serum creatinine <4 mg/dL, urine output <0.3 mL/kg/hr for 24 hr, or anuria for 12 hr or more.
- <u>LOSS</u> is defined as complete loss of kidney function for 1 mo.
- <u>END STAGE</u> is defined as complete loss of kidney function for 3 mo.

AKI, as defined by RIFLE, does not signify damage to the kidney, but instead indicates an impairment of kidney function that comes from increased physiologic demand. AKI is a syndrome that includes interstitial nephritis, prerenal azotemia, obstructive nephropathy, ischemia, toxic injury, etc. The KDIGO board unified the RIFLE and AKIN definitions of AKI and differentiated AKI into three stages, with a higher stage implying worsened kidney outcomes and increased mortality.

- <u>Stage 1</u> – Serum creatinine of 1.5–1.9× baseline, >0.3 mg/dL increase, or urine output <0.5 mL/kg/hr for 6–12 hr
- <u>Stage 2</u> – Serum creatinine of 2–2.9× baseline or urine output <0.5 mL/kg/hr for more than 12 hr
- <u>Stage 3</u> – Serum creatinine of 3× baseline, increased serum creatinine of 4 mg/dL and above, urine output <0.3 mL/kg/hr for more than 24 hr, or initiation of renal replacement therapy

A stage-based management has been recommended. Prevention of AKI and worsening renal function may be achieved by:

- Discontinuing all nephrotoxic drugs when possible. Common nephrotoxic medications commonly used in the ICU include:
  o Diuretics
  o NSAIDs
  o ACE inhibitors and angiotensin receptor blockers (ARBs)
  o Amphotericin B
  o Iodinated contrast
  o Antibiotics (vancomycin, ciprofloxacin, sulfonamides, etc.)
  o Acyclovir
- Ensuring adequate volume status and perfusion pressure
- Monitoring serum creatinine and urine output
- Avoiding hyperglycemia
- Avoiding iodinated radiographic contrast
- Checking for changes in drug dosing according to AKI stage
- Considering renal replacement therapy
- Considering ICU admission and monitoring
- Avoiding subclavian catheters due to the possibility of future arteriovenous fistula for hemodialysis (stenosis or thrombosis of subclavian vein eliminates the possibility of fistula in that arm).

28

Renal replacement therapy (RRT): It is recommended when facing worsening renal dysfunction and oliguria/anuria for >72 hr, BUN level of >80–100, potassium level >6 mmol/L, pH <7.15, or volume overload resulting in pulmonary edema with increased oxygen requirements. RRT options include continuous hemofiltration and hemodialysis, intermittent hemodialysis, and peritoneal dialysis.

Acute Respiratory Distress Syndrome (ARDS)

ARDS is an acute inflammation of the lung in reaction to direct or indirect injury (such as severe pneumonia [viral infections including influenza and COVID-19, sepsis, near drowning, transfusion of multiple units, pancreatitis, many others], trauma, sepsis, aspiration of gastric contents, and many others). This pulmonary injury is manifested by marked respiratory distress and hypoxia. Pulmonary capillaries become more permeable, resulting in noncardiogenic pulmonary edema and protein accumulation in the alveoli. To subclassify different degrees of injury and to eliminate the need for invasive monitoring to diagnose ARDS, the European Society of Intensive Care Medicine endorsed by the American Thoracic Society, and the Society of Critical Care Medicine created the "Berlin Criteria" to define ARDS in three mutually exclusive categories. This differentiation between mild, moderate, and severe ARDS divides patients in groups of increasing mechanical ventilator days and mortality. The Berlin Definition is correlated with mortality with increasing stages of ARDS: mild 27%, moderate 32%, and severe 45%.

Causes: The causes of ARDS are multifactorial and include, but are not limited to:

- Trauma
- Sepsis
- Aspiration
- Pneumonia
- Severe pancreatitis
- Severe burns
- Transfusion-related acute lung injury
- Chemical pneumonitis or inhalational injury

Diagnosis. Based on the Berlin definition of ARDS (Table 28-11).

Treatment: Management of ARDS is generally supportive as there is no specific medication to treat ARDS. The underlying disease that caused the ARDS (i.e., sepsis) should be treated appropriately. Conservative use of IV fluids along with removal of excess fluids with diuretics reduces the need for mechanical ventilation. Efforts focus on preventing secondary insults and avoiding ventilator-associated lung injury via barotrauma. Specific management of COVID-19 patients and ARDS is discussed on pages 934 and 938 and in Figure 28-23, page 935.

Table 28-11. The Berlin Definition of Acute Respiratory Distress Syndrome

1. Onset within 1 week of a known clinical insult or new or worsening respiratory symptoms
2. Bilateral opacities on chest imaging not fully explained by lobar/lung collapse or nodules
3. Respiratory failure not fully explained by cardiac failure or volume overload
4. PaO_2/FIO_2 ratio $\leq$ 300 mm Hg with PEEP $\geq$ 5 cm H_2O
5. Mild PaO_2/FIO_2 200–300 mm Hg
   - Moderate PaO_2/FIO_2 100–200 mm Hg
   - Severe PaO_2/FIO_2 $\leq$ 100 mm Hg

Source: Based on data from Ranieri VM, et al. Acute respiratory distress syndrome. The Berlin Definition. JAMA 2012;307:E1–E8.

COVID-19 Resources: Summary of recommendations on the management of patients with COVID-19 and ARDS

COVID-19 with mild ARDS

DO: Vt 4–8 ml/kg and P_{plat} < 30 cm H_2O

DO: Investigate for bacterial infection

DO: Target SpO2 92–96%

Consider:
- Conservative fluid strategy
- Empiric antibiotics

Uncertain:
- Systemic corticosteroids

COVID-19 with moderate to severe ARDS

DO NOT: Do staircase recruitment maneuvers

Consider:
- Higher PEEP
- NMBA boluses to facilitate ventilation targets
- Traditional recruitment maneuvers **If PEEP responsive**
- Prone ventilation 12–16 hours
- NMBA infusion for 24 hours **If proning, highP_{pl}, asynchrony**
- Short course of systemic corticosteriods

Uncertain:
- Antivirals, chloroquine, anti-IL6

Rescue/adjunctive therapy

Consider:
- NMBA infusion for 24 hours **If proning, highP_{pk}, asynchrony**
- Prone ventilation 12–16 hours
- A trial of inhaled nitric oxide **STOP if no quick response**
- V-V ECMO or referral to ECMO center **Follow local criteria for ECMO**

Uncertain:
- Antivirals, chloroquine, anti-IL6

P_{plat}: Plateau pressure
SpO2: Peripheral capillary oxygen saturation
PEEP: Positive end-expiratory pressure
NMBA: Neuromuscular blocking agents
ECMO: Extracorporeal membrane oxygenation

28

Figure 28-23. Surviving Sepsis Campaign consensus recommendations for patients with COVID-19 and ARDS. (Reproduced with permission from https://www.sccm.org/SurvivingSepsisCampaign/Guidelines/COVID-19. Accessed June 7, 2020.)

Table 28-12. PEEP Ladder Used in the Supportive Management of ARDS

FiO$_2$	30%	40%	50%	60%	70%	80%	90%	100%
PEEP (cm H$_2$O)	5	5–8	8–10	10	10–14	14	14–18	18–22

Source: Based on data from: The Acute Respiratory Distress Syndrome Network. N Engl J Med 2000;342:1301–1308.

- In a few patients with mild ARDS (hemodynamically stable, easily oxygenated, does not meet criteria for immediate intubation), **noninvasive ventilation (NIV)** can be used cautiously (i.e., ventilation via a mask or nasal prongs with breaths delivered by a NIV device, see page 915) and reserved for the occasional patient.

- In patients with ARDS who require mechanical ventilation, the ARDS Network (www.ardsnet.org) advocates a low tidal volume approach (tidal volume of 6 mL/kg of predicted body weight, with respiratory rate adjusted to achieve adequate minute ventilation, known as "lung protective ventilation"). The goal is to achieve plateau pressures of ≤30-cm water. The PEEP ladder in Table 28-12 guides increases or decreases in PEEP settings according to FiO$_2$.

- **Prone ventilation** (sometimes call "proning") is mechanical ventilation that is delivered with the patient lying prone. Prone ventilation is an ARDS strategy to improve oxygenation when more traditional modes of ventilation fail (e.g., lung protective ventilation). Volume-controlled and pressure-controlled modes of ventilation are typically used in the prone position. Physiologically the prone position reduces lung compression and enhances lung perfusion. Contraindications include spinal instability, shock, acute bleeding, pregnancy, raised intracranial pressure, and others. There is no set duration for patients to be placed in the prone position and is also based on local protocols (multiple sessions up to 20 hr/day in the prone position).

- **Extracorporeal membrane oxygenation (ECMO)** is mechanical cardiopulmonary support. It is an option for severe ARDS patients who have uncompensated acidosis (pH <7.15), require high ventilator pressures (plateaus >30 cm H$_2$O) despite lung protective ventilation, and who have a potentially reversible cause of ARDS, such as pneumonia. The types of ECMO include venovenous (VV) ECMO used in patients with respiratory failure and venoarterial (VA) ECMO used in patients with cardiac failure. Anticoagulation is required when patients are using ECMO, thus bleeding is a common complication. ECMO programs are limited to major centers due to the high level of technology, support, and expertise involved. To expand ECMO's availability to COVID-19 patients, the U.S. Food and Drug Administration (FDA) in early 2020 issued a new policy for ECMO as a rescue therapy when ventilator management is insufficient. ECMO should be viewed as providing a period where the heart and the lungs have time to heal and buys time for other therapies to work, such as antibiotics for superimposed bacterial pneumonia and to allow fluid removal in volume-overloaded lungs. Ethics committees are engaged with decisions on which patients are most appropriate for this level of aggressive life support.

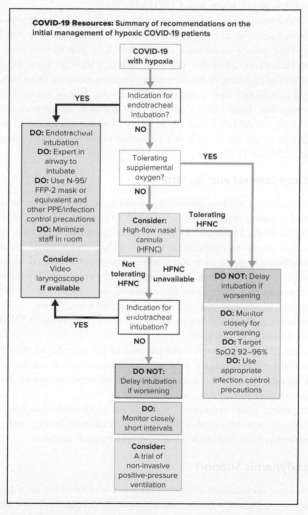

Figure 28-24. Recommendations by the Surviving Sepsis Campaign consensus in the initial management of hypoxic COVID-19 patients. (Reproduced with permission from https://www.sccm.org/SurvivingSepsisCampaign/Guidelines/COVID-19. Accessed June 7, 2020.)

28

COVID-19 ICU Management

Severe acute respiratory syndrome coronavirus 2 (SARS-CoV-2) was the cause of the 2020 COVID-19 pandemic and remains a major health issue pending the development and application of a broad-based vaccine strategy. It is estimated that up to 10% of patients will require ICU admission. The "Surviving Sepsis Campaign" published consensus guidelines on the management of critically ill adults with COVID-19.[12]

The following are high-level summaries of the major recommendations for the management of the COVID-19 positive adult patient in the ICU. Many of the principles are basic to any adult ICU patient with some specific modifications. Note that this information is through June 30, 2020, and subject to updating. Some selected recommendations are listed here, and the level of evidence and strength of the recommendations can be found in the publication. Figure 28-23 outlines recommendations for patients with COVID-19 and ARDS. Figure 28-24 (above) summarizes the initial recommendations by the Surviving Sepsis Campaign in the initial management of hypoxic COVID-19 patients.

Infection Control and Testing

1. For healthcare workers performing aerosol-generating procedures, use of fitted respirator masks is recommended (N95 respirators, FFP2), instead of surgical masks, in addition to other personal protective equipment (PPE). Aerosol-generating procedures in the ICU include endotracheal intubation, bronchoscopy, open suctioning, administration of nebulized treatment, manual ventilation before intubation, physical proning of the patient, disconnecting the patient from the ventilator, noninvasive positive pressure ventilation, tracheostomy, and cardiopulmonary resuscitation.
2. Perform aerosol-generating procedures on ICU patients with COVID-19 in a negative pressure room.
3. For usual care of nonventilated patients, or for performing nonaerosol-generating procedures on patients receiving mechanical ventilation, use of medical masks is recommended, instead of respirator masks, in addition to other PPE.
4. Diagnostic lower respiratory tract samples (endotracheal aspirates) are preferred over bronchial washings, bronchoalveolar lavage, and upper respiratory tract (nasopharyngeal or oropharyngeal) samples.

Hemodynamic Support

1. For acute resuscitation of adults with shock, the following are suggested: measuring dynamic parameters to assess fluid responsiveness, using a conservative fluid administration strategy, and using crystalloids over colloids. Balanced crystalloids are preferred over unbalanced crystalloids.
2. For adults with shock, the following are suggested: using norepinephrine as the first-line vasoactive; use of either vasopressin or epinephrine as the first line if norepinephrine is not available (see Table 28-19). Dopamine

28

is not recommended if norepinephrine is not available. Adding vaso-pressin as a second-line agent is suggested if the target (60–65 mm Hg) mean arterial pressure cannot be achieved by norepinephrine alone. Hydroxyethyl starches are not recommended for the acute resuscitation of adults with COVID-19 in shock.

Ventilatory Support

1. Starting supplemental oxygen is recommended if the SpO_2 is less than 90%. SpO_2 should be maintained no higher than 96%.
2. For healthcare workers performing endotracheal intubation on patients with COVID-19, the use of video-guided laryngoscopy over direct laryngoscopy is preferred.
3. For COVID-19 patients requiring endotracheal intubation, it is recommended that endotracheal intubation be performed by the healthcare worker who is most experienced with airway management in order to minimize the number of attempts and risk of transmission.
4. For acute hypoxemic respiratory failure despite conventional oxygen therapy, use of high-flow nasal cannula (HFNC) is suggested relative to conventional oxygen therapy and noninvasive positive pressure ventilation (NIPPV). If HFNC is not available, a trial of NIPPV is suggested. Close monitoring for worsening of respiratory status and early intubation if worsening occurs is recommended (best practice statement).
5. For adults receiving mechanical ventilation who have ARDS, use of low tidal volume ventilation (4–8 mL/kg of predicted body weight) is recommended and preferred over higher tidal volumes (>8 mL/kg). Targeting plateau pressures of <30 cm H_2O is recommended. Using a higher PEEP strategy over lower PEEP strategy is suggested.
6. For adults receiving mechanical ventilation who have moderate to severe ARDS, prone ventilation for 12–16 hr is suggested over no prone ventilation. Using as-needed neuromuscular blocking agents (NMBAs) instead of continuous NMBA infusion to facilitate protective lung ventilation is suggested.
7. For adults receiving mechanical ventilation who have severe ARDS and hypoxemia despite optimizing ventilation, a trial of inhaled pulmonary vasodilator is suggested. If no rapid improvement in oxygenation is observed, the treatment should be tapered. The use of lung recruitment maneuvers (intended to open otherwise closed lung segments, such as 40 cm H_2O inspiratory hold for 40 s) is suggested, over not using recruitment maneuvers, but using staircase (incremental PEEP) recruitment maneuvers is not recommended. Use of venovenous circulation for extracorporeal membrane oxygenation (ECMO) or referral to an ECMO center is suggested, if available, for selected patients.

28

COVID-19 Therapy

1. In adults receiving mechanical ventilation who do not have ARDS, routine use of systematic corticosteroids is not suggested. In those with ARDS, use of corticosteroids is suggested.

2. In COVID-19 patients receiving mechanical ventilation who have respiratory failure, use of empiric antimicrobial/antibacterial agents is suggested; assess for de-escalation.
3. In critically ill adults with fever, use of pharmacologic agents for temperature control is suggested over nonpharmacologic agents or no treatment. Routine use of standard IV immunoglobulins and convalescent plasma is not suggested. There is insufficient evidence to issue a recommendation on use of any of the following (June 2020): other antiviral agents (besides remdesivir), recombinant interferons, or chloroquine/hydroxychloroquine with or without azithromycin.
4. Although not specifically addressed by the Surviving Sepsis Campaign, hospitalized COVID-19 patients have strong clinical intrinsic and extrinsic risk factors for venous thromboembolism (VTE). In non-ICU patients, a universal strategy of routine thromboprophylaxis with standard-dose unfractionated heparin or UFH or low-molecular-weight heparin (LMWH) should be used after careful assessment of bleed risk, with LMWH as the preferred agent. For the COVID-19 ICU patient, routine thromboprophylaxis with prophylactic-dose UFH or LMWH should be used after careful assessment of bleeding risk. Intermediate-dose LMWH (50% of respondents) can also be considered in high-risk patients. Patients with obesity as defined by actual body weight or BMI should be considered for a 50% increase in the dose of thromboprophylaxis. These recommendations were published by Scientific and Standardization Committee Communication: Clinical Guidance on the Diagnosis, Prevention and Treatment of Venous Thromboembolism in Hospitalized Patients with COVID-19, published online May 27, 2020 in the *Journal of Thrombosis and Haemostasis*.[13]

Deep Venous Thrombosis (DVT) and Pulmonary Embolism (PE)

DVT causes most cases of PE in hospitalized patients. About 90% of cases of PE originate in the femoral–iliac–pelvic veins. DVT is promoted by the **Virchow triad**: endothelial injury, hypercoagulability, and blood stasis.

- **Prevention of DVT:** Risk factors include malignancy, obesity, prior DVT, age >40 yr, extensive abdominal or pelvic surgery, long bone or pelvic fractures, and prolonged immobilization. For surgical patients, prophylaxis should be used in the OR before induction of anesthesia. Use of sequential compression devices and prophylactic anticoagulation has reduced the incidence of DVT.
  - *Physical Methods*: Leg elevation, sequential compression devices, and early postoperative ambulation.
  - *Pharmacologic Methods:*
    1. Heparin (unfractionated heparin or UFH) 5000 units SQ q8h. Monitor platelet count for heparin-induced thrombocytopenia (HIT).
    2. Coumadin for chronic prophylaxis.

28

3. LMWH (e.g., enoxaparin) is considered the agent of choice for high-risk patients.

- **Diagnosis of DVT:**
  - o Signs and symptoms: While the features of lower extremity DVT are nonspecific, patients who present with leg swelling, pain, warmth, and erythema should be suspected of having a DVT.
  - o Doppler ultrasound with compression of the calf or whole leg is the diagnostic test of choice.

- **Diagnosis of PE:**
  - o Signs and symptoms: Dyspnea, tachypnea, tachycardia, chest pain (usually pleuritic), and hypoxia.
  - o Chest radiographs are not sensitive enough to be useful in the diagnosis of PE, but help rule out other causes (e.g., pneumonia, pneumothorax).
  - o Spiral CT: The clinical validity of CT in ruling out PE equals that of pulmonary angiography.

- **Treatment of PE:**
  - o Supportive oxygenation and continuously monitor SpO_2. Intubation may be required.
  - o Anticoagulate with unfractionated or LMWH to prevent clot propagation, decrease inflammation, and allow intrinsic fibrinolysis to lyse the clot.
    - Evidence-based guidelines suggest body weight–adjusted subcutaneous LMWH is the preferred initial therapy for acute, nonmassive PE.
    - If unfractionated heparin is chosen (e.g., patient with severe renal failure), administer bolus with 80 units/kg IV and start an infusion at 18 units/kg/hr. Titrate the infusion to maintain the partial thromboplastin time (PTT) at 2–2.5 × control value. Check the PTT in 6 hr and adjust the rate if needed. Monitor the platelet count for heparin-induced thrombocytopenia.
    - Start oral warfarin (Coumadin) by day 3 of heparin therapy to achieve and maintain an INR of 2–3.
  - o In massive PE, defined by right heart strain and hemodynamic instability, administer thrombolytic therapy (TPA) if not contraindicated.
  - o Consider pulmonary embolectomy for hemodynamically unstable patients with massive PE if medical therapy is not successful.
  - o If anticoagulation is contraindicated (e.g., recent surgery, stroke, GI bleeding) or if PE recurs despite anticoagulation, consider placement of an inferior vena cava filter.

Gastrointestinal Bleeding

28

Critically ill patients are at increased risk of GI hemorrhage secondary to stress-induced mucosal ulceration. Head injury (**Cushing ulcers**); mechanical ventilation; NSAID use; shock, trauma, and burns (**Curling ulcers**); coagulopathy; and a history of peptic ulcer disease or portal hypertension are risk factors for this condition.

- **Prophylaxis:**
  - o Enteral feedings: method of choice to protect the gastric mucosa
  - o Cardiovascular support of visceral perfusion
  - o Acid suppression: prophylaxis with H2-blockers (e.g., famotidine)
  - o Proton-pump inhibitors (e.g., lansoprazole, omeprazole) for refractory bleeding or in patients with adverse reaction to histamine blockade
- **Management of Ulceration:**
  - o Early endoscopy for upper GI bleeding
  - o Endoscopic or surgical intervention for visible bleeding vessel
  - o Aggressive acid suppression for diffuse gastritis and empiric therapy for *Helicobacter pylori* infection
  - o Possible surgical intervention for persistent bleeding from gastritis

Infectious Complications

Catheter-Associated Urinary Tract Infection (CA-UTI)

CA-UTI is defined as infection occurring in a person whose urinary tract is currently catheterized or has been catheterized within the previous 48 hr. CA-UTI is the most common nosocomial infection in the United States, accounting for 40% of hospital-acquired infections and over 80% of the 900,000 cases of bacteriuria annually. (See also Chapter 13, page 389.)

- **Diagnosis:** When infection is suspected, urine culture specimen should be sent from a newly placed catheter or midstream voided specimen. Symptoms may include: chills, rigors, altered mental status, malaise, flank pain, and pelvic discomfort. Many febrile patients in the ICU will be determined to have a febrile event not associated with a CA-UTI. The diagnosis of symptomatic CA-UTI is often a diagnosis of exclusion.
- **Treatment/Prevention:** Most important prevention is adherence to indications for catheter use and prompt removal when no longer indicated. When catheter use is unavoidable, it should be aseptically inserted, maintained in a closed drainage system keeping the bag below the level of the catheter, and the catheter should be removed as early as possible. Treatment should be driven by culture sensitivities and typically last 7–14 days.

Central Line-Associated Blood Stream Infections (CLABSI)

Indwelling venous and arterial catheters are essential, but they can also act as a portal of entry for bacteria. Consider catheter-related sepsis if a fever develops in an ICU patient. The most common mechanism is entry of skin flora along the catheter track. Because prolonged use of polyurethane dressings increases the risk of infection, avoid these dressings. Some ICUs have a policy of routine line changes over a guidewire every 3–4 days. This policy, however, is not supported by evidence in the literature, and the infection rate may increase with this approach. Prevent line sepsis with meticulous aseptic technique during line placement (including full gowning, gloving, and draping) and meticulous care of the line once it is in place. (See also Chapter 13, page 352.)

28

- **Diagnosis:** If the site does not appear infected, the catheter may be changed over a guidewire and the intracutaneous segment and tip sent for culture. A new IV site is chosen if the catheter culture result is positive. Erythema is suggestive of catheter site infection; however, the absence of erythema with a coagulase-negative staphylococcus is common because there is often a minimal inflammatory response.
- **Treatment:** Remove short-term central venous catheters suspected of being infected and culture them. Start empiric antimicrobial therapy, and then tailor the antibiotic regimen based on culture and sensitivity results. A catheter colony count >15 CFU suggests catheter infection.

Ventilator-Associated Pneumonia (VAP)

VAP is clinical pneumonia that develops after 48 hr of mechanical ventilation. Occurs in approximately 25% of intubated ICU patients, with an overall mortality of 20–50%. The strongest risk factor for ICU pneumonia is mechanical ventilation. Other risk factors are age >70 yr, chronic lung disease, nasoenteric tubes, altered mental status, chest trauma or surgery, use of proton pump inhibitors, and frequent transportation of the patient.

- **Diagnosis:** A positive culture (preferably a bronchoalveolar lavage [BAL] specimen with quantitative cultures showing >104 CFU/mL) plus three of the following four:
  - o New, persistent, or progressive CXR infiltrate
  - o Purulent tracheobronchial secretions
  - o Fever
  - o Leukocytosis
- **Treatment of Ventilator-Associated Pneumonia:** *Note:* The Infectious Disease Society of America (IDSA) recommends cultures by noninvasive means as adequate for obtaining cultures. Empiric therapy is customized according to the institution's antibiogram for the ICU and adjusted when culture and sensitivity data become available. Continue therapy for 7 days. Repeat BAL with cultures and special stains as needed if standard antibiotic therapy fails.

Shock

In the simplest terms, shock can be defined as tissue hypoperfusion. Uncorrected shock leads to cellular dysfunction, organ failure, and death. The management of shock is directed at *correcting the underlying problem.* Endogenous compensatory mechanisms directed at reversing shock include the release of catecholamines, endogenous cortisol, and activation of the renin–angiotensin–aldosterone axis. While the morbidity and mortality of shock are related to the underlying cause, it is more closely tied to the degree and duration of circulatory compromise. When the causes are identified and corrected, the patient can be adequately resuscitated to restore tissue perfusion and reverse the effects of shock.

28

Hypovolemic Shock

Inadequate circulating blood volume (at least 20% loss) can be caused by dehydration or acute hemorrhage. Hemodynamic parameters show decreased CVP, PAOP, and end diastolic volume (EDV) with a consequent decrease in CO and increase in SVR. Table 28-13, page 945, lists the current classification and physiologic changes associated with hypovolemic shock.

- **Treatment of hypovolemic shock:**
  - o Control the source of intravascular volume loss
  - o Rapidly replace intravascular volume with isotonic crystalloid, colloid, or blood products as appropriate

Cardiogenic Shock

Cardiogenic shock is caused by cardiac pump failure, either from intrinsic cardiac abnormalities (e.g., severe valvular disease, myocardial infarction, coronary ischemia, arrhythmias) or extrinsic processes (e.g., tension pneumothorax, pericardial tamponade, PE).

- *Treatment of cardiogenic shock:*
  - o Resolve extrinsic processes if present (relieve pneumothorax or tamponade)
  - o Optimize preload for CO (fluid resuscitation, transfusion, etc.)
  - o Decrease afterload (ACE inhibitors, nitrates, etc.)
  - o Improve cardiac contractility with inotropic support (see Table 28-19)
  - o Consider mechanical support (intraaortic balloon pump)
  - o Consider aspirin and heparin therapy

Septic Shock

Septic shock is a clinical syndrome associated with severe infection and is characterized by a systemic inflammatory response with resultant tissue injury. (See also Chapter 13, Clinical Microbiology, page 385.) Previously, sepsis and its corresponding syndromes were defined as **systemic inflammatory response syndrome** (SIRS) (two or more of the following):

- Temperature >38°C or <36°C
- Heart rate >90 beats/min
- Respiratory rate >20 breaths/min or PCO_2 <32 mm Hg
- WBC >12,000/μL or <4000/μL

Sepsis: Refers to an infection with a systemic inflammatory response. Sepsis is a systemic response to the infection. While on the surface identical to SIRS, sepsis must result specifically from infection rather than from any of the noninfectious insults that may also cause SIRS (e.g., pancreatitis, ischemia, multiple trauma). Up to 40% of patients with sepsis will develop septic shock.

Severe Sepsis: Sepsis with organ dysfunction.

Table 28-13. Physiologic Changes Associated with Degree of Hemorrhagic Shock

	Blood Loss (%)	Blood Loss (mL)	Mental Status	Heart Rate	Blood Pressure (SBP/DBP)	Respiratory Rate	Urine Output
Class I	<15	<750	--	--	--/--	--	--
Class II	15–30	750–1500	Anxiety	↑	--/↑	↑	Mild ↓
Class III	30–40	1500–2000	Confusion	↑↑	↓/↓↓	↑↑	Oliguria
Class IV	>40	>2000	Lethargy	↑↑↑	↓↓/↓↓↓	↑↑↑	Anuria

Source: Based on guidelines from the American College of Surgeons Advanced Trauma Life Support (ATLS) courses available at http://bulletin.facs.org/2018/06/atls-10th-edition-offers-new-insights-into-managing-trauma-patients/. Accessed January 21, 2020.

28

Current Definition of Septic Shock: Acute circulatory failure with persistent unexplained hypotension. Clinically, septic shock is identified by requiring a vasopressor to maintain a mean arterial pressure >65 mm Hg with a serum lactate level >2 mmol/L (>18 mg/dL) in the absence of hypovolemia. This is associated with a mortality rate greater than 40%.

Multiple Organ Dysfunction Syndrome (MODS): A clinical syndrome characterized by the development of progressive and potentially reversible physiologic dysfunction in two or more organs or organ systems that is induced by a variety of acute insults, including sepsis.

The 28-day mortality rates are progressive as follows: SIRS 10%, sepsis 20%, severe sepsis 20–40%, and septic shock 40–60%. Currently, sepsis and its corresponding syndromes are defined according to the **Sequential Organ Failure Assessment (SOFA scoring)**, with the diagnosis of sepsis suspected with a documented infection and an acute increase of two or more SOFA points (see Table 28-14). This is associated with a mortality of greater than 10%. A "quick SOFA" (qSOFA) has been described as a rapid bedside test to identify adult patients with suspected infection who are sepsis candidates with at least two of the following criteria: respiratory rate >22/min, altered mentation, or systolic blood pressure of <100 mm Hg. qSOFA is intended to screen patients for ICU admission from out-of-hospital, emergency department, and hospital ward settings.

SOFA can also be used as a measure of mortality with rising scores associated with increasing mortality. SOFA does not specifically diagnose sepsis but rather helps identify patients, as a group, who potentially have a high risk of death from infection.

Tretament of Septic Shock

The following are selected major recommendations from the "**Surviving Sepsis**" Campaign Guidelines developed by the Society of Critical Care Medicine (SCCM) and the European Society of Intensive Care Medicine (ESICM).[14]

- **Resuscitation and management should begin immediately when the diagnosis of sepsis is suspected with these elements ideally completed in the first hour if possible.** (See also Figure 13-5, page 386.)
  o Measure lactate level. Periodically re-measure if initial lactate is >2 mmol/L
  o Obtain blood cultures prior to administration of antibiotics
    ▪ At least two sets, both aerobic and anaerobic
  o Administer broad-spectrum antibiotics within 1 hr of suspected sepsis (some recommendations are in Table 28-15). The Surviving Sepsis consensus has classified antibiotic categories used in this setting (Table 28-16.
    ▪ Antibiotic spectrum of coverage should be narrowed when culture and sensitivity data are available
  o Obtain anatomic source control as rapidly as possible
    ▪ Control the source of the infection and optimize functioning at the site (e.g., incision and drainage of abscesses, remove source of infection such as infected gallbladder or infected hardware)

28

Table 28-14. SOFA Scoring System Based on the European Society of Intensive Care Medicine and the Society of Critical Care Medicine Consensus

System	Score 0	1	2	3	4
Respiration					
Pao$_2$/Fio$_2$, mmHg (kPa)	≥400 (53.3)	<400 (53.3)	<300 (40)	<200 (26.7) with respiratory support	<100 (13.3) with respiratory support
Coagulation					
Platelets, × 10^3/μL	>150	<150	<100	<50	<20
Liver					
Bilirubin, mg/dL (μmol/L)	<1.2 (20)	1.2–1.9 (20–32)	2.0–5.9 (33–101)	6.0–11.9 (102–204)	>12.0 (204)
Cardiovascular	MAP >70 mmHg	MAP <70 mmHg	Dopamine <5 or dobutamine (any dose)[a]	Dopamine 5.1–15 or epinephrine <0.1 or norepinephrine <0.1[a]	Dopamine >15 or epinephringe >0.1 or norepinephrine >0.1[a]
Central Nervous System					
Glasgow Coma Scale[b]	15	13–14	10–12	6–9	<6
Renal					
Creatinine, mg/dL (μmol/L) or urine output, mL/dL	<1.2 (110)	1.2–1.9 (110–170)	2.0–3.4 (171–299)	3.5–4.9 (300–440) or <500	>5.0 (440) or <200

Sources: Adapted from JL Vincent, et al. Working Group on Sepsis-Related Problems of the European Society of Intensive Care Medicine. The SOFA (Sepsis-related Organ Failure Assessment) score to describe organ dysfunction/failure. ntensive Care Med 1996;22(7):707.

Reproduced with permission from Kress JP, Hall JB. Approach to the patient with critical illness. In: Jameson J, Fauci AS, Kasper DL, et al. (eds). Harrison's Principles of Internal Medicine, 20e, New York, NY: McGraw-Hill.

[a]Catecholamine doses are given as mcg/kg/min for at leas 1 hr.

[b]Glasgow Coma Scale scores range from 3 to 15; higher score indicates better neurologic function.

FiO$_2$ = fraction of inspired oxygen; MAP = mean arterial pressure; PaO$_2$ = partial pressure of oxygen.

28

947

Table 28-15. Suggested Initial Empiric Antibiotic Choices for Sepsis
(See also Chapter 13, Table 13-4, pages 332–348.)

Source of Infection	Antimicrobial Choice
Community-acquired pneumonia	Third-generation cephalosporin with a macrolide or respiratory fluoroquinolone. Use cefepime or piperacillin-tazobactam in place of third-generation cephalosporin if risk factors for *Pseudomonas* infection or MDR pathogens
Hospital-acquired pneumonia	Third- or fourth-generation cephalosporin or an extended-spectrum penicillin ± an aminoglycoside or a fluoroquinolone (or: carbapenems, β-lactam–β-lactamase inhibitor); add vancomycin or linezolid if MRSA suspected.
Urinary tract infection	Extended-spectrum β-lactam agent ± aminoglycoside or fluoroquinolone). Use cefepime or a carbapenem if history of, or at risk for MDR organism
Intra-abdominal infection	A carbapenem or piperacillin-tazobactam as monotherapy or a third- or fourth-generation cephalosporin or fluoroquinolone in combination with metronidazole
Neutropenic sepsis	Monotherapy with an antipseudomonal beta-lactam agent, such as cefepime, a carbapenem (meropenem), or piperacilin-tazobactam is recommended (add vancomycin when there is evidence of gram-positive infection or linezolid if MRSA or VRE suspected); add a triazole (voriconazole or fluconazole) or β-glucan inhibitor (e.g., caspofungin or micafungin) if systemic fungal infection suspected.
Necrotizing skin/soft tissue infection	Vancomycin and piperacillin-tazobactam ± clindamycin

Source: Reproduced with permission from McCulloh RJ, Opal SM. Sepsis, septic shock, and multiple organ failure. In: Oropello JM, Pastores SM, Kvetan V (eds.). Critical Care. New York, NY: McGraw-Hill; 2020.
MDR = multiple antibiotic drug resistant; MRSA = methicillin-resistant *Staphylococcus aureus*; VRE = vancomycin resistant enterococcus.

- o Begin rapid administration of 30 mL/kg crystalloid for hypotension or lactate ≥4 mmol/L
  - 30 mL/kg should be provided within the first 3 hr
  - Additional fluid should be given based on frequent reassessment
- o Vasopressors should be used if the patient is hypotensive during or after fluid resuscitation to maintain MAP ≥65 mm Hg (see Table 28-19)
  - Norepinephrine is the vasopressor of choice
  - Vasopressin can be used as an augmenting agent
- o In patients with sepsis-related ARDS, mechanical ventilation should target a tidal volume of 6 mL/kg of predicted body weight, and a plateau pressure of ≤30 cm H_2O
- o Glucose levels in the septic patient should be kept at less than 150 mg/dL.

Table 28-16. Terminology Used by the "Surviving Sepsis" Consensus Concerning Antimicrobial Recommendations

Empiric therapy	Initial therapy started in the absence of definitive microbiologic pathogen identification. Empiric therapy may be mono-, combination, or broad-spectrum, and/or multidrug in nature.
Targeted/definitive therapy	Therapy targeted to a specific pathogen (usually after microbiologic identification). Targeted/definitive therapy may be mono- or combination, but is not intended to be broad-spectrum.
Broad-spectrum therapy	The use of one or more antimicrobial agents with the specific intent of broadening the range of potential pathogens covered, usually during empiric therapy (e.g., piperacillin/tazobactam, vancomycin, and anidulafungin; each is used to cover a different group of pathogens). Broad-spectrum therapy is typically empiric since the usual purpose is to ensure antimicrobial coverage with at least one drug when there is uncertainty about the possible pathogen. On occasion, broad-spectrum therapy may be continued into the targeted/definitive therapy phase if multiple pathogens are isolated.
Multidrug therapy	Therapy with multiple antimicrobials to deliver broad-spectrum therapy (i.e., to broaden coverage) for empiric therapy (i.e., where pathogen is unknown) or to potentially accelerate pathogen clearance (combination therapy) with respect to a specific pathogen(s) where the pathogen(s) is known or suspected (i.e., for both targeted or empiric therapy). This term therefore includes combination therapy.
Combination therapy	The use of multiple antibiotics (usually of different mechanistic classes) with the specific intent of covering the known or suspected pathogen(s) with more than one antibiotic (e.g., piperacillin/tazobactam and an aminoglycoside or fluoroquinolone for gram-negative pathogens) to accelerate pathogen clearance rather than to broaden antimicrobial coverage. Other proposed applications of combination therapy include inhibition of bacterial toxin production (e.g., clindamycin with β-lactams for streptococcal toxic shock) or potential immune modulatory effects (macrolides with a β-lactam for pneumococcal pneumonia).

Source: Reproduced with permission from Rhodes A, et al. Surviving sepsis campaign: International guidelines for management of sepsis and septic shock: 2016. Intensive Care Med 2017;43:304–377.

Neurogenic Shock

28

Caused by loss of sympathetic vascular tone (e.g., high thoracic or cervical spinal cord injury), producing an increase in vascular capacitance.

- *Treatment of neurogenic shock:*
  - Optimize filling pressures by IV fluid administration

o Provide vasopressor support as necessary
o Keep fluid temperature and room temperature warm, as these patients lose the ability of thermoregulation

ICU OUTCOMES AND SEVERITY OF ILLNESS MEASURES

A variety of ICU Severity of Illness (SOI) scoring systems have been developed for defining populations of critically ill patients. These systems may not have utility in predicting the outcome of an individual patient. Commonly utilized ICU scoring systems are the SOFA (Sequential Organ Failure Assessment), the APACHE (Acute Physiology and Chronic Health Evaluation), and the SAPS (Simplified Acute Physiology Score) systems. SOFA has been discussed in relation to defining sepsis and has been used for mortality estimates.

APACHE II Scoring System

The APACHE II system is a commonly used ICU severity scoring system. Age, type of ICU admission (elective surgery vs. nonsurgical or emergency surgery), chronic health problems, and 12 physiologic variables (the worst values for each in the first 24 hr after ICU admission) are used to derive a score. The predicted hospital mortality rate is derived from a formula that takes into account the APACHE II score, the need for emergency surgery, and a weighted, disease-specific diagnostic category (Table 28-17, page 951). Each variable is weighted from 0 to 4, with higher scores denoting an increasing deviation from normal. The APACHE II is determined in the first 24 hr of ICU admission; the maximum score is 71. A score of 25 predicts a 50% mortality with a score >35 representing a predicted mortality of 80%. Updated versions (APACHE III and APACHE IV) have been published and incorporate larger data sets.

SAPS Scoring System

The Simplified Acute Physiology Score (SAPS) is an outcome score more frequently used in Europe than in the United States. The model includes 17 variables. The SAPS II version score can vary between 0 and 163 points. SAPS III, which utilizes a 1-hr rather than a 24-hr window for measuring physiologic derangement scores, was developed in 2005.

Quick Reference to Common ICU Equations

Table 28-18 provides a listing of commonly used ICU equations.

Guidelines for Common Adult Critical Care Drug Infusions

Table 28-19 provides guidelines on commonly used ICU drugs.

Table 28-17. Table for the Calculation of the Acute Physiology and Chronic Health Evaluation II (APACHE II) Score[a]

Acute Physiology Score

Score	4	3	2	1	0	1	2	3	4
Rectal temperature (°C)	≥41	39.0–40.9		38.5–38.9	36.0–38.4	34.0–35.9	32.0–33.9	30.0–31.9	≤29.9
Mean blood pressure (mmHg)	≥160	130–159	110–129		70–109		50–69		≤49
Heart rate (beats/min)	≥180	140–179	110–139		70–109		55–69	40–54	≤39
Respiratory rate (breaths/min)	≥50	35–49		25–34	12–24	10–11	6–9		≤5
Arterial pH	≥7.70	7.60–7.69		7.50–7.59	7.33–7.49		7.25–7.32	7.15–7.24	<7.15
Oxygenation if Fio$_2$ >0.5, use (A-a) Do$_2$ if Fio$_2$ ≤0.5, use Pao$_2$	≥500	350–499	200–349		<200 / >70			55–60	<55
Serum sodium (meq/L)	≥180	160–179	155–159	150–154	130–149	61–70	120–129	111–119	≤110
Serum potassium (meq/L)	≥7.0	6.0–6.9	5.5–5.9		3.5–5.4	3.0–3.4	2.5–2.9		<2.5
Serum creatinine (mg/dL)	≥3.5	2.0–3.4	1.5–1.9		0.6–1.4		<0.6		
Hematocrit (%)	≥60		50–59.9	46–49.9	30–45.9		20–29.9		<20
WBC count (10³/mL)	≥40		20–39.9	15–19.9	3–14.9		1–2.9		<1

[a]The APACHE II score is the sum of the acute physiology score (vital signs, oxygenation, laboratory values), the Glasgow coma scale, age, and chronic health points. The worst values during the first 24 hours should be used.

(Continued)

28

951

Table 28-17. Table for the Calculation of the Acute Physiology and Chronic Health Evaluation II (APACHE II) Score[a] (Continued)

Glasgow Coma Score[b,c]

Eye Opening	Verbal (Nonintubated)	Verbal (Intubated)	Motor Activity
4-Spontaneous	5-Oriented and talks	5-Seems able to talk	6-Verbal command
3-Verbal stimuli	4-Disoriented and talks	3-Questionable ability to talk	5-Localizes to pain
2-Painful stimuli	3-Inappropriate words	1-Generally unresponsive	4-Withdraws from pain
1-No response	2-Incomprehensible sounds		3-Decorticate
	1-No response		2-Decerebrate
			1-No response

Points Assigned to Age and Chronic Disease

Age, Years	Score
<45	0
45–54	2
55–64	3
65–74	5
≥75	6

[b]Glasgow Coma Score (GCS)= eye-opening score + verbal (intubated or non-intubated) score + motor score.
[c]The GCS component of acute physiology score, subtract GCS from 15 to obtain points assigned.

Chronic Health (History of Chronic Conditions)[d]

None	0
If patient is admitted after elective surgery	2
If patient is admitted after emergency surgery or for reason other than after elective surgery	5

[d]Hepatic: cirrhosis with portal hypertension or encephalopathy; cardiovascular: class IV angina, (at rest or minimal self-care activities; pulmonary: chronic hypoxemia, or hypercapnia, polycythemia, ventilator dependence; renal: chronic peritoneal dialysis or hemodialysis; immunocompromised host

Abbreviations: (A - a) Do_2 = alveolar-arterial oxygen difference; Fio_2 = fraction of inspired oxygen; Pao_2 = partial pressure of oxygen; WBC = white blood cell count

Source: Reproduced with permission from Kress JP, Hall JB. Approach to the patient with critical illness. In: Jameson J, Fauci AS, Kasper DL, et al. (eds.). Harrison's Principles of Internal Medicine, 20e, New York, NY: McGraw-Hill.

28

954

Table 28-18. Quick Reference to Common ICU Equations

Determination	Derivation	Normal
RAP-CVP	Measured	2–10 mm Hg
RSVP/RVDP	Measured	15–30/0–5 mm Hg
PAS/PAD	Measured	15–30/8–15 mm Hg
MPAP	$PAD + \dfrac{[PAS - PAD]}{3}$	11–18 mm Hg
PAOP (i.e., PCWP)	Measured	5–16 mm Hg
MAP	$DBP \times \dfrac{(SBP - DBP)}{3}$	85–90 mm Hg
CO	$SV \times HR$	3.5–5.5 L/min
CO	$\dfrac{Vo_2 \times 10}{(1.39[Hgb]) \times (SaO_2 - S\bar{v}O_2)}$	
CI	CO/BSA	2.5–4.2 L/min·m²
SVR	$\dfrac{(MAP - CVP)}{CO} \times 80$	770–1500 dynes × s/cm⁵
SVRI	SVR/BSA	
PVR	$\dfrac{(MPAP - PAOP) \times 80}{CO}$	20–120 dynes × s/cm⁵
PVRI	PVR/BSA	255–285 dynes × s/cm⁵

Alveolar O_2 estimate (PAO_2)	$FiO_2 \times \left(P_{atmospheric} - PH_2O\right) - \dfrac{PaCO_2}{0.8}$	99.7 mm Hg (at sea level)
A-a Gradient	$PAO_2 - PaO_2$	Room air = 12–22 mm Hg
		100% FiO_2 = 10–60 mm Hg
CcO_2 (pulmonary capillary O_2 content)	$(1.39[Hgb] \times ScO_2) + (PcO_2 \times 0.0031)$	18–24 mL O_2/dL blood
CaO_2 (arterial O_2 content)	$(1.39[Hgb] \times SaO_2) + (PaO_2 \times 0.0031)$	16–22 mL O_2/dL blood
$C\bar{v}O_2$ (mixed venous O_2 content)	$(1.39[Hgb] \times S\bar{v}O_2) + (P\bar{v}O_2 \times 0.0031)$	12–17 mL O_2/dL blood
C(a–v) O_2 (A–V O_2 difference)	$(1.39[Hgb] \times (SaO_2 - S\bar{v}O_2)$	3.5–5.5 mL O_2/dL blood
O_2 carrying capacity (CcO_2)	$[Hgb] \times SaO_2 \times CO \times 10$	700–1400 mL/min delivery
O_2 consumption (VO_2)	$(CaO_2 - C\bar{v}O_2) \times CO \times 10$	180–280 mL/min
Qs/Qt (shunt fraction)	$(CcO_2 - CaO_2) / (CcO_2 - C\bar{v}O_2)$	0.05
ICP	Measured	0–20 mm Hg
CPP	MAP – ICP	Ideally > 70 mm Hg

BSA = body surface area (m^2) = height (cm)$^{0.718}$ × weight (kg)$^{0.427}$ × 74.5; CI = cardiac index; CC = cardiac output; CPP = cerebral perfusion pressure; CVP = central venous pressure; DBP = diastolic blood pressure; MPAP = mean pulmonary artery pressure; FiO$_2$ = inhaled O$_2$ concentration; Hgb = hemoglobin concentration; HR = heart rate; ICP = intracranial pressure; MAP = mean arterial pressure; MPAP = mean pulmonary artery pressure; Qs = volume of shunted blood (i.e., blood shunted past nonventilated alveoli not participating in gas exchange); Qt = total cardiac output; RAP = right atrial pressure; RVDP = right ventricular diastolic pressure; RVSP = right ventricular systolic pressure; PaCO$_2$ = partial pressure of CO$_2$ in arterial blood; PAD = pulmonary artery diastolic pressure; PaO$_2$ = partial pressure of O$_2$ in arterial blood; PaO$_2$ = partial pressure in alveolus; PAOP = pulmonary artery occlusion pressure; PAS = pulmonary artery systolic pressure; P$_{atmospheric}$ = atmospheric pressure ~760 torr; PCWP = pulmonary capillary wedge pressure; PH$_2$O = water vapor pressure ~ 47 torr; PVRI = pulmonary vascular resistance; PVRI = pulmonary vascular resistance index; SaO$_2$ = arterial oxygen saturation; SBP = systolic blood pressure; SVR = systemic vascular resistance; SVRI = systemic vascular resistance index; SV = stroke volume; S$\bar{v}$o$_2$ = mixed venous oxygen saturation; VO$_2$ = oxygen consumption.

TABLE 28-19. Guidelines for Common Adult Critical Care Drug Infusions

Drug	Use/Mechanism	Dose Range	Side Effects/Cautions
Amiodarone	Class III antiarrhythmic inhibits adrenergic stimulation (α - and β -blocking properties), affects sodium, potassium, and calcium channels, prolongs the action potential and refractory period in myocardial tissue; decreases AV conduction and sinus node function	Bolus: 150mg over 10 minutes, then 1mg/min for 6 hours Maint: 0.5 mg/min	Central line administration preferred due to phlebitis *Contraindications:* Iodine hypersensitivity Adverse effects: Bradycardia (infusion-rate related); prolonged QT; arrhythmias Long term use: abnormal LFTs; hyper- or hypothyroidism; pulmonary toxicity
Cisatracurium	Nondepolarizing neuromuscular blocker; blocks neural transmission at the myoneural junction by binding with cholinergic receptor sites	Load: 0.1 mg/kg IV push Maint: 1–10 mcg/kg/min titrated to train of four	Patient must be intubated receiving continuous sedation and analgesia Hofmann elimination Adverse effects: Myopathy with prolonged use
Clevidipine	Dihydropyridine calcium channel blocker with potent arterial vasodilating activity. Inhibits calcium ion influx through the L-type calcium channels during depolarization in arterial smooth muscle, producing a decrease in MAP by reducing systemic vascular resistance.	Dose: 1–6 mg/hr titrate to BP goal Maximum Dose: 21 mg/hr	20% lipid emulsion – monitor triglycerides *Contraindications:* Defective lipid metabolism; severe aortic stenosis; acute pancreatitis; egg/ soybean allergies Avoid use in heart failure patients
Dexmedetomidine	Selective α_2-adrenoceptor agonist with anesthetic and sedative properties resulting in inhibition of norepinephrine release; peripheral α_{2b}-adrenoceptors are activated at high doses or with rapid IV administration resulting in vasoconstriction.	Load: 1 mg/kg over 10 minutes Maint: 0.2–1.5 mcg/kg/ hr titrate to RASS	Load associated with bradycardia and hypotension – infusion-related Withdrawal can be seen if abruptly discontinued after 24 hours of infusing Adverse effects: Hypo- or hypertension; bradycardia; tachycardia

Diltiazem	Slow calcium channel blocker; negative inotrope; prolongs AV node refractory time; vasodilates to lower BP without reflex tachycardia	Bolus: 0.25 mg/kg over 2 min (may give second bolus 0.35 mg/kg 15 min after initial dose over 3 minutes) Maint: 5–15 mg/hr titrate to HR goal	*Contraindications*: Wide-complex tachycardia; Wolffe-Parkinson–White syndrome; existing 2nd or 3rd degree AV block; concurrent β-blockade; severe hypotension Adverse effects: Hypotension; AV block; drug-induced hepatitis; flushing
Dobutamine	Racemic mixture (L-isomer: α-agonist/ D-isomer: β-agonist); positive inotrope/ afterload reduction for circulatory failure after AMI, HF, etc.	Dose: 2–20 mcg/kg/min titrate to hemodynamic response Max: 40 mcg/kg/min	*Contraindications*: Hypertrophic cardiomyopathy Adverse effects: May exacerbate ventricular arrhythmias; dose-related tachycardia; can cause myocardial ischemia
Dopamine	Dopamine agonist (0.5–2 mcg/kg/min): renal, cerebral, mesenteric vasodilation β-agonist (2–10 mcg/kg/min): positive inotrope and vasopressor α-agonist (10–20 mcg/kg/min): predominantly vasopressor	Max: 20 mcg/kg/min titrate to hemodynamic response	Central line administration. Urgently treat extravasated drug with phentolamine to prevent skin necrosis *Contraindications*: tachyarrhythmias Adverse effects: Enhances AV conduction, especially with atrial fibrillation; may exacerbate psychosis and arrhythmias
Epinephrine	Nonspecific adrenergic agonist (β > α); potent bronchodilator (β₂ agonist); small doses can cause vasodilation via β₂-vascular receptors; large doses may produce constriction of skeletal and vascular smooth muscle	Shock: 2–10 mcg/min titrate to hemodynamic response	Central line administration Adverse effects: Increases myocardial oxygen consumption; protachyarrhythmia; splanchnic vasoconstrictor (if dose <4 mcg/min); diabetogenic; promotes hypokalemia; increased lactate

(Continued)

28

957

28

Table 28-19. Guidelines for Common Adult Critical Care Drug Infusions (*Continued*)

Drug	Use/Mechanism	Dose Range	Side Effects/Cautions
Esmolol	β_1-selective; very short half-life (9 min); slows AV node conduction; useful to test β-blockade in patients with potential contraindications	Load: 500 mcg/kg over 1 min Maint: 50–200 mcg/kg/min; titrate to HR goal (may need to repeat load)	Large born vein administration due to extravasation risk Adverse effects: Bronchospasm; pallor; nausea; flushing; bradycardia; pulmonary edema (if heart failure occurs); asystole
Fentanyl	Synthetic Mu receptor agonist; increases pain threshold; alters pain reception; inhibits ascending pain pathways	Load: 25–100mcg over 1 to 2 minutes Maint: 50mcg/hr titrate to BPS or CPOT	Preferred agent for hemodynamically unstable patients or those hypotensive on morphine Adverse effects: CNS depression;, respiratory depression; serotonin syndrome; chest wall rigidity (associated with rapid IV push)
Hydromorphone	Mu receptor agonist; causing inhibition of ascending pain pathways; altering the perception of and response to pain; causes cough suppression by direct central action in the medulla; produces generalized CNS depression	Load: 0.25mg–0.5mg every 5–15 minutes over 2 to 3 minutes Maint: 0.2mg–3mg/hr titrate to BPS or CPOT	Adverse effects: CNS depression; respiratory depression; cough suppression
Isoproterenol	Nonspecific β-agonist; potent inotrope/chronotrope for bradycardic states	Dose: 2–20mcg/min titrated to target HR	*Contraindications:* Angina/myocardial ischemia; tachyarrhythmias; digitalis-induced bradycardia Adverse effects: Hypotension; tachycardia; myocardial ischemia; flushing

Lorazepam	Potentiate the effects of GABA, the main inhibitory neurotransmitter; targeting $GABA_A$ receptors which primarily mediate neuronal excitability (seizures), rapid mood changes, clinical anxiety, and sleep	Dose: 0.01–0.1mg/kg/hr titrated to RASS Maximum dose: 10mg/hr	*Contraindications:* Hypersensitivity to polyethylene glycol, propylene glycol, or benzyl alcohol; acute narrow-angle glaucoma Adverse effects: CNS depression; hypotension; propylene glycol toxicity
Midazolam	Potentiate the effects of GABA, the main inhibitory neurotransmitter; targeting $GABA_A$ receptors which primarily mediate neuronal excitability (seizures), rapid mood changes, clinical anxiety, and sleep	Load: 0.01–0.05mg/kg over 2 minutes every 10 to 15 minutes Maint: 0.02–0.1 mg/kg/hr titrated to RASS	Lipophilic drug will store in adipose tissue; metabolized to an active metabolite which accumulates in renal failure due to renal elimination Adverse effects: Cardiorespiratory depression and arrest; CNS depression; hypotension
Milrinone	Phosphodiesterase inhibitor; inotrope and vasodilator (systemic, pulmonary, coronary); used in HF	Dose: 0.375–0.75 mcg/kg/min titrate to hemodynamic response	Renal elimination Adverse effects: Hypotension; tachycardia; aggravates atrial, ventricular arrhythmias; headache
Nicardipine (Cardene IV)	Dihydropyridine calcium channel blocker; producing a relaxation of coronary vascular smooth muscle and coronary vasodilation; increases myocardial oxygen delivery in patients with vasospastic angina	Dose: 5–15 mg/hr; titrate to BP goal	Central line or large peripheral vein; avoid extravasation *Contraindications:* Critical aortic stenosis; will alter cyclosporine levels Adverse effects: Peripheral edema (dose dependent); propylene glycol toxicity (certain formulations); delayed clearance with hepatic and renal insufficiency; may worsen portal hypertension; may cause reflex tachycardia; flushing

(Continued)

28

Table 28-19. Guidelines for Common Adult Critical Care Drug Infusions (*Continued*)

Drug	Use/Mechanism	Dose Range	Side Effects/Cautions
Nitroglycerin	Arterial/venous vasodilator (dose-dependent); coronary vasodilator; primarily reduces cardiac oxygen demand by decreasing preload	Dose: 10–200 mcg/min; titrate to BP goal Maximum dose: 400mcg/min	Hypotension typically seen >200mcg/min *Contraindications*: Increased ICP; narrow-angle glaucoma; pericardial tamponade; concurrent use with phosphodiesterase-5 inhibitors or soluble guanylate cyclase stimulators; cardiomyopathy Adverse effects: Headache (dose related); nausea; vomiting; dizziness; hypotension; bradycardia; increased ICP; propylene glycol toxicity (certain formulations); flushing
Nitroprusside	Arterial/venous vasodilator; donates nitric oxide to interact with vascular smooth muscle >>visceral smooth muscle	Dose: 0.5–10 mcg/kg/min; titrate to goal BP every few min Maximum dose: 10 mcg/kg/min (for a maximum of 10 minutes)	WARNING: (A) EXCESSIVE HYPOTENSION (B) CYANIDE TOXICITY Conversion of Hgb to met-Hgb → cyanide accumulation; keep met-Hgb <10%; detoxified to thiocyanate by liver and kidney – will accumulate in renal failure or prolonged infusions; may shunt blood away from renal/splanchnic beds; increased ICP
Norepinephrine	Potent β_1/α-agonist (low-dose: $\beta > \alpha$) (high-dose: $\alpha > \beta$); use for cardiogenic/septic/neurogenic shock after volume repletion	Dose: 2–4 mcg/min; titrate to hemodynamic response Maximum dose: 12 mcg/min	Central line administration is preferred; urgently treat extravasated drug with phentolamine to prevent skin necrosis Adverse effects: Peripheral A-lines may be dampened by vasoconstriction; may decrease splanchnic blood flow; may cause peripheral gangrene or ischemia

Pentobarbital	Barbiturate depressing the sensory cortex, decreasing motor activity, altering cerebellar function; in high doses, barbiturates exhibit anticonvulsant activity; dose-dependent respiratory depression; reduce brain metabolism and cerebral blood flow in order to decrease intracranial pressure	Load: 5–10mg/kg over 10 minutes Maint: 0.5–4mg/kg/hr	Patient must be intubated with cardiovascular monitoring Central line or large peripheral vein; avoid extravasation Adverse effects: CNS depression; respiratory depression; propylene glycol toxicity (certain formulations); bradycardia; hypotension; hepatoxicity
Phenylephrine	Postsynaptic α-agonist; use for hypotension and shock	Dose: 0.1–10 mcg/kg/ min titrated to BP	Central line administration is preferred; urgently treat extravasated drug with phentolamine to prevent skin necrosis Contraindications: Use reduced doses in patients taking MAO inhibitors Adverse effects: May cause reflex bradycardia (blocked by atropine); constricts coronary, cerebral, and pulmonary vessels; peripheral vasoconstriction; visceral vasoconstriction
Propofol	Short-acting, lipophilic intravenous general anesthetic; CNS depressant, presumably through agonism of GABA_A receptors and perhaps reduced glutamatergic activity through NMDA receptor blockade	Dose: 10–50 mcg/kg/ min titrated to RASS Maximum dose: 100mcg/kg/min	Patient must be intubated; use larger veins of forearm or antecubital fossa 10% fat emulsion – monitor triglycerides Contraindications: Severe allergy to eggs or soy products Adverse effects: Hypotension; PRIS (dysrhythmia, HF, hyperkalemia, lipemia, metabolic acidosis, and/or rhabdomyolysis); exacerbate pancreatitis; pain at injection site; blue/green colored urine

(Continued)

28

Table 28-19. Guidelines for Common Adult Critical Care Drug Infusions *(Continued)*

Drug	Use/Mechanism	Dose Range	Side Effects/Cautions
Rocuronium	Nondepolarizing neuromuscular blocker; blocks acetylcholine from binding to receptors on motor endplate inhibiting depolarization	Load: 0.6mg/kg IV push Maint: 8–12 mcg/kg/min titrated to train of four	Patient must be intubated receiving continuous sedation and analgesia Adverse effects: Myopathy with prolonged use; anaphylaxis; increased peripheral vascular resistance
Vasopressin	Potent vasoconstrictor; anti-diuretic; procoagulant; for vasodilatory shock, stimulates the V1 receptor and increases SVR and MAP; when the V2 receptor is stimulated, cyclic adenosine monophosphate increases water permeability at the renal tubule resulting in decreased urine volume and increased osmolality; for variceal hemorrhage causes smooth muscle contraction in the GI tract by stimulating muscular V1 receptors and release of prolactin and ACTH via V3 receptors.	Shock dose: 0.03 units/min Maximum dose: 0.07 units/min Variceal hemorrhage dose: 0.1–0.4 units/min Maximum dose: 0.8 units/min	Central line administration; urgently treat extravasated drug with nitroglycerin Hepatic/renal metabolism with renal excretion Adverse effects: With variceal bleeding doses, myocardial ischemia due to coronary vasoconstriction; may need to combine with nitroglycerin; SIADH/water intoxication; abdominal cramps; decrease in heart rate and cardiac output; limb ischemia; headache; renal insufficiency
Vecuronium	Nondepolarizing neuromuscular blocker; blocks acetylcholine from binding to receptors on motor endplate inhibiting depolarization	Load: 0.01 mg/kg IV push Maint: 0.8–1.7mcg/kg/min titrated to train of four	Patient must be intubated receiving continuous sedation and analgesia Adverse effects: Myopathy with prolonged use; anaphylaxis; bradycardia

Note: These agents must be administered in the appropriately monitored clinical setting.

ACTH = adrenocorticotropic hormone; AMI = acute myocardial infarction; AV = atrioventricular; BP = blood pressure; BPS = behavioral pain scale; CNS = central nervous system; CPOT = critical care pain observation tool; GABA = gamma-aminobutyric acid; GI = gastrointestinal; HF = congestive heart failure; Hgb = hemoglobin; HR = heart rate; ICP = intracranial pressure; LFTs = liver function tests; MAO = monoamine oxidase; MAP = mean arterial pressure; NMDA = N-methyl-D-aspartate; PRIS = propofol related infusion syndrome; RASS = Richmond agitation sedation scale; SIADH = syndrome of inappropriate antidiuretic hormone; SVR = systemic vascular resistance; V = vasopressin receptor.

References

1. Capuzzo M, et al. Hospital mortality of adults admitted to Intensive Care Units in hospitals with and without Intermediate Care Units: A multicentre European cohort study. *Crit Care* 2014;18(5):551.

2. Blinderman, CD, et al. Comfort care for patients dying in the hospital. *N Engl J Med* 2015;373(26):2549–2561.

3. Barr J, et al. Clinical practice guidelines for the management of pain, agitation, and delirium in adult patients in the intensive care unit. *Crit Care Med* 2013;41:263–306.

4. Pandharipande PP, et al. Long-term cognitive impairment after critical illness. *N Engl J Med* 2013;369(14):1306–1316.

5. Barr J, et al. Clinical practice guidelines for the management of pain, agitation, and delirium in adult patients in the intensive care unit. *Crit Care Med* 2013;41:263–306.

6. American Psychiatric Association. https://www.psychiatry.org/psychiatrists›practice/dsm. Accessed January 20, 2020.

7. Kamdar BB, et al. The effect of a quality improvement intervention on perceived sleep quality and cognition in a medical ICU. *Crit Care Med* 2013;41(3):800–809.

8. Marra A, et al. The ABCDEF bundle in critical care. *Crit Care Clin* 2017;33(2):225–243.

9. Shah MR, et al. Impact of the pulmonary artery catheter in critically ill patients: Meta-analysis of randomized clinical trials, *JAMA* 2005;294.1664–1670.

10. Chatterjee K. The Swan-Ganz catheters: Past, present, and future. *Circulation* 2009;119:147–152.

11. Bellomo R, et al. Acute renal failure— definition, outcome measures, animal models, fluid therapy and information technology needs: the Second International Consensus Conference of the Acute Dialysis Quality Initiative (ADQI) Group. *Crit Care* 2004;8(4):R204–212.

12. Alhazzani W, et al. Surviving Sepsis Campaign: Guidelines on the management of critically ill adults with coronavirus disease 2019 (COVID-19). *Intensive Care Med* 2020;48(6):854–887.

13. https://doi.org/10.1111/jth.14929.

14. https://www.sccm.org/SurvivingSepsisCampaign/Home. Accessed. May 4, 2020.

Common Emergencies

29

Chapter update by Patrick T. Gomella, MD, MPH, EMT-P, Steven A. Haist, MD, MS, and Leonard G. Gomella, MD

OVERVIEW OF EMERGENCY CARDIAC CARE

The algorithms and guidelines of the American Heart Association (AHA) and International Liaison Committee on Cardiac Resuscitation (ILCOR) are routinely updated. The latest guidelines promote the use of automatic external defibrillator (AED) by emergency medical services (EMS), police, and the general public as well as provide an emphasis on high-quality compressions (adequate rate, depth, and recoil while minimizing interruptions) and a team-based approach to resuscitation when available. With the establishment of public access defibrillator (PAD) programs and continued development of EMS protocols, it is essential that receiving providers in emergency departments be knowledgeable about current AHA guidelines regarding the use of the prehospital AEDs as well as for all in-hospital resuscitation guidelines. These recommendations can be found in the most current **Guidelines for Cardiopulmonary Resuscitation and Emergency Cardiovascular Care 2015** and are reviewed in this chapter.[1] In 2017 the American Heart Association (AHA) began moving to a continuous evidence evaluation process and annual Guidelines update. These annual updates allow the rigor of a comprehensive review and expert consensus in as close to real time as possible and can be found at https://eccguidelines.heart.org/circulation/cpr-ecc-guidelines/.

The most recent guidelines emphasize high-quality chest compressions and have notably changed the standard A-B-C (airway-breathing-circulation) to C-A-B (circulation-airway-breathing). This emphasis is primarily focused at lay rescuers to start the CPR sequence with compressions rather than a pulse/breathing check (lay rescuers can frequently misinterpret agonal respirations for spontaneous breathing) to limit delays in adequate chest compressions. In cases of untrained lay rescuers, compression only resuscitation has gained favor as it avoids rescue breathing, which delays chest compressions. Healthcare providers are still expected to check for pulse/breathing. If a person experiences sudden cardiac arrest and a defibrillator or an AED is available, defibrillation can be performed as soon as possible. However, if a person is found unresponsive, prompt initiation of compressions should be performed before defibrillation.

Individuals who experience cardiac arrest and receive immediate defibrillation are more likely to be successfully defibrillated after the first shock. For every minute of circulatory arrest there is an approximately 10% decrease in the likelihood of successful resuscitation. Patients who are subject to delays in receiving resuscitation do not fare as well, unless there has been a brief period of CPR before defibrillation.

Many communities, organizations, and EMS systems participate in **PAD programs**. These programs facilitate early recognition and management by the use of **AEDs**, and some hospitals have AEDs available, so that a patient who suffers cardiac arrest can be defibrillated before the arrival of the code team. The elements of effective CPR are summarized in Table 29-1.

29

Table 29-1. Considerations for Performing High-Quality CPR in Adults

Perform chest compressions at a rate of 100–120/min
Compress to a depth of at least 2.0 inches (5 cm)
Allow for full recoil after each compression
Minimize pauses in compressions
Ventilate adequately (2 breaths after 30 compressions, each breath delivered over 1 second, each causing the chest to rise)

Source: Reproduced with permission from: Cardiopulmonary and Cardiocerebral Resuscitation, Fuster V, Harrington RA, Narula J, Eapen ZJ (eds.). Hurst's The Heart, 14e; 2017, New York, NY: McGraw-Hill.

Interim COVID-19 AHA Guidelines (Released April 2020)

In response to the Global Viral Pandemic that began in December 2019, related to COVID-19, caused by the severe acute respiratory syndrome coronavirus 2 (SARS-CoV-2), the AHA released interim recommendations for BLS and ALS care to help healthcare providers treat victims with cardiac arrest who are suspected or known to be actively infected. Specific algorithms do not change drastically with these interim updates, but instead focus on techniques to balance high-quality resuscitation while also minimizing exposure to the healthcare team given the risk of viral particle aerosolization during various resuscitation maneuvers. While specific to the viral pandemic, they would likely be applicable in any similar potential future event requiring such alterations of the standard resuscitation guidelines. Three general principles were included:

1. "Reduce provider exposure"
2. "Prioritize oxygenation and ventilation strategies"
3. "Consider the appropriateness of starting and continuing resuscitation"

A brief overview of each principle is listed below along with a discussion of in-hospital cardiac arrest and out-of-hospital cardiac arrest.[2]

"Reduce provider exposure"

- All providers should don personal protective equipment (PPE) effective for airborne and droplet precautions. Follow local protocol standards regarding appropriate PPE.
- Limit personnel to essential providers only.

29

- Encourage the use of mechanical CPR devices in appropriate patients (helps reduce the number of healthcare providers).
  - Effective hand-offs between healthcare teams to ensure all new providers are aware of the patient's COVID-19 status.

"Prioritize oxygenation and ventilation strategies"

- Utilize a high-efficiency particulate filter (HEPA) on any ventilation device when providing ventilation support. If using a bag valve mask, maintaining a tight seal is a priority.
- For adults, consider passive oxygenation via a nonrebreather mask (NRB) covered with a standard surgical mask.
- Prioritize intubation with a cuffed tube, preferably attached to a free-standing ventilator with an integrated HEPA filter if available. Intubation attempts should be minimized by assigning most experienced provider to the task while holding chest compressions during the attempt. Video laryngoscopy should be considered, if available. If intubation with a cuffed tube cannot be expeditiously performed, consider a supraglottic airway.
- Minimize disconnections of closed-circuit ventilatory system once established.

"Consider the appropriateness of starting and continuing resuscitation"

- Goals of care should be addressed as soon as possible with the patient or their healthcare proxy.
- Healthcare providers/organizations should adopt policies to guide appropriateness of initiating and terminating CPR in this setting, weighing patient risk factors to determine their likelihood of survival.

Special Scenarios: "In-Hospital Cardiac Arrest"

- Standard recommendations listed above still apply to minimize exposure to the healthcare team (close door to room, don appropriate PPE, limit personnel in room, discuss goals of care).
- Consider leaving patient on mechanical ventilator with HEPA filter if already intubated.
- Ventilator settings—adjust to allow for asynchronous ventilation
  - General ventilator settings suggested: FiO_2—1.0; mode: assist control (patient-controlled ventilation)—turn trigger to off to prevent auto-triggered respirations at time of compression; respiratory rate 10/min for adults.
- For patients who are in prone position at time of arrest, and without advanced airway, attempt to place in supine position for resuscitation.

29

- For patients who are in prone position at time of arrest and have an advanced airway in place, consider placing defibrillator pads in the A-P position and provide compressions over the T7 to T10 vertebral bodies. Can consider moving patient supine if there is no risk of ventilator circuit disconnections and further aerosolization.

Special Scenarios: "Maternal/Neonatal Considerations"

- Routine suction of the neonatal airway should NOT be performed to clear meconium-stained fluid in uncomplicated deliveries.
- IV delivery of epinephrine via an umbilical catheter preferred over ET instillation of an uncuffed tube.
- Use of closed incubators for transfer should be used when possible but does not provide adequate protection of aerosolization. Maintain appropriate distance measures.

Special Scenarios: "Out of Hospital Arrest for Lay Rescuers"

- Adults—Perform at least hands only CPR, especially if someone already exposed to the victim is in close proximity. Consider a face covering for both patient and lay rescuer.
- Children—Perform at least hands only CPR and consider breaths (higher rate of respiratory arrest preceding cardiac arrest than in the adult population) if willing and able (especially if someone already exposed to the victim is in close proximity). Consider a face covering for both patient and lay rescuer.
- Defibrillation is <u>not</u> considered an aerosolizing procedure and should continue to be used by lay rescuers when AEDs are available.

CARDIOPULMONARY RESUSCITATION (CPR)

CPR Basics: CAB (Circulation, Airway, Breathing)

Universal precautions dictate that gowns, gloves, masks, and face shields or goggles be used. Specific considerations for CPR in the pediatric population are summarized in Table 29-6, page 1015.

Unresponsive Adult (Age >8 yr): Witnessed and Unwitnessed Collapse

If a patient becomes unresponsive (no response to verbal or tactile stimuli, i.e., "shake and shout"), call for help (CODE, 911). If an unconscious

29

patient is encountered who is not breathing and has no apparent signs of circulation and the time of onset of symptoms is unknown, the situation is called unwitnessed arrest. In this situation, there may be a benefit for several cycles of high-quality compressions and breaths (breaths if trained rescuers present) prior to attempted defibrillation.

1. Verify scene safety and get a defibrillator or AED to the bedside.
2. Stand or kneel at the patient's shoulder. Position patient on back as a unit, protecting the neck.
3. Simultaneously look for signs of breathing and check a pulse.
4. If a foreign body is visualized in the airway, and can easily be removed, remove it. Blind finger sweeps are no longer recommended.
5. If the patient is breathing and has a pulse, place him or her in the **recovery position:** a stable side-lying position in which the tongue does not block the airway and fluid can drain from the mouth. Call for assistance if not previously done. Continue to monitor the patient for breathing until the next level of care arrives.
6. If there is a definite pulse, provide rescue breaths: give 1 breath every 5–6 s, approximately 10–12 breaths/min, rechecking for a pulse every 2 min. If an advanced airway is placed, ventilate with approximately 1 breath every 6–8 s. In a witnessed adult cardiac arrest situation when an AED is immediately available, it is reasonable that the defibrillator be used as soon as possible. If there is an unmonitored cardiac arrest or when an AED is not immediately available, it is reasonable to begin CPR until the defibrillator equipment is available.
7. If there are no signs of breathing and no palpable pulse, begin chest compressions: Place both hands on the patient's lower sternum, the heel of one hand on top of the heel of the other. Push **fast** and push **hard**, to a depth of at least 2.0 in (5 cm) for the average adult, allowing full recoil of the chest between compressions by not applying any pressure with your hands but maintain contact with the chest. Avoid excessive compression depths greater than 2.4 in (6 cm). Continue compressions until a defibrillator or an AED is brought to the patient's bedside. If a defibrillator is not immediately available, continue chest compressions and ventilations at a ratio of 30:2 at a rate of approximately 100–120 compressions/min. If untrained lay rescuer, compressions only can be performed. Rescuers should attempt to minimize the frequency and duration of interruptions in compressions to maximize the number of compressions delivered per minute.
8. When the defibrillator or AED arrives, attach the two pads to the patient's bare chest. Right-sided sternal pad: right superoanterior infraclavicular position; left-sided apical pad: inferolateral left side of chest

lateral to the left breast. Minimize interruption of chest compressions and compress until the pads are on the chest, if possible.

9. Stop compressions. Analyze the rhythm (or AED automatically identifies rhythm-then follow voice prompts), and if indicated (presence of ventricular fibrillation [VF] or pulseless ventricular tachycardia [VT]), deliver a single shock. If using a manual defibrillator, use manufacturer recommended energy levels if known, but standard levels are biphasic = 200 J and monophasic = 360 J.

10. Immediately resume CPR for another five cycles of 30 compressions/ 2 breaths. Pulse check.

11. If there is no pulse, resume CPR, recharge the defibrillator, and administer another single shock followed by immediate CPR.

12. If unsuccessful, proceed to the **advanced cardiac life support (ACLS) algorithms and guidelines starting on page 981.** Also, see Figure 29-2, page 980.

Note: If the defibrillation results in successful termination of VF, treat the patient by supportively observing for changes in blood pressure, heart rate, and respiratory status.

After successful defibrillation, an unstable rhythm may develop and necessitate intervention. Some patients may arrive in the emergency department with a pulseless rhythm, asystole, pulseless electrical activity, and VT or VF. Other patients may have a slow heart rate incapable of providing good perfusion pressure, i.e., bradycardia (heart rate <60 beats/min) or tachycardia (heart rate >100 beats/min). Proceed to the appropriate ACLS algorithms and guidelines (see below).

CPR of Child (Age 1–Onset of Puberty): Witnessed and Unwitnessed Cardiac Arrest

If a child becomes unresponsive and experiences respiratory arrest, the approach is similar to that for an adult, with slight variations based on the number of rescuers present. (See also Table 29-6, page 1015.)

1. Verify scene safety and get a defibrillator or AED to the bedside.

2. Stand or kneel at the patient's shoulder. Position patient on back as a unit, protecting the neck.

3. Simultaneously look for signs of breathing and check a pulse.

4. If a foreign body is visualized in the airway, and it can easily be removed, remove it. Blind finger sweeps are no longer recommended.

5. If the patient is breathing and has a pulse, call for assistance if not previously done. Continue to monitor the patient for breathing until the next level of care arrives.

29

6. If there is a definite pulse, provide rescue breaths: give 1 breath every 3–5 s, approximately 12–20 breaths/min, rechecking for a pulse every 2 min. If pulse rate is <60 with signs of decreased perfusion, add chest compressions.

7. If there are no signs of breathing and no palpable pulse, begin chest compressions (if a single rescuer, and this was a witnessed arrest, activate the emergency response system and retrieve the defibrillator/AED at this time; if an unwitnessed arrest, immediately begin compressions and if still alone at 2 min, then retrieve AED). Place both hands on the patient's lower sternum, the heel of one hand on top of the heel of the other. Push **fast** and push **hard,** to a depth of 1/3–1/2 of the chest allowing full recoil of the chest. Continue compressions until a defibrillator or an AED is brought to the patient's side. If a single rescuer, provide CPR at a ratio of 30:2; if two rescuers, perform CPR with a ratio of 15:2.

8. As soon as a defibrillator is available, immediately apply the defibrillator or AED pads (pediatric) to the patient's bare chest with minimal interruption in chest compressions. Adult AED pads are acceptable if pediatric pads are not available; however, do not let the pads touch each other on the chest. Pads can be placed in an anterior/posterior configuration on patients with very tiny torsos, with anterior pad below the nipple to the left of the sternum and posterior pad to the left of the spine below the scapula. Minimize interruption of chest compressions and compress until the pads are on the chest, if possible.

9. Stop compressions. Analyze the rhythm (or AED automatically identifies the rhythm—then follow voice prompts), and if indicated (presence of VF or pulseless VT), deliver a single shock. If using a manual defibrillator, use 2 J/kg. For next indicated shock, one can consider increasing energy to 4 J/kg.

10. If unsuccessful, proceed to the **advanced cardiac life support (ACLS) algorithms and guidelines.**

Like adults, children may present in asystole, pulseless electrical activity, or pulseless VT or VF, or these rhythms may develop after defibrillation. Furthermore, children can present with bradycardia or tachycardia. Proceed to the PALS guidelines and attempt to correct the dysrhythmia and determine the cause of the event.

CPR of Unresponsive Infant (Age <1 yr): Witnessed or Unwitnessed Cardiac Arrest

1. Similar to the child algorithm, with modification in hand position. (See also Table 29-6, page 1015.)

2. Look, listen, and feel for breathing and simultaneously check for a pulse (brachial or femoral).

3. If no pulse is present, start chest compressions. Use two or three fingers or a thumb just below the nipple line, and press to 1/3–1/2 the depth of the chest.
4. Use 30 compressions/2 ventilations (single rescuer) or 15 compressions/2 ventilations (two healthcare providers). Rate of compressions is 100/min. Rate of ventilation is 12–20 breaths/min (or ~1 breath/3–5 s).
5. If an advanced airway is present, use 8–10 breaths/min (~1 breath/6–8 s asynchronously).
6. Perform CPR for 2 min or five cycles, then reassess the patient. There are no recommendations regarding defibrillation in this situation. If no success, proceed to the advanced algorithms and guidelines.

Neonatal Resuscitation

Immediately after delivery, a neonate begins to undergo a physiologic transition. (See also Table 29-6, page 1015.) Rapid assessment can determine the need for resuscitation:

1. Was the born baby at term?
2. Is the baby breathing or crying?
3. Does the baby have good muscle tone?

If the answer to all these questions is yes, resuscitation probably is not needed.

It is normal for amniotic fluid to be present in the upper airways of newborns, and this fluid must be cleared. Fluid can be cleared with a bulb syringe or small suction catheter by suctioning the mouth first, followed by the nose. Follow COVID-19 precautions on page 969, Special Scenarios: Maternal/Neonatal Considerations.

If any answer to the above questions is "no," the infant should be placed in a radiant warmer until further stabilization (clear secretions, stimulate). If after basic maneuvers are attempted, and still no breathing, initiate ventilation (after no more than 60 s). If heart rate is below 60/min, initiate compressions, may need IV epinephrine. If after epinephrine and heart rate remains 60/min, consider hypovolemia or pneumothorax.

ADVANCED CARDIAC LIFE SUPPORT (ACLS)

The foundation of ACLS is sound BLS and the integration of airway management, ECG interpretation, cardioversion, defibrillation, and the selective use of medications. In the advanced phase, specific arrhythmias are managed primarily through administration of medications. Rapid reference guides to ACLS and other commonly used emergency medications are on the inside front and back covers of this book with detailed medication listing in Figure 29-9 , p 1019. ECG interpretation is reviewed in Chapter 27, starting on page 951.

29

Cardiac Arrest

Four rhythms can produce pulseless cardiac arrest: ventricular fibrillation (VF), ventricular tachycardia (VT), pulseless electrical activity (PEA), and asystole. See adult ACLS pulseless arrest algorithms pulseless VT/VF, p 981 and asystole/PEA, p 983.

Symptomatic Bradycardia and Tachycardia

Monitor for the development of arrhythmias in any patient with chest pain or who has undergone resuscitation. In addition to the above cardiac arrest arrhythmias, patients may have bradycardia or tachycardia that requires monitoring and intervention if they become symptomatic. Management of bradycardia and tachycardia is based on 2015 Emergency Cardiac Care guidelines outlined in the section on "ACLS Algorithms" starting on page 981.

Emergency Airway and Ventilatory Support

Oxygen administration is often necessary for the management of patients with acute coronary syndromes, pulmonary distress, or stroke. Various devices can deliver supplementary oxygen from 21–100% (see Table 29-2). To maximize oxygenation, administer 100% inspired oxygen during BLS, if available. Airway adjuncts are useful for this purpose and are classified as basic and advanced airway techniques. Make sure suction is readily available. Continuous EtCO$_2$ monitoring should be available if an advanced airway is placed.

Table 29-2. Typical Oxygen Delivery Methods

	Oxygen Flow	Delivered FiO$_2$	Comments
Standard Nasal Cannula	2–6 L/min	24–44%	FiO$_2$ approximate
High-flow Nasal Oxygen	Up to 60 L/min	Up to 100%	Heated, humidified
Simple Face Mask	5–10 L/min	35–50%	FiO$_2$ approximate
Venturi Mask or Equivalent	9–15 L/min*	35–50%	FiO$_2$ more accurate
Non-rebreather Mask	10–15 L/min	Near 100%	Mask fit essential

Abbreviation: FiO$_2$ = fraction of inspired oxygen.
*Required flow rates vary by manufacturer. See individual device specifications.
Source: Reproduced with permission from Glass CM. Blood gases, pulse oximetry, and capnography. In: Tintinalli JE, Ma O, Yealy DM, Meckler GD, Stapczynski J, Cline DM, Thomas SH (eds.). Tintinalli's Emergency Medicine: A Comprehensive Study Guide, 9e, 2020; New York, NY: McGraw-Hill.

Basic Airway Management

Practical aspects of airway management are discussed in Chapter 19, Endotracheal/Tracheal Intubation and Airway Management, starting on page 565.

Bag Mask Ventilation (BMV): Can be supplied with room air or oxygen supplementation; can also be connected to an advanced airway if present. Open the airways adequately with chin lift, lifting the jaw against the mask and maintaining a tight seal. Deliver a tidal volume sufficient to raise the chest over approximately 1–2 cm. Can cause gastric inflation with subsequent complications (e.g., aspiration) if vigorous bag valve mask ventilation is performed. If ventilation is adequate, an advanced airway can be considered only if personnel adequately trained in placement and the interruption to compressions are minimized.

Oropharyngeal Airway: Use only if the patient is unconscious and has no gag reflex.

Nasopharyngeal Airway: Better tolerated by patients who are not deeply unconscious. Useful for patients with tightly clenched jaws; use with caution in craniofacial trauma.

Advanced Airways

Used only by healthcare providers with proper training and frequent practice. Because placement of an advanced airway may require interruption of basic CPR, the risk/benefit ratio must be considered; if adequate ventilations are obtained with a bag-valve-mask (BVM), an advanced airway can be delayed. The bag mask can be connected to an advanced airway for delivery of ventilation. In cases when intubation in an emergency setting is needed and when patients have not been NPO, rapid sequence induction (RSI) can be performed if the provider is adequately trained and comfortable. See Chapter 19, pages 582 and 583, for RSI steps. The following techniques for airway management are discussed in detail in the Chapter 19 section on Endotracheal/Tracheal Intubation and Airway Management, starting on page 565.

Endotracheal Tube (ET): Considered the "gold-standard" of airway management. Unskilled providers can cause more harm than good in attempting ET intubation during resuscitation. Indicated when the rescuer cannot ventilate an unconscious patient with a bag mask and in the absence of airway reflexes. (See Chapter 19, page 565.)

Esophagotracheal Airway (Combitube or ETC): A multilumen airway that consists of a single, dual-lumen tube with two cuffs designed for blind placement. (Chapter 19, page 589.)

Laryngeal Mask Airway (LMA): Inflatable silicone mask and rubber connecting tube. Inserted blindly into the pharynx, a cuff is inflated that forms a low-pressure seal around the laryngeal inlet, allowing gentle positive-pressure ventilation. *Note:* The black line on the airway tube must be oriented toward

29

the upper lip, and a bite block must be in place. Aspiration may be less common with an LMA than with a bag mask. (See Chapter 19, page 589.)

King Systems Airway (King-LT): A single-lumen supraglottic airway designed to be blindly inserted into the pharynx. Choose correct size (sized based on patient height—Yellow 4–5 ft, Red 5–6 ft), and using a lateral approach with dominant hand hold tube at connector. Open airway with chin lift and advance tube behind tongue while rotating tube back to midline so the blue orientation line faces patient's chin. Advance the tube until connector is aligned with teeth or gums and inflate balloon with 60 cm H_2O. Attach BVM, and while gently bagging patient, withdraw King LT until ventilation is easy. Add more air to balloon if needed to maximize seal. (See Chapter 19, page 589.)

Regardless of advanced airway technique used, correct tube placement should be confirmed by auscultation over epigastrium/lung fields and by an $ETCO_2$ monitoring device and when stable, confirmed radiologically.

Automatic External Defibrillation, Defibrillation, Cardioversion

In addition to familiarizing yourself with the location of the code cart, airway supplies, emergency numbers, etc., on each new rotation, become familiar with the defibrillator and automatic external defibrillator (AED). AEDs are small, free-standing, battery-operated defibrillators. Equipped with specialized hardware and software, they are designed to recognize lethal, nonperfusing, and shockable dysrhythmias such as ventricular fibrillation (VF) and ventricular tachycardia (VT). When it recognizes a lethal dysrhythmia, the AED gives visual or voice prompts for the rescuer to press a button and defibrillate the patient. Some models of AED automatically shock the patient after emitting an audible or visual warning to the rescuers to "stand clear." There are monophasic and biphasic defibrillators and AEDs in hospitals. In monophasic shock, the shock is delivered in only one direction passing from one electrode to the other. In the biphasic shock, the direction of shock is reversed by changing the polarity of the electrodes during the shock delivered. In theory, compared to when 360 J are delivered for defibrillation in a monophasic defibrillator, 200 J administered in a biphasic defibrillator reduce the potential heart muscle damage from the higher voltage shocks.

General AED Instructions

1. Place the AED near the patient in such a way that access to the airway and chest is unimpeded.
2. Turn on the AED unit. The majority of current AEDs give auditory and visual prompts such as:
   o "Connect electrodes to AED."
   o "Place electrodes to patient's bare chest." (*Note:* Do not allow the pads to touch each other.)

29

o "Do not touch the patient!"
o "Analyzing rhythm."
o "Shock advised—Do not touch the patient!"
o "Push [flashing button] to shock patient."

3. Check rhythm; if a palpable rhythm is present, check for pulse. If pulse NOT present, resume CPR.

4. Repeat as clinically indicated.

Defibrillation

Defibrillation is used for life-threatening cardiac dysrhythmias, VF, and non-perfusing VT. When defibrillating a patient, follow the updated algorithms.

1. Place pads securely on patient's chest: one to the right of the patient's sternum, just below the clavicle, the other over the left anterior axillary line centered over the 6th rib. Most pads and paddles are labeled to facilitate placement. Make sure there is good contact with the skin to decrease resistance. Some kits include a razor to shave hirsute patients. Most pads can be used for ECG monitoring, defibrillation, cardioversion, and pacing. See Figure 29-1, below.

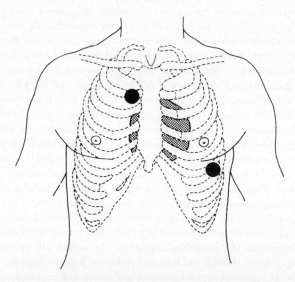

FIGURE 29-1. Contact points for defibrillation electrodes (solid circles). Place one paddle electrode to the right of the sternum in the second or third interspace, and the other paddle should be at the cardiac apex. In children and thin adults, paddles may be placed directly over the heart in anteroposterior orientation. (Reproduced with permission from Stone C, Humphries RL (eds.). CURRENT Diagnosis & Treatment: Emergency Medicine, 8e, 2017; New York, NY: McGraw-Hill.)

29

2. If using paddles, use electrode gel or paste and use at least 25 lb of downward force to enhance contact with the chest. Most paddles can be used for "quick-look" of the rhythm.
3. Charge the defibrillator to the appropriate energy (measured in joules). Adult standard energy levels: biphasic = 200 J and monophasic = 360. Pediatric standard energy levels: 2 J/kg initial, then 4 J/kg.
4. Shout "CLEAR—SHOCKING PATIENT!" Verify that no one (including yourself) is in contact with the patient.
5. Depress both buttons simultaneously on the paddles or "shock" button on the defibrillator panel to deliver the shock.

Cardioversion

There are rapid rhythms (e.g., atrial fibrillation with uncontrolled rates, supraventricular tachycardia [SVT], and Wolff–Parkinson–White [WPW]) that may render a patient's condition unstable with a decrease in blood pressure, change in mentation, etc. These circumstances may necessitate that the rhythm be electrically terminated with cardioversion. Current manual defibrillators include a cardioversion setting. When the cardioversion mode is selected, the machine **synchronizes** the shock automatically with the peak of the R wave on the ECG strip. This step prevents shock delivery during the vulnerable period of the cardiac cycle, which can promote development of a lethal nonperfusing rhythm such as VF (see Figure 29-10B, page 991). The defibrillator hardware and software control the discharge of the shock after the "Shock" button is pressed. The procedure is otherwise as described for defibrillation with the exception that one starts with lower energy levels before reaching typical maximum of 200 J for biphasic and 360 J for monophasic defibrillators. Because cardioversion is done with the patient conscious, consider sedation with a drug such as midazolam, if clinically feasible.

When patients are suffering from rapid arrhythmias but are hemodynamically stable, **chemical cardioversion** may be appropriate. If the patient has a regular narrow complex tachycardia, vagal maneuvers and IV adenosine (6 mg rapid IV push, followed by 12 mg rapid IV push if needed) can be attempted. Wide-complex tachycardias require advanced knowledge of ECG rhythm interpretation and antiarrhythmic therapies. Amiodarone (150 mg IV) is occasionally used for wide-complex tachycardias. AV nodal blocking agents such as adenosine should be avoided in patients with known WPW who have tachyarrhythmias (AV nodal blocking agents can increase HR by changing conduction to go through the accessory pathway). Refer to Figures 29-5 to 29-9 for the suggested steps for various manifestations of tachycardia.

29 Acute Coronary Syndromes and Myocardial Infarction

Perform a 12-lead ECG on any patients experiencing chest pain (see Chapter 19 for ECG procedure and Chapter 27 for ECG interpretation). If the patient has signs of ischemia or has had an acute myocardial infarction (shown in two contiguous leads), a quick decision must be made to administer thrombolytics vs. pursue primary percutaneous coronary intervention. If PCI (Percutaneous Coronary Intervention, formerly known as angioplasty with stenting) can be performed in a timely fashion (90 min or less), then this is usually the preferred therapy. Considerations for patient stability and transport distance to a PCI capable facility are made by prehospital providers for patients with AMI outside a hospital setting or for patients admitted to a smaller hospital without these capabilities. When fibrinolytic therapy is indicated as the primary treatment strategy, the goal for administration is within 30 min of hospital arrival. Absolute contraindications to fibrinolytics include CNS abnormalities (e.g., A–V malformation, tumor, history of intracranial hemorrhage, recent head trauma), suspected aortic dissection, and bleeding diathesis. Relative contraindications include pregnancy, history of severe poorly controlled hypertension, recent (2–4 wk) gastrointestinal or genitourinary bleeding, and recent major surgery. The recommended sequence of acute coronary syndrome management is shown on page 992.

ACLS Algorithms

The following algorithms identify the approach to cardiac arrest, symptomatic bradycardia and tachycardia, and acute coronary syndrome based on the latest "Guidelines for Cardiopulmonary Resuscitation and Emergency Cardiovascular Care 2015."[3] Note that the American Heart Association has transitioned to continuous updates of ECC and ACLS guidelines since 2015 and the most recent yearly updates have been incorporated into the information presented in this chapter.

Table 29-9, page 1019, lists medications used in advanced cardiac life support, and the most commonly used resuscitation medications are also listed on the inside of the front and back covers for convenient reference. The following arrhythmias and management algorithms are included in the AHA ACLS guidelines with selected ECG tracings associated with the algorithm:

- Flowchart for initial steps after BCLS or after being called to evaluate a patient with an arrhythmia (Figure 29-2, page 980).
- Pulseless ventricular tachycardia/ventricular fibrillation (page 981)
- Asystole/pulseless electrical activity (PEA) (page 983)
- Symptomatic bradycardia (page 984)
- Tachycardia: narrow QRS/regular rhythm (page 986)
- Tachycardia: narrow QRS/irregular rhythm (page 987)
- Tachycardia: wide QRS/regular rhythm (page 988)
- Tachycardia: wide QRS/irregular rhythm (page 989)
- Synchronized electrical cardioversion (VT w/pulses in hemodynamic instability) (page 990)
- Acute coronary syndrome: patients with symptoms of ischemia or infarction (page 992)

29

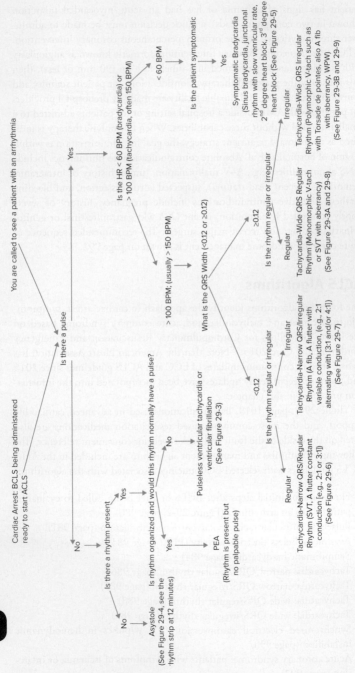

Figure 29-2. Initial approach to a patient in cardiac arrest or who is being evaluated for an arrhythmia. Aberrancy = wide QRS complex.

Initial Steps ACLS

Pulseless Ventricular Tachycardia/Ventricular Fibrillation

(See Figures 29-3 and 29-4.)

1. Perform BLS algorithm
   a. Check for responsiveness/breathing/pulse (no more than 10 s)
   b. Begin 5 cycles of CPR (30:2, 100/min)
   c. Give O_2
   d. Attach monitor/defibrillator

2. Check rhythm
   a. Shockable? Continue CPR, prepare to deliver shock

   b. Not-Shockable (Asystole/PEA)? ⟹ Go to Asystole algorithm on page 983.

3. Deliver shock (based on manufacturer's instructions)
   a. Immediately resume CPR
   b. Check pulse and recheck rhythm every 2 min (about five cycles)

4. Continue CPR/shock sequence and establish at least one IV/IO line.

5. Consider placing an advanced airway if not adequately ventilating with bag valve mask

6. Give medication (Give five cycles and deliver a shock between each medication dose as needed)
   a. Epinephrine 1 mg 1:10,000 IV every 3–5 min until return of spontaneous circulation (ROSC)
   b. Consider an antiarrhythmic (amiodarone, lidocaine, magnesium)
      i. Amiodarone 300 mg IV/IO, may repeat once at 150 mg IV/IO in 5 min
      ii. Lidocaine 1–1.5 mg/kg IV/IO, may repeat at 0.75 mg/kg every 5 min up to a maximum of 3 mg/kg
      iii. Magnesium (for Torsades de pointes/hypomagnesemia) 1–2 g IV/IO in 10 mL NS over 10 min

29

7. Continue CPR/shock sequence until rhythm change, return of spontaneous circulation (ROSC), or resuscitation termination

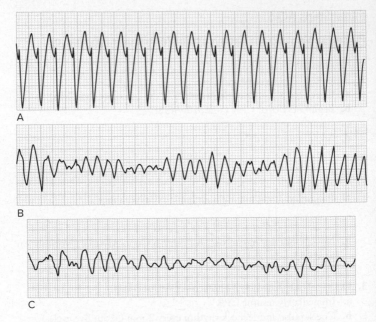

A

B

C

Figure 29-3. **A.** Ventricular tachycardia. **B.** Torsades de pointes is a specific type of polymorphic ventricular tachycardia. **C.** Ventricular fibrillation.

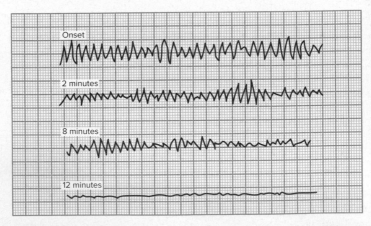

Onset

2 minutes

8 minutes

12 minutes

Figure 29-4. Continuous ECG during an episode of ventricular fibrillation that progresses to fine ventricular fibrillation then asystole (flat line). Note: To ensure that ventricular fibrillation is not masquerading as asystole, switch to another lead whenever a "flat line" is recorded on the ECG during resuscitation. (Reproduced with permission from Up To Date Graphic 67777 Version 3.0.)

29

Asystole/Pulseless Electrical Activity (PEA)

(A rhythm that could normally generate a pulse is present but no palpable pulse is generated)

For asystole, see Figure 29-4, rhythm strip at 12 minutes

1. Perform BLS algorithm
   a. Check for responsiveness/breathing/pulse
   b. Begin CPR (30:2, 100/min)
   c. Give O_2
   d. Attach monitor/defibrillator

2. Check rhythm
   a. Shockable ventricular tachycardia/ventricular fibrillation? ⟹ Go to VT/VF algorithm on page 981
   b. Not-shockable (asystole/PEA)? Continue CPR

3. Continue CPR, establish at least one IV/IO line; consider and correct possible causes
   a. 6 H's and 5 T's (see below)**

4. Consider placing an advanced airway when possible

5. Give medication
   a. Epi 1 mg 1:10,000 IV every 3–5 min until ROSC/termination

6. Continue CPR/medication sequence until rhythm change, ROSC, arrival at the hospital or resuscitation termination

**6 H's and 5 T's
   o Hypovolemia, hypoxia, hydrogen ion (acidosis), hypo/hyperkalemia, hypoglycemia, hypothermia
   o Toxins, tamponade, tension pneumothorax, thrombosis (pulmonary or coronary), trauma

Symptomatic Bradycardia

(See Figure 29-5.)
1. Evaluate airway/breathing/circulation
    a. Give O$_2$

2. Attach and monitor ECG (Obtain 12-lead if available)
    a. Identify rhythm, BP, and oxygen saturation
        i. Signs of instability/poor perfusion? ⟹ Go to step 4

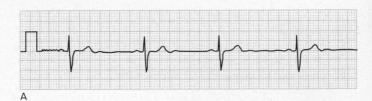

A

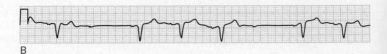

B

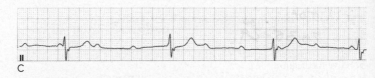

C

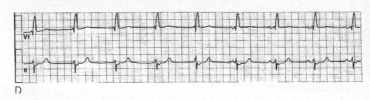

D

Figure 29-5. **A**. Sinus bradycardia. Rate is approximately 38–40 beats/min. **B.** Sinus bradycardia with second-degree AV (4:3 atrial to ventricular conduction), ventricular rate approximately 38 BPM block. **C.** Third-degree AV block (complete heart block), ventricular rate ~ 30 BPM; from C Keith Stone, Roger L Humphries: Current Diagnosis and Treatment: Emergency Medicine, 8th Edition McGraw-Hill; reproduced with permission. **D.** Junctional rhythm, ventricular rate ~ 58 BPM with a transition to sinus bradycardia (P waves emerge at the 6th beat).

29

      1. Signs include acute AMS, angina/MI, hypotension, other signs
         of hemodynamic instability/shock
  b. Establish an IV

3. If adequate perfusion – monitor and transport

  a. Consider medications (i.e., Atropine; see step 5 below)
4. If inadequate perfusion
  a. Atropine; see step 5 below: if IV is not available can go TCP first
  b. Prepare for transcutaneous pacing (TCP) (consider sedation w/ midazolam 1–5 mg IV/IO/IN)

    i. If no IV access and pt is unstable, do not delay TCP for sedation; start IV and provide analgesia/sedation ASAP following initiation of TCP
    ii. Begin pacing rate at 70 bpm at lowest mA setting; ↑voltage until electrical capture is seen
    iii. Confirm presence of mechanical heart activity by checking pulse
    iv. If no IV was established prior to TCP, start one

5. Medications
  a. Atropine—0.5 mg IV; may repeat every 3–5 min until a max of six doses or max dose of 3 mg
  b. Epinephrine or dopamine IV infusion if TCP is not available or is not effective
    i. Epinephrine 2–10 mcg/min
    ii. Dopamine 2–20 mcg/kg/min

6. Monitor pt
  a. If PEA develops ⟹ go to asystole/pulseless electrical activity (PEA), page 983
  b. If VF/VT develops ⟹ go to pulseless ventricular tachycardia/ventricular fibrillation, page 981

29

Tachycardia—Narrow QRS (<0.12 s)/Regular Rhythm

(See Figure 29-6.)

1. Evaluate airway/breathing/circulation
   a. Give O$_2$

   ⇩

2. Attach and monitor ECG (obtain 12-lead if available)
   a. Identify rhythm, BP, and O$_2$ saturation
      i. Signs of instability/poor perfusion? ⇨

> Signs include acute altered mental status, angina/MI, hypotension, other signs of hemodynamic instability/shock

   ⇩

   b. Establish an IV

> At any time, if pt becomes unstable, immediately perform synchronized cardioversion, page 990
>
> If PEA develops, go to page 983

   ⇩

3. Attempt nonpharmaceutical/electrical interventions
   a. Vagal maneuver (pt bears down like they are having a bowel movement, or coughing or gagging)

   ⇩

   b. Carotid sinus massage (check for bruits first)

   ⇩

4. If vagal maneuvers unsuccessful, give medication
   a. Adenosine 6 mg rapid IV push followed with a NS flush; may repeat twice at 12 mg if no conversion
      i. If rhythm converts, ⇨ monitor for recurrence
   b. If rhythm does not convert, ⇨ β-blocker or consider a nondihydropyridine calcium channel blocker (CCBs) (verapamil or diltiazem)

   ⇩

If no conversion with medications, consider elective synchronized cardioversion (50–100 J). ⇨ Go to page 990.

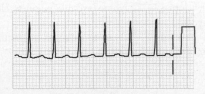

Figure 29-6.   Tachycardia with narrow QRS/regular rhythm, ventricular rate approximately 150 BPM (paroxysmal atrial tachycardia).

29

Tachycardia—Narrow QRS (<0.12 s)/Irregular Rhythm

(See Figure 29-7.)

1. Evaluate airway/breathing/circulation
   a. Give O_2

2. Attach and monitor ECG (obtain 12-lead if available)
   a. Identify rhythm, BP, and saturation
      i. Signs of instability/poor perfusion?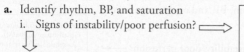

   > Signs include acute altered mental status, angina/MI, hypotension, other signs of hemodynamic instability/shock

   b. Establish an IV

   > NOTE: At any time, if pt becomes unstable, immediately perform synchronized cardioversion (go to page 990)
   > If PEA develops, go to page 983

3. Give medication
   a. If probable Afib, atrial flutter with variable block or multifocal atrial tachycardia, control w/ diltiazem (0.25cmg/kg IV over 2 min, may repeat in 15 min at 0.35 mg/kg) or use β-blockers (BBs) IV
      i. Use BBs w/ caution in pts with COPD, asthma, pulmonary edema/CHF

4. If no conversion with medications, consider elective synchronized cardioversion (120–200 J biphasic or 200 J monophasic). ⟹ Go to page 990.

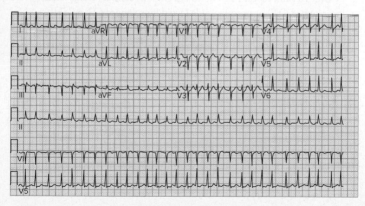

Figure 29-7. Example of atrial fibrillation with a fast ventricular rate (179 BPM), a rhythm and rate that could require immediate cardioversion if there is decompensation such as hypotension, pulmonary edema, or angina. (Reproduced with permission from Gupta D, Roistacher N. Arrhythmia diagnosis and management. Oropello JM, Pastores SM, Kvetan V (eds.). In: Critical Care. New York, NY: McGraw-Hill; 2017.)

29

Tachycardia—Wide QRS (>0.12 s)/Regular Rhythm

(See Figures 29-3A and 29-8.)
1. Evaluate airway/breathing/circulation
   a. Give O_2

   ⇩

2. Attach and monitor ECG (obtain 12-lead if available)
   a. Identify rhythm, BP, and oxygen saturation

   ⇩

      i. Signs of instability/poor perfusion?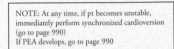

   ⇩

   b. Establish an IV

> Signs include acute altered mental status, angina/MI, hypotension, other signs of hemodynamic instability/ shock

⇩

> NOTE: At any time, if pt becomes unstable, immediately perform synchronized cardioversion (go to page 990)
> If PEA develops, go to page 990

3. If supraventricular tachycardia (SVT) with aberrancy (aberrancy = wide QRS, usually with an SVT rhythm, expect a wide QRS interval)

   ⇩

   a. Adenosine 6mg rapid IV followed with a NS flush; may repeat twice at 12 mg if no conversion
      i. If rhythm converts ⇨ monitor for recurrence

   ⇩

4. If ventricular tachycardia or uncertain rhythm, ⇨ use amiodarone 150 mg IV over 10 min, repeat PRN up to 2.2 g/24 hr; consider using sotalol (avoid if prolonged QT) or procainamide (avoid if prolonged QT or CHF)
5. If no conversion with medications, ⇨ consider elective synchronized cardioversion (100 J). Go to page 990.

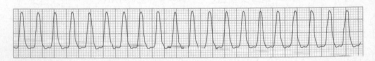

Figure 29-8. Ventricular tachycardia with wide QRS and regular rhythm.

Tachycardia—Wide QRS/Irregular Rhythm

(See Figure 29-9.)

1. Evaluate airway/breathing/circulation
   a. Give O_2

   ⬇

2. Attach and monitor ECG (obtain 12-lead if available)
   a. Identify rhythm, BP, and oxygen saturation

   ⬇

   i. Signs of instability/poor perfusion? ⟹

   ⬇

   > Signs include altered mental status, chest pain, hypotension, other signs of hemodynamic instability/shock

   ⬇

   b. Establish IV access

   ⬇

   > NOTE: At any time, if pt becomes unstable, immediately perform synchronized cardioversion (go to page 990)
   > If PEA develops, go to page 983

3. If atrial fibrillation (Afib) with aberrancy (aberrancy = wide QRS, usually with an SVT rhythm, expect a normal QRS interval):

   ⬇

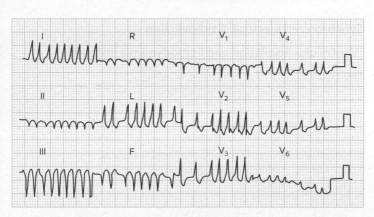

Figure 29-9. **A.** Rhythm strip of atrial fibrillation with left bundle branch, ventricular rate of ~ 155 BPM. **B.** This 12-lead electrocardiogram shows a rapid irregular rhythm with broad QRS complex. This is pathognomonic of atrial fibrillation in a patient with Wolff–Parkinson–White syndrome. This arrhythmia requires urgent treatment. (Reproduced with permission from Atrial fibrillation, Crawford MH. CURRENT Diagnosis & Treatment: Cardiology, 5e. New York, NY: McGraw-Hill Education; 2017.)

29

a. Use diltiazem (0.25 mg/kg IV over 2 min, may repeat in 15 min at 0.35 mg/kg) or beta-blockers (BBs)
   i. Use BBs w/ caution in pulm/CHF pts

4. If Afib with Wolf Parkinson White (WPW):

a. Consider amiodarone (150 mg over 10 min)
b. Do not use adenosine, diltiazem, or verapamil (may increase the HR by blocking conduction through the AV node and then conduction goes through the by-pass track)

5. If Torsades de pointe (see Figure 29-3B, page 982):
a. Use magnesium; 1–2 g IV/IO in 10 mL NS over 5–60 min (DO NOT routinely use magnesium except for Torsades de pointes/hypomagnesemia)

6. If recurrent polymorphic VT, may be secondary to myocardial ischemia, ⟹ consider amiodarone and/or β-blocker

7. If no conversion with medications, ⟹ consider elective cardioversion (120–200 J, **NOT synchronized**). See below.

Synchronized Electrical Cardioversion
(Ventricular fibrillation and hemodynamic instability)

(See Figure 29-10.)

1. Evaluate airway/breathing/circulation
a. Give O₂

2. Attach and monitor ECG (obtain 12-lead if available)
a. Identify rhythm, BP, and saturation
b. Establish an IV

3. Prepare suction and intubation equipment

4. Premedicate when possible (diazepam, midazolam)
a. Diazepam *Adults* 5–10 mg IV
b. Midazolam *Adults* 1–5 mg IV

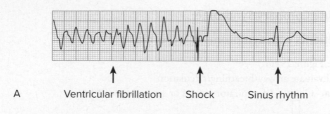

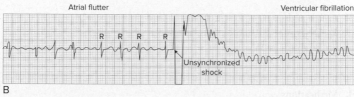

A   Ventricular fibrillation   Shock   Sinus rhythm

Figure 29-10.   **A**. Ventricular fibrillation converting to sinus rhythm after a shock (cardioversion). (In: Principles and Practice of Hospital Medicine, 2e. New York, NY: McGraw-Hill Education; 2017.) **B**. A complication of cardioversion: induction of ventricular fibrillation. The ventricular arrhythmia occurred because the operator failed to enable the synchronizer, resulting in an inadvertent delivery of the shock on the vulnerable T wave instead of the intended delivery on the R wave. This complication is preventable by enabling the synchronizer and checking that it is properly functioning before shock delivery. (Reproduced with permission from Pacemakers, defibrillators, and cardiac resynchronization devices in hospital medicine. McKean SC, Ross JJ, Dressler DD, Scheurer DB [eds.]. In: Principles and Practice of Hospital Medicine, 2e. New York, NY: McGraw-Hill Education; 2017.)

5. Select cardioversion mode on monitor/defibrillator

6. Depress "synchronize" button to allow machine to sync w/ R waves (if unable to synchronize—typically when wide-complex irregular arrhythmias are present—perform defibrillation)

7. Confirm that markers are synched to R waves

8. Set energy level (common energies listed—use manufacturer recommended energies for your defibrillator)
   a. Atrial fibrillation—biphasic/monophasic 120–200/200 J
   b. Paroxysmal supraventricular tachycardia (PSVT)—biphasic/monophasic 50–100/100 J
   c. VT w/pulses—biphasic/monophasic 100/200 J
   d. Increase energy for subsequent shocks based on manufacturer's recommendation

29

9. Reevaluate ABCs and cardiac rhythm

Acute Coronary Syndrome

(Patients with symptoms of ischemia or infarction)

(See Figure 29-11.)

1. Evaluate airway/breathing/circulation
   a. Give O_2 (if respiratory issues or saturation <94%)

2. Attach and monitor ECG; obtain 12-lead
   a. Determine BP and oxygen saturation
   b. Establish an IV

3. Medications
   a. Aspirin: 325 mg, chewable
   b. Nitroglycerin 0.4 mg/SL, one pill Q 5 min up to three doses; OR 1–2 sprays translingual Q 3–5 min, max three doses; can also be given topically or IV (close monitoring required, setting is ICU or ER)
   c. IV morphine 1–4 mg (if pain not relieved by nitroglycerin)

4. Interpret ECG rhythm ⟶ a. If ECG rhythm Normal /nondiagnostic
   i. consider serial troponin monitoring

b. If ST depression
   i. STAT cardiology evaluation
   ii. Consider adjunctive treatments such as heparin (unfractionated or low molecular weight)
   iii. Admit/transfer to monitored bed
   iv. Consider additional antiplatelet medicines (clopidogrel) and glycoprotein IIb/IIIa inhibitors
   v. Consider β-blocker
   vi. Consider statin therapy, ACE inhibitors

c. If ST elevation
   i. STAT cardiology evaluation, including interventional cardiology, if available
   ii. If < 12 hrs from symptom onset, consider fibrinolysis or percutaneous coronary intervention depending on center availability
   iii. If > 12 hr from symptom onset, start initial adjunctive treatments such as listed under ST depression MI and admit/transfer to monitored bed.

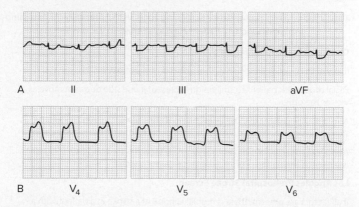

Figure 29-11. **A**. ST segment depression in leads II, III, and aVF in a patient with ischemic ECG changes. **B**. ST elevation in leads V₄, V₅, and V₆ in a patient with acute anterolateral myocardial injury.

STROKE, INITIAL MANAGEMENT

Stroke is also called "brain attack." Early activation of the facility stroke protocol/response team is imperative. Signs and symptoms of a stroke include:

- Facial droop
- Change in mental status
- Pronator drift (see page 62)
- Unilateral motor weakness
- Slurred speech
- Syncope
- Difficulty swallowing
- Confusion

Several stroke assessment scales exist. In the prehospital setting, EMS personnel typically use tools such as the **Cincinnati Prehospital Stroke Scale** or other prehospital stroke screening tools to determine the likelihood that a patient is having a stroke. **FAST** (**F**ACE, **A**RM, **S**PEECH, **T**IME) has been used in many public campaigns as a simplified approach for the lay public to help recognize early symptoms in order to get patients to medical care quickly. While originally designed for research, the NIH Stroke Scale (NIHSS) has become widely used in hospitals to evaluate the acuity of patients, guide treatment, and predict patient outcomes. See Table 29-3, page 994, for an overview of several common stroke scales. (Refer to stroke.nih.gov for details regarding the NIHSS.) Carefully determine time of symptom onset. This step is crucial in decision making regarding the use of thrombolytics in a stroke patient without bleeding. Measure a finger stick glucose level to detect possible hypo- and hyperglycemia as the cause of the

29

Table 29-3. Prehospital Stroke Screening Tools Useful Clinically for Assessing Likelihood of a Patient Having a Stroke in Various Settings

Cincinnati Prehospital Stroke Scale
If any of these signs are present, the probability of a stroke is 72%:
Facial droop: Ask patient to smile; sign is present if one side does not move as well as the other
Arm drift: Ask patient to close eyes and hold arms out with palms up for 10 s; sign is present if one arm drifts downward or both arms do not move equally
Abnormal speech: Have patient say "you can't teach an old dog new tricks." Sign is present if the patient slurs speech or uses wrong words
Los Angeles Prehospital Stroke Screen
If all factors are present, there is high likelihood of a stroke in a patient with a nontraumatic neurologic concern:
Age >45 yr
No seizure or epilepsy history
Symptoms present <24 hr
Patient not wheelchair bound or bedridden at baseline
Blood glucose 60–400 mg/dL
Asymmetry of face, grip, or arm strength

Source: https://www.stroke.org › media › stroke-files › ems-resources ›) Los Angeles Prehospital Stroke Screen – Internet Stroke Center (www.strokecenter.org › wp-content › uploads › 2011/08 › LAPSS). Accessed April 24, 2020.

symptoms. If present, correct it immediately. **Activate the stroke team if not done already.** Perform a neurologic screening exam, obtain blood for lab work, order an emergency CT scan to assess for active bleeding, obtain a 12-lead ECG, and take the patient to the CT suite. If no intracranial hemorrhage, no contraindications to fibrinolytics, and no improvement in repeat neurologic exams, the goal is to initiate therapy within 1 hr of hospital arrival and 3 hr of symptom onset.

OTHER COMMON EMERGENCIES

Regardless of the acute emergency cause, a basic approach should be undertaken. Considerations activating rapid response protocols if in a healthcare facility or calling 911 if outside the hospital, as well as performing a general assessment and work-up including vital signs with initial patient contact, include the following.

Adrenal Crisis

Definition: Acute physiological changes (see below) that result from an underproduction of cortisol can result in death if not recognized

(~5%). The patient may produce enough cortisol under normal conditions that the adrenal insufficiency goes unrecognized without testing. When this patient is physiologically stressed, they are unable to increase their cortisol production unlike someone with an intact hypothalamic–pituitary–adrenal axis. In these patients, surgery or an acute infection such as bacterial pneumonia or pyelonephritis could precipitate adrenal crisis. Causes of adrenal insufficiency can be categorized as either primary (adrenal gland), secondary (pituitary), or tertiary (hypothalamus). Infection, metastatic carcinoma, trauma/surgery, hemorrhage or infarction, and hypotension can cause primary, secondary, or tertiary adrenal insufficiency. Autoimmune adrenalitis is a common primary cause. Suppression of cortisol production can result from exogenous corticosteroid use with doses higher than physiologic production, dosing more than once a day, and prolonged administration (more than 2–3 wk). Even inhaled steroids for asthma can cause adrenal suppression. Other medications can cause adrenal suppression either directly (e.g., ketoconazole, aminoglutethimide, etomidate) or indirectly by increasing cortisol metabolism (e.g., phenytoin).

History: Common symptoms include severe fatigue and weakness, nausea, vomiting, abdominal pain, mental status changes, and dizziness with standing.

Physical: Orthostatic hypotension, hypotension, fever, hyperpigmentation (especially in the creases of the palms—a sign of chronic primary adrenal insufficiency), abdominal tenderness to palpation, guarding, and mental status changes (confusion, stuporous, and coma)

Laboratory: ↑ K^+, ↓ HCO_3^-, ↓Na^+, ↓ glucose, ↑ Ca^{++}, anemia, ↑eosinophils

Diagnosis: Must have a high index of suspicion especially if the patient has been on exogenous steroids. Adrenal crisis should always be in your differential in someone who is hypotensive without an obvious cause especially if there is a potential precipitating event (surgery, pneumonia, etc.). Do not delay treatment in order to establish a definitive diagnosis. Obtain baseline cortisol, ACTH, aldosterone, renin, and ACTH stimulation test with 250 mcg of Cortysyn and measure cortisol at 30 and 60 mins. Adrenal insufficiency/crisis is ruled out with a cortisol >20 mcg/dL and the diagnosis suggested by an 8 A.M. cortisol of <5 mcg/dL. An elevated ACTH suggests a primary adrenal etiology.

Treatment: The mainstay of therapy is IVFs for hypotension and corticosteroids for replacement. Monitor serum electrolytes with treatment and follow serum sodium closely (see Chapter 15, page 432). You should never delay treatment because of pending laboratory results.

- 100 mg hydrocortisone given immediately as IV bolus or IM
- 200–400 mg/day in four divided doses or as a continuous infusion for 2–3 days and then taper to physiologic doses

29

Anaphylaxis

Allergic Reaction with Systolic BP <90 mm Hg or Airway Failure

- **Epinephrine:** Drug of choice; IM/SubQ route typically first; then IV infusion if multiple IM doses fail. **Dose:** *Adults.* 0.3–0.5 mL SQ/IM of 1 mg/mL, repeat PRN q5–15 min, or 0.5–1.0 mg (0.1 mg/mL) IV if SQ dose ineffective, then IV inf: 1–4 mcg/min. *Peds.* 0.01 mg/kg (1 mg/mL) IM, repeat PRN; max single dose 0.3 mg (0.1 mg/mL) IV then inf: 0.1–0.3 mcg/kg/min, max 1.5 mcg/kg/min

Allergic Reaction with Systolic BP >90 mm Hg

- **Epinephrine dose:** *Adults.* 0.3–0.5 mL (1 mg/mL) SQ. *Peds.* 0.01 mL/kg (1 mg/mL) SQ, max 0.3 mg

Supplemental drugs for anaphylaxis may include:

- **Diphenhydramine dose:** *Adults.* IV/IM/PO 25–50 mg. *Peds.* IV/IM/PO 1 mg/kg (max 30 mg in children)
- **Methylprednisolone dose:** *Adults.* 125–250 mg IV/IM. *Peds.* 1–2 mg/kg
- **Ranitidine (Zantac) dose:** *Adults.* 50 mg IV in 20 mL 5% dextrose over 5 min. *Peds.* 0.5 mg/kg IV over 5 min (max 50 mg)
- **Albuterol dose:** *Adults.* 2.5 mg nebulized. *Peds.* 1.25 mg nebulized

Asthma, Acute Attack

Acute asthma exacerbation can be classified as mild, moderate, or severe based on guidelines from the National Heart, Lung, and Blood Institute.[4]

Asthma Attack: Mild Dyspnea only with activity; prompt relief with inhaler typical; peak expiratory flow >70% predicted
- **Albuterol (Nebulized) dose:** *Adults.* 1.25–5.0 mg, can repeat at 20 min for up to three doses in first hour. *Peds.* 0.05 mg/kg (max 2.5 mg), can repeat at 20 min for up to three doses in first hour. **Supplemental oxygen to keep saturation >90%**

Asthma Attack: Moderate (Dyspnea interferes/limits activity; peak expiratory flow 40–69% predicted) **to Severe** (Dyspnea at rest, interferes with conversation; peak expiratory flow <40% predicted)
- **Ipratropium bromide (nebulized) dose:** *Adults.* 0.5 mg combined with first albuterol treatment. *Peds.* 125–250 mcg with first albuterol treatment. Give continuously or every 20 min for first hour
- **Levalbuterol (Xopenex) dose:** *Adults.* 0.63–1.25 mg neb q6–8h PRN. *Peds.* 6–11 yr 0.31–0.63 mg neb q6–8h. *Peds.* >11 yr same as adult dose

29

- **Methylprednisolone dose:** *Adults.* 125–250 mg IV/IM. *Peds.* 1–2 mg/kg IV. **Supplemental oxygen to keep saturation >90%**

Asthma Attack: Severe/Life-Threatening (Too dyspneic to speak; perspiration; peak expiratory flow <25% predicted)
- Administer aerosolized beta-agonists with anticholinergic continuously. Intubate and ventilate with 100% oxygen if impending or respiratory arrest. **Methylprednisolone dose:** *Adults.* 125–250 mg IV/IM. *Peds.* 1–2 mg/kg IV

Anticholinergic Toxicity

Usually related to drug overdose. Medications that possess anticholinergic properties include antidepressants, antihistamines, anti-Parkinson agents, antipsychotics, antispasmodics, and mydriatics. Patients present "Hot as Hades, Blind as a Bat, Dry as a Bone, Red as a Beet, Mad as a Hatter." (See also Table 29-5, page 1008.)

Physostigmine is only to be used when seizures, coma, hypotension, and agitation are refractory to conventional therapy. **Dose:** Adults: 0.5–2.0 mg IV or IM q20 min. Peds: 0.01–0.03 mg/kg/dose IV q15–30 min up to 2 mg. *Note:* **ADMINSTER** S-L-O-W-L-Y (can cause seizures if given rapidly). Have cardiac monitor attached and resuscitation equipment at the bedside.

Organophosphate, Insecticide Poisoning

Due to the muscarinic effects of the poison in adults consider using these mnemonics to identify the symptoms: *DUMBELS:* (**D**efecation/**D**iaphoresis; **U**rination; **M**iosis; **B**ronchospasm; **E**mesis; **L**acrimation; **S**alivation) or *SLUDGE* (**S**alivation; **L**acrimation; **U**rination; **D**efecation; **G**astrointestinal motility; **E**mesis). Also, other common symptoms/signs are confusion, anxiety, circulatory and respiratory depression, tachycardia, weakness, hypertension, and muscle fasciculations.

If respiratory depression is present, the patient may need 100% oxygen and endotracheal intubation.

Atropine: Adults: 1–2 mg IV, repeat q3–5min. Peds: <12 yr 0.02–0.05 mg/kg IV/IO, repeat PRN q20–30 min; >12 yr 2 mg IV/IO, then 1–2 mg IV/IO PRN

Pralidoxime: Atropine should be given first or the two drugs given concurrently. Adults: Loading dose of 1–2 g IV mixed with 250–500 mL NS, may repeat once after 1 hr; or 0.6–1.8 g IM, max dose 1.8 g, may repeat once. Peds: 20–50 mg/kg IV over 30 min, 10–20 mg/mL over 15–30 min.

Available with atropine and pralidoxime in combined autoinjector kits (DuoDote and Mark 1Injector)

29

Coma

1. Establish and secure airway (protect cervical spine if trauma has occurred).
2. Assess for respiratory failure and shock; use BLS and ACLS protocols as appropriate.
3. Supply oxygen, IV access, cardiac monitor, and pulse oximetry.
4. Administer 1 amp (50 mL) of D_{50} IV manually; consider checking a stat glucose first. If not hypoglycemic, may worsen stroke outcomes.
5. Administer 100 mg thiamine IV.
6. Give 0.4 mg naloxone (Narcan) IV (see Opioid Overdose, page 1011).
7. Obtain finger stick glucose, SMA, CBC, urinalysis, and ABG. Consider ECG, CT of head (see page 1007 for management of Seizures, Status Epilepticus).

Dental Emergencies

Not including facial fractures, the most common dental emergencies include: toothaches with associated abscesses, avulsed (knocked-out) or fractured teeth, postextraction complications, and mandibular dislocation. Most **toothaches** can be managed with antibiotics (usually amoxicillin or penicillin-V 500 mg q6h) and analgesics (acetaminophen 650–1000 mg q6h, ibuprofen 400–800 mg q6h, or a combination of ibuprofen 600 mg and acetaminophen 500 mg) until proper dental attention can be obtained. **Drain fluctuant abscesses** if convenient. The exception to this rule is submandibular or infraorbital swelling. With **submandibular infections, Ludwig angina, a life-threatening condition, can develop.** Observe these patients while treating with IV antibiotics, paying special attention to maintaining the airway until a dental consult can be obtained. Infraorbital infections can lead to cavernous sinus thrombosis if allowed to progress.

Avulsed teeth may or may not have an associated dentoalveolar fracture. Reposition the displaced tooth in the socket within 30 min or as soon as possible. If the tooth root is dirty, wash it gently with sterile saline solution. Do not scrub or scrape the root. Obtain a dental consult to arrange to have the tooth splinted back in the socket. Systemic antibiotics (usually 7-day penicillin or amoxicillin course) are recommended following replantation. Follow-up with a dentist within 7–10 days is required for possible root canal therapy of the replanted tooth. Primary teeth should not be replanted due to risk of necrosis and interference with permanent tooth eruption, but dental follow-up is recommended.

Fractured teeth can be divided by depth of fracture. If the fracture only involves the enamel, patients are typically asymptomatic and should be told to follow up with a dentist for elective smoothing/reshaping of the fractured surface. If the fracture involves the dentin (vital yellow tissue beneath the enamel), patients will typically have sensitivity to cold air/water. Analgesic and referral to dentist is recommended for restoration of the tooth. If the fracture extends to the pulp, the tooth will bleed, and dental referral is urgent. Treatment usually involves root canal therapy. Root fractures are not

29

visible clinically but may involve tooth mobility/sensitivity to percussion. In this case, dental referral is urgent for extraction or stabilization. With this type of trauma, the exam must include checking for a dentoalveolar fracture by palpating for movement of the alveolar bone and by imaging. The lips must also be examined for any embedded tooth fragments.

Postextraction problems include swelling, pain, bleeding, postextraction alveolitis (dry socket), osteomyelitis, and osteonecrosis. Some swelling is normal following oral surgery and ice should be used to control swelling for the first day. If there is no reduction in swelling by the third postoperative day, antibiotic therapy with amoxicillin (500 mg, q6h) or clindamycin (300 mg, q6h) should be considered. Postextraction bleeding is typically managed with a folded gauze pad which the patient bites down on for 1 hr following the procedure. Tea bags (which contain tannins) can also be held onto the socket to encourage clotting. If bleeding persists, the site can be anesthetized and local hemostatic agents such as topical thrombin or oxidized cellulose can be placed into the socket.

- **Postextraction alveolitis** occurs when the socket's blood clot is lost or fails to form, causing inflammation of the alveolar bone. While usually self-limiting, the condition causes severe pain and can be treated by irrigating the socket with saline and placing a palliative medicament into the socket (often eugenol or iodoform saturated gauze). Dental referral is recommended for treatment and follow-up.
- **Osteomyelitis**, which is rare in the head and neck, can be distinguished from alveolitis by the presence of fever and swelling and usually occurs in immunocompromised patients. Osteomyelitis requires long-term follow-up and treatment with broad spectrum antibiotics.
- **Osteonecrosis of the jaw (ONJ)** is a condition where exposed bone becomes necrotic and usually occurs following dental extractions. Patients taking antiresorptive agents, such as bisphosphonates for osteoporosis, have a higher risk of ONJ. Treatment of ONJ is difficult and usually involves conservative treatment with rinses, antibiotics, and analgesics. Immediate oral surgery referral is required.

Mandibular dislocation can occur in patients with a history of spontaneous dislocation and typically results from trauma or wide opening (such as yawning). Patients present with an open mouth and inability to close. Manual reduction is usually indicated and should be performed as soon as possible to prevent complications. To perform reduction, the patient's head is stabilized, and the operator's thumbs are placed outside the mandibular molars on the buccal shelf. The remaining fingers are curled around the mandible downward, and forward force is applied to the mandible until the mandible reduces. The mandible may snap back into position, which is why the thumbs are not placed on top of the molars. A Barton bandage may be indicated for several days to stabilize the reduced mandible. The patient should be instructed to avoid wide mouth opening for 6 wk and to support

29

the underside of the chin while yawning for this period. Further treatment and follow-up may be necessary if frequent dislocations occur.

Hypercalcemia

See Chapter 15, Fluids and Electrolytes, page 441.

Hyperglycemia

Diabetic Ketoacidosis (DKA)[5]

Definition: DKA is caused by absolute insulin deficiency that results in hyperglycemia and metabolic gap acidosis from an accumulation of ketones. DKA is a complication of type 1 diabetes mellitus (DM) and is often the presenting manifestation of DM. About 20% of cases are seen with type 2 DM. There are multiple factors that can precipitate DKA including an acute infection, the most common cause (i.e., pneumonia, sepsis), insulin noncompliance (second most common cause), myocardial infarction, trauma, pancreatitis, acute gastroenteritis, drug or alcohol use/misuse, and others.

History: Symptoms include polyuria, polydipsia, dizziness (especially with standing), fatigue, nausea, vomiting, abdominal pain (may mimic an acute abdomen), and altered mental status.

Physical: Tachycardia, hypotension, orthostatic hypotension from volume depletion, tachypnea, deep and labored breathing to compensate for the metabolic acidosis (Kussmaul respirations), fruity odor on breath (from ketones), dry mucosal membranes, and tenting of the skin from volume depletion.

Laboratory: $\uparrow\uparrow$ glucose (at least 250 mg/dL, can be 400–600 mg/dL); pH <7.30, presence of serum ketones (β-hydroxybutyrate and acetoacetate); $\downarrow HCO_3^-$; $\uparrow$ anion gap (nl ~ 10 mmol/L); $\downarrow Na^+$ (expect $\downarrow$ of 1.6–2.1 mg/dL for every 100 mg/dL $\uparrow$ in glucose above 100 mg/dL); $\uparrow K^+$ but may be nl or $\downarrow$ (often total body stores are severely depleted despite $\uparrow K^+$); $\downarrow$, nl, or $\uparrow PO4^{-3}$ (total body stores are often severely depleted); $\downarrow Mg^{++}$ (total body stores are often depleted); $\uparrow$ BUN and $\uparrow$ creatinine from volume depletion; $\uparrow$ amylase (usually unrelated to pancreatitis); $\uparrow$ WBC (often NOT from an infection). The HCO_3^- should equal to 26 (normal HCO_3^-) minus the increase in anion gap above normal (10 mmol/L = normal) (see Chapter 14, pages 405 and 406), otherwise you may have a secondary acid–base disturbance, which could point toward a precipitating cause.

Diagnosis: pH <7.30, glucose >250 mg/dL, serum ketones, always look for a precipitating cause of the DKA.

Treatment:

- **IVFs:** 0.9% NaCl, 1–1.5 L during the first hour; then continue 0.9% NaCl; IVF rate will depend on the degree of volume and sodium depletion; if $\uparrow Na^+$ then switch to 0.45% NaCl after the initial bolus.

- **Insulin:** Initially 0.1 u/kg IV bolus; then 0.1 u/kg/hr continuous infusion; when glucose is 200–250 mg/dL, change IVFs to D5½NS and insulin drip to 0.05 u/kg/hr (often the glucose will normalize before the ketones are "cleared"; IVF with dextrose allows insulin to continue to decrease ketones through preventing further lipolysis, decrease continued ketone formation, and metabolize remaining ketones without causing hypoglycemia). Also, too rapid a decrease in glucose can cause cerebral edema. Do NOT begin insulin if K^+ is below 3.3 mmol/L (see below).

- **Potassium:** Total body K^+ stores are markedly depleted, the K^+ may be nl or high initially because of the acidosis; when K^+ <5.3 begin replacement (20–30 mmol/L of IVFs). Initially, if K^+ is <3.3 mmol/L, you risk life-threatening hypokalemia with insulin therapy (insulin drives the K^+ into the cells, as does correction of the acidosis). Begin IVFs with K^+ supplementation and once K^+ is >3.3 mmol/L, then begin insulin therapy. Initially check K^+ every 1 hr in severe DKA.

- **Phosphate:** Deficits can be severe in DKA; replace IV if PO_4^{-3} <1 mg/dL or with end-organ manifestations such as respiratory or cardiac dysfunction. See Chapter 14, page 447.

- **Magnesium:** See Chapter 14, page 445.

- **Correction of pH:** If pH <6.90, then 100 mmol $NaHCO_3$ added to 400 cc sterile H_2O and add 20 mmol KCl, give over 2 hr. Repeat if pH <7.0. Some experts will give $NaHCO_3$ for pH 6.90–7.10.

Hyperglycemia Hyperosmolar State (HHS)[5]

Definition: Relative insulin deficiency may lead to a markedly elevated glucose (600–1000 mg/dL) that leads to symptoms from the hyperosmolar state such as altered mental status. Enough insulin is present to prevent lipolysis and ketogenesis. As with DKA, there is usually a precipitating event (infections including pneumonia and UTIs, trauma, MI, CVA, and noncompliance with insulin).

History: Symptoms include polyuria, polydipsia, dizziness (especially with standing), fatigue, and decreased sensorium that may progress to coma. More insidious onset than DKA and more often in the elderly where there is a decreased thirst response to the dehydration and/or a decreased access to fluids.

Physical: Tachycardia, hypotension, orthostatic hypotension from volume depletion, dry mucosal membranes, and tenting of the skin from volume depletion.

Laboratory: ↑↑↑ glucose (600–1000 mg/dL); pH >7.30; HCO_3^- 20–28 mg/dL; normal anion gap; ↓ Na^+ (expect a ↓ of 1.6–2.1 mg/dL for every 100 mg/dL ↑ above 100 mg/dL); ↑ osm (>320 mOsm/kg); ↑ K^+ but may be nl or ↓ (often total body stores are severely depleted despite ↑ K^+; deficit is generally greater with HHS than DKA); ↓, nl, or ↑ PO_4^{-3} (total body stores are often severely depleted); ↓ or nl Mg^{++} (total body stores are often depleted); ↑ BUN and ↑ creatinine from volume depletion.

29

Diagnosis: pH $\geq$7.30, glucose $\geq$600 mg/dL, negative serum and urine ketones, and always look for a precipitating cause of the HHS.

Treatment:

- **IVF:** Primary goal is volume replacement. In HHS, volume replacement will go a long way in treating the hyperglycemia. Initially 1000 cc of 0.9% NaCl and then 250–500 mg/dL if there is normal cardiac and kidney function. If ↑ Na^+, IVFs should be changed to 0.45% NaCl. Be careful not to lower the serum Na^+ and osmolality too quickly; glucose should decrease no more than 70–100 mg/dL/hr and plasma osmolality by 3–8 mOsmol/kg/hr.
- **Insulin:** See DKA.
- **Potassium:** 20–30 mmol/L add to IVFs when K^+ <5.2 mg/dL; as with DKA, DO NOT begin insulin if K^+ is <3.3 mg/dL, begin insulin when K^+ is >3.3 mg/dL (see DKA, *Treatment*, page 439).
- **Phosphate:** See Chapter 15, page 447.
- **Magnesium:** See Chapter 15, page 445.

Hyperkalemia

See Chapter 15, Fluids and Electrolytes, page 436.

Hypermagnesemia

See Chapter 15, Fluids and Electrolytes, page 444.

Hypernatremia

See Chapter 15, Fluids and Electrolytes, page 431.

Hyperphosphatemia

See Chapter 15, Fluids and Electrolytes, page 447.

Hypertensive Crisis

Definition: Urgent management is required for systolic blood pressure (SBP) >220 or diastolic blood pressure (DBP) >110 without signs of end-organ damage. Emergency management is only for the above BP findings AND evidence of end-organ damage. Only emergency treatment is indicated for hypertensive emergency. Patients may require ICU care for arterial line placement, intravenous medications, and monitoring. Goal is to reduce MAP (mean arterial pressure) by 25% over approximately 24 hr.

Treatment:

- **Labetalol dose:** 20–40 mg IV bolus, then 2 mg/min IV to target BP
- **Sodium nitroprusside dose:** 0.5 mcg/kg/min to max of 10 mcg/kg/min
- **Special circumstances:** Pregnancy: use labetalol (see page 1024) and/or hydralazine (5–10 mg IV q20 min). Catecholamine producing tumor such as a pheochromocytoma: use phentolamine (alpha-blockade) 5–15 mg IV.

Hyperthyroidism

See Thyroid: Thyroid Storm, page 1014.

Hypocalcemia

See Chapter 15, Fluids and Electrolytes, page 442.

Hypoglycemia

Definition: Hypoglycemia unrelated to exogenous insulin therapy is an uncommon clinical syndrome characterized by low plasma glucose level, symptomatic sympathetic nervous system stimulation, and central nervous system dysfunction. Many drugs and disorders cause it. Diagnosis requires blood tests done at the time of symptoms. Verification is that a low plasma glucose level (<50 mg/dL [<2.8 mmol/L]) exists at the time of hypoglycemic symptoms.

Treatment:

1. Draw a stat serum glucose. **Do not wait for result before treating if hypoglycemia is suspected.** A finger stick (point of care test) can be obtained quickly.
2. Give orange juice with sugar if the patient is awake and alert; if not, give *Adults:* 1 amp of D_{50} IV. *Peds:* 1 mL/kg (use D_{10} for newborn).
3. If IV access is not possible, give glucagon 0.5–1 mg IM or SubQ; repeat in 20 min PRN; Peds: Neonates, 0.3 mg/kg/dose SQ, IM, or IV q4h PRN; Children, 0.025–0.1 mg/kg/dose SQ, IM, or IV; repeat in 20 min PRN (onset w/in 5–20 min)

Hypokalemia

See Chapter 15, Fluids and Electrolytes, page 439.

Hypomagnesemia

See Chapter 15, Fluids and Electrolytes, page 445.

Hyponatremia

See Chapter 15, Fluids and Electrolytes, page 432.

Hypophosphatemia

See Chapter 15, Fluids and Electrolytes, page 447.

29

Hypothyroidism

See Thyroid: Myxedema Coma, page 1013.

Medication-Induced Syndromes

Adverse drug reactions can occur in up to 1% of patients taking systemic medications. Some common iatrogenic and life-threatening syndromes are listed in Table 29-4, page 1005.

Overdose, Opioid

Opioids include three categories of pain-relieving drugs: (1) natural opioids (also called opiates) which are derived from the opium poppy (morphine, codeine); (2) semisynthetic opioids (hydrocodone, oxycodone, and heroin); (3) synthetic opioids (methadone, tramadol, and fentanyl). Fentanyl is 50–100 times more potent than morphine. Fentanyl analogues, such as carfentanil, are 100 times more potent than fentanyl and 10,000 times more potent than morphine. Overdose deaths from fentanyl have greatly increased since 2013 with the introduction of illicitly manufactured fentanyl entering the drug supply [MMWR 65(33):837–843]. **Common findings include:** Low to normal heart rate and blood pressure, altered mental state (mild euphoria or lethargy or coma), hypoventilation, miotic pupils, and reduced bowel sounds.

    Naloxone (Narcan): *Adults:* 0.4–2.0 mg IV or IM, repeat as needed. *Note:* If you suspect the patient is addicted to narcotics, give 0.4 mg and repeat PRN to avoid severe withdrawal. Available as autoinjector (2mg SQ or IM) known as EVZIO and as intranasal spray (4 mg/dose). *Peds:* 0.01–0.1 mg/kg IV or IM, repeat PRN.

1. Observe patient for at least 6 hr after naloxone treatment.
2. Confirm adequate ventilation (respiratory rate is ≥ 12/min, O_2 saturation $>90\%$ on room air, and observe the patient closely. End-tidal CO_2 monitoring (capnography) is an excellent means to monitor ventilation. Manage airway by intubation if not immediately responsive to naloxone. (See Coma, page 998.)
3. Naloxone is now available as autoinjector and nasal forms for improved access to address the opioid crisis in the community.

Overdose, Benzodiazepine

A common feature of benzodiazepine overdose is excessive sedation with unremarkable vital signs and anterograde amnesia; larger doses can cause coma and respiratory depression. **Flumazenil** (Romazicon) is given as follows:

- Adults: 0.2 mg IV over 30 s; repeat PRN, up to 3 mg max (give just enough to reverse respiratory depression).
- Peds: 0.01 mg/kg (0.2 mg/dose max) IV over 30 s.

29

Note there are risks from using flumazenil that may outweigh the benefits in reversing acute toxicity; flumazenil is not recommended for routine reversal. Side effects of flumazenil include: seizures, cardiac dysrhythmias, and fatalities have been reported. The drug can also precipitate acute withdrawal syndromes.

Table 29-4. Three Potentially Life-Threatening Medication-Induced Syndromes

Medical Emergency	Symptoms	Management Pearls	Treatment
Malignant hyperthermia	Muscle rigidity, which may lead to rhabdomyolysis (↑CK, myoglobinuria, hyperkalemia), fever, increased pCO_2 (most common), and arrhythmias; from general anesthetic (often succinylcholine) in the presence of a genetic skeletal muscle receptor defect.	Suspect with an increasing end-tidal CO_2 without another cause especially if CO_2 is still increasing after an increase in minute ventilation.	Supportive care including 100% O_2, discontinue potential offending agents; Dantrolene 1 mg/kg IV push, continue dosing until symptoms subside or a total dose of 10 mg/kg is given. Peds dose is the same as adults. Oral doses 1–2 mg/kg/ Q6h for 1–3 days should be given to prevent recurrence.
Neuroleptic syndrome (Neuroleptic malignant syndrome)	Mental status changes (including coma), muscle rigidity, fever, normal to decreased bowel sounds, hyporeflexia.	Usually occurs within 1–2 weeks of beginning an antipsychotic; can be differentiated from serotonin syndrome by normal pupils, decreased reflexes, normal or decreased bowel sounds.	Muscle relaxants (dantrolene or benzodiazepines); bromocriptine, a dopamine agonist, can be used to restore dopamine homeostasis.

(Continued)

Table 29-4. Three Potentially Life-Threatening Medication-Induced Syndromes (*Continued*)

Medical Emergency	Symptoms	Management Pearls	Treatment
Serotonin syndrome	Agitation, ataxia, fever, tremor, hyperreflexia, clonus, muscle rigidity, mydriasis, diaphoresis, hyperactive bowel sounds, hypertension, tachycardia, seizures, arrhythmias, coma, rhabdomyolysis (↑ CK, myoglobinuria, hyperkalemia), DIC; results from ↑ 5-hydroxytryptamine (5HT) (serotonin) levels from a variety of mechanisms; overdose of selective serotonin reuptake inhibitors (SSRIs) or serotonin-norepinephrine reuptake inhibitors (SNRIs), or other antidepressants, or therapeutic dosing of SSRIs or SNRIs plus another drug such as monoamine oxidase inhibitors (MAOIs) including linezolid, tricyclic or other antidepressants, amphetamines, tryptophans, some pain meds (tramadol, fentanyl, meperidine), illicit drugs (ecstasy, cocaine), many others including drugs or substrates of the same CYP450 microsomal oxidase enzyme associated with metabolizing the specific SSRI or SNRI used.	Unexplained muscle rigidity, mental status changes, or fever in a patient on a SSRI or SNRI; use of a SSRI or SNRI and another recently started medication that alters 5HT metabolism; rapid onset (<24 hr); can be differentiated from neuroleptic syndrome by mydriasis, hyperreflexia, clonus, hyperactive bowel sounds.	Discontinue all potential offending agents and supportive care including IVFs; benzodiazepines can be used to treat muscle rigidity; for hyperthermia, treat with external cooling and benzodiazepines; for temperature over 105°F, consider neuromuscular paralysis (and intubation); cyproheptadine and olanzapine or chlorpromazine can be used.

Poisoning (Common Agents)

See Table 29-5 for common poisoning agents and antidotes.
1. Support airway, respiration, and circulation, as needed. *Note:* Ipecac syrup to induce vomiting is no longer a recommended treatment.
2. Determine ingested substance; give specific antidote, if available. **Call Regional Poison Center for assistance (1-800-222-1222).** Some common poisons with their symptoms and antidotes (adult doses, unless specified) are in Table 29-5, page 1005.
3. Prevent further absorption as described for consciousness level.

Unconscious Poisoning

1. Protect airway with an endotracheal tube.
2. Gastric lavage has high complication rate (e.g., esophageal perforation) and is generally not recommended unless ingestion occurred within the last hour with a potentially lethal agent. Use large bore (28 Fr or larger) NG tube. Use a series of 300-mL NS boluses through the NG for adults and 20-mL/kg boluses for children.
3. Consider using activated charcoal with sorbitol unless an oral antidote is to be given.

Conscious Poisoning

1. Consider giving activated charcoal 1 g/kg; contraindicated for iron, lithium, lead, alkali, and acid poisoning. In adults, one can also consider sorbitol solution in addition to charcoal for cathartic effect. Monitor any patient given sorbitol for hypokalemia and hypomagnesemia. If only combined charcoal/sorbitol solutions available, can provide to children for a single dose only.
2. Promote excretion through IV hydration.
3. Administer alkalinization (0.5–1 mEq/kg/L in IV fluids) for salicylates, barbiturates, and tricyclics.

Seizures, Status Epilepticus

Status epilepticus refers to 30 min or more of continuous seizure activity or two or more seizures without recovery of consciousness between seizures.

Initial Supportive Care

1. Maintain airway with cervical spine precautions.
2. Deliver oxygen by nasal cannula.
3. Monitor ECG and blood pressure.
4. Maintain normal temperature.

29

29

Table 29-5. List of Common Poisoning Substances with Management Overview and Specific Antidotes (Adult Doses)

Medication/Substance	Toxicity Presentation	Management Pearls	Antidote
Acetaminophen	N, V, pallor, tachycardia, RUQ pain	Symptomatic/Supportive	N-acetylcysteine(Acetadote) w/in 8 hr 140 mg/kg po load, then 70 mg/kg every 4 hr for 17 doses OR 150 mg/kg IV load over 60 min then 50 mg/kg over 4 hr, then 100 mg/kg over 16 hr
Anticholinergics	**"Red as a beet, dry as a bone, blind as a bat, mad as a hatter".** * Signs/Symptoms opposite of SLUDGE (see page 997)	Symptomatic/Supportive, can be caused by medications or certain natural substances (i.e., jimsonweed)	Physostigmine 0.5–2 mg IV over 5 min
Antifreeze (Ethylene glycol)	Inebriation similar to EtOH; N, V, altered mental status, lethargy, flank pain, hematuria, metabolic acidosis (Kussmaul respirations), renal failure, respiratory failure	Airway management key due to risk of aspiration, determine blood glucose level	Fomepizole, loading dose of 15 mg/kg, followed by doses of 10 mg/kg every 12 hours for 4 doses, then 15 mg/kg every 12 hours until ethylene glycol concentration is undetectable or has been reduced below 20 mg/dL, and the patient is asymptomatic with normal pH; Ethanol 10% IV; also give thiamine, folate, and pyridoxine; consider hemodialysis especially with renal failure and metabolic acidosis with high anion gap
Arsenic	Garlic smell (breath, tissues), N/V/Severe D, dehydration, cardiac arrhythmias, Mees lines	Symptomatic/Supportive	Dimercaprol, succimer
Aspirin (Salicylate)	N, V, hyperventilation, noncardiac pulmonary edema, tinnitus, tachycardia, hypotension, tremors, blurred vision; can cause mixed metabolic acidosis and respiratory alkalosis	Symptomatic/Supportive	Urine alkalinization (Sodium bicarbonate)

Benzodiazepines	AMS, slurred speech, ataxia, respiratory depression, hypotension, hallucinations	O_2	Flumazenil 0.2 mg/kg IV, repeat PRN, up to 3 mg max (max dose)
Beta-blockers	Bradycardia, hypotension, shock, seizures, bronchospasm (rare)	O_2, IV boluses, charcoal	Glucagon (primary) 0.05 mg/kg IV bolus (may repeat every 10 min); atropine, calcium chloride/gluconate, vasopressors
Calcium channel blockers	Bradycardia, hypotension, heart block, altered mental state, seizures, decreased mesenteric perfusion	O_2, charcoal, glucagon, calcium (if known CCB OD), atropine, or vasopressor	Calcium chloride 10% 0.2–0.25 mL/kg IV Insulin 1 unit/kg bolus w/50 mL 50% dextrose followed by 1 unit/kg/hr w/ D10 W 200 mL/hr Glucagon 0.05 mg/kg IV bolus, repeat every 10 min Lipid emulsion 20% IV 100 mL IV over 1 min, then 400 ml IV over 20 min
Carbon monoxide	Dull headache; weakness; dizziness; nausea or vomiting; shortness of breath; confusion; blurred vision; loss of consciousness	Immediate removal from the source of the poisoning	High-dose oxygen 100%; may need hyperbaric oxygen depending on the severity of the CO poisoning
Cyanide and nitroprusside	Bitter almond smell on breath, cherry red skin color, mydriasis, confusion, convulsion, hypotension	O_2, IV fluid, vasopressors, cyanide antidote kit or cyanokit, sodium bicarb, anticonvulsants for Szs	Hydroxocobalamin sodium thiosulfate (25%) 70 mg/kg IV (max 5 g over 15 min) can repeat X 1 dose over 15 to 120 min

(Continued)

29

Table 29-5. List of Common Poisoning Substances with Management Overview and Specific Antidotes (Adult Doses) *(Continued)*

Medication/Substance	Toxicity Presentation	Management Pearls	Antidote
Digoxin	N/V, lethargy, cardiac arrythmias, acute CHF, PVCs, heart block, visual changes	O₂, charcoal, atropine (for bradycardia), antiarrhythmic (lidocaine, amiodarone)	Digoxin-Fab (Digibind) 5–10 vials IV
Heparin	Massive hemorrhage (GI; bruising; epistaxis; hematuria) or intracranial hemorrhage	O₂, IV fluid, control external bleeding	Protamine 25–50 mg IV
Iron	**Stage 1:** w/in 6 hr GI effects (N/V/D, hypovolemia), **Stage 2:** 6–24 hr latent period (GI effects disappear), **Stage 3:** Metabolic/CV (acidosis, stupor, coma), **Stage 4:** Hepatic (hypoglycemia, jaundice), **Stage 5:** Delayed (lasting GI effects with tissue fibrosis)	O₂, IVF boluses of NS or LR solution	Deferoxamine (Desferal) 2 g IM, or 15 mg/kg/hr IV (max dose, 6–8 g/day)
Lead	Hyperactivity/lethargy, pale skin from anemia	Protect airway	Dimercaprol, edetate calcium disodium, D-penicillamine, succimer
Mercury	Tremors, gingivitis, erethism (shyness, timidity, social phobia), HA, tunnel vision, salivation, ataxia	O₂, charcoal	Dimercaprol, D-penicillamine, succimer

29

Methanol	Inebriation similar to EtOH; N, V, abdominal pain, visual changes including blurred vision, sluggish pupils, blindness, mydriasis, hyperemia of optic disk, altered mental state, metabolic acidosis, coma, respiratory and circulatory failure, and death	Airway management key due to risk of aspiration, O_2	Fomepizole, loading dose of 15 mg/kg, followed by doses of 10 mg/kg every 12 hours for 4 doses, then 15 mg/kg every 12 hours, until methanol concentration is undetectable or has been reduced below 20 mg/dL, and the patient is asymptomatic with normal pH; Ethanol 10% IV; also give thiamine, folate, and pyridoxine; consider hemodialysis (indicated in the presence of metabolic acidosis or visual impairment, and relative indications include lethal ingestion [1 gm/kg] or methanol concentration ≥50mg/dL)
Opioids	Slow shallow breathing, confusion, lessened alertness, loss of consciousness, respiratory failure, small pupils, unresponsiveness	Support and protect airway. Goal of naloxone administration is NOT a normal level of consciousness, but adequate ventilation	Naloxone 0.1–2 mg IV, titrate to response; over dosing can precipitate withdrawal in the opioid dependent individual; nasal 2–4 mg
Organophosphate/ Insecticide	SLUDGE * , DUMBELS **	O_2, atropine, pralidoxime	Atropine 2–5 mg IV followed by pralidoxime 30 mg/kg bolus then 8 mg/kg/hr infusion

(Continued)

29

Table 29-5. List of Common Poisoning Substances with Management Overview and Specific Antidotes (Adult Doses) (Continued)

Medication/Substance	Toxicity Presentation	Management Pearls	Antidote
Tricyclic antidepressants	Anticholinergic effects, tachycardia, prolonged QT interval, arrhythmias, hypotension, extrapyramidal symptoms, seizures	O_2, IV fluid, cardiac monitoring, anticonvulsants (for seizures)	Sodium bicarbonate 1–2 mEq/kg IV bolus, repeat as needed
Warfarin	Massive hemorrhage (GI, bruising, epistaxis, hematuria) or intracranial hemorrhage; may not appear for up to 24 hr; coagulopathy INR >1.4; toxicity INR >3.0 or 3.5 with mechanical heart valve	O_2, IV fluid, charcoal, control external bleeding; for patients on coumadin, if INR is > therapeutic and <5.0, hold or reduce dose	Vitamin K 10 mg and fresh frozen plasma with active bleeding only; if on warfarin for Tx, lower doses of vitamin K may be given to allow restarting warfarin for treatment

* **SLUDGE** (salivation, lacrimation, urination, defecation, gastrointestinal motility, emesis)
** **DUMBELS** (defecation/diaphoresis, urination, miosis, bronchospasm, emesis, lacrimation, salivation)

29

Pharmacologic Therapy

1. Establish IV, administer thiamine 100 mg IV.
2. Administer 1 amp of D_{50} IV in an adult (2 mL/kg D_{25} in children) unless obviously hyperglycemic. Consider checking a stat glucose first. If not hypoglycemic, administration of D_{50} can worsen CVA outcomes (and a new CVA can cause seizures).
3. Administer IV lorazepam (0.1 mg/kg IV) or diazepam (0.15 mg/kg IV) initially; can use midazolam 10 mg IM if no IV access.
4. If seizures persist, give one of the following: fosphenytoin, phenytoin, valproic acid, or levetiracetam.
5. If still no response, obtain emergency neurology/neurosurgery and anesthesiology consultations; propofol and pentobarbital infusions can be used for refractory cases.

Thyroid Emergencies

Myxedema Coma[6,7]

Definition: Severe hypothyroidism with four key features: (1) hypothermia (the lower the temperature the worse the prognosis), (2) mental status changes (lethargy, somnolence, stupor, coma), (3) severe bradycardia, and (4) a precipitating cause (exposure to cold temperatures, acute infection/sepsis, surgery, trauma, CVA, MI, PE, others). Mortality rate is very high.

History: More often in the elderly. Symptoms of hypothyroidism may be long-standing and include fatigue, cold intolerance, weight gain without increasing caloric intake, constipation, deep coarse voice, dry skin, hair loss, slowly perform daily activities compared to the past, depression.

Physical: ↓ HR, ↑ BP (diastolic), ↓ temperature, ↓ respiratory rate, cool and dry skin, lateral thinning of the eyebrows, periorbital edema, goiter, delayed relaxation phase of the reflexes (best observed with the Achilles' reflex with the leg parallel to the floor; neutralize gravity).

Laboratory: ↑↑ TSH (could be ↓↓ if a pituitary or a hypothalamic cause), ↓↓ free T_4; ↓ Na^+ (from impaired water excretion), ↓ glucose, ↑ cholesterol, ↑ LDL-cholesterol.

Diagnosis: ↑↑ TSH and ↓↓ free T_4, ↓ temperature, ↓ HR, mental status changes/coma, and a precipitating event.

Treatment:

- **ICU admission**
- **Thyroid hormone replacement:** Levothyroxine (T_4) 200–400 mcg IV followed by 1.6 mcg/kg PO per day. In addition, many experts will give liothyronine (T_3) because of the decreased conversion of T_4 to T_3 (initially 5–25 mcg IV then 2.5–10 mcg PO Q8 hr until clinical improvement). In the elderly or in patients with known ASCVD, consider beginning with lower maintenance doses (T_4 25–50 mcg PO per day and slowly titrate upwards).
- **Stress dose of glucocorticoid:** ALWAYS give stress doses of a glucocorticoid (hydrocortisone 50–100 mg Q6 hr); hypothyroidism may mask

29

adrenal insufficiency and correcting the hypothyroidism first may precipitate adrenal crisis. Assess adrenal function.
- **Supportive care:** May include intubation, mechanical ventilation, warming, IVFs, and supplemental glucose.

Thyroid Storm[8,9]

Definition: Severe thyrotoxicosis with five key features: (1) hyperthermia ($\geq$ 100.4° F, can be as high as 106° F), (2) mental status changes (restlessness, delirium, psychosis, lethargy, coma), (3) cardiac involvement (tachycardia, pulmonary edema, cardiogenic shock), (4) GI/hepatic involvement (nausea, vomiting, diarrhea, abdominal pain, hepatic failure), and (5) precipitating cause (discontinuing antithyroid medications, acute infection, surgery, trauma, CVA, MI, others). Mortality rate is 10–20%.

History: Typical hyperthyroid symptoms include weight loss despite normal caloric intake, palpitations, diaphoresis, heat intolerance, frequent bowel movements (from increased peristalsis-decreased transient time), tremor; acutely with thyroid storm may have nausea, vomiting, diarrhea, abdominal pain, dyspnea on exertion or at rest, and leg swelling. May have a history of hyperthyroidism with noncompliance of thyroid medication(s).

Physical: Typical symptoms of hyperthyroidism including ↑ HR (irregularly irregular if Afib), ↑ BP (systolic); lid lag, proptosis, thyroid bruit, and nonpitting skin changes over the shins (all 4 seen in Grave disease), ↑ bowel sounds, decreased relaxation phase in reflexes, fine tremor, signs of CHF (elevated JVD, inspiratory crackles, pitting edema).

Laboratory: TSH < lower limits of normal; ↑↑ free T_4 and ↑↑ free T_3, ↑ glucose, ↑ liver function studies (↑ ALT, AST, alk phos, T bili).

Diagnosis: High index of suspicion when TSH <lower limits of normal; ↑↑ free T_4 and ↑↑ free T_3 and symptoms and signs listed in *Definition*, above.

Treatment: Goals of initial therapy:

- **Decrease thyroid hormone synthesis:** Methimazole or propylthiouracil (PTU)
- **Decrease thyroid hormone release:** Iodide PO or IV; ALWAYS give methimazole or PTU before administering iodine.
- **Block conversion of T_4 to T_3:** Propranolol, glucocorticoid, and PTU all block conversion of T_4 to T_3.
- **Decrease HR (goal is <100 BPM):** IV β-blocker or if β-blocker contraindicated, then IV nondihydropyridine calcium channel blocker (diltiazem or verapamil).
- **Supportive care:** Include treating the precipitating event.

29 PEDIATRIC EMERGENCY CARE CONSIDERATIONS

Basic cardiac life support for the pediatric population can be found starting on page 971. Table 29-6, page 1015, provides guidelines on the different approaches to BCLS in this population. Table 29-7, page 1016 lists emergency equipment

Table 29-6. CPR Guidelines in Pediatric Basic Life Support

Maneuver	Newborn	Infant <1 Y	Child 1 Y to Puberty	Onset of Puberty to Adult
Airway	Head tilt/chin lift	Head tilt/chin lift	Head tilt/chin lift	Head tilt/chin lift
If trauma	Jaw thrust	Jaw thrust	Jaw thrust	Jaw thrust
If foreign body—conscious	Suction	Back blows and chest thrusts	Abdominal thrusts	Abdominal thrusts
If foreign body—unconscious	Suction	Chest compressions	Abdominal thrusts	Abdominal thrusts
Breathing rate	30–60/min (every 1–2s)	12–20/min (every 3s)	12–20/min (every 3s)	10–12/min (every 5s)
Circulation Pulse check	Umbilical	Brachial	Carotid or femoral	Carotid or femoral
Compression	One finger below intermammary line	One finger below intermammary line or lower half of sternum	Lower half of sternum	Lower half of sternum
Location	Two fingers or two thumbs	Two fingers or two thumbs	Heel of one hand or two hands	Two hands
Method	One-third of chest	One-third to one-half of chest	One-third to one-half of chest 100/min	One-third of chest
Depth Rate	120/min	100/min		100/min
Compression-to-ventilation ratio	3:1	15:2 (single rescuer—30:2)	15:2 (single rescuer—30:2)	30:2

Source: Reproduced with permission from Tintinalli JE, Ma O, Yealy DM, Meckler GD, Stapczynski J, Cline DM, Thomas SH. (eds). Tintinalli's Emergency Medicine: A Comprehensive Study Guide, 9e, 2020; New York, NY: McGraw-Hill.

29

Table 29-7. Listing for Emergency Equipment Sizes Based on Estimated Weight and Age

Age (y)	Weight (kg)	Laryngeal Mask Airway (LMA) Size	Endotracheal Tube Size (mm)[a,b]	Laryngoscope Blade Size	Chest Tube (Fr)	Foley (Fr)
Premature	1–2.5	1	2.5 (uncuffed only)	0	8	5
Term newborn	3	1	3.0 (uncuffed only)	0–1	10	8
1	10	1.5	3.5–4.0	1	18	8
2	12	2	4.5	1	18	10
3	14	2	4.5	1	20	10
4	16	2	5.0	2	22	10
5	18	2	5.0–5.5	2	24	10
6	20	2–2.5	5.5	2	26	12
7	22	2.5	5.5–6.0	2	26	12
8	24	3	6.0	2	28	14
10	32	4	6.0–6.5	2–3	30	14
Adolescent	50	4	7.0	3	36	14
Adult	70		8.0	3	40	14

[a]Internal diameter.

[b]Decrease tube size by 0.5 mm if using a cuffed tube.

Note: Items addressed include LMA, endotracheal tubes, laryngoscope blade, chest tubes, and Foley urinary catheters.

Source: Reproduced with permission from Current Diagnosis & Treatment: Pediatrics, 25e, Hay WW, Levin MJ, Abzug MJ, Bunik M (eds.), 2020; New York, NY: McGraw Hill-Medical.

Table 29-8. Important Emergency Pediatric Drugs

Drug	Indications	Dosage and Route	Comment
Epinephrine	1. Bradycardia, especially hypoxic-ischemic 2. Hypotension (by infusion) 3. Asystole 4. Fine ventricular fibrillation refractory to initial defibrillation 5. Pulseless electrical activity 6. Anaphylaxis (IM)	Bradycardia and cardiac arrest: ● 0.01 mg/kg of 1:10,000 solution IV/IO; ● 0.1 mg/kg of 1:1000 solution ET Anaphylaxis ● 0.01 mg/kg of 1:1000 solution SC/IM ● Maximum dose: 0.3 mg. ● May repeat every 3–5 min. ● Constant infusion by IV drip; 0.1–1 mcg/kg/min	Epinephrine is the single most important drug in pediatric resuscitation. Recent pediatric studies have shown no added advantage to high-dose epinephrine in terms of survival to discharge or neurologic outcome. Because other studies have indicated adverse effects, including increased myocardial oxygen consumption during resuscitation and worsened postarrest myocardial dysfunction, high-dose epinephrine is no longer recommended.
Glucose	1. Hypoglycemia 2. Altered mental status (empirical) 3. With insulin, for hyperkalemia	0.5–1 g/kg IV/IO. Continuous infusion may be necessary.	2–4 mL/kg D_{10}W, 1–2 mL/kg D_{25}W.
Naloxone	1. Opioid overdose 2. Altered mental status (empirical)	0.1 mg/kg IV/IO/ET; maximum single dose, 2 mg. May repeat as necessary	Side effects are few. A dose of 2 mg may be given in children ≥5 years or >20 kg. Repeat as necessary, or give as constant infusion in opioid overdoses.

(Continued)

Table 29-8. Important Emergency Pediatric Drugs (*Continued*)

Drug	Indications	Dosage and Route	Comment
Sodium bicarbonate	1. Documented metabolic acidosis 2. Hyperkalemia	1 mEq/kg or IO; by arterial blood gas: $0.3 \times kg \times$ base deficit. May repeat every 5 min.	Infuse slowly. Sodium bicarbonate will be effective only if the patient is adequately oxygenated, ventilated, and perfused. Some adverse side effects.
Calcium chloride 10%	1. Documented hypocalcemia 2. Calcium channel blocker overdose 3. Hyperkalemia, hypermagnesemia	20 mg/kg slowly IV, preferably centrally, or IO with caution. Maximum single dose 2 g.	Calcium is no longer indicated for asystole. Potent tissue necrosis results if infiltration occurs. Use with caution and infuse slowly.

D_5W would be 10 mL/kg; $D_{10}W$ would be 1 mL/kg; $D_{50}W$, $10\%/25\%$ glucose in water; ET, endotracheally; IO, intraosseously; IV, intravenously; SC, subcutaneously; $D_{50}W$ is not recommended PIV and use caution with D_{25}. D_{10} is preferred for neonates (newborn – 1 month of age).

Source: Reproduced with permission from Tintinalli JE, Ma O, Yealy DM, Meckler GD, Stapczynski J, Cline DM, Thomas SH. (eds). Tintinalli's Emergency Medicine: A Comprehensive Study Guide, 9e, 2020; New York, NY: McGraw-Hill.

sizes based on estimated weight and age. Commonly used emergency medications in pediatrics are found in Table 29-8, above on pages 1017–1018.

ADULT EMERGENCY CARDIAC CARE (ECC) MEDICATIONS

Table 29-9. ECC Medications Used in Adults Based on American Heart Association Guidelines (See Footnote).

Generic (Trade)	Adult Dose
Adenosine (Adenocard)	**Tachycardia (regular, monomorphic or paroxysmal SVT):**
	First dose: 6 mg rapid IV push, follow with 20 mL NS flush and elevation of extremity.
	Second dose: 12 mg IV (if required); may repeat X 1.
Alteplase (Activase)	**STEMI (accelerated regimen):**
	Maximum dose 100 mg.
	Patients ≤67 kg: 15 mg IV bolus over 1–2 min followed by infusions of 0.75 mg/kg (not to exceed 50 mg) over 30 min then 0.5 mg/kg (not to exceed 35 mg) over 1 hr.
	Patients >67 kg: 15 mg IV bolus over 1–2 min followed by infusions of 50 mg over 30 min then 35 mg over 1 hr.
	Acute ischemic stroke (within 3 hr of symptom onset):
	Total dose 0.9 mg/kg (max 90 mg)
	Patients <100 kg: Load with 0.09 mg/kg (10% of 0.9 mg/kg dose) as an IV bolus over 1 min, followed by 0.81 mg/kg (90% of 0.9 mg/kg dose) as continuous infusion over 60 min.
	Patients ≥100 kg: Load with 9 mg (10% of 90 mg) as an IV bolus over 1 min, followed by 81 mg (90% of 90 mg) as a continuous infusion over 60 min.
Amiodarone (Nexterone, Pacerone)	**Pulseless VF/pVT unresponsive to defibrillation, CPR, and epinephrine:**
	First dose: 300 mg IV/IO bolus.
	Second dose: 150 mg IV (if required).
	Stable wide-QRS tachycardia:
	First dose: 150 mg IV over 10 min. Repeat as needed to a total of 2.2 g IV over the first 24 hr.
	Follow by maintenance infusion: 1 mg/min for first 6 hr then 0.5 mg/min for 18 hr or more.

29

(Continued)

Table 29-9. ECC Medications Used in Adults Based on American Heart Association Guidelines (See Footnote). (*Continued*)

Generic (Trade)	Adult Dose
Aspirin	**ACS:**
	Immediate release: 162–325 mg PO nonenteric-coated chewed and swallowed at time of diagnosis or if high clinical suspicion.
	Rectal (alternative route): 600 mg once at time of diagnosis (if oral not feasible).
Atenolol (Tenormin)	**Angina pectoris:**
	50 mg PO QD (may increase to 100 mg PO QD).
	MI (STEMI or NSTE-ACS):
	5 mg IV over 5 min, followed by an additional 5 mg over 10 min; if tolerated, start 50 mg PO, titrate PRN
Atropine	**Bradycardia:**
	0.5–1.0 mg IV bolus, repeat q3–5 min (max: 3 mg).
Bivalirudin (Angiomax)	**Acute STEMI (treated with primary PCI):**
	Initial 0.75 mg/kg IV bolus followed by IV infusion of 1.75 mg/kg/hr.
	Can be discontinued after PCI.
	NSTE-ACS (invasive approach):
	If given in ED, 0.1 mg/kg IV bolus and infusion of 0.25 mg/kg/hr before angiography.
	If PCI performed, additional 0.5 mg/kg IV bolus given and infusion rate increased to 1.75 mg/kg/hr.
Calcium chloride	**Cardiac arrest or cardiotoxicity (in the presence of hyperkalemia, hypocalcemia, or hypermagnesemia):**
	500–1000 mg IV over 2–5 min, repeat PRN.
	Routine use in cardiac arrest not recommended.
	Beta-blocker overdose; CCB overdose:
	Initial: 20 mg/kg IV (10% solution) over 5–10 min (max: 1–2 g/dose).
	May repeat q10–20m for 3–4 additional doses or initiate continuous infusion of 20–40 mg/kg/hr titrated to improve hemodynamic response.
Clopidogrel (Plavix)	**STEMI (treated with fibrinolytic therapy):**
	Age ≤75 years: 300 mg PO loading dose with 75 mg PO QD.
	Age >75 years: 75 mg PO QD.

Table 29-9. ECC Medications Used in Adults Based on American Heart Association Guidelines (See Footnote). *(Continued)*

Generic (Trade)	Adult Dose
	STEMI (treated with primary PCI):
	600 mg PO (in patients at high risk of bleeding or cannot take prasugrel or ticagrelor), followed by 75 mg PO QD after PCI.
	NSTE-ACS (invasive approach):
	300–600 mg PO followed by 75 mg PO QD.
Diltiazem (Cardizem, Cartia)	**Rate control (e.g., AF):**
	15–20 mg IV over 2 min, followed by 20–25 mg IV after 15 min.
	Maintenance infusion: 5–15 mg/hr IV (titrated to AF HR).
Dobutamine (Dobutrex)	**Cardiac decompensation:**
	Initial dose: 0.5–1 mcg/kg/min, with titration to effect.
	Maintenance dose: 2–20 mcg/kg/min with maximum dose of 20 mcg/kg/min.
	Immediate postcardiac arrest care setting:
	IV infusion 5–10 mcg/kg/min; titrate to effect.
Dopamine (Intropin)	**Symptomatic bradycardia following atropine:**
	2–20 mcg/kg/min; titrated to patient's response and maximum dose of 50 mcg/kg/min; taper slowly.
Enoxaparin (Lovenox)	**STEMI (treated with fibrinolysis); STEMI (no reperfusion therapy):**
	Age <75 years: loading dose 30 mg IV bolus followed by 1 mg/kg SQ q12h (max 100 mg for first two doses). The first SQ dose should be administered with the IV bolus.
	Dose adjustment for CrCl <30 mL/min: Loading dose of 30 mg IV followed by 1 mg/kg SQ q24h. First SQ dose should be administered with IV bolus.
	Age ≥75 years: No IV loading dose. 0.75 mg/kg SQ q12h (max 75 mg for first two doses).
	Dose adjustment for CrCl <30 mL/min: No IV loading dose. Administer 1 mg/kg SQ q24h.
	NSTE-ACS (noninvasive approach):
	1 mg/kg SQ q12h.
	Dose adjustment for CrCl <30 mL/min: 1 mg/kg SQ q24h.

29

(Continued)

Table 29-9. ECC Medications Used in Adults Based on American Heart Association Guidelines (See Footnote). *(Continued)*

Generic (Trade)	Adult Dose
Epinephrine	**Asystole/pulseless arrest, pVT/VF:**
	IV/IO: 1 mg (using **0.1 mg/mL solution**) q3–5m until return of spontaneous circulation.
	Endotracheal (alternative route): 2–2.5 mg diluted in 5–10 mL NS or sterile water q3–5m until IV/IO access established or return of spontaneous circulation.
	Bradycardia (unresponsive to atropine or pacing):
	IV infusion: 2–10 mcg/min or 0.1–0.5 mcg/kg/min; titrate to desired response.
	Inotropic support:
	IV infusion: 0.01–0.5 mcg/kg/min; titrate to desired response.
	Hypersensitivity reaction (anaphylaxis):
	IM (anterolateral aspect of the middle third of the thigh): 0.3–0.5 mg using **1 mg/mL solution**; repeat q5–15m in absence of clinical improvement.
Eptifibatide (Integrilin)	**STEMI/NSTEMI:**
	180 mcg/kg IV bolus (max 22.6 mg) followed by continuous infusion of 2 mcg/kg/min (max 15 mg/hr).
	Repeat bolus in 10 min. May continue infusion for up to 18–24 hr after PCI.
Esmolol (Brevibloc)	**Rate control (e.g., SVT and AF/AFl or noncompensatory sinus tachycardia):**
	IV loading dose 500 mcg/kg (0.5 mg/kg) over 1 min, followed by infusion of 50 mcg/kg/min (0.05 mg/kg/min) for 4 min.
	If response inadequate, infuse second bolus of 0.5 mg/kg over 1 min and increase maintenance infusion to 100 mcg/kg/min (0.1 mg/kg/min) with increment increase to max infusion rate of 300 mcg/kg/min (0.3 mg/kg/min).
Fondaparinux (Arixtra)	**STEMI (treated with fibrinolysis):**
	2.5 mg IV, followed by 2.5 mg SQ q24h.
	Drug should be avoided in CrCl <30 mL/min.

Table 29-9. ECC Medications Used in Adults Based on American Heart Association Guidelines (See Footnote). (*Continued*)

Generic (Trade)	Adult Dose
	NSTE-ACS (noninvasive approach):
	2.5 mg SQ q24h.
	Drug should be avoided in CrCl <30 mL/min.
Glucagon	**Beta-blocker or CCB overdose:**
	3–10 mg IV bolus over 3–5 min. If no clinical response, may repeat bolus dose.
	If clinical response with bolus, start continuous infusion at 3–5 mg/h; titrate to achieve adequate hemodynamic response.
	Hypoglycemia:
	Injection: 1 mg IV, IM, or SQ. May repeat 15 min PRN.
	Intranasal: 3 mg (one actuation) into a single nostril. May repeat 15 min PRN.
	Anaphylaxis (refractory to epinephrine) in patients on beta-blocker therapy:
	1–5 mg IV bolus over 5 min followed by infusion of 5–15 mcg/min; titrate.
Heparin – unfractionated	**STEMI (treated with primary PCI):**
	Initial 50–70 U/kg IV bolus (max 5000 U).
	Additional UFH may be given in the cath lab based on results of ACT monitoring.
	STEMI (treated with fibrinolysis):
	60–100 U/kg IV bolus (max 4000 U), followed by IV infusion of 12U/kg/hr (max 1000 U/hr), adjusted to achieve goal aPTT of approximately 50–70 s (1.5–2× control).
	STEMI (no reperfusion therapy):
	50–70 U/kg IV bolus (max 5000 U), followed by IV infusion 12 U/kg/hr adjusted to achieve goal aPTT of approximately 50–70 s (1.5–2× control).
	NSTE-ACS (invasive approach):
	60–70U/kg IV bolus (max 5000 U), followed by IV infusion 12 U/kg/hr adjusted to achieve goal of aPTT of approximately 50–70 s (1.5–2× control).

(*Continued*)

29

Table 29-9. ECC Medications Used in Adults Based on American Heart Association Guidelines (See Footnote). (*Continued*)

Generic (Trade)	Adult Dose
Ibutilide (Corvert)	**AF/AFl:**
	<60 kg: 0.01 mg/kg over 10 min.
	≥60 kg: 1 mg over 10 min.
Labetalol	**Acute aortic syndromes/acute aortic dissection:**
	Intermittent IV: Initial 20 mg over 2 min followed by 20–80 mg q10m until target HR and BP reached; may transition to continuous infusion if unable to obtain target goals.
	Continuous IV infusion: Initial loading dose 20 mg over 2 min (optional if intermittent dosing used), followed by 0.5–2 mg/min (may titrate to 10 mg/min).
	Emergency blood pressure management: (NOT pregnant and NOT postpartum women):
	Intermittent IV: Initial 10–20 mg over 1–2 min followed by 20–80 mg q10m until target HR and BP reached; may transition to continuous infusion if unable to obtain target goals.
	Continuous IV infusion: Initial loading dose 10–20 mg over 2 min (optional if intermittent dosing used), followed by 0.5–2 mg/min (may titrate to 10 mg/min).
	Emergency blood pressure management in pregnant and postpartum women:
	Intermittent IV: Initial 20 mg over 1–2 min ; if blood pressure exceeds threshold after 10 min, increase dose in increments of 20–40 mg every 10 min (max dose 80 mg).
	Continuous IV infusion: Initial loading dose 20 mg over 2 min (optional if intermittent dosing used), followed by 1–2 mg/min (may titrate to response). Max total dose 300 mg/24 hr
Lidocaine	**VF/pVT unresponsive to defibrillation, CPR, and epinephrine:**
	First dose: 1–1.5 mg/kg IV/IO bolus.
	Second dose: 0.5–0.75 mg/kg IV/IO q5–10m (max cumulative dose 3 mg/kg)
	Follow with continuous infusion (1–4 mg/min) after return of perfusion.

29

Table 29-9. ECC Medications Used in Adults Based on American Heart Association Guidelines (See Footnote). (*Continued*)

Generic (Trade)	Adult Dose
	Hemodynamically stable monomorphic VT:
	1–1.5 mg/kg IV. Repeat with 0.5–0.75 mg/kg q5–10m (max cumulative dose 3 mg/kg).
	Follow with continuous infusion (1–4 mg/min) after return of perfusion.
Magnesium sulfate	**Torsades de pointes:**
	1–2 g IV push (2–4 mL 50% solution) in 10 mL D5W. If pulse present, then 1–2 g in 50–100 mL D5W over 5–60 min. Routine use for cardiac arrest without Torsades de pointes is **NOT** advised.
Metoprolol (Lopressor, Toprol)	**AMI:**
	Oral (preferred): Metoprolol tartrate 25–50 mg PO q6–12h.
	IV (if indicated): 5 mg slow IV (over 1–2 min) q5 min, total initial dose of 15 mg.
	If tolerated, initiate early oral therapy with metoprolol succinate 25–50 mg PO QD with careful up-titration to as much as 200 mg PO QD or metoprolol tartrate 25–50 mg PO BID-QID beginning 15–30 min after last IV dose.
	Goal discharge HR of approximately 70 bpm.
	Irregular narrow-complex tachycardia (acute rate control):
	5 mg IV for 3 doses q2–5m.
Morphine	**ACS:**
	2–4 mg IV initially, then q5–15 min PRN.
Nitroglycerin	**ACS:**
	Sublingual 0.4 mg q5 min or one aerosol spray under tongue q5 min for total 3 doses.
	If persistent chest pain, IV infusion: initial 5–10 mcg/min, gradually increased at approximately 10-min intervals by 5–10 mcg/min. Usual dose 50–200 mcg/min (dose should not exceed 400 mcg/min).
Nitroprusside (Nipride)	**Acute hypertension:**
	Initial: 0.3–0.5 mcg/kg/min IV; may be titrated by 0.5 mcg/kg/min every few min (max dose 10 mcg/kg/min for max 10 min).

29

(*Continued*)

Table 29-9. ECC Medications Used in Adults Based on American Heart Association Guidelines (See Footnote). (*Continued*)

Generic (Trade)	Adult Dose
	Acute decompensated heart failure:
	Initial: 5–10 mcg/min IV; titrate to effect.
Prasugrel (Effient)	**PCI for ACS; STEMI (if PCI performed >24 hr after fibrin-specific thrombolytic):**
	60 mg PO loading dose.
	Maintenance dose: 10 mg PO QD (in combination with ASA).
	NSTE-ACS (invasive approach after diagnostic coronary angiography):
	60 mg PO loading dose.
	Maintenance dose: 10 mg PO QD (in combination with ASA).
Procainamide	**Stable monomorphic VT, refractory reentry SVT, stable wide-complex tachycardia, AF w/ WPW:**
	Loading dose: 10–17 mg/kg IV at rate of 20–50 mg/min or 100 mg every 5 min.
	Continue until arrhythmia controlled, hypotension occurs, or QRS widens > 50% of original width.
	Not recommended for use in ongoing VF/pVT.
	Maintenance infusion: 1–4 mg/min IV.
Propranolol (Inderal)	**SVT:**
	1 mg IV over 1 min; repeat PRN q2 min up to max 3 doses.
	VT (hemodynamically stable):
	1–3 mg IV q5m up to total 5 mg in combination with an IV antiarrhythmic.
Reteplase (Retavase)	**STEMI:**
	10 U IV over 2 min, then repeat 10 U IV bolus at 30 min.
Sodium bicarbonate	**Cardiac arrest:**
	1 mEq/kg/dose IV; repeat doses guided by ABGs.
	Routine use **NOT** recommended. Considered in setting of prolonged cardiac arrest only after adequate alveolar ventilation has been established and effective cardiac compressions.

Table 29-9. ECC Medications Used in Adults Based on American Heart
Association Guidelines (See Footnote). (*Continued*)

Generic (Trade)	Adult Dose
	QRS widening (OD of TCAs, cocaine, anticholinergics):
	1–2 mEq/kg rapid IV push through large bore IV catheter. If no response, may repeat after 5 min.
	Follow with continuous IV infusion (150 mEq in 1 L D5W, infuse at 250 mL/hr).
	Alkalization of serum and urine (OD of ASA):
	Target urine pH 7.5–8.8. Use ABG to guide treatment. Correct and avoid hypokalemia.
Sotalol (Betapace)	**Stable wide-QRS tachycardia:**
	100 mg (1.5 mg/kg) IV over 5 min.
	Avoid if prolonged QT.
Streptokinase	**AMI:**
	1.5 million U over 60 min.
Tenecteplase (TNKase)	**STEMI:**
	Single IV bolus over 5–10 s based on body weight. Maximum dose: 50 mg.
	<60 kg: 30 mg
	≥60 to <70 kg: 35 mg
	≥70 to <80 kg: 40 mg
	≥80 to <90 kg: 45 mg
	≥90 kg: 50 mg
Ticagrelor (Brilinta)	**Acute STEMI (treated with no reperfusion therapy or with primary PCI):**
	180 mg PO loading dose. Maintenance dose 90 mg q12h.
	NSTE-ACS:
	180 mg PO loading dose. Maintenance dose 90 mg q12h.
Tirofiban (Aggrastat)	**NSTE-ACS:**
	Loading dose: 25 mcg/kg IV over 5 min or less.
	Maintenance infusion: 0.15 mcg/kg/min continued for up to 18 hr.

(*Continued*)

29

Table 29-9. ECC Medications Used in Adults Based on American Heart Association Guidelines (See Footnote). (*Continued*)

Generic (Trade)	Adult Dose
	STEMI undergoing primary PCI:
	Loading dose: 25 mcg/kg IV over 5 min or less at time of PCI.
	Maintenance infusion: 0.15 mcg/kg/min in combination with heparin or bivalirudin in selected patients (continued for 18–24 hr).
	Stable ischemic heart disease (high-risk features) undergoing primary PCI:
	Loading dose: 25 mcg/kg IV over 5 min or less at time of PCI.
	Maintenance infusion: 0.15 mcg/kg/min continued for up to 48 hr.
	Reserved for patients not pretreated with clopidogrel or who are undergoing elective PCI with stent implantation with adequate clopidogrel pretreatment.
Verapamil (Calan, Verelan)	**Rate control (e.g., AF):**
	5–10 mg (0.075–0.15 mg/kg) IV over 2 min, followed by 10 mg IV 15–30 min after initial dose. If response, then infusion at 5 mg/hr and titrate to goal, max dose 20 mg/hr.
	SVT:
	5–10 mg (0.075–0.15 mg/kg) IV over 2 min, followed by 10 mg (0.15 mg/kg) IV 30 min after initial dose. If response, then infusion at 0.005 mg/kg/min.

(Commonly used emergency cardiac care medications are summarized inside the front and back covers.)

ABG: arterial blood gas, ACS: acute coronary syndrome, ACT: activated clotting time, AF: atrial fibrillation, AFl: atrial flutter, AMI: acute myocardial infarction, CCB: calcium channel blocker, ED: emergency department, NSTE-ACS: non-ST-segment elevation acute coronary syndromes, PCI: percutaneous coronary intervention, pVT: pulseless ventricular tachycardia, QRS: electrocardiogram complex, STEMI: ST-elevation myocardial infarction, SVT: supraventricular tachycardia, UFH: unfractionated heparin, VF: ventricular fibrillation, VT: ventricular tachycardia, TCA: tricyclic antidepressant.

Sources: AHA transitioned to continuous updates of guidelines since 2015 and yearly updates have been incorporated in the listed medications. Based on data from: 2019 American Heart Association Focused Update on Advanced Cardiovascular Life Support: Use of Advanced Airways, Vasopressors, and Extracorporeal Cardiopulmonary Resuscitation During Cardiac Arrest: An Update to the American Heart Association Guidelines for Cardiopulmonary Resuscitation and Emergency Cardiovascular Care. Circulation. 2019;140:e881–e894. Available online at: https://www.ahajournals.org/doi/10.1161/CIR.0000000000000732 "Annual updates published in Circulation from 2010 through 2018 have been incorporated in this section."

References

1. American Heart Association Guidelines for Cardiopulmonary Resuscitation and Emergency Cardiovascular Care. Circulation 2015;18 [suppl 2]. Available online at: https://www.ahajournals.org/toc/circ/132/18_suppl_2. Accessed June 29, 2020.
2. https://www.ahajournals.org/doi/pdf/10.1161/CIRCULATIONAHA.120.047463. Accessed 5/22/2020.
3. https://www.ahajournals.org/toc/circ/132/18_suppl_2. Accessed May 25, 2020.
4. National Asthma Education and Prevention Program. Expert panel report 3: Guidelines for the diagnosis and management of asthma; 2007:375. Available at http://www.nhlbi.nih.gov/guidelines/asthma/asthgdln.htm. Accessed May 10, 2020.
5. French EK, et al. Diabetic ketoacidosis and hyperosmolar hyperglycemia syndrome: Review of acute decompensated diabetes in adult patients. The *BMJ* 2019;365:1114.
6. Wiersinga WM. Myxedema and Coma. In: Feingold KR, et al. (eds.). Endotext [Internet]. South Dartmouth (MA): MDText.com, Inc.; 2000–2020.
7. Jameson JL, et al. Hypothyroidism. In: Jameson JL, Fauci AS, Kasper DL, Hauser SL, Longo DL, Loscalzo J (eds.). Harrison's Principles of Internal Medicine, 20e. New York, NY: McGraw-Hill Education; 2018.
8. McDermott MT. In the Clinic® Hyperthyroidism. *Ann Intern Med.* 2020;172(7): ITC49 -ITC64.
9. De Leo S, et al. Hyperthyroidism. The *Lancet* 2016;388:906–918.

Mastering the Clinical History and Physical

30

- ➤ Rules for Clinicians in Daily Practice
- ➤ Observation: An Invaluable Asset for the Clinician
- ➤ Rules for Doing a History and Physical Examination
- ➤ The Stethoscope
- ➤ Vital Signs
- ➤ Assessing for Pain

- ➤ Cardiac History and Physical Examination
  - ➢ Cardiac Exam Important Clinical Points
- ➤ Pulmonary History and Physical Examination
- ➤ Gastrointestinal Tips and Pearls
- ➤ Oncologic Tips and Pearls
- ➤ Endocrine Tips and Pearls

RULES FOR CLINICIANS IN DAILY PRACTICE

1. Never let the situation, the procedure, and the moment take control of you. You are in control.
2. You will not find it unless you look for it. Anticipation is key and comes from taking a focused (chief concern directed) history.
3. An easy admission is only one in retrospect.
4. Going into a patient's room is like going into a darkened hallway. You never know where it will lead you.
5. Never take for granted what a patient does not tell you, never assume. Always ASK!
6. If a patient tells you they feel like impending doom, admit them and watch them closely.
7. Trust no one. Doubt and verify everything.

Chapter update by Joseph F. Majdan, MD, FACP, FCPP; Dr. Majdan is a senior clinician in the Department of Medicine and responsible for Clinical Remediation at Sidney Kimmel Medical College. Here he shares his experience with tips, pearls, and words of wisdom to help learners "master" the clinical history and physical examination. This chapter builds upon the information in Chapter 6, "History and Physical Examination."

8. A laboratory result is not attached to a patient; it is the patient and their HISTORY that gives meaning to the laboratory result.
9. One of the marks of a true physician is knowing what she/he does not know and being able to admit it to yourself, your colleagues, and your patients.

OBSERVATION: AN INVALUABLE ASSET FOR THE CLINICIAN

1. The art of observation is an essential clinical tool that each physician must master and develop. Observation in its purest form is what is before you without inserting judgment, prejudice, or a preconceived diagnosis.
2. Observation entails using all of your inherent senses: smell, touch, sight, hearing, and gestalt (one's overall perception). It is a bridge between the history and the physical examination that leads us ultimately to the diagnosis.

RULES FOR DOING A HISTORY AND PHYSICAL EXAM

1. Why am I doing this?
2. What am I looking for?
3. Has my physical examination explored all of the essential elements being considered in my differential diagnosis?

THE STETHOSCOPE

1. Developed by Rene Laennec in 1816. Its name is derived from two Greek words: stethos = chest and scopia = to listen.
2. It has two key components: the diaphragm and the bell.
3. Diaphragm: Useful for a majority of sounds evaluated. Reveals high-frequency sounds.
4. Bell: Useful for hearing bruits, gallops, mitral stenosis, and the last Korotkoff sound when taking a blood pressure. Reveals low-frequency sounds.
5. Earpieces commonly are repositories of pocket lint, earwax, and food crumbs. Important to clean them every couple of months.
6. Always place your stethoscope *directly* on the skin: never listen through clothing or a gown. This allows the best chance to hear all possible sounds present.
7. When listening for carotid bruits, have the patient hold their breath for 2 sec. Otherwise, the breath sounds could mask a significant bruit.

VITAL SIGNS

1. **Pulse:** Assess not only the rate but also its characteristics:
   - o Regular or irregular: Remember, you cannot evaluate a cardiac rhythm just by the pulse.
   - o Intensity: A bounding pulse (Corrigan pulse or water-hammer pulse) is associated not only with aortic regurgitation but also with any hyperdynamic state, i.e., hyperthyroidism, severe anemia, AV fistula, others.
   - o Consistency: Alternating pulse intensity (pulsus alternans) is associated with left or right ventricular failure.

2. **Respirations:** Assess not only the rate but also observe for patterns:
   - o Cheyne-Stokes respirations: A roller-coaster breathing pattern starting with a short apneic episode followed by a gradual increase in the depth and frequency of breathing and then a decrease in depth and frequency with another apneic episode, and this pattern is repeated. Associated with congestive heart failure and suggests a worse prognosis; also associated with cerebrovascular accident, brain tumor, and increased intracerebral pressure.
   - o Biot respirations: Erratic, chaotic alternating deep/superficial respirations. Associated with meningitis.
   - o Kussmaul respirations: Deep sighing, regular respirations. Associated with diabetic ketoacidosis as well as with other causes of ketoacidosis.

3. **Blood Pressure: All patients with chest pain *must* have BP taken in both arms.**
   - o Must always consider aortic dissection with any patient who presents with chest pain.
   - o Blood pressure cuff width should never be less than half the length of the arm. This avoids fictitious blood pressure readings.
   - o A palpable pulse implies a systolic BP ≥50 mm Hg.
   - o Systolic hypertension: Systolic BP ≥130 mm Hg with normal diastolic BP (<80 mm Hg). Common causes: atherosclerosis, hyperthyroidism, anxiety, aortic regurgitation, and arteriovenous fistula.
   - o Hypotension: Both the systolic and diastolic BP are significantly lower than the standard normal of 120/70. This can result from volume loss (GI bleed, dehydration), cardiac failure (myocardial infarction, congestive heart failure, pericardial tamponade), iatrogenic, or sepsis. Clinical differentiation is made first by, as always, the **history**, and then by the following: hypotension caused by cardiac or volume loss will have cold extremities due to secondary vascular contraction; hypotension caused by sepsis is usually initially associated with warm extremities.
   - o Orthostatic hypotension: This should be assessed in patients presenting with vomiting, GI bleeding, syncope, dizziness, and certain neurologic diseases such as Parkinson disease. Appropriate technique: (1) After 2-3 minutes in the supine position, take the patient's BP. (2) Sit

the patient up with the LEGS DANGLING, then after at least 1 min repeat the BP. A decrease of the systolic BP of 20 mm Hg or more or a decrease of the diastolic BP of 10 mm Hg or more defines orthostatic hypotension. If the blood pressure does not change and the clinical situation warrants, have the patient stand up for a minute and repeat the blood pressure. An increase in HR by 20–30 BPM accompanies the change in BP due to volume depletion. The HR change due to volume depletion usually occurs at lesser degrees of volume depletion than the BP changes.

o Widened pulse pressure: Pulse pressure is the difference between the systolic and diastolic blood pressure. Normal pulse pressure is 30–40 mm Hg. Widened pulse pressure is seen with aortic regurgitation, arteriovenous fistula, hyperthyroidism, severe anemia, and pregnancy.

o Narrowed pulse pressure is defined as a pulse pressure of <30 mm Hg. It is associated with cardiogenic shock, aortic stenosis, cardiac tamponade, and constrictive pericarditis.

ASSESSING FOR PAIN

1. Use the mnemonic "O-P-Q-R-S-T"
   o **O**nset: When did it start?
   o **P**alliative: What makes it better?/**P**rovocative: What makes it worse?
   o **Q**uality: Is the pain sharp, dull, or like a pressure on the chest?
   o **R**egion/**R**adiation: Where does it start/does it radiate? If so, where?
   o **S**everity: Grade the pain on a scale of 0–10, 0 being no pain, 10 being the worst pain they have ever had.
   o **T**ime: How long does it last when it occurs?
2. Fleeting pain, i.e., 1–2 sec in duration, is usually not from serious underlying pathology.
3. Pain is often not verbalized by stoic individuals. Thus, during the physical examination look for any other "signs" of pain such as pursing of lips, eyebrow movement, or clenching of fingers as subtle manifestations.

CARDIAC HISTORY AND PHYSICAL EXAM

1. **Cardiac History:**
   o Angina pectoris is a *clinical* diagnosis defined as any substernal chest, arm, jaw, or intrascapular discomfort brought on with exercise and relieved with rest. William Heberden first described it in 1768.
   o Levine sign: Clenching of a patient's fist over the sternum is suggestive of coronary artery disease.
   o Pericarditis pain: Chest pain worsens with lying down and decreases with sitting up and leaning forward.
   o Aortic stenosis when symptomatic, classic symptoms are "ASH": **A**ngina, **S**yncope, and **H**eart failure.

2. Cardiac Physical:

Consider this novel approach to the diagnosis of heart sounds and murmurs (see Figure 30-1). (See also Chapter 6, pages 58 and 59, for additional details on heart sounds and murmurs.) Heart sounds and murmurs are not always heard best over the four heart valves. They can migrate due to body habitus, age, natural history of a heart murmur, or direction of blood flow through the valve. To fully explore and assess murmurs as well as gallops and clicks in an adult, use this approach:

o Draw an imaginary transverse line through the midpoint of the patient's sternum.
o Now listen and determine if the murmur is heard loudest above or below that line (remember that murmurs can radiate but it is *where* it is heard the **loudes**t that is most important).
o If the murmur is heard loudest **above** that midpoint sternal line, the murmur originates from the aortic valve, pulmonic valve, or an atrial septal defect.
o If the murmur is heard loudest **below** that midpoint sternal line, it originates from the mitral valve, tricuspid valve, or a ventricular septal defect.

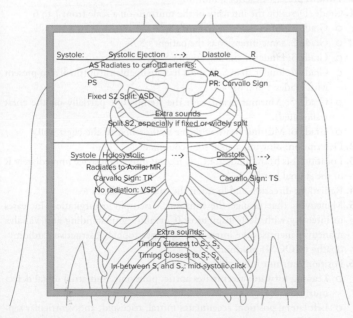

Figure 30-1. The process for possible origin of the murmur.

o Does the murmur occur in systole or diastole?

o If the murmur is loudest in systole above the line, it is a stenosis murmur: aortic stenosis, pulmonary stenosis, and atrial septal defect (functional stenosis).

o If the murmur is loudest in systole below the line, it is a leaking murmur: mitral regurgitation, tricuspid regurgitation, and ventricular septal defect.

o If the murmur is loudest in diastole above the line, it is a leaking murmur: aortic regurgitation and pulmonary regurgitation.

o If the murmur is heard loudest in diastole below the line, it is a stenotic murmur: mitral stenosis and tricuspid stenosis.

This approach allows you to consider only three cardiac structures and not six as the possible origin for the murmur. Figure 30-1, page 1035 summarizes this process:

- How to differentiate a systolic ejection murmur from a holosystolic murmur:
  o Guilt by location: Draw a line through the midportion of the patient's sternum and if the systolic murmur is heard loudest ABOVE that midsternal line, it must be a systolic ejection murmur (SEM). If the systolic murmur is heard loudest below that midsternal line, it must be a holosystolic murmur. There are no holosystolic murmurs heard above the midsternal line. There are no systolic ejection murmurs heard loudest below the midsternal line.
- How to present/describe a murmur:
1. Grade: Describe the intensity of the murmur on a scale from 1 to 6
   o Grade 1: softer than the patient's S_1/S_2
   o Grade 2: same intensity as the patient's S_1/S_2
   o Grade 3: louder than the patient's S_1/S_2
   o Grade 4: louder than S_1/S_2 plus has a palpable thrill (thrill also present with grades 5 and 6)
   o Grade 5: Murmur heard with the stethoscope partially off the chest wall (tilted).
   o Grade 6: Murmur heard with the stethoscope off the chest wall.
2. Description: blowing, harsh, soft, cooing, etc.
3. Location it is heard loudest, i.e., R second intercostal space immediately R of the sternal border
4. Radiation: direction and location the murmur radiates to
5. Maneuvers that change the murmur: Tricuspid regurgitation increases in intensity with deep inspiration (Carvallo sign); standing and Valsalva maneuver increases the intensity of a hypertrophic obstructive cardiomyopathy (HOCM) murmur.
6. Position murmur is heard loudest in:
   o Leaning forward: accentuates aortic, pulmonic, and atrial septal defect murmurs
   o Left lateral position: accentuates mitral, tricuspid, and ventricular septal defect murmurs

- Pericardial friction rub:
  - ○ Can have one, two, or three components (corresponding to atrial systole, ventricular systole, and early ventricular diastole [ventricular] filling) and best heard along the lower left sternal border. The rub is harsh in quality and is often fleeting.
  - ○ In caring for patients with pericarditis, always be mindful to look for the potential complications of pericarditis such as pericardial tamponade.
  - ○ Clinical findings of pericardial tamponade: **Beck triad** (distended neck veins, sinus tachycardia, and hypotension).
  - ○ BE CAREFUL: **Hamman crunch** is a crunchy, scratchy sound heard along the left sternal to apical region that mimics pericardial rub sounds. Palpable subcutaneous emphysema is often found with this auscultatory finding. It is produced by a pneumomediastinum, usually caused by either a ruptured pulmonary bleb or trauma (accidental or iatrogenic).

Cardiac Exam Important Clinical Points

1. All regurgitation murmurs require that their origin be evaluated and defined.
2. Mitral valve prolapse is associated with migraine headaches, type A personalities, and is more prevalent in women.
3. The commonest cause of aortic dissection in a premenopausal woman is pregnancy.
4. A palpable right ventricle (RV heave/lift) implies pulmonary hypertension and RV enlargement.
5. Shortening of the duration of an aortic regurgitation murmur defines significant worsening of the regurgitation warranting further assessment immediately.
6. The auscultatory hallmark of tricuspid regurgitation is Carvallo sign: an increase in intensity with inspiration and decrease with expiration.
7. Although the descriptions of the pressure changes seen by looking at the internal jugular vein are well known, a wave, c wave (never seen), v wave, and the x and y descent, the truth is that they are only seen in 5–10% of all patients.

PULMONARY HISTORY AND PHYSICAL

1. **Pulmonary History:**
   - ○ Differentiation of symptoms originating from cardiac pathology must always be considered.
   - ○ A history suggestive of allergen induction, i.e., cold, dust, and pets, implies a primary pulmonary process.
   - ○ With wheezing, you must always differentiate primary end expiratory wheezes, which imply a distal tubular constrictive process, i.e., asthma,

30

from primary inspiratory wheezes, i.e., an upper airway constrictive process (angioedema, upper airway obstructive tumors, etc.).

o Nighttime cough can be caused by left-side heart failure, esophageal reflux, chronic bronchitis, and sinus congestion.

o Hemoptysis raises consideration of the following etiologies: infectious, cardiac, iatrogenic, neoplastic, and rheumatologic.

o Rusty-colored sputum is associated with a *Streptococcus pneumoniae* pneumonia.

o Currant jelly sputum is a thick red sputum that is associated with a *Klebsiella pneumoniae* pneumonia.

o Green sputum is associated with pneumonia from *Hemophilus influenzae* and *Pseudomonas aeruginosa*.

o Foul-smelling sputum raises the possibility of pneumonia from an anaerobic infection from aspiration.

2. **Pulmonary Physical Exam:**

o Many times, clinicians tell the patient to take a deep breath every time they place their stethoscope on the chest. A more fluent way to achieve this and improve the assessment of lung sounds is to tell the patient "Every time you feel my stethoscope touch your chest, please take one breath in and out through your mouth."

o In the examination of the lungs, visualize where the various lobes of the lungs would lie anteriorly, posteriorly, and in both axillae. Once you do this, you can proceed with doing a thorough lung examination.

o In differentiating pneumothorax, consolidation, or pleural effusion, the pulmonary examination must include the following three maneuvers: palpation (tactile fremitus), percussion, and auscultation (see Table 30-1).

o **Egophony** is a sign associated with consolidation. Egophony is identified with the patient saying the letter "EEEEEE" and it sounds like a goat making the sound of "AAAAAA" when the examiner is listening over the consolidated area of the lung. "Egos" is Greek for "goat." Laennec, who developed the stethoscope, coined the term.

o To completely examine the lungs, the anterior, posterior, and axillary areas must be assessed.

Table 30-1. Clinical Differentiation of Pulmonary Diseases

	Percussion	*Auscultation*	*Tactile Fremitus*
Pneumothorax	Tympanic	Absent	Diminished
Consolidation	Dull	Bronchial breath sounds, crackles	Increased
Pleural effusion	Dull	Decreased breath sounds	Absent or diminished, may be increased at the top of the fluid level

o Several physical barriers to fully evaluate the lungs must be realized and addressed. The first is in examining the posterior lung fields; the scapulae obstruct appropriate examination of the upper lung fields by auscultation, percussion, and tactile fremitus. The examiner must have the patient cross their arms and lean forward. This moves the scapula away from the vertebrae and opens the upper lung fields to being appropriately assessed.

o Another barrier is associated with examining the anterior chest. Examination of this region using palpation (tactile fremitus), percussions, and auscultation should be done at the midclavicular line bilaterally. To examine medial to the left midclavicular line, the examiner would listen over the heart and hilum and this would not allow a true analysis of the lung fields.

o Any true examination of the lungs must include examination of both axillae, otherwise a right middle lobe pneumonia can be missed.

o With any patient who presents with symptoms suggestive of bronchitis or lung infection, you must consider sinusitis as the primary source of the symptoms. Thus, a careful examination of the sinuses and nose should be included.

o **Dahl sign** is thickened (hyperkeratotic) elbows occurring with patients with chronic obstructive lung disease (COPD). This occurs because such patients sit forward leaning on their elbows to improve their ability to breathe.

o Patients with COPD are also found to have indentations of the anterior portion of both thighs. To assist in breathing, they lean forward by putting their elbows on their thighs.

o In the evaluation of the lungs, one should check for clubbing. The normal angle of the base of the nail with the finger, called **Lovibond angle**, is 160 degrees. This is assessed by having the patient place the DIPs and the extensor surface of the tips of the corresponding fingers together. If there is a normal angle, a diamond-shaped space can be seen between the digits. However, if the angle is increased, that diamond-shaped space will be lost. This is called **Shamroth sign**. It is associated with lung cancer, interstitial lung disease, cyanotic heart disease, and inflammatory bowel disease.

o Anxiety and restlessness, along with rapid respirations, intercostal retractions, use of accessory muscles to breathe, and audible, moist crackles and wheezing are signs of respiratory distress.

o Signs of hypoxia include not only cyanosis of the lips but also of the nose and ears. A more subtle manifestation is the appearance of the patient being "dusky" (imagine a patient being painted with charcoal gray paint). These are late and ominous signs of advanced lung disease, hypoxia, and impending arrest.

o The onset of weight loss in patients with chronic obstructive lung disease is a poor prognostic sign. Worsening of this disease produces a

30

continued hyperinflation of the lungs resulting in pressure from the diaphragm on the stomach, lessening its capacity for food. This and the increased work of breathing lead to weight loss.

GASTROINTESTINAL TIPS AND PEARLS

1. The examiner may at times be presented with patients who are "faking" abdominal pain. A maneuver to rule this out is to establish where the patient is having pain by first palpating the abdomen and then observing their response. After this, the patient is then told that you have to listen to their abdomen with your stethoscope. However, during this maneuver, the examiner places pressure on the abdomen with the stethoscope in the area(s) of the pain. If the patient does not express pain with pressure of the stethoscope over the area the patient previously had pain with hand palpation, consideration must be made that the pain is fictitious. This is, however, a diagnosis of exclusion.

2. A clinician is sometimes faced with a patient who is very ticklish. This makes examination of the abdomen difficult. This is overcome by doing the following maneuver. Have the patient place and move their hand over your hand while you palpate the abdomen. This alleviates the ticklish response because people are never ticklish to themselves. By having the patient place their hand on the examiner's hand, the patient senses they are touching their own abdomen and will remain calm.

3. The first area of the body to show jaundice is the sublingual region.

4. Sometimes patients with excess intake of carrots can present with hypercarotenemia that mimics jaundice. A physical examination finding that helps in distinguishing this from jaundice is that the sclera are clear in hypercarotenemia but yellow in true jaundice.

5. Jaundice is best seen under regular sunlight. It is more difficult to see under artificial lighting, especially with milder degrees of jaundice (bilirubin 5 mg/dL).

6. Patients with an abnormal metallic taste (dysgeusia) should be assessed for possible liver disease. Other unsuspected potential causes are lung cancer, DM, GERD, Crohn disease, irradiation of the head and neck, pregnancy, sinus infection, chemotherapy, and esophageal reflux.

7. In assessing the liver, the contour of the liver's edge yields clinical insight: a sharp edge is associated with a normal liver, a blunted edge with chronic disease, and a hard edge with cancer.

8. Normal liver span is determined by measuring its length at the right midclavicular line. The normal mean size is 10 cm. Physical examination maneuvers used to determine liver size are either by percussion or by using the scratch test. Of these two maneuvers, the scratch test appears to be the easier to perform and is less subjective. The scratch test is also easier to perform on patients who are obese or with other

physically challenging characteristics. In the end, it is a personal preference.

9. The presence of a palpable periumbilical nodule is called a **Sister Mary Joseph nodule**. It is associated with gastrointestinal cancers such as pancreatic cancer, gastric cancer, and colonic cancer as well as with uterine and ovarian cancer. It is named after Sister Mary Joseph Dempsey, who was the nursing supervisor at Saint Mary's Hospital, which became the world-famous Mayo Clinic. She was a surgical assistant to Dr. Mayo and was well known for her clinical and observational skills.

10. **Virchow node** is a palpable sentinel lymph node in the left supraclavicular fossa and is associated with gastric cancer as well as other cancers of the abdomen. It is named after the German pathologist, Rudolph Virchow, MD.

ONCOLOGIC TIPS AND PEARLS

1. In elderly patients with nocturnal generalized pruritus, you must rule out malignancy.
2. A negative or very low anion gap is suggestive of multiple myeloma.
3. The finding of leukemia cutis implies the presence of extramedullary disease and is a poor prognosis.
4. A palpable, right supraclavicular node implies the presence of thoracic malignancies such as breast, lung, and esophageal cancer as well as lymphoma.
5. Ascending colon cancers present at times with iron-deficiency anemias.
6. Descending colon cancers present at times with changes in bowel habits as well as colicky abdominal pain and abdominal distension.
7. Cancers of the rectum often present with rectal pain and tenesmus.
8. Depression can be seen in the early stages of pancreatic cancer.
9. **Lambert-Eaton syndrome** is associated with small-cell lung cancer. This syndrome is manifest in the following ways: peripheral paresthesia, weakness, difficulty in walking, and dry mouth. The weakness improves with repetitive movement (the opposite of myasthenia gravis). It is an autoimmune response affecting the nervous system, most commonly associated with small-cell lung cancer.
10. **Trousseau syndrome** or migratory thrombophlebitis is associated with pancreatic cancer in 50% of all cases. It is also associated with lung, prostate, and colon cancers.

ENDOCRINE TIPS AND PEARLS

1. Only three disease processes are associated with a normal/increased appetite and weight loss: diabetes mellitus, hyperthyroidism, and malabsorption.

30

2. Patients can present with peripheral neuropathies up to 1 year prior to manifesting other symptoms and signs of diabetes mellitus. As such, any patient presenting with a peripheral neuropathy should have laboratory testing to rule out diabetes mellitus.

3. Another potential early sign of diabetes mellitus is blurred vision and impairment of the extraocular muscles.

4. Thyroid disease, i.e., thyrotoxicosis, thyroid cancer, MUST always be assessed and ruled out in any patient presenting with unilateral or bilateral ear pain and no defined otic pathology. Thyroid pathologic processes can often present as referred ear pain.

5. A bruit is sometimes heard over the thyroid with Graves disease.

6. A deepened or husky voice is often a subtle presentation of hypothyroidism.

7. Patients with hypothyroidism often have a loss of or lateral thinning of the outer one-third of their eyebrows. This is called **Queen Anne's sign**. Allegedly, Queen Anne of England had a habit of removing the outer third of her eyebrows.

8. Patients with hypothyroidism have an abnormal reflex response; contraction or the initial phase of the reflex is normal and the relaxation phase of the reflex is delayed.

9. Patients with hyperthyroidism often have a fine tremor that is at times difficult to see. This can be brought out by asking the patient to raise their arms in front of them and then placing a piece of paper over their hands. If there is a fine tremor, the paper will vibrate.

10. Patients with hyperthyroidism from Graves disease can present with lid lag, **von Graefe sign**. This is elicited by having the patient follow the examiner's finger first from neutral to an upward extreme gaze, then following the examiner's finger rapidly downward. Patients with hyperthyroidism will have a delay in the eyelid moving downward in relation to the eyeball itself. There will be white from the conjunctiva seen initially with the rapid downward gaze, and the white will decrease or disappear as the lid catches up.

11. **Chvostek sign** is associated with hypocalcemia. This is done by repeated tapping over the facial nerve located anterior to the ear and just below the zygomatic arch. A positive sign is when facial twitching is elicited. It has a low level of sensitivity and specificity, particularly in children.

12. **Trousseau sign** is a test for hypocalcemia. It is performed by placing a blood pressure cuff over the patient's arm and blowing the cuff up approximately 20 mm Hg above the patient's systolic blood pressure for approximately 3 min. A positive test results in wrist flexion, finger contractions, and adduction of the thumb. It has higher sensitivity and specificity than Chvostek sign.

Appendix

APGAR SCORES

Apgar scores (Table A-1, page 1044) are a numerical expression of a newborn infant's physical condition. Usually determined 1 min after birth and again at 5 min, the score is the sum of points (0–10) gained on assessment of color, heart rate, reflex irritability, muscle tone, and respirations. Apgar conveniently

Appendix update by Lydia Glick, MD, Timothy Han, MD, Steven A. Haist, MD, MS and Leonard G. Gomella, MD

Table A-1. Apgar Scores

Sign	Score		
	0	**1**	**2**
Appearance (color)	Blue or pale	Pink body with blue extremities	Completely pink
Pulse (heart rate)	Absent	Slow (< 100/min)	>100/min
Grimace (reflex irritability)	No response	Grimace	Cough or sneeze
Activity (muscle tone)	Limp	Some flexion	Active movement
Respirations	Absent	Slow, irregular	Good, crying

stands for "Appearance, Pulse, Grimace, Activity, and Respiration" and was actually developed by Dr. Virginia Apgar in 1952 (https://medlineplus.gov/encyclopedia.html. Accessed June 1, 2020).

BODY SURFACE AREA FOR ADULTS AND CHILDREN

Figure A-1, page 1045. Nomogram for determining the body surface area of an adult.
Figure A-2, page 1046. Nomogram for determining the body surface area of children.

BODY MASS INDEX (BMI)

Table A-2, page 1047. Body mass index (BMI) is a measurement based on height in relation to weight, and is closely linked to a person's body fat. BMI is designed to give patients and health professionals a way to measure when a person's weight is hazardous and there is a potential risk of developing health conditions based on excess weight (obesity and other health-related risks). See discussion in Chapter 17, Nutritional Assessment, Therapeutic Diets and Infant Feeding, page 465. Calculators for adult, child, and teen BMI are available on the CDC website: https://www.cdc.gov/widgets/healthyliving/index.html (accessed June 2, 2020).

CANCER SCREENING

Some general recommendations for the early detection of common cancers in average-risk asymptomatic persons from two major organizations who influence cancer screening activities in the United States, the American Cancer Society and

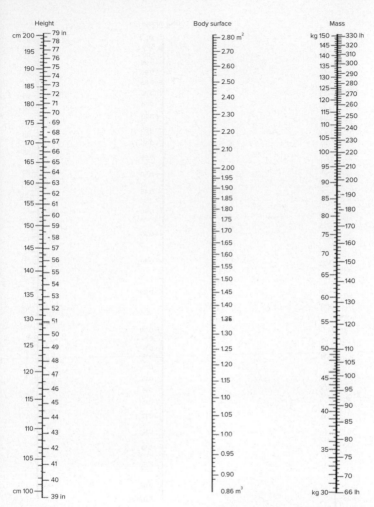

FIGURE A-1. Body surface area: Adult. Use a straight edge to connect the height and mass. The point of intersection on the body surface line gives the body surface area (in m²). (Reprinted, with permission, from: Lentner C (ed.). Geigy Scientific Tables, Vol. 1, 8e. San Francisco, CA: Ciba-Geigy; 1981, p. 226.)

the United States Preventative Services Task Force (see Table A-3, page 1048). Other groups or specialty societies may vary from these commonly cited sources.

CHILD-PUGH SCORE

The Child-Pugh (AKA Child-Turcotte-Pugh [CTP] score was originally developed to evaluate the risk of portocaval shunt procedures for portal

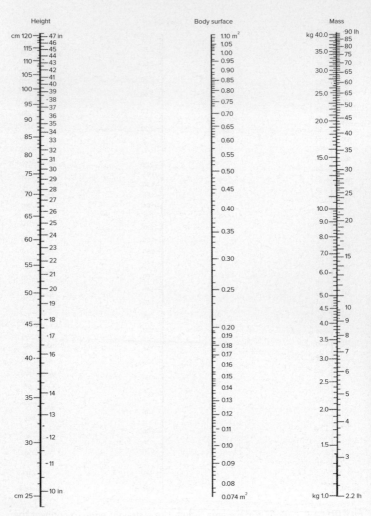

Height | Body surface | Mass

FIGURE A-2. Body surface area: Child. Use a straight edge to connect the height and mass. The point of intersection on the body surface line gives the body surface area (in m²). (Reprinted, with permission, from: Lentner C (ed.). Geigy Scientific Tables, Vol. 1, 8e. San Francisco, CA: Ciba-Geigy: 1981, p. 226.)

hypertension (see Table A-4, page 1054). It has been shown to be useful in predicting surgical risks of other intraabdominal operations on cirrhotic patients. Overall surgical mortality rates are 10% for patients with class A cirrhosis, 30% for those with class B cirrhosis, and 75–80% for those with class C cirrhosis. (Tsoris A, Marlar C. Use of the Child Pugh Score in Liver Disease, https://www.ncbi.nlm.nih.gov/books/NBK542308/.)

Table A-2. Body Mass Index (BMI) in Adults

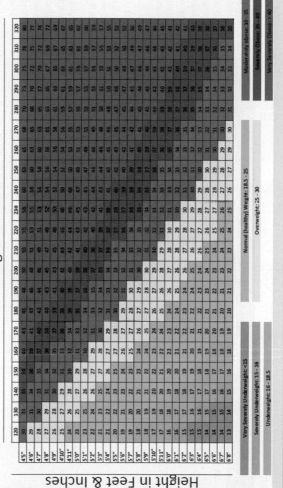

Table A-3. Cancer Screening

Cancer Site (Incidence[a])	Population	Test or Procedure	American Cancer Society[b]	U.S. Preventative Services Task Force (USPSTF)[c]
Breast (127.5 per 100,000)	Women, age ≥20 yr	Breast self-examination (BSE)	Not regularly recommended, but does not mean that these exams should never be performed. People should be encouraged to be familiar with how their breasts normally look and feel, and report any changes to a healthcare provider immediately.	Teaching breast self-exam is not recommended. However, patients should be encouraged to be aware of any changes in their body and to discuss these changes with clinicians.
		Clinical breast examination (CBE)	Not regularly recommended, but this does not mean that these exams should never be performed. Some patients may prefer having them performed.	If clinicians chose to perform this exam, it should be done in a structured and systematic fashion at periodic health examinations.
		Mammography	Annual mammography from 45 to 54 yr (women 40–44 yr should have the opportunity to begin screening earlier). Biennial screening (or continued annual screening) for women ≥55 yr. Continue screening as long as overall health is good and life-expectancy is 10+ yr.	Begin biennial (every other year) mammography at age 50 yr and continue through 74 yr. Women with a first-degree relative with breast cancer or for whom the perceived benefits outweigh the harms of biennial screening may start at age 40–49 yr.

Cervical (7.3 per 100,000)	Women, age ≥21 yr	Pap (Papanicolaou) test	Screening for ages 25–65 yr. Screen every 5 yr with a primary HPV test or a combination of HPV test and Pap test, or every 3 yr with a Pap test alone. Women >65 yr with regular screening in the past 10 yr with normal results and no history of CIN2 or higher diagnosis in the past 25 yr should stop screening. Women with a total hysterectomy should stop cervical cancer screening (unless it was done for treatment of cervical cancer or serious precancer).	Screening should occur every 3 yr with cervical cytology from 21 to 29 yr. In women 30–65 yr, screen every 3 yr with cervical cytology, or every 5 yr with HPV testing, or every 5 yr with HPV and cytology co-testing. Stop screening in women older than 65 yr who have adequate screening and are not at high risk for cervical cancer (high risk: those diagnosed with a high-grade precancerous lesion – CIN 2 or 3, cervical cancer, who have a compromised immune system, or were exposed in-utero to diethylstilbestrol). Do not screen women who have undergone hysterectomy and removal of the cervix who do not have a history of a high-grade lesion or cervical cancer.

(Continued)

Table A-3. Cancer Screening (Continued)

Cancer Site (Incidence[a])	Population	Test or Procedure	American Cancer Society[b]	U.S. Preventative Services Task Force (USPSTF)[c]
Ovarian (11.4 per 100,000)	Asymptomatic women, without a high-risk hereditary cancer syndrome	Transvaginal ultrasound, or CA-125	Do not perform screening for ovarian cancer in asymptomatic women.	Do not perform screening for ovarian cancer in asymptomatic women.
Endometrial (27.5 per 100,000)	Asymptomatic women		At menopause, women should be informed of the symptoms and risks factors for endometrial cancer, and strongly encouraged to report unusual vaginal bleeding or spotting to a physician.	No recommendations.
Prostate (109.5 per 100,000)	Men, age ≥40 yr	Digital rectal examination (DRE) and prostate-specific antigen test (PSA)	Men at age 40 yr with >1 first-degree relative with prostate cancer at an early age, age 45 yr who are African American or have a first-degree relative with prostate cancer at an early age, or age 50 who are at average risk for prostate cancer and with a 10+ yr life-expectancy should make an informed decision with healthcare providers about prostate cancer screening after learning about the potential benefits, risks, and uncertainties associated with prostate cancer screening.	The PSA test and DRE may be offered periodically for men aged 55–69 yr. The decision to screen is patient-specific, and the patient must weigh the benefits of screening against the harms involved in biopsy and treatment (overscreening, overdiagnosis, excessive treatment, and complications of all of the above). Men ≥70 yr should not receive a PSA screening test.

Lung (54.9 per 100,000)	Adults ≥50 yr with a smoking history	Low-dose helical CT	Annual screening from age 55 to 74 yr in adults with a 30+ pack-year smoking history AND currently smoke or have quit in the past 15 yr, after having undergone informed decision making about the benefits, limitations, and harms of screening with low-dose CT. People undergoing screening should have access to a high-volume, high-quality center for screening and treatment. Current smokers should receive evidence-based smoking cessation counseling.	Annual screening from age 50 to 80 yr in adults with a 20+ pack-year smoking history AND currently smoking or who have quit smoking within 15 yr. Stop screening after a person discontinued smoking more than 15 yr ago, or in whom there is another health concern that limits life expectancy or candidacy for curative surgery.
Thyroid (15.8 per 100,000)	Asymptomatic adults	Neck ultrasound	Screening for thyroid cancer is not recommended in asymptomatic adults.	Screening for thyroid cancer is not recommended in asymptomatic adults.
Pancreatic (12.9 per 100,000)	Asymptomatic adults	Abdominal imaging	Screening for pancreatic cancer is not recommended in asymptomatic adults.	Screening for pancreatic cancer is not recommended in asymptomatic adults.
Colorectal (38.6 per 100,000)	Men and women, age ≥45 yr	Fecal occult blood test (FOBT)[a] or fecal immunochemical test (FIT), or multitarget stool DNA test (mt-sDNA), or	Annual testing starting at 45 yr. Every 3 yr, starting at 45 yr.	Testing starting at 45 yr. Annual FIT OR high-sensitivity guaiac fecal occult blood test (HSgFOBT) OR stool DNA-FIT every 1-3 yr

(Continued)

Table A-3. Cancer Screening (*Continued*)

Cancer Site (Incidence[a])	Population	Test or Procedure	American Cancer Society[b]	U.S. Preventative Services Task Force (USPSTF[c])
		Flexible sigmoidoscopy, or	Every 5 yr, starting at 45 yr.	Every 5 yr, starting at 45 yr.
		Fecal occult blood test (FOBT)[a] and flexible sigmoidoscopy,[b] or		OR flexible sigmoidoscopy Q 10 yr + annual FIT starting at 45 yr
		CT colonography or colonoscopy	CT colonography Q 5 yr, starting at 45 yr. Colonoscopy every 10 yr, starting at 45 yr.	CT colonography Q 5 yr or colonoscopy Q 10 yr starting at 45 yr
			All positive results of noncolonoscopy tests should be followed up with timely colonoscopy, and screening should continue to 75 yr in patients with a life expectancy of 10+ yr. Adults 76–85 yr should make screening decisions based on patient preferences, life expectancy, and health status. Over the age of 85 yr, individuals should be discouraged from colon cancer screening.	Screen all adults ages 45–75 yr and selectively screen adults 76–85 yr based on patient's overall health, prior screening, and patient preferences. Screening benefits are small ages 76–85 yr.
Renal (16.1 per 100,000)	Asymptomatic adults	Urine dipstick, microscopic urinalysis, or abdominal imaging	Screening for renal cancer is not recommended in asymptomatic adults.	No recommendations.

Bladder (20.1 per 100,000)	Asymptomatic adults	Urine dipstick, microscopic urinalysis, urine cytology, or urine biomarkers	Screening for bladder cancer is not recommended in asymptomatic adults.	Insufficient evidence for screening recommendations in asymptomatic adults.

All guidelines up to date as of December 2020.[a]Incidence: Number of new cases per people per year, 2012–2016; National Cancer Institute, National Institutes of Health. Guidelines are from the American Cancer Society and the United States Preventative Services Task Force. There are also society-specific guidelines not listed here that may have different recommendations.

[b]https://www.cancer.org/health-care-professionals/american-cancer-society-prevent-on-early-detection-guidelines.html. Accessed December 15, 2020.

[c]https://www.uspreventiveservicestaskforce.org/Page/Name/recommendations. Accessed December 15, 2020, for details.

Table A-4. Child-Pugh Score

Component	Points Scored		
	1	2	3
Encephalopathy[a]	None	Grade 1–2	Grade 3––4
Ascites	None	Mild or controlled by diuretics	Moderate or refractory despite diuretics
Albumin	>3.5 g/dL	2.8–3.5 g/dL	<2.8 g/dL
Total Bilirubin, *or*	<2 mg/dL(<34 μmol/L)	2–3 mg/dL (34–50 μmol/L)	>3 mg/dL (>50 μmol/L)
Modified Total Bilirubin[b]	<4 mg/dl	4–7 mg/dL	>7 mg/dL
Prothrombin Time (Seconds Prolonged), *or*	<4	4–6	>6
International Normalized Ratio (INR)	<1.7	1.7–2.3	>2.3
Child-Pugh Classification	**Total Child-Pugh Score**[c]		
Class A	5–6 points		
Class B	7–9 points		
Class C	>9 points		

[a]Encephalopathy Grades
> *Grade 1:* Mild confusion, anxiety, restlessness, fine tremor, slowed coordination
> *Grade 2:* Drowsiness, disorientation, asterixis
> *Grade 3:* Somnolent but reusable, marked confusion, incomprehensible speech, incontinence, hyperventilation
> *Grade 4:* Coma, decerebrate posturing, flaccidity

[b]Modified total bilirubin used for patients who have Gilbert's syndrome or who are taking indinavir or atazanavir.
[c]Sum of points for each component of the Child-Pugh Score.
Source: StatPearls [Internet]. Treasure Island (FL): StatPearls Publishing; 2021 Jan. 2021 Mar 22 available on line at: https://www.ncbi.nlm.nih.gov/books/NBK542308/.

CHOLESTEROL GUIDELINES AND MANAGEMENT

The United States Preventive Services Task Force (USPSTF) recommends screening for lipid disorders in all men 35 years and older and women 45 years and older who are at increased risk for coronary heart disease. Additionally, they recommend screening men 20–35 years and women 20–45 years who are at increased risk for atherosclerotic cardiovascular disease (ASCVD). They recommend screening every 5 years with a fasting or nonfasting total cholesterol, LDL-cholesterol, and HDL. The ACC and AHA recommends screening all adults 20 years and older (who are not on lipid Tx) with a fasting or nonfasting lipid profile. They recommend assessing adults without ASCVD for risk factors every 4–6 years starting at the age of 20 years. Additionally, for those patients who are started on drug treatment, they recommend a lipid profile 4–12 wk after initiation of treatment and then every 3–12 mo thereafter. Follow-up for patients on statins should always include questions regarding potential side effects (myalgias, myositis, new onset of DM type 2, and liver inflammation [increase in AST/ALT up to 3X upper limits of normal]/liver failure).

Treatment decisions regarding total cholesterol, as well as lipoproteins including low-density lipoprotein (LDL) cholesterol, high-density lipoprotein (HDL), triglycerides, lipoprotein (a) [Lp(a)], and apolipoprotein B (apoB) should never be made in isolation. For instance, an LDL cholesterol level in one patient may be "normal" and thus, does not need treatment; whereas, the same level of cholesterol in another patient may need to be aggressively treated. See Chapter 10, page 195 for cholesterol laboratory testing.

The 2018 cholesterol clinical practice guidelines published by the American College of Cardiology (ACC) and American Heart Association (AHA) Task Force drastically changed the approach to and management of cholesterol as a risk factor for ASCVD. The initial question is whether you are assessing the patient for primary prevention (Figure A-5, page 1064) or secondary prevention (Figure A-3, page 1060 and Figure A-4, page 1061). The treatment plan for every patient should always include lifestyle/behavioral changes to reduce the risk of an ASCVD event. Additionally, shared decision-making regarding treatment, whether it involves lifestyle/behavioral changes or starting the patient on a medication, should always include a discussion of the risks and benefits of the proposed treatment as well as the risks of no treatment.

Secondary Prevention

In patients with any condition secondary to atherosclerosis such as history of MI, stable or unstable angina, coronary artery revascularization, stroke, TIA(s), PVD, or aortic aneurysm, the goal of treatment is to prevent a second ASCVD event. The number needed to treat to prevent one event or one death will be much lower when treating patients who have had a history of MI, etc., (secondary prevention) compared to patients who have not yet had an event (primary prevention). For secondary prevention, the treatment will vary depending on whether the patient is deemed very high risk or NOT very high risk. For those deemed NOT very high risk, the recommendations are based on the patient's age (75 years and younger or greater than 75 years). Criteria for very high risk and NOT very high risk are included in secondary prevention (Figure A-3, page 1060 and Figure A-4, page 1061).

The initial treatment for the very high risk is with a high-intensity statin* with the goal to decrease the LDL by at least 50% (the lower the better) and to have the LDL <70 mg/dL. There are only two statins that should be used in this setting, atorvastatin or rosuvastatin. For the very high-risk group, ezetimibe and then proprotein convertase subtilisin/kexin type 9 (PCSK9) inhibitors can be added to the high-intensity statin* if LDL ≥70 mg/dL, or if the non-HDL cholesterol ≥100 mg/dL.

For those patients who need secondary prevention and are at NOT very high risk and age less than 75 years, they should be started on high-intensity statin* therapy and if they do not tolerate the high-intensity statin they should be changed to a moderate-intensity statin**. On either the high*- or moderate**-intensity statin, if the LDL is ≥70 mg/dL, consider adding ezetimibe. For those patients NOT very high risk and greater than 75 years of age, start a moderate**- or high-intensity statin*. If the patient was on a high-intensity statin* when they were <75 years, maintaining the patient on the high-intensity statin* is reasonable.

Primary Prevention

For a vast majority of patients, primary prevention for ASCVD begins with counseling to change or to modify behavior/lifestyle as well as modify other cardiovascular risk factors. Lifestyle changes are effective in reducing risk and should begin when the patient is relatively young (20–30 years old). The counseling is dependent upon the individual patient and may include smoking-cessation counseling; aerobic exercise; weight loss; dietary counseling to reduce total fat and saturated fats, and increase fiber, fruits, and vegetables; decrease blood pressure in patients with hypertension (reduce dietary sodium, aerobic exercise, weight loss, and review and adjust antihypertensive medications, if indicated); control of glucose for patients with diabetes (weight loss, aerobic exercise, dietary counseling, and review and adjust their diabetic medications, if indicated).

In primary prevention (see Figure A-5, page 1064), the first decision is whether the patient has one of three major risk factors: an LDL ≥190 mg/dL, diabetes mellitus, and is 40–75 years of age. The patients with an LDL ≥ 190 mg/dL should be started on a high-intensity statin* and if the LDL is ≥ 50% of baseline or if the LDL ≥100 mg/dL on maximally tolerated statin, then ezetimibe should be added. A bile sequestrant can then be added if the LDL is still >50% of the baseline as long as the triglycerides are <300 mg/dL. For patients 30–75 years old who still have an LDL ≥100 mg/dL on a high-intensity statin and ezetimibe, consider adding a PCSK9 inhibitor. Also, for those 40–75 years old whose baseline LDL was ≥220 mg/dL and with a treated LDL of ≥130 mg/dL, consider adding PCSK9 inhibitor to the high-intensity statin plus ezetimibe.

Patients ages 40–75 years with diabetes mellitus should be started on a moderate-intensity statin** and the treatment could be escalated to a high-intensity statin* based on other risk factors including DM-risk enhancers^^ and/or ASCVD-risk enhancers.^^^ If the 10-year risk of an ASCVD event is ≥20% (see below), initiate therapy with a high-intensity statin* and if the LDL is not reduced by at least 50%, add ezetimibe to the maximally tolerated dose of statin. For patients with DM who are 20–39 years of age, if they have any DM-risk enhancers^^, such as ≥30 mcg albumin/mg creatinine, it is reasonable to recommend a statin.

For all other patients age 40–75 and for the subset of patients with diabetes mellitus above, primary prevention is guided by the 10-year risk of a cardiovascular event. To determine this risk, one must use a cardiovascular risk calculator because of the number of variables that are included and the different weights for each variable.

Four commonly used calculators are:

(1) ASCVD Risk Predictor Plus Assessment calculator: http://tools.acc.org/ASCVD-Risk-Estimator-Plus/#!/calculate/estimate/
(2) Framingham risk calculator: https://globalrph.com/medcalcs/framingham-10-year-risk-calculator/
(3) Reynolds risk score calculator (for patients without DM): http://www.reynoldsriskscore.org/
(4) Multiethnic study on atherosclerosis calculator: https://ebmcalc.com/MESA.htm/

The clinical data that may be required with various calculators include **age, gender**, ethnicity, **systolic blood pressure**, diastolic blood pressure, history or treatment for hypertension, **active smoker**, history of diabetes mellitus, whether the patient is taking aspirin or a statin, **total cholesterol**, LDL cholesterol, triglycerides, **HDL cholesterol**, high-sensitivity C-reactive protein, family history of a premature myocardial infarction, and CT coronary artery calcium score. The above bolded clinical data are used in all four of the risk calculators listed. Be sure to identify and obtain the clinical information required for the calculator you are using.

Once the 10-year risk is determined, the patient can be classified into one of four levels of risk:

(1) <5.0% low risk
(2) 5.0–7.4% borderline risk
(3) 7.5–19.9% intermediate risk
(4) ≥20% high risk

For low-risk patients, counseling should stress a healthy lifestyle such as aerobic exercise, maintaining or achieving a healthy BMI, and a diet low in fats and high in fruits and vegetables.

For patients in the borderline-risk or intermediate-risk group, ASCVD-risk enhancers^^^ may argue to recommend more aggressive treatment. For borderline-risk patients, if there are ASCVD-risk enhancers^^^, then discussion should include treatment with a moderate-intensity statin** with the goal to reduce the LDL by at least 30%.

For intermediate-risk patients, the discussion should include the potential use of moderate-intensity statin** to reduce LDL by at least 30% and if there are ASCVD-risk enhancers^^^, then the goal is to reduce the LDL by at least 50% which could include changing from a moderate-intensity** to high-intensity statin* and, if needed, the addition of ezetimibe.

For intermediate-risk patients, and in some instances, certain borderline-risk patients, CT coronary artery calcium (CAC) score can be used to influence recommendations. With a CAC score of 0, the recommendation of no statin therapy is reasonable; a score of 1–99 pushes one to recommend a statin, especially for patients ≥ 55 years; and for scores of ≥ 100, a statin should be recommended regardless of age.

For primary prevention of high-risk patients (10-year risk $\geq 20\%$), statin therapy to reduce LDL by at least 50% should be recommended. Begin with a moderate-intensity statin** and if needed to achieve the goal of at least a 50% reduction in LDL, change to a high-intensity statin*. Ezetimibe can be added to the maximally tolerated dose of statin, if the goal has not been met.

For patients 20–39 years old who have an LDL-cholesterol of 160–189 mg/dL or a family history of a premature ASCVD event, consider recommending a statin. Otherwise for patients 20–39 years of age without DM and an LDL <160 mg/dL, encourage changes in lifestyle to reduce their risk.

References

Grundy SM, Stone NJ, Bailey AL, et al. 2018 AHA/ACC/AACVPR/AAPA/ABC/ ACPM/ADA/AGS/ APhA/ASPC/NLA/PCNA Guideline on the Management of Blood Cholesterol: A Report of the American College of Cardiology/American Heart Association Task Force on Clinical Practice Guidelines. *Circulation*. 2019;139:e1082–e1143. DOI: 10.1161/CIR.0000000000000625.

Grundy SM, Stone NJ; for the Guideline Writing Committee for the Cholesterol Guidelines. 2018 Cholesterol Clinical Practice Guidelines: Synopsis of the 2018 American Heart Association/American College of Cardiology/Multisociety Cholesterol Guideline. Ann Intern Med. 2019;170:779–783.

Correction to: 2018 AHA/ACC/AACVPR/AAPA/ABC/ ACPM/ADA/AGS/APhA/ ASPC/NLA/PCNA Guideline on the Management of Blood Cholesterol: A report of the American College of Cardiology/American Heart Association Task Force on clinical practice guidelines. *Circulation*. 2019;139:e1182–e1186.

https://www.uspreventiveservicestaskforce.org/Page/Document/Recommendation StatementFinal/lipid-disorders-in-adults-cholesterol-dyslipidemia-screening (accessed April 20, 2020).

Key to Symbols Used in Text

***High-intensity statins** = atorvastatin 80 mg or rosuvastatin 20 mg

****Moderate-intensity statin** = atorvastatin 10 mg, rosuvastatin 10 mg, simvastatin 20–40 mg, pravastatin 40 mg, lovastatin 40 mg or fluvastatin 20 mg BID

^**High-risk conditions** = age equal to or >65 yr, Hx of CABG or PCI, Hx of CHF, DM, ↑BP, stage 3 or 4 chronic kidney disease, current smoker, heterozygote for familial hypercholesterolemia, LDL ≥ 100 mg/dL despite max does of tolerated statin plus ezetimibe

^^**DM-risk enhancers** = >10 yr DM type 1 or >20 years DM type 2; ≥30 mcg of albumin/mg of creatinine; GFR <60 mL/min/1.73 m^2; ankle/brachial arterial BP ratio <0.9; neuropathy; retinopathy

^^^**ASCVD-risk enhancers** = baseline LDL of 160–189 mg/dL, ethnicity (South Asian), family Hx of premature ASCVD event (males <55 yr and females <65 yr), chronic infections or rheumatologic conditions causing inflammation (HIV, RA, SLE, etc.), stage 3 or 4 chronic kidney disease, premature menopause, Hx of preeclampsia, metabolic syndrome (3 or more of the following: triglycerides ≥150, HLD <40 mg/dL for men and <50 mg/dL for women, BP ≥130/85 or Tx for hypertension, glucose ≥100 mg/dL or drug Tx for elevated glucose, waistline circumference ≥40 inches for men and ≥35 inches for women), and if measured biomarkers for ASCVD risk (ankle/brachial arterial BP ratio <0.9, persistent triglycerides ≥175 mg/dL, highly sensitive CRP ≥2.0 mg/dL, Lp(a) ≥50 mg/dL, and apoB ≥130 mg/dL)

Key to Symbols Used in Figure A-3

#**Secondary prevention:** indicated if there is a Hx of MI, stable or unstable angina, coronary artery revascularization, stroke, TIA(s), PVD, or aortic aneurysm (all secondary to atherosclerosis)

##**Very high risk** = Hx of >1 ASCVD event or 1 event and multiple high-risk conditions^

ASCVD events = ACS within the last 12 mo (unstable angina, non–ST-segment elevation myocardial infarction, and ST-segment elevation myocardial infarction), Hx of MI (other than recent event), Hx of ischemic stroke, or PVD (Hx of claudication with ABI <0.85 or revascularization or amputation secondary to PVD)

^**High-risk conditions** = age equal to or ≥65 yr, Hx of CABG or PCI, Hx of CHF, DM, ↑BP, stage 3 or 4 chronic kidney disease, current smoker, heterozygote for familial hypercholesterolemia, LDL ≥ 100 mg/dL despite max does of tolerated statin plus ezetimibe

***High-intensity statin** = atorvastatin 80 mg (40 mg), rosuvastatin 20 mg (40 mg)

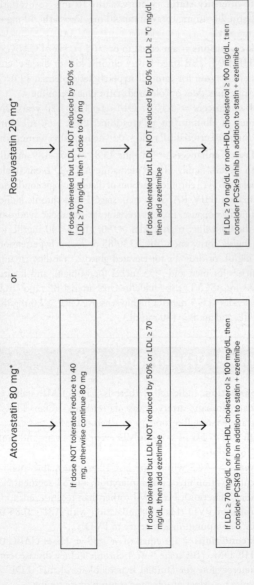

Secondary Prevention#, Very high-risk##

Atorvastatin 80 mg*   or   Rosuvastatin 20 mg*

↓

If dose NOT tolerated reduce to 40 mg, otherwise continue 80 mg

If dose tolerated but LDL NOT reduced by 50% or LDL ≥ 70 mg/dL, then ↑ dose to 40 mg

↓

If dose tolerated but LDL NOT reduced by 50% or LDL ≥ 70 mg/dL, then add ezetimibe

If dose tolerated but LDL NOT reduced by 50% or LDL ≥ 70 mg/dL, then add ezetimibe

↓

If LDL ≥ 70 mg/dL or non-HDL cholesterol ≥ 100 mg/dL, then consider PCSK9 inhib in addition to statin + ezetimibe

If LDL ≥ 70 mg/dL or non-HDL cholesterol ≥ 100 mg/dL, then consider PCSK9 inhib in addition to statin + ezetimibe

Figure A-3.   Cholesterol management: Secondary prevention of ASCVD, very high risk.

Secondary Prevention#, NOT Very High Risk###

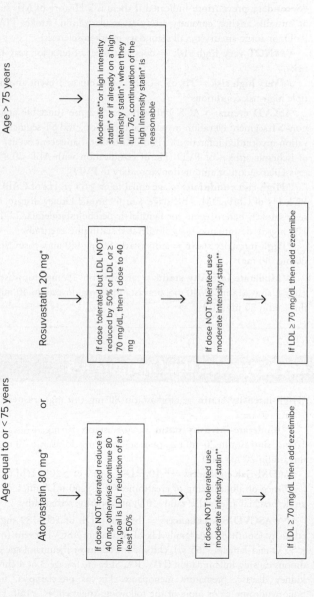

Age equal to or < 75 years

| Atorvastatin 80 mg* | or | Rosuvastatin 20 mg* |

→ If dose NOT tolerated reduce to 40 mg, otherwise continue 80 mg, goal is LDL reduction of at least 50%

→ If dose tolerated but LDL NOT reduced by 50% or LDL ≥ 70 mg/dL, then ↑ dose to 40 mg

→ If dose NOT tolerated use moderate intensity statin**

→ If LDL ≥ 70 mg/dL then add ezetimibe

Age > 75 years

→ Moderate**or high intensity statin* or if already on a high intensity statin*, when they turn 76, continuation of the high intensity statin* is reasonable

Figure A-4. Cholesterol management: Secondary prevention of ASCVD, not very high risk.

Key To Symbols Used In Figure A-4

#Secondary prevention: indicated if there is a History of MI, stable or unstable angina, coronary artery revascularization, stroke, TIA(s), PVD, or aortic aneurysm (all secondary to atherosclerosis)

###NOT very high risk = does not meet criteria for very high risk##

##Very high risk = Hx of >1 ASCVD event or 1 event and multiple high-risk conditions^

ASCVD events = ACS within the last 12 mo (unstable angina, non–ST-segment elevation myocardial infarction, and ST-segment elevation myocardial infarction), Hx of MI (other than recent event), Hx of ischemic stroke, or PVD (Hx of claudication with ABI <0.85 or revascularization or amputation secondary to PVD)

^High-risk conditions = age equal to or ≥65 yr, Hx of CABG or PCI, Hx of CHF, DM, ↑BP, stage 3 or 4 chronic kidney disease, current smoker, heterozygote for familial hypercholesterolemia, LDL ≥ 100 mg/dL despite max does of tolerated statin plus ezetimibe

*High-intensity statin = atorvastatin 80 mg (40 mg), rosuvastatin 20 mg (40 mg)

**Moderate-intensity statin = atorvastatin 10 mg, rosuvastatin 10 mg, simvastatin 20–40 mg, pravastatin 40 mg, lovastatin 40 mg, or fluvastatin 20 mg BID

Key to Symbols Used in Figure A-5

*High-intensity statin = atorvastatin 80 mg (40 mg), rosuvastatin 20 mg (40 mg)

**Moderate-intensity statin = atorvastatin 10 mg, rosuvastatin 10 mg, simvastatin 20–40 mg, pravastatin 40 mg, lovastatin 40 mg, or fluvastatin 20 mg BID

^^DM-risk enhancers = >10 yr DM type 1 or >20 yr DM type 2; ≥30 mcg of albumin/mg of creatinine; GFR <60 mL/min/1.73 m²; ankle/brachial arterial BP ratio <0.9; neuropathy; retinopathy

^^^ASCVD-risk enhancers = baseline LDL of 160–189 mg/dL, ethnicity (South Asian), family Hx of premature ASCVD event (males <55 yr and females <65 yr), chronic infections or rheumatologic conditions causing inflammation (HIV, RA, SLE, etc.), stage 3 or 4 chronic kidney disease, premature menopause, Hx of preeclampsia, metabolic syndrome (3 or more of the following: triglycerides ≥150, HLD <40 mg/dL for men and <50 mg/dL for women, BP ≥130/85 or Tx for hypertension, glucose ≥100 mg/dL or drug Tx for elevated glucose, waistline circumference ≥40 inches for men and ≥35 inches for women), and if measured biomarkers for ASCVD risk (ankle/brachial arterial BP ratio <0.9, persistent triglycerides ≥175 mg/dL, highly-sensitive CRP ≥2.0 mg/dL, Lp(a) ≥50 mg/dL, and apoB ≥ 130 mg/dL)

DEVELOPMENTAL MILESTONES

Used in pediatrics to assesses whether the child has achieved developmental milestones within appropriate range (see Table A-5, page 1065). These milestones include assessment of gross and fine motor skills, expressive and receptive speech.

EPIDEMIOLOGY BASICS

$$\text{Prevalance} = \frac{\text{Number of persons who have a disease at one point in time}}{\text{Number of persons at risk at thatpoint}}$$

$$\text{Incidence} = \frac{\text{Number of new cases of a disease over a period of time}}{\text{Number of persons at risk during that period}}$$

Sensitivity = Proportion of subjects with the disease who have a positive test
$$= (A / A = C)$$

Specificity = Proportion of subjects without the disease who have a negative test
$$= (d / b + d)$$

Positive predictive value: = likelihood of a positive test indicates disease
$$= (A / A + b)$$
Negative predictive value: = likelihood of a negative test indicates lack of disease
$$= (d / C + d)$$

		Disease is	
		Present	Absent
Test Result	+	A	b
Test Result	−	C	d

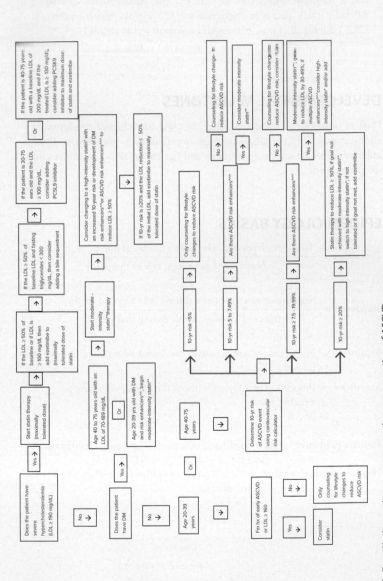

Figure A-5. Cholesterol management primary prevention of ASCVD.

Table A-5. Developmental Milestones from the CDC (Centers for Disease Control and Prevention)

	Social/Emotional	Language/ Communication	Cognitive (Learning, Thinking, Problem-Solving)	Movement/Physical Development
2 Mo	Begins to smile at people Can briefly calm herself (hands to mouth and suck on hand) Tries to look at parent	Coos, makes gurgling sounds Turns head toward sounds	Pays attention to faces Begins to follow things with eyes/ recognize people at a distance Begins to act bored (cries, fussy) if activity doesn't change	Can hold head up and begins to push up when lying on tummy Makes smoother movements with arms and leg
4 Mo	Smiles spontaneously, especially at people Likes to play with people and might cry when playing stops Copies movements and facial expressions (smiling or frowning)	Begins to babble Babbles with expression and copies sounds he hears Cries in different ways to show hunger, pain, or being tired	Lets you know if he is happy or sad Responds to affection Reaches for toy with one hand Uses hands and eyes together, such as seeing a toy and reaching for it Follows moving things with eyes from side to side Watches faces closely Recognizes familiar people and things at a distance	Holds head steady, unsupported Pushes down on legs when feet are on a hard surface May be able to roll over from tummy to back Can hold a toy and shake it and swing at dangling toys Brings hands to mouth When lying on stomach, pushes up to elbows

(Continued)

Table A-5. Developmental Milestones from the CDC ((Centers for Disease Control and Prevention) *(Continued)*

	Social/Emotional	Language/Communication	Cognitive (Learning, Thinking, Problem-Solving)	Movement/Physical Development
6 Mo	Knows familiar faces and begins to know if someone is a stranger Likes to play with others, especially parents Responds to other people's emotions and often seems happy Likes to look at self in a mirror	Responds to sounds by making sounds Strings vowels together when babbling ("ah," "eh," "oh") and likes taking turns with parent while making sounds Responds to own name Makes sounds to show joy and displeasure Begins to say consonant sounds (jabbering "m," "b")	Looks around at things nearby Brings things to mouth Shows curiosity about things and tries to get things that are out of reach Begins to pass things from one hand to the other	Rolls over in both directions (front to back, back to front) Begins to sit without support When standing, supports weight on legs and might bounce Rocks back and forth, sometimes crawling backward before moving forward
9 Mo	May be afraid of strangers May be clingy with familiar adults Has favorite toys	Understands "no" Makes a lot of different sounds like "mamamama" and "babababa" Copies sounds and gestures of others Uses fingers to point at things	Watches the path of something as it falls Looks for things she sees you hide Plays peek-a-boo Puts things in his mouth Moves things smoothly from one hand to the other Picks up things like cereal o's between thumb and index finger	Stands, holding on Can get into sitting position Sits without support Pulls to stand Crawls

(Continued)

| **1 y** | Is shy or nervous with strangers
Cries when mom or dad leaves
Has favorite things and people
Shows fear in some situations
Hands you a book when he wants to hear a story
Repeats sounds or actions to get attention
Puts out arm or leg to help with dressing
Plays games such as "peek-a-boo" and "pat-a-cake" | Responds to simple spoken requests
Uses simple gestures, like shaking head "no" or waving "bye-bye"
Makes sounds with changes in tone (sounds more like speech)
Says "mama" and "dada" and exclamations like "uh-oh!"
Tries to say words you say | Explores things in different ways, like shaking, banging, throwing
Finds hidden things easily
Looks at the right picture or thing when it's named
Copies gestures
Starts to use things correctly; for example, drinks from a cup, brushes hair
Bangs two things together
Puts things in a container, takes things out of a container
Lets things go without help
Pokes with index (pointer) finger
Follows simple directions like "pick up the toy" | Gets to a sitting position without help
Pulls up to stand, walks holding on to furniture ("cruising")
May take a few steps without holding on
May stand alone |
| **18 mo** | Likes to hand things to others as play
May have temper tantrums
May be afraid of strangers
Shows affection to familiar people
Plays simple pretend, such as feeding a doll
May cling to caregivers in new situations
Points to show others something interesting
Explores alone but with parent close by | Says several single words
Says and shakes head "no"
Points to show someone what he wants | Knows what ordinary things are for; for example, telephone, brush, spoon
Points to get the attention of others
Shows interest in a doll or stuffed animal by pretending to feed
Points to one body part
Scribbles on his own
Can follow 1-step verbal commands without any gestures; for example, sits when you say "sit down" | Walks alone
May walk up steps and run
Pulls toys while walking
Can help undress herself
Drinks from a cup
Eats with a spoon |

Table A-5. Developmental Milestones from the CDC ((Centers for Disease Control and Prevention) *(Continued)*

	Social/Emotional	Language/Communication	Cognitive (Learning, Thinking, Problem-Solving)	Movement/Physical Development
2 yr	Copies others, especially adults and older children Gets excited when with other children Shows more and more independence Shows defiant behavior (doing what he has been told not to) Plays mainly beside other children, but is beginning to include other children, such as in chase games	Points to things or pictures when they are named Knows names of familiar people and body parts Says sentences with 2–4 words Follows simple instructions Repeats words overheard in conversation Points to things in a book	Finds things even when hidden under two or three covers Begins to sort shapes and colors Completes sentences and rhymes in familiar books Plays simple make-believe games Builds towers of 4 or more blocks Might use one hand more than the other Follows two-step instructions such as "Pick up your shoes and put them in the closet." Names items in a picture book such as a cat, bird, or dog	Stands on tiptoe Kicks a ball Begins to run Climbs onto and down from furniture without help Walks up and down stairs holding on Throws ball overhand Makes or copies straight lines and circles

3 yr	Copies adults and friends	Follows instructions with 2 or 3 steps	Can work toys with buttons, levers, and moving parts	Climbs well
	Shows affection for friends without prompting	Can name most familiar things	Plays make-believe with dolls, animals, and people	Runs easily
	Takes turns in games	Understands words like "in," "on," and "under"	Does puzzles with 3 or 4 pieces	Pedals a tricycle (3-wheel bike)
	Shows concern for crying friend	Says first name, age, and sex	Understands what "two" means	Walks up and down stairs, one foot on each step
	Understands the idea of "mine" and "his" or "hers"	Names a friend	Copies a circle with pencil or crayon	
	Shows a wide range of emotions	Says words like "I," "me," "we," and "you" and some plurals (cars, dogs, cats)	Turns book pages one at a time	
	Separates easily from mom and dad	Talks well enough for strangers to understand most of the time	Builds towers of more than 6 blocks	
	May get upset with major changes in routine	Carries on a conversation using 2–3 sentences	Screws and unscrews jar lids or turns door handle	
	Dresses and undresses self			

(Continued)

Table A-5. Developmental Milestones from the CDC (Centers for Disease Control and Prevention) *(Continued)*

	Social/Emotional	Language/ Communication	Cognitive (Learning, Thinking, Problem-Solving)	Movement/Physical Development
4 yr	Enjoys doing new things Plays "Mom" and "Dad" Is more and more creative with make-believe play Would rather play with other children than by himself Cooperates with other children Often can't tell what's real and what's make-believe Talks about what she likes and what she is interested in	Knows some basic rules of grammar, such as correctly using "he" and "she" Sings a song or says a poem from memory such as the "Itsy Bitsy Spider" or the "Wheels on the Bus" Tells stories Can say first and last name	Names some colors and some numbers Understands the idea of counting Starts to understand time Remembers parts of a story Understands the idea of "same" and "different" Draws a person with 2 to 4 body parts Uses scissors Starts to copy some capital letters Plays board or card games Tells you what he thinks is going to happen next in a book	Hops and stands on one foot up to 2 seconds Catches a bounced ball most of the time Pours, cuts with supervision, and mashes own food

5 yr	Wants to please friends Wants to be like friends More likely to agree with rules Likes to sing, dance, and act Is aware of gender Can tell what's real and what's make-believe Shows more independence (for example, may visit a next-door neighbor by himself [adult supervision is still needed]) Is sometimes demanding and sometimes very cooperative	Speaks very clearly Tells a simple story using full sentences Uses future tense; for example, "Grandma will be here." Says name and address	Counts 10 or more things Can draw a person with at least 6 body parts Can print some letters or numbers Copies a triangle and other geometric shapes Knows about things used every day, like money and food	Stands on one foot for 10 s or longer Hops; may be able to skip Can do a somersault Uses a fork and spoon and sometimes a table knife Can use the toilet on her own Swings and climbs

Source: https//www.cdc.gov/ncbddd/actearly/milestones/index.html. Accessed May 17, 2020.

GLASGOW COMA SCALE

The Glasgow Coma Scale (sometimes called the EMV Scale) is a fairly reliable, objective way to monitor changes in levels of consciousness. It is based on **Eye opening, Motor responses, and Verbal responses.** A person's score is based on the total of the three responses. The score ranges from 3 (lowest) to 15 (highest) (Table A-6, page 1073) (www.glasgowco mascale.org/downloads/GCS-Assessment-Aid-English.pdf?v=3, accessed May 15, 2020).

GROWTH CHARTS

Growth charts consist of a series of percentile curves that illustrate the distribution of selected body measurements in children. Pediatric growth charts have been used by pediatricians, nurses, and parents to track the growth of infants, children, and adolescents in the United States since 1977. Growth charts are not intended to be used as a sole diagnostic instrument. Instead, growth charts are tools that contribute to forming an overall clinical impression for the child being measured.

CDC recommends that healthcare providers:

- Use the **WHO growth charts** to monitor growth for infants and children ages 0–2 yr of age in the United States (https://www.cdc.gov/growth-charts/who_charts.htm#The%20WHO%20Growth%20Charts).
- Use the **CDC growth charts** to monitor growth for children age 2–20 yr in the United States (https://www.cdc.gov/growthcharts/clinical_charts.htm).

Figures A-6 to A-9 are the WHO growth charts for infants up to 2 years of age as this is a common clinical assessment of growth rates in that age range. CDC growth charts for older children can be found online as noted above. Percentile curves (2–98) are shown on each chart and values are commonly reported in terms of percentile vs the absolute values.

Figure A-6, page 1074 **Birth to 24-mo boys:** Head circumference-for-age and weight-for-length percentiles

Figure A-7, page 1075 **Birth to 24-mo boys:** Length-for-age and weight-for-age percentiles

Figure A-8, page 1076 **Birth to 24-mo girls:** Head circumference-for-age and weight-for-length percentiles

Figure A-9, page 1077 **Birth to 24-mo girls:** Length-for-age and weight-for-age percentiles

Table A-6. Glasgow Coma Scale

Parameter	Response		Score
Eyes	Open	Spontaneously	4
		To verbal command	3
		To pain	2
		No response	1
Best motor response	To verbal command	Obeys	6
	To painful stimulus*	Localizes pain	5
		Flexion-withdrawal	4
		Decorticate (flex)	3
		Decerebrate (extend)	2
		No response	1
Best verbal response		Oriented, converses	5
		Disoriented, converses	4
		Inappropriate responses	3
		Incomprehensible sounds	2
		No response	1

*Painful stimuli include finger-tip pressure, trapezius pinch, or thumb pressure in the supraorbital notch.

Source: Adapted from www.glasgowcomascale.org.

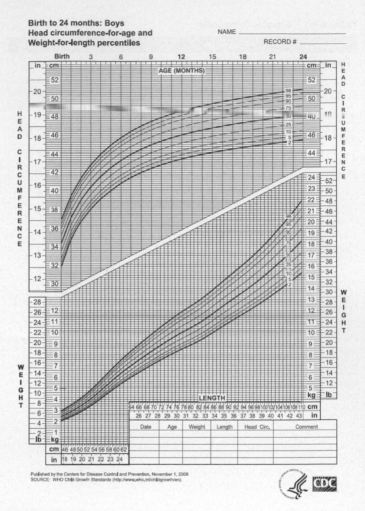

Figure A-6. Birth to 24-mo boys: Head circumference-for-age and weight-for-length percentiles.

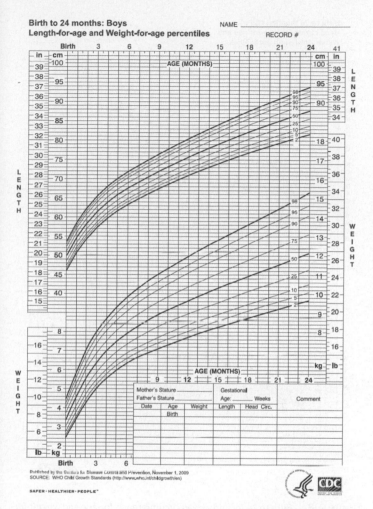

Figure A-7. Birth to 24-mo boys: Length-for-age and weight-for-age percentiles.

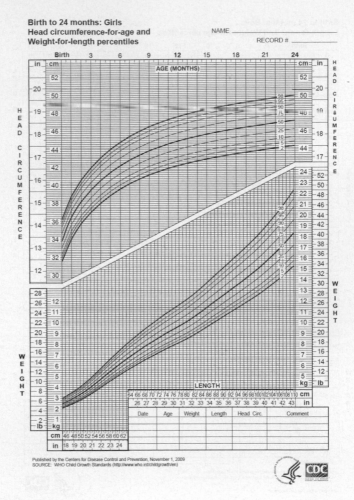

Birth to 24 months: Girls
Head circumference-for-age and
Weight-for-length percentiles

NAME _____

RECORD # _____

Published by the Centers for Disease Control and Prevention, November 1, 2009
SOURCE: WHO Child Growth Standards (http://www.who.int/childgrowth/en)

Figure A-8. Birth to 24-mo girls: Head circumference-for-age and weight-for-length percentiles.

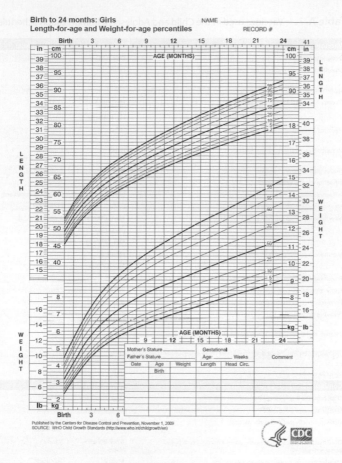

Birth to 24 months: Girls
Length-for-age and Weight-for-age percentiles

NAME _____

RECORD # _____

Published by the Centers for Disease Control and Prevention, November 1, 2009
SOURCE: WHO Child Growth Standards (http://www.who.int/childgrowth/en)

Figure A-9. Birth to 24-months girls: Length-for-age and weight-for-age percentiles.

IMMUNIZATION GUIDELINES (ADULTS AND CHILDREN)

Each year the Advisory Committee on Immunization Practices (ACIP), a federal advisory committee within the CDC, provides expert advice and guidance on use of vaccines and related agents for the control of vaccine-preventable diseases in the civilian population of the United States. These recommendations are typically widely endorsed by other professional societies. For a listing see the CDC ACIP web site. (www.cdc.gov/vaccines/acip) Complete updated information is published annually in MMWR and can be found at http://www.cdc.gov/vaccines/schedules/. All information presented here is from that source as of February 22, 2022. These tables only provide general guidance on the recommended vaccines. It is essential to assess for medical conditions and be familiar with the indications and contraindications for each vaccine product.

Table A-7. Vaccines used in the Child and Adolescent Immunization Schedule.

Vaccine	Abbreviation(s)	Trade name(s)
Dengue vaccine	DEN4CYD	Dengvaxia®
Diphtheria, tetanus, and acellular pertussis vaccine	DTaP	Daptacel® Infanrix®
Diphtheria, tetanus vaccine	DT	No trade name
Haemophilus influenzae type b vaccine	Hib (PRP-T) Hib (PRP-OMP)	ActHIB® Hiberix® PedvaxHIB®
Hepatitis A vaccine	HepA	Havrix® Vaqta®
Hepatitis B vaccine	HepB	Engerix-B® Recombivax HB®
Human papillomavirus vaccine	HPV	Gardasil 9®
Influenza vaccine (inactivated)	IIV4	Multiple
Influenza vaccine (live, attenuated)	LAIV4	FluMist® Quadrivalent
Measles, mumps, and rubella vaccine	MMR	M-M-R II®
Meningococcal serogroups A, C, W, Y vaccine	MenACWY-D MenACWY-CRM MenACWY-TT	Menactra® Menveo® MenQuadfi®
Meningococcal serogroup B vaccine	MenB-4C MenB-FHbp	Bexsero® Trumenba®
Pneumococcal 13-valent conjugate vaccine	PCV13	Prevnar 13®
Pneumococcal 23-valent polysaccharide vaccine	PPSV23	Pneumovax 23®
Poliovirus vaccine (inactivated)	IPV	IPOL®
Rotavirus vaccine	RV1 RV5	Rotarix® RotaTeq®
Tetanus, diphtheria, and acellular pertussis vaccine	Tdap	Adacel® Boostrix®
Tetanus and diphtheria vaccine	Td	Tenivac® Tdvax™
Varicella vaccine	VAR	Varivax®
Combination vaccines *(use combination vaccines instead of separate injections when appropriate)*		
DTaP, hepatitis B, and inactivated poliovirus vaccine	DTaP-HepB-IPV	Pediarix®
DTaP, inactivated poliovirus, and *Haemophilus influenzae* type b vaccine	DTaP-IPV/Hib	Pentacel®
DTaP and inactivated poliovirus vaccine	DTaP-IPV	Kinrix® Quadracel®
DTaP, inactivated poliovirus, *Haemophilus influenzae* type b, and hepatitis B vaccine	DTaP-IPV-Hib-HepB	Vaxelis®
Measles, mumps, rubella, and varicella vaccine	MMRV	ProQuad®

Based on data from: https://www.cdc.gov/vaccines/schedules/hcp/imz/child-adolescent.html (Accessed February 22, 2022)

Table A-8. Recommended Child and Adolescent Immunization Schedule for ages 18 years or younger, United States, 2022. ACIP recommends use of COVID-19 vaccines for everyone ages 5 and older. COVID-19 vaccine and other vaccines may be administered on the same day. Recommended Catch-up Immunization Schedule for Children and Adolescents Who Start Late or Who Are More than 1 month Behind, or for Immunization Schedule by Medical Indication refer to the CDC website. This is for guidance only and the specific notes references can be found on the CDC website https://www.cdc.gov/vaccines/schedules/hcp/imz/child-adolescent.html (Accessed February 22, 2022).

Vaccine	Birth	1 mo	2 mos	4 mos	6 mos	9 mos	12 mos	15 mos	18 mos	19–23 mos	2–3 yrs	4–6 yrs	7–10 yrs	11–12 yrs	13–15 yrs	16 yrs	17–18 yrs
Hepatitis B (HepB)	1st dose	←2nd dose→			←————— 3rd dose —————→												
Rotavirus (RV): RV1 (2-dose series), RV5 (3-dose series)			1st dose	2nd dose	See Notes												
Diphtheria, tetanus, acellular pertussis (DTaP <7 yrs)			1st dose	2nd dose	3rd dose			←——— 4th dose ———→				5th dose					
Haemophilus influenzae type b (Hib)			1st dose	2nd dose	See Notes		←— 3rd or 4th dose, See Notes —→										
Pneumococcal conjugate (PCV13)			1st dose	2nd dose	3rd dose		←——— 4th dose ———→										
Inactivated poliovirus (IPV <18 yrs)			1st dose	2nd dose	←————— 3rd dose —————→							4th dose					
Influenza (IIV4)							Annual vaccination 1 or 2 doses						Annual vaccination 1 dose only				
Influenza (LAIV4)							Annual vaccination 1 or 2 doses						Annual vaccination 1 dose only				
Measles, mumps, rubella (MMR)					See Notes		←— 1st dose —→					2nd dose					
Varicella (VAR)					See Notes		←— 1st dose —→					2nd dose					
Hepatitis A (HepA)					See Notes		2-dose series, See Notes										
Tetanus, diphtheria, acellular pertussis (Tdap ≥7 yrs)														1 dose			
Human papillomavirus (HPV)														See Notes			
Meningococcal (MenACWY-D ≥9 mos, MenACWY-CRM ≥2 mos, MenACWY-TT ≥2years)								See Notes						1st dose		2nd dose	
Meningococcal B (MenB-4C, MenB-FHbp)														See Notes			
Pneumococcal polysaccharide (PPSV23)														See Notes			
Dengue (DEN4CYD; 9-16 yrs)														Seropositive in endemic areas only (See Notes)			

Range of recommended ages for all children
Range of recommended ages for catch-up vaccination
Range of recommended ages for certain high-risk groups
Recommended vaccination can begin in this age group
Recommended vaccination based on shared clinical decision-making
No recommendation/ not applicable

Table A-9. Vaccines in the Adult Immunization Schedule.

Vaccine	Abbreviation(s)	Trade name(s)
Haemophilus influenzae type b vaccine	Hib	ActHIB® Hiberix® PedvaxHIB®
Hepatitis A vaccine	HepA	Havrix® Vaqta®
Hepatitis A and hepatitis B vaccine	HepA-HepB	Twinrix®
Hepatitis B vaccine	HepB	Engerix-B® Recombivax HB® Heplisav-B®
Human papillomavirus vaccine	HPV	Gardasil 9®
Influenza vaccine (inactivated)	IIV4	Many brands
Influenza vaccine (live, attenuated)	LAIV4	FluMist® Quadrivalent
Influenza vaccine (recombinant)	RIV4	Flublok® Quadrivalent
Measles, mumps, and rubella vaccine	MMR	M-M-R II®
Meningococcal serogroups A, C, W, Y vaccine	MenACWY-D MenACWY-CRM MenACWY-TT	Menactra® Menveo® MenQuadfi®
Meningococcal serogroup B vaccine	MenB-4C MenB-FHbp	Bexsero® Trumenba®
Pneumococcal 15-valent conjugate vaccine	PCV15	Vaxneuvance™
Pneumococcal 20-valent conjugate vaccine	PCV20	Prevnar 20™
Pneumococcal 23-valent polysaccharide vaccine	PPSV23	Pneumovax 23®
Tetanus and diphtheria toxoids	Td	Tenivac® Tdvax™
Tetanus and diphtheria toxoids and acellular pertussis vaccine	Tdap	Adacel® Boostrix®
Varicella vaccine	VAR	Varivax®
Zoster vaccine, recombinant	RZV	Shingrix

Based on data from https://www.cdc.gov/vaccines/schedules/hcp/imz/adult.html; accessed February 22, 2022.

Table A–10. Recommended Adult Immunization Schedule by Age Group, United States, 2022. ACIP recommends use of COVID-19 vaccines for everyone ages 5 and older. COVID-19 vaccine and other vaccines may be administered on the same day. See Table A-9 for additional vaccine details. (https://www.cdc.gov/vaccines/schedules/downloads/adult/adult-combined-schedule.pdf, Accessed February 22, 2022).

Vaccine	19–26 years	27–49 years	50–64 years	≥65 years
Influenza inactivated (IIV4) or Influenza recombinant (RIV4)	1 dose annually			
Influenza live, attenuated (LAIV4)	1 dose annually			
Tetanus, diphtheria, pertussis (Tdap or Td)	1 dose Tdap each pregnancy; 1 dose Td/Tdap for wound management (see notes)			
	1 dose Tdap, then Td or Tdap booster every 10 years			
Measles, mumps, rubella (MMR)	1 or 2 doses depending on indication (if born in 1957 or later)			
Varicella (VAR)	2 doses (if born in 1980 or later)		2 doses	
Zoster recombinant (RZV)	2 doses for immunocompromising conditions (see notes)		2 doses	
Human papillomavirus (HPV)	2 or 3 doses depending on age at initial vaccination or condition	27 through 45 years		
Pneumococcal (PCV15, PCV20, PPSV23)	1 dose PCV15 followed by PPSV23 OR 1 dose PCV20 (see notes)			1 dose PCV15 followed by PPSV23 OR 1 dose PCV20
Hepatitis A (HepA)	2 or 3 doses depending on vaccine			
Hepatitis B (HepB)	2, 3, or 4 doses depending on vaccine or condition			
Meningococcal A, C, W, Y (MenACWY)	1 or 2 doses depending on indication, see notes for booster recommendations			
Meningococcal B (MenB)	19 through 23 years	2 or 3 doses depending on vaccine and indication, see notes for booster recommendations		
Haemophilus influenzae type b (Hib)	1 or 3 doses depending on indication			

Recommended vaccination for adults who meet age requirement, lack documentation of vaccination, or lack evidence of past infection

Recommended vaccination for adults with an additional risk factor or another indication

Recommended vaccination based on shared clinical decision-making

No recommendation/ Not applicable

Table A-11. Recommended Adult Immunization Schedule by Medical Condition or Other Indication, United States, 2022. ACIP recommends use of COVID-19 vaccines for everyone ages 5 and older. COVID-19 vaccine and other vaccines may be administered on the same day. See table A-9 for additional vaccine details. (https://www.cdc.gov/vaccines/schedules/downloads/adult/adult-combined-schedule.pdf, Accessed February 22, 2022).

Vaccine	Pregnancy	Immunocompromised (excluding HIV infection)	HIV Infection CD4 percentage and count <15% or <200 mm³	HIV Infection CD4 percentage and count ≥15% and ≥200 mm³	Asplenia, complement deficiencies	End-stage renal disease, or on hemodialysis	Heart or lung disease; alcoholism¹	Chronic liver disease	Diabetes	Health care personnel²	Men who have sex with men
IIV4 or RIV4 *or*	1 dose annually										
LAIV4	Precaution	Contraindicated	Contraindicated		Precaution					1 dose annually	
Tdap or Td	1 dose Tdap each pregnancy	1 dose Tdap, then Td or Tdap booster every 10 years									
MMR	Contraindicated*	Contraindicated	Contraindicated		1 or 2 doses depending on indication						
VAR	Contraindicated*	Contraindicated	Contraindicated		2 doses						
RZV		2 doses at age ≥19 years			2 doses at age ≥50 years						
HPV	Not Recommended*	3 doses through age 26 years			2 or 3 doses through age 26 years depending on age at initial vaccination or condition						
Pneumococcal (PCV15, PCV20, PPSV23)		1 dose PCV15 followed by PPSV23 OR 1 dose PCV20 (see notes)									
HepA							2 or 3 doses depending on vaccine				
HepB	3 doses (see notes)	2, 3, or 4 doses depending on vaccine or condition									
MenACWY		1 or 2 doses depending on indication, see notes for booster recommendations									
MenB	Precaution	2 or 3 doses depending on vaccine and indication, see notes for booster recommendations									
Hib		3 doses HSCT³ recipients only			1 dose						

Legend:
- Recommended vaccination for adults who meet age requirement, lack documentation of vaccination, or lack evidence of past infection
- Recommended vaccination for adults with an additional risk factor or another indication
- Recommended vaccination based on shared clinical decision-making
- Precaution—vaccination might be indicated if benefit of protection outweighs risk of adverse reaction
- Contraindicated or not recommended—vaccine should not be administered. *Vaccinate after pregnancy.
- No recommendation/Not applicable

1. Precaution for LAIV4 does not apply to alcoholism. 2. See notes for influenza; hepatitis B; measles, mumps, and rubella; and varicella vaccinations. 3. Hematopoietic stem cell transplant.

Table A-12 A, B, C   Interim COVID-19 vaccine dosing and schedule as of February 22, 2022. For primary and booster vaccination for all populations, an mRNA COVID-19 vaccine series (Pfizer-BioNTech/COMIRATY™ or Moderna/SPIKEVAX™) is preferred over the Janssen COVID-19 Vaccine (recombinant adenovirus type). Details on COVID-19 vaccination can be found on the CDC website (https://www.cdc.gov/vaccines/covid-19/clinical-considerations/covid-19-vaccines-us.html, Accessed February 22, 2022).

Table A-12 A.   COVID-19 vaccine formulations currently approved or authorized in the United State

Vaccine manufacturer	Age indication	Vaccine vial cap color	Dilution required	Primary Series		Booster dose	
				Dose	Injection volume	Dose	Injection volume
Pfizer-BioNTech	5–11 years	Orange	Yes	10 µg	0.2 mL	NA	NA
Pfizer-BioNTech	≥12 years	Purple	Yes	30 µg	0.3 mL	30 µg	0.3 mL
Pfizer-BioNTech	≥12 years	Gray	No	30 µg	0.3 mL	30 µg	0.3 mL
Moderna	≥18 years	NA	No	100 µg	0.5 mL	50 µg	0.25 mL
Janssen	≥18 years	NA	No	5×10¹⁰ viral particles	0.5 mL	5×10¹⁰ viral particles	0.5 mL

Table A-12 B.   COVID-19 vaccination schedule for the primary series in the general population

Primary series vaccine manufacturer	Age group	Number of doses in primary series	Number of booster doses	Interval between 1st and 2nd dose	Interval between primary series and booster dose
Pfizer-BioNTech	5–11 years	2	NA	3 weeks	NA
Pfizer-BioNTech	≥12 years	2	1	3-8 weeks*	≥5 months
Moderna	≥10 years	7	1	4-8 weeks*	≥5 months
Janssen	≥18 years	1	1	NA	≥2 months

Table A-12 C.   COVID-19 vaccination schedule for people with moderate or severe immunocompromise

Primary vaccination	Age group	Number of primary vaccine doses	Number of booster doses	Interval between 1st and 2nd dose	Interval between 2nd and 3rd dose	Interval between 3rd and 4th dose
Pfizer-BioNTech	5–11 years	3	NA	3 weeks	≥4 weeks	N/A
Pfizer-BioNTech	≥12 years	3	1	3 weeks	≥4 weeks	≥3 months
Moderna	≥18 years	3	1	4 weeks	≥4 weeks	≥3 months
Janssen	≥18 years	1 Janssen, followed by 1 mRNA	1	4 weeks	≥2 months	N/A

MEASUREMENT EQUIVALENTS (APPROXIMATE)

Length	Household
1 centimeter (cm) = 0.4 in	1 teaspoon (tsp) = 5 mL
1 meter (m) = 39.4 in	1 tablespoon (tbsp) = 15 mL
	1 ounce (oz) = 30 mL
Apothecary	8 ounces (oz) = 1 cup = 240 mL
1 grain (gr) = 60 mg	1 quart (qt) = 946 mL
30 g = 1 oz	
1 g = 15 gr	

MEASUREMENT PREFIXES AND SYMBOLS

Factor	Prefix	Symbol
10^9	giga	G
10^6	mega	M
10^3	kilo	k
10^2	hecto	h
10^1	deka	da
10^{-1}	deci	d
10^{-2}	centi	c
10^{-3}	milli	m
10^{-6}	micro	μ
10^{-9}	nano	n
10^{-12}	pico	p
10^{-15}	femto	f

PERFORMANCE STATUS SCALES

Patient performance status is used commonly in cancer care. These scales are often used for assessments of patient's progress, eligibility for clinical trials, and in guidelines for standard treatments. Performance status estimates the patient's ability to perform certain activities of daily living (ADLs) without the help of others. These ADLs include getting dressed, eating, and bathing, as well as more complex activities such as cleaning the house and working. There are several commonly used scales. The Zubrod or ECOG (Eastern

Cooperative Oncology Group) scale ranges from 0 to 4, with 0 being fully functional and asymptomatic, and 4 being bedridden. The other common scale is the Karnofsky scale that ranges from 10 (moribund) to 100 (no limitations). See Figure A-10.

Performance Status Scales

Karnofsky Scale		Zubrod Scale (ECOG)	
100	Normal; no complaints; no evidence of disease	0	Fully active, able to carry on all pre-disease performance without restriction
90	Able to carry on normal activity; minor signs or symptoms of disease		
80	Normal activity with effort; some signs or symptoms of disease	1	Restricted in physically strenuous activity but ambulatory and able to carry out work of a light or sedentary nature
70	Cares for self; unable to carry on normal activity or do active work		
60	Requires occasional assistance but is able to care for most needs	2	Ambulatory and capable of all self-care but unable to carry out any work activities. Up and about >50% of waking hours
50	Requires considerable assistance and frequent medical care		
40	Disabled; requires special care and assistance	3	Capable of only limited self-care, confined to bed or chair > 50% of waking hours
30	Severely disabled; hospitalization is indicated, although death is not imminent		
20	Very sick; hospitalization is necessary; active supportive treatment is necessary	4	Completely disabled. Cannot carry on any self-care. Totally confined to bed or chair
10	Moribund, fatal processes progressing rapidly		
0	Dead	5	Dead

Figure A-10. Commonly used performance scales. Zubrod scale is also known as the ECOG scale (Reproduced with permission from West H, Jin J. Performance status in patients with Cancer. JAMA Oncol. 2015;1(7):998.

RADIATION TERMINOLOGY

Measure	Old Term	SI Unit
Activity	Curie	Becquerel (Bq)
Absorbed dose	rad	gray (Gy)

RULE OF NINES

Used in the assessment of the total body surface area that has been burned. Using the "rule of nines," (sometimes referred to as the "Wallace rule of Nine") the adult body is partitioned into areas and each region constitutes approximately 9% of the total body surface area (TBSA, Figure A-11). Regions on the adult that constitutes 9% of the TBSA include the head and arms, while the legs, anterior trunk, and posterior trunk account for 18% of TBSA each. In children, the arms each account for 9% of the TBSA, while the legs account for 14%. The head and neck region, the anterior trunk, and the posterior trunk each account for 18% in children. Careful estimation of TBSA is essential for proper early management of burn patients, as patients who have burns of more than 20% TBSA commonly require significant IV fluid resuscitation.

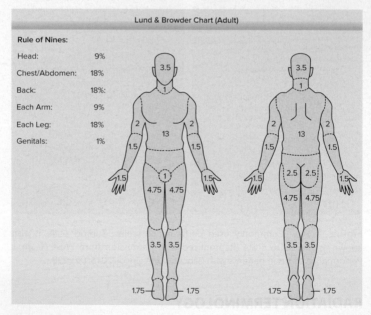

Figure A-11. Rule of nines and the Lund & Browder Chart are methods commonly employed to estimate the total body surface area (TBSA) of a burn. Numbers in Lund & Browder Chart indicate percent TBSA of body region. (Reproduced with permission form Levi B, Wang S. Burns. In: Kang S, Amagai M, Bruckner AL, et al. (eds.). Fitzpatrick's Dermatology, 9e. 2019; New York, NY: McGraw-Hill.)

TEMPERATURE CONVERSION

Table A-13, gives information for converting temperature in Fahrenheit to Celsius and vice versa.

Table A-13. Temperature Conversion Table

F	C	C	F
0	−17.7	0	32.0
95.0	35.0	35.0	95.0
96.0	35.5	35.5	95.9
97.0	36.1	36.0	96.8
98.0	36.6	36.5	97.7
98.6	37.0	37.0	98.6
99.0	37.2	37.5	99.5
100.0	37.7	38.0	100.4
101.0	38.3	38.5	101.3
102.0	38.8	39.0	102.2
103.0	39.4	39.5	103.1
104.0	40.0	40.0	104.0
105.0	40.5	40.5	104.9
106.0	41.1	41.0	105.8
$C = (F-32) \times 5/9$		$F = (C \times 9/5) + 32$	

WEIGHT CONVERSION

Table A-14, gives information for converting weight in pounds (lb) to weight in kilograms (kg) and vice versa.

Table A-14. Weight Conversion Table

lb	kg	kg	lb
1	0.5	1	2.2
2	0.9	2	4.4
4	1.8	3	6.6
6	2.7	4	8.8
8	3.6	5	11.0
10	4.5	6	13.2
20	9.1	8	17.6
30	13.6	10	22.0
40	18.2	20	44.0
50	22.7	30	66.0
60	27.3	40	88.0
70	31.8	50	110.0
80	36.4	60	132.0
90	40.9	70	154.0
100	45.4	80	176.0
150	68.2	90	198.0
200	90.8	100	220.9
kg = lb × 0.454		lb = kg × 2.2	

Index

Page numbers followed by *f* refer to figures.
Page numbers followed by *t* refer to tables.